Get Ready for a Whole New
Mastering Health Experience

P9-DUC-623

New! **Ready-to-Go Teaching Modules** help you find the best assets to use before, during, and after class to teach the toughest topics in Personal Health. These curated sets of teaching tools save you time by highlighting the most effective and engaging videos, quizzing, coaching, self-assessment, and behavior change activities to assign within **Mastering™ Health**.

Donatelle, *Health The Basics*, 13/e
Ready-To-Go Teaching Modules

Ready-To-Go Teaching Modules make use of teaching tools for before, during, and after class, including new ideas for in-class activities.

The modules incorporate the best that the text, Mastering Health, and Learning Catalytics have to offer and guide instructors through using these resources in the most effective way.

Health

Psychological Health	Stress
Reproductive Choices	Addiction and Drug Abuse
Alcohol and Tobacco	Nutrition
Fitness	CVD and Cancer
Infectious Conditions	Violence and Unintentional Injuries

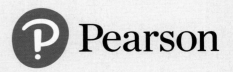

Connecting Cutting Edge Content to Enact

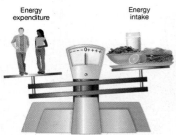

Energy expenditure = Energy intake

FIGURE 11.5 The Concept of Energy Balance If you consume more calories than you burn, you gain weight. If you burn more calories than you consume, you lose weight. If your consumption and burning of calories are equal, your weight will not change.

consume 140 calories (the amount in one can of regular soda) more than you need every single day and make no other changes in diet or activity, you would gain 1 pound in 25 days (3,500 calories ÷ 140 calories per day = 25 days). Conversely, if you walk for 30 minutes each day at a pace of 15 minutes per mile (172 calories burned) in addition to your regular activities, you would lose 1 pound in 20 days (3,500 calories ÷ 172 calories per day = 20.3 days). FIGURE 11.5 illustrates the concept of energy balance.

Diet and Eating Behaviors

Successful weight loss requires shifting your energy balance. The first part of the equation is to reduce calorie intake through modifying eating behaviors using a variety of strategies.

Being Mindful of Your Eating Triggers

When you sit down to eat, is your mind actually "out to lunch"? If you are like the 66 percent of American adults who eat in front of the TV or computer, it should be no surprise that you are eating faster and eating more, with more awareness of the TV than of your food.[54] *Mindless eating*, or putting food in your mouth that you don't really taste or notice while consuming more than you should, may be a key contributor to excess calorie consumption and weight gain. When we eat mindlessly, we may miss feelings of satiety and ignore tendencies we might have to use restraint in shoving potato chips into our mouths.

▶ SEE IT! VIDEOS

Do you snack like crazy when you're watching an exciting movie? Watch **Fast-Paced Movies, Television Shows May Lead to More Snacking** in the Study Area of Mastering Health.

Eating mindfully means eating with awareness— awareness of *why* we are eating (was it a trigger, or are we really hungry?), *what* we are eating (should we really be eating this?), and *how much* we are eating (stop! put it down!).

Before you can change an unhealthy eating habit, you must first determine what triggers you to eat. Keeping a log of eating triggers—*when, what, where,* and *how much* you eat—for 2 to 3 days can help you identify what is pushing those "eat everything in sight" buttons for you.

Typically, dietary triggers center on patterns and problems in everyday living rather than real hunger pangs. Many people eat compulsively when stressed; however, for other people, the same circumstances diminish their appetite, causing them to lose weight. When your mind wanders, you may find yourself grazing in the refrigerator or pulling into a fast-food drive-through. Ask yourself: Are you really hungry, or are you eating

NEW! A Mindfulness Theme throughout the book relates mindfulness research and practices to topics ranging from relationships to mindful eating to stress management and more. Mindfulness coverage is flagged by an icon next to all applicable passages in the text.

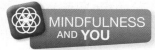

MINDFULNESS AND YOU

MINDFULNESS FOR SMOKING CESSATION

NEW! Mindfulness and You feature boxes cover topics such as mindfulness and smoking cessation, technostress, relapse prevention, etc. and are featured throughout the book.

More people are addicted to nicotine than to any other drug in the United States. Research suggests that nicotine maybe as addictive as heroin, cocaine, or alcohol. Successfully quitting smoking is a challenge that often requires more than one attempt. About 70 percent of adult smokers report wanting to quit smoking completely. Fifty-five percent tried to stop smoking for more than one day in the past year.

Recently, mindfulness-based therapies have been found to offer greater chances of success for those attempting to quit smoking. Mindfulness interventions have also been shown to decrease negative affect and craving in smokers.

Dr. Judson Brewer, the Director of Research at the Center for Mindfulness at the University of Massachusetts, has found that people who use mindfulness training

may have better outcomes than those who use standard methods of quitting. Dr. Brewer uses the acronym RAIN to help people manage their nicotine cravings.

- **R**ecognize the craving that is occurring, and relax with it.
- **A**ccept the moment. Pay attention to how your body is feeling.
- **I**nvestigate the experience. Ask yourself what is happening to your body in this moment.
- **N**ote what is happening. As you acknowledge anxiousness, irritability, and other feelings, realize that they are nothing more than body sensations that will pass.

Using mindfulness techniques in this way will help the body become familiar with the cravings and learn that it can adapt.

Cravings usually last from 90 seconds to 3 minutes. Simply using the acronym above helps many smokers to acknowledge and get through the craving, which should then become weaker over time.

Sources: J. Brewer, "A Randomized Controlled Trial of Smartphone-Based Mindfulness Training for Smoking Cessation: A Study Protocol," *BMC Psychiatry* 15, no. 83 (2015): 2–7; J. Brewer, "A Simple Way to Break A Habit," TED TalkMED, November, 2015; Centers for Disease Control and Prevention, "Smoking & Tobacco Use: Quitting Smoking," February 1, 2017, https://www.cdc.gov/tobacco/data_statistics/fact_sheets/cessation/quitting; L. Peltz, "Practicing Mindfulness to Help You Break the Habit of Smoking," Expert Beacon, 2016, https://expertbeacon.com/practicing-mindfulness-help-you-break-habit-smoking/#.WM2YbhAfSPV; A. Ruscio et al., "Effect of Brief Mindfulness Practice on Self-Reported Affect, Craving and Smoking: A Pilot Randomized Controlled Trial Using Ecological Momentary Assessment," *Nicotine Tobacco Research* 18, no. 1 (2016): 64–73.

Positive Change in Students' Lives

NEW! Focus on Difference, Disparity, and Health chapter looks at health equity as a critical issue in 21st century America. Coverage includes specific actions to take to promote health equity on campus, in the community, and individually, and systemic changes needed for the U.S. to progress towards better health for all.

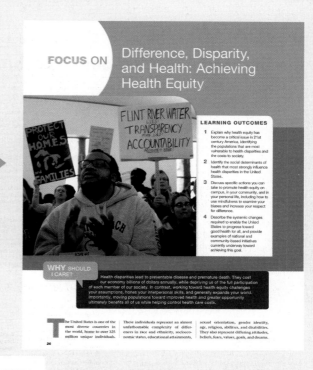

FOCUS ON Difference, Disparity, and Health: Achieving Health Equity

LEARNING OUTCOMES

1. Explain why health equity has become a critical issue in 21st century America, identifying the populations that are most vulnerable to health disparities and the costs to society.

2. Identify the social determinants of health that most strongly influence health disparities in the United States.

3. Discuss specific actions you can take to promote health equity on campus, in your community, and in your personal life, including how to use mindfulness to examine your biases and increase your respect for difference.

4. Describe the systemic changes required to enable the United States to progress toward good health for all, and provide examples of national and community-based initiatives currently underway toward achieving this goal.

WHY SHOULD I CARE?
Health disparities lead to preventable disease and premature death. They cost our economy billions of dollars annually, while depriving us of the full participation of each member of our society. In contrast, working toward health equity challenges your assumptions, hones your interpersonal skills, and generally expands your world. Importantly, moving populations toward improved health and greater opportunity ultimately benefits all of us while helping control health care costs.

NEW! Full Chapter on Sleep more thoroughly examines the connections between sleep and stress, sleep and nutrition, and much more.

UPDATED! Why Should I Care? features open each chapter, engaging students and helping them recognize the relevance of health issues to their own lives.

WHY SHOULD I CARE?
If you think cardiovascular disease and cancer are just things [ ] grandparents develop, think again! Increasing rates of obes[ ] levels of stress and anxiety, as well as a penchant for sitting t[ ] adults and adolescents at risk.

Continuous Learning
Before, During, and After Class

BEFORE CLASS

Mobile Media and Reading Assignments Ensure Students Come to Class Prepared

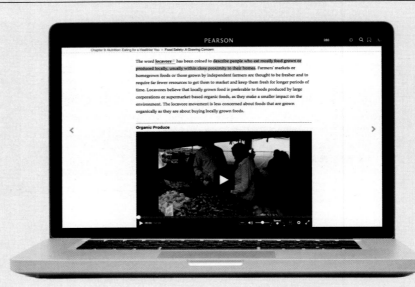

NEW! Interactive Pearson eText gives students access to their text, anytime, anywhere. Pearson eText features include:

- Offline access on smartphones/tablets

- Seamlessly integrated videos and other rich media.

- Interactive Self-Assessment Worksheets

- Accessible (screen-reader ready).

- Configurable reading settings, including resizable type and night reading mode.

- Instructor and student note-taking, highlighting, bookmarking, and search.

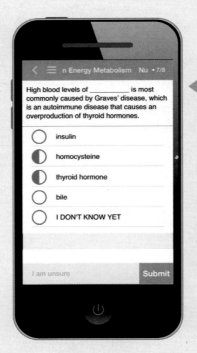

UPDATED! Dynamic Study Modules help students study effectively by continuously assessing student performance and providing practice in areas where students struggle the most. Each Dynamic Study Module, accessed by computer, smartphone or tablet, promotes fast learning and long-term retention.

Lecture Reading Quizzes are easy to customize and assign

...ng Questions ensure that students complete the assigned reading before class. Reading ...ns can be completed by students on any mobile device.

with Mastering Health

DURING CLASS

Engage Students with Learning Catalytics

Learning Catalytics, a "bring your own device" student engagement, assessment, and classroom intelligence system, allows students to use their smartphone, tablet, or laptop to respond to questions in class.

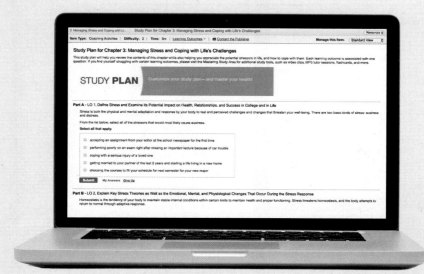

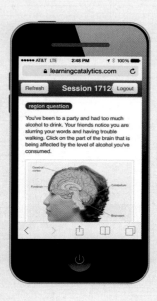

AFTER CLASS

Mastering Health Delivers Automatically Graded Health and Fitness Activities

Interactive Behavior Change Activities—Which Path Would You Take? Have students explore various health choices through an engaging, interactive, low-stakes, and anonymous experience. These activities show students the possible consequences of various choices they make today on their future health and are made assignable in Mastering Health with follow-up questions.

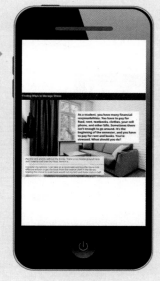

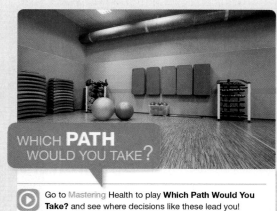

WHICH **PATH** WOULD YOU TAKE?

Go to Mastering Health to play **Which Path Would You Take?** and see where decisions like these lead you!

Continuous Learning
Before, During, and After Class

AFTER CLASS

Easy to Assign, Customize, Media-Rich, and Automatically-Graded Assignments

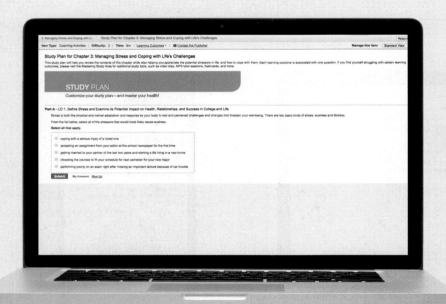

UPDATED! Study Plans tie all end-of-chapter material (including chapter review, pop quiz, and Think About It questions) to specific numbered Learning Outcomes and Mastering assets. Assignable study plan items contain at least one multiple choice question per Learning Outcome and wrong-answer feedback.

Video Tutors highlight a book figure or discussion point in an engaging video, covering key concepts such as how drugs act on the brain, reading food labels, and the benefits of regular exercise. All Video Tutors include assessment activities and are assignable in Mastering Health.

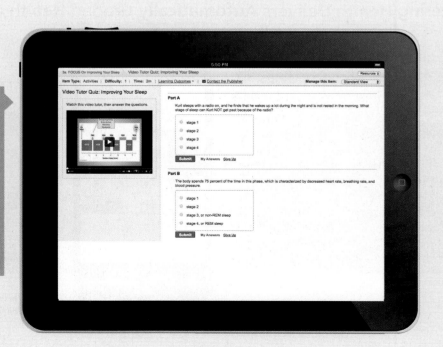

with Mastering Health

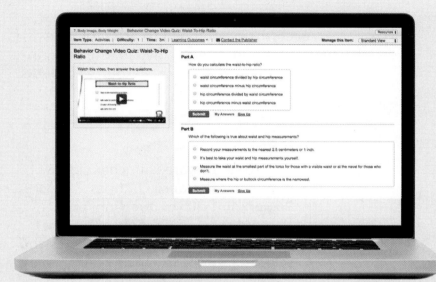

HALLMARK! **Behavior Change Videos** are concise whiteboard-style videos that help students with the steps of behavior change, covering topics such as setting SMART goals, identifying and overcoming barriers to change, planning realistic timelines, and more. Additional videos review key fitness concepts such as determining target heart rate range for exercise. All videos include assessment activities and are assignable in **Mastering Health**.

ABC News Videos spark discussions with up-to-date hot topics. The videos can be used to launch lectures or can be assigned in Mastering Health, with multiple choice questions that include wrong-answer feedback.

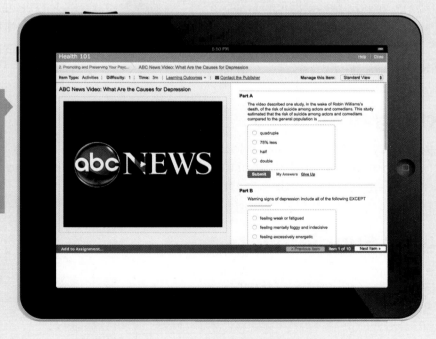

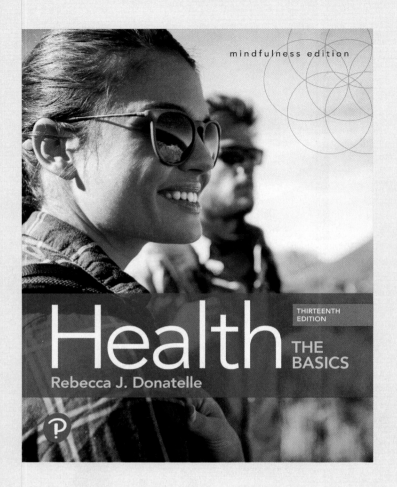

mindfulness edition

THIRTEENTH
EDITION

Health THE BASICS

Rebecca J. Donatelle

Mastering Health provides you with everything you need to prep for your course and deliver a dynamic lecture, in one convenient place. Resources include:

Media Assets For Each Chapter

- *ABC News* Lecture Launcher videos
- PowerPoint Lecture Outlines
- PowerPoint clicker questions and Jeopardy-style quiz show questions
- Files for all illustrations and tables and selected photos from the text

Test Bank

- Test Bank in Microsoft, Word, PDF, and RTF formats
- Computerized Test Bank, which includes all the questions from the printed test bank in a format that allows you to easily and intuitively build exams and quizzes.

Teaching Resources

- **New!** Ready-to-Go Teaching Modules
- Instructor Resource and Support Manual in Microsoft Word and PDF formats
- Learning Catalytics: Getting Started
- Getting Started with Mastering Health

Student Supplements

- Take Charge of Your Health Worksheets
- Behavior Change Log and Wellness Journal
- Eat Right!
- Live Right!
- Food Composition Table

Measuring Student Learning Outcomes?
All of the Mastering Health assignable content is tagged to book content and to Bloom's Taxonomy. You also have the ability to add your own learning outcomes, helping you track student performance against your learning outcomes. You can view class performance against the specified learning outcomes and share those results quickly and easily by exporting to a spreadsheet.

mindfulness edition

Health

THIRTEENTH EDITION

THE BASICS

Rebecca J. Donatelle

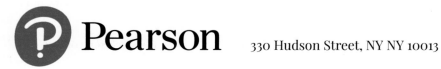

Pearson

330 Hudson Street, NY NY 10013

Courseware Portfolio Manager: Michelle Yglecias
Content Producer: Deepti Agarwal
Managing Producer: Nancy Tabor
Courseware Director, Content Development: Barbara Yien
Development Editor: Nic Albert
Courseware Editorial Assistants: Nicole Constantine, Crystal Trigueros
Rich Media Content Producers: Timothy Hainley, Lucinda Bingham
Full-Service Vendor: SPi Global
Copyeditor: Barbara Willette
Art Project Manager: Morgan Eawald, Lachina Publishing Services
Design Manager: Mark Ong
Interior Designer: Elise Lansdon
Cover Designer: Elise Lansdon
Rights & Permissions Project Manager: Donna Kalal, Cenveo Publisher Services
Rights & Permissions Management: Ben Ferrini
Photo Researcher: Kathleen Olson
Manufacturing Buyer: Stacey Weinberger, LSC Communications
Product Marketing Manager: Alysun Burns
Field Marketing Manager: Mary Salzman

Cover Photo Credit: Ammentorp Photography/Alamy Stock Photo.

Library of Congress Cataloging-in-Publication Data

Names: Donatelle, Rebecca J., 1950- author.
Title: Health : the basics / Rebecca J. Donatelle.
Description: 13th edition. | New York : Pearson, [2019] | Includes
    bibliographical references and index.
Identifiers: LCCN 2017044704| ISBN 9780134709680 (student edition) | ISBN
    9780134842790 (instructor's review copy)
Subjects: | MESH: Hygiene | Health Behavior
Classification: LCC RA776 | NLM QT 180 | DDC 613—dc23 LC record
available at https://lccn.loc.gov/2017044704

ISBN 10: 0-13-470968-3
(Student edition)
ISBN 13: 978-0-13-470968-0
(Student edition)
ISBN 10: 0-13-484279-0
(Instructor's Review Copy)
ISBN 13: 978-0-13-484279-0
(Instructor's Review Copy)

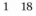

1   18

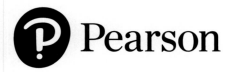

www.pearson.com

BRIEF CONTENTS

CONTENTS

PART THREE | **AVOIDING RISKS FROM HARMFUL HABITS**

8 Recognizing and Avoiding Addiction and Drug Abuse   209

9 Drinking Alcohol Responsibly and Ending Tobacco Use   238

PART FOUR | BUILDING HEALTHY LIFESTYLES

10 Nutrition: Eating for a Healthier You 270

11 Reaching and Maintaining a Healthy Weight 300

FOCUS ON Enhancing Your Body Image 325

12 Improving Your Personal Fitness 337

FEATURE BOXES

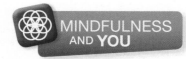
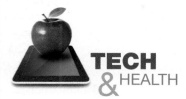
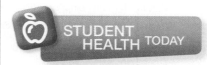

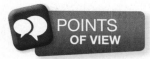

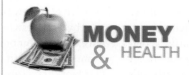

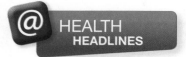

PREFACE

Today, threats to our health and the health of our planet dominate the media and affect our lives on a daily basis. Water shortages, polluted air, food safety concerns, violence and the threat of terrorism, diseases, and other concerns have us wondering about our ability to survive and thrive. The issues often seem so overwhelming, that you might wonder whether there is anything you can do to make a difference—to ensure your health, and a planet that is preserved for future generations. You are not alone! The good news is that you can do things to improve your health while being an agent for change with your loved ones and the greater community. It can start now, and it can start with you!

After years of teaching and working with students of all ages and stages of life and careers, I am encouraged by the fact that so many people, particularly younger adults, are "tuned in" to health. The problem is that with so much talk about health on so many platforms, sifting through the "junk information" and making the right choices based on good science and good sense can be difficult. My goals in writing *Health: The Basics, the Mindfulness Edition*, were to build on the strengths of past editions; to utilize the most current, scientifically valid research; and to examine key issues and potential solutions. We face increasing levels of stress, mental and emotional health problems, and real and perceived threats. As such, I have taken an exciting new Mindfulness approach to this edition. Mindfulness strategies are found in new "mindfulness and you" feature boxes and throughout the chapter text, flagged by a new icon.

Another ground-breaking and essential area of focus is our new chapter on *difference, disparity*, and *health equity*. Clearly, we face challenges in adapting to large and growing demographic shifts in the United States, complete with lingering stereotypes, distrust, anger, misperceptions, and other potentially destructive consequences. I challenge students to think about these issues and to explore actions that can be taken as individuals and as a society to begin to remove barriers and promote health equity for all.

As part of the process, I have worked hard to provide students with essential tools and resources to empower them to examine their behaviors and the factors that contribute to those behaviors, and to prioritize health now rather than next week or in some distant future. My other goal is to challenge students to also think globally as they consider health risks and seek creative solutions, both large and small, to address complex health problems. There is no one-size-fits-all recipe for health. You can do it your way, whether that means starting slowly with "baby steps" designed to change deeply engrained behaviors or gearing up for major changes that all happen at once. Remember, you didn't develop your behaviors overnight. Being patient but persistent with yourself is often part of the process. This book is designed to help students quickly grasp the information, focusing on key objectives that have relevance to their own lives. Importantly, encourage students to think about the issues, and help students answer these questions: What is the issue and why should I care? What are my options for action? When and how do I get started?

With each new edition of *Health: The Basics*, I have been gratified by the overwhelming success that this book has enjoyed. I am excited about making this edition the best yet—more timely, more relevant, and more interesting for students. Let's be real: Our world faces unprecedented challenges to individual and community health. Understanding these challenges and having a personal plan to preserve, protect, and promote health will help to ensure our healthful future!

NEW TO THIS EDITION
Chapter 1: Accessing Your Health

- Updated research linking poor diet to poor health
- Additional coverage of rising rates of prescription and illegal drug abuse, particularly opioids
- New stats on American insurance status
- A new focus on mindfulness, including an entire section on why mindfulness is so important to health, how to practice mindfulness, and potential current and long-range benefits of mindfulness.

Focus On: Difference, Disparity, and Health: Achieving Health Equity

This exciting new chapter, "Focus On: Difference, Disparity, and Health: Achieving Health Equity," looks at:

- What we mean by the terms *difference, disparity*, and *health equity* and why these are critical issue in America today
- The populations that are most vulnerable to health disparities as well as societal costs
- The social determinants of health that most strongly influence health disparities in the United States.
- Specific actions to take to promote health equity on campus, in community, and individually
- Systemic changes needed for the United States to progress toward better health for all, as well as examples of national and community-based initiatives focused on this goal

Chapter 2: Promoting and Preserving Your Psychological Health

- Updated research on all mental health issues with comprehensive research on contributors to these issues
- An enhanced section on self-esteem that addresses growing concerns about people who seem to be overdosing on self-esteem. Can you have too much of a good thing?

- A new section on defense mechanisms and how they can work to protect you or hold you back
- A new section on lifespan, maturity and health
- Updated and expanded information about the growing mental health crisis among young adults today and college students are particularly vulnerable to problems such as depression and anxiety
- A new **Mindfulness and You** box on potential positive effects of mindfulness practice and mental health problems

Focus On: Cultivating Your Spiritual Health

- Enhanced discussion of what it means to be spiritually healthy, the difference between being spiritual and being religious, and trends in spirituality based on age, with an emphasis on college students and Millennials
- Updated information on the physical, social, and psychological benefits of spiritual health
- New information on mindfulness as it relates to spiritual health, particularly environmental mindfulness

Chapter 3: Managing Stress and Coping with Life's Challenges

- A revised figure focusing on stress levels by age
- New coverage of the transactional model of stress and coping
- Expanded coverage of stress, immunity, and susceptibility to infectious diseases
- New minority-stress theory and it's importance.
- New coverage of the Yerkes-Dodson Law of arousal
- A new **Mindfulness and You** box on technostress and what you can do about it
- Updated coverage of stress related to relationships and money
- New coverage of stress-induced cardiomyopathy and new research on broken heart syndrome
- New coverage of dispositional mindfulness and ways to mindfully assess your stressors

Chapter 4: Improving Your Sleep

- New information on the growing recognition of how sleep affects health, sleep in the U.S., and reasons why so many people are sleep deprived.
- Updated information on the role of sleep in coping with life's challenges, maintaining your immune system, reducing your risks for CVD and Alzheimer's, and contributing to cognitive functioning
- New coverage of the "short sleeper" who needs less sleep
- A new **Mindfulness and You** box on how mindfulness strategies can improve your sleep
- New information on technology's effect on sleep and how to reduce risks

Chapter 5: Preventing Violence and Injury

- Expanded coverage of trends in violence in the United States and whether we are experiencing an epidemic of meanness?
- New trends and statistics on violent crimes in the United States
- Updated statistics on campus violence, new definitions on sexual assault, and enhanced overage of new legal implications related to sexual assault and rape on campus.

- Updated information on factors contributing to various forms of violence
- A new section on the growing problem of cybercrime and what you can do to protect yourself
- An expanded section on reducing rape on campus, with coverage of the "It's on Us" program
- New information on tech-facilitated stalking
- Updated information on the prevalence of unintentional injuries, particularly distracted driving crashes.
- A new **Mindfulness and You** box on anger, reactivity, and mindful cooling-off strategies

Chapter 6: Connecting and Communicating in the Modern World

- Updated statistics and information on the various types of relationships, how they are changing, and how they may differ on the basis of selected variables.
- Enhanced information on the criteria for healthy versus unhealthy relationships and the impact of each on overall health
- Updated information on the benefits of intimate relationships, friendships, social capital, and family relationships and how each is important to overall health
- Updated and expanded information about social media and how social media interactions can be stressful
- A new **Mindfulness and You** box covering how mindfully listening can improve your relationships

Focus On: Understanding Your Sexuality

- Updated information on trends in hormone replacement therapy and potential risks versus benefits.
- A new **Mindfulness and You** box on mindfulness as a way to manage some forms of sexual dysfunction
- Updated information on the correlation between drinking and unprotected sex among college students
- Updated coverage of gender identity, including transgender and cisgender individuals

Chapter 7: Considering Your Reproductive Choices

- Updated statistics on contraceptive usage rates and effectiveness among American college students
- Updated statistics on percentages of Americans who consider themselves pro-choice or pro-life.
- Updated information on lack of abortion availability for low-income populations
- A new **Mindfulness and You** box on coping with depression during pregnancy

Chapter 8: Recognizing and Avoiding Addiction and Drug Abuse

- Expanded coverage of addictions, psychological dependence, and health risks
- Expanded coverage of gambling disorder, particularly the four common phases individuals pass through
- Expanded coverage of compulsive buying disorder, particularly as it relates to the impact of the Internet
- Updated information on illicit drug use on campus and overall in the United States, including the growing threat of heroin addiction in many areas.

- Updated information on the status of legalized marijuana, the impact of legalization, and the pros and cons of a legal marijuana society
- A new **Mindfulness and You** box on mindfulness-based relapse prevention methods and the effectiveness of selected intervention strategies
- A new section on recovery coaching and its effectiveness

Chapter 9: Drinking Alcohol Responsibly and Ending Tobacco Use

- Updated and enhanced statistics on drinking prevalence, at-risk individuals, abstinence, and overall trends in alcohol use and abuse in America.
- Updated information on the long-term effects of alcohol use, particularly the possible correlation with cancer and other health risks
- Updated information on alcohol use in college, particularly high-risk drinking behaviors such as pregaming, binge drinking, and calorie "saving"
- New sections on alcohol inhalation
- Updated data on the social, health care, employee, and safety costs of alcohol misuse and abuse
- Updated statistics on trends in tobacco use and economic, health, and social costs to society
- Expanded coverage of e-cigarettes and their use
- Expanded coverage of drugs that play a role in tobacco cessation and reduction
- A new **Mindfulness and You** box on how mindfulness can help in quitting smoking

Chapter 10: Nutrition: Eating for a Healthier You

- New and expanded coverage of dietary trends in consumption in the United States and how these changes are related to changes in health status, particularly trends in obesity
- Updated information on the benefits and risks of fiber, protein, fats, carbohydrates, and other nutrients
- Updated information on the risks of *trans* fats and partially hydrogenated oils. Is butter better?
- Updated information on dietary fats, changes in recommendations for eggs and other products, and their potential roles in health and disease
- Overview of the New Dietary Guidelines for Americans
- A new **Mindfulness and You** box on mindful eating

Chapter 11: Reaching and Maintaining a Healthy Weight

- New statistics and trends in overweight, obesity, and super obesity in the United States and globally and the importance of these changes in overall risks to health
- New research on the potential role of genetics, hormones, and other factors in appetite
- Expanded discussion of psychosocial and socioeconomic factors in weight problems
- A new section on emerging theories on obesity risk, including discussions of pathogens and environmental toxins, drugs, and sleep deprivation
- A new section on mindful eating and eating triggers
- Updated coverage of weight loss interventions and treatments, including drugs and new surgical techniques

Focus On: Enhancing Your Body Image

- Updated tips for helping a friend with disordered eating
- Updated research throughout

Chapter 12: Improving Your Personal Fitness

- New material on how mindfulness strategies can help you make better use of your physical and social environments and enhance your activity levels
- New information on green exercise as a way to get physical and mental health benefits
- New information on assessing your social environment

Chapter 13: Reducing Your Risk of Cardiovascular Disease and Cancer

- Complete revision of trends, statistics, and risk factors for cardiovascular disease and cancer in the United States.
- New and updated information on the prevalence of coronary heart disease and hypertension and increased risks among young adults
- New information on preventricular contractions and other arrhythmias among young, apparently healthy adults
- New trends and statistics on smoking prevalence, at-risk populations, and long-term consequences
- A new section on *Helicobacter pylori* and stomach cancer
- A new **Mindfulness and You** box on ways of coping with the emotional side effects of cancer diagnoses

Focus On: Minimizing Your Risk for Diabetes

- New **Mindfulness and You** box on mindfulness-based interventions for controlling Type 2 Diabetes
- Updated information around global prevalence of Diabetes
- New information on diabetic neuropathy

Chapter 14: Protecting Against Infectious Diseases and Sexually Transmitted Infections

- New statistics and information on infectious diseases and the threat of strains of bacteria that are resistant to antibiotics and antimicrobials
- New information on a new tuberculosis vaccine
- A new and expanded section on the rising threats of tick-borne diseases, including coverage of the Powassan virus in the upper Midwest and northeastern United States
- Updated information on flu vaccination rates and the importance of vaccination for high-risk groups
- Expanded coverage of the Zika virus and continuing efforts to diagnose and treat the disease and prevent its spread.
- A new section on the potential role of mindfulness in reduced infectious disease risk
- Updated information on the latest HIV/AIDS trends and new diagnostic tests, treatments, and prevention methods

Focus On: Reducing Risks for Chronic Diseases and Conditions

- New **Mindfulness and You** box on using mindfulness and manage chronic pain
- New coverage of new guidelines surrounding LBP and treatment
- Update research throughout

Chapter 15: Making Smart Health Care Choices

- Updated information on current trends, issues, and concerns regarding consumer use of health care system and prescription drug use problems
- An updated and expanded section on various health care systems and services, the Affordable Care Act, and current Medicaid and Medicare concerns
- Updated information on the costs of the U.S. health care system, uninsured and underinsured populations, and potential health care changes that will affect young and old in the United States

Focus On: Understanding Complementary and Integrative Health

- New and expanded information on the increasing role of complementary and integrative medicine in the United States and the potential risks and benefits of selected treatments
- Added information on how mindfulness-based meditation has been shown to increase patients' sense of control over their symptoms and treatment
- A new **Mindfulness and You** box on the unexpected academic benefits of mindfulness
- Updated information on the benefits of acupuncture
- Added information on recalls of certain natural products

Focus On: Aging, Death, and Dying

- Updated data and information on U.S. aging
- Updated information on the prevalence of hospice facilities in the United States
- Updated figure on living arrangements of Americans age 65 and older
- Updated exercise recommendations for adults over age 65

Chapter 16: Promoting Environmental Health

- New and expanded coverage of the threats and challenges to the environment caused by human populations, including key contributors and potential risks of too little action to intervene
- New information and a new figure illustrating how we typically use water each day in our homes, with suggestions for reduction
- New information and trends on species extinction, natural resource depletion, and accelerations in both resulting from human activity and climate change
- New dire predictions involving unchecked population growth, depletion of resources, and the need for more planets to supply life in the future at current rates of use
- Updated information on energy consumption
- A new **Mindfulness and You** environmental mindfulness box
- Updated information and strategies for preserving and protecting our environment and all living creatures
- Updated information on food waste and strategies to preserve resources

TEXT FEATURES AND LEARNING AIDS

Health: The Basics includes the following special features, all of which have been revised and improved for this edition:

- **Chapter Learning Outcomes** summarize the main competencies students will gain from each chapter and alert students to the key concepts and are now explicitly tied to chapter sections. Focus On mini-chapters now also include learning outcomes.
- **Study Plans** tie all end-of-chapter material (including Chapter Review, Pop Quiz, and Think About It questions) to specific numbered Learning Outcomes and Mastering Health assets.
- **What Do You Think?** critical-thinking questions appear throughout the text, encouraging students to pause and reflect on material they have read.
- A **Why Should I Care?** feature now opens each chapter, presenting students with information about the effects poor health habits have on students in the here and now, engaging them at the onset of the chapter and encouraging them to learn more.
- **Assess Yourself** boxes help students evaluate their health behaviors. The **Your Plan for Change** section within each box provides students with targeted suggestions for ways to implement change.
- **Skills for Behavior Change** boxes focus on practical strategies that students can use to improve health or reduce their risks from negative health behaviors.
- **Mindfulness and You** boxes focus on mindfulness research and applications in relation to high-interest topics such as sleep, technostress, mental health, and sexual dysfunction.
- **Tech & Health** boxes cover the new technology innovations that can help students stay healthy.
- **Money & Health** boxes cover health topics from the financial perspective.
- **Points of View** boxes present viewpoints on a controversial health issue and ask students *Where Do You Stand?* questions, encouraging them to critically evaluate the information and consider their own opinions.
- **Health Headlines** boxes highlight new discoveries and research, as well as interesting trends in the health field.
- **Student Health Today** boxes focus attention on specific health and wellness issues that affect today's college students.
- **Health in a Diverse World** boxes expand discussion of health topics to diverse groups within the United States and around the world.
- A **running glossary** in the margins defines terms where students first encounter them, emphasizing and supporting understanding of material.
- A **Behavior Change Contract** for students to fill out is included at the back of the book.

SUPPLEMENTARY MATERIALS

Instructor Supplements

- **Mastering Health** (www.masteringhealthandnutrition.com or www.pearsonmastering.com). Mastering Health coaches students through the toughest health topics. A variety of **Coaching Activities** guide students through key health concepts with interactive mini-lessons, complete with hints and wrong-answer feedback. **Reading Quizzes** (20 questions per chapter) ensure that students have completed the assigned reading before class. ABC News **videos** stimulate classroom discussions and include multiple-choice questions with feedback for students. Assignable **Behavior Change Video Quiz** and **Which Path Would You Take?** activities ensure that students complete and reflect on behavior change and health choices. **NutriTools** in the nutrition chapter allow students to combine and experiment with different food options and learn firsthand how to build healthier meals. **MP3 Tutor Sessions** relate to chapter content and come with multiple-choice questions that provide wrong-answer feedback. **Learning Catalytics** provides open-ended questions that students can answer in real time. **Dynamic Study Modules** enable students to study effectively in an adaptive format. Instructors can also assign these for completion as a graded assignment before class.

- **Ready to Go Teaching Modules** are a new tool designed to save instructors valuable course preparation time. These ten online modules are much like a visual Instructor's Resource Manual in which each module includes recommendations for materials, activities, and resources instructors can use to prepare for their course and deliver a dynamic lecture in one convenient place. Each module has paired student assignments in Mastering Health that instructors can deploy before, during, and after lecture.

- **Digital Instructional Resources: Download Only.** All book- and course-specific teaching resources are downloadable from the Instructor Resources tab in Mastering Health as well as from Pearson's Instructor Resource Center (www.pearson.com). Resources include *ABC News* videos; Health Video Tutor videos; clicker questions; Quiz Show questions; PowerPoint lecture outlines; all figures and tables from the text; PDF and Microsoft Word files of the *Instructor Resource and Support Manual*; and PDF, RTF, and Microsoft Word files of the Test Bank, the Computerized Test Bank, the User's Quick Guide, *Teaching with Student Learning Outcomes*, *Teaching with Web 2.0*, *Great Ideas! Active Ways to Teach Health and Wellness*, *Behavior Change Log Book and Wellness Journal*, *Eat Right!*, *Live Right!*, and *Take Charge of Your Health* worksheets.

- **ABC News Videos** and **Health Video Tutors.** New *ABC News* videos, each 3 to 8 minutes long, and 26 Health Video Tutors flagged by the play icon in the text help instructors to stimulate critical discussion in the classroom. Videos are embedded within PowerPoint lectures and are assignable through Mastering Health.

- ***Instructor Resource and Support Manual.*** This teaching tool provides chapter summaries, outlines, integrated *ABC News* video discussion questions, tips and strategies for managing large classrooms, ideas for in-class activities, and suggestions for integrating Mastering Health into your course.

- **Test Bank.** The Test Bank incorporates Bloom's Taxonomy, or the higher order of learning, to help instructors create exams that encourage students to think analytically and critically. Test Bank questions are tagged to global and book-specific student learning outcomes.

Student Supplements

- **The Study Area of Mastering Health** is organized by learning areas. *Read It* houses the Pearson eText as well as the Chapter Objectives and up-to-date health news. *See It* includes *ABC News* videos and the Behavior Change videos. *Hear It* contains MP3 Tutor Session files and audio-based case studies. *Do It* contains the choose-your-own-adventure-style Interactive Behavior Change Activities—Which Path Would You Take?, interactive NutriTools activities, critical-thinking Points of View questions, and Web links. *Review It* contains Practice Quizzes for each chapter, Flashcards, and Glossary. *Live It* will help to jump-start students' behavior change projects with interactive Assess Yourself Worksheets and resources to plan change.

- **Pearson eText** comes complete with embedded *ABC News* videos and Health Video Tutors. The Pearson eText is mobile friendly and ADA accessible, is available on smartphones and tablets, and includes instructor and student note-taking, highlighting, bookmarking, and search functions.

- ***Behavior Change Log Book and Wellness Journal.*** This assessment tool helps students track daily exercise and nutritional intake and suggests topics for journal-based activities.

- ***Eat Right! Healthy Eating in College and Beyond.*** This booklet provides students with practical nutrition guidelines, shopper's guides, and recipes.

- ***Live Right! Beating Stress in College and Beyond.*** This booklet gives students tips for coping with stress during college and for the rest of their lives.

- **Digital 5-Step Pedometer.** This pedometer measures steps, distance (miles), activity time, and calories and provides a time clock.

- **MyDietAnalysis** (www.mydietanalysis.com). Powered by ESHA Research, Inc., this tool features a database of nearly 20,000 foods and multiple reports. It allows students to track their diet and activity using up to three profiles and to generate and submit reports electronically.

ACKNOWLEDGMENTS

It is hard for me to believe that *Health: The Basics* is in its 13th edition! Who could have envisioned the evolution of health texts even a decade ago? With the nearly limitless resources of the Internet, social networking sites and national databases, finding the most appropriate information for today's students is challenging. Each step in planning, developing, and translating that information to students and instructors requires a tremendous amount of work from many dedicated people, and I cannot help but think how fortunate I have been to work with the gifted publishing professionals at Pearson. Through time constraints, decision making, and computer meltdowns, this group handled every issue, every obstacle with patience, professionalism, and painstaking attention to detail.

Some key individuals who have made this 13th edition have moved on to other positions; however, I would be remiss in not acknowledging Susan Malloy and Kari Hopperstead, who were the internal "life blood" of my texts for many years and were instrumental in their successes. Their efforts and the efforts of Sandy Lindelof as editor and Neena Bali as marketing manager for previous editions are also noteworthy. These two individuals helped to promote my books and keep them vibrant and ahead of the competition in a field of outstanding personal health books.

Many others have been key to each of my book successes. One person in particular is Courseware Portfolio Director Barbara Yien. Regardless of her roles and responsibilities, she has been the glue that holds these books together. She is hardworking and highly skilled, "gets it" when it comes to the health marketplace, is a skilled problem solver, and worries the details in producing high-quality products. Importantly, she is also fun and has a wonderful approach to working with those of us who can sometimes be challenging. In short, she is the managerial, development, and editorial expert/leader who any author dreams of having on their books. THANK you, Barbara!

Another person I'd like to acknowledge in particular is Nic Albert, developmental editor, writer, and contributor. Nic did a fantastic job of providing guidance and editorial assistance streamlining page length, and fine-tuning the many aspects of each chapter to maximize impact in a relatively short space. Thank you, Nic!

I would also like to provide a special thank you to Deepti Agarwal, who has worked tirelessly and efficiently on both *Access to Health*, 15th edition, and *Health: The Basics*, 13th edition. Not only is Deepti a creative, highly skilled, hard-working, and well-organized content producer; she also has the temperament and professionalism to help move a project through time constraints, deadlines, and challenges and to make sure that all of the great work from so many people comes to fruition in a top-notch product. Her skills in navigating production pitfalls, keeping the author and contributors on task, and meeting production deadlines are truly exemplary.

Further praise and thanks go to the highly skilled and hard-working, creative, and charismatic Courseware Portfolio Manager Michelle Yglecias, who has helped to catapult this book into the competitive twenty-first century. Michelle's fresh approach and enthusiasm for the work are much appreciated, and Pearson is fortunate to have someone with her experience and competence at the helm. Michelle has consistently been a key figure in moving the college/university health text to the next level. When I first proposed adding a new chapter on difference, disparity, and health and taking a mindfulness approach to this edition, she listened, made suggestions, did a market analysis, and enthusiastically took on this project to help bring it to fruition.

Although these individuals were key contributors to the finished work, there were many other people who worked on this revision of *Health: The Basics*. At every level, I was extremely impressed by the work of key individuals. Thanks also to Michelle Gardner and the hard-working staff at SPi Global, who put everything together to make a polished finished product. The talented artists at Lachina deserve many thanks for making an innovative art program a reality. Timothy Hainley, Senior Rich Media Content Producer, and Lucinda Bingham, Rich Media Content Producer, put together our most innovative and comprehensive media package yet. Additional thanks go to the rest of the team at Pearson.

The editorial and production teams are critical to a book's success, but I would be remiss if I didn't thank another key group who ultimately helps to determine a book's success: the textbook representative and sales group and their hard-working, top-notch marketers Executive Product Marketing Manager Allison Rona and Product Marketer Alysun Burns. From directing an outstanding marketing campaign to the everyday tasks of being responsive to instructor needs, Allison, Alysun, and Field Marketing Manager Mary Salzman do a superb job of making sure that *Health: The Basics* gets into instructors' hands and that adopters receive the service they deserve. In keeping with my overall experiences with Pearson, the marketing and sales staffs are among the best of the best. I am very lucky to have them working with me on this project, and I want to extend a special thanks to all of them!

CONTRIBUTORS TO THE 13TH EDITION

Many colleagues, students, and staff members have provided the feedback, reviews, extra time, assistance, and encouragement that have helped me meet the rigorous demands of publishing this book over the years. Whether acting as reviewers, generating new ideas, providing expert commentary, or revising chapters, each of these professionals has added his or her skills to our collective endeavor.

To make a book like this happen on a relatively short timeline, the talents of many specialists in the field must be combined. Whether contributing creative skills in writing, envisioning areas that will be critical to the current and future health needs of students, using their experiences to make topics come alive for students, or utilizing their professional expertise to ensure scientifically valid information, each of these individuals was carefully selected to help make this text the best that it can be. I couldn't do it without their help! As always, I would like to give particular thanks to Dr. Patricia Ketcham of Western Oregon University and past president of the American College Health Association, who has helped with the *Health: The Basics* series since its earliest beginnings. As the former associate director of health promotion at Oregon State University and current role at WOU, Dr. Ketcham has excellent background and experience with the myriad of health issues and the key challenges facing today's students. She contributed to revisions of Chapter 8, "Recognizing and Avoiding Addiction and Drug Abuse"; Chapter 9, "Drinking Alcohol Responsibly and Ending Tobacco Use"; Chapter 15, "Making Smart Health Care Choices"; and "Focus On: Aging, Death, and Dying." Dr. Susan Dobie, associate professor in the School of Health, Physical Education, and Leisure Services at University of Northern Iowa, used her background in health promotion and health behavior and in teaching a diverse range of students to provide a fresh approach to revisions of Chapter 6, "Connecting and Communicating in the Modern World"; "Focus On: Understanding Your Sexuality"; and Chapter 7, "Considering Your Reproductive Choices." Dr. Erica Jackson, associate professor in the Department of Public & Allied Health Sciences at Delaware State University, applied her wealth of fitness knowledge to update and enhance "Focus On: Enhancing Your Body Image" and Chapter 12, "Improving Your Personal Fitness." Amber Emanuel utilized her extensive background in counseling, relationships, and spirituality to provide a fresh and engaging update to Chapter 2, "Promoting and Preserving Your Psychological Health." Dr. Disa Cornish at the University of Northern Iowa has used her considerable knowledge and expertise to revise "Focus On: Cultivating Your Spiritual Health." With her outstanding background in nutrition science and applied dietary behavior, Dr. Kathy Munoz, professor in the Department of Kinesiology and Recreation Administration at Humboldt State University, provided an extensive revision and updating of Chapter 10, "Nutrition: Eating for a Healthier You." Laura Bonazzoli, who has been a key part of developing and refining many aspects of this book over the last editions, used her considerable knowledge and skills in providing major revisions of Chapter 1, "Accessing Your Health"; "Focus On: Difference, Disparity, and Health: Achieving Health Equity"; and "Focus On: Understanding Complementary and Integrative Health." Although Laura has done a tremendous job in providing high-quality, scientifically accurate and thoughtful revisions to several chapters over the years, her development and authorship on the new, much needed chapter on difference, diversity and health exemplifies her excellent writing ability and intellectual creativity. Laura does an outstanding job and is a pleasure to work with!

REVIEWERS FOR THE 13TH EDITION

With each new edition of *Health: The Basics*, we have built on the combined expertise of many colleagues throughout the country who are dedicated to the education and behavioral changes of students. We thank the many reviewers who have made such valuable contributions to the past 12 editions of *Health: The Basics*. For the 13th edition, reviewers who have helped us continue this tradition of excellence include the following:

Natascha Romeo, Wake Forest University
Dina Hayduk, Kutztown University
Julie Kuykendall, Georgia Southern University
Amber Emanuel, University of Florida
Patricia Hardin, William Paterson University
Dara Vanzin, Cal State Fullerton
Sharon Woodard, Wake Forest University
Timothy Garcia, Butte College
Holly Moses, University of Florida
Paul Greer, San Diego Mesa College
Holly Aguila, Arizona State University

REVIEWERS FOR MASTERING HEALTH

We continue to thank the following members of the Faculty Advisory Board, who offered us valuable insights that helped develop Mastering Health in previous editions: Steve Hartman (Citrus College), William Huber (County College of Morris), Kris Jankovitz (Cal Poly), Stasi Kasaianchuk (Oregon State University), Lynn Long (University of North Carolina Wilmington), Ayanna Lyles (California University of Pennsylvania), Steven Namanny (Utah Valley University), Karla Rues (Ozarks Technical Community College), Debra Smith (Ohio University), Sheila Stepp (SUNY Orange), and Mary Winfrey-Kovell (Ball State University). For the 13th edition, the following people contributed content to Mastering Health:

Timothy Garcia, Butte College
Jen Henderson, West Los Angeles Community College
Sharon Woodard, Wake Forest University

Many thanks to all!
Rebecca J. Donatelle, PhD

1

Accessing Your Health

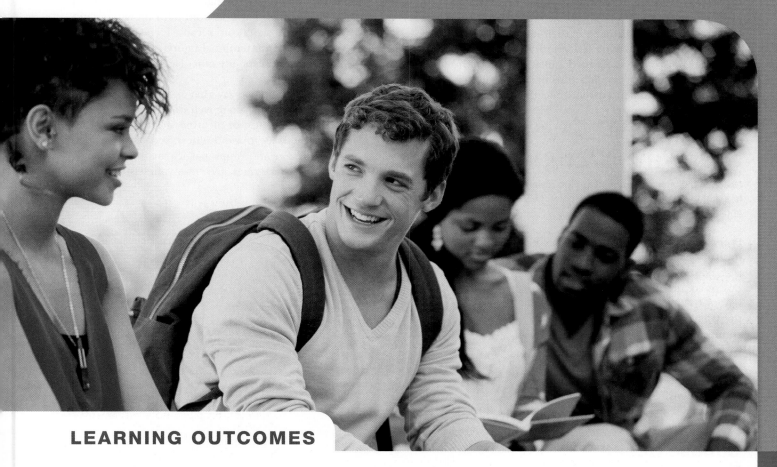

LEARNING OUTCOMES

LO 1 Describe the immediate and long-term rewards of healthy behaviors and the effects that your health choices may have on others.

LO 2 Compare and contrast the medical model of health and the public health model, and discuss the six dimensions of health.

LO 3 Classify factors that influence your health status into one of five broad categories identified by *Healthy People 2020* as determinants of health.

LO 4 Describe mindfulness, identifying its health benefits and ways to incorporate it into your life.

LO 5 Compare and contrast the health belief model, the social cognitive model, and the transtheoretical model of behavior change, and explain how you might use them in making a specific behavior change.

LO 6 Identify your own current risk behaviors, the factors that influence those behaviors, and the strategies you can use to change them.

By being a savvy health consumer and improving and maintaining your health, you will reap many benefits. Academic and career success, healthy relationships, a zest for living, and reduced risks for disease and disability can help you maximize your healthy years. Much of who you are and what you will become is in *your* hands!

Got health? That might sound like a simple question, but it isn't. Health is a process, not something we just "get." People who are healthy in their fifties, sixties, and beyond aren't just lucky or the beneficiaries of hardy genes. In most cases, those who are healthy and thriving in their later years set the stage for good health by making it a priority in their early years. Whether your coming decades are filled with good health, a productive career, strong relationships, and fulfillment of your life goals is influenced by the health choices you make—beginning right now.

LO 1 | WHY HEALTH, WHY NOW?

Describe the immediate and long-term rewards of healthy behaviors and the effects that your health choices may have on others.

Every day, the media remind us of health challenges facing the world, the nation—maybe even your campus or community. You might want to ignore these issues, but you can't. In the twenty-first century, your health is connected to the health of people with whom you directly interact as well as to that of people you've never met and the well-being of your local environment and of the entire planet. Let's take a look at how.

Choose Health Now for Immediate Benefits

Almost everyone knows that overeating leads to weight gain and that driving after drinking increases the risk of motor vehicle accidents. But other choices you make every day may influence your well-being in ways you're not aware of. For instance, did you know that the amount of sleep you get each night could affect your body weight, your ability to ward off colds, your mood, your interactions with others, and your driving? What's more, inadequate sleep is one of the

most commonly reported impediments to academic success (**FIGURE 1.1**). Similarly, drinking alcohol impairs your immediate health and your academic performance. It also sharply increases your risk of unintentional injuries—not only from motor vehicle accidents, but also from falls, drowning, and burns. This is especially significant because for people between the ages of 15 and 44, unintentional injury—whether related to drowsiness, alcohol use, or any other factor—is the leading cause of death (**TABLE 1.1**).

It isn't an exaggeration to say that healthy choices have immediate benefits. When you're well nourished, fit, rested, and free from the influence of nicotine, alcohol, and other drugs, you're more likely to avoid illness, succeed in school, maintain supportive relationships, participate in meaningful work and community activities, and enjoy your leisure time.

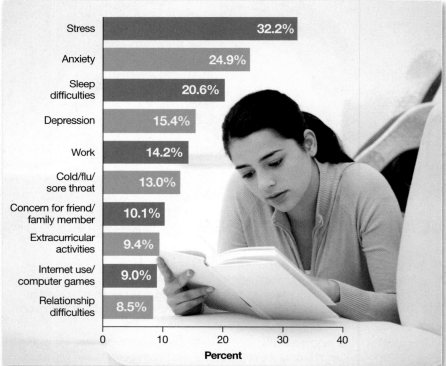

Impediment	Percent
Stress	32.2%
Anxiety	24.9%
Sleep difficulties	20.6%
Depression	15.4%
Work	14.2%
Cold/flu/sore throat	13.0%
Concern for friend/family member	10.1%
Extracurricular activities	9.4%
Internet use/computer games	9.0%
Relationship difficulties	8.5%

FIGURE 1.1 Top Ten Reported Impediments to Academic Performance—Past 12 Months In a recent survey by the National College Health Association, students indicated that stress, anxiety, poor sleep, and other factors had prevented them from performing at their academic best.

Source: Data are from American College Health Association, *American College Health Association—National College Health Assessment II (ACHA-NCHA II) Reference Group Data Report, Fall 2016* (Baltimore, MD: ACHA, 2017).

TABLE 1.1 | Leading Causes of Death in the United States in 2014, Overall and by Age Group (15 and older)

All Ages	Number of Deaths
Diseases of the heart	614,348
Malignant neoplasms (cancer)	591,699
Chronic lower respiratory diseases	147,101
Accidents (unintentional injuries)	136,053
Cerebrovascular diseases (stroke)	133,103
Aged 15–24	
Accidents (unintentional injuries)	11,836
Suicide	5,079
Assault (homicide)	4,144
Malignant neoplasms (cancer)	1,569
Diseases of the heart	953
Aged 25–44	
Accidents (unintentional injuries)	63,225
Malignant neoplasms (cancer)	14,891
Diseases of the heart	13,709
Suicide	13,275
Assault (homicide)	6,747
Aged 45–64	
Malignant neoplasms (cancer)	160,116
Diseases of the heart	109,264
Accidents (unintentional injuries)	38,640
Chronic liver disease and cirrhosis	21,419
Chronic lower respiratory diseases	20,894
Aged 65+	
Diseases of the heart	489,722
Malignant neoplasms (cancer)	413,885
Chronic lower respiratory diseases	124,693
Cerebrovascular diseases	113,308
Alzheimer's disease	92,604

Source: Data from M. Heron, "Deaths: Leading Causes for 2014, Table 1," *National Vital Statistics Reports* 65, no. 5 (June 2016), www.cdc.gov/nchs/data/nvsr/nvsr65/nvsr65_05.pdf.

Choose Health Now for Long-Term Rewards

Successful aging starts now. The choices you make today are like seeds: If you plant good seeds and tend them well, you're more likely to enjoy the fruits of a longer and healthier life. In contrast, failure to plant the seeds or to nurture them will increase the likelihood of a shorter life as well as persistent illness, addiction, and other limitations on quality and quantity of life.

Personal Choices Influence Life Expectancy According to current **mortality** rates—the proportion of deaths within a population—the average **life expectancy** at birth in the United States is projected to be 78.8 years for a child born in 2015.[1] In other words, we can expect that Americans born today will live much longer than people born in the early 1900s, whose average life expectancy was 47 years. But life expectancy a century ago was determined largely by our susceptibility to infectious disease. In 1900, over 30 percent of all deaths occurred among children younger than 5 years old, and the number one cause of death was infection.[2] Even among adults, infectious diseases such as tuberculosis and pneumonia were the leading causes of death, and widespread epidemics of infectious diseases such as influenza crossed national boundaries, killing millions.

With the development of vaccines and antibiotics, life expectancy increased dramatically as premature deaths from infectious diseases decreased. As a result, **chronic diseases** such as heart disease, cerebrovascular disease (which leads to strokes), cancer, and chronic lower respiratory diseases became leading causes of death. Advances in diagnostic technologies, heart and brain surgery, radiation and other cancer treatments, and new medications have continued the trend of increasing life expectancy into the twenty-first century.

78.8 YEARS

is the **LIFE EXPECTANCY** in the United States.

Unfortunately, life expectancy in the United States is several years below that of many other nations. Factors contributing to premature mortality and thus limiting U.S. life expectancy include obesity, tobacco and alcohol abuse, and drug overdose, which is now the leading cause of accidental death.[3] Our highly fragmented system of health care and lower quality of care for chronic disease are also part of the complex, multifactorial influences on our lower life expectancy.[4] For more, see the Health Headlines box.

Personal Choices Influence Healthy Life Expectancy Healthful choices increase your **healthy life expectancy**—the number of years of full health you enjoy without disability, chronic pain, or significant illness. One aspect of healthy life expectancy is **health-related quality of life (HRQoL)**, a concept

mortality The proportion of deaths to population.

life expectancy The expected number of years of life remaining at a given age, such as at birth.

chronic disease A disease that typically begins slowly, progresses, and persists, with a variety of signs and symptoms that can be treated but not cured by medication.

healthy life expectancy The expected number of years of full health remaining at a given age, such as at birth.

health-related quality of life (HRQoL) Assessment of impact of health status—including elements of physical, mental, emotional, and social function—on overall quality of life.

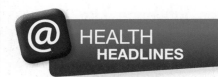

SHORTER LIVES, POORER HEALTH

In 2013, the Institute of Medicine (now the National Academy of Medicine) published a report comparing health and longevity in the United States to that of 16 peer countries—high-income democracies including Canada, Australia, Japan, and 13 countries in Western Europe. Its sobering finding was that, for decades, Americans have been dying at earlier ages than people in peer countries and experiencing poorer health at all life stages, from birth through older adulthood.

An intriguing aspect of the findings is that Americans' reduced longevity reverses after age 75; that is, an American who reaches age 75 can actually expect to live longer than a 75-year-old from a peer country. This advantage is thought to be due to lower cancer death rates as well as better management of blood pressure and blood lipids, two factors in heart disease. Our reduced longevity overall, therefore, must be due to factors affecting us earlier in life. For example, the United States has a higher infant mortality rate than that of the peer countries. We also have a higher rate of homicides and accidental injury deaths, especially drug-related deaths, which are more common in young or middle adulthood. Americans also have higher rates of HIV/AIDS, obesity, and diabetes, conditions that reduce the likelihood that people will reach age 75.

The Institute of Medicine report identified four general factors for our high rates of life-threatening diseases and injuries:

- **Our troubled health care system.** Americans are more likely to be uninsured and underinsured
- **Our unequal society.** The United States has a high level of poverty and income inequality as well as lower levels of social services.
- **Our car culture.** The infrastructure in communities throughout the United States tends to be designed for driving rather than for walking or cycling, discouraging physical activity.
- **Our poor behaviors.** Although our rates of smoking are lower, we're more likely to abuse drugs, use firearms, drive while intoxicated, and fail to wear a safety belt. We also consume the most calories per person.

If citizens of 16 peer countries can enjoy better health and longer lives, Americans can as well. Get involved by supporting increased access to health care and social services and pedestrian-friendly community redevelopment. As you learn about health-promoting behaviors in this text, be sure to put them into practice.

Source: Institute of Medicine, "U.S. Health in International Perspective: Shorter Lives, Poorer Health," January 2013, www.iom.edu/~/media/Files /Report%20Files/2013/US-Health-International -Perspective/USHealth_Intl_PerspectiveRB.pdf.

---

well-being An assessment of the positive aspects of a person's life, such as positive emotions and life satisfaction.

that focuses on the impact of health on physical, mental, emotional, and social function. Closely related to this is **well-being**, which assesses the positive aspects of a person's life, such as positive emotions and life satisfaction.[5]

the public indirectly through reduced tax revenues because of income lost from absenteeism and premature death, increased disability payments because of an inability to remain in the workforce, and increased health insurance rates as claims rise for treatment of obesity and associated diseases.

Your Health Is Linked to Societal Health

Our personal health choices affect the lives of others because they contribute to national health and the global burden of disease. For example, overeating and inadequate physical activity contribute to obesity, but obesity isn't a problem only for the individual. Along with its associated health problems, obesity affects the U.S. health care system and the overall U.S. economy. According to the U.S. Centers for Disease Control and Prevention, the medical costs of obesity in the United States are nearly $150 billion each year.[6] Obesity also costs

⊙ SEE IT! VIDEOS

Can simply being kind improve your health? Watch **Helping Others Could Be Good for Your Health** in the Study Area of Mastering Health.

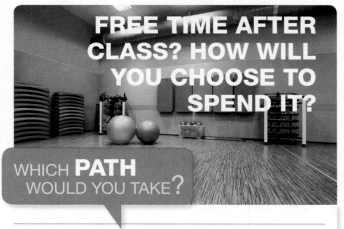

FREE TIME AFTER CLASS? HOW WILL YOU CHOOSE TO SPEND IT?

WHICH **PATH** WOULD YOU TAKE?

⊙ Go to Mastering Health to see how your actions today affect your future health.

Models of Health

Over the centuries, different ideals—or models—of human health have dominated. Our current model of health has broadened from a focus on the physical body to an understanding of health as a reflection not only of ourselves, but also of our communities.

Medical Model Before the twentieth century, perceptions of health were dominated by the **medical model**, in which health status focused primarily on the individual and his or her tissues and organs. The surest way to improve health was to cure the individual's disease, either with medication to treat the disease-causing agent or through surgery to remove or repair the diseased tissues. Therefore, government resources focused on initiatives that led to treatment, rather than prevention, of disease.

Public Health Model Not until the early decades of the 1900s did researchers begin to recognize that the health of entire populations of poor people, particularly those living in certain locations, was affected by environmental factors over which the people had little control: polluted water and air, a low-quality diet, poor housing, and unsafe work settings. As a result, researchers began to focus on an **ecological or public health model**, which views diseases and other negative health events as a

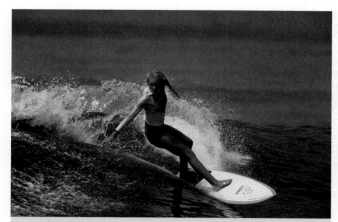

What is meant by *quality of life*? Hawaiian surfer Bethany Hamilton lost her arm in a shark attack while surfing at age 13, but that hasn't prevented her from achieving her goals as a professional surfer.

▶ **SEE IT!** VIDEOS

What can one person do to fight childhood hunger? Watch **Viola Davis Fights to End Child Hunger**, available on Mastering Health.

Smoking, excessive alcohol consumption, and illegal drug use also place an economic burden on our communities and society. Moreover, these behaviors have social and emotional consequences, such as the effects on people who lose their loved ones to these choices. The burden on caregivers who personally sacrifice to take care of people disabled by diseases is another part of this problem.

At the root of concerns about what individual health choices cost society is an ethical question: To what extent should the public bear the brunt of an individual's unhealthy choices? Should we require individuals to pay somehow for their poor choices? In some cases, we already do. We tax cigarettes and alcohol, and several cities now tax sweetened soft drinks, which have been blamed for rising obesity rates. On the other side of the debate are those who argue that smoking, drinking, and overeating are behaviors that require treatment, not punishment. Are seemingly personal choices that influence health always entirely within our control? Before we can explore these questions further, we need to understand what health actually is.

> **health** The ever-changing process of achieving individual potential in the physical, social, emotional, mental, spiritual, and environmental dimensions.
>
> **medical model** A view of health in which health status focuses primarily on the individual and a biological or diseased organ perspective.
>
> **ecological or public health model** A view of health in which diseases and other negative health events are seen as a result of an individual's interaction with his or her social and physical environment.

LO 2 | WHAT IS HEALTH?

Compare and contrast the medical model of health and the public health model, and discuss the six dimensions of health.

For some people, the word **health** simply means the antithesis of sickness. For others, it means fitness, wellness, or well-being. As our collective understanding of illness has improved, so has our ability to understand health's many nuances.

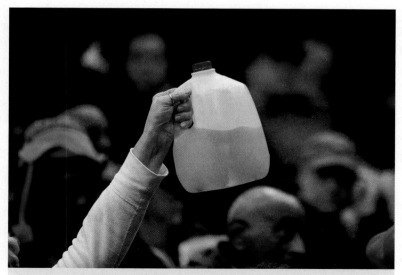

Negative health events can be caused by people's interaction with the physical environment. High levels of lead in the tap water in Flint, Michigan, have made water in that city largely undrinkable and put the health and wellness of many children and families at risk.

disease prevention Actions or behaviors designed to keep people from getting sick.

health promotion The combined educational, organizational, procedural, environmental, social, and financial supports that help individuals and groups to reduce negative health behaviors and promote positive change.

risk behaviors Actions that increase susceptibility to negative health outcomes.

wellness The achievement of the highest level of health possible in each of several dimensions.

result of an individual's interaction with his or her social and physical environment.

Recognition of the public health model led health officials to move to control contaminants in water, for example, by building adequate sewers, and to control burning and other forms of air pollution. In the early 1900s, colleges began offering courses in health and hygiene. Over time, public health officials began to recognize and address many other forces that affect human health, including hazardous work conditions; pollution; negative influences in the home and social environment; abuse of drugs and alcohol; stress; unsafe behavior; diet; sedentary lifestyle; and cost, quality, and access to health care.

By the 1940s, progressive thinkers began calling for policies, programs, and services to improve individual health and that of the population as a whole, shifting the focus from treatment of individual illness to **disease prevention**. For example, childhood vaccination programs reduced the incidence and severity of infectious disease; safety features such as seatbelts and airbags in motor vehicles and helmet laws for cyclists reduced traffic injuries and fatalities; and laws governing occupational safety reduced injuries and deaths among American workers. In 1947, at an international conference focusing on global health issues, the World Health Organization proposed a new definition of health: *"Health is the state of complete physical, mental, and social well-being, not just the absence of disease or infirmity."*[7] This new definition prompted a global movement to expand our concept of health.

The public health model also began to emphasize **health promotion**—policies and programs that promote behaviors known to support good health. Health promotion programs identify people engaging in **risk behaviors** (behaviors that increase susceptibility to negative health outcomes) and motivate them to change their actions by improving their knowledge, attitudes, and skills. Numerous public policies and services, technological advances, and individual actions have worked to improve our overall health status greatly in the past 100 years. FIGURE 1.2 lists the ten greatest public health achievements of the twentieth century.

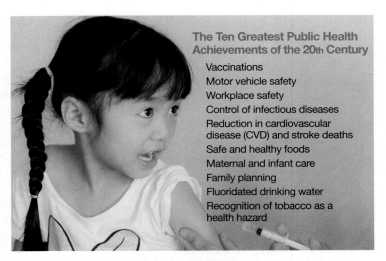

The Ten Greatest Public Health Achievements of the 20th Century

Vaccinations
Motor vehicle safety
Workplace safety
Control of infectious diseases
Reduction in cardiovascular disease (CVD) and stroke deaths
Safe and healthy foods
Maternal and infant care
Family planning
Fluoridated drinking water
Recognition of tobacco as a health hazard

FIGURE 1.2 The Ten Greatest Public Health Achievements of the Twentieth Century

Source: Adapted from Centers for Disease Control and Prevention, "Ten Great Public Health Achievements in the 20th Century," April 26, 2013, www.cdc.gov/about/history /tengpha.htm.

Pulitzer Prize–winning book *So Human an Animal*, Dubos defined health as *"a quality of life, involving social, emotional, mental, spiritual, and biological fitness on the part of the individual, which results from adaptations to the environment."*[8] This concept of *adaptability*, or the ability to cope successfully with life's ups and downs, became key to our overall understanding of health.

Later, the concept of **wellness** enlarged Dubos's definition of health by recognizing levels—or gradations—of health (FIGURE 1.3). To achieve *high-level wellness*, a person must move progressively higher on a continuum of positive health indicators. People who fail to achieve these levels may slip into illness, disability, or premature death.

Today, the words *health* and *wellness* are often used interchangeably to describe the dynamic, ever-changing process of trying to achieve one's potential in each of six interrelated dimensions (FIGURE 1.4):

- **Physical health.** This dimension includes features such as the shape and size of your body, how responsive and acute your senses are, and your body's ability to function at optimum levels with adequate sleep and rest, nutrition, and physical activity. It also includes your ability to avoid, manage, or heal from injury or illness. More recent definitions of physical health encompass a person's ability to perform

Wellness and the Dimensions of Health

In 1968, biologist, environmentalist, and philosopher René Dubos proposed an even broader definition of health. In his

| Irreversible disability and/or death | Chronic illness | Signs of illness | Signs of health/ wellness | Improved health/ wellness | Optimal wellness/ well-being |

▲
Neutral
point

FIGURE 1.3 The Wellness Continuum

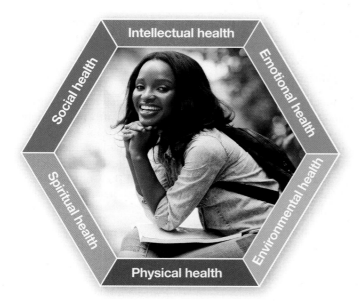

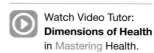

FIGURE 1.4 The Dimensions of Health When all dimensions are balanced and well developed, they support an active, thriving lifestyle.

Watch Video Tutor:
Dimensions of Health
in Mastering Health.

activities of daily living (ADLs), which are the activities that are essential to function normally in society—including things like getting up out of a chair, bathing and dressing yourself, cooking, toileting, and walking.

- **Social health.** The ability to have a broad social network and maintain satisfying interpersonal relationships with friends, family members, and partners is a key part of overall wellness. Successfully interacting and communicating with others, adapting to various social situations, and being able to give and receive love are all part of social health.

- **Intellectual health.** The ability to think clearly, reason objectively, analyze critically, and use brainpower effectively to meet life's challenges are all part of this dimension. This includes learning from successes and mistakes, making sound decisions, and having a healthy curiosity about life.

- **Emotional health.** This is the feeling component—being able to express emotions when appropriate and to control them when not. Self-esteem, self-confidence, trust, and love are all part of emotional health.

- **Spiritual health.** This dimension involves creating and expressing meaning and purpose in your life. This may include believing in a supreme being, following a particular religion's rules and customs, or simply feeling that

you are part of a greater spectrum of existence. The capacities to contemplate life's experiences and to care about and respect all living things are aspects of spiritual health.

- **Environmental health.** This dimension entails understanding how the health of the environments in which you live, work, and play can affect you; protecting yourself from hazards in your own environment; and working to preserve, protect, and improve environmental conditions for everyone.

Achieving wellness means attaining the optimal level of well-being for your unique limitations and strengths. For example, a physically disabled person may function at his or her optimal level of physical and intellectual performance, enjoy satisfying relationships, and be engaged in environmental concerns. In contrast, someone who spends hours lifting weights but pays little attention to others may lack social or emotional health. The perspective we need is *holistic*, emphasizing the balanced integration of mind, body, and spirit.

LO 3 | WHAT INFLUENCES YOUR HEALTH?

Classify factors that influence your health status into one of five broad categories identified by *Healthy People 2020* as determinants of health.

If you're lucky, aspects of your world conspire to promote your health: Everyone in your family is fit and has a weight appropriate to age and build; there are fresh vegetables on sale at the neighborhood farmer's market; and a new bike trail has opened along the river (and you have a bike!). If you're not so lucky, aspects of your world discourage health: Everyone in your family is overweight and nobody gets much exercise;

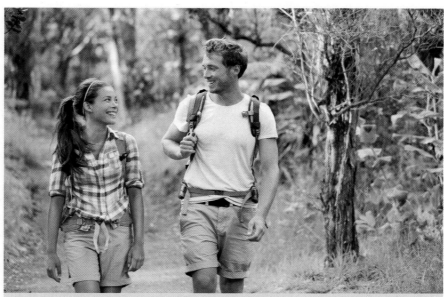

Today, health and wellness mean taking a positive, proactive attitude toward life and living it to the fullest.

determinants of health The range of personal, social, economic, and environmental factors that influence health status.

health disparities Differences in the incidence, prevalence, mortality, and burden of diseases and other health conditions among specific population groups.

your peers urge you to keep up with their drinking; the corner market has only cigarettes, alcohol, and junk food for sale; and you wouldn't dare walk or ride alongside the river for fear of being mugged. In short, seemingly personal choices are not always totally within an individual's control.

Public health experts refer to the factors that influence health as **determinants of health**, a term the U.S. Surgeon General defines as "the range of personal, social, economic, and environmental factors that influence health status."[9] The Surgeon General's health promotion plan, called *Healthy People*, has been published every ten years since 1990 with the goal of improving the quality and years of life for all Americans. The overarching goals set out by the newest version, *Healthy People 2020*, are as follows:

- Attain high-quality, longer lives free of preventable diseases.
- Achieve health equity, eliminate disparities, and improve health of all groups.
- Create social and physical environments that promote good health for all.
- Promote good quality of life, healthy development, and healthy behaviors across all life stages.

Healthy People 2020 classifies health determinants into five categories: individual behavior, biology and genetics, social factors, health services, and policymaking (**FIGURE 1.5**). It also includes strong language about reducing **health disparities** that exist between populations based on racial or ethnic background, sex and gender, income and education, health insurance status, geographic location, sexual orientation, and disability.[10] See the Focus On: Difference, Disparity, and Health: Achieving Health Equity for more on health disparities.

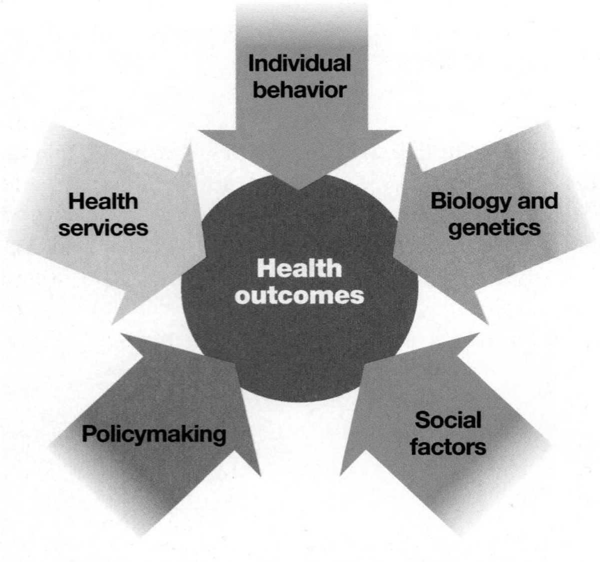

FIGURE 1.5 *Healthy People 2020* **Determinants of Health** The determinants of health often overlap with one another. Collectively, they affect health of individuals and communities.

Individual Behavior

Individual behaviors can help you attain, maintain, or regain good health, or they can undermine your health and promote disease. Health experts refer to behaviors within your power to change as *modifiable determinants*. Modifiable determinants significantly influence your risk for chronic disease, which is responsible for seven out of ten deaths in the United States.[11] Incredibly, just four modifiable determinants are responsible for most chronic disease (**FIGURE 1.6**):[12]

- **Lack of physical activity.** Low levels of physical activity contribute to over 200,000 deaths in the United States annually.[13]
- **Poor nutrition.** Multiple studies have linked diets low in fruits and vegetables with an increased risk of death by any cause.[14]
- **Excessive alcohol consumption.** Alcohol causes 88,000 deaths in adults annually through cardiovascular disease, liver disease, cancer, and other diseases, as well as motor vehicle accidents and violence.[15]
- **Tobacco use.** Tobacco smoking and the cancer, high blood pressure, and respiratory disease it causes are responsible for about one in five deaths of American adults.[16]

On the flip side, a recent study tracking more than 2,100 young adults (aged 18 to 30 years) found that those who maintained a healthful body weight, ate a nourishing diet, engaged in physical activity, and did not smoke were about twice as likely to maintain normal blood pressure and other indicators of cardiovascular health 25 years later than were those who did not practice these behaviors.[17]

7 OUT OF 10

deaths are caused by **CHRONIC DISEASE.**

Another major contributor to disease and mortality among Americans is our rising abuse of prescription and illegal drugs, especially opioid pain relievers and heroin. Between 1999 and 2015, the number of overdose deaths involving these drugs quadrupled. Every day, 142 Americans die from an opioid overdose.[18]

Other modifiable determinants include stress levels, exposure to toxic chemicals in the home and work environments, use of over-the-counter medications, sexual behaviors and use of contraceptives, sleep habits, and hand hygiene and other simple infection control measures. In addition, climate change, which has contributed to a rise in emerging infectious diseases, malnutrition, and many other global health problems, is modifiable with individual behavior change and with changes in policies and programs.

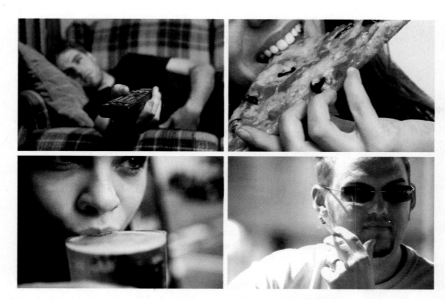

FIGURE 1.6 Four Leading Causes of Chronic Disease in the United States Lack of physical activity, poor nutrition, excessive alcohol consumption, and tobacco use—all modifiable health determinants—are the four most significant factors leading to chronic disease among Americans today.

occupational hazards, the quality of air, soil, and water, and even climate are all examples.

Economic Factors Even in affluent nations such as the United States, people in lower socioeconomic brackets have, on average, substantially shorter life expectancies and more illnesses than do people who are wealthy.[19] Economic disadvantages that can impair health include the following:

- Lacking access to high-quality education from early childhood through adulthood
- Living in poor housing with potential exposure to asbestos, lead, dust mites, rodents and other pests, inadequate sanitation, unsafe drinking water, and high levels of crime
- Being unable to pay for nourishing food, warm clothes, and sturdy shoes; heat and other utilities; medications and medical supplies; transportation; and counseling, fitness classes, and other wellness measures.

Biology and Genetics

Biological and genetic determinants are things that typically can't be changed or modified. Health experts frequently refer to these factors as *nonmodifiable determinants*. Genetically inherited traits include genetic disorders such as sickle cell disease, hemophilia, and cystic fibrosis, as well as predispositions to certain conditions—such as allergies and asthma, cardiovascular disease, diabetes, and certain cancers—that are linked to multiple gene variants in combination with environmental factors. Although we cannot influence the structure of our genes, the emerging field of *epigenetics* is increasingly linking aspects of our diet, physical activity, and other behavioral choices to our cells' ability to use our genes to build proteins that influence our health. In the future, research into epigenetics might help us gain more control over our genetic inheritance.

Nonmodifiable determinants also refer to certain innate characteristics, such as your age, race, ethnicity, metabolic rate, and body structure. Your sex is another key biological determinant: As compared to men, women have an increased risk for low bone density and autoimmune diseases (in which the body attacks its own cells), whereas men have an increased risk for heart disease compared to women. Your own history of illness and injury also classifies as biology. For instance, if you had a serious knee injury in high school, it may still cause pain with walking and exercise, which in turn may predispose you to weight gain.

Social Factors

Social factors include both the social and physical conditions in the environment where people are born or live. Disparities in income and education, exposure to crime and violence, the availability of healthful foods, the state of buildings and roads,

The Built Environment

As the name implies, the *built environment* includes anything created or modified by human beings, including buildings, roads, recreation areas, transportation systems, electric transmission lines, and communications cables.

Researchers in public health have increasingly been promoting changes to the built environment that can improve the health of community members.[20] These include increased construction of parks, sidewalks, pedestrian-only areas, bike paths, and public transit systems to which commuters typically walk or bike. Some communities are enticing supermarkets to open in underserved neighborhoods to increase residents' access to fresh fruits and vegetables.

Pollutants and Infectious Agents Physical conditions also include the quality of the air we breathe, our land, our water, and our foods. Exposure to toxins, radiation, and infectious agents via the environment can cause widespread harm in a region and, with the rise of global travel and commerce, can affect the health of people around the world. Recent outbreaks of the Ebola and Zika viruses, for example, are grim reminders of the need for a proactive international response for disease prevention and climate change.

Access to High-Quality Health Services

The health of individuals and communities is also determined by whether they have access to high-quality health care, including not only services for physical and mental health, but also accurate and relevant health information and products such as eyeglasses, medical supplies, and medications.

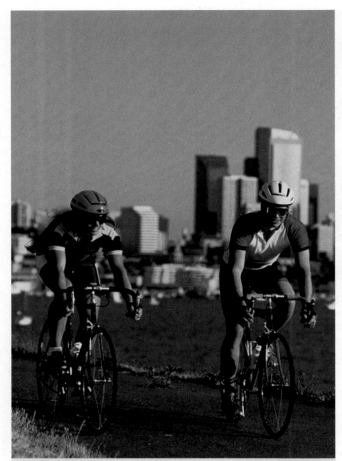

The built environment of your community can promote positive health behaviors. Wide bike paths, good signage and lighting, and major thoroughfares that are closed to automobile traffic encourage residents to safely incorporate healthy physical activity into their daily lives.

policies that require people to be vaccinated before enrolling in classes or to wear helmets while riding bicycles or motorcycles, and laws that ban cell phone use, drinking, and pot smoking while driving. Health policies serve a key role in protecting public health and motivating individuals and communities to change.

Access to high-quality, low-cost health services is also affected by policymaking, including health insurance legislation.

LO 4 | HOW DOES MINDFULNESS INFLUENCE HEALTH?

Describe mindfulness, identifying its health benefits and ways to incorporate it into your life.

A veritable explosion of media outlets have been promoting a shift to *mindful* behavior as a path to optimum health. If you have seen these claims, you may be wondering whether or not they're backed by evidence and, if so, how to practice mindfulness in your own life. In this section, we explore definitions of mindfulness, provide an overview of scientific evidence linking it to health, and introduce simple strategies for living more mindfully. In later chapters of this text, we will provide further research, resources, and tips for how to include mindfulness as part of a comprehensive plan for living your best, most healthful life.

Definitions of Mindfulness

Definitions of **mindfulness** vary, but most share certain essential components. These include being present in the moment through greater awareness of yourself—your sensations, thoughts, and feelings—and your environment. Some proponents have called mindfulness an extended "stop and smell the roses" moment—one that can become a total approach to daily life. Others describe it as a way of looking at yourself and the world with gentleness and compassion rather than judgment. Key to mindfulness is focusing—bringing your complete attention to the present rather than rehashing the past or dwelling on future fears. In fact, one of the clearest descriptions found in popular media is "Keep your feet in the now!"

Although mindfulness has become increasingly popular recently, it is not new. It is believed to have originated around 1500 B.C.E. or earlier as an element of the Hindu practices of yoga and meditation. Buddhism, which evolved from Hinduism around 600 B.C.E., incorporated mindfulness as a core practice. Today, individuals who practice mindfulness may follow one of these religions, another religion, or no religion at all.

mindfulness Awareness of the present moment, including sensations, thoughts, feelings, and the environment, without evaluation, qualification, or judgment.

Although the 2010 Affordable Care Act had reduced the numbers of uninsured Americans by 20 million people by the end of 2016, millions remained without insurance, and the current status of health insurance coverage in the United States is uncertain.[21] In addition to the uninsured, there are millions of underinsured—individuals who have some coverage but not enough. They may have plans with a high annual deductible or a high copayment for services; as a result, they cannot afford to pay the difference between what their insurance covers and what their providers and medications cost. People who are uninsured or underinsured tend to delay care or try other cost-saving measures, such as taking only half of the prescribed dose of their medications, that may put their health at risk.

Policymaking

Public policies and interventions can have a powerful and positive effect on the health of individuals and communities. Examples include policies that ban smoking in public places,

Health Benefits of Mindfulness

The current surge in interest in mindfulness can be explained in part by the growing body of research evidence linking the practice to improved health. Studies associate mindfulness with pain relief, for example, as well as stress reduction, lower levels of anxiety and depression, improved memory and attention, weight loss, improved sleep, reduced risks for cardiovascular disease, and more satisfying relationships. In later chapters of this book, we will discuss specific studies linking mindfulness to these improvements in health.

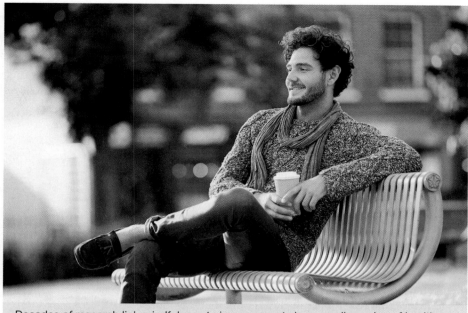

Decades of research link mindfulness to improvements in every dimension of health.

How to Practice Mindfulness

How many times have you walked to class and never noticed anything in your path as your mind rehashed the quarrel you just had with your roommates or a romantic encounter the night before? You reach your destination but couldn't have explained how you got there or what you passed along the way. In class, you hear the instructor talking, but afterwards you have no idea what was said. Sound familiar? If so, there are steps you can take to tune in to life around you and gain a greater appreciation for yourself and your place in the world. The following is a brief introduction to mindfulness strategies. Each chapter of the book will provide specific skills for helping you develop mindfulness.

You can practice mindfulness at any time, in any place. According to mindfulness guru Jon Kabat-Zinn, it requires only a willingness to examine who you are, your view of the world and your place in it and to cultivate an appreciation for the fullness of each moment you live.[22] However, the path to mindfulness is different for everyone. It might include formal actions, such as carving out times to meditate or perform yoga. Alternatively, it might comprise informal actions, such as increasing your attention in your relationships, your food choices, your regard for the environment, or your compassion for others, or pausing to acknowledge the things in your life that you're thankful for. The following are some basic mindfulness skills.

Cultivate Compassion The word *compassion*, derived from the Latin phrase "to suffer together," is a recognition of another's pain and a sincere desire to help. You cultivate compassion for others by supporting loved ones who are going through difficult times or by volunteering to help others who are less fortunate. You cultivate compassion for yourself by learning to recognize critical or judgmental thoughts—thoughts that tell you you're not good enough, smart enough, or attractive enough—and then setting them aside. You may then remind yourself of your positive qualities, achievements, and loving relationships. Practicing yoga can help you to silence your internal critic and develop self-confidence. You might also take a vow to avoid engaging in negative thinking about yourself and others for a single day. Throughout that day, replace negativity with intentions of kindness. Meet other people's eyes as you pass, acknowledging that you're aware of their presence. Smile. When friends criticize others, try to listen fully to what's behind the words, and respond with gentleness and honesty.

Start Each Day with Intention What are your values, and how do your values guide your actions? What might you wish to do differently today? What will success look like? Each morning, jot down some intentions—perhaps to listen more, to stop procrastinating, or to think before you act. During the day, try to stay mindful of how your actions align with these intentions. Then, before bed each night, take a moment to consider—without judgment—how well you lived your intentions that day.

Examine the Way You Deal with Life's Challenges Perhaps you became angry with a friend, felt upset about a critique of your work, or just got stressed out by an enormous load of homework. One method for confronting challenges with mindfulness is to acknowledge what you felt, then try to determine why. Was the event really as negative as you felt it to be at the time? Could you have responded differently? In the future, would you prefer to let go of your attachment to particular outcomes, say "It is what it is," and move on? One way to do this is to acknowledge that nothing in life—and no one—is perfect, including you. For yourself and for others, seek goodness rather than perfection.

For more information on the benefits and practices of mindfulness, check out the **Mindfulness and You** features throughout this text.

LO 5 | HOW DOES BEHAVIOR CHANGE OCCUR?

Compare and contrast the health belief model, the social cognitive model, and the transtheoretical model of behavior change, and explain how you might use them in making a specific behavior change.

Now that you've read about some of the health benefits of mindfulness, perhaps you would like to become more mindful in your daily life. Or maybe your dream is to stop smoking, cut down on your alcohol intake, or lose weight. The question is: How? Over the years, social scientists and public health researchers have developed a variety of models to illustrate how individual behavior change occurs. We explore three of those here.

Health Belief Model

We often assume that when rational people recognize that their behaviors put them at risk, they will change the behaviors to reduce that risk. It doesn't always work that way. Consider the number of health professionals who smoke, consume junk food, or text while driving. They surely know better, but their "knowing" is disconnected from their "doing." One classic model of behavior change suggests that our beliefs may help to explain why this occurs.

A **belief** is an appraisal of the relationship between some object, action, or idea (e.g., smoking) and some attribute of that object, action, or idea (e.g., "Smoking is expensive and dirty and causes cancer" or "Smoking is relaxing, and I'm too young to get cancer"). Psychologists studying the relationship between beliefs and health behaviors have determined that, although beliefs may subtly influence behavior, they may or may not cause people to change their actions. In the 1950s, psychologists at the U.S. Public Health Service developed the **health belief model (HBM)**, which describes the ways in which beliefs affect behavior change.[23] The HBM holds that several factors must support a belief before change is likely:

- **Perceived seriousness of the health problem.** The more serious the perceived effects are, the more likely action will be taken.
- **Perceived susceptibility to the health problem.** People who perceive themselves to be at high risk are more likely to take preventive action.
- **Perceived benefits.** People are more likely to take action if they believe that this action will benefit them.
- **Perceived barriers.** Even if a recommended action is perceived to be effective, the individual may believe it is too expensive, difficult, inconvenient, or time-consuming. These perceived barriers must be overcome or acknowledged as less important than the benefits.

belief Appraisal of the relationship between some object, action, or idea and some attribute of that object, action, or idea.

health belief model (HBM) A model for explaining how beliefs may influence behaviors.

social cognitive model (SCM) A model of behavior change that emphasizes the role of social factors and thought processes (cognition) in behavior change.

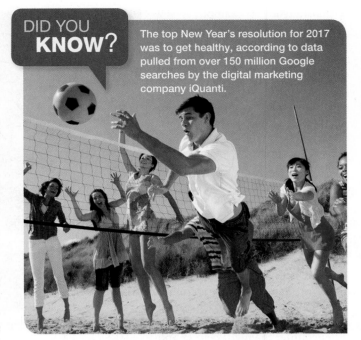

Source: N. Spector, "2017 New Year's Resolutions: The Most Popular and How to Stick to Them," *NBC News*, January 1, 2017, https://www.nbcnews.com/business/consumer/2017-new-year-s-resolutions-most-popular-how-stick-them-n70.

- **Cues to action.** A person who is reminded or alerted about a potential health problem—by anything from early symptoms to an e-mail from a health care provider—is more likely to take action.

Let's return to our example of smokers. Older people are likely to know smokers who have developed serious heart or lung disease and are therefore more likely to perceive tobacco as a threat to their health than are teenagers. The greater the perceived threat of health problems caused by smoking, the greater is the chance that a person will avoid it. However, many chronic smokers know the risks yet continue to smoke. Why? If they do not believe they are susceptible to a smoking-related disease, they would be unlikely to quit. Or they may feel that the immediate pleasure outweighs the long-range cost.

Social Cognitive Model

Developed from the work of several researchers over decades, the **social cognitive model (SCM)** is most closely associated with the work of psychologist Albert Bandura.[24] Fundamentally, the model proposes that three factors interact in a reciprocal fashion to promote and motivate change: the *social environment* in which we live, *our thoughts or cognition*, and *our behaviors*. We change our behavior in part by observing models in our environments, reflecting on our observations, and regulating ourselves accordingly. For instance, if we observe a family member successfully quitting smoking, we are more apt to believe we can do it too. In addition, when we succeed in changing ourselves, we change our thoughts about ourselves, potentially promoting further behavior change: After we have successfully quit smoking, we may feel empowered to increase our level of physical activity.

SEE IT! VIDEOS

How can you change your habits and stick with it? Watch **Life-Changing Resolutions** in the Study Area of Mastering Health.

Moreover, as we change ourselves, we become a model for others to observe. Thus, we are not just products of our environments, but also producers.

The SCM is often used to design health promotion programs. For example, one public health initiative in the southeastern United States used the SCM to develop a nutrition and physical activity afterschool program for preteens. The program supported participants in mastering certain physical activities and self-regulation of eating habits. Participants improved not only their eating and activity patterns, but also their body weight, cardiovascular endurance, mood, and ability and confidence in regulating their behaviors.[25]

Transtheoretical Model

Why do so many New Year's resolutions fail before Valentine's Day? According to Drs. James Prochaska and Carlos DiClemente, it's because most of us aren't really prepared to take action. Their research indicates that behavior changes usually do not succeed when we start with the change itself. Instead, we must go through a series of stages to adequately prepare ourselves for that eventual change.[26] According to Prochaska and DiClemente's **transtheoretical model** of behavior change (also called the *stages of change model*), our chances of keeping those New Year's resolutions will be greatly enhanced if we have proper reinforcement and help during each of the following stages:

1. **Precontemplation.** People in the precontemplation stage have no current intention of changing. They may have tried to change a behavior before and given up, or they may be in denial and unaware of any problem.
2. **Contemplation.** In this phase, people recognize that they have a problem and begin to contemplate the need to change. Despite this acknowledgment, people can languish in this stage for years, realizing that they have a problem but lacking the time or energy to make the change.
3. **Preparation.** Most people at this point are close to taking action. They've thought about what they might do and may even have a plan.
4. **Action.** In this stage, people begin to follow their action plans. Those with a plan of action are more ready for action than are those who have given it little thought.
5. **Maintenance.** During the maintenance stage, a person continues the actions begun in the action stage and works toward making these changes a permanent part of his or her life. In this stage, it is important to be aware of the potential for relapses and to develop strategies for dealing with such challenges.
6. **Termination.** By this point, the behavior is so ingrained that constant vigilance may be unnecessary. The new behavior has become an essential part of daily living.

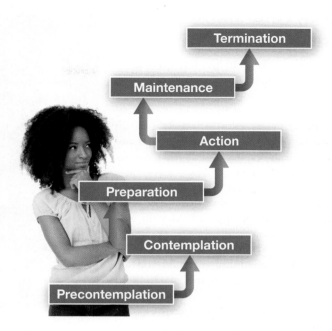

FIGURE 1.7 Transtheoretical Model People don't move through the transtheoretical model stages in sequence. We may make progress in more than one stage at one time, or we may shuttle back and forth from one to another—say, from contemplation to preparation, then back to contemplation—before we succeed in making a change.

We don't necessarily go through these stages sequentially. They may overlap, or we may shuttle back and forth from one to another—say, from contemplation to preparation, then back to contemplation—for a while before we become truly committed to making the change (**FIGURE 1.7**). Still, it's useful to recognize "where we are" with a change so that we can consider the appropriate strategies to move us forward.

LO 6 | HOW CAN YOU IMPROVE YOUR HEALTH BEHAVIORS?

Identify your own current risk behaviors, the factors that influence those behaviors, and the strategies you can use to change them.

Clearly, change is not always easy. To successfully change a behavior, you need to see change not as a singular *event* but as a *process* by which you substitute positive patterns for new ones—a process that requires preparation, has several stages, and takes time to occur. Whether you are working to become more mindful or deciding to eat more healthfully or exercise, the following four-step plan integrates ideas from each of the above behavior change models into a simple guide to moving forward.

transtheoretical model A model of behavior change that identifies six distinct stages people go through in altering behavior patterns; also called the *stages of change model*.

Step One: Increase Your Awareness

Before you make a change, it helps to learn what researchers know about behaviors that contribute to and detract from good health. Each chapter in this book provides a foundation of information focused on these factors. Check out the Table of Contents to locate chapters with the information you're looking for.

This is also a good time to take stock of the health determinants in your life: What aspects of your biology and behavior support your health, and which are obstacles to overcome? What elements of your social and physical environment could you tap into to help you change, and which might hold you back? Making a list of all of the health determinants that affect you—both positively and negatively—should greatly improve your understanding of what you might want to change and what to do to make that change happen.

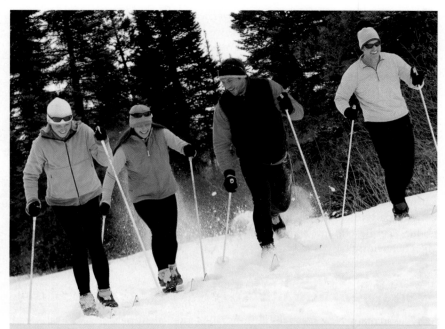

Your friends can help you stay motivated by modeling healthy behaviors, offering support, joining you in your change efforts, and providing reinforcement.

Step Two: Contemplate Change

With increased awareness of the behaviors that contribute to wellness and the specific health determinants affecting you, you may be contemplating change. In this stage, the following strategies may be helpful.

Examine Your Current Health Habits and Patterns

Do you routinely stop at fast-food restaurants for breakfast? Smoke when you're feeling stressed? Party too much on the weekends? Get to bed way past 2 A.M.? When considering a behavior you might want to change, ask yourself the following:

- How long has this behavior existed, and how frequently do I do it?
- How serious are the long- and short-term consequences of the habit or pattern?
- What are some of my reasons for continuing this problematic behavior?
- What kinds of situations trigger the behavior?
- Are other people involved in this behavior? If so, how?

Health behaviors involve elements of personal choice, but they are also influenced by other determinants. Some are *predisposing factors*—for instance, if your parents smoke, you're more likely to start smoking than is someone whose parents don't smoke.

Some determinants are *enabling factors*—for example, peers who smoke enable one another's smoking. In such cases, it can be helpful to employ the social cognitive model and deliberately change your social environment by spending more time with nonsmoking friends who model the behavior you want to emulate.

Various *reinforcing factors* can support or undermine your effort to change. If you decide to stop smoking but, when you do stop, notice that you begin to gain weight, you may lose your resolve. In contrast, noticing that you're breathing more easily when you walk up a flight of stairs can powerfully motivate you to continue to avoid smoking.

Identify a Target Behavior

To clarify your thinking around the various behaviors you might target for change, ask yourself these questions:

- **What do I want?** Is your ultimate goal to lose weight? To exercise more? To reduce stress? To have a lasting relationship? You need a clear picture of your target outcome.
- **Which change is the greatest priority at this time?** Rather than saying, "I need to eat less *and* start exercising," identify one specific behavior that contributes significantly to your greatest problem and tackle that first.
- **Why is this important to me?** Think through why you want to change. Are you doing it because of your health? To improve your academic performance? To look better? To win someone else's approval? It's best to target a behavior for a reason that's right for you rather than because you think it will help you win someone else's approval.

Learn More about the Target Behavior

Once you have clarified what behavior you would like to change, you're ready to learn more about that behavior. This text will help, and this is a great time to learn how to find accurate and reliable health information on the Internet (see the **Tech & Health** box).

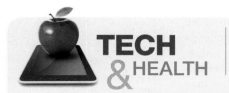

TECH & HEALTH | SURFING FOR THE LATEST IN HEALTH

The Internet can be a wonderful resource for quickly finding answers to your questions, but it can also be a source of much misinformation. To ensure that the sites you visit are reliable and trustworthy, follow these tips:

- Look for websites sponsored by an official government agency, a university or college, or a hospital or medical center. Government sites are easily identified by their *.gov* extensions, college and university sites typically have *.edu* extensions, and many hospitals have an *.org* extension (e.g., the Mayo Clinic's website is www.mayoclinic.org). Major philanthropic foundations, such as the Robert Wood Johnson Foundation, the Kellogg Foundation, and others, often provide information about selected health topics. National nonprofit organizations, such as the American Heart Association and the American Cancer Society, are often good, authoritative sources of information. Foundations and nonprofits usually have URLs ending with an *.org* extension.

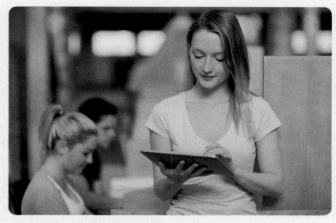

Find reliable health information at your fingertips!

- Search for well-established, professionally peer-reviewed journals such as the *New England Journal of Medicine* (http://content.nejm.org) or the *Journal of the American Medical Association* (http://jama.ama-assn.org). Although some of these sites require a fee for access, you can often locate concise abstracts and information that can help you conduct a search. Your college may make these journals available to students for no cost.
- Consult the Centers for Disease Control and Prevention (www.cdc.gov) for consumer news, updates, and alerts.

- For a global perspective on health issues, visit the World Health Organization website (www.who.int/en).
- Other sites offering reliable health information include the following:
  1. For College Women: www.4collegewomen.org
  2. Young Men's Health: www.youngmenshealthsite.org
  3. MedlinePlus: www.nlm.nih.gov/medlineplus
  4. Go Ask Alice!: www.goaskalice.columbia.edu
- The nonprofit health care accrediting organization Utilization Accreditation Review Commission (URAC; www.urac.org) has devised more than 50 criteria that health sites must satisfy to display its seal. Look for the "URAC Accredited Health Web Site" seal on websites you visit.
- Finally, gather information from two or more reliable sources to see whether facts and figures are consistent. Avoid websites that try to sell you something, whether products such as dietary supplements or services such as medical testing. When in doubt, check with your own health care provider, health education professor, or state health division website.

As you conduct your research, don't limit your focus to the behavior and its health effects. Learn all you can about aspects of your world that might support or pose obstacles to your success. For instance, let's say you decide you want to meditate for 15 minutes a day. Are there other people in your dorm or neighborhood who might be interested in meditating with you? What about classes or a meditation group? On the other hand, do you live in a super-noisy dorm? Are you afraid your friends might think meditating is weird? In short, learn everything you can about your target behavior now, and you'll be better prepared for change.

Assess Your Motivation and Your Readiness to Change
Wanting to change is an essential prerequisite of the change process, but to achieve change, you need more than desire. You need real **motivation**, which isn't just a feeling, but a social and cognitive force that directs your behavior. To understand what goes into motivation, let's return for a moment to two models of change discussed earlier: the health belief model (HBM) and the social cognitive model (SCM).

Remember that, according to the HBM, your beliefs affect your ability to change. For example, when reaching for another cigarette, smokers sometimes tell themselves, "I'll stop tomorrow" or "They'll have a cure for lung cancer before I get it." These beliefs allow them to continue what they're doing because they dampen motivation. As you contemplate change, consider whether your beliefs are likely

motivation A social, cognitive, and emotional force that directs human behavior.

to motivate you to achieve lasting change. Ask yourself the following questions:

- **Do you believe that your current pattern could lead to a serious problem?** The more severe the consequences are, the more motivated you'll be to change the behavior. For example, smoking can cause cancer, emphysema, and other deadly diseases. The fear of developing those diseases can help you stop smoking. But what if cancer and emphysema were just words to you? In that case, you could study up on these disorders and the suffering they cause. Doing so might increase your motivation: Over 70 countries have laws requiring cigarette packages to display graphic warning labels (GWLs) with images of the physical effects of smoking, from diseased organs to chests sawed open for autopsy. Research clearly shows that these GWLs have reduced the adoption of smoking among adolescents and young adults and have increased smoking cessation among established smokers. Countries have reported that 25, 50, and even 60 percent of current smokers have attempted to quit as a result of the GWLs.[27]
- **Do you believe that you are personally likely to experience the consequences of your behavior?** If you don't, try employing the social cognitive model by interviewing people who are struggling with the consequences of the same behavior. Ask them what their life is like and whether, when they were engaging in the behavior, they believed that it would harm them. Your health care provider may be able to put you in touch with patients who would be happy to support your behavior change plan in this way. And don't ignore the motivating potential of positive role models.

Another key to boosting your motivation to change may well be mindfulness. A recent study of physical activity among adults found that mindfulness practices increased study participants' exercise motivation and participation.[28]

Even though motivation is powerful, to achieve change, it has to be combined with common sense, commitment, and a realistic understanding of how best to move from point A to point B. *Readiness* is the state of being that precedes behavior change. People who are ready to change possess the knowledge, skills, and external and internal resources that make change possible.

Develop Self-Efficacy

One of the most important factors influencing health status is **self-efficacy**, an individual's belief that he or she is capable of achieving certain goals or of performing at a level that may influence events in life. In general, people who exhibit high self-efficacy approach challenges with a positive attitude and are confident that they can succeed. In turn, they may be more motivated to change and more likely to succeed. Prior success can lead to expectations of success in the future.

Conversely, someone with low self-efficacy or with self-doubts may give up easily or never even try to change a behavior. These people tend to shy away from difficult challenges. They may have failed before, and when the going gets tough, they are more likely to give up or revert to old patterns of behavior. A number of methods for developing self-efficacy follow.

> **self-efficacy** Belief in one's ability to perform a task successfully.
>
> **locus of control** The location, *external* (outside oneself) or *internal* (within oneself), that an individual perceives as the source and underlying cause of events in his or her life.

WHAT DO YOU THINK?

Do you have an internal or an external locus of control?

- Can you think of some friends whom you would describe as more internally or externally controlled?
- How do people with these different views deal with similar situations?

Cultivate an Internal Locus of Control

The conviction that you have the ability to change is a powerful motivator. People who have a strong *internal* **locus of control** believe that they have power over their own actions. They are more driven by their own thoughts and are more likely to state their opinions and be true to their own beliefs. In contrast, people who believe that external circumstances largely control their situation have an *external* locus of control. They may easily succumb to feelings of anxiety and disempowerment and give up. For example, a recent study of cancer patients found that, compared to those with a high internal locus of control, people with an external locus of control were more likely to perceive their cancer as a threat that they felt unable to manage and more likely to respond with depression to their diagnosis.[29]

Having an internal or external locus of control can vary according to circumstance. For instance, someone who learns that diabetes runs in his family may resign himself to facing the disease one day instead of actively working to minimize his risk. On this front, he would be demonstrating an external locus of control. However, the same individual might exhibit an internal locus of control when resisting a friend's pressure to smoke.

Step Three: Prepare for Change

You've contemplated change for long enough! Now it's time to set a realistic goal, anticipate barriers, reach out to others, and commit. Here's how.

Set SMART Goals

Unsuccessful goals are vague and open-ended—for instance, "Get into shape by exercising more." In contrast, SMART goals are have the following characteristics:

- **S**pecific. "Attend a Tuesday/Thursday aerobics class at the YMCA."
- **M**easurable. "Reduce my alcohol intake on Saturday nights from three drinks to two."
- **A**ction oriented. "Volunteer at the animal shelter on Friday afternoons."
- **R**ealistic. "Increase my daily walk from 15 to 20 minutes."
- **T**ime-oriented. "Stay in my strength-training class for the full ten-week session, then reassess."

Knowing that your SMART goal is attainable—that you can achieve it within the current circumstances of your life—increases your motivation. This, in turn, leads to a better chance of success and to a greater sense of self-efficacy, which can motivate you to succeed even more.

Use Shaping
Shaping is a process that involves taking a series of small steps toward a goal. Suppose you want to start jogging 3 miles every other day, but right now you get tired and winded after half a mile. Shaping would dictate a process of slow, progressive steps, such as walking 30 minutes every other day at a relaxed pace for the first week, walking at a faster pace the second week, and speeding up to a slow run the third week.

Regardless of the change you plan to make, start slowly to avoid causing yourself undue stress. Master one small step before moving on to the next. Be willing to change the original plan if it proves to be ineffective.

Anticipate Barriers to Change
Recognizing possible stumbling blocks in advance will help you prepare fully for change. Besides negative social determinants, aspects of the built environment, or lack of adequate health care, a few general barriers to change include the following:

To reach your behavior change goals, you need to take things one step at a time.

- **Overambitious goals.** Even with the strongest motivation, overambitious goals can undermine self-efficacy and derail change. Habits are best changed one small step at a time.
- **Self-defeating beliefs and attitudes.** As the health belief model explains, believing that you're immune to the consequences of a bad habit can keep you from making a solid commitment to change. Likewise, thinking that you're helpless to change your habits can undermine your efforts.
- **Failure to accurately assess your current state of wellness.** You might assume that you will be able to walk 2 miles to campus each morning, for example, only to discover that you're winded after 1 mile. Make sure that the planned change is realistic for *you*.
- **Lack of support and guidance.** If you want to cut down on your drinking, socialize with peers who drink moderately, if at all. Remember that positive role models and social support are key aspects of the social cognitive model of behavior change.
- **Emotions that sabotage your efforts and sap your will.** Sometimes the best-laid plans go awry because you're having a bad day. Emotional reactions to life's challenges are normal, but don't let them sabotage your efforts to

change. If you're experiencing severe psychological distress, seek counseling before trying to change other aspects of your health.

Enlist Others as Change Agents
The social cognitive model recognizes the importance of social contacts in successful change. Most of us are highly influenced by other people's approval or disapproval (real or imagined). In addition, **modeling**—learning by observing and imitating role models—can give you practical strategies, inspiration, and confidence for making your own changes. Observing a friend who is a good conversationalist, for example, can help you improve your communication skills. Change agents commonly include the following:

- **Family members.** Positive family units provide care and protection, are dedicated to the healthful development of all family members, and work together to solve problems. If loving family members are not available to support your efforts to change, turn to friends and professionals.
- **Friends.** If your friends offer encouragement or express interest in joining with you in the behavior change, you are more likely to remain motivated. Thus, friends who share your personal values can greatly support your behavior change.
- **Professionals.** Consider enlisting support from professionals such as your health or PE instructor, coach, health care provider, or other adviser. As appropriate, consider the counseling services offered on campus as well as community services such as smoking cessation programs, support groups, and your local YMCA.

Sign a Contract
It's time to get it in writing! A formal *behavior change contract* serves many powerful purposes. It functions as a promise to yourself and as an organized plan that lays out your goals, start and end dates, daily actions, and any barriers you anticipate. Writing a contract also gives you an opportunity to brainstorm strategies, list sources of support, and remind yourself of the benefits of sticking with the program. To get started, fill out the Behavior Change Contract at the back of this book. FIGURE 1.8 shows an example of a completed contract.

Step Four: Take Action to Change

As you begin to put your plan into action, the following behavior change strategies can help.

shaping Using a series of small steps to gradually achieve a particular goal.

modeling Learning and adopting specific behaviors by observing others perform them.

Behavior Change Contract

My behavior change will be:
To snack less on junk food and more on healthy foods.

My long-term goal for this behavior change is:
Eat junk food snacks no more than once a week.

These are three obstacles to change (things that I am currently doing or situations that contribute to this behavior or make it harder to change):
1. The grocery store is closed by the time I come home from school.
2. I get hungry between classes, and the vending machines only carry candy bars.
3. It's easier to order pizza or other snacks than to make a snack at home.

The strategies I will use to overcome these obstacles are:
1. I'll leave early for school once a week so I can stock up on healthy snacks in the morning.
2. I'll bring a piece of fruit or other healthy snack to eat between classes.
3. I'll learn some easy recipes for snacks to make at home.

Resources I will use to help me change this behavior include:
a friend/partner/relative: my roommates: I'll ask them to buy healthier snacks instead of chips when they do the shopping.
a school-based resource: The dining hall: I'll ask the manager to provide healthy foods we can take to eat between classes.
a community-based resource: The library: I'll check out some cookbooks to find easy snack ideas.
a book or reputable website: The USDA nutrient database at www.ars.usda.gov: I'll use this site to make sure the foods I select are healthy choices.

In order to make my goal more attainable, I have devised these short-term goals:
short-term goal Eat a healthy snack 3 times per week   target date September 15   reward new CD
short-term goal Learn to make a healthy snack   target date October 15   reward concert tickets
short-term goal Eat a healthy snack 5 times per week   target date November 15   reward new shoes

When I make the long-term behavior change described above, my reward will be:
ski lift tickets for winter break   target date: December 15

I intend to make the behavior change described above. I will use the strategies and rewards to achieve the goals that will contribute to a healthy behavior change.

Signed: Elizabeth King   Witness: Susan Bauer

FIGURE 1.8 Example of a Completed Behavior Change Contract A blank version is included in the back of the book and in Mastering Health for you to fill out.

Visualize New Behavior
Athletes and others often use a technique known as **imagined rehearsal** to reach their goals. Careful mental and verbal rehearsal of how you intend to act will help you anticipate problems and greatly improve your chances of success.

Learn to Counter
Countering means substituting a desired behavior for an undesirable one. If you want to stop eating junk food on your break, for example, toss a banana in your backpack to eat instead.

Control the Situation
Any behavior has both antecedents and consequences. *Antecedents* are the aspects of the situation that come beforehand; these cue or stimulate a person to act in certain ways. *Consequences*—the results of behavior—affect whether a person will repeat that action. Both antecedents and consequences can be physical events, thoughts, emotions, or the actions of other people.

Once you recognize the antecedents of a given behavior, you can employ **situational inducement** to modify the ones that are working against you—you can seek settings, people, and circumstances that support your efforts to change, and you can avoid those likely to derail your change.

Change Your Self-Talk
There is a close connection between what people say to themselves, known as **self-talk**, and how they feel. According to psychologist Albert Ellis, most emotional problems and related behaviors stem from irrational statements that people make to themselves when events in their lives are different from what they would like them to be.[30]

For example, suppose that after doing poorly on a test, you say to yourself, "I can't believe I flunked that easy exam. I'm so stupid!" Now change this irrational, negative self-talk into rational, positive statements about what is really going on: "I really didn't study enough for that exam. I'm certainly not stupid; I just need to prepare better for the next test." Changing negative self-talk can help you recover from disappointment and take positive steps to correct the situation.

Another technique for changing self-talk is to practice blocking and stopping. For example, suppose you are preoccupied with thoughts of your ex-partner, who has recently left you. You can block those thoughts by focusing on the actions you're taking right now to help you move forward. The Skills for Behavior Change box offers more strategies for changing self-talk.

Reward Yourself
Another way to promote positive behavior change is to reward yourself for it. This is called **positive reinforcement**. Types of positive reinforcement can be classified as follows:

- *Consumable reinforcers* are edible items, such as your favorite snack.
- *Activity reinforcers* are opportunities to do something enjoyable, such as going on a hike or taking a trip.
- *Manipulative reinforcers* are incentives such as the promise of a better grade for doing an extra-credit project.
- *Possessional reinforcers* are tangible rewards, such as a new electronic gadget.
- *Social reinforcers* are signs of appreciation, approval, or love, such as affectionate hugs and praise.

The difficulty with employing positive reinforcement often lies in determining which incentive will be most effective. Your reinforcers may initially come from other

imagined rehearsal Practicing, through mental imagery, to become better able to perform an event in actuality.

countering Substituting a desired behavior for an undesirable one.

situational inducement Attempt to influence a behavior through situations and occasions that are structured to exert control over that behavior.

self-talk The customary manner of thinking and talking to oneself, which can affect one's self-image.

positive reinforcement Presenting something positive following a behavior that is being reinforced.

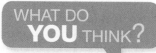

WHAT DO YOU THINK?

What type of reinforcers would most likely get you to change a behavior?

- Why would it motivate you?
- Can you think of options to reinforce behavior changes?

BEHAVIOR CHANGE

Challenge the Thoughts that Sabotage Change

Are any of the following thought patterns and beliefs holding you back? Try these strategies to combat self-sabotage:

- **"I don't have enough time!"** Chart your hourly activities for 1 day. What are your highest priorities and what can you eliminate? Plan to make time for a healthy change next week.

- **"I'm too stressed!"** Assess your major stressors right now. List those you can control and those you can change or avoid. Then identify two things you enjoy that can help you reduce stress now.

- **"I'm worried about what others may think."** Ask yourself how much other people influence your decisions about drinking, sex, eating habits, and the like. What is most important to you? What actions can you take to act in line with these values?

- **"I don't think I can do it."** Just because you have never done something before doesn't mean you can't do it now. To develop some confidence, take baby steps and break tasks into small segments of time.

- **"I can't break this habit!"** Habits are difficult to break but not impossible. What triggers your behavior? List ways you can avoid these triggers. Ask for support from friends and family.

people (*extrinsic* rewards), but as you see positive changes in yourself, you will begin to reward and reinforce yourself (*intrinsic* rewards). Keep in mind that reinforcers should immediately follow a behavior, but beware of overkill. If you reward yourself with a movie every time you go jogging, this reinforcer will soon lose its power. It would be better to give yourself this reward after, say, a full week of adherence to your jogging program.

Journal Writing personal experiences, interpretations, and results in a journal, notebook, or blog is an important skill for behavior change. You can log your daily activities, monitor your progress, record how you feel about it, and note ideas for improvement.

> **relapse** Returning to a pattern of negative behavior after a period of successfully avoiding that behavior.

Deal with Relapse Relapse is often defined as a return of symptoms in a person thought to have been successfully treated for a serious disease. But relapse can also be defined as a return to a previous pattern of negative behavior (drinking, binge eating, etc.) after a period of successfully avoiding that behavior. For example, an estimated 40 to 60 percent of people recovering from a substance abuse disorder suffer a relapse.[31] It doesn't mean that your program of change is a failure: Behavior change is a process, and setbacks are part of learning to change.

A few simple strategies can help you can get back on track after a relapse. First, figure out what went wrong. Every relapse begins with a slip—a one-time mistake.[32] What triggered that slip, and how can you modify your personal choices or the aspects of your environment that contributed to it? Second, use countering: If you've been overeating ever since your relationship ended, identify and choose other behaviors that comfort you. Third, a relapse might be telling you that you need some assistance with making this change; consider getting some professional help.

Let's Get Started!

After you acquire the skills to support successful behavior change, you're ready to apply those skills to your target behavior. Place your behavior change contract where you will see it every day and where you can refer to it as you work through the chapters in this text. Consider it a visual reminder that change doesn't "just happen." Reviewing your contract helps you to stay alert to potential problems, consider your alternatives, and stick to your goals under pressure.

ASSESS YOURSELF

How Healthy Are You?

LIVE IT! ASSESS YOURSELF

An interactive version of this assessment is available online in Mastering Health.

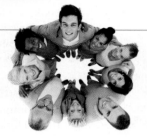

Although we all recognize the importance of being healthy, sorting out which behaviors are most likely to cause problems or pose great risk can be a challenge. Before you decide where to start, it is important to evaluate your current health status.

Completing the following assessment will give you a clearer picture of health areas in which you excel, as well as those that could use some work. Answer each question, then total your score for each section and fill it in on the Personal Checklist at the end of the assessment. Think about the behaviors that influenced your score in each category. Would you like to change any of them? Choose the area in which you'd like to improve, and then complete the

Behavior Change Contract at the back of your book. Use the contract to think through and implement a behavior change over the course of this class.

Each of the categories in this questionnaire is an important aspect of the total dimensions of health, but this is not a substitute for the advice of a qualified health care provider. Consider scheduling a thorough physical examination by a licensed physician or setting up an appointment with a mental health counselor at your school if you need help making a behavior change.

For each of the following, indicate how often you think the statements describe you.

1 Physical Health

	Never	Rarely	Some of the Time	Usually or Always
1. I am happy with my body size and weight.	1	2	3	4
2. I engage in vigorous exercises such as brisk walking, jogging, swimming, or running for at least 30 minutes per day, three to four times per week.	1	2	3	4
3. I get at least 7 to 8 hours of sleep each night.	1	2	3	4
4. My immune system is strong, and my body heals itself quickly when I get sick or injured.	1	2	3	4
5. I listen to my body; when there is something wrong, I try to make adjustments to heal it or seek professional advice.	1	2	3	4

Total score for this section: _____

2 Social Health

1. I am open and honest, and I get along well with others.	1	2	3	4
2. I participate in a wide variety of social activities and enjoy being with people who are different from me.	1	2	3	4
3. I try to be a "better person" and decrease behaviors that have caused problems in my interactions with others.	1	2	3	4

	Never	Rarely	Some of the Time	Usually or Always
4. I am open and accessible to a loving and responsible relationship.	1	2	3	4
5. I try to see the good in my friends and do whatever I can to support them and help them feel good about themselves.	1	2	3	4

Total score for this section: _____

3 Emotional Health

1. I find it easy to laugh, cry, and show emotions such as love, fear, and anger, and I try to express these in positive, constructive ways.	1	2	3	4
2. I avoid using alcohol or other drugs as a means of helping me forget my problems.	1	2	3	4
3. I recognize when I am stressed and take steps to relax through exercise, quiet time, or other calming activities.	1	2	3	4
4. I try not to be too critical or judgmental of others and try to understand differences or quirks that I note in others.	1	2	3	4
5. I am flexible and adapt or adjust to change in a positive way.	1	2	3	4

Total score for this section: _____

4 Environmental Health

	Never	Rarely	Some of the Time	Usually or Always
1. I buy recycled paper and purchase biodegradable detergents and cleaning agents, or I make my own cleaning products whenever possible.	1	2	3	4
2. I recycle paper, plastic, and metals; purchase refillable containers when possible; and try to minimize the amount of paper and plastics that I use.	1	2	3	4
3. I try to wear my clothes for longer periods between washing to reduce water consumption and the amount of detergents in our water sources.	1	2	3	4
4. I vote for pro-environment candidates in elections.	1	2	3	4
5. I minimize the amount of time that I run the faucet when I brush my teeth, shave, or shower.	1	2	3	4

Total score for this section: _____

5 Spiritual Health

	Never	Rarely	Some of the Time	Usually or Always
1. I take time alone to think about what's important in life—who I am, what I value, where I fit in, and where I'm going.	1	2	3	4
2. I have faith in a greater power, be it a supreme being, nature, or the connectedness of all living things.	1	2	3	4
3. I engage in acts of caring and goodwill without expecting something in return.	1	2	3	4
4. I sympathize and empathize with people who are suffering and try to help them through difficult times.	1	2	3	4
5. I go for the gusto and experience life to the fullest.	1	2	3	4

Total score for this section: _____

6 Intellectual Health

	Never	Rarely	Some of the Time	Usually or Always
1. I carefully consider my options and possible consequences as I make choices in life.	1	2	3	4
2. I learn from my mistakes and try to act differently the next time.	1	2	3	4
3. I have at least one hobby, learning activity, or personal growth activity that I make time for each week, something that improves me as a person.	1	2	3	4
4. I manage my time well rather than letting time manage me.	1	2	3	4
5. My friends and family trust my judgment.	1	2	3	4

Total score for this section: _____

Although each of these six aspects of health is important, there are some factors that don't readily fit in one category. As college students, you face some unique risks that others may not have. For this reason, we have added a section to this self-assessment that focuses on personal health promotion and disease prevention. Answer these questions, and add your results to the Personal Checklist in the following section.

7 Personal Health Promotion/Disease Prevention

	Never	Rarely	Some of the Time	Usually or Always
1. If I were to be sexually active, I would use protection such as latex condoms, dental dams, and other means of reducing my risk of sexually transmitted infections.	1	2	3	4
2. I can have a good time at parties or during happy hours without binge drinking.	1	2	3	4
3. I eat when I am hungry and stop eating when I am full. I do not try to lose weight by starving or forcing myself to vomit.	1	2	3	4
4. If I were to get a tattoo or piercing, I would go to a reputable person who follows strict standards of sterilization and precautions against bloodborne disease transmission.	1	2	3	4
5. I do not engage in extreme sports that risk bodily injury.	1	2	3	4

Total score for this section: _____

Personal Checklist

Now total your scores for each section and compare them to what would be considered optimal scores. Are you surprised by your scores in any areas? Which areas do you need to work on?

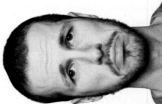

	Ideal Score	Your Score
Physical health	20	_____
Social health	20	_____
Emotional health	20	_____
Environmental health	20	_____
Spiritual health	20	_____
Intellectual health	20	_____
Personal health promotion/ disease prevention	20	_____

Scores of 10–14:

Your health risks are showing! Find information about the risks you are facing and why it is important to change these behaviors. Perhaps you need help in deciding how to make the changes you desire. Assistance is available from this book, your professor, and student health services at your school.

Scores of 15–20:

Outstanding! Your answers show that you are aware of the importance of these behaviors in your overall health. More important, you are putting your knowledge to work by practicing good health habits that reduce your overall risks. Although you earned a very high score, still consider areas in which your scores could be improved.

Scores below 10:

You may be taking unnecessary risks with your health. Perhaps you are not aware of the risks and what to do about them. Identify each risk area, and make a mental note as you read the associated chapter in the book. Whenever possible, seek additional health resources, either on your campus or through your local community, and make a serious commitment to behavior change. If any area is causing you to be less than functional in your class work or personal life, seek professional help. Remember that these scores are only indicators, not diagnostic tools.

YOUR PLAN FOR **CHANGE**

The **ASSESS YOURSELF** activity gave you the chance to gauge your total health status. Now that you have considered these results, you can take steps toward changing certain behaviors that may be detrimental to your health.

TODAY, YOU CAN:

- ☐ Evaluate your behavior and identify patterns and specific things you are doing.
- ☐ Select one pattern of behavior that you want to change.
- ☐ Fill out the Behavior Change Contract at the back of your book. Be sure to include your long- and short-term goals for change, the rewards you'll give yourself for reaching these goals, the potential obstacles along the way, and the strategies for overcoming these obstacles. For each goal, list the small steps and specific actions that you will take.

WITHIN THE NEXT TWO WEEKS, YOU CAN:

- ☐ Start a journal and begin charting your progress toward your behavior change goal.
- ☐ Tell a friend or family member about your behavior change goal, and ask this person to support you along the way.
- ☐ Reward yourself for reaching your short-term goals, and reevaluate your goals as needed.

BY THE END OF THE SEMESTER, YOU CAN:

- ☐ Review your journal entries, and consider how successful you have been in following your plan. What helped you be successful? What made change more difficult? What will you do differently next week?
- ☐ Revise your plan as needed: Are the goals attainable? Are the rewards satisfying? Do you have enough support and motivation?

STUDY **PLAN**

Visit the Study Area in Mastering Health to enhance your study plan with MP3 Tutor Sessions, Practice Quizzes, Flashcards, and more!

CHAPTER **REVIEW**

LO **1** | Why Health, Why Now?

- Choosing good health has immediate benefits, such as reducing the risk of injury and illnesses and improving academic performance; long-term rewards, such as disease prevention, longevity, and improved quality of life; and societal benefits, such as reducing the public costs of disability and disease.
- The average life expectancy at birth in the United States is 78.8 years. This has increased greatly over the past century; however, unhealthy behaviors continue to contribute to chronic diseases such as heart disease and stroke, among the leading causes of death for Americans.

LO **2** | What Is Health?

- The definition of *health* has changed over time. The medical model focused on physical aspects of health and treatment of disease, whereas the current ecological or public health model focuses on social, environmental, economic, and other factors contributing to health, disease prevention, and health promotion.
- Health can be seen as existing on a continuum and encompassing the dynamic process of fulfilling one's potential in the physical, social, intellectual, emotional, spiritual, and environmental dimensions of life. Wellness means achieving the highest possible level of health in each of the health dimensions.

LO **3** | What Influences Your Health?

- Health is influenced by factors called *determinants*. The Surgeon General's health promotion plan, *Healthy People*, classifies determinants as individual behavior, biology and genetics, social factors, policymaking, and health services. Disparities in health among different groups contribute to increased risks.

LO **4** | How Does Mindfulness Influence Health?

- Mindfulness—giving nonjudgmental attention to the present moment—enhances health in all dimensions. Formal activities such as meditation can help you develop mindfulness. Informal actions such as paying attention while eating or accepting your partner's anger without judgment are also effective.

LO **5** | How Does Behavior Change Occur?

- Models of behavior change include the health belief model, the social cognitive model, and the transtheoretical (stages of change) model. A person can increase the chance of successfully changing a health-related behavior by viewing change as a process containing several steps and components.

LO **6** | How Can You Improve Your Health Behaviors?

- When you are contemplating a behavior change, it is helpful to examine current habits, learn about a target behavior, and assess motivation and readiness to change. Developing self-efficacy and having an internal locus of control are essential for maintaining motivation. When you are preparing to change, it is helpful to set SMART goals that employ shaping, anticipate barriers to change, enlist the help and support of other people, and sign a behavior change contract. When you take action to change, it is helpful to visualize the new behavior; practice countering; control the situation; change self-talk; reward oneself; and keep a log, blog, or journal.

POP **QUIZ**

LO **1** | Why Health, Why Now?

1. What term is used to describe the expected number of years of full health remaining at a given age, such as at birth?
   a. Healthy life span
   b. Healthy life expectancy
   c. Health-related quality of life
   d. Wellness

2. What statistic is used to describe the number of deaths from heart disease this year?
   a. Morbidity
   b. Mortality
   c. Incidence
   d. Prevalence

LO **2** | What Is Health?

3. Everyday tasks, such as walking up the stairs or tying your shoes, are known as
   a. wellness behaviors.
   b. healthy life expectancy.
   c. cues to action.
   d. activities of daily living.

4. Janice describes herself as confident and trusting, and she displays both high self-esteem and high self-efficacy. The dimension of health to which these qualities relate is the
   a. physical dimension.
   b. emotional dimension.
   c. spiritual dimension.
   d. intellectual dimension.

5. *Healthy People 2020* is a(n)
   a. blueprint for health actions designed to improve health in the United States.
   b. projection for life expectancy rates in the United States in the year 2020.
   c. international plan for achieving health priorities for the environment by the year 2020.
   d. set of specific goals that states must achieve in order to receive federal funding for health care.

LO **4** | **How Does Mindfulness Influence Health?**

6. Which of the following statements about mindfulness is true?
   a. The technique of mindfulness was discovered and developed by Jon Kabat-Zinn in the late 1970s.
   b. Although there has been a surge of interest in mindfulness in the last decade, very little research links the practice to improved health.
   c. Meditation is a helpful but not essential tool for developing mindfulness.
   d. One technique that is recommended for developing mindfulness is to contemplate your perfection.

LO **5** | **How Does Behavior Change Occur?**

7. The social cognitive model of behavior change suggests that
   a. understanding the seriousness of a health problem and our susceptibility to it motivates change.
   b. contemplation is an essential step to adequately prepare ourselves for change.
   c. behavior change usually does not succeed if it begins with action.
   d. the environment in which we live, from childhood to the present, influences change.

LO **6** | **How Can You Improve Your Health Behaviors?**

8. Suppose you want to lose 20 pounds. To reach your goal, you take small steps. You start by joining a support group and counting calories. After 2 weeks, you begin an exercise program and gradually build up to your desired fitness level. What behavior change strategy are you using?
   a. Shaping
   b. Visualization
   c. Modeling
   d. Reinforcement

9. After Kirk and Tammy pay their bills, they reward themselves by watching TV together. The type of positive reinforcement that motivates them to pay their bills is a(n)
   a. activity reinforcer.
   b. consumable reinforcer.
   c. manipulative reinforcer.
   d. possessional reinforcer.

10. The aspects of a situation that cue or stimulate a person to act in certain ways are called
    a. antecedents.
    b. setting events.
    c. consequences.
    d. active inducements.

Answers to the Pop Quiz questions can be found on page A-1. If you answered a question incorrectly, review the section identified by the Learning Outcome. For even more study tools, visit MasteringHealth.

THINK ABOUT IT!

LO **1** | **Why Health, Why Now?**

1. How healthy is the U.S. population today? What factors influence today's disparities in health?

LO **2** | **What Is Health?**

2. How are the words *health* and *wellness* similar? What, if any, are important distinctions between these terms? What is health promotion? What is disease prevention?

LO **3** | **What Influences Your Health?**

3. What are some of the health disparities that exist in the United States today? Why do you think these differences exist? What policies do you think would most effectively address or eliminate health disparities?

LO **4** | **How Does Mindfulness Influence Health?**

4. Could mindfulness help you improve your academic performance this semester? If not, why not? If so, how?

LO **5** | **How Does Behavior Change Occur?**

5. What is the health belief model? How may this model be working when a young woman decides to smoke her first cigarette? Her last cigarette?

LO **6** | **How Can You Improve Your Health Behaviors?**

6. Using our four-step plan for behavior change, discuss how you might act as a change agent to help a friend stop smoking. Why is it important that your friend be ready to change before trying to change?

ACCESS YOUR HEALTH ON THE INTERNET

Visit Mastering Health for links to the websites and RSS feeds.

The following websites explore further topics and issues related to personal health.

CDC Wonder. This is a clearinghouse for comprehensive information from the Centers for Disease Control and Prevention (CDC), including special reports, guidelines, and access to national health data. **http://wonder.cdc.gov**

Mayo Clinic. This reputable resource for specific information about health topics, diseases, and treatment options is provided by the staff of the Mayo Clinic. It is easy to navigate and is consumer friendly. **www.mayoclinic .org**

National Center for Health Statistics. This resource contains links to key reports; national survey information; and information on mortality by age, race, gender, geographic location, and other important information about health status in the United States. **www.cdc .gov/nchs**

National Health Information Center. This is an excellent resource for consumer information about health. **www.health.gov/nhic**

World Health Organization. This resource for global health information provides information on the current state of health around the world, such as illness and disease statistics, trends, and illness outbreak alerts. **www.who.int/en**

Difference, Disparity, and Health: Achieving Health Equity

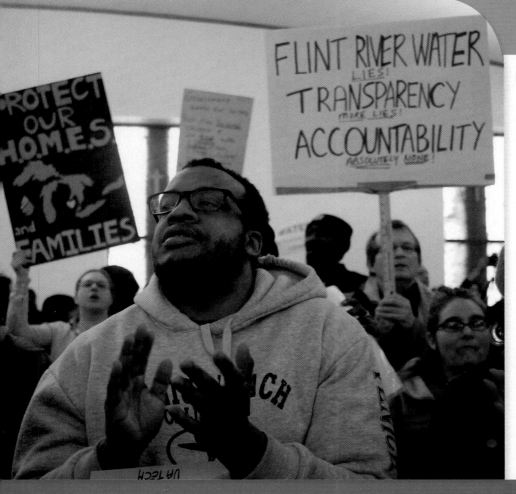

LEARNING OUTCOMES

1 Explain why health equity has become a critical issue in 21st century America, identifying the populations that are most vulnerable to health disparities and the costs to society.

2 Identify the social determinants of health that most strongly influence health disparities in the United States.

3 Discuss specific actions you can take to promote health equity on campus, in your community, and in your personal life, including how to use mindfulness to examine your biases and increase your respect for difference.

4 Describe the systemic changes required to enable the United States to progress toward good health for all, and provide examples of national and community-based initiatives currently underway toward achieving this goal.

WHY SHOULD I CARE?

Health disparities lead to preventable disease and premature death. They cost our economy billions of dollars annually, while depriving us of the full participation of each member of our society. In contrast, working toward health equity challenges your assumptions, hones your interpersonal skills, and generally expands your world. Importantly, moving populations toward improved health and greater opportunity ultimately benefits all of us while helping control health care costs.

The United States is one of the most diverse countries in the world, home to over 325 million unique individuals. These individuals represent an almost unfathomable complexity of differences in race and ethnicity, socioeconomic status, educational attainments, sexual orientation, gender identity, age, religion, abilities, and disabilities. They also represent differing attitudes, beliefs, fears, values, goals, and dreams.

These individuals live in a country where our founders proclaimed, in the *Declaration of Independence*, that we are all created equal. It is ironic, then, that the United States has consistently ranked lowest in *health equity* among the world's eleven wealthiest industrialized nations.[1] What is health equity, and why are we so low on the health equity scale? Why should we care? This chapter explores how differences can lead to health disparities and profound inequities in health. It explores why some of us live longer and thrive in life while others barely survive. Furthermore, it challenges us to think about what we can do individually and collectively to move toward health equity.

LO 1 | WHY HAS HEALTH EQUITY BECOME A CRITICAL ISSUE IN AMERICA?

Explain why health equity has become a critical issue in 21st century America, identifying the populations that are most vulnerable to health disparities and the costs to society.

In Chapter 1, you learned that one of the primary goals of the U.S. Surgeon General's health promotion plan *Healthy People 2020* is to achieve health equity, eliminate disparities, and improve the health of all groups.[2] What does this mean, and why does it matter?

Health Equity Is Attainment of the Highest Level of Health for All

The World Health Organization defines *equity* as "the absence of avoidable or remediable differences among groups of people."[3] A society characterized by **health equity** has worked to prevent or reverse conditions such as persistent

poverty and discrimination that undermine health. Informed by the values of fairness and justice, such a society values health as an essential resource for each individual's development, and as an important public good.[4] *Healthy People 2020* states that health equity is attainment of the optimal level of health for all people.[5]

Clearly, then, a society lacking health equity has a high level of health disparities. Recall from Chapter 1 that health disparities are differences in health that are "closely linked with social, economic, and/or environmental disadvantages."[6] These differences result from an unequal distribution of social resources, from education to housing to jobs that provide adequate health insurance and a living wage.[7] Thus, health disparities are fundamentally unjust, reflecting an unfair distribution of health risks and health resources.[8]

America: A Country of Increasing Diversity

America is a country of increasing **diversity**. In 2014, 62.2 percent of Americans were non-Hispanic whites (referred to in some research as Caucasians); 17.4 percent were Hispanic or Latino; 12.4 percent were non-Hispanic blacks (African Americans); 5.2 percent were Asians; and the rest were Native Americans and others.[9] About 27 percent of all people living in the United States today are immigrants, including their U.S.-born children.[10]

Immigration is expected to continue to diversify the U.S. population throughout the 21st century. The U.S. Census Bureau projects that between 2014 and 2060, as the population grows by about 98 million, the percentage of non-Hispanic whites will decline by more than a quarter (**FIGURE 1**). During the same period, the Hispanic population will more than double, and the non-Hispanic black, Asian American, and mixed-race populations will increase modestly. In 2044, a "majority-minority crossover" will occur,

health equity A condition characterized by an absence of avoidable or remediable differences in health and the attainment of optimal health for all.

diversity A condition characterized by varied composition, especially in terms of culture, race/ethnicity, religion, sexual orientation, and the like.

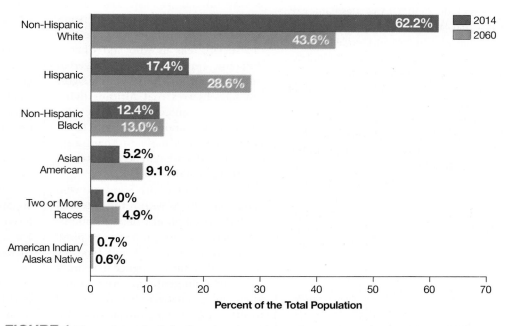

FIGURE 1 The racial and ethnic diversity of the United States population is expected to increase between 2014 and 2060.

Source: S.L. Colby and J. M. Ortman, "Projections of the Size and Composition of the U.S. Population: 2014–2060," U.S. Census Bureau, March 2015, Available at www.census.gov/content/dam/Census/library/publications/2015/demo/p25-1143.pdf.

and non-Hispanic white Americans will make up less than 50 percent of the U.S. population.[11]

America's age composition is also changing. The population of Americans under age 18, for example, is expected to increase only slightly between 2014 and 2060, from 74 million to 82 million. In contrast, the population of Americans age 65 or older is expected to more than double, from 46 million to 98 million.[12] These increasing numbers of older adults will challenge us to expand age-appropriate health care and other social and community services from transportation to nutritious meals to programs that encourage social interaction and reduce isolation. Without these supports, many older people will move farther away from health equity.

Americans are diversifying in self-identity as well. According to phone surveys, the percentage of Americans identifying as LGBT (lesbian, gay, bisexual, transgender) more than doubled between 2000 and 2017, from 2 percent to 4.1 percent, and among Millennials (born between 1980 and 1998), the percentage is now 7.3 percent.[13, 14] The LGBT category has itself diversified, especially on U.S. college campuses, to include LGBTQIAA+ (lesbian, gay, bisexual, transgender, queer, intersex, asexual, ally, inclusive). Gender identity itself is in flux: Americans are identifying as bigender, gender fluid, or gender queer or are rejecting the concept of gender altogether (agender).

Religious identity is also diversifying. The percentage of Americans who identify as Christian has been declining for decades, while those who identify as non-Christian religious have increased. In 2007, Muslims represented just 0.4 percent of the U.S. population. Now, nearly 1 percent of Americans are Muslim.[15] The percentage of Americans who are religiously unaffiliated (atheists, agnostics, or "nothing in particular") has been rising as well, from about 15 percent in 2007 to 22.8 percent in 2015.[16,17] About 36 percent of young Millennials are unaffiliated, and this generational trend is expected to continue.[18]

What are the implications of America's increasing diversity for our health and well-being? That depends in part on our response.

Our Response to Difference Can Lead to Disparities in Health

Our differences have the potential to enrich us, enabling us to learn from each other and pool our resources to meet the complex challenges of our changing world. However, our differences also have the potential to divide us. In social psychology, **difference** is the recognition of another person as being unlike us in some important way. Because we can never fully know another as he or she really is, this ability to recognize difference is very limited: We can base it only on our observations of the person's appearance and behavior. Notice that our society tells us who and what is different. For example, the Nigerian American author Chimamanda Ngozi Adichie observes that Africans living in many African countries do not distinguish one another by skin color. Only when they move to America do Africans with dark skin become "black" and therefore different.[19]

Any encounter with someone who is different brings with it the potential for false assumptions, misperceptions, unrecognized biases, and **stereotyping**, in which a generalized and typically negative attribute is assigned to an individual of a different population group. These thought patterns in turn can lead to **othering**, that is, interacting with people who are different as if they were intrinsically inferior to us in ways that make them less deserving of our respect and care. Such ways of thinking can also contribute to discrimination and other social injustices; trigger struggles for power and control; increase the threat of violence; and reduce every American's potential to thrive physically, emotionally, intellectually, and socially. Consider how misperceptions and unrecognized biases might influence our choices as individuals. For example, how might they influence whether to rent an apartment to a lesbian couple, hire an older adult, or even converse with a classmate wearing a headscarf? They also inform the actions we take as a society; for example, community members may oppose a measure to invest in high-quality low-income housing in their neighborhood because of unrecognized biases against people they consider "others." In these ways, our individual and collective responses to difference can reduce opportunities, lead to injustices, and create a society characterized by health disparities.

Certain Population Groups Are More Vulnerable to Health Disparities

Healthy People 2020 Identifies the people who are especially vulnerable to health disparities as those "who have systematically experienced greater obstacles to health based on their racial or ethnic group; religion; socioeconomic status; gender; age; mental health; cognitive, sensory, or physical disability; sexual orientation or gender identity; geographic location; or other characteristics historically linked to discrimination or exclusion."

Within each of the above categories, certain populations tend to have higher levels of disease, disability, and death. For example, non-Hispanic blacks tend to experience greater health disparities than non-Hispanic whites overall, as you will note in many areas covered in this text. They are more likely to die from heart disease, stroke, and most cancers; they are more apt to die of gun-related violence; and they have a lower average life expectancy (75.6 years versus 79.0 years for whites).[20,21] However, many exceptions to this

---

difference The recognition of another person as being unlike oneself in some important way.

stereotyping Assigning a generalized and typically negative attribute to an individual of a different population group.

othering Interacting with people who are different as if they were intrinsically inferior, less deserving of respect, or even threatening.

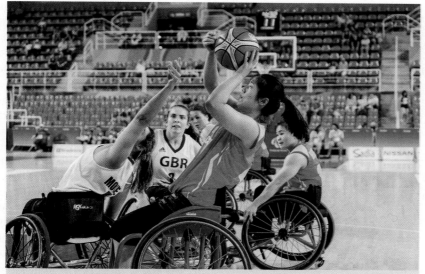
The experiences of each individual in a population group are unique.

general tendency exist. Non-Hispanic whites, for example, experience more suicides and drug overdose deaths than non-Hispanic blacks; in fact, largely because of these deaths, the mortality rate among middle-age non-Hispanic whites increased between 1999 and 2013 while it declined among all other racial and ethnic groups.[22] On the other hand, disparities often cross populations; for example, both black and white Americans who live in the Southeast have a much lower life expectancy than those who live in other parts of the country.[23]

Disparities occur not only between populations, but also between subgroups within a population. Consider the LGBT population, for example. Smoking rates are higher among lesbian, gay, and bisexual Americans (20.6 percent) than among heterosexuals (14.9 percent), but rates are highest among transgender Americans (35.5 percent), possibly because of higher levels of stress in the transgender population.[24] Similarly, clinical depression and suicide are more common among transgender individuals than within the non-transgender LGB population.[25]

There are also innumerable differences between people *within* groups. We may speak of "the Jewish experience" or "the experience of poverty," but the lives of individuals within any population group are unique and can vary

dramatically. Because our assumptions about different populations are typically based on limited exposure to individuals from those populations, they are likely be inaccurate. Even health statistics from government agencies such as the Centers for Disease Control and Prevention (CDC) are only averages and, as such, do not reflect the vast differences between the people those statistics represent.

Health Disparities Incur Enormous Costs

> *"Every person who dies young, is avoidably disabled, or is unable to function at their optimal level not only represents a personal and family tragedy but also impoverishes our communities and our country. We are all deprived of the creativity, contributions, and participation that result from disparities in health status."*[26]

The above quotation from the director of the CDC can only begin to encompass the human costs of health disparities in the United States. Disparities in health also have significant financial costs. Racial and ethnic health disparities alone are estimated to cost the U.S. economy an estimated $35 billion in direct medical expenditures, $10 billion

in lost productivity, and nearly $200 billion in premature deaths.[27] These costs occur when chronic diseases such as type 2 diabetes are neither prevented nor appropriately managed; when patients without access to primary care seek treatment in the most costly type of medical facility—the hospital emergency department; when inadequate health education contributes to unprotected sex, tobacco use, and other risky health behaviors; and when people with substance abuse and mental health disorders are not able to access treatment programs and therefore leave the workforce, never enter the workforce, or become victims of overdose or suicide.

Again, health disparities—and their accompanying costs—are avoidable. If as a society we are to reduce them, we need to understand the social, economic, and environmental disadvantages to which they are closely linked.[28]

LO 2 | HOW DO THE SOCIAL DETERMINANTS OF HEALTH INFLUENCE HEALTH DISPARITIES IN AMERICA?

Identify the social determinants of health that most strongly influence health disparities in the United States.

Indicators of health disparities, such as rates of disease and death, are outcomes of a system that doesn't value individuals equally. This inequity in valuing increases the health risks to certain populations while decreasing their access to the resources that could help them to thrive. In contrast, certain other populations have **privilege**, that is, resources and rights, that are denied or are not as available to others. For example, children born into affluent families may have a nourishing diet, excellent educational opportunities, and access to high-quality health

privilege Advantages and rights, often unearned, that are available to only some members of a society.

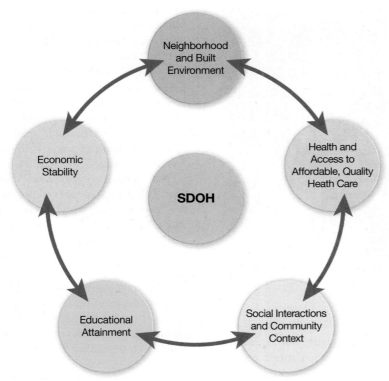

FIGURE 2 Social determinants of health (SDOH).

care. These resources support health. Children born into families where they are valued and nurtured, even if they are not wealthy, also have resources that support health, including social connectedness and an overall sense of safety and security.

Conditions that affect—positively or negatively—access to and distribution of health-related resources are known as the **social determinants of health (SDOH)**.[29] You encountered them in Chapter 1. Here, we'll take a closer look at how they influence health and health disparities (**FIGURE 2**) both directly and indirectly A low-income individual, for example, may be unable to afford a prescription for a drug to treat his asthma. Less directly, the individual's

housing options may be limited to neighborhoods with high levels of air pollution that exacerbate the asthma. The SDOH are interconnected. Discrimination, for example, can influence educational attainment, housing, employment options and thus income, and other SDOH.[30]

Economic Stability and Educational Attainment

In the decades after World War II, income gains were broadly shared throughout American society. However, between 1980 and 2013, the gap between the rich and the poor widened dramatically, contributing to what has been called "the disappearance of the middle class."[31] In 2014, the richest 20 percent of households had an average income of $194,053, nearly 17 times the average income of $11,676 for the bottom 20 percent of households.[32]

In 2015, the U.S. Census Bureau defined poverty as a household income of $12,331 a year for a single person and

$18, 871 for a family of three. A single parent with two children working full-time at the federal minimum wage ($7.25 an hour) would earn $15,080 a year—well below the poverty line. Although a majority of U.S. states have set their minimum wage above $7.25 an hour, many states abide by the federal minimum wage. To learn the minimum wage in your state, search for the "state minimum wage chart" at www.ncsl.org.

Decades of research support a close association between poverty and poor health.[33] Many poor Americans, for example, experience hunger; in 2015, nearly 13 percent of U.S. households were **food insecure**, meaning that they lacked access to sufficient food for all household members.[34] In addition, poor Americans are more likely to reside in **food deserts**, communities with low or no access to food stores that sell fresh fruits and vegetables, whole-grain breads, fish, and other nutritious foods. Living in a food desert increases the risk for health problems such as obesity and obesity-related diseases. Low-income communities may also have low walkability, lower-performing schools, poorer-quality health care facilities, and higher than average levels of pollution and violence.[35]

---

social determinants of health Social, economic, and physical conditions in the environments in which people live that affect a range of health, functioning, and quality-of-life outcomes and risks.

food insecure Lacking reliable access to sufficient food for all household members.

food desert A community in which residents lack ready access to fresh, healthful, and affordable food.

43.1 MILLION AMERICANS

live in **POVERTY**

Nearly 13% of U.S. households lack sufficient food. Many poor Americans in both cities and rural communities live in food deserts.

Low educational attainment—a distinct SDOH—increases with increasing poverty; as compared to middle-income Americans, the poorest Americans have triple the rate of noncompletion of high school. Education enhances health in multiple ways: It directly increases access to information about nutrition, physical activity, alcohol use, and other lifestyle choices that influence health. It also leads to better job opportunities and, in turn, better working conditions, sick leave, paid vacation, health insurance coverage, and other benefits, including the ability to afford good-quality housing, food, and other essentials.[36] Income stability and educational attainment provide emotional, social, and material resources that promote health throughout life.[37]

By reducing access to society's resources, poverty contributes to significant and chronic stress, which leads to physical and mental health problems that begin in childhood and typically persist throughout the lifespan.[38] One of the most striking poverty-related health disparities is in life expectancy. Males in the lowest 10 percent of income have an average life expectancy 14 years below that of males with income in the top 10 percent; for females, the gap is 13 years.[39] Other disparities linked to poverty include an increased risk for preterm birth and infant mortality;[40] impaired neurological development in children[41]; reduced access to needed medical care, dental care, and prescription drugs[42]; and higher rates of chronic disease and disability.[43] In 2014, over 37 percent of impoverished Americans age 18 to 64 living at or below the poverty line had at least one disability, compared to 17 percent of middle-income or affluent Americans.[44]

Social Interactions and Community Context

Our social interactions and community environment strongly influence our health. Such factors include our level of social support, social norms and attitudes (including prejudice, discrimination, racism, and bullying), cultural influences, language barriers and

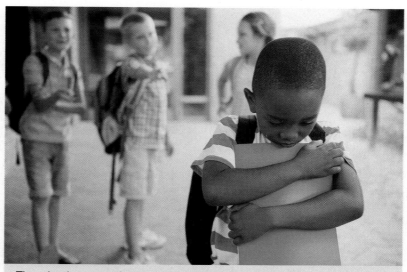

The minority-stress theory attempts to explain the link between stress and the discrimination experienced by members of minority groups. According to this theory, even the anticipation of discrimination can trigger the stress response.

levels of literacy, incarceration rates, and availability of community-based resources.[45]

Among these factors, discrimination has emerged as a key contributor to stress and stress-related symptoms and poor health.[46] A recent report from the American Psychological Association identified an increased risk for discrimination among members of the following five groups: the poor, the disabled, racial/ethnic minorities, LGBT Americans, and older Americans.[47] The *minority-stress theory* attempts to explain the link between frequent exposure to discrimination—such as being stopped unfairly by police, passed over for a job promotion, discouraged by a teacher, or even treated discourteously—and stress levels that reduce health. Even the anticipation of discrimination increases stress; for example, an older worker who is accustomed to being honest might feel the need to lie about age on a job application to get hired. Americans who report experiencing extreme levels of stress are twice as likely to also report fair or poor health, compared to those with low stress levels.[48] (See Chapter 3 for more on the link between stress and health.)

Culture—the attitudes, beliefs, values, and behaviors characteristic of a group of people—can also influence

health. Culture is transmitted through language, material objects, art, rituals, institutions, and other modes and is passed from generation to generation as people adapt to social and environmental changes. Individuals may hold culturally based beliefs about what causes disease, what is appropriate treatment, or whether to seek care at all. Culturally based behavior patterns can also affect trust of and communication with health care providers and health-related lifestyle choices such as diet and levels of physical activity. Although culture is a widely acknowledged determinant of health, it's important to recognize that we are all individuals engaging in complex and varied behaviors, any one of which may or may not be culturally influenced.

Language barriers and illiteracy can also affect health. **Health literacy** is the ability to obtain, process, and understand health information and services needed to make appropriate health decisions.[49] It includes the ability to understand, for example, instructions

culture The collective attitudes, beliefs, values, and behaviors that distinguish one group of people from another.

health literacy The ability to obtain, process, and understand health information and services needed to make appropriate health decisions.

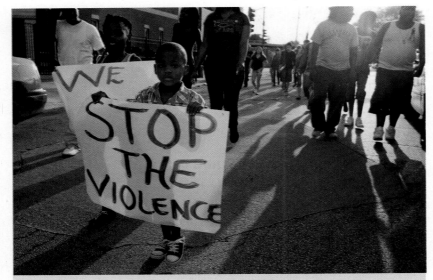
Exposure to neighborhood violence is another powerful social determinant of health.

about prescription drugs, appointment slips, health education brochures, physician instructions, and insurance and consent forms.[50] People with low health literacy also may have problems communicating with health care providers and may be less able to make informed health care decisions. In consequence, they are more likely not to obtain recommended vaccinations, cancer screenings, and other types of preventive care; may make medication errors; may suffer complications from poor disease management; and may be more likely to be hospitalized. They also have a higher mortality rate.[51]

Neighborhood and Built Environment

Neighborhood characteristics, such as walkability, the presence of food stores that offer plenty of healthy choices, and density of recreational facilities, also influence health.[52] Multiple studies have linked rural environments with reduced opportunities for physical activity and increased levels of obesity.[53]

Another aspect of the built environment that can contribute to health disparities is the level of industrial and traffic pollution in air, water, and soil.[54,55] After the Environmental Protection Agency's discovery in 2015 of lead contamination in the public water supply in Flint, Michigan—where over 40 percent of the population lives below the poverty line—municipal water systems in other low-income communities across the United States also were found to be contaminated with lead.[56]

Exposure to neighborhood violence is another powerful SDOH, contributing directly to traumatic injuries and deaths and indirectly to disparities in mental and physical health as well as increased risks for several chronic diseases.[57,58,59,60,61]

LO 3 | HOW CAN YOUR ACTIONS CONTRIBUTE TO HEALTH EQUITY?

Discuss specific actions you can take to promote health equity on campus, in your community, and in your personal life, including how to use mindfulness to examine your biases and increase your respect for difference.

The factors that contribute to health disparities are complex and interconnected, and solutions can seem overwhelming, especially when viewed from a systems perspective. But health disparities can be addressed on a smaller scale—in your own neighborhood and your own mind.

Use Mindfulness to Examine Your Assumptions and Biases

As we discussed in Chapter 1, a highly effective strategy for challenging the beliefs and attitudes that limit us is to cultivate mindfulness. Participants in a recent mindfulness training program enhanced their ability to pay attention to their own unconscious biases, increased their insights into and understanding of the unconscious aspects of other people's behavior, and adopted less of an "us" versus "them" approach to interactions with others.[62] Another study offering a single session of mindfulness training to college students found that those who received the training demonstrated reduced racial and age biases and fewer negative behaviors that commonly result from such biases.[63] The researchers attributed this reduction in bias to a dampening of the brain's activation of automatic negative associations. In other words, when we pay close attention to what is actually occurring in our mind and our surroundings, we disable previously established, habitual neurological pathways by which we perceive, interpret our perceptions, and respond.[64]

The Assess Yourself at the end of this chapter offers steps for examining your assumptions, perceptions, and biases.

Affirm the Benefits of Diversity

Were you raised in a region with a population largely sharing the same language, culture, religion, and race or ethnicity? Even if you're from a tremendously diverse area, did you stick to your own group most of the time? If so, you might find the diversity of campus life exhilarating—or challenging. It can be stressful to take a class with an instructor whose primary language isn't English or to work on a team project with people of different ages, backgrounds, or abilities. Understanding and affirming the benefits of diversity can help.

Diversity is a teacher. Interacting every day with other people who are different from you challenges your assumptions; exposes you to new ideas, values, and experiences; and generally expands your world. The skills you develop in working across differences are likely to improve your career prospects, perhaps even preparing you for international job opportunities. As you compare and contrast your values, beliefs, and personal history with those of other people, you discover more about yourself. This deeper self-awareness can in turn support you in making decisions about your coursework, social life, and future plans.[65] Finally, building relationships with people who are different from you can expose you to new foods, new sports, new music, new authors—and a lot of fun!

Learn to Communicate across Differences

Even among people who habitually examine their biases and practice mindfulness, miscommunications can occur. The following techniques can help you communicate effectively across real and imagined differences.[66]

A first step is to establish some rules for the dialogue, creating a shared agreement about the values and goals of your communication. For example, do you both commit to civility, honesty, and mutual respect? What do you hope to gain from your dialogue?

When the other person is speaking, stop your inner monologue and truly listen. Pay attention not only to the content of the person's message, but also to the way the person is saying it. Each time your mind begins to wander, return it to what the other person is saying. After the person has finished speaking, paraphrase back what you believe you heard. Check in: Was your paraphrase close to what the person actually said? If not, respectfully ask for clarification.

Aim for full disclosure. In other words, admit that your age, gender identity, race or ethnicity, abilities and disabilities, life experiences, and countless other factors have contributed to who you are in this moment of dialogue, including how you perceive other people and how they perceive you.

When things get tense, hit the pause button. Take time to reflect on the factors that have contributed to the differences between you.

Close with a dialogue about the dialogue; that is, share your observations about your process of communication and questions and suggestions for future conversations.

Advocate for Yourself and Others

In addition to practicing mindfulness and communicating across differences, you can contribute to health equity by advocating for yourself and others. To do that, it helps to be able to recognize othering and discrimination when it happens to you and to take action to protect your health and change your interactions in the future. For strategies, see the Skills for Behavior Change box on this page.

LO 4 | HOW CAN SYSTEMIC CHANGE LEAD TO HEALTH FOR ALL?

Describe the systemic changes required to enable the United States to progress toward good health for all, and provide examples of national and community-based initiatives currently underway toward achieving this goal.

"Health for all" means living in communities that offer opportunities to thrive, physically, mentally, economically, and socially. It means access to healthy nutrition, physical activity, safe and affordable housing, education from early childhood through adulthood, jobs that pay living wages, career opportunities, social support, community resources, freedom from discrimination, high-quality health care, and other social resources. This is where, as a society, we want to go. The question is: How do we get there?

SKILLS FOR
BEHAVIOR CHANGE

Becoming Your Own Advocate

If you have experienced othering, stereotyping, or discrimination, you might be tempted simply to accept the situation and move on. But a more healthy way to respond is to become your own advocate. Here are some suggestions:

- Actively reject the negative messages you've received. Remind yourself of your goodness, your core values, and your life purpose.

- Discuss the experience with family members, friends, members of student diversity groups, and leaders at campus diversity centers or with a mental health professional.

- If you are likely to engage in the future with an individual who has treated you unfairly, decide in advance how you would like your interactions to change. Make mental or written notes about the message you want to communicate and how to do it calmly, clearly, and effectively.

- Remember that you have a right to speak up for your interests. Someone else disagreeing with you or becoming defensive does not negate the importance of your needs or your right to make them known.

- If you believe you have been discriminated against in housing or employment, file a complaint. For example, for job discrimination, contact the U.S. Equal Opportunity Employment Commission at www.eeoc.gov.

- Remember that you are helping others by speaking out.

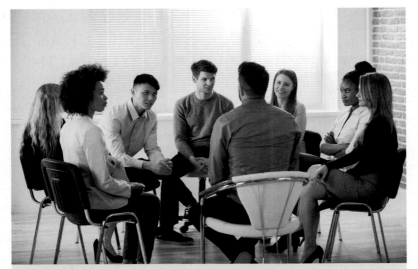

Civility, honesty, and mutual respect are necessary to successful communication.

Increase Access to Health Care

In 2014, the U.S. Surgeon General published a National Prevention Strategy on the elimination of health disparities. One of its key recommendations was to increase access to health care, especially among the communities at greatest health risk.[67]

Public health experts have proposed the following initiatives to achieve a more equitable distribution of health care:

■ **Increase minority providers.** Members of minorities are more likely to seek care from health care providers of their own race or ethnicity.[68] Educational programs and policies should encourage minority Americans (racial or ethnic minorities, LGBT Americans, and disabled Americans) to pursue careers in the health professions.[69]

■ **Increase diversity training.** All health care providers should be required to undergo diversity training to improve their ability to communicate health information in the language and at the appropriate literacy level of the client they are serving.[70] Whether a person is young or old, thin or overweight, gay or straight, able or disabled—regardless of differences—high-quality care delivered promptly and with respect should be the goal.

■ **Increase preventive services.** Municipalities, employers, school districts, and health care organizations should partner to offer preventive services such as mental health services, dental exams and cleanings, vision care, vaccinations, blood pressure screenings, and other services for underserved populations.

■ **Expand access to health insurance.** The national initiative that has had perhaps the greatest effect on increasing access to health care for all population groups is the Affordable Care Act (ACA), which was signed into law in 2010 and implemented in stages. Under the ACA, the percentage of poor and near-poor Americans who are uninsured dropped from 27 percent and 29 percent, respectively, in 2013 to 17 percent and 18 percent, respectively, in 2015.[71] Currently, provisions of the ACA are being questioned, as some members of Congress say it goes too far and others say it doesn't go far enough. Stay tuned!

Reduce the Social Determinants That Contribute to Health Disparities

In addition to increasing access to high-quality care, we must reduce the SDOH that significantly contribute to health disparities. Because these determinants are intertwined, they must be counteracted by systemic measures such as social programs, economic investment, reform of public education, improvements in mental health programs, reform of our criminal justice system, decreased segregation in our communities and institutions, and more funding for inclusive research into health care disparities.[72]

The Surgeon General's National Prevention Strategy recommends, for example, that key community representatives

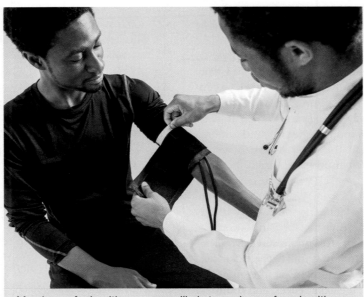

Members of minorities are more likely to seek care from health care providers of their own race or ethnicity.

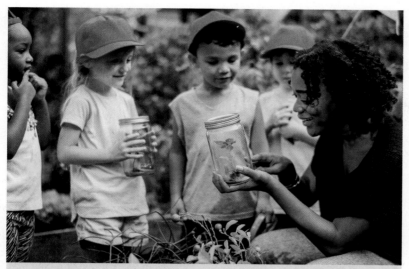

Community gardens can help to increase access to nourishing food and reduce health disparities.

meet with professionals from a range of community organizations to identify the community's health needs and the barriers to meeting those needs.[73] Specific strategies to reduce SDOH affecting the physical environment include construction of high-quality, safe, and affordable housing; identifying and working to remediate sources of pollution; increasing neighborhood walkability; building parks and playgrounds; establishing after-school programs for tutoring, physical activity, and social support; offering incentives to chain grocers to open food stores that provide plenty of healthy options; building community gardens; supporting meetings between law enforcement officers and community members to foster collaboration and establish neighborhood watch programs; and using libraries and community centers to increase health literacy. Each of these strategies has the potential to reduce health disparities. Together, they could be transformative.

Examples of Initiatives to Increase Health for All

In the latter decades of the 20th century, recognizing that health disparities exist, several national and community-level initiatives were implemented to improve "health for all." Here, we review some of the most significant.

National Initiatives

In 1979, the Healthy People initiative was launched with the publication of *Healthy People: The Surgeon General's Report on Health Promotion and Disease Prevention*, a document that established national goals for reducing injuries, preventable disease, and premature death.[74] Other initiatives have followed, including the creation in 1985 of the U.S. Department of Health and Human Services Task Force on Black and Minority Health[75] and new reports on health disparities from the Surgeon

General, the Institute of Medicine, and the CDC. Although these reports set goals and objectives for reducing health disparities, only minimal progress has been made toward meeting those goals because accountability and funding have been inadequate.

City, County, and State Initiatives

City, county, and state governments can employ a variety of approaches to improve health equity. These efforts include improvements in standards for construction of public housing and businesses; changes to zoning ordinances to avoid the release of pesticides and other pollutants within a reasonable distance of residential neighborhoods; support for public transportation to increase accessibility to supermarkets, health care facilities, and schools and colleges; and policies or legislation to increase the minimum wage, ban environmental tobacco smoke in public spaces; build and staff community health care facilities; improve neighborhood walkability; or support famers markets or community gardens.

Initiatives on Campus

College can provide unique opportunities to students from underserved communities to develop more healthful habits via access to the student health center, healthy meal options in the student union and the dorms, fitness facilities, and security services. Some campuses have food service providers that are committed to offering healthy foods, others have community gardens, and some have a food pantry for student use. Conduct some research on campus-based programs to advance health equity, and recommend model programs for your own campus.

ASSESS YOURSELF

LIVE IT! ASSESS YOURSELF
An interactive version of this assessment is available online in Mastering Health.

Examining Assumptions, Perceptions, and Biases

Our beliefs affect how we interact with others. Unexamined assumptions, perceptions, and biases can cause us to engage in stereotyping, othering, and discrimination. Think through the following questions to discover how your biases may be affecting your health and the health of others.

1. In what type of community (e.g., urban, rural, suburban, small, large) were you raised? List some ways in which it was diverse. In what ways might aspects of your community or home life have affected your health?

2. How would you characterize yourself in terms of being "different"? Have you felt that you belong to a particular group or groups? Why or why not? Do your differences or similarities make you feel as if you fit in to society at large, or not? Explain.

3. Would you describe your family, friends, and community as accepting of or biased against other populations or groups? How does that acceptance or bias play out in terms of people you associate with, your compassion for other people, and your concerns about the treatment of those who are different?

4. Do your interactions with other people tend to include diverse populations? Do you actively seek out people who are different from you, or do you prefer interactions with people who are like you?

5. Some people would say, "Everyone is biased—they just don't realize it." Do you agree with this statement? Why or why not? Give an example of a bias that you may hold against a person from a different population. Why do you think you have that bias? What could you do to explore those feelings and work to change them?

6. What are some ways in which your assumptions, misperceptions, and biases might affect the health of someone other than yourself?

YOUR PLAN FOR CHANGE

The ASSESS YOURSELF activity gave you the chance to create your own family health history and identify the health risks present in your family. Now you can take steps to help you take charge of your destiny!

TODAY, YOU CAN:

☐ Review your responses to the questions in the Assess Yourself, and identify any aspects of them that might contribute to health disparities.

☐ Consider discussing your answers with a classmate or close friend and asking for feedback, including insights that you might not have addressed.

WITHIN THE NEXT TWO WEEKS, YOU CAN:

☐ Increase your awareness of your automatic responses to people you see as different from you. Think about what triggers the response, and assess whether the response is appropriate.

☐ Increase your awareness of messages from family members, friends, community members, and media that either promote or challenge prejudice, and think about how these messages can either contribute to or reduce health disparities. Strive to adopt attitudes that promote health for all.

BY THE END OF THE SEMESTER, YOU CAN:

☐ List the values you hold that support health equity.

☐ Take at least one action at the local level to promote health equity, such as writing about the issue on your social networking site, volunteering at a food pantry or homeless clinic, or joining the local chapter of a social justice group.

☐ Join a national or international health equity or antidiscrimination group such as Doctors Without Borders or Feeding America.

STUDY **PLAN**

Visit the Study Area in Mastering Health to enhance your study plan with MP3 Tutor Sessions, Practice Quizzes, Flashcards, and more!

CHAPTER **REVIEW**

LO **1** Why Has Health Equity Become a Critical Issue in America?

■ Health equity, which is informed by the values of fairness and justice, is attainment of the optimal level of health for all people. Health disparities are differences in health that are tied to persistent and unjust social, economic, and/or environmental disadvantages. Our society's evolving diversity brings with it an increased potential for false assumptions, misperceptions, unrecognized biases, discrimination, and stereotyping.

LO **2** How Do the Social Determinants of Health Influence Health Disparities in America?

■ Conditions that affect—positively or negatively—access to and distribution of health-related resources are known as the social determinants of health. Some of the most significant are persistent poverty, low educational attainment, discrimination and minority stress, and health-related neighborhood characteristics such as walkability and the presence of food stores that offer plenty of healthy choices, level of pollution, and neighborhood violence.

LO **3** How Can Your Actions Contribute to Health Equity?

■ The practice of mindfulness can help you pay close attention to what is occurring in your mind and your surroundings and thereby reduce bias. Learning techniques to

communicate across difference— such as establishing shared rules, values, and goals of the dialogue, listening and paraphrasing, and fully disclosing—can help you communicate more effectively with people of different population groups.

LO **4** What Systemic Changes Support Health for All?

■ Increasing health equity will require increasing everyone's access to high-quality health care. We must also implement systemic solutions to reduce the social determinants of health that contribute most significantly to health disparities, including poverty, low educational attainment, discrimination, pollution, and violence. National, state, county, and local initiatives are also important.

POP **QUIZ**

LO **1** Why Has Health Equity Become a Critical Issue in America?

1. Assigning a generalized and typically negative attribute to an individual of a different population group is known as
   a. othering.
   b. stereotyping.
   c. negating.
   d. discriminating.

LO **2** How Do the Social Determinants of Health Influence Health Disparities in America?

2. Which of the following social determinants of health contributes significantly to chronic stress?

a. Poverty
b. Discrimination
c. Exposure to neighborhood violence
d. All of the above

LO **3** How Can Your Actions Contribute to Health Equity?

3. Which of the following is thought to be an effect of mindfulness training?
   a. It can more effectively activate previously established neurological pathways by which we perceive and respond to others.
   b. It can help reinforce negative stereotypes.
   c. It can reduce the brain's activation of automatic negative associations.
   d. It can increase negative behaviors that result from biases.

LO **4** What Systemic Changes Support Health for All?

4. Which of the following initiatives would be most likely to achieve a more equitable distribution of health care?
   a. Conduct research into the root causes of neighborhood violence.
   b. Increase taxes on tobacco products.
   c. Establish educational programs and policies to encourage members of minority groups to pursue careers in the health professions.
   d. Raise the age for Medicare eligibility to 75 years.

2 Promoting and Preserving Your Psychological Health

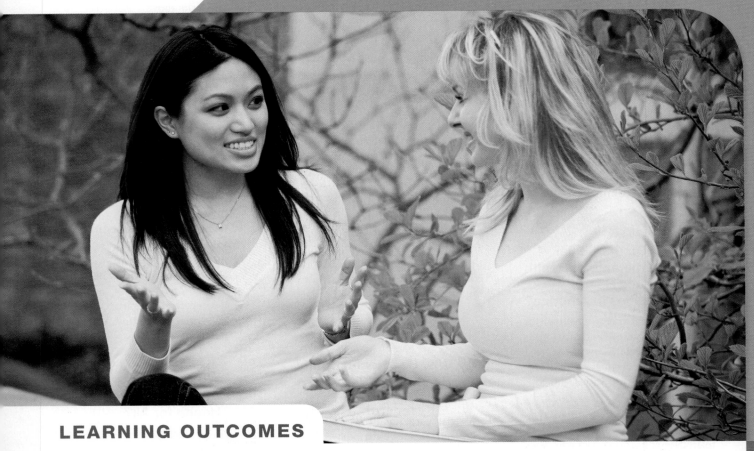

LEARNING OUTCOMES

LO **1** Define each of the four components of psychological health, and identify basic traits shared by psychologically healthy people.

LO **2** Discuss the roles of self-efficacy and self-esteem, emotional intelligence, personality, maturity, and happiness in psychological well-being.

LO **3** Describe and differentiate psychological disorders, including mood disorders, anxiety disorders, obsessive-compulsive disorder, posttraumatic stress disorder, personality disorders, and schizophrenia, and explain their causes and treatments.

LO **4** Discuss risk factors and possible warning signs of suicide, as well as actions that can be taken to help a person contemplating suicide.

LO **5** Explain the different types of treatment options and professional services available to people experiencing mental health problems.

Most students describe their college years as among the best of their lives, but they may also find the pressure of grades, finances, and relationships, along with the struggle to find themselves, to be extraordinarily difficult. Psychological distress caused by relationship issues, family concerns, academic competition, financial pressures, career worries, and adjusting to college life is common. Experts believe that the anxiety-inducing campus environment is a major contributor to poor health decisions such as high levels of alcohol consumption and overeating. These, in turn, can affect academic success and overall health.

LO 1 | WHAT IS PSYCHOLOGICAL HEALTH?

Define each of the four components of psychological health, and identify basic traits shared by psychologically healthy people.

Psychological health is the sum of how we think, feel, relate, and exist in our day-to-day lives. Our thoughts, perceptions, emotions, motivations, interpersonal relationships, and behaviors are a product of our experiences and the skills we have developed to meet life's challenges. Psychological health includes mental, emotional, social, and spiritual dimensions and can be influenced by physical health (**FIGURE 2.1**).

Most experts identify several basic elements that psychologically Healthy people regularly display:

- **They feel good about themselves.** They are not typically overwhelmed by fear, love, anger, jealousy, guilt, or worry. They know who they are, have a realistic sense of their capabilities, and respect themselves.
- **They feel comfortable with other people, respect others, and have compassion for others.** They enjoy satisfying and lasting personal relationships and do not take advantage of other people or allow others to take advantage of them. They can give love, consider other people's interests, take time to help others, and respect personal differences.
- **They are "self-compassionate."** Being kind and understanding of their own imperfections and weaknesses, they acknowledge their "humanness." They are mindful of the problems in life, and work to be the best that they can be, given their limitations and things they can't control. They are not self-absorbed, narcissistic, or overly critical of themselves.[1]

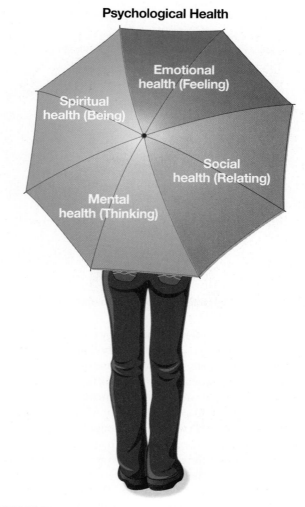

Psychological Health

Emotional health (Feeling)

Spiritual health (Being)

Social health (Relating)

Mental health (Thinking)

FIGURE 2.1 Psychological health is a complex interaction of the mental, emotional, social, and spiritual dimensions of health. Possessing strength and resiliency in these dimensions can help you maintain your overall well-being and weather the storms of life.

- **They control tension and anxiety.** They recognize the underlying causes and symptoms of stress and anxiety in their lives and consciously avoid irrational thoughts, hostility, excessive excuse making, and blaming other people for their problems. They use resources and learn skills to control reactions to stressful situations.

psychological health The mental, emotional, social, and spiritual dimensions of health.

Psychologically unhealthy			Psychologically healthy
No zest for life; pessimistic/cynical most of the time; spiritually down	Shows poorer coping than most, often overwhelmed by circumstances	Works to improve in all areas, recognizes strengths and weaknesses	Possesses zest for life; spiritually healthy and intellectually thriving
Laughs, but usually at others, has little fun	Has regular relationship problems, finds that others often disappoint	Healthy relationships with family and friends, capable of giving and receiving love and affection	High energy, resilient, enjoys challenges, focused
Has serious bouts of depression, "down" and tired much of time; has suicidal thoughts	Tends to be cynical/critical of others; tends to have negative/critical friends	Has strong social support, may need to work on improving social skills but usually no major problems	Realistic sense of self and others, sound coping skills, open-minded
A "challenge" to be around, socially isolated	Lacks focus much of the time, hard to keep intellectual acuity sharp	Has occasional emotional "dips", but overall good mental/emotional adaptors	Adapts to change easily, sensitive to others and environment
Experiences many illnesses, headaches, aches/pains, gets colds/infections easily	Quick to anger, sense of humor and fun evident less often		Has strong social support and healthy relationships with family and friends

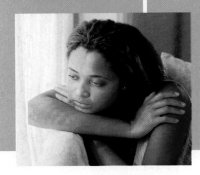
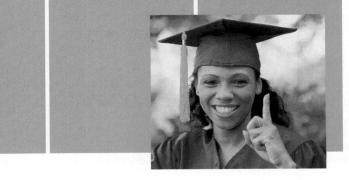

FIGURE 2.2 Characteristics of Psychologically Healthy and Unhealthy People Where do you fall on this continuum?

- **They meet the demands of life.** They try to solve problems as they arise, accept responsibility, and plan ahead. They set realistic goals, think for themselves, and make independent decisions. Acknowledging that change is inevitable, they welcome new experiences.
- **They curb hate and guilt.** They acknowledge and combat tendencies to respond with anger, thoughtlessness, selfishness, vengefulness, or feelings of inadequacy. They do not try to knock other people aside to get ahead but rather reach out to help others.
- **They maintain a positive outlook.** They approach each day with a presumption that things will go well. They look to the future with enthusiasm rather than dread. Having fun and making time for themselves are integral parts of their lives.
- **They value diversity.** They do not feel threatened by people of a different gender, religion, sexual orientation, race, ethnicity, age, or political party. They are nonjudgmental and do not force their beliefs and values on other people.
- **They appreciate and respect the world around them.** They take time to enjoy their surroundings, are conscious of their place in the universe, and act responsibly to preserve their environment.

resiliency The ability to adapt to change and stressful events in healthy and flexible ways.

In sum, psychologically healthy people possess emotional, mental, social, and spiritual **resiliency**. Resilient individuals have the ability to overcome challenges from major tragedies to minor disappointments and typical life obstacles we often face. They usually respond to challenges and frustrations in appropriate ways, despite occasional slips (see **FIGURE 2.2**). When they do slip, they recognize it, are kind to themselves rather than engaging in endless self-recrimination, and take action to rectify the situation.

Psychologists have long argued that before we can achieve any of the above characteristics of psychological health, we must meet certain basic human needs. In the 1960s, humanistic theorist Abraham Maslow developed a *hierarchy of needs* to describe this idea (**FIGURE 2.3**): At the bottom are basic *survival needs*, such as food, sleep, and water; at the next level are *security needs*, such as shelter and safety; at the third level, *social needs* include a sense of belonging and affection; at the fourth level are *esteem needs*, self-respect and respect for other people; and at the top are needs for *self-actualization* and self-transcendence.

According to Maslow, a person's needs must be met at each of these levels before the person can be truly healthy. Failure to meet needs at a lower level will interfere with a person's ability to address higher-level needs. For example, someone who is homeless or worried about threats from violence will be unable to focus on fulfilling social, esteem, or actualization needs.[2]

Self-Actualization
creativity, spirituality,
fulfillment of potential

Esteem Needs
self-respect, respect for others,
accomplishment

Social Needs
belonging, affection, acceptance

Security Needs
shelter, safety, protection

Survival Needs
food, water, sleep, exercise, sexual expression

FIGURE 2.3 **Maslow's Hierarchy of Needs** To be psychologically healthy, basic needs must be met. Without these, life challenges can be difficult.

Source: From A.H. Maslow, *Motivation and Personality*, 3rd ed., eds. R.D. Frager and J. Fadiman (Upper Saddle River, NJ: Pearson Education, Inc., 1987). Reprinted by permission.

▶ Watch Video Tutor: **Maslow's Hierarchy of Needs** in Mastering Health.

fashion or behaving inconsistently or offensively, they express their feelings, communicate with other people, and show emotions in appropriate ways. In contrast, emotionally unhealthy people are much more likely to let their feelings overpower them. They may be highly volatile and prone to unpredictable emotional responses.

> **mental health** The thinking part of psychological health; includes your values, attitudes, and beliefs.
> **emotional health** The feeling part of psychological health; includes your emotional reactions to life.
> **emotions** Intensified feelings or complex patterns of feelings.
> **social health** The aspect of psychological health that includes interactions with other people, ability to use social supports, and ability to adapt to various situations.

Social Health

Social health includes interactions with other people, ability to use social resources and social support in times of need, and ability to adapt to a variety of social situations. Typically, socially healthy individuals can listen, express themselves, form healthy attachments, act in socially acceptable and responsible ways, and adapt to an ever-changing society. Numerous studies document the importance of positive relationships and support from family members, friends, coworkers, community groups, and significant others to overall well-being. In addition, social support has been shown

Mental Health

The term **mental health** is used to describe the "thinking" or "rational" dimension of our health. A mentally healthy person perceives life in realistic ways, can adapt to change, can develop rational strategies to solve problems, and can carry out personal and professional responsibilities. In addition, a mentally healthy person has the intellectual ability to learn and use information effectively and to strive for continued growth. This is often referred to as *intellectual health*, a subset of mental health.[3]

Emotional Health

The term **emotional health** refers to the feeling, or subjective, side of psychological health. **Emotions** are intensified feelings or complex patterns of feelings that we experience on a regular basis; they include love, hate, frustration, anxiety, and joy, among others. Typically, emotions are described as the interplay of four components: physiological arousal, feelings, cognitive (thought) processes, and behavioral reactions. As rational beings, we are responsible for evaluating our individual emotional responses, their causes, and the appropriateness of our actions.

Emotionally healthy people usually respond appropriately to upsetting events. Rather than reacting in an extreme

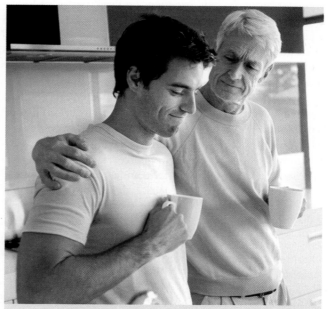

Your family members play an important role in your psychological health. As you were growing up, they modeled behaviors and skills that helped you develop cognitively and socially. Their love and support can give you a sense of self-worth and encourage you to treat other people with compassion and care.

to moderate the effects of stress, reduce risks of depression, and improve overall longevity.[4]

Families have a significant influence on psychological development. Healthy families model and help to develop the cognitive and social skills necessary to solve problems, express emotions in socially acceptable ways, manage stress, and develop a sense of self-worth and purpose. In adulthood, family support is one of the best predictors of health and happiness.[5] Children brought up in **dysfunctional families**—in which there is violence, distrust, anger, dietary deprivation, drug abuse, significant parental discord, or abuse—may run an increased risk of psychological problems.[6]

The concept of **social support** refers to the people and services with which we interact and share social connections. (See Chapter 6 for more information on the importance of social networks and social bonds.) These people and services can provide *tangible support*, such as babysitting services or money to help pay the bills, or *intangible support*, such as encouraging you to share your concerns. Research shows that college students with adequate social support have higher GPAs, higher perceived ability in math and science courses, less stress and depression, less peer pressure for binge drinking, lower rates of suicide, and higher overall life satisfaction.[7]

The communities we live in can provide social support, as can religious institutions, schools (including your own campus community), clinics, public health programs and services, social services, and local businesses that work to provide support for those in need.

Loneliness Happiness is most closely connected to having friends and family. Even so, you could have people around you constantly and still experience a deep, pervasive loneliness. Loneliness is not the same as being alone. Loneliness is a feeling of emptiness or hollowness, causing people to feel alone and unwanted. Approximately 61 percent of college students reported feeling lonely in the past year.[8] See Chapter 6 for more on loneliness and social media relationships.

Several factors may contribute to increased reports of loneliness in modern society. These factors include divorce and death; living longer and losing most of our close friends; connecting with more people on social media but having fewer close social relationships; a more mobile workforce, in which people may telecommute or change jobs and locations frequently; and many other causes of *social isolation*.[9] A recent study of twins raised apart and together provides preliminary evidence that genetics may play a role in risk for loneliness. More research on the potential role of genetics and loneliness is necessary.[10]

Some of the health risks of loneliness are depression and suicide, increased stress levels, antisocial behavior, and alcohol and drug abuse.[11] Finding ways to change feelings of loneliness is key. The first step is to recognize the feelings of loneliness and find ways to express them. Becoming engaged in a campus activity or club provides an opportunity to meet with other people who have similar interests, which will often mitigate loneliness.

Spiritual Health

It is possible to be mentally, emotionally, and socially healthy and still not achieve optimal psychological well-being. For many people, the difficult-to-describe element that gives life purpose is the *spiritual dimension*.

The term *spirituality* is defined as an individual's sense of purpose and meaning in life; it involves a sense of peace and connection to other people.[12] Spirituality may be practiced in many ways, including through religion; however, religion does not have to be part of a spiritual person's life. **Spiritual health** refers to the sense of belonging to something greater than the purely physical or personal dimensions of existence. For some people, this unifying force is nature; for others, it is a feeling of connection to other people; for still others, it may be a god or higher power. (**Focus On: Cultivating Your Spiritual Health** explores the role spirituality plays in your overall health.)

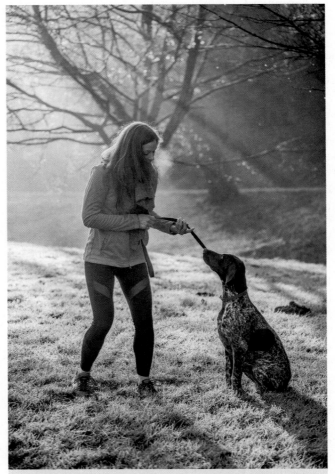

Spending time in the fresh air with your best friend is a simple thing you can do to improve psychological health.

dysfunctional families Families in which there is violence; physical, emotional, or sexual abuse; significant parental discord; or other negative family interactions.

social support A network of people and services with which you share ties and from which you get support.

spiritual health The aspect of psychological health that relates to having a sense of meaning and purpose to one's life as well as a feeling of connection with other people and with nature.

Discuss the roles self-efficacy and self-esteem, emotional intelligence, personality, maturity, and happiness in psychological well-being.

Psychological health is the product of many influences, including family, social supports, and community. Your psychological health is also shaped by your sense of *self-efficacy* and *self-esteem, your personality*, and your *maturity*.

Self-Efficacy and Self-Esteem

During our formative years, successes and failures in every aspect of life subtly shape our beliefs about our personal worth and abilities. These beliefs become internal influences on our psychological health.

Self-efficacy describes a person's belief about whether he or she can successfully engage in and execute a specific behavior. **Self-esteem** refers to one's realistic sense of self-respect or self-worth. People with high levels of self-efficacy and self-esteem tend to express a positive outlook on life. Self-esteem results from the relationships we have with our parents and family growing up; with friends as we grow older; with our significant others as we form intimate relationships; and with our teachers, coworkers, and other people throughout our lives.

While psychologists support the idea that self-esteem is important for positive growth and development, it may be possible to have too much of it. Preliminary research indicates that people who have been protected from failure (perhaps by well-meaning parents and teachers) and have extremely high levels of self-esteem might be more prone to anger, aggression, and other negative behaviors when other people don't praise them or meet their needs for instant gratification. Second, learning to lose can teach us valuable lessons.[13] Carol Dweck, a psychology professor at Stanford University, found that after a steady diet of praise, kids collapsed at the first experience of difficulty.[14] Failure can teach us to keep trying—and that just showing up is not enough to excel. More research is needed to examine potential risks of too much self-esteem and the best ways to deal with it.

Learned Helplessness versus Learned Optimism

Psychologist Martin Seligman proposed that people who continually experience failure may develop a pattern of response known as **learned helplessness** in which they give up and fail to take action to help themselves.[15] Seligman ascribes this response in part to society's tendency toward *victimology*—blaming one's problems on other people and circumstances. Although viewing ourselves as victims can make us feel better temporarily, it does not address the underlying causes of a problem. Ultimately, it can erode self-efficacy by making us feel that we cannot improve a situation.

Today, many self-help programs use elements of Seligman's principle of **learned optimism**. The idea is that we can teach ourselves to be optimistic. By changing our self-talk, examining our reactions, and blocking negative thoughts, we can "unlearn" habitual negative thought processes. Some programs practice positive affirmations with clients, teaching them the habit of acknowledging positive things about themselves.

Defense Mechanisms

Freud proposed that, to deflect negative emotions and stress, we develop defense mechanisms, strategies we unconsciously use to distort our present reality to help avoid anxiety. While defense mechanisms can be pathological if taken to an extreme; fantasizing about a vacation to cope with work stress or rationalizing why a selection for the lead role in a play did not go as planned can help relieve stress and disappointment.[16]

Emotional Intelligence

Intelligence has long been regarded as key to a successful career and healthy social life. In the 1990s, two leading psychologists, Peter Salavey and John Mayer, championed a more comprehensive view of intelligence, known as **emotional intelligence (EI)**.[17] EI is our ability to identify, use, understand, and manage our own emotions and those of other people. Reacting to and channeling those emotions in positive and constructive ways has been shown to improve well-being.[18] Your *emotional intelligence quotient (EQ)* is an indicator of social and interpersonal skills—your ability to successfully maneuver in sometimes emotionally charged settings. Emotional intelligence typically consists of the following:

- **Self-awareness.** The ability to recognize your own emotions, moods, and reactions, as well as have an awareness of how other people perceive or react to you.
- **Self-regulation/self-management.** The ability to control your emotional impulses, think before responding, and express yourself appropriately.
- **Internal motivation.** A drive for learning about things, being able to take initiative and follow through, as well as being trustworthy, stable, and consistent.
- **Empathy.** An awareness of what other people might be going through rather than being so engrossed in yourself that you are oblivious to others. Not being judgmental and rigid in thinking and reacting appropriately to other people's little "mental moments" is part of this element.
- **Social skills.** Abilities that include identifying social cues, being able to listen and respond appropriately, and knowing how to work with other people for the common good and to avoid conflicts with others.

Proponents of EI suggest that developing or increasing your emotional intelligence can help you build stronger relationships, succeed at work, and achieve your goals.[19]

self-efficacy A person's belief about whether he or she can successfully engage in and execute a specific behavior.

self-esteem One's realistic sense of self-respect or self-worth.

learned helplessness A pattern of responding to situations by giving up because of repeated failure in the past.

learned optimism Teaching oneself to think positively.

emotional intelligence (EI) A person's ability to identify, understand, use, and manage emotional states in positive and constructive ways.

Personality

Your personality is the unique mix of characteristics that distinguishes you from other people. Heredity, environment, culture, and experience influence how each person develops. Personality determines how we react to the challenges of life, interpret our feelings, and resolve conflicts. A leading personality theory called the *five-factor model* distills personality into five traits, often called the "Big Five":[20]

- **Agreeableness.** People who score high are trusting, likable, and demonstrate friendly compliance and love; low scorers are critical and suspicious.
- **Openness.** People who score high demonstrate curiosity, independence, and imagination; low scorers are more conventional and down-to-earth.
- **Neuroticism.** People who score high in neuroticism are anxious and insecure; those who score low show the ability to maintain emotional control.
- **Conscientiousness.** People who score high are dependable and demonstrate self-control, discipline, and a need to achieve; low scorers are disorganized and impulsive.
- **Extroversion.** People who score high adapt well to social situations, demonstrate assertiveness, and draw enjoyment from the company of other people; low scorers are more reserved and passive.

Scoring high on agreeableness, openness, conscientiousness, and extroversion while scoring low on neuroticism is often related to psychological well-being.

Most recent schools of psychological theory indicate that we have the power to understand our behavior and change it, thus molding our own personalities, even as adults.[21] Although inhospitable social environments make it more difficult, there are opportunities for making changes and improving our long-term psychological well-being.

Lifespan and Maturity

Although our temperaments are largely determined by genetics, we learn to channel our feelings in acceptable ways as we age. Transition periods—such as the college years—are easier for people who have successfully accomplished earlier developmental tasks such as learning how to solve problems, define and adhere to personal values, and establish relationships. Graduating from college can also be another transition for many into adulthood and further independence. Anticipating an adjustment period and exploring campus resources for new graduates can help in developing autonomy after graduation.

Happiness and the Mind–Body Connection

Can negative emotions make a person physically ill? Can positive emotions help us stay well? At the core of the mind–body connection is **psychoneuroimmunology (PNI)**, the study of the interactions of behavioral, neural, and endocrine functions and the functioning of the body's immune system.

One area of study that appears to be particularly promising in enhancing health is **positive psychology**. According to psychologist Martin Seligman, who is seen as its founder, positive psychology is the scientific study of human strengths and virtues.[22] People who are described as mentally healthy have certain strengths and virtues in common:

- They have high self-esteem.
- They are realistic.
- They value close relationships with other people.
- They approach life with excitement and energy.
- They think things through and examine things from all sides.

Positive psychology interventions have proven effective in enhancing emotional, cognitive, and physical health, reducing depression, lessening disease and disability, and increasing longevity.[23]

Seligman suggests that we can develop well-being by practicing positive psychological actions. He describes five elements of well-being—**P**ositive emotion, **E**ngagement, **R**elationships, **M**eaning, and **A**ccomplishment (PERMA)—that help humans flourish.[24] The Skills for Behavior Change box provides some suggestions for things you can do to incorporate PERMA principles in your own life.

The study of **happiness**—a collective term for several positive states in which individuals actively embrace the world around them—is part of the study of positive psychology.[25] Happy people share four characteristics: *health* (knowing and

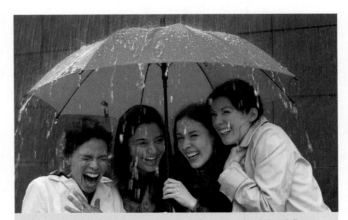

Research suggests that laughter can increase blood flow, boost the immune response, lower blood sugar levels, and facilitate better sleep. Additionally, sharing laughter and fun with other people can strengthen social ties and bring joy to your everyday life.

partaking in healthy habits), *intimacy* (being able to enjoy the company of friends and family, as well as practice empathy), *resources* (possessing a certain agency over one's conditions in life), and *competence* (the knowledge of and ability to learn new skills).[26] People who experience more feelings of happiness have fewer mental health issues (depression, anxiety, and obsessive-compulsive disorders), behavioral health issues, and physical health (e.g., cardiovascular disease, obesity, cancer) issues.[27] However, some of the newest research shows that being happy or unhappy has no direct effect on mortality and suggested that earlier studies had mixed up cause and effect.[28]

LO 3 | WHEN PSYCHOLOGICAL HEALTH DETERIORATES

Describe and differentiate psychological disorders, including mood disorders, anxiety disorders, obsessive-compulsive disorder, post-traumatic stress disorder, personality disorders, and schizophrenia, and explain their causes and treatments.

Mental illnesses are disorders that disrupt thinking, feeling, moods, and behaviors and cause varying degrees of impaired functioning in daily living. They are believed to be caused by a variety of biochemical, genetic, and environmental factors.[29] Among the most common risk factors are a genetic or familial predisposition and excessive unresolved stress, particularly due to trauma or war or devastating natural or human-caused disaster. Changes in biochemistry due to illness, drug use, or other imbalances may trigger unusual mental disturbances. Car accidents or occupational injuries that cause physical brain trauma are among common threats to brain health. In addition, a mother's exposure to viruses or toxic chemicals while pregnant may play a part, as can having a history of child abuse or neglect.[30] Mental illnesses can range from mild to severe and can exact a heavy toll on quality of life, both for people with the illnesses and for those who interact with them.

Mental disorders are common in the United States and worldwide. The basis for diagnosing mental disorders in the United States is the fifth edition of the *Diagnostic and Statistical Manual of Mental Disorders (DSM-5)*. An estimated 17.9 percent of Americans age 18 years and older—just slightly under 1 in 5 adults—suffer from a diagnosable mental disorder in a given year, and nearly half of them have more than one mental illness at the same time.[31] About 4 percent, or approximately 1 in 20, suffer from a serious mental illness requiring close monitoring, residential care in many instances, and medication.[32] Mental disorders are the leading cause of disability worldwide for people age 15 to 44 years, costing more than $464 billion annually in the United States alone.[33]

Mental Health Threats to College Students

Mental health problems among college students are increasing in both number and severity.[34] The most recent National College Health Assessment survey found that approximately 38 percent of undergraduates reported "feeling so depressed it was difficult to function" at least once in the past year, and 10.4 percent of students reported "seriously considering attempting suicide" in the past year.[35] In all, more than 1 in 4 college students are diagnosed or treated by a professional for a mental health issue each year.[36] Anxiety is the most common (17.0 percent), with depression (13.9 percent) not far behind.[37] Although these data may appear alarming, it is important to note that increases in help-seeking behavior, in addition to actual increases in overall prevalence

mental illnesses Disorders that disrupt thinking, feeling, moods, and behaviors and impair daily functioning.

chronic mood disorder A disorder involving persistent emotional states, such as sadness, despair, hopelessness, or euphoria.

major depression A severe depressive disorder with physical effects such as sleep disturbance and exhaustion, and mental effects such as the inability to concentrate; also called *clinical depression*.

of disorders, may contribute to these trends. FIGURE 2.4 shows the mental health concerns reported by American college students.

Although there are many types of mental illnesses, we will focus on the disorders that are most common among college students: mood disorders, anxiety disorders, obsessive-compulsive disorder (OCD), posttraumatic stress disorder (PTSD), personality disorders, and schizophrenia. See the Health Headlines box for information on other brain-based disorders in young adults. (For coverage of addiction, which is classified as a mental disorder, see Chapter 8.)

Mood Disorders

Chronic mood disorders affect how you feel, such as persistent sadness or feelings of euphoria. Key examples are major depression, persistent depressive disorder, bipolar disorder, and seasonal affective disorder. In any given year, approximately 10 percent of Americans age 18 or older suffer from a mood disorder.[38]

Major Depression We've all had days when life's challenges push us over the proverbial edge, but short periods of feeling down are not the same as major depression. **Major depression** or *clinical depression* is a common mood disorder, affecting approximately 9 percent of the adult U.S. population in a given year.[39]

Major depression is characterized by a combination of symptoms that interfere with work, study, sleep, appetite, relationships, and enjoyment of life. Symptoms can last for weeks, months, or years and vary in intensity.[40] Sadness and despair are the main symptoms of depression.[41] Other common signs include:

- Loss of motivation or interest in pleasurable activities
- Preoccupation with one's failures or inadequacies; concern over what other people are thinking
- Difficulty concentrating, indecisiveness, memory lapses
- Loss of sex drive or lack of interest in being close to other people
- Fatigue, oversleeping, insomnia, and loss of energy

- Feeling anxious, worthless, or hopeless
- Significant weight loss or gain due to appetite changes
- Recurring thoughts that life isn't worth living; thoughts of death or suicide

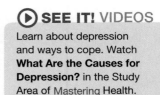
SEE IT! VIDEOS

Learn about depression and ways to cope. Watch **What Are the Causes for Depression?** in the Study Area of Mastering Health.

Depression in College Students Mental health problems, particularly depression, have gained increased recognition as obstacles to healthy adjustment and success in college. Students who have weak communication skills, who find that college isn't what they expected, or who lack motivation often have difficulties. Stressors such as anxiety over relationships, pressure to get good grades and win social acceptance, abuse of alcohol and other drugs, poor diet, and lack of sleep can overwhelm even the most resilient students. Being far from home without the security of family and friends can exacerbate problems. International students are particularly vulnerable. In a recent survey by the American College Health Association, 13.9 percent of college students reported having been diagnosed with or treated for depression in the past 12 months.[42]

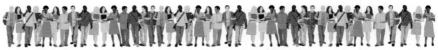

Felt overwhelmed by all they needed to do: 86%

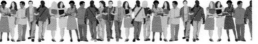

Felt things were hopeless: 50.9%

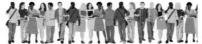

Felt so depressed that it was difficult to function: 38.2%

Seriously considered suicide: 10.4%

Intentionally injured themselves: 6.9%

Attempted suicide: 1.9%   **= 2%**

FIGURE 2.4 Mental Health Concerns of American College Students, Past 12 Months

Source: Data from American College Health Association, *American College Health Association, National College Health Assessment II (ACHA-NCHA II): Reference Group Data Report, Fall 2016* (Hanover, MD: American College Health Association, 2017).

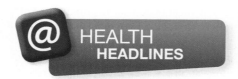

COLLEGE SUCCESS WITH LEARNING DISABILITIES AND NEURODEVELOPMENTAL DISORDERS

Some brain-based disorders are not mental illnesses. Just as people living with mental illness can be successful with appropriate counseling, medication, and/or accommodations, people living with learning disabilities (LDs) and neurodevelopmental disorders can also be successful with proper support.

Attention-deficit (hyperactivity) disorder (ADD/ADHD) is a learning disability usually associated with school-age children, but it can persist into adulthood. People with ADD/ADHD are often distracted. Even when they try to concentrate, they find it difficult. Organizing things, listening to instructions, and remembering details are especially hard. About 4 percent of the adult population, or slightly over 12 million adults, are living with ADHD. Recent studies indicate that ADHD affects somewhere between 2 and 8 percent of college students. Left untreated, ADHD can disrupt everything from careers to relationships to financial stability. Key areas of disruption might include:

- **Health.** Alcohol and drug abuse, compulsive eating, and forgetting to take important medications are all ways in which ADHD can affect health.
- **Work and finances.** Difficulty concentrating, completing tasks, listening, and relating to other people can lead to trouble at work and at school. A person with ADHD may also struggle to pay bills on time, lose paperwork, miss deadlines, or spend impulsively, resulting in debt.
- **Relationships.** If you have ADHD, it might feel as though your friends and loved ones regularly prod you to be tidy and to get things done. If your partner has ADHD, you might be hurt

that your loved one doesn't seem to listen to you, blurts out hurtful things, and leaves you with the bulk of organizing and planning.

Dyslexia is a language-based learning disorder that can pose problems for reading, writing, and spelling. Lesser known, but equally challenging, are **dyscalculia** (a learning disability involving math) and **dysgraphia** (a learning disability involving writing). People with dysgraphia may have difficulty putting letters, numbers, and words on a page in order.

Autism spectrum disorder (ASD) is not a learning disability but an impairment in brain development. People with an ASD continue to learn and grow intellectually but struggle to master communication and social behavior skills, which affects their performance in school and work. Some adults with an ASD (especially those with high-functioning autism, also known as **Asperger syndrome**) attend college and go on to succeed in the workforce.

Universities regularly offer a variety of support services to help students with learning disabilities. These may include testing and diagnosis for LDs; reading and writing supports; exam accommodations, such as extra time or a quiet location; and classes on study skills and test anxiety. These supports are generally offered at no cost through an office of disability services or health center. Some campuses have developed programs specifically targeted toward students on the autism spectrum. Students with ASD usually need a significant amount of support to be successful in college. In addition to the free services offered to students with LDs, some schools offer additional fee-based assistance including tutoring, help with financial management, and support groups for social interaction and leisure activities.

Disorder and chaos can be headaches for us all, but ADHD sufferers may find them insurmountable obstacles.

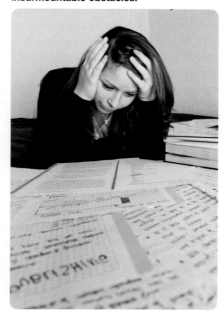

Sources: Centers for Disease Control and Prevention, "Attention-Deficit Hyperactivity Disorder," January 2016, www.cdc.gov/ncbddd/adhd/facts.html; Healthline, "ADHD by the Numbers: Facts, Statistics, and You," September 2014, www.healthline.com/health/adhd/facts-statistics-infographic#1; Helpguide.org, "Adult ADD/ADHD: Signs, Symptoms, Effects, and Treatment," December 2014, www.helpguide.org/articles/add-adhd/adult-adhd-attention-deficit-disorder; National Center for Learning Disabilities, "Types of LD," Accessed February 2014, www.ncld.org/types-learning-disabilities; M. Gormley et al., "First-Year GPA and Academic Service Use among College Students with and without ADHD," *Journal of Attention Disorders* (2016), doi:10.1177/1087054715623046; P. Pedrelli et al., "College Students: Mental Health Problems and Treatment Considerations," *Academic Psychiatry* 39 no. 5 (2015): 503–11; A. Fleming et al., "Pilot Randomized Controlled Trial of Dialectical Behavior Therapy Group Skills Training for ADHD Among College Students," *Journal of Attention Disorders* 19, no. 3 (2015): 260–71.

Persistent Depressive Disorder

Persistent depressive disorder (PDD), formerly called *dysthymic disorder* or *dysthymia*, is a less severe form of chronic mild depression. Individuals with PDD may appear to function well but may lack energy or fatigue easily; may be short-tempered, overly pessimistic, and ornery; or may not feel quite up to par but not have any significant overt symptoms. Genetics and a history of abuse, neglect, or trauma as well as high stress levels are among suspected causes. People with PDD may cycle into major depression over time. For a diagnosis, symptoms must persist for at least 2 years in adults (1 year

attention-deficit (hyperactivity) disorder (ADD/ADHD) A learning disability that is usually associated with school-aged children, often involving difficulty concentrating, organizing things, listening to instructions, and remembering details.

in children). This disorder affects approximately 1.5 percent of the adult population in the United States in a given year.[43]

Bipolar Disorder People with **bipolar disorder** (also known as *manic-depressive illness*) often have severe mood swings, ranging from extreme highs (mania) to extreme lows (depression). Sometimes these swings are dramatic and rapid; other times they are slow and gradual. When in the manic phase, the person may be overactive and talkative and typically has tons of energy; in the depressed phase, the person may experience some or all of the symptoms of major depression. Bipolar disorder affects approximately 2.6 percent of the adult population in the United States and 11.2 percent of 13- to 18-year-olds in the United States.[44]

Although the cause of bipolar disorder is unknown, biological, genetic, and environmental factors, such as drug abuse and stressful or psychologically traumatic events, seem to be involved in triggering episodes. Once diagnosed, people with bipolar disorder have several counseling and pharmaceutical options, and most can live a healthy, functional life while being treated.

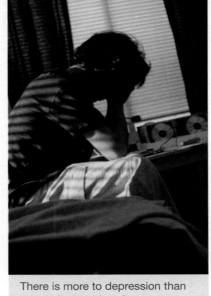

There is more to depression than simply feeling blue. A person who is clinically depressed finds it difficult to function, sometimes struggling just to get out of bed in the morning or to follow a conversation.

dyslexia A language-based learning disorder that can pose problems for reading, writing, and spelling.

dyscalculia A learning disability involving math.

dysgraphia A learning disability involving writing; individuals may have difficulty putting letters, numbers, and words on a page into order.

autism spectrum disorder (ASD) A neurodevelopmental disorder (an impairment in brain development) in which individuals learn and grow intellectually throughout their lives, but struggle to master communication and social behavior skills, affecting school and work performance.

Asperger syndrome A form of high-functioning autism.

persistent depressive disorder A type of depression that is milder and harder to recognize than major depression; chronic; and often characterized by fatigue, pessimism, or a short temper; formerly known as *dysthymic disorder*.

Seasonal Affective Disorder *Seasonal depression*, typically referred to as **seasonal affective disorder (SAD)**, strikes during the fall and winter months and is associated with reduced exposure to sunlight. People with SAD suffer from extreme fatigue, irritability, apathy, carbohydrate craving and weight gain, increased sleep time, and general sadness. Several factors are implicated in SAD development, including disruption in the body's natural circadian rhythms and changes in levels of the hormone melatonin and the brain chemical serotonin.[45] Over 500,000 people in the United States suffer from SAD. Nearly three-fourths of those with SAD are women in early adulthood, particularly those living at high latitudes with long winter nights.[46]

The most beneficial treatment for SAD is light therapy, which exposes patients to lamps that simulate sunlight. Other treatments include diet change (such as eating more complex carbohydrates), increased exercise, stress-management techniques, sleep restriction (limiting the number of hours slept in a 24-hour period), psychotherapy, and prescription medications.

What Causes Mood Disorders? Mood disorders are caused by multiple factors, including biological differences, hormones, inherited traits, life events, and early childhood trauma.[47] The biology of mood disorders is related to individual levels of brain chemicals called *neurotransmitters*. Several types of depression, including bipolar disorder, appear to have a genetic component. Depression can also be triggered by a serious loss, difficult relationships, financial problems, and pressure to succeed. Early childhood trauma, such as loss of a parent, may cause permanent changes in the brain, making one more prone to depression. Changes in the body's physical health can be accompanied by mental changes, particularly depression. Stroke, heart attack, cancer, Parkinson's disease, chronic pain, type 2 diabetes, certain medications, alcohol, hormonal disorders, and a wide range of other afflictions can cause a person to become depressed, frustrated, or angry. When this happens, recovery is often more difficult, as a person who feels exhausted and defeated may lack the will to fight illness and do what is necessary to optimize recovery.

Anxiety Disorders

Anxiety disorders are characterized by persistent feelings of threat and worry and include generalized anxiety disorder, panic disorders, and phobic disorders. The largest mental health problem in the United States, anxiety disorders affect more than 40 million adults in any given year. Anxiety disorders are most prevalent among 13- to 17-year-olds, with a median age of onset of 6 years.[48] Approximately 19 percent of U.S. undergraduates report having been diagnosed with or treated for anxiety in the past year.[49]

Generalized Anxiety Disorder One common form of anxiety disorder, **generalized anxiety disorder (GAD)**, is severe enough to interfere significantly with daily life. To be diagnosed with GAD, one must exhibit at least three of the following symptoms for more days than not during a 6-month period: restlessness or feeling keyed up or on edge, being easily fatigued, difficulty concentrating or mind going blank, irritability, muscle tension, and/or sleep disturbances.[50]

Panic Disorder Panic disorder is characterized by the occurrence of **panic attacks**, an acute feeling of anxiety causing an intense physical reaction. Approximately 8.4 percent of college students report having been diagnosed or treated for panic attacks in the last year.[51] Panic attacks and disorders are increasing in incidence, particularly among young women.

Although highly treatable, panic attacks may become debilitating and destructive, particularly if they happen often or cause a person to avoid going out in public or interacting with other people. Panic attacks typically begin abruptly, peak within 10 minutes, last about 30 minutes, and leave the person tired and drained. Symptoms include increased respiration, chills, hot flashes, shortness of breath, stomach cramps, chest pain, difficulty swallowing, and a sense of doom or impending death.[52]

Phobic Disorders **Phobias**, or phobic disorders, involve a persistent and irrational fear of a specific object, activity, or situation, often out of proportion to the circumstances. Between 5 and 12 percent of American adults suffer from specific phobias, such as fear of spiders, snakes, or riding in elevators.[53]

Another 7.4 percent of American adults suffer from **social anxiety disorder**, also called *social phobia*.[54] Social anxiety disorder is characterized by a persistent fear and avoidance of social situations. Essentially, a person with social anxiety disorder dreads these situations for fear of being humiliated, embarrassed, or even looked at. These disorders vary in scope. Some individuals experience difficulties only in specific situations, such as getting up in front of the class to give a presentation. In extreme cases, a person avoids all contact with other people.

What Causes Anxiety Disorders? Because anxiety disorders vary in complexity and degree, it is not yet clear why one person develops them and another doesn't. The following factors are often cited as possible causes:[55]

- **Biology.** Some scientists trace the origin of anxiety to the brain and its functioning. Using sophisticated positron-emission tomography (PET) scans, scientists can analyze areas of the brain that react during anxiety-producing events. Families appear to display similar brain and physiological reactivity, so we may inherit tendencies toward anxiety disorders.
- **Environment.** Anxiety can be a learned response. Experiencing a repeated pattern of reaction to certain situations can program the brain to respond in a certain way. For example, if one of your siblings had a huge fear of spiders and screamed whenever one crawled into sight during your childhood, you might develop similar anxieties.

- **Social and cultural roles.** Because men and women are taught to assume different roles, women may find it more acceptable to scream, tremble, or otherwise express extreme anxiety. Men, in contrast, may have learned to repress anxious feelings rather than act on them.

Obsessive-Compulsive Disorder

People who feel compelled to perform rituals over and over again; who are fearful of dirt or contamination; who have an unnatural concern about order, symmetry, and exactness; or who have persistent intrusive thoughts may be suffering from **obsessive-compulsive disorder (OCD)**. Approximately 1 percent of Americans 18 years of age and over have OCD.[56]

Not to be confused with being a perfectionist, a person with OCD often knows that the behaviors are irrational yet is powerless to stop them. According to the DSM-5, a diagnosis of OCD applies when obsessions consume more than 1 hour per day and interfere with normal social or life activities. Although the exact cause of OCD is unknown, genetics, biological abnormalities, learned behaviors, and environmental factors have all been considered. OCD usually begins in childhood or the teen years; most people are diagnosed before age 20.[57]

Although OCD is highly treatable, only one-third of individuals with the disorder receive treatment. Treatments vary by disorder type, severity, and other factors. The most effective treatments tend to be a combination of psychotherapy and medications designed to treat symptoms, such as antidepressants or antianxiety medication.[58]

Posttraumatic Stress Disorder

People who have experienced or witnessed a traumatic event may develop

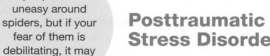

Many people are uneasy around spiders, but if your fear of them is debilitating, it may be a phobia.

---

bipolar disorder A form of mood disorder characterized by alternating mania and depression; also called *manic-depressive illness*.

seasonal affective disorder (SAD) A type of depression that occurs in the winter months, when sunlight levels are low.

anxiety disorders A mental illness characterized by persistent feelings of threat and worry in coping with everyday problems.

generalized anxiety disorder (GAD) A constant sense of worry that may cause restlessness, difficulty in concentrating, tension, and other symptoms.

panic attack A severe anxiety reaction in which a particular situation, often for unknown reasons, causes terror.

phobia Deep and persistent fear of a specific object, activity, or situation that results in a compelling desire to avoid the source of the fear.

social anxiety disorder A phobia characterized by fear and avoidance of social situations; also called *social phobia*.

obsessive-compulsive disorder (OCD) A form of anxiety disorder characterized by recurrent, unwanted thoughts and repetitive behaviors.

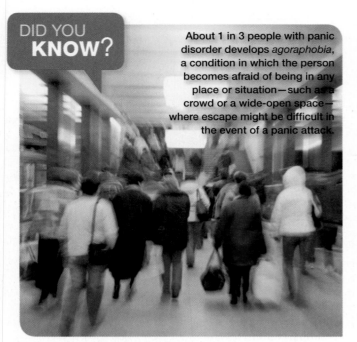

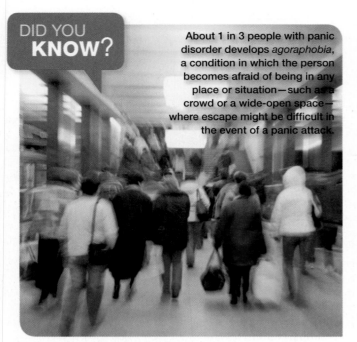

DID YOU KNOW?

About 1 in 3 people with panic disorder develops *agoraphobia*, a condition in which the person becomes afraid of being in any place or situation—such as a crowd or a wide-open space— where escape might be difficult in the event of a panic attack.

Sources: Anxiety and Depression Association of America, "Panic Disorder and Agoraphobia," Accessed February 2016, https://www.adaa.org/understanding-anxiety/panic-disorder-agoraphobia.

posttraumatic stress disorder (PTSD). About 4 percent of Americans suffer from PTSD each year, and about 7 percent will experience PTSD in their lifetimes; women experience PTSD at rates twice as high as those of men.[59] Fourteen percent of U.S. combat veterans who fought in Iraq and Afghanistan have experienced PTSD.[60] However, the worst stressful experiences that are reported most frequently by people with PTSD are not war-related but rather the unexpected death, serious illness, or injury of someone close and sexual assault. PTSD in women appears related to a history of abuse, rape, or assault. Natural disasters, serious accidents, violent assault, and terrorism are all causes of PTSD in both men and women.[61] PTSD is not rooted in weakness or an inability to cope; traumatic events can actually cause chemical changes in the brain, leading to PTSD.[62]

Symptoms of PTSD include the following:

- Dissociation, or perceived detachment of the mind from the emotional state or even the body
- Intrusive recollections of the traumatic event, such as flashbacks, nightmares, and recurrent thoughts or images
- Acute anxiety or nervousness, in which the person is hyperaroused, may cry easily, or experiences mood swings
- Insomnia and difficulty concentrating
- Intense physiological reactions, such as shaking or nausea, when something reminds the person of the traumatic event.

posttraumatic stress disorder (PTSD) A collection of symptoms that may occur as a delayed response to a traumatic event or series of events.

personality disorder A mental disorder characterized by inflexible patterns of thought and beliefs that lead to socially distressing behavior.

PTSD may be diagnosed if a person experiences symptoms for at least 1 month following a traumatic event. However, in some cases, symptoms don't appear until months or even years later. Treatment for PTSD may involve psychotherapy, as well as medications to help with depression, anxiety, and sleep. Group therapy and individual talk therapy are also often recommended, depending on the nature and severity of PTSD.

Personality Disorders

According to the DSM-5, a **personality disorder** is an "enduring pattern of inner experience and behavior that deviates markedly from the expectation of the individual's culture and is pervasive and inflexible."[63] It is estimated that at least 10 percent of adults in the United States have some form of personality disorder as defined by the DSM-5.[64] People who live, work, or are in relationships with individuals suffering from personality disorders often find interactions with them to be challenging and destructive.

One common type of personality disorder is *paranoid personality disorder*, which involves pervasive, unfounded suspicion and mistrust of other people; irrational jealousy; and secretiveness. People with this illness have delusions of being persecuted by everyone, from family members and loved ones to the government.

Narcissistic personality disorder involves an exaggerated sense of self-importance and self-absorption. People with narcissistic personalities are preoccupied with fantasies of how wonderful they are. Typically, they are overly needy and demanding and believe that they are entitled to nothing but the best.

People with *antisocial personality disorder* display a long-term pattern of manipulation and taking advantage of other people, often in a criminal manner. Symptoms include disregard for the safety of others, lack of remorse, arrogance, and anger. Men with antisocial personality disorder far outnumber women, and it remains one of the hardest to treat of all personality disorders.[65]

Borderline personality disorder (BPD) is characterized by severe emotional instability, impulsiveness, mood swings, and poor self-image.[66] High suicide rates, unpredictable mood swings, and erratic and risky behaviors, including gambling, unsafe sex, illicit drug use, daredevil driving, and self-mutilation, are typical.[67] (For more about self-mutilation, see Student Health Today.) Although causation is not clear, genetics and environment appear to converge to increase risks for BPD. About 1.6 million adults in the United States have BPD in a given year. BPD usually begins to manifest during adolescence or early adulthood.[68]

For treating personality disorders, individual and group psychotherapy, skill development, family education, support from peers, and medications can lead to a good long-term prognosis.[69]

Schizophrenia

Schizophrenia is a severe psychological disorder that affects about 1 percent of the U.S. population.[70] Schizophrenia is

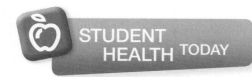
CUTTING THROUGH THE PAIN

Some people, unable to deal with pain, pressure, or stress, may resort to self-harm to cope. **Self-injury**, also termed *self-mutilation*, *self-harm*, or *nonsuicidal self-injury (NSI)*, is the act of deliberately harming one's body tissue without suicidal attempt and for purposes that are not socially supported.

The most common method of self-harm is cutting (with razors, glass, knives, or other sharp objects). Other methods include burning, bruising, excessive nail biting, breaking bones, pulling out hair, and embedding sharp objects under the skin.

Approximately 4 to 6 percent of adults in the United States have engaged in NSI at least once. However, the occurrence of NSI is much higher in young adults and adolescents. The prevalence of NSI in college students is approximately 6 percent. NSI more commonly occurs in female college students, approximately 7 percent in the past 12 months, compared to approximately 4 percent in males. Estimates are higher in the high school population; the majority of studies report that between 14 and 18 percent of adolescents and young adults engaging in self-injury at least once. Many people who harm themselves suffer from other mental health conditions and have experienced sexual, physical, or emotional abuse. Self-harm is also commonly associated with mental illnesses such as borderline personality disorder, depression, anxiety disorders, substance abuse disorders, posttraumatic stress disorder, and eating disorders.

Signs of self-injury include multiple scars, current cuts and abrasions, and implausible explanations for wounds and ongoing injuries. A self-injurer may attempt to conceal scars and injuries by wearing long sleeves and pants. Other symptoms can include difficulty handling anger, social withdrawal, sensitivity to rejection, or body alienation. If you or someone you know engages in self-injury, seek professional help. Treatment is challenging; not only must the self-injurious behavior be stopped, but the sufferer must also learn to recognize and manage the feelings that trigger it.

If you are a recovering self-injurer, these steps may be part of your treatment:

1. Start by being aware of feelings and situations that trigger you.
2. Identify a plan of what you can do instead when you feel the urge.
3. Create a list of alternatives, including:

   - Things that might distract you
   - Things that might calm you
   - Things that might help you express yourself
   - Things that might help release physical tension and distress
   - Things that might help you feel supported and connected
   - Things that might substitute for the cutting sensation.

For more information, visit these resources: S.A.F.E. Alternatives, www.selfinjury.com, and Help Guide, www.helpguide.org/mental/self_injury.htm.

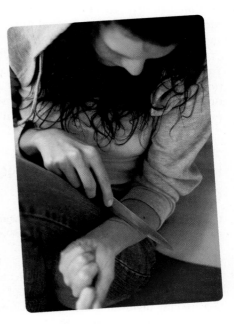

In self-injury, cutting and scratching behaviors are more common in females, while burning and hitting behaviors are more common in males.

---

characterized by alterations of the senses; the inability to sort and process incoming stimuli and make appropriate responses; an altered sense of self; and radical changes in emotions, movements, and behaviors. Typical symptoms include fluctuating courses of delusional behavior, hallucinations, incoherent and rambling speech, inability to think logically, erratic movement, odd gesturing, and difficulty with activities of daily living.[71] Symptoms usually appear in men during the late teen years and twenties, while women generally show symptoms in their late twenties and early thirties.[72] Often regarded as odd or dangerous, schizophrenic individuals can have difficulties in social interactions and may withdraw.

For decades, scientists believed that schizophrenia was a form of madness provoked by the environment in which a child lived. In the mid-1980s, magnetic resonance imaging (MRI) and PET scans began allowing scientists to study brain function more closely; that knowledge indicated that schizophrenia is a biological disease of the brain. The brain damage occurs early in life, possibly as early as the second trimester of fetal development. Fetal exposure to toxic substances, infections, and medications have been studied as a possible risk, and hereditary links are being explored.

schizophrenia A mental illness with biological origins that is characterized by irrational behavior, severe alterations of the senses, and often an inability to function in society.

self-injury Intentionally causing injury to one's own body in an attempt to cope with overwhelming negative emotions; also called *self-mutilation*, *self-harm*, or *nonsuicidal self-injury (NSSI)*.

Even though theories that blame abnormal family life or childhood trauma for schizophrenia have been discarded in favor of biological theories, a stigma remains. Families of people with schizophrenia frequently experience anger and guilt. They often need counseling on how to meet the schizophrenic person's needs for shelter, medical care, vocational training, and social interaction.

At present, schizophrenia is treatable but not curable. Treatments usually include some combination of hospitalization, medication, and psychotherapy. With proper medication, public understanding, support of loved ones, and access to therapy, many people with schizophrenia lead normal lives.

LO 4 | SUICIDE: GIVING UP ON LIFE

Discuss risk factors and possible warning signs of suicide, as well as actions that can be taken to help a person who is contemplating suicide.

"Every 40 seconds a person dies of suicide somewhere in the world . . . another 20 or so more attempt suicide." These grim statistics highlight the growing international toll of suicide.[73] Each year, over 800,000 deaths are reported internationally. Individuals 15 to 29 years of age are particularly vulnerable, suicide being the second leading cause of death internationally in this group.[74] In some of the richest countries, more than three times as many men die of suicide as women. However, in low- and middle-income countries, the male-to-female suicide ratio is only 1.5 men to every woman. Globally, suicides make up 50 percent of all violent deaths for men and over 71 percent for women. The highest rates of suicide are among individuals aged 70 years and older.[75]

In the United States, older adults' suicide rates are comparable to overall international rates in this age group. Suicide is the second leading cause of death for 15- to 19-year-olds and the second leading cause of death for 20- to 24-year-olds.[76] The pressures, disappointments, challenges, and changes of the college years may contribute to the emotional turmoil that can lead a young person to contemplate suicide. According to the 2016 National College Health Assessment, approximately 9 percent of students had seriously considered suicide at some point

in their life, and 1.9 percent had attempted to kill themselves in the past year.[77] However, young adults who do not attend college are also at risk; in fact, suicide rates are higher for young adults in the general population than for college students.[78]

Risk Factors for Suicide

Risk factors include a family history of suicide, previous suicide attempts, excessive drug and alcohol use, prolonged depression, financial difficulties, serious illness in oneself or a loved one, and loss of a loved one through death or rejection. Recent research indicates that lesbian, gay, bisexual, and transgender (LGBT) people are significantly more likely to have thought about or attempted suicide than their heterosexual counterparts; transgender individuals have the highest rates.[79] Those raised in home and school environments where homophobic teasing is not condoned had significantly lower rates of suicide attempts, whereas those from low-income homes with less than high school education and with the presence of substance abuse had significantly more suicide attempts.[80]

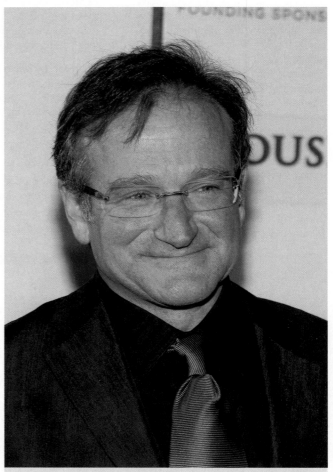

Suicide symptoms are not always obvious. It was only after his suicide in August 2014 that comedian and actor Robin Williams's struggles with severe depression became widely known.

APPROXIMATELY 9.3 MILLION

adults seriously CONSIDERED SUICIDE in the past year.

Whether they are more likely to attempt suicide or are more often successful, nearly four times as many men die by suicide as women.[81] The most commonly used method of suicide among men is firearms; for women, the most common method is poisoning.[82]

Warning Signs of Suicide

People who commit suicide usually indicate their intentions, although other people do not always recognize the warnings.[83] Anyone who expresses a desire to kill himself or herself or who has made an attempt is at risk. Common signs a person may be contemplating suicide include:[84]

- Recent loss and a seeming inability to let go of grief
- History of depression
- Change in personality, such as sadness, withdrawal, irritability, anxiety, tiredness, indecisiveness, apathy
- Change in behavior, such as inability to concentrate, loss of interest in classes or work, unexplained demonstration of happiness following a period of depression, or risk-taking behavior
- Change in sexual interest
- Change in sleep patterns and/or eating habits
- A direct statement (including statements posted on social media) about committing suicide, such as "I might as well end it all"
- An indirect statement (including statements posted on social media), such as "You won't have to worry about me anymore"
- Final preparations such as writing a will, giving away prized possessions, or writing revealing letters or social media posts
- Preoccupation with themes of death
- Marked changes in personal appearance

Preventing Suicide

Most people who attempt suicide really want to live but see death as the only way out of an intolerable situation. Crisis counselors and suicide hotlines may help temporarily, but the best way to prevent suicide is to get rid of conditions and substances that may precipitate attempts, including alcohol, drugs, loneliness, isolation, and access to guns.

If someone you know threatens suicide or displays warning signs, get involved. Ask questions and seek help. Specific actions you can take include:[85]

- **Monitor the warning signals.** Keep an eye on the person, or make sure that someone else is present. Don't leave the person alone.
- **Take threats seriously.** Don't brush talk of suicide off as "cries for attention." Act now.
- **Let the person know how much you care.** State that you are there to help.
- **Ask directly.** Ask "Are you thinking of hurting or killing yourself?" Don't be judgmental. Let them share their thoughts.

- **Take action.** Remove any firearms or objects that could be used for suicide from the area.
- **Help the person think about alternatives to suicide.** Offer to go for help along with the person. Call your local suicide hotline, and use all available community and campus resources.
- **Tell the person's spouse, partner, parents, siblings, or counselor.** Do not keep suspicions to yourself. Don't let a suicidal friend talk you into keeping your discussions confidential. If your friend succeeds in a suicide attempt, you may blame yourself.

LO 5 | SEEKING PROFESSIONAL HELP

Explain the different types of treatment options and professional services available to people who are experiencing mental health problems.

A physical ailment will readily send most people to the nearest health professional, but many view seeking help for psychological problems as an admission of personal failure. Although estimates show that while about 20 percent of adults have some kind of mental disorder, only 13 percent of adults use mental health counseling services.[86]

Consider seeking help in any of the following situations:

- You feel out of control.
- You experience wild mood swings or inappropriate emotional responses to normal stimuli.
- Your fears or feelings of guilt frequently distract your attention.
- You begin to withdraw from other people.
- You have hallucinations.
- You feel inadequate or worthless or that life is not worth living.
- Your daily life seems to be a series of repeated crises.
- You are considering suicide.
- You turn to drugs or alcohol to escape your problems.

Low-cost or free counseling sessions or support groups are often available on college campuses to help students deal with all types of issues, including mental illness. Investigate options on your campus.

Mental Illness Stigma

A **stigma** is a negative perception about groups of people or certain situations or conditions. Common stigmas about people with mental illness are that they are dangerous, irresponsible, and require constant care or that they "just need to get over it." In truth, only 3 to 5 percent of all violent acts are attributed to people with serious mental illness. It is no more likely for most people with mental health problems to be violent than it is for anyone else, even though the mentally ill are ten

stigma Negative perception about a group of people or a certain situation or condition.

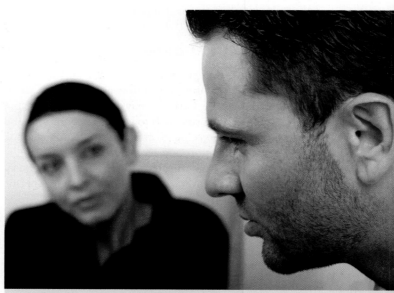

WHAT DO YOU THINK?

Do you notice a stigma associated with mental illness in your community?

- How often do you hear terms such as "crazy" or "whacko" used to describe people who appear to have a mental health problem or a situation in general? Why are such expressions harmful?

- Why do so many people hide their mental illnesses and/or refuse to seek treatment? What can be done to reduce the fear of mental illness disclosure?

times more likely to become victims of violence. Most hold regular jobs, are productive members of society, and lead normal lives.[87]

The stigma of mental illness often leads to feelings of shame and guilt, a loss of self-esteem, and a sense of isolation and hopelessness. Many people who have successfully managed their mental illness report that the stigma was more disabling at times than the illness itself.[88] Stigma may cause people who are struggling with a mental illness to hide their difficulties from friends, delay seeking treatment, or avoid care that could dramatically improve their symptoms and quality of life.

Getting Evaluated for Treatment

If you are considering treatment, schedule a complete evaluation first. Consult a credentialed health professional for a thorough examination, including:

- A physical checkup, which will rule out thyroid disorders, viral infections, and anemia—all of which can result in depression-like symptoms—and a neurological check of coordination, reflexes, and balance to rule out brain disorders

- A psychiatric history, which will trace the course of the apparent disorder, genetic or family factors, and any past treatments

- A mental status examination, which will assess thoughts, speaking processes, and memory and will include an in-depth interview with tests for other psychiatric symptoms.

Once physical factors have been ruled out, you may decide to consult a professional who specializes in psychological health.

Mental Health Professionals

Several types of mental health professionals are available; **TABLE 2.1** provides information on the most common types of practitioners. In choosing a therapist, it is important to verify that he or she has the appropriate training and certification. The most important factor is whether you feel that you can work with the therapist. A qualified mental health professional should be willing to answer all your questions during an initial consultation. Questions to ask the therapist or yourself include:

- **Can you interview the therapist before starting treatment?** An initial meeting can help you determine whether this person will be a good fit.

- **Do you like the therapist as a person?** Can you talk to him or her comfortably?

- **Is the therapist watching the clock or easily distracted?** You should be the focus of the session.

- **Does the therapist demonstrate professionalism?** Be concerned if your therapist is frequently late or breaks appointments, suggests social interactions outside your therapy sessions, talks inappropriately about himself or herself, has questionable billing practices, or resists releasing you from therapy.

- **Will the therapist help you set your own goals and timetables?** A good professional should evaluate your general situation and help you set goals to work on between sessions.

Note that the use of the title *therapist* or *counselor* is not nationally regulated. Check credentials and make your choice carefully.

What to Expect in Therapy

Most people have misconceptions about what therapy is and what it can do. Do not expect the therapist to tell you what to do or how to behave. The responsibility for improved behavior lies with you.

Before making an appointment, call for information and briefly explain your needs. Ask about office hours, policies and procedures, fees, and insurance participation. The first visit serves as a sizing-up between you and the therapist. If after your first visit (or even after several visits), you feel that you cannot work with this person, say so. You will at least have learned how to present your problem and what qualities you need in a therapist. The therapist may even be able to refer you to someone who will be a better fit for you.

When you begin seeing a mental health professional, you enter into a relationship with that person, and just as with any person, you will connect better with some therapists than others. If your connection with one therapist or counselor doesn't "feel right," trust your instincts and look for someone else.

TABLE 2.1 | Mental Health Professionals

What Are They Called?	What Kind of Training Do They Have?	What Kind of Therapy Do They Do?	Professional Association
Psychiatrist	Medical doctor degree (MD), followed by 4 years of mental health training	Can prescribe medications and may have admitting privileges at a local hospital	American Psychiatric Association www.psych.org
Psychologist	Doctoral degree in counseling or clinical psychology (PhD) plus several years of supervised practice to earn license	Various types, such as cognitive-behavioral therapy and specialties including family or sexual counseling	American Psychological Association www.apa.org
Clinical/psychiatric social worker	Master's degree in social work (MSW), followed by 2 years of experience in a clinical setting to earn license	May be trained in certain specialties, such as substance abuse counseling or child counseling	National Association of Social Workers www.socialworkers.org
Counselor	Master's degree in counseling, psychology, educational psychology, or related human service; generally must complete at least 2 years of supervised practice to obtain a license	Many are trained to provide individual and group therapy; may specialize in one type of counseling, such as family, marital, relationship, children, or substance abuse	American Counseling Association www.counseling.org
Psychoanalyst	Postgraduate degree in psychology or psychiatry (PhD or MD), followed by 8 to 10 years of training in psychoanalysis, which includes undergoing analysis themselves	Based on the theories of Freud and other psychologists, focuses on patterns of thinking and behavior and recalling early traumas that block personal growth. Treatment lasts 5 to 10 years, with three to four sessions per week.	American Psychoanalytic Association www.apsa.org
Licensed marriage and family therapist (LMFT)	Master's or doctoral degree in psychology, social work, or counseling, specializing in family and interpersonal dynamics; generally must complete at least 2 years of supervised practice to obtain a license	Treats individuals or families who want relationship counseling. Treatment is often brief and focused on finding solutions to specific relational problems.	American Association for Marriage and Family Therapy www.aamft.org

ABOUT 50%
of students with mental health problems **RECEIVE TREATMENT**.

Treatment Models

Many different types of counseling exist, including psychodynamic therapy, interpersonal therapy, and cognitive-behavioral therapy.

Psychodynamic therapy focuses on the psychological roots of emotional suffering. It involves self-reflection, self-examination, and the use of the relationship between therapist and patient as a window into problematic relationship patterns in the patient's life. Its goal is not only to alleviate the most obvious symptoms, but also to help people lead healthier lives.[89]

Interpersonal therapy focuses on social roles and relationships. The patient works with a therapist to evaluate specific problem areas, such as conflicts with family and friends or significant life changes or transition. Although past experiences help to inform the process, interpersonal therapy focuses mainly on improving relationships in the present.[90]

Treatment for mental disorders can include various cognitive-behavioral therapies. *Cognitive therapy* focuses on the impact of thoughts and ideas on feelings and behavior. It helps a person to look at life rationally and correct habitually pessimistic or faulty thinking patterns. *Behavioral therapy* focuses on what we do. Behavioral therapy uses the concepts of stimulus, response, and reinforcement to alter behavior patterns. With cognitive-behavioral therapy, you work with a mental health professional in a structured way, attending a limited number of sessions to become aware of inaccurate or negative thinking. Cognitive-behavioral therapy enables you to view challenging situations more clearly and respond to them more effectively. It can be very helpful for treating anxiety or depression.[91]

Current research also shows that mindfulness may have positive effects on treating mental health problems. See the **Mindfulness and You** box for more.

Pharmacological Treatment

Treatment for some conditions combines cognitive-behavioral therapies with psychoactive medication. Psychoactive drugs

▶ SEE IT! VIDEOS
When should you consider professional psychological help? Watch **Psychological Disorders** in the Study Area of Mastering Health.

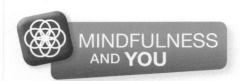
MINDFULNESS AS MENTAL HEALTH TREATMENT

Imagine going to the doctor's office and being prescribed mindfulness instead of medication. This may happen in the future, as research shows that mindfulness practices have positive effects on treating mental health problems.

Millions of Americans have mental health issues, anxiety and depression being among the most common. Today, some mindfulness training, such as Mindfulness Based Stress Reduction (MBSR) and Mindfulness Based Cognitive Therapy (MBCT), show promising results as therapies to treat anxiety and depression. Mindfulness therapies emphasize an acceptance of the present moment without ruminating over past events or catastrophizing over future events.

In a recent study comparing the efficacy of mindfulness-based therapy to that of the standard cognitive-based therapy for individuals with depression and anxiety, mindfulness-based therapy was determined to be as effective as traditional therapy in reducing depression and anxiety. The authors of that study concluded that mindfulness-based therapy is a viable alternative to more traditional therapies and may be less expensive and easier to implement. It may also be very helpful

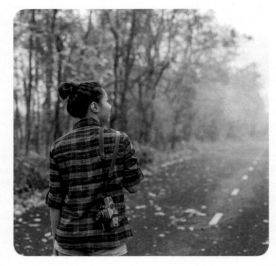

for individuals who do not respond to medications.

Mindfulness practice shows lasting changes in the brain. After an 8-week MBSR course, participants showed increased gray matter volume in some parts of the brain (such as the hippocampus) and decreased gray matter volume in other areas (such as the amygdala), supporting the idea that mindfulness increases the encoding of current experiences and decreases

automatic responses to immediate emotional events.

If you're interested in mindfulness-based therapy, contact your school's counseling center. Some centers have their own mindfulness group sessions; other centers can refer you to a counselor that specializes in mindfulness-based therapy.

Sources: National Institute of Mental Health, "Major Depression among Adults," Accessed April 2017, https://www.nimh.nih.gov/health/statistics/prevalence/major-depression-among-adults.shtml; National Institute of Mental Health, "Any Anxiety Disorder among Adults," Accessed April 2017, https://www.nimh.nih.gov/health/statistics/prevalence/any-anxiety-disorder-among-adults.shtml; National Institute of Mental Health, "Any Anxiety Disorder among Children," Accessed April 2017, https://www.nimh.nih.gov/health/statistics/prevalence/any-anxiety-disorder-among-children.shtml; N. Farm et al., "The Mindful Brain and Emotion Regulation in Mood Disorders," *Canadian Journal of Psychiatry* 57, no. 2 (2012): 70–7; J. Vollestad et al., "Mindfulness- and Acceptance-Based Interventions for Anxiety Disorders: A Systematic Review and Meta-analysis," *British Journal of Clinical Psychology* 51, no. 3 (2012): 239–60; J. Sundquist et al., "Mindfulness Group Therapy in Primary Care Patients with Depression, Anxiety and Stress and Adjustment Disorders: Randomised Controlled Trial," *British Journal of Psychiatry* 206, no. 2 (2015): 128–35.

require a doctor's prescription and carry approval from the U.S. Food and Drug Administration (FDA). Common side effects of psychoactive drugs include dry mouth, headaches, nausea, sexual dysfunction, and weight gain. Additionally, the FDA requires warnings for antidepressant medications, including a black box label (black box warnings are the FDA's most stringent a drug can carry) that warns of increased risks of suicidal thinking and behavior during initial treatment with the medication in young adults 18 to 24 years of age.[92]

Potency, dosage, and side effects of psychoactive medications can vary greatly. It is vital to talk to your health care provider and completely understand the risks and benefits of any prescribed medication. Likewise, your doctor needs to be notified of any adverse effects you may experience. With some drug therapies, such as antidepressants, you might not feel the therapeutic

effects for several weeks, so patience is important. Finally, be sure to follow your doctor's recommendations for beginning or ending a course of any medication.

To avoid the side effects of psychoactive drugs, some patients choose complementary or alternative therapies such as St. John's wort or omega-3 fatty acids for depression and kava or acupuncture for anxiety. Although the efficacy of these therapies has not yet been determined, the National Center for Complementary and Integrative Health continues to invest in research to explore alternatives to prescription drugs. Some therapies, such as St. John's wort, can be life threatening when combined with traditional depression medications. Much research is still needed on both traditional and alternative therapies for mental illness, so it is essential to talk to a medical professional when you are considering any new treatment or change in treatment.

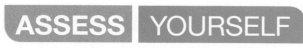

LIVE IT! ASSESS YOURSELF
An interactive version of this assessment is available on Mastering Health.

How Psychologically Healthy Are You?

Being psychologically healthy requires both introspection and the willingness to work on areas that need improvement. Begin by completing the following assessment scale. Use it to determine how well each statement describes you. When you're finished, ask someone who is very close to you to take the same test, responding with his or her own perceptions of you.

	Never	Rarely	Fairly frequently	Most of the time	All the time
1. My actions and interactions indicate that I am confident in my abilities.	1	2	3	4	5
2. I am quick to blame other people for things that go wrong in my life.	1	2	3	4	5
3. I am spontaneous and like to have fun with other people.	1	2	3	4	5
4. I am able to give love and affection to other people and show my feelings.	1	2	3	4	5
5. I am able to receive love and signs of affection from other people without feeling uneasy.	1	2	3	4	5
6. I am generally positive and upbeat about things in my life.	1	2	3	4	5
7. I am cynical and tend to be critical of other people.	1	2	3	4	5
8. I have a large group of people whom I consider to be good friends.	1	2	3	4	5
9. I make time for other people in my life.	1	2	3	4	5
10. I take time each day for myself for quiet introspection, having fun, or just doing nothing.	1	2	3	4	5
11. I am compulsive and competitive in my actions.	1	2	3	4	5
12. I handle stress well and am seldom upset or stressed out by other people.	1	2	3	4	5
13. I try to look for the good in everyone and every situation before finding fault.	1	2	3	4	5

	Never	Rarely	Fairly frequently	Most of the time	All the time
14. I am comfortable meeting new people and interact well in social settings.	1	2	3	4	5
15. I would rather stay in and watch TV or read than go out with friends or interact with other people.	1	2	3	4	5
16. I am flexible and can adapt to most situations even if I don't like them.	1	2	3	4	5
17. Nature, the environment, and other living things are important aspects of my life.	1	2	3	4	5
18. I think before responding to my emotions.	1	2	3	4	5
19. I tend to think of my own needs before those of other people.	1	2	3	4	5
20. I am consciously trying to be a better person.	1	2	3	4	5
21. I like to plan ahead and set realistic goals for myself.	1	2	3	4	5
22. I accept other people for who they are.	1	2	3	4	5
23. I value diversity and respect other people's rights, regardless of their culture, race, sexual orientation, religion, or other differences.	1	2	3	4	5
24. I try to live each day as if it might be my last.	1	2	3	4	5
25. I have a great deal of energy and appreciate the little things in life.	1	2	3	4	5
26. I cope with stress in appropriate ways.	1	2	3	4	5
27. I get enough sleep each day and seldom feel tired.	1	2	3	4	5

	Never	Rarely	Fairly frequently	Most of the time	All the time
28. I have healthy relationships with my family.	1	2	3	4	5
29. I am confident that I can do most things if I put my mind to them.	1	2	3	4	5

	Never	Rarely	Fairly frequently	Most of the time	All the time
30. I respect other people's opinions and believe that other people should be free to express their opinions, even when the opinions differ from mine.	1	2	3	4	5

Interpreting Your Scores

Look at items 2, 7, 11, 15, and 19. Add up your score for these five items, and divide by 5. ____

Is your average for these items above or below 3? Did you score a 5 on any of these items? Do you need to work on any of these areas?

Now look at your scores for the remaining items (there should be 25 items). Total these scores and divide by 25. ____

Is your average above or below 3? On which items did you score a 5? Obviously, you're doing well in these areas. Now remove these items from this grouping of 25 (scores of 5), and add up your scores for the remaining items. Then divide your total by the number of items included. Now what is your average? ____

Do the same for the scores completed by your friend or family member. Which scores, if any, are different, and how do they differ? Which areas do you need to work on? What actions can you take now to improve your ratings in these areas?

YOUR PLAN FOR **CHANGE**

The **ASSESS YOURSELF** activity "How Psychologically Health Are You?" gives you the chance to look at various aspects of your psychological health and compare your self-assessment with a friend's perceptions. After considering these results, you can take steps to change behaviors that may be harmful.

TODAY, YOU CAN:

☐ Evaluate your behavior and identify patterns and specific things you are doing that negatively affect your psychological health. What can you change now? What can you change in the near future?

☐ Start a journal and list people you can rely on and trust in life. How do these individuals contribute to your overall life satisfaction? What can you do to make more room for the people who contribute to your happiness?

WITHIN THE NEXT TWO WEEKS, YOU CAN:

☐ Visit your campus health center's website and find out about counseling services they offer. If you are feeling overwhelmed, depressed, or anxious, make an appointment with a counselor.

☐ Pay attention to negative thoughts that pop up throughout the day. Note times when you find yourself undermining your abilities and notice when you project negative attitudes. Bringing awareness to these thoughts gives you an opportunity to stop and reevaluate them. Try to block negative thoughts and focus on the positives in your life.

BY THE END OF THE SEMESTER, YOU CAN:

☐ Make a commitment to an ongoing practice aimed at improving your psychological health. Depending on your current situation, this could mean anything from seeing a counselor, taking time to be more supportive of people who enhance your life, or taking time to help other people who are lonely, need help, or are facing challenges.

☐ Volunteer regularly with a local organization you care about. Focus your energy and gain satisfaction by helping to improve other people's lives or the environment.

STUDY PLAN

CHAPTER REVIEW

LO 1 | What Is Psychological Health?

- Psychological health is a complex phenomenon involving mental, emotional, social, and spiritual dimensions.

LO 2 | Keys to Enhancing Psychological Health

- Developing self-esteem and self-efficacy, enhancing emotional intelligence, cultivating healthy personality traits, and pursuing happiness are key to enhancing psychological health. The mind–body connection is an important link in overall health and well-being.

LO 3 | When Psychological Health Deteriorates

- The college years are a high-risk time for developing disorders such as depression or anxiety because of high stress levels, pressures for grades, and financial problems, among others.
- Mood disorders include major depression, persistent depressive disorder, bipolar disorder, and seasonal affective disorder. Anxiety disorders include generalized anxiety disorder, panic disorders, and phobic disorders. People with obsessive-compulsive disorder often have irrational concern about order, symmetry, or exactness or have persistent intrusive thoughts.
- PTSD is caused by experiencing or witnessing a traumatic event, such as those that occur in war, natural disasters, or the loss of a loved one. Personality disorders include paranoid, narcissistic, and borderline personality disorders. Schizophrenia is often characterized by visual and auditory hallucinations, an altered sense of self, and radical changes in emotions, among others.

LO 4 | Suicide: Giving Up on Life

- Suicide is a result of negative psychological reactions to life. People who intend to commit suicide often give warning signs of their intentions and can often be helped. Suicide prevention involves eliminating the conditions that may lead to attempts.

LO 5 | Seeking Professional Help

- Mental health professionals include psychiatrists, psychoanalysts, psychologists, social workers, and counselors or therapists. Many therapy methods exist, including psychodynamic, interpersonal, and cognitive-behavioral therapy.
- Treatment of mental disorders can combine talk therapy and drug therapy using psychoactive drugs such as antidepressants.

POP QUIZ

LO 1 | What Is Psychological Health?

1. All of the following traits have been identified as characterizing psychologically healthy people *except*
   a. conscientiousness.
   b. understanding.
   c. openness.
   d. agreeableness.

LO 2 | Keys to Enhancing Psychological Health

2. A person with high self-esteem
   a. possesses feelings of self-respect and self-worth.
   b. believes that he or she can successfully engage in a specific behavior.
   c. believes that external influences shape one's psychological health.
   d. has a high altruistic capacity.

3. People who have experienced repeated failures at the same task may eventually give up and quit trying altogether. This pattern of behavior is termed
   a. posttraumatic stress disorder.
   b. learned helplessness.
   c. self-efficacy.
   d. introversion.

4. The initial "A" in PERMA represents which concept?
   a. Activity
   b. Advocacy
   c. Acceptance
   d. Accomplishment

LO 3 | When Psychological Health Deteriorates

5. Which of the following statements is *false*?
   a. One in five adults in the United States suffers from a diagnosable mental disorder in a given year.
   b. Mental disorders are the leading cause of disability in the United States.
   c. Dysthymia is an example of an anxiety disorder.
   d. Bipolar disorder can also be referred to as manic-depressive illness.

6. Which of the following statements is *false*?
   a. *Seasonal depression* and *seasonal affective disorder* are terms that are used interchangeably.
   b. Persistent depressive disorder is actually major depression that lasts a long time.
   c. Bipolar disorder has historically been referred to as manic-depressive illness.
   d. Many more women than men suffer from depression.

7. What is the most common mental health problem in the United States?
   a. Depression
   b. Anxiety disorders
   c. Alcohol dependence
   d. Schizophrenia

8. The disorder that is characterized by a need to perform rituals over and over again; fear of dirt or contamination; or an unnatural concern with order, symmetry, and exactness is
   a. personality disorder.
   b. obsessive-compulsive disorder.
   c. phobic disorder.
   d. posttraumatic stress disorder.

LO 4 | Suicide: Giving Up on Life

9. For 15- to 29-year-olds in the United States, suicide is the ___ leading cause of death.
   a. first
   b. second
   c. third
   d. fourth

LO 5 | Seeking Professional Help

10. A person with a Ph.D. in counseling psychology and training in various types of therapy is a
    a. psychiatrist.
    b. psychologist.
    c. social worker.
    d. psychoanalyst.

NOTE Answers to the Pop Quiz can be found on page A-1. If you answered a question incorrectly, review the section identified by the Learning Outcome. For even more study tools, visit MasteringHealth.

THINK ABOUT IT!

LO 1 | What Is Psychological Health?

1. What is psychological health? What indicates that a person is or is not psychologically healthy? Why might the college environment provide a challenge to psychological health?

LO 2 | Keys to Enhancing Psychological Health

2. Consider the factors that influence your overall level of psychological health. Which factors can you change? Which ones may be more difficult to change?

3. Which psychological dimensions do you need to work on? Which are most important to you and why? What actions can you take today?

LO 3 | When Psychological Health Deteriorates

4. What proportion of the student population suffers from some type of mental illness? What type of support networks exist on your campus?

5. What are the symptoms of major depression? Anxiety disorders? Panic attacks? What are risk factors for each and how are they treated?

LO 4 | Suicide: Giving Up on Life

6. What are the warning signs of suicide? Why are some people more vulnerable to suicide than others? What could you do if you heard a classmate say to no one in particular that he was going to "do the world a favor and end it all"?

LO 5 | Seeking Professional Help

7. Describe the various types of mental health professionals and types of therapies. If you felt depressed about breaking off a long-term relationship, which professional and which therapy do you think would be most beneficial to you?

ACCESS YOUR HEALTH ON THE INTERNET

Visit Mastering Health for links to the websites and RSS feeds.

The following websites explore further topics related to psychological health.

Active Minds. A campus education and advocacy/volunteer organization that was formed to combat the stigma of mental illness, educate the campus community, encourage students who need help to seek it early, and prevent tragedies related to untreated mental illness. www.activeminds.org

American Foundation for Suicide Prevention. Provides resources for suicide prevention and support for family and friends of people who have committed suicide. Includes information on the National Suicide Prevention Hotline, 1-800-273-TALK (8255). www.afsp.org

American Psychological Association Help Center. Includes information on psychology at work, the mind-body connection, understanding depression, psychological responses to war, and other topics. www.apa.org/helpcenter/wellness

National Alliance on Mental Illness. Support and advocacy organization of families and friends of people with severe mental illnesses. www.nami.org

National Institute of Mental Health (NIMH). Provides an overview of mental health information and new research. www.nimh.nih.gov

Helpguide. Resources for improving mental and emotional health as well as specific information on topics such as self-injury, sleep, depressive disorders, and anxiety disorders. www.helpguide.org

Cultivating Your Spiritual Health

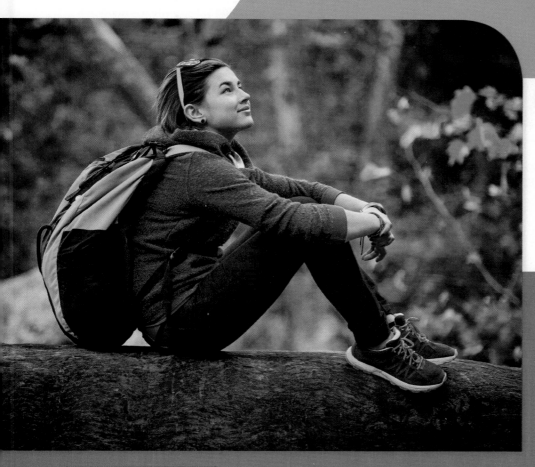

LEARNING OUTCOMES

1 Define spirituality, describe its three facets, and distinguish between religion and spirituality.

2 Describe the evidence that spiritual health has physical benefits, has psychological benefits, and lowers stress.

3 Describe three ways in which you can develop your spiritual health.

WHY SHOULD I CARE?

Spirituality can provide physical and psychological benefits to individuals (such as lowering blood pressure and decreasing stress and anxiety) and can also help communities become stronger and more connected—all important factors for healthy students and a healthy campus. Spiritual practices such as meditation can improve concentration and the brain's ability to process information. It can also reduce stress, anxiety, and depression—all important for managing classes and handling daily demands.

Lia's favorite spot on campus is the secluded Japanese garden on the south side of the library. Whether she's feeling stressed about exams or is mulling over an important decision, a few minutes alone in the garden always seem to help. Sometimes she sits quietly and watches the birds come and go. Sometimes she gets out her camera and photographs particularly brilliant blossoms. Often, she simply rests, eyes closed, feeling the sun's warmth on her face, and lets her thoughts turn to gratitude for her health, her loving family, and her opportunity to be in college. However she spends it, her "garden break" leaves Lia feeling refreshed and refocused,

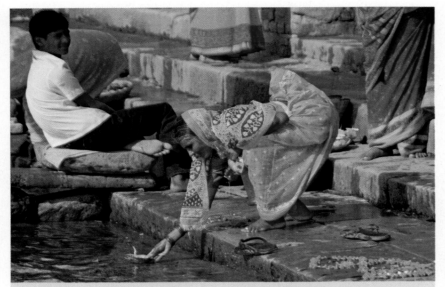
Spirituality and religion are not the same. Many people find that religious practices, for example, attending services or making offerings—such as the small lamp this Hindu woman is placing in the sacred Ganges River—help them to focus on their spirituality. However, religion does not have to be part of a spiritual person's life.

with greater confidence in her ability to tackle the challenges of her day.

Lia's desire to find a sense of purpose, meaning, and harmony in her life is shared by a majority of American college students, according to UCLA's Higher Education Research Institute.[1] Of the 1.5 million freshmen surveyed as they arrived on campuses in 2015, most reported a spiritual and/or religious interest; in fact, over 37 percent rated themselves as above average in spirituality when asked to compare themselves to the average person their age.[2]

Spiritual health is one of six key dimensions of health (see Figure 1.4 in Chapter 1). This chapter will look at what spiritual health is and provide the tools for enhancing your own spiritual health.

LO 1 | WHAT IS SPIRITUALITY?

Define spirituality, describe its three facets, and distinguish between religion and spirituality.

From one day to the next, many of us attempt to satisfy our needs for belonging and self-esteem by acquiring

---

spirituality An individual's sense of peace, purpose, and connection to other people and beliefs about the meaning of life.

---

material possessions, hanging with the "right crowd," and being the "best" at everything we do. But new "toys" and keeping up with other people don't necessarily bring happiness or improve our sense of self-worth or well-being, nor do they protect us from life's ups and downs. Friends and family can disappoint; relationships can falter; and even the best-laid plans can fail. Buffeted by life, many of us begin seeking more answers, hoping to grow and develop in a way that helps us cope. With this seeking, our quest for spirituality begins.

But what is spirituality? Let's begin by exploring its root, the word *spirit*, which in many cultures refers to *breath*, or the force that animates life. When you're "inspired," you are filled with energy. You're not held back by doubts about the purpose or meaning of your work and life. Indeed, many definitions of spirituality incorporate this sense of transcendence, focused on the way our work and life mesh with our psychological and emotional well-being. **Spirituality** has been defined as an internal, or personal, search for meaning and answers about life, the sacred, or the transcendent.[3] The sacred or transcendent could be thought of as a higher power or being, or it could refer to the essential goodness of life or our relationship with nature or forces we cannot explain.

Spirituality and Religion

Spirituality and religion are not the same thing. Religion is a set of rituals, beliefs, symbols, and practices intended to enable a feeling of connection to the holy or divine, often represented by one or more specific deities (such as God, Allah, or Buddha, among many others). It is possible to be spiritual and not religious, to be religious and not spiritual, and to be both spiritual and religious. In fact, while one global survey revealed that 4 out of 5 people worldwide are religiously affiliated, it also showed that 16 percent (1.1 billion) are not affiliated, making them the third largest group surveyed.[4] Many people without religious affiliation still have some religious or spiritual beliefs.[5] Research suggests that so-called Millennials, the people born roughly between the years 1981 and 1996, are less likely than older Americans to say that religion is very important to them. In contrast, they are just as likely as older Americans to report that spirituality is important.[6] Spirituality is the belief in the interconnectedness between people and recognition of forces greater than individuals; this can be accessed via traditional religious worship or via spending time in nature.[7] Spirituality is not bound by affiliation with a religious denomination, ceremony, building, or doctrine; individuals have the option to choose whatever path or paths that allows them to find meaning and a sense of purpose in life. **TABLE 1** identifies some characteristics that can help to distinguish between religion and spirituality.

29.5%

of first-year students marked "agnostic," "atheist," or "none" as their **RELIGIOUS PREFERENCE,** nearly double the 15.4% who indicated no religious preference in 1971.

TABLE 1 | Characteristics Distinguishing Religion and Spirituality

Religion	Spirituality
Observable, measurable, objective	Less measurable, more subjective
Formal, orthodox, organized	Less formal, less orthodox, less systematic
Behavior-oriented, outward practices	Emotionally oriented, inwardly directed
Authoritarian in terms of behaviors	Not authoritarian, little accountability
Doctrine separating good from evil	Unifying, not doctrine oriented

Source: R.F. Paloutzian and C.L. Park, *Handbook of the Psychology of Religion and Spirituality*, 2nd ed. (New York: Guilford Press, 2013); National Center for Complementary and Integrative Health, "Prayer and Spirituality in Health: Ancient Practices, Modern Science," *CAM at the NIH* 12, no. 1 (2005): 1–4.

Relationships, Values, and Purpose

Another definition of spirituality integrates three facets: relationships, values, and purpose in life (FIGURE 1).[8] Questions arising in these three domains prompt many of us to look for spiritual answers.

Relationships

Have you ever wondered whether someone you were attracted to is right for you? Conversely, have you wondered whether you should break off a long-term relationship? Have you ever wished you had more friends or that you were a better friend to yourself? For many people, such questions and yearnings are natural triggers for spiritual growth: As we contemplate who we should choose as a life partner or how to mend a quarrel with a friend, we begin to foster our own inner sense of what is right for us as individuals and to understand how to reflect on our choices mindfully. At the same time, healthy relationships are a sign of spiritual well-being. When we think well of ourselves and treat other people with respect, honesty, integrity, and love, we are manifesting our spiritual health.

Values

Our personal **values** are our principles—the set of fundamental rules by which we conduct our lives. Our values are what we stand for. When we attempt to clarify our values and then live according to those values, we're moving closer to a spiritually healthy life. Spiritual health is characterized by a personal understanding of one's own values, as well as a respect and curiosity about the values of others in our community.

Purpose in Life

What things make you feel complete? How do you hope to find meaning in your life? Is there some wrong in the world that you would like to help make right? How do these choices reflect what you hold as your purpose in life? How will the way you live your life contribute to your community and society?

Spiritual growth is fostered by contemplating questions like these—questions about our place in the world rather than our individual gains and material possessions. People who are spiritually healthy are able to articulate their search for purpose and to make choices that manifest that purpose.

Picture in your mind someone you think has made the world a better place—perhaps by volunteering in their community, working with youth, or finding other ways of improving the quality of life of those around them. This person may be someone close to you or someone like Gandhi, Martin Luther King, Jr., or Mother Theresa—people whose spiritual quests took on a life-size view of a better world. Each of these individuals devoted his or her life's work to helping make the world be a better place for others. They fought the "good fight" to improve social

values Principles that influence our thoughts and emotions and guide the choices we make in our lives.

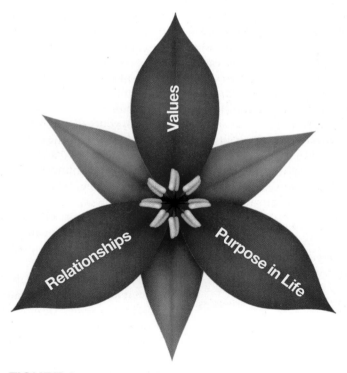

FIGURE 1 **Three Facets of Spirituality** Most of us are prompted to explore our spirituality because of questions relating to our relationships, values, and purpose in life. At the same time, these three facets together constitute spiritual well-being.

Watch Video Tutor: **Facets of Spirituality** in Mastering Health.

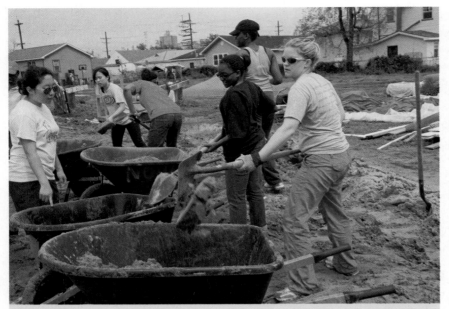
Spiritual and ethical concerns are important to most American college students. One of the ways in which students express their spirituality is by working to reduce suffering in the world. Many students contribute their time and skills to volunteer organizations such as Habitat for Humanity.

and political injustice and did so in a peaceful yet powerful way. Their lives had meaning, and each of them had a unique purpose in life and a path toward achieving it. Think about something you would like to do that would make a difference in the lives of other people or in the world more generally. Besides family, career, and other life course events, what would make your life more meaningful? Allow yourself to see your life as having its own mission and purpose.

How can you bring spirituality into your own life, work, and experiences? Spirituality may take different forms for different people. However, there are often several common elements, including:

- **Actively searching for meaning in your life.** What purpose do your actions serve in your community?
- **Finding a way to give back, knowing that service to others is a source of true happiness.** Is there a volunteering hub on your campus that can connect you with organizations that need assistance?

- **Understanding the interconnectedness of humanity, nature, and the universe and respecting all elements.** Do you spend time outside, respecting and appreciating the way nature can affect your emotional state? Do you take actions to protect and preserve the environment and all living things as part of an interconnected universe?
- **Nurturing loving relationships with yourself and others.** Do your relationships bring you joy? Are they based on mutual respect and love?
- **Living with intention, as if every day matters.** Do you have a sense that even small things (such as your attitude toward a task or a brief interaction with a classmate) can have a positive impact on the world around you?
- **Developing a philosophy of life that guides your daily attitudes and decisions.** Are most of your actions and decisions guided by a belief system about what is truly right and wrong?
- **Accepting your limitations as well as your strengths.** How can you use your strengths to have a positive impact on your surroundings? How can you work with other people to build on the strengths of the group?

spiritual intelligence (SI) The ability to access higher meanings, values, abiding purposes, and unconscious aspects of the self, a characteristic that helps us find a moral and ethical path to guide us through life.

Essentially, spirituality is about actively paying attention to our relationships, our community, and our selves, emphasizing respect and awareness while considering the impact our actions have on our communities.

Spiritual Intelligence

Our relationships, values, and sense of purpose together contribute to our overall **spiritual intelligence (SI)**. This term was introduced by physicist and philosopher Danah Zohar, who defined it as "an ability to access higher meanings, values, abiding purposes, and unconscious aspects of the self."[9] Humility, the capacity to consider ideas that fall "outside the box," and tapping into energies outside the ego all fit in her definition. SI allows us to utilize values, meanings, and purposes to be more creative and enrich our lives.

Since Zohar introduced the idea of SI, a number of psychologists, clerics, and even business consultants have taken the liberty of expanding the definition of the term. For example, spiritual intelligence expert Cindy Wigglesworth explains that SI helps us find compassion and wisdom to guide us through life.[10] SI also helps us maintain our peaceful center. To find out your own spiritual IQ, see the Assess Yourself activity on page 70.

LO 2 | THE BENEFITS OF SPIRITUAL HEALTH

Describe the evidence that spiritual health has physical benefits, has psychological benefits, and lowers stress.

A broad range of large-scale surveys have documented the importance of the mind–body connection to human health and wellness.

Physical Benefits

The emerging science of mind–body medicine is a research focus of the National Center for Complementary and Integrative Health (NCCIH) and an important objective of the organization's 2016 strategic plan. One area under study is the ways in which mind–body interventions affect well-being and general health, with specific attention to the impact on the brain and nervous system. The NCCIH is researching how these interventions (mindfulness, acupuncture, meditation, massage, etc.) can change our perceptions and control of pain in addition to other health outcomes.[11] Increasing numbers of studies are examining the effect that certain spiritual practices, such as yoga, deep meditation, and prayer, have on the mind, body, social and emotional health, and behavior and how these practices may improve health and promote healthy behaviors.[12]

The National Cancer Institute (NCI) contends that when we get sick, our spiritual or religious well-being may help restore our health and improve our quality of life in the following ways:[13]

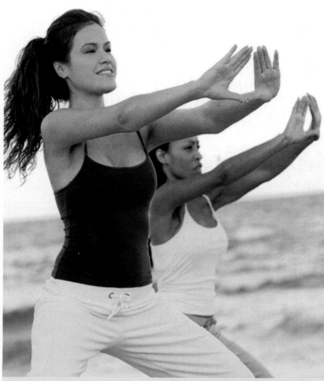

Spirituality is widely acknowledged to have a positive impact on health and wellness, from reductions in overall morbidity and mortality to improved abilities to cope with illness and stress. These students are using the movement techniques of tai chi to improve their spiritual health.

- Decreasing anxiety, depression, anger, discomfort, and feelings of isolation
- Decreasing alcohol and drug abuse
- Decreasing blood pressure and the risk of heart disease
- Increasing the person's ability to cope with the effects of illness and with medical treatments
- Increasing feelings of hope and optimism, freedom from regret, satisfaction with life, and inner peace.

Several studies show an association between spirituality and/or religion and a person's ability to cope with a variety of physical illnesses, including cancer.[14] However, other research has questioned the efficacy of many of these studies, citing small sample sizes and methodological issues.[15]

One recent study of over 33,000 adults found that indicators of "social capital" such as visiting friends or relatives, visiting neighbors, attending church, belonging to clubs, and attending club meetings were associated with

improved biomarkers such as cholesterol and blood pressure.[16] Another recent review of literature found that measures of spirituality were related to biomarkers such as blood pressure, immune factors, cardiac reactivity, and the progression of disease.[17] In addition, spiritual well-being and spiritual growth has been shown to be associated with reports of overall physical health.[18] Recent studies of college students found a relationship between personal spirituality and healthy college behaviors such as physical activity, reduced alcohol use, and reduced non-suicidal self-harm behaviors.[19]

Psychological Benefits

Current research also suggests that spiritual health contributes to psychological health. For instance, the NCI and independent studies have found that spirituality reduces levels of anxiety, stress, and depression.[20] In the case of student outcomes, practices that

enhance spirituality may provide a protective factor against burnout. For example, a review of meditation interventions in schools showed modest effects of meditation on student outcomes including well-being, social competence, and academic achievement.[21]

When people undergo psychological trauma, the meaning of life can be severely challenged. Counselors work with trauma survivors to help them find meaning in their trauma, to change their ways of thinking, and move them toward involvement in meaningful life experiences. Psychologists at the U.S. Department of Veterans Affairs have done extensive clinical work with veterans who are experiencing *posttraumatic stress disorder (PTSD)* as a result of their combat service. Research suggests that, following trauma, powerful emotions such as anger, rage, and wanting to get even are moderated, or softened, by psychological or emotional actions such as forgiveness or the application of other spiritual beliefs and practices.[22]

People who have found a **spiritual community**—a group of people meeting together for the purpose of enriching and expanding their spirituality—also benefit from increased social support. For instance, participation in charitable organizations, religious groups, book clubs, meditation circles, social gatherings, fund raising to help people in trouble, or spiritual learning experiences can help members think critically about their values and actions and avoid isolation. A community may include retired members who offer child care for working parents, support for individuals with addictions or mental health problems, shelter and food for homeless individuals, or transportation to medical appointments. Spiritually

spiritual community A group of people who meet together for the purpose of enriching and expanding their spirituality.

active members may volunteer or receive help from other volunteers, all of which may enhance feelings of self-worth, security, and belonging. This benefits the individual participants as well as the community as a whole.

Additionally, the NCI cites stress reduction as one probable mechanism among spiritually healthy people for improved health and longevity and for better coping with illness.[23] Chapter 3, "Managing Stress and Coping with Life's Challenges," goes into more detail on this topic.

LO 3 | CULTIVATING YOUR SPIRITUAL HEALTH

Describe three ways in which you can develop your spiritual health.

Cultivating your spiritual side takes just as much work as becoming physically

---

contemplation The practice of concentrating the mind on a spiritual or ethical question or subject, a view of the natural world, or an icon or other image representative of divinity.

mindfulness The practice of purposeful, nonjudgmental observation in which the person is fully present in the moment.

---

fit. Ways to develop your spiritual health include tuning in to yourself, training your body, and reaching out.

Tune in to Yourself and Your Surroundings

Focusing on your spiritual health can be likened to tuning in to a station on a radio: Spirituality is perpetually available to us, but if we fail to tune our "receiver" to it, we won't be able to get it through all the "static" of daily life. Fortunately, four ancient practices that are still in use today can help you focus specifically on spirituality in daily life. These are *contemplation* (studying), *mindfulness* (observing), *meditation* (quieting), and *prayer* (communing with the divine).

Contemplation

The word *contemplation* means a study of something—whether a candle flame or a theory of quantum mechanics. In the domain of spirituality, **contemplation** refers to concentrating the mind on a spiritual or ethical question or subject, a view of the natural world, or an icon or other image representative of divinity. Most religious and spiritual

WHAT DO YOU THINK?

Why do you think mindfulness practices are gaining more recognition?

■ What are benefits of mindfulness?

■ In today's fast-paced, multitasking world, what are the challenges to practice mindfulness on a regular basis?

traditions advocate engaging in the contemplation of gratitude, forgiveness, and unconditional love. This engagement can take many forms, such as journaling or blogging.

Mindfulness

A practice of focused, nonjudgmental observation, **mindfulness** is the ability to be fully present in the moment (**FIGURE 2**). "The moment" could include listening to music, having friends around you, attending religious services, or volunteering your time in the community. Mindfulness is an awareness of present-moment reality—a holistic sensation of being totally involved in the moment rather than focusing on some worry or being on "autopilot."[24] The range of opportunities to practice mindfulness is as plentiful as the moments of our lives. Living mindfully means allowing ourselves to be wholly aware of what we are experiencing at any given time.[25]

Pursuing almost any endeavor that requires close concentration can help you develop mindfulness. Linked to activities that help to cultivate spirituality, mindfulness can be used to intentionally foster healthy relationships and engage in activities that underscore our life philosophies. Mindfulness can also be a healing practice, allowing us to give emotional and mental space to the practice of facing the many daily challenges of life. The difficult work of continuing on our path when obstacles (emotions, events, people, etc.) are in the way is "spirit work" that builds our resiliency and allows us to grow alongside other people. Mindfulness is a way to acknowledge our emotions, feelings, and experiences without allowing them to define us.[26]

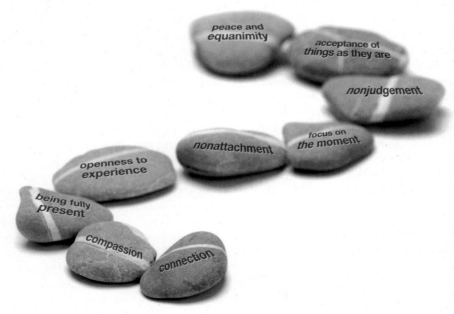

FIGURE 2 Qualities of Mindfulness

Source: M. Greenberg, "Nine Essential Qualities of Mindfulness," *Psychology Today*, February 22, 2012, www.psychologytoday.com/blog/the-mindful-self-express/201202/nine-essential-qualities-mindfulness.

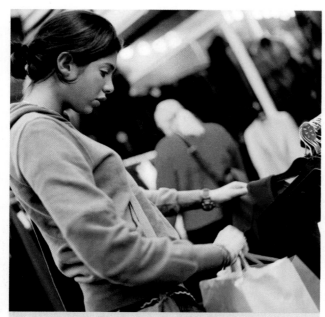

To be mindfully green requires us to ask ourselves some tough questions, such as "What is my fair share?" and "How much do I really need?"

Meditation

Meditation is a practice of cultivating a still or quiet mind. Although the precise details vary with different schools of meditation, the fundamental task is the same: to quiet the mind's noise (variously referred to as "chatter," "static," or "monkey mind"). In many ways, meditation and mindfulness go hand in hand.

For thousands of years, humans of different cultures and traditions have found that achieving periods of meditative stillness each day enhances their spiritual health. Today, researchers are beginning to discover why. Studies suggest that people who engage in mindfulness and compassion meditation show a significantly increased level of *empathy*—the ability to understand and share another person's experience—as well as an increased level of compassion toward other people.[27] Studies also suggest that mindfulness meditation improves

⏵ **SEE IT!** VIDEOS

Can meditation help reduce your stress and improve your grades? Watch **Meditation Becoming More Popular among Teens** in the Study Area of Mastering Health.

the brain's ability to process information; reduces stress, anxiety, and depression; reduces insomnia; improves concentration; and lowers blood pressure.[28]

The physiological processes that produce these effects are only partially understood. One theory suggests mindfulness meditation works by reducing the body's stress response. People who engage in this practice seem to promote activity in the body's systems, leading to a sense of peacefulness and subjective well-being and to physical relaxation that may slow breathing, lower blood pressure, improve sleep, and reduce symptoms of digestive problems.[29]

New research has shown actual differences in the brain structures of experienced meditators compared to those of people with no history of meditation.[30] Other studies have shown mindfulness meditation to boost gray matter density in parts of the brain critical to learning and memory and improved psychological and emotional health, compassion, and introspection.[31] At the same time, mindfulness meditation may decrease gray matter areas of the brain known to play key roles in anxiety and stress.[32]

So how do you meditate? Detailed instructions are beyond the scope of this text, but most teachers suggest beginning by sitting in a quiet place with low lighting where you won't be interrupted. Many advocate assuming a full lotus position, with legs bent fully at the knees, each ankle over the opposite knee. If this is impossible or uncomfortable, you may want to assume a modified lotus position, with your legs simply crossed in front of you. Rest your hands on your knees, palms upward. Beginners usually find it easier to meditate with their eyes closed.

Once you're in position, it's time to start emptying your mind. The various schools of meditation teach different methods to achieve this. Some options include:

- **Mantra meditation.** Focus on a *mantra*, a single word such as *Om*, *Amen*, *Love*, or *God*, and repeat this word silently. When a distracting thought arises, simply set it aside. It may help to imagine the thought as a leaf, and visualize placing it on a gently flowing stream. Do not fault yourself for becoming distracted. Simply notice the thought, release it, and return to your mantra.
- **Breath meditation.** Count each breath: Pay attention to each inhalation, the brief pause that follows, and the exhalation. Together, these equal one breath. When you have counted ten breaths, start over, counting from 1. As with mantra meditation, release distractions as they arise, and return to following the breath.
- **Color meditation.** When your eyes are closed, you may perceive a field of color, such as a deep, restful blue. Focus on this color. Treat distractions as in other forms of meditation.
- **Candle meditation.** With your eyes open, focus on the flame of a candle. Allow your eyes to soften as you meditate on this object. Treat distractions as in the other forms of meditation.

With practice, you may, after several minutes of meditation, come to experience a sensation sometimes described as "dropping down," in which you feel yourself release into the meditation. In this state, which can be likened to a wakeful sleep, distracting thoughts are far less likely to arise, yet you may receive surprising insights.

Initially, try meditating for just 10 to 20 minutes once or twice a day. In time, you can increase your sessions to 30 minutes or more. As you meditate

meditation The practice of concentrated focus on a sound, object, visualization, the breath, movement, or attention itself in order to increase awareness of the present moment, reduce stress, promote relaxation, and enhance personal and spiritual growth.

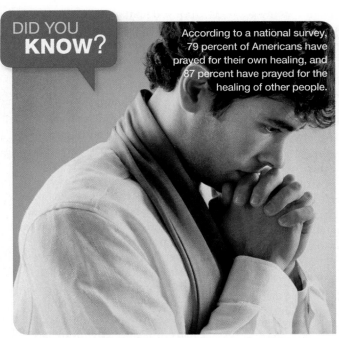

According to a national survey, 79 percent of Americans have prayed for their own healing, and 87 percent have prayed for the healing of other people.

Source: J. Levin, "Prevalence and Religious Predictors of Healing Prayer Use in the USA: Findings from the Baylor Religion Survey," *Journal of Religion and Health* 55, no. 4 (2016): 1136–58, doi:10.1007/s10943-016-0240-9.

prayer Communication with a transcendent presence.

yoga A system of physical and mental training involving controlled breathing, physical postures (*asanas*), meditation, chanting, and other practices that are believed to cultivate unity with the *Atman*, or spiritual life principle of the universe.

for longer periods, you will likely find yourself feeling more rested and less stressed, and you may begin to experience the increased levels of empathy that have been recorded among expert meditators.

Prayer

In **prayer**, an individual focuses the mind in communication with a transcendent presence. For many people, prayer offers a sense of comfort, a sense that we are not alone. It can be the means of expressing concern for other people, for admission of transgressions, for seeking forgiveness, and for renewing hope and purpose. Focusing on the things we are grateful for can move people to look to the future with hope and give them the strength to get through the most challenging

times. Research has shown that spiritual practices can increase the ability to cope and decrease stress among cancer patients.[33]

You can expand your awareness of different spiritual practices further by taking classes in spiritual or religious subjects, attending religious meetings or services, or studying sacred texts. In each case, evaluate the messages and ideas you encounter and decide which practices or beliefs hold meaning for you.

Train Your Body

For thousands of years, in regions throughout the world, spiritual seekers have pursued transcendence through physical means. One of the foremost examples is the practice of **yoga**. Although many people in the West tend to picture yoga as having to do with a number of physical postures and some controlled breathing, more traditional forms tend to also emphasize chanting, meditation, and other techniques

31 MILLION

U.S. adults have **PRACTICED YOGA**, and 21 million have practiced yoga in the past 12 months. Of these, 18- to 29-year-olds were most likely to practice yoga.

believed to encourage unity with the *Atman*, or spiritual life principle of the universe.

If you are interested in exploring yoga, sign up for a class. Choose a form that seems right to you: Some, such as *hatha yoga*, focus on developing flexibility, deep breathing, and tranquility; others, such as *ashtanga yoga*, are fast-paced and demanding and thus more focused on developing physical fitness. See Chapter 3 and Chapter 12 for more on various styles of yoga.

The Eastern meditative movement practices of tai chi or qigong can also increase physical activity and mental focus. With roots in Chinese medicine, both have been shown to have beneficial effects on bone health, stress,

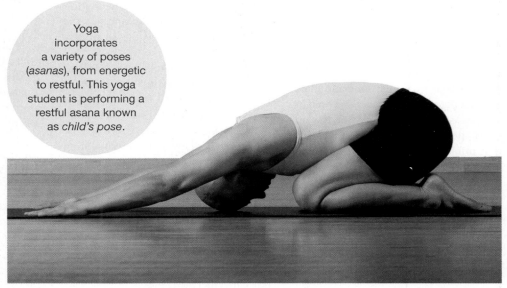

Yoga incorporates a variety of poses (*asanas*), from energetic to restful. This yoga student is performing a restful asana known as *child's pose*.

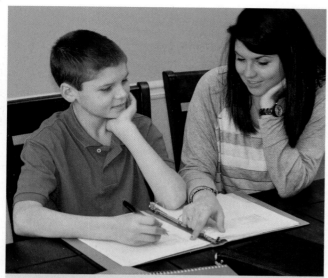

Volunteering can be a fun and fulfilling way to broaden your experience, connect with your community, and focus on your spiritual health.

cardiopulmonary fitness, mood, balance, and quality of life.[34] See Chapter 3 for more on tai chi and qigong.

Training your body to improve your spiritual health doesn't necessarily require you to engage in a formal practice. By energizing your body and sharpening your mental focus, jogging, biking, aerobics, dance, or any other regular exercise can contribute to your spiritual health. In particular, mindfulness *while* exercising or engaging in physical pursuits can enhance the physical benefits.

Reach Out to Other People

Altruism, the giving of oneself out of genuine concern for other people, is a key aspect of a spiritually healthy lifestyle. Volunteering time, donating money or other resources to a food bank or other program, even spending an afternoon picking up litter in your neighborhood—all are ways to serve other people and simultaneously enhance your own spiritual and overall health. Researchers have referred to the benefits of volunteering as a "helper's high," a specific feeling connected with helping other people.[35] Altruism, in the form of volunteering, can benefit the individual helper, the people who receive the help, and the community in which they live through increased satisfaction and interconnectedness of residents.[36]

For more strategies to enhance your spiritual health by reaching out to other people, refer to the Skills for Behavior Change box.

SKILLS FOR
BEHAVIOR CHANGE

Finding Your Spiritual Side Through Service

Recognizing that we are all part of a greater system with responsibilities to and for other people is a key part of spiritual growth. Volunteering your time and energy is a great way to connect with other people and help make the world a better place while improving your own health. Here are a few ideas:

- Offer to help elderly neighbors with lawn care or simple household repairs.
- Volunteer with Meals on Wheels, a local soup kitchen, a food bank, or another program that helps people obtain adequate food.
- Organize or participate in an after-school or summertime activity for neighborhood children.
- Participate in a highway, beach, or neighborhood cleanup; restoration of park trails and waterways; or other environmental preservation projects.
- Volunteer at the local humane society or animal shelter.
- Apply to become a Big Brother or Big Sister, and mentor a child who may face significant challenges or have poor role models.
- Join an organization working on a cause such as global warming or hunger, or start such an organization yourself. Check out these inspiring examples: Students Against Global Apathy (SAGA), Students for the Environment (S4E), and the National Student Campaign Against Hunger and Homelessness.
- Volunteer in a neighborhood challenged by poverty, low literacy levels, or a natural disaster. Or volunteer with an organization such as Habitat for Humanity to build homes or provide other aid to developing communities.

To find out more information on service, the following are some online resources:

Locates service opportunities: **www.volunteermatch.org**

Lists overseas volunteer opportunities: **www.projects -abroad.org**

Oriented toward students: **www.dosomething.org**

Competition for money for service projects: **www.truehero.org**

altruism The giving of oneself out of genuine concern for other people.

ASSESS YOURSELF

What's Your Spiritual IQ?

LIVE IT! ASSESS YOURSELF

An interactive version of this assessment is available online in Mastering Health.

Many tools are available for assessing your SI. Although the tools differs significantly according to the target audience (e.g., therapy clients, business executives, church members), most share certain underlying principles reflected in the questionnaire below. Answer each question as follows:

0 = not at all true for me
1 = somewhat true for me
2 = very true for me

___ 1. I frequently feel gratitude for the many blessings of my life.

___ 2. I am often moved by the beauty of the earth, music, poetry, or other aspects of my daily life.

___ 3. I readily express forgiveness toward people whose missteps have affected me.

___ 4. I recognize in other people qualities that are more important than their appearance and behaviors.

___ 5. When I do poorly on an exam, lose an important game, or am rejected in a relationship, I am able to know that the experience does not define who I am.

___ 6. When fear arises, I am able to know that I am eternally safe and loved.

___ 7. I meditate or pray daily.

___ 8. I frequently and fearlessly ponder the possibility of an afterlife.

___ 9. I accept total responsibility for the choices I have made in building my life.

___ 10. I feel that I am on the earth for a unique and sacred reason.

Scoring

The higher your score on this quiz, the higher is your SI. To improve your score, apply the suggestions for spiritual practices from this chapter.

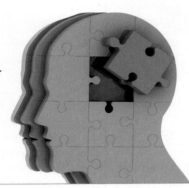

YOUR PLAN FOR CHANGE

The **ASSESS YOURSELF** activity gives you the chance to evaluate your spiritual intelligence, and the text introduced you to some practices that millions of people have used successfully over many generations to enhance their spiritual health. If you are interested in further cultivating your spirituality, consider some of the small but significant steps listed below.

TODAY, YOU CAN:

☐ Find a quiet spot, turn off your cell phone, close your eyes, and contemplate, meditate, or pray for 10 minutes, or spend 10 minutes in quiet mindfulness of your surroundings.

☐ In a journal or on your computer, compose a list of at least ten things you are grateful for. Include people, pets, talents and abilities, achievements, places, foods—whatever comes to mind.

WITHIN THE NEXT TWO WEEKS, YOU CAN:

☐ Explore the options on campus for beginning psychotherapy, joining a spiritual or religious group, or volunteering with an organization working for positive change.

☐ Think of a person in your life with whom you have experienced conflict.

Spend a few minutes contemplating forgiveness toward this person, and then write a letter or e-mail apologizing for any offense and offering your forgiveness in return. Wait a day or two before deciding whether you are truly ready to send the message.

☐ Take a time out. Focus on the things around you— the sounds, sights, and smells. Take time to look at people as you pass them, saying "hello" or merely nodding to indicate that you notice their existence. Write down the things you noticed today that were beautiful or that you never noticed before.

BY THE END OF THE SEMESTER, YOU CAN:

☐ Develop a list of several spiritual texts you would like to read during your break.

☐ Begin exploring options for volunteer work that would serve other people and have meaning for you.

STUDY **PLAN**

Visit the Study Area in Mastering Health to enhance your study plan with MP3 Tutor Sessions, Practice Quizzes, Flashcards, and more!

CHAPTER **REVIEW**

LO **1** | What Is Spirituality?

- Although spirituality is hard to define and can mean different things to different people, it encompasses an individual's sense of peace, purpose, connection to other people, and beliefs about the meaning of life. It involves a person's values and way of viewing life and behaving in the world, and is often guided by a sense of connection to a higher presence.

LO **2** | The Benefits of Spiritual Health

- Because of the diversity of human spiritual experience and the overlap of spirituality with religious practice, it is often hard to delineate the exact impact of spiritual beliefs and actions. However, in recent years, a number of studies of specific practices such as mindfulness, meditation, and prayer have shown that good spiritual health reduces stress, decreases anxiety and depression, increases a person's ability to heal from illness and cope with medical treatment, and increases feelings of hope and optimism, among other positive benefits.

LO **3** | Cultivating Your Spiritual Health

- Similar to developing physical fitness, developing spiritual health takes knowledge, guidance, commitment, and consistency. Learning practices such as mindfulness, meditation, contemplation, right-mindedness, prayer, and service and doing them regularly will help to build a foundation of spiritual health.

POP **QUIZ**

LO **1** | What Is Spirituality?

1. Spirituality could be characterized by all of the following, except
   a. bringing greater awareness to the present moment, such as in the practice of mindfulness.
   b. focusing on relationships, values, and finding meaningful purpose in life.
   c. participating in psychotherapy using a short-term, problem-solving model.
   d. studying teachings from ancient spiritual traditions.

LO **2** | The Benefits of Spiritual Health

2. Benefits of spiritual health have been shown in all of the following except
   a. decreases in blood pressure and risk of heart disease.
   b. an increase in muscle mass during regular resistance exercise.
   c. an increase in the ability to heal from illness.
   d. a decrease in drug and alcohol use.

LO **3** | Cultivating Your Spiritual Health/

3. All of the following are purposeful ways to cultivate spiritual health except
   a. taking a course on improving relationships that is offered at the university ecumenical ministry center.
   b. volunteering to help build a Habitat for Humanity home because you want to meet the cute guy or girl in charge of the project.
   c. taking a hatha yoga class.
   d. browsing Amazon for books written by spiritual teachers of our time.

*Answers to the Pop Quiz questions can be found on page A-1. If you answered a question incorrectly, review the section identified by the Learning Outcome. For even more study tools, visit **MasteringHealth**.*

3

Managing Stress and Coping with Life's Challenges

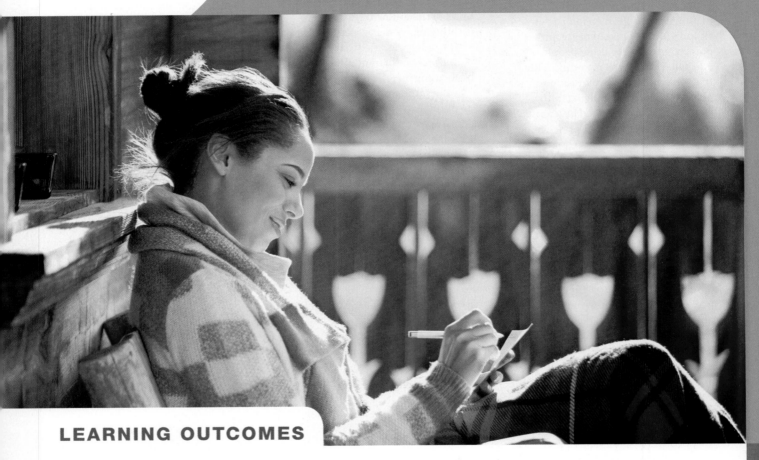

LEARNING OUTCOMES

LO 1 Define *stress*, and examine its potential impact on health, relationships, and success in college and life.

LO 2 Explain key stress theories as well as the emotional, mental, and physiological changes that occur during the stress response.

LO 3 Examine the physical health risks that may occur with chronic stress.

LO 4 Examine the intellectual and psychological effects of stress and their impacts on college students.

LO 5 Discuss sources of stress, and examine the unique stressors that affect young adults, particularly college students.

LO 6 Explain key individual factors that may influence whether or not a person is able to cope with stressors.

LO 7 Explore stress management and stress reduction strategies, ways you can cope more effectively with stress, and mindfulness strategies that can enrich your life experiences and reduce health risks.

Your stress level right now may be having a significant effect on your sleep, your relationships, and the ability of your immune system to ward off infectious diseases. Your stress level may be contributing to lower grades and poor performance, or it may be limiting your career options. In the long term, chronic stress may affect your risks of high blood pressure, heart arrhythmias and CVD, diabetes, and many other health-related problems. Stress effects are cumulative, and you have only one body. Think about ways to prevent and control your perceptions and reactions before you become a victim of "overwhelm."

n today's fast-paced, 24/7-connected world, stress can cause us to feel overwhelmed and zap our energy. It can also cause us to push ourselves to improve performance, bring excitement, and help us thrive.

Chronic stress inhibits normal functioning for prolonged periods and is a growing public health crisis among people of all ages. According to recent studies by the American Psychological Association, the health care system is not giving Americans the support they need to cope with stress and build healthy lifestyles. Here are some key findings:[1]

- Americans consistently report high stress levels (20 percent report extreme stress), and teenagers report stress levels on par with those of adults.
- Among those likely to report high levels of stress are lower-income populations, Blacks, Latinos, Millennials, Gen-Xers, and women (see **Focus On: Difference, Disparity, and Health: Achieving Health Equity** for more).
- Only about half of all teens say they feel confident in their ability to handle personal problems.
- The biggest sources of stress for adults aged 18 to 32 years are work, relationships, money, and job stability. When all adults report their sources of stress, money tops the list, followed by work, family, and health.

While key sources of stress are similar for men and women (money, work, and health), huge gender differences exist in how people experience, report, and cope with stress. Both men and women report above average levels of stress, but women are more likely to report stress levels that are on the rise and more extreme.[2] Women are also more likely to report experiencing negative stress symptoms that affect their eating habits and prevent them from making lifestyle changes.[3] Additionally, although men may recognize and report stress, they are much less likely to take action to reduce it.[4] Being stressed out can take a major toll on people at all ages and stages of life (**FIGURE 3.1**).

Stress isn't always a bad thing. In fact, it's part of our natural physiological response—a "revving up" designed to put body systems on alert. In the short term, this heightened response not only increases energy levels, but can also improve performance. How we react to real and perceived threats often determines whether stressors

are enabling or debilitating. Especially when a feeling of being overwhelmed persists—as in those unrelenting weeks of academic demands punctuated by negative interactions with others, financial worries, and other life challenges—stress can become a looming, slow-motion assault on our systems that drains our reserves and can result in serious health problems. Learning to be mindful of our perceptions and reactions—to anticipate, avoid, and develop skills to reduce or better manage stressors and refocus our energies—is key. The first step in controlling or reducing stress is to understand what stress is, how it affects the body, and why we may be particularly vulnerable.

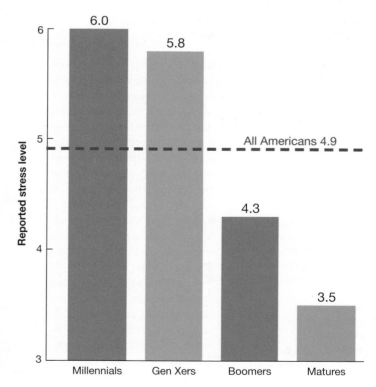

FIGURE 3.1 **Stress Levels by Age** Stress levels for Gen-Xers and Millennials are above average, particularly compared to those of older generations.

SOURCE: American Psychological Association, "Stress in America, The Impact of Discrimination," March 2016, http://www.apa.org/news/press/releases/stress/2015/impact-of-discrimination.pdf.

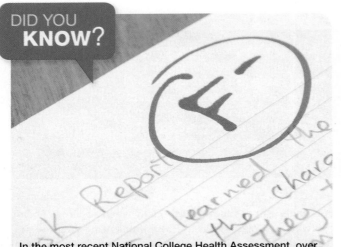

In the most recent National College Health Assessment, over 32 percent of students reported that stress was the factor that most negatively affected their grade on an exam or course or caused them to drop a course, followed by nearly 25 percent reporting anxiety and nearly 21 percent reporting sleep problems as the culprits.

Source: Data are from American College Health Association, *American College Health Association–National College Health Assessment II (ACHA-NCHA II): Reference Group Data Report Fall, 2016.* (Hanover, MD: American College Health Association, 2017).

LO 1 | **WHAT** IS STRESS?

Define stress, and examine its potential impact on health, relationships, and success in college and life.

Most current definitions of **stress** describe it as the mental and physical response and adaptation by our bodies to real or perceived change and challenges. A **stressor** is any real or perceived physical, social, or psychological event or stimulus that causes the body to react or respond. Several factors influence one's response to stressors, including *characteristics of the stressor* (How traumatic is it? Can you control it? Did it surprise you?), *biological factors* (e.g., your age, gender, or health status or whether you've had enough sleep recently), and *past experiences* (e.g., things that have happened to you, their consequences, and how you felt or responded). Stressors may be *tangible*, such as a failing grade, or *intangible*, such as the angst associated with meeting your significant other's parents for the first time. *Change* can also be a major stressor.

Generally, positive stress is called **eustress**. Eustress presents the opportunity for personal growth and satisfaction and can actually improve health. Getting married, the excitement of a first date, or winning a major competition can give rise to the pleasurable rush associated with eustress.

Distress, or negative stress, is more likely to occur when you are tired; under the influence of alcohol or other drugs; under pressure to do well; or coping with an illness, financial trouble, or relationship problems. There are several kinds of distress. The most common type, **acute stress**, comes from demands and pressures of the recent past and near future.[5] Usually, acute stress is intense, lasts for a short time, and disappears quickly without permanent damage to your health. Seeing someone you have a crush on could cause your heart to race and your muscles to tense while you may appear cool, calm, and collected on the outside. If you have a positive reaction to this acute stress, you rise to the occasion and put your most charming self forward. In contrast, if you do not enjoy performing in front of other people, anticipating a class presentation could cause shaking hands and voice, nausea, headache, cramping, or diarrhea along with a galloping heartbeat and forgetfulness. **Episodic acute stress** is the state of regularly reacting with wild, acute stress to various situations. Individuals who experience episodic acute stress may complain about all they have to do and focus on negative events that may or may not occur. These "awfulizers" are often reactive and anxious, constantly complaining about their lack of sleep and all they have to do— habits that are so much a part of these individuals that they seem normal. Others may respond to stress with a hyperactive, chirpy, "happy-happy" persona.

Acute stress and episodic acute stress can both involve physical and emotional reactions, but they may or may not result in negative physical or emotional outcomes. In fact, they may serve as a form of self-protection.

In contrast, **chronic stress** can linger indefinitely and wreak silent havoc on body systems. Caregivers are especially vulnerable to prolonged physiological stress as they watch a loved one struggle with illness while having the increased

stress A series of mental and physiological responses and adaptations to a real or perceived threat to one's well-being.

stressor A physical, social, or psychological event or condition that upsets homeostasis and produces a stress response.

eustress Stress that presents opportunities for personal growth; positive stress.

distress Stress that can have a detrimental effect on health; negative stress.

acute stress The short-term physiological response to an immediate perceived threat.

episodic acute stress The state of regularly reacting with wild, acute stress about one thing or another.

chronic stress An ongoing state of physiological arousal in response to ongoing or numerous perceived threats.

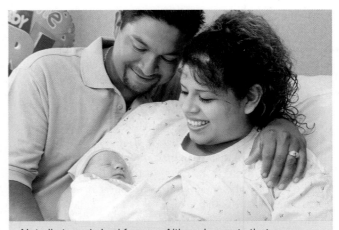

Not all stress is bad for you. Although events that cause prolonged *distress*, such as a natural disaster, can undermine your health, events that cause *eustress*, such as the birth of a child or the excitement of a new love, can have positive effects on your personal growth and well-being.

responsibilities of caring for the ill person along with the other aspects of their own lives. When a loved one dies, the survivors may struggle to balance the need to process emotions with the need to stay caught up in classes, work, and everyday life.

Another type of stress, **traumatic stress**, is a form of acute stress that is often a result of witnessing or experiencing events such as major accidents, violence and war, or being caught in a natural disaster. Effects of traumatic stress may be felt for years after the event and cause significant disability, potentially leading to *posttraumatic stress disorder*, or PTSD (see Chapter 2 for a discussion of PTSD).[6]

LO 2 | **YOUR** BODY'S STRESS RESPONSE

Explain key stress theories as well as the emotional, mental, and physiological changes that occur during the stress response.

Over the years, several theories have evolved to explain what happens (physiologically and psychologically) when a person perceives or experiences a stressor, as well as why some people thrive in stressful situations and others suffer debilitating consequences. In this section, we'll look at some of the key theories.

Physiology/Systems Theory: The General Adaptation Syndrome

When stress levels are low, the body is often in a state of **homeostasis**, or balance; all body systems are operating smoothly to maintain equilibrium. Stressors trigger a crisis-mode physiological response, after which the body attempts to

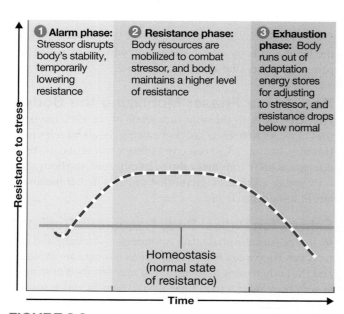

① **Alarm phase:** Stressor disrupts body's stability, temporarily lowering resistance

② **Resistance phase:** Body resources are mobilized to combat stressor, and body maintains a higher level of resistance

③ **Exhaustion phase:** Body runs out of adaptation energy stores for adjusting to stressor, and resistance drops below normal

Resistance to stress

Homeostasis (normal state of resistance)

Time

FIGURE 3.2 The General Adaptation Syndrome (GAS) The GAS is the body's method of coping with prolonged stress.

return to homeostasis by means of an **adaptive response**. First characterized by Hans Selye in 1936, the internal fight to restore homeostasis in the face of a stressor is known as the **general adaptation syndrome (GAS)** (**FIGURE 3.2**). The GAS has three distinct phases: alarm, resistance, and exhaustion.[7]

Alarm Phase: The Body in "Protect Mode"

Suppose you are walking home after a night class on a dimly lit campus. You hear someone cough behind you and sense the person approaching rapidly. You walk faster, only to hear the other person's footsteps quicken. Your senses go on high alert, you start breathing faster, your heart races, and you begin to perspire. In desperation, you stop, pull off your backpack, and prepare to fling it at your would-be attacker. You turn around, arms flailing, and let out a blood-curdling yell. To your surprise, the would-be-attacker screeches in alarm. It's just one of your classmates trying to stay close to you out of her own fear of being alone in the dark! You have just experienced the alarm phase of GAS. Also known as the **fight-or-flight response**, this physiological reaction is one of our most basic, innate survival instincts [8] (**FIGURE 3.3**).

When the mind perceives a real or imaginary stressor, the cerebral cortex, the region of the brain that interprets the nature of an event, triggers an **autonomic nervous system (ANS)** response that prepares the body for action. The ANS is the portion of the nervous system that regulates body functions that we do not normally consciously control, such as heart and glandular functions and breathing.

The ANS has two branches: sympathetic and parasympathetic. The **sympathetic nervous system** energizes the body for fight or flight, while the **parasympathetic nervous system** slows systems the stress response stimulates.

The sympathetic nervous system's responses to stress involve a series of biochemical exchanges between different parts of the body. The **hypothalamus**, a structure in the brain, functions as the control center of the sympathetic nervous system and determines the overall reaction to stressors. When the hypothalamus perceives that extra energy is needed to fight a stressor, it stimulates the adrenal glands, located near

traumatic stress A physiological and mental response that occurs for a prolonged period of time after a major accident, war, assault, or natural disaster or an event in which one may have been seriously hurt or witnessed horrible things.

homeostasis A balanced physiological state in which all the body's systems function smoothly.

adaptive response The physiological adjustments the body makes in an attempt to restore homeostasis.

general adaptation syndrome (GAS) The pattern followed in the physiological response to stress, consisting of the alarm, resistance, and exhaustion phases.

fight-or-flight response Physiological arousal response in which the body prepares to combat or escape a real or perceived threat.

autonomic nervous system (ANS) The portion of the peripheral nervous system that regulates body functions that a person does not normally consciously control.

sympathetic nervous system Branch of the autonomic nervous system responsible for stress arousal.

parasympathetic nervous system Branch of the autonomic nervous system responsible for slowing systems stimulated by the stress response.

hypothalamus A structure in the brain that controls the sympathetic nervous system and directs the stress response.

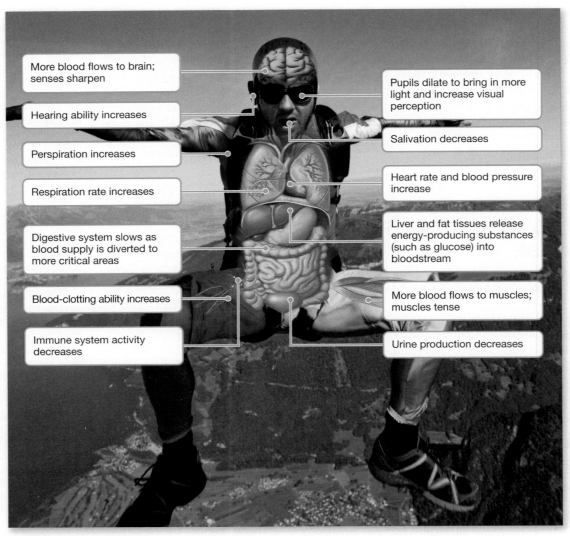

More blood flows to brain; senses sharpen

Hearing ability increases

Perspiration increases

Respiration rate increases

Digestive system slows as blood supply is diverted to more critical areas

Blood-clotting ability increases

Immune system activity decreases

Pupils dilate to bring in more light and increase visual perception

Salivation decreases

Heart rate and blood pressure increase

Liver and fat tissues release energy-producing substances (such as glucose) into bloodstream

More blood flows to muscles; muscles tense

Urine production decreases

FIGURE 3.3 **Fight or Flight: The Body's Acute Stress Response** Exposure to stress of any kind causes a complex series of involuntary physiological responses.

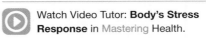 Watch Video Tutor: **Body's Stress Response** in Mastering Health.

the top of the kidneys, to release the hormone **epinephrine**, also called *adrenaline*. Epinephrine "kicks" the body into gear, causing more blood to be pumped with each beat of the heart, dilates the airways in the lungs to increase oxygen intake, increases the breathing rate, stimulates the liver to release more glucose (which fuels muscular exertion), and dilates the pupils to improve visual sensitivity. In addition to the fight-or-flight response, the alarm phase can trigger a longer-term reaction to stress. The hypothalamus uses chemical messages to trigger the pituitary gland within the brain to release a powerful hormone, *adrenocorticotropic hormone (ACTH)*. ACTH signals the adrenal glands to release **cortisol**, a key hormone that makes stored nutrients more readily available to meet energy demands. Finally, other parts of the brain and body release *endorphins*, which can relieve the pain and anxiety that a stressor may cause.

Resistance Phase: Mobilizing the Body's Resources
In the resistance phase of the GAS, the body tries to return to homeostasis by resisting the alarm responses. However, because some perceived stressor still exists, the body does not achieve complete calm or rest. Instead, the body stays activated or aroused at a level that causes a higher metabolic rate in some organ tissues.

Exhaustion Phase: Body Resources Depleted
In the exhaustion phase, the hormones, chemicals, and systems that trigger and maintain the stress response are depleted, and the body returns to balance. You may feel tired or drained as your body returns to normal. In situations in which stress is *chronic*, triggers may reverberate in the body, keeping body systems in a heightened arousal state. The prolonged effort to adapt to the stress response leads to **allostatic load**, or exhaustive wear

epinephrine Also called *adrenaline*, a hormone that stimulates body systems in response to stress.

cortisol Hormone released by the adrenal glands that makes stored nutrients more readily available to meet energy demands.

allostatic load Wear and tear on the body caused by prolonged or excessive stress responses.

and tear on the body. As the body adjusts to chronic unresolved stress, the adrenal glands continue in resistance mode; a steady stream of cortisol is released and remains in the bloodstream for longer periods of time as a result of slower metabolic responsiveness. Over time, cortisol can reduce **immunocompetence**—the ability of the immune system to respond to attack—and can increase the risk of health problems such as depression, diabetes, heart arrhythmias, cancer, inflammatory responses, cardiovascular disease (CVD), digestive diseases, weight gain, insomnia, and many other health problems.[9]

Psychological Theory: The Transactional Model of Stress and Coping

In the **transactional model of stress and coping**, psychologist Richard Lazarus proposed that our reaction to stress is not so much about the nature of a stressor as about the interaction between a person's *perception*, his or her *coping ability*, and *the environment*. In other words, your history, experience, and beliefs about a stressor will influence your perceptions about whether you should worry or jump into action, remain calm and unreactive, or utilize coping strategies that have worked in the past. According to Lazarus, the transactional model consists of four stages: (1) *appraisal*, in which you size up whether the stressor is a real threat; (2) *secondary appraisal*, in which you assess whether your actions might reduce the threat with the resources you have; (3) *coping*, in which you take action to reduce the threat; and (4) *postassessment*, in which you examine what happened and decide whether you need to take more action. In this model, your perceptions are key to your stress response. By changing your perceptions, you can reduce the stress effect.

Minority Stress Perspective

Another theory explaining the role of negative stressors relates to the role that stress plays in the lives of minority populations. According to the **minority stress perspective**, there are unresolved conflicts between minority and dominant group members. In this view, minority stress may be explained in large part by disparities and the chronic stress inherent in populations that experience persistent rejection, alienation, and hostility. This is especially true when there has been a long history of harassment, maltreatment, discrimination, and victimization.[10]

Yerkes-Dodson Law of Arousal

According to the **Yerkes-Dodson law of arousal**, when arousal or stress increases, performance improves—but only to a point. Too much stress can drive performance down. For example, a college athlete who does a great job passing the football in regular season games might choke during the conference championship when NFL scouts are on the field. On the other end, if you cram for four exams in just two days before you have to take them, you may find yourself so wound up that you do horribly on all of the exams. You may be tired and listless, find it hard to concentrate, and watch helplessly as your grade plummets.

This stress response is often depicted as a bell-shaped curve. As your stress increases, you move upward on the performance curve; however, once you reach a certain level of stress, your performance levels off. If stress persists and increases beyond this point, your performance can drop precipitously.[11]

Do Men and Women Respond Differently to Stress?

Walter Cannon's landmark studies in the 1930s suggested that humans and many species of animals respond similarly to stressful events. However, newer research indicates that men and women may actually respond very differently to stressors. While men may be prone to fighting or fleeing, women may be more likely to "tend and befriend" to ease stress-related reactions.[12] Many researchers believe that the neurotransmitter *oxytocin* is key to this response. Essentially, women under stress appear to have higher levels of oxytocin than men in similar circumstances and are more likely to form tight social alliances, be empathic, and seek out friends for support when stress levels are high. In contrast, men are more likely to withdraw when highly stressed.[13]

LO 3 | PHYSICAL EFFECTS OF STRESS

Examine the physical health risks that may occur with chronic stress.

Researchers have only recently begun to untangle the complex web of responses that can take a toll on a person's physical, intellectual, and emotional well-being. Stress is often described as a disease of prolonged arousal that leads to a cascade of negative health effects. Some warning symptoms of prolonged stress are shown in **FIGURE 3.4**.

The higher the levels of stress you experience and the longer that stress continues, the greater is the likelihood of damage to your physical health.[14] A recent international study indicated a universal tendency toward heart attack and stroke among people with chronically high stress in their lives.[15] New research indicates that the more **cumulative adversity** (total stressor exposure, including complex trauma) some groups experience, the greater is their risk of psychopathology and developmental problems as well as increased risk for a wide range of social, emotional, and psychological problems.[16]

immunocompetence The ability of the immune system to respond to attack.

transactional model of stress and coping A theory proposed by psychologist Richard Lazarus, saying that our reaction to stress is about the interaction between perception, coping ability, and environment.

minority stress perspective A theory positing that minority stress may be partially explained by disparities and the chronic stress inherent in populations in which rejection, alienation, and hostility persist.

Yerkes-Dodson law of arousal A theory suggesting that when arousal or stress increases, performance goes up to a point, after which performance declines.

cumulative adversity Total stressor exposure, including complex trauma.

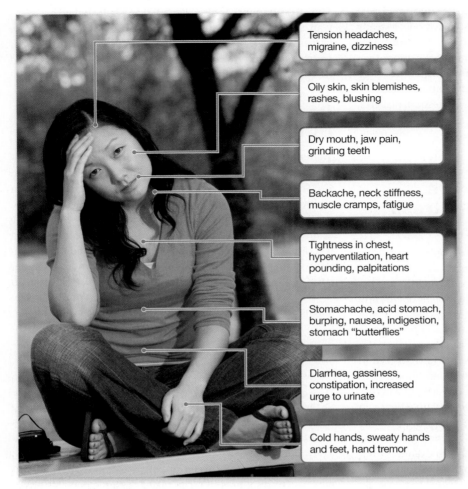

The labeled callouts in the figure read:

- Tension headaches, migraine, dizziness
- Oily skin, skin blemishes, rashes, blushing
- Dry mouth, jaw pain, grinding teeth
- Backache, neck stiffness, muscle cramps, fatigue
- Tightness in chest, hyperventilation, heart pounding, palpitations
- Stomachache, acid stomach, burping, nausea, indigestion, stomach "butterflies"
- Diarrhea, gassiness, constipation, increased urge to urinate
- Cold hands, sweaty hands and feet, hand tremor

FIGURE 3.4 Common Physical Symptoms of Stress Sometimes you might not notice how stressed you are until your body starts sending you signals. Do you frequently experience any of these physical symptoms of stress?

when you are extremely stressed, you didn't imagine it. Higher stress levels may increase cortisol levels in the bloodstream, which contributes to increased hunger and seems to activate fat-storing enzymes. Animal and human studies, including those in which subjects suffer from posttraumatic stress, seem to support the theory that cortisol plays a role in laying down extra belly fat and increasing eating behaviors.[19]

Stress and Hair Loss: A Little Known Fact

Too much stress can lead to thinning hair and even baldness in men and women. The most common type of stress-induced hair loss is *telogen effluvium*. Often seen in individuals who have lost a loved one or those who have experienced severe weight loss or other trauma, this condition pushes groups of hair follicles into a resting phase. Over time, hair falls out. Typically, this is not a permanent condition and the hair will begin to grow again. A similar stress-related condition known as *alopecia areata* occurs when stress triggers white blood cells to attack and destroy hair follicles, usually in patches.[20]

Stress and Cardiovascular Disease

Perhaps the most studied and documented health consequence of unresolved stress is cardiovascular disease (CVD). Recent research indicates that chronic stress plays a significant role in increased risk of heart arrhythmias, high blood pressure, hardening of the arteries, inflammation in blood vessels that increases risks of atherosclerosis, and several other CVD risks.[17]

In recent decades, research into the relationship between stress and CVD has shown direct links between the incidence and progression of CVD and stressors such as job strain, caregiving, bereavement, and natural disasters.[18] (For more on CVD, see Chapter 13.)

Stress and Weight Gain

Are you a "stress eater" or "emotional eater"? Do you run for the refrigerator when you are under pressure or feeling anxious or down? If you think you tend to eat more and gain weight

Stress and Diabetes

New guidelines from the American Diabetes Association highlight the importance of stress management in reducing the risk of type 2 diabetes and helping with short- and long-term diabetes prognosis.[21] People who are under a lot of stress often don't get enough sleep, may be depressed or suffer from anxiety, might not eat well, and may drink or take other drugs to help them get through a stressful time. All of these behaviors can alter blood sugar levels and appear to increase the risks of type 2 diabetes.[22] Stress hormones, particularly cortisol, may affect blood glucose levels directly.[23] (For more, see **Focus On: Minimizing Your Risk for Diabetes**.)

Stress and Digestive Problems

Digestive disorders are physical conditions for which causes are often unknown. It is widely assumed that an underlying illness, pathogen, injury, or inflammation is already present when stress triggers nausea, vomiting, stomach cramps and

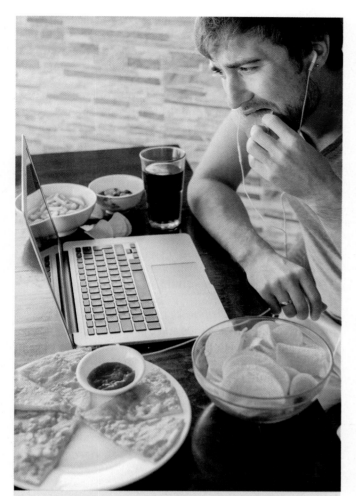

High stress levels may increase cortisol levels in the bloodstream, increasing hunger and encouraging stress eating.

gut pain, or diarrhea. Although stress doesn't directly cause these symptoms, it is clearly related to them and may make your risk of having symptoms worse.[24] For example, people with depression or anxiety or who feel tense, angry, or overwhelmed are more susceptible to dehydration, inflammation, and other digestive problems.[25]

Stress and Impaired Immunity

A growing area of scientific investigation known as **psychoneuroimmunology** analyzes the intricate relationship between the mind's response to stress and the immune system's ability to function effectively. Several recent research reviews suggest that too much stress over a long period can negatively affect various aspects of the cellular immune response. This increases risks for upper respiratory infections and certain chronic conditions, increases adverse fetal development and birth outcomes in pregnant women, and exacerbates problems for children and adults suffering from posttraumatic stress.[26] More prolonged stressors, such as the loss of a loved one, caregiving, living with a handicap, and unemployment, also have been shown to impair the natural immune response over time.[27]

LO 4 | WHEN OVERWHELM STRIKES: THREATS TO MENTAL HEALTH

Examine the intellectual and psychological effects of stress and their impacts on college students.

In a recent national survey of college students, 56 percent of respondents (43 percent of men and 61 percent of women) said they felt overwhelmed by all that they had to do within the past 2 weeks, and a similar number reported feeling exhausted.[28] Nearly 56 percent of students reported more than average or tremendous stress in the last year. Not surprisingly, these same students rated stress as their number one impediment to academic achievement.[29] Stress can play a huge role in whether students stay in school, get good grades, and succeed on their career path. It can also wreak havoc on students' ability to concentrate, understand, and retain information.

Stress, Memory, and Concentration

Although the exact ways in which stress affects grades and job performance are complex, new research provides possible clues. Animal studies suggest that *glucocorticoids*—stress hormones released from the adrenal cortex—may affect cognitive functioning and overall mental health. In humans, memory is impaired when acute stress bombards the brain with hormones and neurotransmitters, affecting the way we think, make decisions, and respond in stressful situations.[30] Recent laboratory studies have linked prolonged exposure to cortisol to actual shrinking of the hippocampus, the brain's major memory center.[31] Other research indicates that prolonged exposure to high levels of stress hormones may actually predispose women, in particular, to Alzheimer's disease.[32] More research is needed to determine the validity of these theories.

Psychological Effects of Stress

Stress may be one of the single greatest contributors to mental disability and emotional dysfunction in industrialized nations. Studies have shown that chronic stress may cause structural degeneration and impaired function of the brain, leading to depression, dementia, and Alzheimer's disease as well as an overactive *amygdala* (the region of the brain associated with emotional responses), which may increase rates of violence.[33]

LO 5 | WHAT CAUSES STRESS?

Discuss sources of stress, and examine the unique stressors that affect young adults, particularly college students.

Stress comes from a wide range of sources. The American Psychological Association annually conducts one of the most

psychoneuroimmunology The study of the interrelationship between mind and body on immune system functioning.

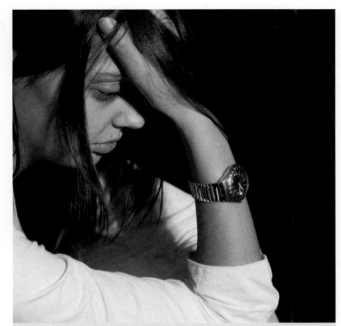

Stress, anxiety, and depression have complicated interconnections based on emotional, physiological, and biochemical processes. Prolonged stress can trigger depression in susceptible people, and prior periods of depression can leave individuals more susceptible to stress.

comprehensive studies examining sources of stress among various populations. The 2015 survey found that concerns over money, work, family responsibilities, and personal and family health and the economy were the biggest reported causes of stress for American adults (**FIGURE 3.5**).[34] Younger adults and women are more likely to struggle with stress.[35] The good news is that increasing numbers of Americans recognize the physical and mental effects of stress on health and are seeking psychological help for problems as well as engaging in mindfulness-related activities to avoid, prevent, or control stress.[36]

College Students: Adjusting to Change

College students face a number of stressors—from both internal sources and external ones, particularly around succeeding in what can be a competitive environment. Unfortunately, although your first days on campus can be exciting, they can also be among the most stressful you will face in your life. Moving away from home, trying to fit in and make new friends, adjusting to a new schedule, and learning to live with strangers in housing that often lacks the comforts of home can all cause sleeplessness and anxiety and may keep your body in a continual fight-or-flight mode.

Hassles: Little Things That Bug You

A growing chorus of psychologists propose that the little stressors, frustrations, and petty annoyances, known collectively as *hassles*, can eventually be just as stressful and damaging to your physical and mental health as major life changes.[37] Cumulative hassles add up, increasing allostatic load and resulting in wear and tear on body systems. Listening to others monopolize class time, long lines, hunting for parking, loud music while you are trying to study, and a host of other irritants can push your buttons, triggering fight-or-flight responses. A lifetime of hassles can wreak havoc on the body, triggering mental health issues, high blood pressure, and other chronic health problems.[38] In addition to life and work stressors, electronic devices pose increased stress load for many. See the **Mindfulness and You** box for more on technostress.

Stress: The Toll of Relationships

Let's face it: Relationships can trigger some of the biggest fight-or-flight reactions of all. Although romantic relationships are the ones we often think of first, relationships with other people in our lives, particularly coworkers, can lead to high stress. Characteristics of the job such as job insecurity, jobs with high demands and low control, jobs in which people must compete for promotions and raises, and jobs in which there are unrelenting performance expectations increase health risk. New research points to personality characteristics that may exacerbate high-stress health risks, particularly for people who are driven and are constantly overcommitting on what they can accomplish.[39] Competition for rewards and systems that favor certain classes of employees or pit workers against one another are among the most stressful job situations.

Money and Stress

College and university students face a number of difficulties managing ever-increasing tuition, housing costs, and general expenses of college life. Many students must hold jobs to

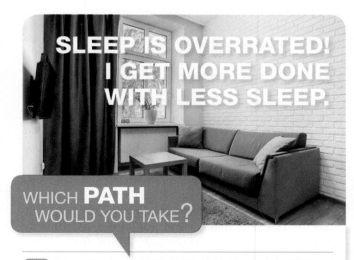

SLEEP IS OVERRATED! I GET MORE DONE WITH LESS SLEEP.

WHICH **PATH** WOULD YOU TAKE?

Go to Mastering Health to play Which Path Would You Take? and see where decisions like these lead you!

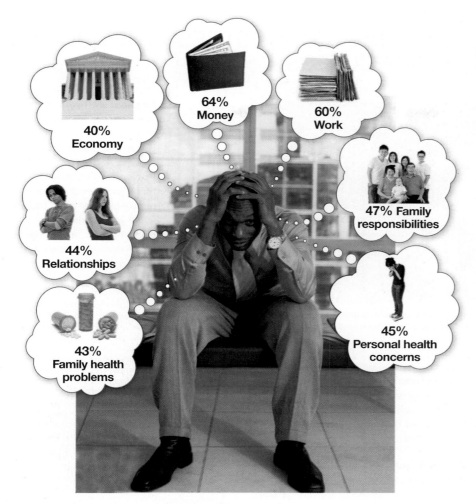

FIGURE 3.5 What Do We Say Stresses Us? These data represent the percentage of American adults who reported each category as a very significant or somewhat significant source of stress in their lives. Money, work, family responsibilities, and health are the top stressors.

Source: Data from American Psychological Association, "Stress in America: Paying with Our Health," 2015, http://www.apa.org/news/press/releases/stress/2014/stress-report.pdf.

Like other forms of acute and chronic stress, money worries are among the biggest sources of stress in the United States and can lead to many health problems.[42]

Stress, Frustration, and Conflict

Whenever there is a disparity between our goals (what we hope to obtain in life) and our behaviors (actions that may or may not lead to these goals), frustration can occur. Conflicts occur when we are forced to decide among competing motives, impulses, desires, and behaviors (for example, to party or study) or when we are forced to face pressures or demands that are incompatible with our values and sense of importance (for example, pressure to get good grades or compete in college athletics). College students may face a variety of conflicts among their parents' values, their own beliefs, and the beliefs of people who are different from themselves.

Overload

Overload occurs when we are overextended and, try as we might, there are not enough hours in the day to do everything we need to do. Students suffering from overload may experience depression, sleeplessness, mood swings, frustration, anxiety, or a host of other symptoms. Binge drinking and high consumption of junk food—

stay afloat, and some incur huge student loan debt. According to recent estimates, the 2016 graduating class was the most indebted class ever, with over 70 percent of students graduating with staggering debts, averaging over $37,000. This occurred at a time when the job market had tightened and the price of housing had skyrocketed. Over 11 percent of these students are likely to default on these loans, and another 39 percent will move back in with their parents or already have. Statistics are even worse among private and for-profit online graduate programs.[40] Worries over finding a job after graduation coupled with the need to repay student loans underscore the fact that finances are a major source of stress for most students.[41]

What's more, because money is often seen as an indicator of status and success, individuals with long-term financial insecurity may experience increased feelings of inferiority, low self-esteem, and self-doubt. These feelings are in part due to **relative deprivation**—the inability of lower-income groups to sustain the same lifestyle as higher-income groups in the same community.

often coping strategies for stress overload—catch many in a downward spiral as their negative behaviors actually add to their stress load. Unrelenting stress and overload can lead to a state of physical and mental exhaustion known as **burnout**.

Stressful Environments

For many students, their living environment causes significant levels of stress. Perhaps you cannot afford safe, comfortable housing; perhaps a troublesome or incompatible roommate constantly makes your life miserable; or perhaps loud neighbors prevent you from sleeping at night. Noise,

relative deprivation The inability of lower-income groups to sustain the same lifestyle as higher-income groups in the same community, often resulting in feelings of anxiety and inferiority.

overload A condition in which a person feels overly pressured by demands.

burnout A state of physical and mental exhaustion resulting from unrelenting stress.

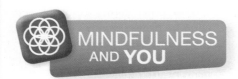

MINDFULNESS AND YOU

BEATING TECHNOSTRESS THROUGH MINDFULNESS

If you become anxious when you get to class and realize that you forgot your phone, you may need to think about why even an hour unplugged is more than you can take. *High-frequency cell phone* use is on the rise, and with it comes a variety of problems. According to a new study, college students who can't keep their hands off their mobile devices are reporting higher levels of anxiety, less satisfaction with life, and lower grades than peers who use their devices less often. The average student surveyed spent nearly 5 hours per day using their cell phones. Are you surprised?

Technostress refers to stress created by a dependence on technology and the constant state of connection, which can include a perceived obligation to respond, chat, or tweet. Some have likened this obsession to a form of *technology addiction*, whereby individuals may check their phones 35 to 50 times on an average day, even waking in the night to respond. Such obsessive behavior can sap energy, lead to insomnia/sleep disorders, damage relationships and normal in-person interactions, and hurt grades. The negative consequences of these addictive behaviors, which are sometimes labeled *iDisorders*, are on the rise. If you

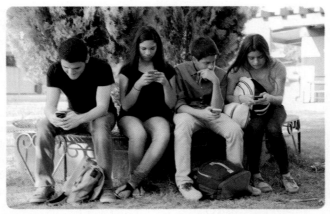

Technology may keep you in touch, but it can also add to your stress and take you away from healthful real-world interactions.

find yourself in an unhealthy relationship with your smartphone or tablet, it may be time to unplug. Here are some mindful strategies that may help you live more in the moment:

- **Schedule screen time**. Set aside time to check e-mail, text messages, and your Facebook and Twitter feeds. Resist the urge to check if you're outside this set time frame. NO reading messages in the middle of the night!
- **Unfriend the annoying and offensive**. Lighten your load by focusing only on the people who really matter to you and add to your day in a positive way.

- **Connect with your friends in real time**. Socialize with friends in person. And while you're at it, put your phone away.
- **Power devices down**. Turn off all your devices completely (not just silent mode) when you're driving, in class, at work, in bed, having dinner with friends, or on vacation.

Sources: S. Deatherage, H. Servaty-Seib, and I. Aksoz, "Stress, Coping and the Internet Use of College Students," *Journal of American Health* 62, no. 1 (2014): 40–46; Y. Lee et al., "The Dark Side of Smartphone Usage: Psychological Traits, Compulsive Behavior and Technostress," *Computers in Human Behavior* 31 (2014): 373–81; A. Lepp, J. Barkley, and A. Karpinski, "The Relationship between Cell Phone Use, Academic Performance, Anxiety, and Satisfaction with Life in College Students," *Computers in Human Behavior* 31 (2014): 343–50; G. Guitierez, et al."Cell Phone Addiction: A Review. 7(2016).https://www.ncbi.nlm.nih.gov/pmc/articles/PMC5076301/. H. Elgendi. "The Effect of Facebook on College Students" *International Journal of Networks and Communications*, Vol. 5 No. 2. 2015, pp. 37-40. doi: 10.5923/j.ijnc.20150502.03. T. Panova and A. Lleras. "Avoidance or boredom: Negative mental health outcomes associated with use of Information and Communication Technologies depend on users' motivations." *Computers in Human Behavior*, 2016; 58: 249 DOI: 10.1016/j.chb.2015.12.06.

pressure of people in crowded living situations, and uncertainties over food and housing can keep even the most resilient person on edge.

Natural disasters can cause tremendous stress both when they occur and for years afterwards. Typhoons and hurricanes, earthquakes and tsunamis, and killer tornadoes as well as human-generated disasters such as the *Exxon Valdez* and Gulf oil spills, terrorist attacks, and the devastation of war have disrupted millions of lives and damaged ecosystems. Even after the initial images of suffering pass and the crisis has subsided, shortages of vital resources such as gasoline, clean water, food, housing, health care, sewage disposal, and other necessities, as well as electricity outages and transportation problems, can devastate local communities and campuses.

background distressors
Environmental stressors of which people are often unaware.

72%

of adults report feeling **STRESSED ABOUT MONEY** at least some of the time; 26 percent report feeling stressed about money *all* the time.

Background distressors in the environment, such as noise, air, and water pollution; allergy-aggravating pollen and dust; unsafe food; or environmental tobacco smoke can also be incredibly stressful. As with other challenges, our bodies respond to environmental distressors with the GAS. People

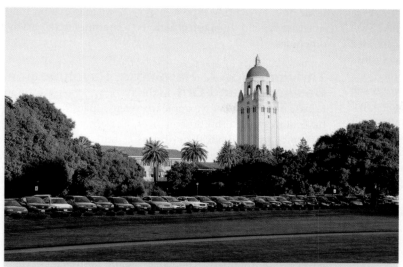

Although campus parking fees have increased, finding parking can be a major stressor, as permits often amount to "hunting licenses" rather than parking permits.

real and perceived experiences. Low self-esteem, negative appraisal, lack of self-compassion, fears and anxiety, narcissistic tendencies, and other learned behaviors and coping mechanisms can increase stress levels.

Appraisal

A lot of times, our **appraisal** of life's demands, not the demands themselves, result in experiences of stress. Appraisal is defined as the interpretation and evaluation of information provided to the brain by the senses. As new information becomes available, appraisal helps us recognize stressors, evaluate them on the basis of past experiences and emotions, and decide whether we can cope. When you feel that the stressors of life are overwhelming and you lack control, you're more likely to feel strain and distress.

Self-Esteem

Recall that *self-esteem* refers to your sense of self-worth—how you judge yourself in comparison to others. Research on adolescents and young adults indicates that high stress and low self-esteem significantly predict **suicidal ideation**, a desire to die and thoughts about suicide. Fortunately, research has shown that you can improve your ability to cope with stress by increasing self-esteem.[43]

While a healthy dose of self-esteem has long been regarded as necessary for mental health, new research also points to a potential dark side. Critics of the self-esteem movement point

WHAT DO YOU THINK?

Do you get stressed out by things in your home or school environment?

- Which environmental stressors bug you the most?
- When you encounter these environmental stressors, what actions do you take, if any?

who cannot escape background distressors may exist in a constant resistance phase.

Bias and Discrimination

Racial and ethnic diversity of students, faculty members, and staff enriches everyone's educational experience on campus. It also challenges us to examine our personal attitudes, beliefs, and biases. Today's campuses include a diverse cultural base of vastly different life experiences, languages, and customs. Bias and discrimination based on race, ethnicity, religious affiliation, age, sexual orientation, or other real or perceived differences—whether in viewpoints, appearance, behaviors, or backgrounds—can take the form of bigotry, insensitivity, harassment, hostility, or simply ignoring a person or group and can have major effects on health. (see **Focus On: Difference, Disparity, and Health: Achieving Health Equity** for more).

LO 6 | INDIVIDUAL FACTORS THAT AFFECT YOUR STRESS RESPONSE

Explain key individual factors that may influence whether or not a person is able to cope with stressors

Although stress can come from the environment and external sources, it can also be a result of internal or individual factors—the "baggage" that we carry with us from a lifetime of

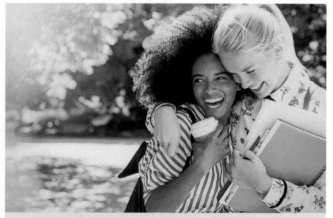

New research indicates that hugging doesn't just feel good, it can also buffer the effects of stress in your life. Hug more, and pay attention to how hugs make you feel. Hugging may just be one of the easiest stress reducers in your day!

Source: S. Cohen, et al., "Does Hugging Provide Stress-Buffering Social Support? A Study of Susceptibility to Upper Respiratory Infection and Illness," *Psychological Science* 26, no. 2 (2015): 135–47.)

to the fact that today's college students have the highest level of narcissism ever recorded and that quests to have thousands of "friends" on Facebook or huge Twitter followings can be significant stressors.[44] Environments in which individuals are always compared to others as indicators of self-worth may contribute to more elitism, more bullying in a quest for power, more prejudice between groups, and more difficulties in working with other people after graduation.[45]

Self-Efficacy

Research has shown that people with high levels of confidence in their skills and ability to cope with life's challenges tend to feel more in control of stressful situations and report fewer stress effects.[46] Self-efficacy is considered one of the most important personality traits that influences psychological and physiological stress responses.[47] Developing self-efficacy is also vital to coping with and overcoming academic pressures and worries.[48] High test anxiety has been shown to account for up to 15 percent of the variance in student performance on exams.[49] Research suggests that if you learn to handle test anxiety, your confidence may increase and your test scores will improve, leading to improved performance overall.[50] Tips on how to deal with test anxiety and build your testing self-efficacy can be found in the Skills for Behavior Change box.

Type A and Type B Personalities

It's no surprise that personality can have affect whether you are happy and socially well adjusted or sad and socially isolated. But personality may also be a critical factor in determining your stress levels and your risk for CVD, cancer, and other chronic and infectious diseases.

In 1974, physicians Meyer Friedman and Ray Rosenman published a book indicating that so-called Type A individuals had a greatly increased risk of heart disease due to increased physiological reactivity and prolonged activation of the stress response, including increased heart rate and blood pressure.[51] *Type A* personalities have been defined as hard-driving, competitive, time-driven perfectionists. In contrast, *Type B* personalities are described as being relaxed, noncompetitive, and more tolerant of others. Today, most researchers recognize that

How daunting that pile of books and homework is depends on your appraisal of it.

none of us are wholly Type A or Type B; we may exhibit traits of either type in different situations, sometimes with varying outcomes.

Thriving Type A: Hardiness, Psychological Resilience, and Grit

In the 1970s, psychologist Susan Kobasa noted that many people who were super stressed didn't have negative health consequences. She aptly described the theory of **psychological hardiness** as indicating that hardy individuals were unique in their *control, commitment,* and *willingness to embrace challenges* in life rather than succumbing to them.[52] Today, Kobasa's work has been expanded and refined to suggest that some individuals even seem to thrive on their supercharged lifestyles, at least in the short term. These individuals are described as having **psychological resilience**—a dynamic process in which people exposed to sustained adversity or traumatic challenges adapt positively.[53] These high-achieving *thrivers* often demonstrate (1) a positive and proactive personality; (2) experience and learning history that contributes to self-efficacy; (3) a sense of control, flexibility, and adaptability—an ability to "go with the flow"; (4) balance and perspective in their reactions; and (5) a perceived safety net of social support.[54] Newer researchers have focused their attention on another factor that contributes to thriving and resilience despite stress: **grit**, which is a combination of passion and perseverance in striving for a singularly important goal that high achievers demonstrate in all walks of life.[55] Studies of youth have shown that stress management and mindfulness training may help people develop resilience and grit, particularly if they have strong social support, healthy family environments, and community supports during the stress management programming.[56]

Type A and a Toxic Core

In contrast to those who thrive, some Type A individuals exhibit a "toxic core" made up of a disproportionate amount of negative emotions, including anger, fear, volatility, distrust, grief, and a cynical, glass-half-empty approach to life—a set of characteristics referred to as **hostility**. These individuals have an increased risk for heart disease and a host of other health issues.[57]

Broken Heart Syndrome

Also known as stress-induced cardiomyopathy, *broken heart syndrome* is the very real heart damage experienced by some people as a result of chronic, debilitating stress; depression; loss; a breakup; betrayal; or another major emotional blow. The resulting overload of stress hormones, such as adrenaline, can lead to short-circuiting of the heart's electrical system (including serious arrythmias) or damage to the heart muscle (cardiomyopathy), interfering with the heart's ability to move blood. With symptoms similar to those of a heart attack, this syndrome can lead to heart failure and even death if untreated.[58]

Type C and Type D Personalities

In addition to CVD, personality types have often been linked to increased risk for a variety of other illnesses. A third personality type is the *Type C* personality, characterized as stoic, with a tendency to stuff feelings down and conform to the wishes of others. Preliminary research suggests that Type C individuals may be more susceptible to illnesses such as asthma, multiple sclerosis, autoimmune disorders, and cancer; however, more research is necessary to support this relationship.[59]

A more recently identified personality type is *Type D* (distressed), which is characterized by a tendency toward excessive negative worry, irritability, gloom, and social inhibition. Several recent studies have indicated that Type D people may be up to eight times more likely to die of a heart attack or sudden death.[60]

Shift and Persist

Some young people who face extreme poverty, abuse, and unspeakable living conditions as they grow up seem to thrive, despite bleak conditions. Why? An emerging body of sociological research proposes that in the midst of extreme, persistent adversity, young people—often with the help of positive role models in their lives—are able to reframe appraisals of current stressors more positively (*shifting*) while *persisting* in focusing on the future. This outlook enables people to endure the present by adapting, holding onto meaningful things in their lives, and staying optimistic and positive. These **shift and persist** strategies are among the most recently identified factors that protect against the negative effects of stress in our lives.[61]

LO 7 | MANAGING STRESS IN COLLEGE: DEALING WITH OVERWHELM

Explore stress management and stress reduction strategies, ways you can cope more effectively with stress, and mindfulness strategies that can enrich your life experiences and reduce health risks.

College students thrive under a certain amount of stress; however, excessive stress can leave them overwhelmed and unable to cope. Recent studies of college students indicate that the emotional health self-rating of first-year college students compared to their peers is at an all-time low. In fact, researchers report that the emotional health of students has declined precipitously since surveys were first conducted in 1985 and that increasing numbers of these students frequently feel overwhelmed.[62] They spend more time studying and less time socializing with friends, and nearly 10 percent report that they are driven to succeed and are frequently depressed.[63] In contrast, sophomores and juniors reported fewer problems with these issues, and seniors reported the fewest problems. This may indicate students' progressive emotional growth through experience, maturity, increased awareness of support services, and more social connections.[64] It is also possible that some of the highly stressed first-year students did not continue their college education.

Although you can't eliminate all life stressors, you can train yourself to recognize the events that cause stress and to anticipate your reactions to them. **Coping** is the act of managing events or conditions to lessen the physical or psychological effects of excess stress.[65] One of the most effective ways to combat stressors is to build coping strategies and skills, known collectively as *stress management techniques*. Training in mindfulness strategies, particularly **dispositional mindfulness**—an acute "tuning in" to and awareness of your thoughts, feelings, and reaction, focused on finding nonjudgmental views of situations—may significantly improve your overall stress responses.[66]

shift and persist A strategy of reframing appraisals of current stressors and focusing on a meaningful future that protects a person from the negative effects of too much stress.

coping Managing events or conditions to lessen the physical or psychological effects of excess stress.

dispositional mindfulness An acute tuning in and awareness of your thoughts, feelings, and reactions, focused on finding nonjudgmental views of situations.

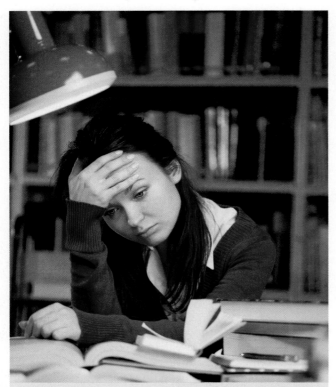

Studies suggest that college students are more stressed out than other groups. The combination of a new environment, peer and parent pressures, and juggling the demands of work, school, and a social life likely contribute to this phenomenon.

A Mindful Approach to Stress

Stress management isn't something that just happens. It calls for getting a handle on what is going on in your life, taking a careful look at yourself, and coming up with a personal plan of action.

One useful way of coping with your stressors is to consciously anticipate and prepare for specific ones, a technique known as **stress inoculation**. For example, if speaking in front of a class scares you, practice in front of friends or a video camera to prevent freezing up on the day of the presentation.

Because your perceptions are often part of the problem, assessing your self-talk, beliefs, and actions are good first steps. The tools in this section will help you.

Assess Your Stressors to Solve Problems

Mindfully Before you can prevent or control your life stressors, you must first analyze them. Several quick mindfulness assessments—which may help you look at your daily experiences and whether you are tuned in or merely reacting to circumstances—are available online. Beyond self-assessments, here are some more suggestions for ways to de-stress:

- **Start a journal.** Track your worries and the factors that seem to trigger stress every

stress inoculation Stress management technique in which a person consciously anticipates and prepares for potential stressors.

day for 1 week. Think about when your stress is greatest, who is around you, and how you respond. Do you move on, or do you tend to dwell on things?

- **Examine the causes of your stress.** Which are tangible? Which are intangible?
- **Think about what is going on with you right now.** Are you wound up and edgy? Tired? A bit ticked at someone? Focus on your body. Are you tense? Sweating? Exhausted? Breathe deeply several times, and focus on your breath. Take a moment that is all about you. Tune in in you, and tune out whatever is bothering you.
- **Take a 10-minute break.** Go for a walk. Focus on the smells in the air, the colors of the landscape, or anything that takes you away from your worries. If you hear yourself being judgmental, either aloud or in your thoughts, stop. Focus on one good thing about someone near you. Smile at a stranger.
- **Focus on your stressor.** Whether it's unnecessary clutter, conflict with friends and family, or chaotic world events putting you over the edge, jot down three things you will change, starting now—and then *act!* Limit your exposure to unsettling news to no more than 30 minutes a day. Take care of clutter. Focus on something positive.

A mindful action plan—in which you increase your self-awareness, tune in to your body and surroundings, and assess your stressors and how to avoid them—can help to reduce stress. There's a lot here, but it doesn't take earth-shattering changes to help you cope. Making small changes now—and focusing in on your life and reactions—can really make a difference.

Change Your Inner Voice: Be Compassion-

ate Often we are our own worst enemies—nicer to strangers than we are to ourselves or to people we care about. Remember that *compassion* includes kindness, empathy, tolerance, concern for others, sensitivity, and a desire to help someone who needs emotional or tangible help. Unfortunately, many of us grieve for hurt animals but walk right past homeless people without looking at them, treating them as objects. Likewise, our biases, beliefs, and values can keep us from being compassionate toward certain groups. We can also be our own worst critics and show little compassion for ourselves.

A good place to begin is with *self-compassion*. Start each day with two or three things you are thankful for—the good things in your life or something you like about yourself—instead of seeing only faults. Practicing mindfulness can help to reduce your stress interactions, help you become less sensitive to potential criticisms, and let you look at your day in a more positive light.

Several types of negative self-talk exist. Among the most common are *pessimism*, or focusing on the negative; *perfectionism*, or expecting superhuman standards; "*should-ing*," or reprimanding yourself for things that you should have done; *blaming* yourself or others for circumstances and events; and *dichotomous thinking*, in which everything is either black or white (good or bad). To combat negative self-talk, we must first become aware of it, then stop it, and finally replace the negative thoughts with positive ones—a process called **cognitive restructuring**. Once you realize that some of your thoughts may be negative, irrational, or overreactive or reflect a bias, interrupt this self-talk by saying, "Stop" (under your breath or aloud), and make a conscious effort to think positively. See the Skills for Behavior Change box for other suggestions of ways to mindfully rethink your thinking.

Developing a Support Network

As you plan a stress management program, remember the importance of social networks and social bonds. Friendships are important for inoculating yourself against harmful stressors. Studies of college students have demonstrated the importance of social support, particularly from trusted friends and family in *buffering* individuals from the effects of adverse childhood stressors.[67] Most colleges and universities offer counseling services at no cost for short-term crises when the pressures of life seem overwhelming. Clergy, instructors, and residence hall supervisors also may be excellent resources.

To have a healthy social support network, you have to invest time and energy. Cultivate and nurture the relationships that matter: those built on trust, mutual acceptance and understanding, honesty, and genuine caring. If you want others to

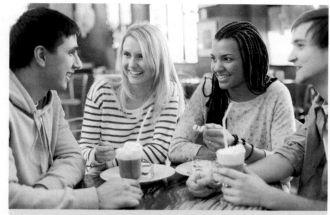

Face-to-face socializing is an important part of a healthy social life. How often recently have you had dinner with friends and everyone was talking to each other instead of checking their phones?

be there for you to help you cope with life's stressors, you need to be there for them. Spend more time in face-to-face interactions.

> **cognitive restructuring** The modification of thoughts, ideas, and beliefs that contribute to stress.

Cultivating Your Spiritual Side

One of the most important factors in reducing stress in your life is taking the time to cultivate your spiritual side: finding your purpose and living your days more fully. Spiritual health and practice can be vital components of your support system, often linking you to a community of like-minded individuals and giving you perspective. (For more, see **Focus On: Cultivating Your Spiritual Health**.)

Managing Emotional Responses

Have you ever been upset by something only to find that your perceptions were wrong? We often get upset not by realities, but by our faulty perceptions. In digital communications, it is too easy to read meaning into things that are said and perceive issues that don't exist. Interactions in which body language, voice intonation, and opportunities for clarification are present are much better for interpreting true meanings than are cryptic texts or e-mails.

Stress management requires examining your emotional responses. With any emotional response, you are responsible

43%

of people with no emotional support report significant **INCREASES IN OVERALL STRESS** levels in last year.

SKILLS FOR
BEHAVIOR CHANGE

A Mindful Rethinking of Your Thinking Habits

Sometimes, our own thinking habits can contribute to stress. Here are a few ways to rethink those stressful habits:

- Reframe a distressing event from a positive perspective. Change your perspective on the issue to highlight your strengths.

- Remember that nobody is perfect. Tolerate mistakes. Change your focus and self-talk. Take yourself less seriously, and cut the judgment.

- Let things be. Learn to accept what you cannot change, and remember that you don't always have to be in control.

- Break the worry habit. If you are preoccupied with what-ifs and worst-case scenarios, the following suggestions can help to slow the worry drain:

  - If you must worry, create a 20-minute "worry period" when you can journal or talk about your worrying each day. After that, block the worry if it pops up again.

  - Try to focus on what is going right rather than what *might* go wrong.

  - Seek help. Talk with a trusted friend or family member, or make an appointment with a counselor.

for the emotion and the resulting behaviors. Learning to tell the difference between normal emotional responses and emotions that are based on irrational beliefs or seem excessive can help you stop the emotion or express it in a healthy way.

Fight the Anger Urge Major sources of anger include (1) perceived *threats* to self or others we care about; (2) *reactions to injustice*, such as unfair actions, policies, or behaviors; (3) *fear*, which leads to negative responses (for more on this topic, see the Health Headlines box); (4) *faulty emotional reasoning*, or misinterpretation of normal events; (5) *low frustration tolerance*, often fueled by stress, drugs, lack of sleep, and other factors; (6) *unreasonable expectations* about ourselves and others; and (7) *people rating*, or applying derogatory ratings to others.

There are three main approaches to dealing with anger: *expressing it, suppressing it*, or *calming it*. You may be surprised to find out that expressing anger is probably the healthiest thing to do in the long run if you express it in an assertive rather than an aggressive way. There are several strategies you can use to keep aggressive reactions at bay:[68]

- **Identify your anger style.** Do you express anger passively or actively? Do you hold anger in, or do you explode?
- **Learn to recognize patterns in your anger responses and how to de-escalate them.** For one week, keep track of everything that angers you or keeps you stewing. What thoughts or feelings lead up to your boiling point? Explore ways to interrupt patterns of anger, such as counting to ten, getting a drink of water, or taking some deep breaths.
- **Find the right words to de-escalate conflict.** When conflict arises, be respectful and state your needs or feelings rather than shooting zingers at the other person. Avoid *"you* always" or *"you* never" and instead say, *"I* feel ___ when you ___" or *"I* would really appreciate it if you could ___." If you find yourself continually revved up for battle, consider taking a class or workshop on assertiveness training or anger management.
- **Plan ahead.** Explore options to minimize your exposure to anger-provoking situations, such as traffic jams.
- **Vent to your friends.** Find a few close friends you trust and who can be honest with you. Allow them to listen and give their perspectives on things, but don't wear down your supporters with continual rants.
- **Develop realistic expectations of yourself and others.** Are your expectations of yourself and others realistic? Try talking about your feelings with the people involved at a time when you are calm.
- **Turn complaints into requests.** When you are frustrated or angry with someone, try reworking the problem into a request. Instead of screaming and pounding on the wall because your neighbors are blaring music at 2 A.M., talk with them. Think about the words you will use, and try to reach an agreement that works for everyone.
- **Leave past anger in the past.** Learn to resolve issues and not bring them up over and over. Let it go. If you can't seem to do that, seek the counsel of a professional to learn how.

Learn to Laugh, Be Joyful, and Cry Adages such as "Laughter is the best medicine" and "Smile and the world smiles with you" didn't come from nowhere. Humans have long recognized that actions such as smiling, laughing, singing, and dancing can elevate our moods, relieve stress, and improve our relationships. Crying can have similar positive physiological effects. Preliminary research indicates that laughter and joy may increase endorphin levels, increase oxygen levels in the blood, decrease stress levels, relieve pain, help in recovery from cardiovascular disease, improve relationships, and even reduce risks of chronic disease. However, evidence for long-term effects requires more rigorous study.[69]

Taking Physical Action

Do you often feel sluggish and ready to nap? Or do you tend to feel wired, restless, and ready to explode? Either could be the result of too much stress.

Get Enough Exercise Remember that the human stress response is intended to end in physical activity (fight or flight). Exercise "burns off" existing stress hormones by directing them toward their intended metabolic function.[70]

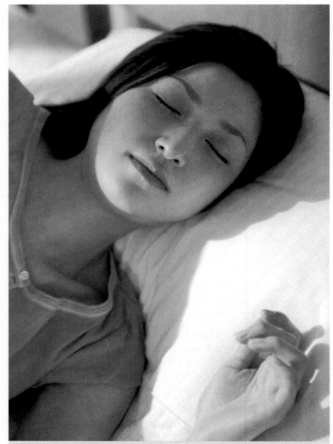

Taking care of your physical health—through good-quality sleep, sufficient exercise, and healthful nutrition—is a crucial component of stress management.

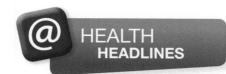

AN EPIDEMIC OF FEAR IN AMERICA
Stressing Ourselves Out Needlessly, Or Real Threat?

If someone were to ask you what you were most afraid of—what your greatest fear was right now—what would you respond? It may not surprise you, but when a sample of Americans was asked to rate their top 10 fears in 2015, these things were rated highly by significant percentages of respondents:

- Corruption of government officials (58.0%)
- Cyber-terrorism (44.8%)
- Corporate tracking of personal information (44.6%)
- Terrorist attacks (44.4%)
- Government tracking of personal information (41.4%)
- Bio-warfare (40.9%)
- Identity theft (39.6%)
- Economic collapse (39.2%)
- Running out of money in the future (37.4%)
- Credit card fraud (36.9%)

Consider the following "selfchecks" whenever your fears seem to be hindering your behaviors:

1. Are my fears rational or irrational? Where is the evidence that because a shooting took place in Florida, that I will be shot at a concert or football game in my community? What is the threat to me here and now based on statistics? What safety nets are in place to protect me?
2. Can I do anything about it? Are there things I can do to protect myself?

Four-legged friends can be great stress relievers as they allow you to focus on something besides yourself and can add laughter to your life.

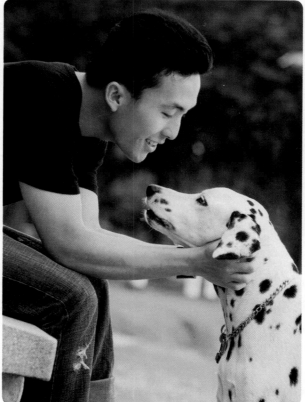

3. Where is the evidence that government officials are corrupt? Is it real or just part of the growing viciousness of political campaigns and ways that people discredit others in the media to gain advantage. Am I being manipulated by myths/misperceptions about situations to win votes? Even if part of the corruption in politics is true, are

there things I can do to change the situation?

4. Have I educated myself about the facts? Is the Zika Virus present in my area right now? Because a restaurant had a foodborne outbreak, should I avoid similar restaurants? What can I do to ensure my safety? What can I do to find out more about a situation and actions I can take?
5. Have I thought about what is triggering my fears? Is there anyone I can talk to about it? Are there any support groups or speakers in my area where I can go to discuss issues, vent and express my concerns?
6. Have my fears prevented me from doing something I really like to do or from going places I would love to go? If so, answering items 1-5 above might help me get a grip on my fears and better understand that my beliefs are unrealistic and causing me to alter my lifestyle in negative and unnecessary ways. If you find out that your fears are real, take action to stay safe, seek support from others.

Source: S. Ledbetter, "America's Top Fears, 2015," The Chapman University Survey of American Fears, 2015, October 13, 2015, https://blogs.chapman.edu/wilkinson/2015/10/13/americas-top-fears-2015/.

Exercise can also help combat stress by raising levels of endorphins—mood-elevating, painkilling hormones—in the bloodstream, increasing energy, reducing hostility, and improving mental alertness. Still, according to a recent meta-analysis of stress and exercise research, the people who would benefit most—particularly sedentary, overweight individuals—are more likely to eat when they are stressed and less likely to exercise. Motivating reluctant people to exercise for health and stress relief is a major challenge that could reap huge rewards.[71] (For more on the beneficial effects of exercise, see Chapter 12.)

Get Enough Sleep Adequate amounts of sleep allow you to refresh your vital energy, cope with multiple stressors more effectively, and be productive when you need to be. In fact, sleep is one of the biggest stress busters of them all.

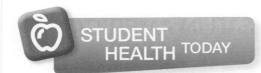

FENG SHUI FOR STRESS RELIEF

Today, many interior designers are trying to create peaceful "me caves" for reducing the stress of harried lives. *Feng shui* (translation: "wind and water") is part of an ancient Chinese art designed to restore balance of *chi* and create peace and harmony with help from the built environment. Several feng shui tips can help reduce stress in your bedroom area:

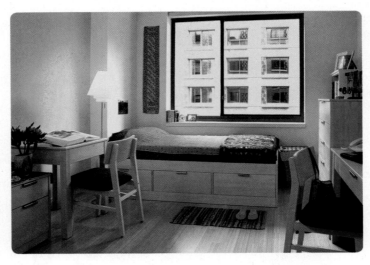

Keeping your room clear of clutter and well organized using feng shui techniques can reduce stress.

- **De-clutter.** Get rid of any extra material objects in your space. Pick up and put things away each day.
- **Beautify.** Paint your room with peaceful, welcoming colors. Coordinate the colors of your walls and linens to enhance warmth. Include objects that make you feel peaceful.

- **Relocate.** Your bed should never be in line with the door. Nightstands should be balanced on either side of bed, and mirrors should never reflect the bed.
- **Shut out the world.** Use shades that allow you to dim or darken the room. If you can't get rid of a desk covered in work, use a curtain to keep it out of sight.
- **Invest.** Get a set of soft sheets, duvet covers, and blankets. Plump and soften pillows.
- **Refresh.** Open windows to remove stale odors. Consider using relaxing fragrances such as lavender.

(These benefits of sleep and others are discussed in much more depth in Chapter 4.)

Eat Healthfully

It is clear that eating a balanced, healthy diet can stress-proof you in ways that are not fully understood. Research has also shown that undereating, overeating, and eating the wrong kinds of foods can create distress in the body. In particular, avoid **sympathomimetics**, substances in foods that produce (or mimic) stresslike responses, such as caffeine. (For more information about the benefits of sound nutrition, see Chapter 10.)

Managing Your Time

Have you ever put off writing a paper until the night before it was due? We all **procrastinate**, or voluntarily delay some task, despite expecting to be worse off for the delay. Procrastination can result in academic difficulties, financial problems, relationship problems, and a multitude of stress-related ailments.

How can you avoid the temptation to procrastinate? According to recent research focused on university students, the key is setting clear **implementation intentions**, a series of goals to accomplish toward a specific end.[72] Having a plan that includes specific behaviors or deadlines (and rewards for meeting goals can help you stay on task). The following time management tips can help:

- **Do one thing at a time.** Don't multitask. Instead of watching TV, doing laundry, and writing your term paper all at once, schedule uninterrupted time for work. Break overwhelming tasks into smaller pieces.
- **Clean off your desk.** Sort the items on your desk, tossing unnecessary paper and mail and filing the important papers in labeled folders. (For more on organizing to de-stress, see the Student Health Today box.)
- **Prioritize your tasks.** Make a daily "to do" list, and stick to it. Categorize what you must do today, what must eventually get done, and what it would be nice to do. Consider the "nice to do" items only if you finish the others and have the luxury of extra time.
- **Work when you're at your best.** If you're a morning person, study and write papers in the morning, and take breaks when you start to slow down. If you're a night person, use the daytime hours for less demanding tasks.
- **Remember that time is precious.** Many people learn to value their time only when they face a terminal illness. Try to value each day. To avoid overcommitment, learn to say "no," sympathetically but firmly.

sympathomimetics Food substances that can produce stresslike physiological responses.

procrastinate To intentionally put off doing something.

implementation intentions A series of goals to accomplish toward a specific end.

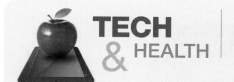
Consider Downshifting

Today's lifestyles are hectic, and stress often comes from trying to keep up. Many people are questioning whether "having it all" is worth it, if it can be done at all, and are working to simplify their lives. This trend has been labeled **downshifting**, or *voluntary simplicity*. Moving out of metropolitan areas and into smaller homes in smaller towns, giving up high-stress jobs for ones you enjoy, house decluttering, and making other life changes is part of downshifting.

Deciding what is most important in life, cutting down on material things and considering your environmental footprint are part of downshifting. When you contemplate any form of downshifting—or perhaps even start your career this way—it's important to move slowly and have a plan.

Relaxation Techniques for Stress Management

Relaxation techniques to reduce stress have been practiced for centuries and offer opportunities for calming your nervous energy and coping with life's challenges. Some common techniques include yoga, qigong, tai chi, deep breathing, meditation, visualization, progressive muscle relaxation, massage therapy, biofeedback, and hypnosis, many of which incorporate mindfulness strategies. Newer forms of relaxation may be found in the latest technology; see the Tech & Health box for more information.

▶ **SEE IT! VIDEOS**

Can a test identify your risk for stress-related illnesses? Watch **Stress Can Damage Women's Health**, available on Mastering Health.

Yoga Yoga is an ancient practice that combines meditation, stretching, and breathing techniques designed to relax, refresh, and rejuvenate. Practice of yoga began about 5,000 years ago in India and has been evolving ever since. Over 80 million Americans (34 percent of the population) say that, over the next year, they are very likely or somewhat likely to practice yoga.[73] People are flocking to yoga as part of a mindfulness lifestyle designed to reduce stress, increase balance and flexibility, and enhance overall health and fitness.

Classical yoga is the ancestor of nearly all modern forms of yoga. Breathing, poses, and verbal mantras are often part of classical yoga. Of the many branches of classical yoga, *hatha yoga* is the best-known; it is body focused, involving the practice of breath control and *asanas*—held postures and choreographed movements that enhance strength and flexibility. Recent research shows increased evidence of benefits of hatha yoga in reducing inflammation, boosting mood, increasing relaxation, and reducing stress among those who practice regularly.[74] Although studies have shown yoga to have similar benefits in treating insomnia and PTSD, reducing anxiety, lowering heart rate and blood pressure, improving fitness and flexibility, reducing pain, and other benefits, much of this research is still in its infancy and could benefit from more rigorous investigation. (See **Focus On: Cultivating Your Spiritual Health** for more.)

Qigong and Tai Chi *Qigong* (pronounced "chee-kong"), one of the fastest-growing, most widely accepted forms of mind-body health exercise, is used by some of the country's largest health care organizations, particularly for people suffering from chronic pain or stress. An ancient Chinese practice, qigong involves awareness and control of vital body energy known as *qi* or *chi* (pronounced "chee"). A complex system of internal pathways called *meridians* are believed to carry *qi* throughout your body. If *qi* becomes stagnant or blocked, you'll feel sluggish or powerless. Qigong incorporates

> **downshifting** Taking a step back and simplifying a lifestyle that is hectic, packed with pressure and stress, and focused on trying to keep up; also known as *voluntary simplicity*.

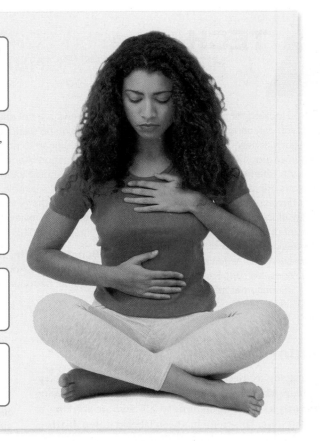

1 Assume a natural, comfortable position either sitting up straight with your head, neck, and shoulders relaxed or lying on your back with your knees bent and your head supported. Close your eyes and loosen binding clothes.

2 To feel your abdomen moving as you breathe, place one hand on your upper chest and the other just below your rib cage.

3 Breathe in slowly and deeply through your nose. Feel your stomach expanding into your hand. The hand on your chest should move as little as possible.

4 Exhale slowly through your mouth. Feel the fall of your stomach away from your hand. Again, the hand on your chest should move as little as possible.

5 Concentrate on the act of breathing. Shut out external noise. Focus on inhaling and exhaling, the route the air is following, and the rise and fall of your stomach.

FIGURE 3.6 **Diaphragmatic Breathing** This exercise will help you learn to breathe deeply as a way to relieve stress. Practice it for 5 to 10 minutes several times a day, and diaphragmatic breathing will soon become natural for you.

▶ SEE IT! VIDEOS

Looking for ways to relax and reduce stress? Watch **Generation Stress: Tips for Millennials to Reduce Stress** in the Study Area of Mastering **Health.**

mindful techniques including a series of flowing movements, breath techniques, mental visualization exercises, and vocalizations of healing sounds that are designed to restore balance and integrate and refresh the mind and body.

Another popular form of mind-body exercise is *tai chi* (pronounced "ty-chee"), often described as "meditation in motion." Originally developed in China over 2,000 years ago, this graceful form of exercise began as a form of self-defense. Noncompetitive and self-paced, tai chi involves a defined series of postures or movements done in a slow, graceful manner. Each movement or posture flows into the next without pause. Tai chi has been widely practiced in China for centuries and is becoming increasingly popular around the world, both as a basic exercise program and as a key component of stress reduction and balance and flexibility programs. Research demonstrating the effectiveness of these benefits is only in its infancy.

Diaphragmatic or Deep Breathing Typically, we breathe using only our upper chest and thoracic region. Simply stated, diaphragmatic breathing is deep breathing that maximally fills the lungs by involving the movement of the diaphragm and lower abdomen. This technique is commonly used in yoga exercises and other meditative practices. Try the diaphragmatic breathing exercise in **FIGURE 3.6** right now. Do you feel more relaxed?

Meditation Emerging evidence suggests that individuals who meditate may reap significant health rewards. Increasing numbers of Americans are meditating to relieve stress, improve their overall health, and aid in relaxation. Meditators are most likely to be female between the ages of 40 and 64 years, live in the western United States, have at least a college education, and not be involved in a relationship. They are also more likely to have one or more chronic health conditions.[75] Although there are many different forms of meditation, most involve sitting quietly for 15 to 20 minutes, focusing one's thoughts, blocking the "noise" in one's life, controlling one's breathing, and ultimately relaxing.

According to a recent review of key *randomized controlled trials (RCTs)* by the American Heart Association, *transcendental meditation (TM)*—in which one sits in lotus position, internally chants a mantra, and focuses on rising above the negative in one's life—appeared to be most effective in lowering blood pressure, overall mortality, and CVD events. Other forms of meditation appeared to have little or no effect on these health

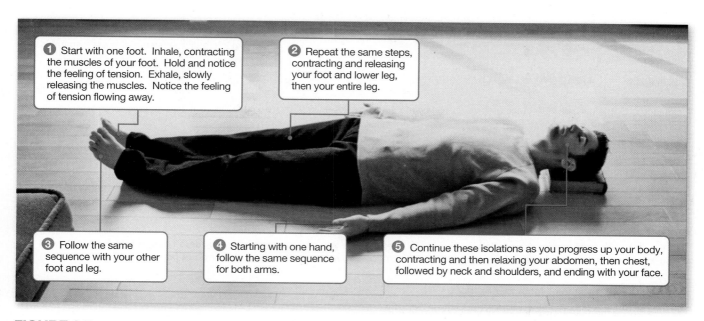

① Start with one foot. Inhale, contracting the muscles of your foot. Hold and notice the feeling of tension. Exhale, slowly releasing the muscles. Notice the feeling of tension flowing away.

② Repeat the same steps, contracting and releasing your foot and lower leg, then your entire leg.

③ Follow the same sequence with your other foot and leg.

④ Starting with one hand, follow the same sequence for both arms.

⑤ Continue these isolations as you progress up your body, contracting and then relaxing your abdomen, then chest, followed by neck and shoulders, and ending with your face.

FIGURE 3.7 Progressive Muscle Relaxation Sit or lie down in a comfortable position, and follow the steps described to increase your awareness of tension in your body and your ability to release it.

risks.[76] More rigorous, controlled research must be done to better understand the potential benefits of meditation. (See **Focus On: Cultivating Your Spiritual Health**.)

Progressive Muscle Relaxation

Progressive muscle relaxation involves teaching awareness of the feeling of tension and release by systematically focusing on areas of the body, contracting and relaxing different muscle groups while breathing in deeply and exhaling slowly. The standard pattern is to begin with your feet and work your way up your body, contracting and releasing as you go (**FIGURE 3.7**). With practice, you can quickly identify tension in your body and consciously release that tension to calm yourself.

Massage Therapy

Massage not only feels great, it is also an excellent way to relax. Techniques vary from deep-tissue massage to the gentler acupressure, use of hot rocks on tense muscle groups, and a wide range of other techniques. Although a variety of studies have been carried out to assess the health effects of massage, much of this research is poorly controlled and lacks sufficient sample size, and the results are preliminary or conflicting. However, a growing body of evidence indicates that massage may ease back pain, reduce anxiety, and potentially improve quality of life for cancer patients as well as those with HIV/AIDS and depression.[77] Though promising, this research is in its infancy. (See **Focus On: Understanding Complementary and Integrative Health** for more on the benefits of massage and other body-based methods.)

Biofeedback

Biofeedback is a technique in which a person learns to use the mind to consciously control bodily functions such as heart rate, body temperature, and breathing rate. Using devices as simple as stress dots that change color with body temperature variation or as sophisticated as electrical sensors, individuals learn to pay close attention to their bodies and make necessary adjustments, such as relaxing certain muscles, changing their breathing, or concentrating to slow their heart rate and relax. Eventually, individuals develop the ability to recognize and lower stress responses without machines and can practice biofeedback techniques anywhere.

biofeedback A technique in which a machine is used to self-monitor physical responses to stress.

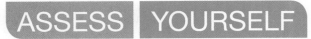

ASSESS YOURSELF

How Stressed Are You?

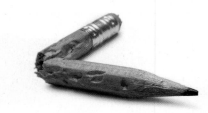

Let's face it: Some periods in life, including your college years, can be especially stressful. Learning to "chill" starts with an honest examination of your life experiences and your reactions to stressful situations. Respond to each section, assigning points as directed. Total the points from each section, then add them and compare them to the life stressor scale.

 Recent History

In the last year, how many of the following major life events have you experienced? (Give yourself five points for each event you experienced; if you experienced an event more than once, give yourself five points for each occurrence.)

1. Death of a close family member or friend _____
2. Ending a relationship (whether by your choice or not) _____
3. Major financial upset jeopardizing your ability to stay in college _____
4. Major move, leaving friends, family, and/or your past life behind _____
5. Serious illness (you) _____
6. Serious illness (someone you're close to) _____
7. Marriage or entering a new relationship _____
8. Loss of a beloved pet _____
9. Involvement in a legal dispute or issue _____
10. Involvement in a hostile, violent, or threatening relationship _____

Total: _____

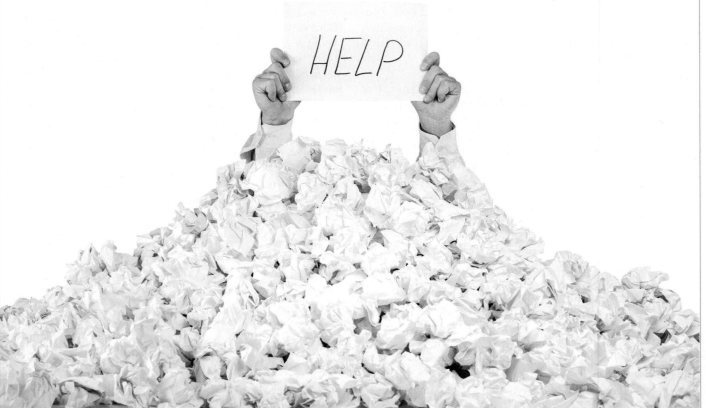

2 Self-Reflection

For each of the following, indicate where you are on the scale of 0 to 5.

		Strongly Disagree					Strongly Agree
1.	I have a lot of worries at home and at school.	0	1	2	3	4	5
2.	My friends and/or family put too much pressure on me.	0	1	2	3	4	5
3.	I am often distracted and have trouble focusing on schoolwork.	0	1	2	3	4	5
4.	I am highly disorganized and tend to do my schoolwork at the last minute.	0	1	2	3	4	5
5.	My life seems to have far too many crisis situations.	0	1	2	3	4	5
6.	Most of my time is spent sitting; I don't get much exercise.	0	1	2	3	4	5
7.	I don't have enough control in decisions that affect my life.	0	1	2	3	4	5
8.	I wake up most days feeling tired/as though I need a lot more sleep.	0	1	2	3	4	5
9.	I often have feelings that I am alone and that I don't fit in very well.	0	1	2	3	4	5
10.	I don't have many friends or people I can share my feelings or thoughts with.	0	1	2	3	4	5
11.	I am uncomfortable in my body, and I wish I could change how I look.	0	1	2	3	4	5
12.	I am very anxious about my major and whether I will get a good job after I graduate.	0	1	2	3	4	5
13.	If I have to wait in a restaurant or in lines, I quickly become irritated and upset.	0	1	2	3	4	5
14.	I have to win or be the best in activities or in classes or I get upset with myself.	0	1	2	3	4	5
15.	I am bothered by world events and am cynical and angry about how people behave.	0	1	2	3	4	5
16.	I have too much to do, and there are never enough hours in the day.	0	1	2	3	4	5
17.	I feel uneasy when I am caught up on my work and am relaxing or doing nothing.	0	1	2	3	4	5
18.	I sleep with my cell phone near my bed and often check messages, tweets, and/or texts during the night.	0	1	2	3	4	5
19.	I enjoy time alone but find that I seldom get enough alone time each day.	0	1	2	3	4	5
20.	I worry about whether or not other people like me.	0	1	2	3	4	5
21.	I am struggling in my classes and worry about failing.	0	1	2	3	4	5
22.	My relationship with my family is not very loving and supportive.	0	1	2	3	4	5
23.	When I watch people, I tend to be critical and think negatively about them.	0	1	2	3	4	5
24.	I believe that people are inherently selfish and untrustworthy, and I am careful around them.	0	1	2	3	4	5
25.	Life is basically unfair, and most of the time there is little I can do to change it.	0	1	2	3	4	5
26.	I give more than I get in relationships with people.	0	1	2	3	4	5
27.	I tend to believe that what I do is often not good enough or that I should do better.	0	1	2	3	4	5
28.	My friends would describe me as highly stressed and quick to react with anger and/or frustration.	0	1	2	3	4	5
29.	My friends are always telling me that I need a vacation to relax.	0	1	2	3	4	5
30.	Overall, the quality of my life right now isn't all that great.	0	1	2	3	4	5

Total: _____

Scoring Total your points from sections 1 and 2.

Although the following scores are not meant to be diagnostic, they do serve as an indicator of potential problem areas. If your scores are:

0–50, your stress levels are low, but it is worth examining areas where you did score points and taking action to reduce your stress levels.

51–100, you may need to reduce certain stresses in your life. Long-term stress and pressure from your stresses can be counterproductive. Consider what you can do to change your perceptions of things, your behaviors, or your environment.

100–150, you are probably pretty stressed. Examine what your major stressors are, and come up with a plan for reducing your stress levels right now. Don't delay or blow this off because your stress could lead to significant problems, affecting your grades, your social life, and your entire future!

151–200, you are carrying high stress, and if you don't make changes, you could be heading for some serious difficulties. Find a counselor on campus to talk with about some of the major issues you identified as causing stress. Try to get more sleep and exercise, and find time to relax. Surround yourself with people who are supportive of you and make you feel safe and competent.

YOUR PLAN FOR **CHANGE**

The **ASSESS YOURSELF** activity gave you the chance to look at your sources of chronic stress, identify major stressors that you experienced in the last year, and see how you typically respond to stress. Now that you are aware of these patterns, you can focus on developing behaviors that lead to reduced stress.

TODAY, YOU CAN:

☐ Practice one new stress management technique. For example, you could spend 10 minutes doing a deep-breathing exercise or find a good spot on campus to meditate.

☐ In a journal, list the five most significant situations that you believe are current stressors in your life. Try to focus on intense emotional experiences and explore how they affect you.

WITHIN THE NEXT TWO WEEKS, YOU CAN:

☐ Attend a class or workshop in yoga, tai chi, qigong, meditation, or some other stress-relieving activity. Look for beginner classes offered on campus or in your community.

☐ Make a list of the papers, projects, and tests that you will have over the coming semester, and create a schedule for them. Break projects and term papers into small, manageable tasks with a plan for completing each. Be realistic about how much time you'll need to get these tasks done.

☐ Chart your day. Keep track of how much time you spend on Facebook, on Twitter, or surfing the Internet and how much you spend on schoolwork, exercise, and watching TV. Set time aside for you, but limit your nonproductive time each day.

BY THE END OF THE SEMESTER, YOU CAN:

☐ Keep track of the money you spend and where it goes. If your spending is out of control, your credit and savings will quickly be depleted, adding to your stress levels. Track your daily spending. Establish a realistic budget for necessities with an affordable amount for fun, and stick to it.

☐ Find some form of exercise you can do regularly. You may consider joining a gym or just arranging regular walk dates or bike rides with your friends. Try to exercise at least 30 minutes every day, making sure that strength training is part of this regimen. (See Chapter 11 for more information about physical fitness.)

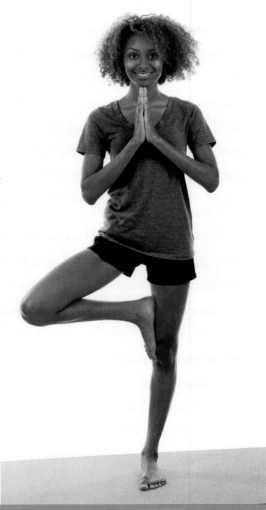

STUDY **PLAN**

CHAPTER **REVIEW**

LO **1** | What Is Stress?

■ Stress is inevitable. *Eustress* is associated with positive events; *distress* is associated with negative events. Both can have negative effects on your health.

LO **2** | Body Responses to Stress

■ The alarm, resistance, and exhaustion phases of general adaptation syndrome (GAS) involve physiological responses to real or imagined stressors and cause complex hormonal reactions. The transactional theory, the minority stress theory, and the Yerkes-Dodson law of arousal help to explain other factors that influence how stress is perceived, how people cope, and how health disparities can influence stress levels.

LO **3** | Physical Effects of Stress

■ Experiencing undue stress for extended periods of time can compromise the immune system. Stress has been linked to cardiovascular disease, weight gain, hair loss, diabetes, digestive problems, and increased susceptibility to infectious diseases. *Psychoneuroimmunology* analyzes the relationship between the mind's reaction to stress and immune system function.

LO **4** | When Overwhelm Strikes: Threats to Mental Health

■ Stress can negatively impact your intellectual and psychological health, including impaired memory, poor concentration, depression, anxiety, and other disorders.

LO **5** | What Causes Stress?

■ Sources of stress include change, hassles, relationships, academic and financial pressure, frustrations and conflict, overload, bias/discrimination, and environmental stressors.

LO **6** | Individual Factors that Affect Your Stress Response

■ Some sources of stress are internal and are related to appraisal, self-esteem, self-efficacy, personality types, hardiness, resilience, and shift and persist factors.

LO **7** | Managing Stress in College: Dealing with Overwhelm

■ Managing emotional responses, taking action, developing a support network, cultivating spirituality, downshifting, learning time management, managing finances, or learning relaxation techniques—will help you better cope with stress in the long run. An emphasis on mindfulness can help you focus.

POP **QUIZ**

LO **1** | What Is Stress?

1. Even though Andre experienced stress when he graduated from college and moved to a new city, he viewed these changes as an opportunity for growth. What is Andre's stress called?
   a. Strain
   b. Distress
   c. Eustress
   d. Adaptive response

LO **2** | Body Responses to Stress

2. In which stage of the general adaptation syndrome does the fight-or-flight response occur?
   a. Exhaustion stage
   b. Alarm stage
   c. Resistance stage
   d. Response stage

3. The branch of the autonomic nervous system that is responsible for energizing the body to either fight or flee is the
   a. central nervous system.
   b. parasympathetic nervous system.
   c. sympathetic nervous system.
   d. endocrine system.

LO **3** | Physical Effects of Stress

4. The area of scientific investigation that analyzes the relationship between the mind's response to stress and the immune system's ability to function effectively is
   a. psychoneuroimmunology.
   b. immunocompetence.
   c. psychoimmunology.
   d. psychology.

LO **4** | When Overwhelm Strikes: Threats to Mental Health

5. When Jessie encounters a stressful situation, she adapts well and bounces back easily. What protective factor is Jessie exhibiting to deal with stress?
   a. Cognitive restructuring
   b. Type A personality
   c. High self-esteem
   d. Psychological resilience

6. Losing your keys is an example of what psychosocial source of stress?
   a. Cumulative adversity
   b. Relative deprivation
   c. Hassles
   d. Conflict

7. A state of physical and mental exhaustion caused by excessive stress is called
   a. conflict.
   b. overload.
   c. hassles.
   d. burnout.

LO **6** | Individual Factors That Affect Your Stress Response

8. Kindness, empathy, tolerance, concern for others, sensitivity, and a desire to help are examples of which element of mindfulness?
   a. Reinforcing factors
   b. Adaptive thermogenesis
   c. Compassion
   d. Psychological resilience

LO **7** | Managing Stress in College: Dealing with Overwhelm

9. Which of the following is the best strategy to avoid test-taking anxiety?
   a. Do most studying the night before the exam so the material is fresh in your mind.
   b. Study over a period of time with a thorough review the night before.
   c. Drink a caffeinated beverage before the exam because sympathomimetics reduce stress.
   d. Take the exam as quickly as possible so you don't dwell on potential mistakes.

10. After 5 years of 70-hour work weeks, Tom decided to leave his high-paying, high-stress law firm and lead a simpler lifestyle. What is this trend called?
    a. Adaptation
    b. Conflict resolution

    c. Burnout reduction
    d. Downshifting

*Answers to the Pop Quiz questions can be found on page A-1. If you answered a question incorrectly, review the section identified by the Learning Outcome. For even more study tools, visit **MasteringHealth**.*

THINK ABOUT IT!

LO **1** | What Is Stress?

1. Define stress. What are some examples of situations in which you might feel distress? Eustress?

LO **2** | Body Responses to Stress

2. Describe the alarm, resistance, and exhaustion phases of the general adaptation syndrome and the body's physiological response to stress. Does stress lead to more irritability or emotionality, or does irritability or emotionality lead to stress? Provide examples.

LO **3** | Physical Effects of Stress

3. What are some of the health risks that result from chronic stress? How does the study of psychoneuroimmunology link stress and illness?

LO **4** | When Overwhelm Strikes: Threats to Mental Health

4. Why might stress and mental disorders be correlated?

LO **5** | What Causes Stress?

5. Why are the college years often high-stress times for many students? What factors increase stress risks?

LO **6** | Individual Factors That Affect Your Stress Response

6. What predisposing, reinforcing, and enabling factors influence your ability to cope with stress?

LO **7** | Managing Stress in College: Dealing with Overwhelm

7. How does anger affect the body? Discuss the steps you can take to manage your own anger.

8. What sorts of situations make you most likely to be a procrastinator? What could you do to reduce the likelihood of procrastinating?

ACCESS YOUR HEALTH ON THE INTERNET

Visit Mastering Health for links to the websites and RSS feeds.

The following websites explore further topics and issues related to stress.

American College Counseling Association. The website of the professional organization for college counselors offers useful links and articles. **www.collegecounseling.org**

American College Health Association. This site provides yearly information and data from the National College Health Assessment survey, which covers stress, anxiety, and other health issues for students. **www.acha.org**

American Psychological Association. Here, you can find current information and research on stress and stress-related conditions as well as an annual survey. **www.apa.org**

Higher Education Research Institute. This organization provides annual surveys of first-year and senior college students that cover academic, financial, and health-related issues and problems. **www.heri.ucla.edu**

National Institute of Mental Health. A resource for information on all aspects of mental health, including the effects of stress. **www.nimh.nih.gov**

4 Improving Your Sleep

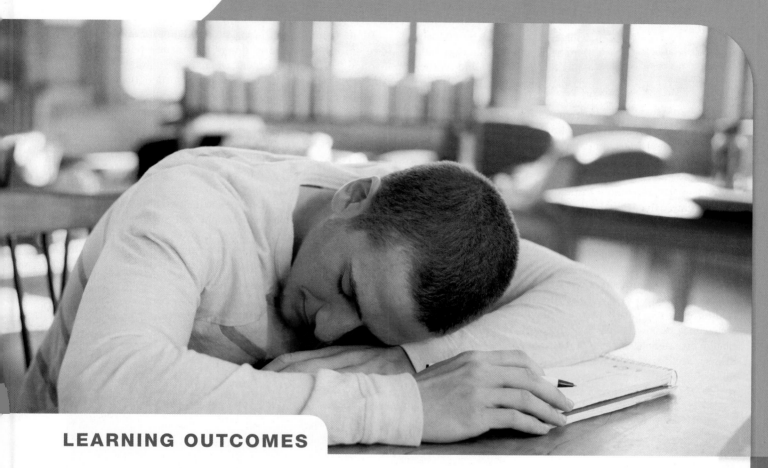

LEARNING OUTCOMES

LO 1 Describe the problem of sleep deprivation in the United States, including the unique challenges of sleep deprivation on campus.

LO 2 Explain why we need sleep and what happens if we don't get enough sleep, including potential physical, emotional, social, and safety threats to health.

LO 3 Explain the processes of sleep, including the two-stage model, circadian rhythm, and the sleep-wake cycle, as well as how they work and their importance for restful sleep.

LO 4 Describe some common sleep disorders, including risk factors and what can be done to prevent or treat them.

LO 5 Explore ways to improve your sleep through changing daily habits, modifying your environment, avoiding sleep disruptors, adopting mindfulness sleep strategies, and using other sound sleep hygiene approaches.

sleep deprivation A condition that occurs when sleep is insufficient.

somnolence Drowsiness, sluggishness, and lack of mental alertness that can affect your daily performance and lead to life-threatening sleepiness while driving.

Nearly every night, we leave our waking world and slide into a series of sleep stages, punctuated by changes in heart rate, respiration rate, blood pressure, and other bodily processes. We all need sleep; we need the stages and changes that allow the body to repair, restore, and refresh itself. However, over 83 million people in the United States don't get the sleep they need, and as many as 70 million of these individuals suffer from an actual sleep disorder.[1]

Inadequate sleep isn't just an American problem. The United States, the United Kingdom, Germany, Canada, and Japan have the dubious distinction of being the most sleep-deprived countries in the world. Overall, poor sleep affects the quality of life, productivity, physical and mental health, and social interactions of 45 percent of the world's population, and those numbers are increasing.[2] Sleep deprivation has been linked to seven of the fifteen leading causes of death in the United States, including cardiovascular disease, malignant neoplasm, cerebrovascular disease, accidents, diabetes, and hypertension.[3] **FIGURE 4.1** compares average nightly sleep times across a number of countries.

LO 1 | SLEEPLESS IN AMERICA

Describe the problem of sleep deprivation in the United States, including the unique challenges of sleep deprivation on campus.

Just how serious is **sleep deprivation**, a condition that occurs when sleep is insufficient for a given person? How many Americans suffer from **somnolence**—drowsiness, sluggishness, and a lack of mental alertness that can affect daily performance?[4] Although recent surveys of nearly 450,000 U.S. adults' self-reported sleep habits indicate that just over 65 percent had slept the recommended 7 hours in the last 24 hours, the other 35 percent—over 83 million people—did not. Over 38 percent of Americans reported unintentionally falling asleep during the day at least once in the last month.[5]

While falling asleep in class or studying for an exam can have serious implications, one of the greatest potential risks involving drowsiness occurs when a tired individual gets behind the wheel of a motor vehicle. Although many people think drowsy driving means actually falling asleep at the wheel, significant numbers of drowsy drivers are profoundly impaired, unable to react quickly, or so sleepy that miles pass without them even noticing—yet, they don't actually fall asleep. This is comparable to a drunk driver who, while awake, should not be driving. In a research survey, over 5 percent of respondents reported falling asleep at the wheel in the previous month, and 1 in 25 reported actually falling asleep at the wheel![6] Drowsy driving was responsible for nearly 100,000 police-reported crashes, 71,000 injuries, and 1500 deaths in the United States in 2015 and nearly $14 billion dollars in losses.[7]

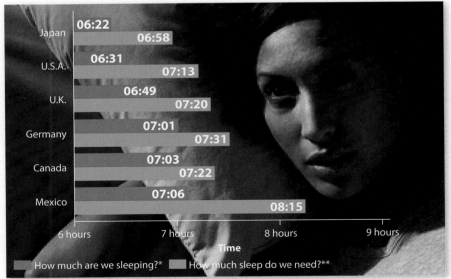

	How much are we sleeping?*	How much sleep do we need?**
Japan	06:22	06:58
U.S.A.	06:31	07:13
U.K.	06:49	07:20
Germany	07:01	07:31
Canada	07:03	07:22
Mexico	07:06	08:15

Time: 6 hours — 7 hours — 8 hours — 9 hours

* Represents workdays. All slept an average of 45 minutes more on weekends.
** Represents the number of hours needed for respondents to function at their best the next day (self-reported).

FIGURE 4.1 International Sleep Statistics

Source: Data from National Sleep Foundation, *2013 International Sleep Poll: Summary of Findings* (Arlington, VA: National Sleep Foundation, 2014), Available at http://sleepfoundation.org/sites/default/files/RPT495a.pdf.

Sleepless on Campus: Tired and Dragged-Out Students?

College students seem to be particularly vulnerable to sleep problems. In a recent survey by the American College Health Association, only 10.6 percent of students reported getting enough sleep to feel well rested in the morning 6 or more days a week.[8] Nearly 63 percent of students say they feel tired, dragged out, or sleepy during the day 3 to 7 days each week.[9] Sixty-one percent of students aged 18 to 29 years say that they often stay awake late and get up early.[10] They also indicated that sleep was more than a little problem (26 percent), a big problem (13.3 percent), or a very big problem (5.5 percent) in the last week.[11] Sleep deficiencies have been linked to a host of issues for students, including poor academic performance, weight gain, increased alcohol abuse, accidents, daytime drowsiness, relationship issues, and depression.[12] Despite large numbers of students reporting sleep problems, fewer than 5 percent have sought treatment for insomnia, and just over 2 percent have sought treatment for other sleep problems.[13] Clearly, there is room for greater awareness about possible resources and easier access to sleep resources on America's campuses.

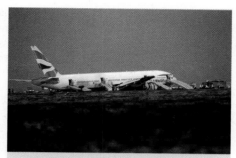

Many major transportation and industrial accidents occur among shift workers or those who suffer from chronic sleep deprivation.

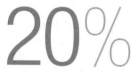

20%

of all crashes result in fatality due to **DROWSY DRIVING**. The less the sleep, the greater the risk.

Approximately 20 percent of the U.S. population suffers from a condition known as **excessive daytime sleepiness or excessive sleepiness**—a major compulsion to sleep, along with persistent sluggishness and fatigue, that can cause individuals to nod off at inopportune times and interfere with most aspects of life.[14] Adults aged 16 to 24 years are twice as likely to be drowsy at the time of crashes as 40- to 59-year-olds and are the most likely to nod off during the day (see **TABLE 4.1**).[15] In clinical terms, **primary idiopathic hypersomnia** refers to excessive daytime sleepiness without narcolepsy or the associated features of other sleep disorders.[16]

Why Are We So Sleep Deprived?

Several factors can lead to sleep deprivation:

■ **Shift work.** Work shifts that change from one day to the next and shifts that are outside the normal 9-to-5 work schedule can disrupt biological clocks and lead to sleeplessness, insomnia, and a host of other problems.[17] Chronic insomnia and disruptions in biological clocks can result in high levels of on-the-job errors; in fact, sleepy workers are 70 percent more likely to be involved in accidents than are those who get enough sleep.[18] Some train crashes, cruise ship crashes, and other serious accidents appear to be sleep-related. Drowsy driving is a major public health issue, particularly affecting the 9.5 million shift workers who routinely drive without adequate sleep and have a significantly higher risk of accidents in the 30 minutes after they get off their shift.[19] Short sleepers or drowsy workers are also more likely to be depressed, miss work, and have increased on-the-job accidents and worker's compensation claims.[20]

■ **Long-haul driving.** Sixty-five percent of all fatal truck crashes involve long-haul trucks. More than one in four truck drivers report that they have fallen asleep behind the wheel in the last month. Over two thirds of all long-haul drivers are obese and many have sleep apnea. Sleep deprivation is common among truckers, particularly those who drive commercially over 60 hours per week and drive alone.[21]

■ **Drugs and medications.** As noted on their warning labels, many prescription drugs and over-the-counter

> ▶ **SEE IT!** VIDEOS
>
> How you can avoid nodding off behind the wheel? Watch **Dozing and Driving**, available on Mastering Health.

excessive daytime sleepiness or excessive sleepiness A condition in which a person feels a major compulsion to sleep during normal waking hours along with persistent sluggishness and fatigue.

primary idiopathic hypersomnia Excessive daytime sleepiness without narcolepsy or the associated features of other sleep disorders.

TABLE **4.1** | Adults Reporting Selected Sleep Behaviors in 12 States

Age (Years)	Unintentionally Fell Asleep during the Day at Least Once in the Past Month	Nodded Off or Fell Asleep While Driving in the Past Month
18 to 25	43.7%	4.5%
25 to 35	36.1%	7.2%
35 to 45	34.0%	5.7%
45 to 55	35.3%	3.9%
55 to 65	36.5%	3.1%
>65	44.6%	2.0%

Source: Centers for Disease Control and Prevention, "Insufficient Sleep is a Public Health Problem," September 3, 2015, www.cdc.gov/features/dssleep.

$411 BILLION

is the amount that **LACK OF SLEEP** could cost Americans each year through either low productivity or use of sick days.

drugs can lead to excessive sleepiness, as can some illicit drugs. Antihistamines, anxiety drugs, Parkinson's medications, antidepressants, certain blood pressure and antinausea drugs, muscle relaxants, alcohol, and marijuana, are among key culprits.

- **Pain.** Excessive pain can keep you tossing and turning through the night, and the enormous amounts of pain medications given to relieve pain can cause millions of people to feel sleepy during the day. People who experience chronic or acute pain along with high stress levels are more likely to report worse quality of life, more depression, and more physical and mental health problems. Add poor environmental conditions such as excessive noise, too much light, temperature extremes, and uncomfortable mattresses, and you have a perfect storm of sleeplessness.[22]

- **Sleep habits.** Burning the candle at both ends, exercising before bed, and hours of time spent on smartphones or tablets can lead to excess sleepiness. See the **Tech & Health** box for more on the adverse effects of too much screen time.

- **Gender.** Although men and women have the same sleep needs, they face different sleep challenges throughout life. Women have twice the sleep difficulties of men, believed to be caused by hormonal factors, pregnancy, menopause, and psychological issues such as anxiety and depression.[23] Women are more likely to face problems with insomnia, particularly during midlife and later life as hormones may change dramatically. Estrogen influences how long it takes to fall asleep, soundness of sleep, and sleep duration as well as temperature regulation. Disrupt estrogen levels, and sleep is likely to suffer. Testosterone levels fluctuate in both men and women, typically rising at night during REM sleep and falling during the day. If testosterone levels are low, it can affect more than sexual activity; it can lead to chronic fatigue and disinterest in sex. Low testosterone can also increase the risk of sleep apnea and cardiovascular diseases. Men are significantly more likely to suffer from sleep-disordered breathing such as snoring and sleep apnea, which can raise risks for cardiovascular disease and a variety of other health problems. Although men are at greater risk for sleep-disordered breathing, they are less likely to seek help for sleep problems and often are diagnosed later in life with conditions that might have been prevented.[24]

- **Sleep disorders.** Any chronic disruptions in circadian rhythms can pose major risks for psychiatric, cardiovascular, metabolic, and hormonal diseases and can have far-reaching effects on social health, relationships, and emotional health. Additionally, excessive daytime sleepiness can affect cognitive function and professional efficiency, increase error rates and accidents, and have a significant effect on direct and indirect health care costs.[25]

LO 2 | THE IMPORTANCE OF SLEEP

Explain why we need sleep and what happens if we don't get enough sleep, including potential physical, emotional, social, and safety threats to health.

When there just aren't enough hours in the day, sleep can get short-changed. Because Americans are managing to function with less sleep, you might conclude that the recommended amount of sleep isn't all that necessary. In fact, evidence for the importance of adequate sleep to overall health and daily functioning grows daily. Sleep serves to maintain your physical health, affects your ability to function effectively, and enhances your intellectual, social, emotional, and psychological health in several ways:

- **Sleep restores you both physically and mentally.** Certain reparative chemicals are released while you sleep. There is also evidence that during sleep, the brain is cleared of daily minutiae, learning is synthesized, and memories are consolidated.

- **Sleep conserves body energy.** When you sleep, your core body temperature and the rate at which you burn calories drop. This leaves you with more energy to perform activities throughout your waking hours.

- **Sleep helps you cope with life's challenges.** Sleep refreshes you; it helps you consolidate cognitive, physiological, and emotional processes and autonomic functions. Well-rested individuals tend to be happier, have more vigor in their lives, and have a more positive outlook than do those who are sleep deprived. People who get enough rest are also more likely to control their emotions and have more positive social interactions.[26]

Sleep and Health

Sleep has beneficial effects on most body systems. That's why, when you consistently don't get a good night's rest, your body doesn't function as well and you become more vulnerable to a wide variety of health problems.[27] Researchers are just beginning to explore the physical benefits of sleep. The following is a brief summary of these physical benefits:

- **Sleep helps to maintain your immune system.** The common cold, strep throat, flu, mononucleosis, cold sores, and a variety of other ailments are more common when your immune system is depressed. If you aren't getting enough sleep, your body's immune response is weakened. Twin studies have provided strong evidence that habitually sleep-deprived adults are much more susceptible to diseases such as the common cold, inflammatory responses, and other risks than their twins who habitually slept the

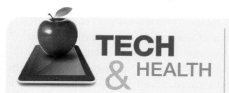

TECH & HEALTH

TECHNOLOGY'S TOLL ON OUR SLEEP
Why You Should be Dreaming rather than Streaming

If you have ever crawled into bed only to find yourself switching on the TV and staying awake for hours when you should be sleeping, you are not alone. If you find that the next day you tend to doze or can't focus on your instructor's lecture, you shouldn't be surprised. When you find yourself constantly turning to your smartphone to see what's happening in the outside world, you may be like many of your peers. Cyberloafing (the classroom equivalent of slacking on the student job of being engaged in learning) while your instructor is lecturing is increasingly common. According to recent research, college students are more distracted than ever, checking their digital devices, particularly their smartphones, nearly 12 times during a typical class or texting, e-mailing, or posting on Facebook instead of taking notes. In fact, only about 3 percent of students are *not* sneaking peeks at their electronic devices throughout a lecture. College students aren't unique. The average person in the United States has nearly four connected devices at any given time. Although 16- to 24-year-olds tend to use their devices the most, 25- to 44-year-olds have the most devices of any age group. We sleep with phones a few inches from our heads, check texts during sleep time, and grab our phones as soon as we wake up. Sleep disruptions are one of the major consequences of our seemingly insatiable need to stay connected.

Why is too much time spent "connected" potentially hazardous to our sleep, our health, and our academic success? Numerous studies indicate that technology can affect our health in several ways:

- Light, particularly the blue light of LED screens found in most electronic devices and in homes, wakes the brain up, telling it that it's daytime. Particularly when we are getting ready for bed, this light can suppress melatonin, a hormone that helps you fall asleep and stay asleep. The screen size, your proximity to the screen, and the number of devices turned on can all affect how significant your wake-up call is. Long-term melatonin deficiencies can increase your risk for type 2 diabetes, heart arrhythmias, migraines, and many other problems, in addition to making you feel like a zombie when you're awake.
- Being connected can make you wired and stimulate your brain just when it should be slowing down. Anyone who has ever received an upsetting text or e-mail late in the day will tell you that communication can have a major effect on your wakefulness. Also, using your laptop or tablet late at night or lying in bed reading that chapter you should have read last week can create a pattern of behavior that associates bed with work rather than sleep. Turn off the TV by 10 P.M. Keep work out of the bedroom. Turn off your phone ringer after a set time. And don't log in during the night for any reason.

Here are a few ways to avoid the melatonin-draining effects of blue light on your sleep and health and to create a healthy sleep environment:

- Ideally, you should not have a TV, computer, or laptop in your bedroom. If you must have a device in your room, stick to small screens, and keep them far away from your eyes. Dim your screen as bedtime approaches, and turn off LED lighting.
- Have no violent video games or deep discussions with friends after dusk. Change your music to soothing classical or new age as you prepare for sleep.
- When buying glasses or sunglasses, purchase protection from blue lights as your glasses are ordered. If you can't afford prescription blue light blockers, purchase amber-tinted glasses that block blue light.
- Allow yourself only an hour or two of screen time after dark. Record your favorite shows and watch them during the day—and not in the bedroom.

Sources: L. Rosen et al., "Sleeping with Technology: Cognitive, Affective, and Technology Usage Predictors of Sleep Problems among College Students," *Sleep Health* 2, no. 1 (2016): 49–56; S. Gokcearslan et al., "Modeling Smartphone Addiction: The Role of Smartphone Usage, Self-regulation, General Self-efficacy and Cyberloafing in University Students," *Computers in Human Behavior* 63 (2016): 639–49; F. Yilmaz, "Cyberloafing as a Barrier to the Successful Integration of Information and Communication Technologies into Teaching and Learning Environments," *Computers in Human Behavior* 45 (2015): 290–98; C Buckle, "Digital Consumers Own 3.64 Connected Devices," Global Webindex, February 18, 2016, https://www.globalwebindex.net/blog/digital-consumers-own-3.64-connected-devices; C. Czeisler et al., "Problems Associated with Use of Mobile Devices in the Sleep Environment—Streaming Instead of Dreaming," *JAMA Pediatrics* 170, no. 12 (2016):1146–47; M. Grandner et al., "The Use of Technology at Night: Impact on Sleep and Health," *Journal of Clinical Sleep Medicine* 9, no. 12 (2013) :1301–02; B. McCoy, "Digital Distractions in the Classroom Phase II: Student Classroom Use of Digital Devices for Non Class-related Activity," *Journal of Media Education* 7, no. 11 (2016): 5–11.

recommended number of hours per night.[28] Other studies have shown that sleep disruption, particularly when circadian rhythms are disturbed repeatedly, disrupts overall immune function.[29] In contrast, adolescents getting more than 9 hours of sleep per night showed improvements in markers of immune functioning.[30]

- **Sleep helps to reduce your risk for cardiovascular disease.** Several recent studies suggest a link between short sleep duration and chronic inflammation, increased risk of coronary artery disease, risk of stroke, hypertension, metabolic syndrome, obesity, and decreases in high-density lipoprotein ("good cholesterol") levels and other disruptions in cholesterol metabolism, as well as increases in other cardiovascular risks.[31] Among people with untreated or noncompliant sleep apnea and nighttime oxygen deprivation, autonomic nervous system dysfunction, heart arrhythmias, and heart failure risks increase dramatically in all age groups—even among those who have otherwise healthy hearts.[32] Newer research points to a strong association between short-duration sleep and increased risk of developing and/or dying from cardiovascular disease.[33]

- **Sleep contributes to a healthy metabolism.** Chemical reactions in your body's cells break down food and synthesize compounds that the body needs. The sum of all these reactions is called *metabolism*. Several recent studies suggest that sleep contributes to healthy metabolism and possibly to a healthy body weight. In fact, people who sleep less than 5 hours per night have a 40 percent higher risk of developing obesity than do those who sleep 7 to 8 hours per night.[34] Sleeping less is associated with eating more—particularly high-fat, high-protein foods—and exercising less.[35]

- **Short sleep increases the risk of type 2 diabetes.** There is evidence that sleep deficiencies, particularly sleep disorders such as sleep apnea, can increase the risk of *type 2 diabetes*, a disorder of glucose metabolism.[36]

- **Sleep may be a factor in male reproductive health.** Although issues with sexual interest and sexual performance are common problems for tired people, new research suggests that sleep deprivation may affect males more than they realize. Young males who suffered from chronic sleep deficits were shown to have reduced semen concentration, reduced sperm quality and motility, and smaller testicular size than men with higher sleep levels. Women have increased issues with conception and overall fertility.[37] More research is necessary to determine the mechanisms contributing to these problems.

- **Sleep contributes to neurological/mental/cognitive functioning.** Restricting sleep can cause a wide range of neurological problems, including lapses of attention, slowed or poor memory, reduced cognitive ability, difficulty concentrating, and a tendency for thinking to get "stuck in a rut."[38] Studies of college students consistently show pulling an all-nighter to be a bad idea if you want to perform well on exams or be productive. Sleep before and after a task improves performance and is important to memory consolidation and retention.[39] New research at Oregon Health and Science University indicates that chronic lack of sleep may lead to early dementia and set the stage for Alzheimer's disease. On the basis of MRI brain scans, they hypothesize that during deep sleep, the brain is working to remove toxins from the brain. If you are awake, the brain is busy with other activity, and toxins that cause problems may increase.[40] Several studies have shown that chronic lack of sleep can also affect memory, particularly for simple tasks. Poor sleep is also a major contributor to depression, anxiety, and tobacco use—all factors that may result in exacerbated risks for a wide range of social, emotional, and physical health risks.[41]

- **Sleep improves motor tasks, particularly driving.** Sleep also has a restorative effect on motor function, that is, the ability to perform tasks such as shooting a basket, playing a musical instrument, or driving a car. Motor function is affected by sleep throughout the life span among otherwise healthy individuals.[42] Some researchers contend that drivers who have had only 4 to 5 hours of sleep or less have vehicle crash rates that are four times the rates for drivers who get the recommended 7 hours of sleep—comparable to crash rates of those who are driving drunk![43] In fact, drivers who get only 5 to 6 hours of sleep instead of the recommended 7 to 8 hours have over twice the risk of a crash. Last year, over 35,000 people died in auto crashes. Between 7 and 20 percent of those deaths are thought to involve a drowsy driver.[44] A recent survey found that, in the last month, nearly one third of drivers drove when they were struggling to keep their eyes open.[45] Drivers under the age of 26 are the most likely of any age group to report falling asleep at the wheel within the last year, and men of all ages are more likely to fall asleep than are women.[46]

- **Sleep plays a role in stress management and mental health.** The relationship between sleep and stress is highly complex: Stress can cause or contribute to sleep problems, and sleep problems can cause or increase your level of stress. The same is true of depression and anxiety disorders: Reduced or poor-quality sleep can trigger these disorders, but it's also a common symptom resulting from them. Individuals who suffer from chronic insomnia have over twice the risk of developing depression.[47]

LO 3 | THE PROCESSES OF SLEEP

Explain the processes of sleep, including the two-stage model, circadian rhythm, and the sleep-wake cycle, as well as how they work and their importance for restful sleep.

If you have ever taken an airplane flight that crossed two or more time zones, you've probably experienced *jet lag*, a feeling that your body's "internal clock" is out of sync with the hours of daylight and darkness at your destination. Jet lag happens because the new day/night pattern disrupts the 24-hour biological clock by which you are accustomed to going to sleep,

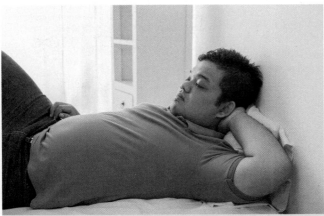

Obesity is a significant risk for diabetes-related excessive daytime sleepiness as well as a variety of sleep disorders.

waking up, and performing habitual behaviors throughout your day. This cycle, known as your **circadian rhythm**, is regulated by a master clock that coordinates the activity of nerve cells, protein, and genes. The hypothalamus and a tiny gland in your brain called the *pineal body*, which is responsible for producing the drowsiness-inducing hormone called **melatonin**, are key to these cyclical rhythms.[48] See **FIGURE 4.2** for more on brain structures involved in sleep.

Stages and Cycles of Sleep

Humans should spend roughly one third of every day asleep. Sleep researchers generally distinguish between two primary sleep stages. During **REM sleep**, rapid eye movement and dreams occur, and brain-wave activity appears similar to that when you are awake. **Non-REM (NREM) sleep**, in contrast, is the period of restful sleep with slowed brain activity that does *not* include rapid eye movement. During the night, you alternate between periods of NREM and REM sleep, repeating one full cycle about once every 90 minutes.[49] Overall, you spend about 75 percent of each night in NREM sleep and 25 percent in REM sleep (**FIGURE 4.3**).

Non-REM Sleep Is Restorative
During non-REM (NREM) sleep, the body rests. Both your body temperature and your energy use drop; sensation is dulled; and your brain waves, heart rate, and breathing slow. In contrast, digestive processes speed up, and your body stores nutrients. During NREM sleep—also called *slow-wave sleep*—you do not typically dream. Four distinct stages of NREM sleep have been distinguished by their characteristic brain-wave patterns as shown on an electroencephalogram (EEG), a test that detects electrical activity in the brain.

Stage 1 is the lightest stage of sleep, lasts only a few minutes, and involves the transition between waking and sleep.

Your brain begins to produces *theta waves* (slow brain waves), and you may experience sensations of falling with quick, jerky muscle reactions. During *stage 2*, your eyes close, body movement slows, and you disengage from your environment. During *stages 3* and *4*, your brain generates slow, large-amplitude *delta waves*. Your blood pressure drops, your heart rate and respiration slow considerably, and you enter deep sleep. The hypothalamus stimulates the pituitary gland to release human growth hormone, signaling the body to repair worn tissues. Speech and movement are rare during the final stage (but sometimes people sleepwalk, cook, clean, or drive during this stage).

REM Sleep Energizes
Dreaming takes place primarily during REM sleep. On an EEG, a REM sleeper's brain-wave activity is almost indistinguishable from that of someone who is wide awake, and the brain's energy use is higher than that of a person performing a difficult math problem.[50] The *pons*, one of the smallest areas of the brain, is a major message transmitter and is responsible for much of what happens in the sleep-wake cycle. Unless disrupted, the pons helps you enter REM sleep and keeps you down and out, with muscles essentially immobilized. You may dream that you're rock climbing, but your body is incapable of movement. Almost the only exceptions are your respiratory muscles, which allow you to breathe, and the tiny muscles of your eyes, which move your eyes rapidly as if you were following the scenario of your dream. This *rapid eye movement* gives REM sleep its name.

circadian rhythm The 24-hour cycle by which you are accustomed to going to sleep, waking up, and performing habitual behaviors.

melatonin A hormone that affects sleep cycles, increasing drowsiness.

REM sleep A period of sleep characterized by brain-wave activity similar to that seen in wakefulness; rapid eye movement and dreaming occur during REM sleep.

non-REM (NREM) sleep A period of restful sleep dominated by slow brain waves; during non-REM sleep, rapid eye movement is rare.

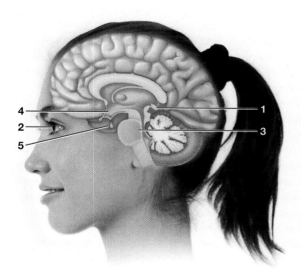

1. Pineal Body
Responsible for releasing the drowsiness-inducing hormone called melatonin as light dims and the sun goes down. During the day, the pineal gland is inactive and you remain awake.

2. Retina
Light travels through the retina and triggers the regulation of melatonin, slowing its production in daylight and encouraging it in darkness, helping to regulate the sleep cycle.

3. Pons
The *pons*, one of the smallest areas of the brain, is a major message transmitter and is responsible for much of what happens in our sleep-wake cycle. Unless disrupted, the pons helps you enter REM sleep and keeps you down and out, with muscles essentially immobilized.

4. Hypothalamus
With parts that function as your body's clock, regulating your circadian rhythm, the hypothalamus stimulates the pineal gland to secrete melatonin.

5. Pituitary gland
After being stimulated by the hypothalamus, the pituitary gland releases human growth hormone, signaling the body to repair worn tissues.

FIGURE 4.2 Parts of the Brain Involved in Sleep

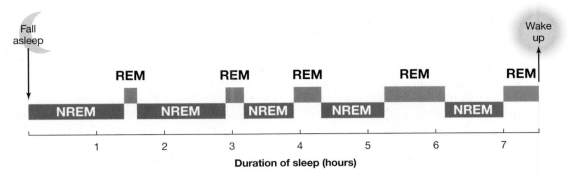

FIGURE 4.3 The Nightly Sleep Cycle As the number of hours you sleep increases, your brain spends more and more time in REM sleep. Thus, sleeping for too few hours could mean that you're depriving yourself primarily of essential REM sleep.

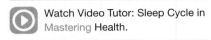
Watch Video Tutor: Sleep Cycle in Mastering Health.

Research indicates that deep phases of slow-wave sleep consolidate and organize the day's information, while REM sleep stabilizes consolidated memory.[51] Without adequate slow-wave sleep and REM sleep, your short-term memory may suffer.

Your Sleep Needs

Recently, a major U.S. consensus statement was published, providing guidelines for how much sleep a healthy adult should get each night. The key recommendations are as follows:[52]

- Adults should sleep 7 or more hours each night to promote optimal health.
- Getting fewer than 7 hours of sleep per night on a regular basis increases risks of adverse health outcomes.
- Regularly getting more than 9 hours of sleep may be appropriate for young adults, people trying to recover from sleep debt, and those recovering from illness. For others, it's not clear whether getting that much sleep is associated with health risks.

Keep in mind that sleep needs vary from person to person. Your gender, health, and lifestyle will also affect how much rest your body demands. For example, women need more sleep than men, overall.[53]

It is worth noting that sleep patterns change over the lifespan. Newborns need 16 to 18 hours of sleep daily, and teens and younger adults need 8 to 9 hours per night, slightly more than the adult average. Older adults may experience sleep difficulties that result in fewer hours of rest per night, owing to health conditions, pain, and the need to use the bathroom more frequently.[54]

Of concern for young adults are the results of a recent study of healthy undergraduate males indicating that short sleep cycles resulted in significant prolonged elevations in heart rate and diastolic pressure recovery after exposure to stressful stimuli as compared to those with longer sleep cycles.[55] Many scientists believe that diabetes, obesity, and other metabolic disorders may be linked with biological clock activity.[56] In general, people who get adequate sleep live longer and enjoy more good-quality days than those who don't.[57]

Sleep Debt In addition to your body's physiological need, consider your current **sleep debt**. That's the total number of hours of missed sleep you're carrying around with you. Let's say that last week you managed just 4 to 5 hours of sleep a night Monday through Thursday. Even if you get 7 to 8 hours a night Friday through Sunday, your unresolved sleep debt of 8 to 12 hours will leave you feeling tired and groggy when you start the week again. Research has consistently showed that accruing several days of sleep deprivation can not only make you sleepy, it can also affect your performance over a wide range of activities, lead to inflammation, and negatively affect the immune system. People with chronic sleep debt may have up to four times the risk of catching the common cold or other illnesses.[58]

Can you make up for lost sleep by sleeping in on the weekend? Some research shows that you *can* catch up if you go about it sensibly. Trying to catch up may make you feel more wide awake, as well as reducing those dark circles and eye bags. It also may reduce stress-related cortisol levels that shoot up while you are sleep deprived. On the other side of the coin, that catch-up sleep is not likely to make much difference in your performance levels, won't restore your functioning, and is likely to disrupt your circadian rhythm. It's best to work on establishing good sleep hygiene to help ensure that you get a healthy amount of sleep throughout the week.[59]

WHAT DO YOU THINK?

Do you find it difficult to get 7 or 8 hours of sleep each night?

- Do you think you are able to catch up on sleep you miss? What is the best way to erase a sleep debt?
- Have you noticed any negative consequences in your own life when you get too little sleep?

sleep debt The difference between the number of hours of sleep an individual needed in a given time period and the number of hours he or she actually slept.

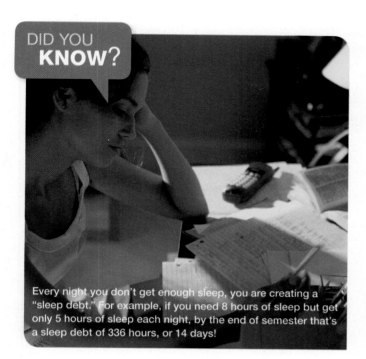

Every night you don't get enough sleep, you are creating a "sleep debt." For example, if you need 8 hours of sleep but get only 5 hours of sleep each night, by the end of semester that's a sleep debt of 336 hours, or 14 days!

Is Napping a Good Idea? Speaking of catching up, do naps count? Although naps can't entirely cancel out a significant sleep debt, they can improve your mood, alertness, and possibly performance if your sleep debt is more an occasional deficit than a chronic problem. Regular naps may also improve immune functioning and help ward off infections as well as improving performance and reducing sleepiness.[60] It's best to nap in the early afternoon to midafternoon, when the pineal body in your brain releases a small amount of melatonin and your body experiences a natural dip in its circadian rhythm. Never nap in the late afternoon, as that could interfere with your ability to fall asleep that night. Keep your naps short, because a nap of more than 30 minutes can leave you in a state of **sleep inertia**, which is characterized by cognitive impairment, grogginess, queasiness, and a disoriented feeling.

The Rare "Short Sleeper" Although many people who don't get enough sleep suffer the consequences, a small group of people—perhaps fewer than 1 percent—seem to thrive on less than 6 hours of sleep per night. Recent research points to a possible gene—the *DEC2 gene*—that affects circadian rhythms and changing normal day/night cycles. Individuals with this gene sleep less and seem to have few adverse affects. They do not accrue the negative consequences of typical sleep debt and are considered to be unique in the sleep literature.[61]

LO 4 | SLEEP DISORDERS

Describe some common sleep disorders, including risk factors and what can be done to prevent or treat them.

Sleep disorders, also known as **somnipathy** or **dyssomnia**, are any medical disorders with a negative effect on sleep patterns. While millions of people don't get enough sleep on any given night, as many as 70 million people suffer from an actual sleep-related disorder.[62] Over 61 percent of college students aged 18 to 29 years report staying awake late and getting up early—a recipe for sleep deprivation.[63] Although more than 4 percent of college students report having been treated for insomnia, the vast majority go it alone when trying to get enough sleep.[64] Nearly 2.5 percent of students report having sleep disorders other than insomnia.[65] Nearly 29 percent of students say that they have had sleep difficulties in the last year that were traumatic or difficult to handle.[66] If you're following the advice in this chapter and still aren't sleeping well, it's time to visit your health care provider. To aid in diagnosis, you will probably be asked to keep a sleep diary like the one in FIGURE 4.4. You may also be referred to a sleep disorders center for an overnight clinical **sleep study**. While you are asleep in the sleep center, sensors and electrodes record data that will be reviewed by a sleep specialist, who will work with you and your doctor to diagnose and treat your sleep problem.

The American Academy of Sleep Medicine identifies more than 80 sleep disorders. The most common disorders in adults are *insomnia*, *sleep apnea*, *restless legs syndrome*, and *narcolepsy*.

Insomnia

Insomnia—difficulty in falling asleep, frequent arousals during sleep, or early morning awakening—is the most common sleep complaint. Young adults aged 18 to 29 years experience the most insomnia, with 68 percent reporting symptoms, often relating to depression, stress, and anxiety.[67] Somewhat fewer adults (59 percent) aged 30 to 64 years experience regular symptoms, and only 44 percent of those over age 65 have regular symptoms.[68] Adults with children in the household tend to report more insomnia symptoms than do those without children.[69] Approximately 10 to 15 percent of Americans have experienced chronic insomnia that lasts longer than a month; nearly twice as many women as men experience symptoms of insomnia.[70] Although nearly 21 percent of students report that sleep difficulties are affecting their academic performance, only about 5 percent of them report having been treated for insomnia.[71]

Symptoms and Causes of Insomnia Symptoms of insomnia include difficulty falling asleep, waking up frequently during the night, difficulty returning to sleep, waking up too early in the morning, unrefreshing sleep, daytime sleepiness, trouble focusing, and irritability. Sometimes

	Day 1	Day 2	Day 3
Fill out in morning			
Bedtime	11 pm	11:30 pm	
Wake time	7:30 am	8:30 am	
Time to fall asleep	45 min	30 min	
Awakenings (how many and how long?)	2 times 1 hour	1 time 45 min	
Total sleep time	6.75 hrs	7.75 hrs	
Feeling at waking (refreshed, groggy, etc.)	Still tired	Energized	
Fill out at bedtime			
Exercise (what, when, how long?)	Jog at 2 pm 30 min	Soccer practice at 4 pm; 2 hrs	
Naps (when, where, how long?)	4 pm, my bed 30 min	2 pm, library 1 hour	
Caffeine (what, when, how much?)	2 cups coffee at 8 am	1 latte at 10 am; 1 soda at 9 pm	
Alcohol (what, when, how much?)	1 beer at 8 pm	None	
Evening snacks (what, when, how much?)	Bag of popcorn at 10 pm	Chips and soda at 9 pm	
Medications (what, when, how much?)	None	None	
Feelings (happiness, anxiety, major cause, etc.)	Stressed about paper	Worried about sister	
Activities 1 hour before bed (what and how long?)	Wrote paper	Watched TV	

FIGURE 4.4 **Sample Sleep Diary** Using a sleep diary can help you and your health care provider discover behavioral factors that might be contributing to your sleep problem.

insomnia is related to stress and worry. In other cases, it may be related to disrupted circadian rhythms, which can occur with travel across time zones, shift work, and other major schedule changes. Left untreated, long-term insomnia may be associated with depression, drug and alcohol use, and heart disease.[72]

Treatment for Insomnia Sometimes, hormonal changes or issues with the gastrointestinal tract or bladder may be underlying causes of insomnia. Excess stress can also be a key factor, and strategies designed to treat or control the underlying contributors can be helpful in reducing insomnia.

A major new "study of studies" indicates that **cognitive-behavioral therapy for insomnia (CBT-I)** is one of the best first-line defenses for people who can't get to sleep or who wake up during the night and can't get back to sleep.[73] Essentially, CBT-I helps people better understand the thoughts and feelings that influence their behaviors and focuses on changing the habits that disrupt sleep. Strategies such as thought blocking, thought refocusing, learning to meditate, listening to relaxing music, biofeedback, deep breathing, and other actions can all help turn an anxiety-prone bedroom experience into a calm setting for sleep. Today, increasing numbers of sleep therapists are helping to coach people on better sleep hygiene, including examining the environmental factors that may prevent deep sleep.

Relaxation strategies, including yoga and meditation, can be helpful in preparing the body to sleep. Exercise, done early in the day, can also help reduce stress and promote deeper sleep. Talk to a health professional if you experience insomnia that is unresolved in spite of your best efforts to make changes.

cognitive-behavioral therapy for chronic insomnia (CBT-I) A form of therapy that helps people better understand the thoughts and feelings that influence their behaviors and focus on changing habits that disrupt sleep.

Sleep Apnea

Sleep apnea is a disorder in which breathing is briefly and repeatedly interrupted during sleep.[74] *Apnea* refers to a breathing pause that lasts at least 10 seconds. Sleep apnea affects more than 18 million Americans, or 1 in every 15 people.[75]

Symptoms and Causes of Sleep Apnea There are two major types of sleep apnea: central and obstructive. *Central sleep apnea* occurs when the brain fails to tell the respiratory muscles to initiate breathing. Consumption of alcohol, certain illegal drugs, and certain medications can contribute to central sleep apnea.

Obstructive sleep apnea (OSA) is more common and occurs when air cannot move into and out of a person's nose or mouth even though the body tries to breathe. Typically, OSA occurs when a person's throat muscles and tongue relax during sleep and block the airway, causing snorting, snoring, and gagging. These sounds occur because falling oxygen saturation levels in the blood stimulate the body's autonomic nervous system to trigger inhalation, often via a sudden gasp of breath. This

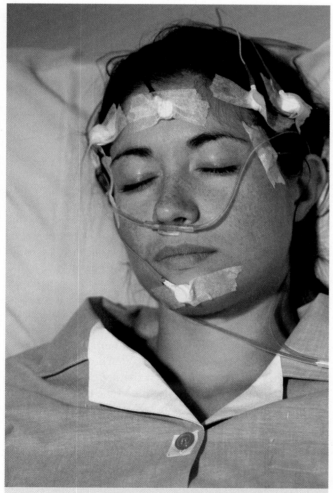

There are more than 80 different clinical sleep disorders affecting as many as 70 million Americans. One of the most common disorders is sleep apnea, which typically requires a sleep study for a definitive diagnosis.

response may wake the person, preventing deep sleep and causing the person to awaken in the morning feeling as though he or she hasn't slept.

People who are overweight often have sagging internal throat tissue, which puts them at higher risk for sleep apnea. Other risk factors include smoking and alcohol use, being 40 years of age or older, and ethnicity—sleep apnea occurs at higher rates in African Americans, Pacific Islanders, and Hispanics.[76] Anatomical risk factors for OSA can include a small upper airway (or large tongue, tonsils, or uvula), a recessed chin, a small jaw or a large overbite, and a large neck size. Because OSA runs in some families, genetics may also play a role.[77] OSA is associated with higher risks for chronic high blood pressure, irregular heartbeats, heart attack, and stroke. Apnea-associated sleeplessness may also increase the risk of type 2 diabetes, immune system deficiencies, and a host of other problems.[78]

Treatment for Sleep Apnea For those who are overweight, the most effective method for preventing and treating sleep apnea is to lose weight, along with avoiding factors that appear to increase risk. The most commonly prescribed therapy for OSA is *continuous positive airway pressure (CPAP)*, which involves uses of a machine consisting of an airflow device, a long flexible tube, and a mask (see **FIGURE 4.5**). People with sleep apnea wear the mask during sleep, and air is forced into the nose to keep the airway open. The FDA recently approved an implantable *upper airway stimulator (UAS)* called Inspire for use by people who cannot tolerate CPAP devices. Implanted under the skin in the upper chest, Inspire is a small pulsing device that stimulates airway muscle action and improved breathing and can be programmed remotely by a doctor. It is turned on before bed each night and turned off in the morning.[79]

Other methods for treating OSA include dental appliances, which reposition the lower jaw and tongue, and surgery to remove tissue in the upper airway. In general, these approaches are most helpful for mild disease or snoring; they may not be as effective with severe sleep apnea.

Restless Legs Syndrome

Restless legs syndrome (RLS) is a neurological disorder characterized by unpleasant sensations in the legs when at rest combined with an uncontrollable urge to move in an effort to relieve these feelings. The sensations range in severity from mildly uncomfortable to painful. Some researchers estimate that RLS affects over 10 percent of the U.S. population, with increasing diagnosis in all age groups.[80]

Symptoms and Causes of Restless Legs Syndrome The sensations of restless legs syndrome are often described as burning, creeping, or tugging or like insects crawling inside the legs. In general, symptoms are

sleep apnea A disorder in which breathing is briefly and repeatedly interrupted during sleep.

restless legs syndrome (RLS) A neurological disorder characterized by an overwhelming urge to move the legs when they are at rest.

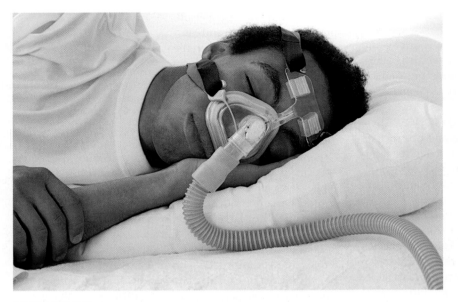

FIGURE 4.5 **Continuous Positive Airway Pressure (CPAP) Device** People with sleep apnea can get a better night's sleep by wearing a CPAP device. A gentle stream of air flows continuously into the nose through a tube connected to a mask, helping to keep the sleeper's airway open.

narcolepsy A neurological disorder that causes people to fall asleep involuntarily during the day.

parasomnias All of the abnormal things that disrupt sleep, not including some of the major problems such as sleep apnea.

more pronounced in the evening or at night. Lying down or trying to relax activates the symptoms, and moving the legs relieves the discomfort, so people with RLS often have difficulty falling and staying asleep.

In most cases, the cause of RLS is unknown. A family history of the condition is seen in approximately 50 percent of cases, suggesting some genetic link. In other cases, RLS appears to be related to other conditions, including Parkinson's disease, kidney failure, diabetes, peripheral neuropathy, and anemia. Pregnancy or hormonal changes can worsen symptoms.[81]

Treatment of Restless Legs Syndrome
If there is an underlying condition, treatment of that condition may provide relief. Other treatment options include use of prescribed medications, decreasing tobacco and alcohol use, and applying heat to the legs. For some people, relaxation techniques or stretching exercises can alleviate symptoms.

Narcolepsy

Narcolepsy is a neurological disorder caused by the brain's inability to properly regulate sleep-wake cycles. The result is excessive, intrusive sleepiness and daytime sleep attacks. Narcolepsy occurs in about 1 of every 3,000 people.[82] Narcolepsy is not rare, but it is an underrecognized and underdiagnosed condition.

Symptoms and Causes of Narcolepsy
Narcolepsy is characterized by overwhelming and uncontrollable sleepiness during the day. Narcoleptics are prone to falling asleep at inappropriate times and places—in class, at work, while driving or eating, or even in the middle of a conversation. These sleep attacks can last from a few seconds to several minutes. Other symptoms include *cataplexy* (the sudden loss of voluntary muscle tone, often triggered by emotional stimuli), hallucinations during sleep onset or on awakening, and brief episodes of paralysis during sleep-wake transitions.

In most cases, narcolepsy appears to be caused by a deficiency of sleep-regulating chemicals in the brain. Genetics may also play a role.[83] Other possible factors include having another sleep disorder, using certain medications, or having a mental disorder or substance abuse disorder.

Treatment for Narcolepsy
Narcolepsy is commonly treated with medications that improve alertness, and antidepressants may be prescribed to treat cataplexy, hallucinations, and sleep paralysis. Behavioral therapy can help narcoleptics cope with their condition. Some lifestyle changes, such as scheduling brief naps during the day or eating smaller meals on a regular schedule may be helpful.

Other Parasomnias

Parasomnias include all of the abnormal things that disrupt sleep outside the major problems such as sleep apnea. Among the most common parasomnias are *circadian rhythm disorder*, in which there are abnormalities in the sleep-wake cycle due to jet lag and adjustments to shift work; *sleep phase disorder*, in which the person either wakes up or goes to sleep too early; *sleep-related eating disorder*, in which the person may be found munching away in the kitchen but later has no memory of eating an entire cake or bucket of ice cream; *sleepwalking*, in which the individual may wander around the house or even go for a drive and not remember it; *night terrors*, in which the person wakes up frightened and screaming, often without knowing why (probably because this often occurs in non-REM sleep cycles); *sexsomnia*, in which the person may have sex while asleep and have no recollection of the event; *bedwetting* or *enuresis*, in which the person wets the bed without being aware of it; and *snoring*, in which inhaled air passes over loose tissue in the back of the throat or nasal passages and causes a rattling sound. Snoring, by itself, is not a problem unless the loose tissue interferes with breathing. In many cases, prescription sleep aids and other drugs can contribute to some of these parasomnias (see the Student Health Today box for the truth about sleeping pills). Trauma, underlying illnesses, or other neurological conditions may also be factors. For others, the causes are unknown. With many sleep disorders, the

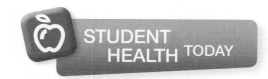
SLEEPING PILLS *A Cautionary Tale*

Tired, irritable, and frustrated by hours of tossing and turning when you should be sleeping? Thinking about taking a sleeping pill? If so, you're not alone. Between 37 and 42 percent of Americans have used over-the-counter (OTC) or prescription sleep aids in the last year. Like any other medication, these can lead to potential health risks. And guess what? They might not be as helpful as you think.

Results of a new study showed that people who took newer classes of prescription sleep medications such as Belsomra, Lunesta, Sonata, Ambien CR, and some OTC sleeping aids, slept only 6 to 20 minutes longer than those who took a placebo. Older medications such as Sominex and Tylenol PM don't perform any better, and melatonin, a popular OTC supplement that is promoted as easing sleep deprivation among shift workers, results in only a 7-minute faster "fall asleep" time and an 8-minute longer sleep time in users compared to nonusers.

What do you get besides an extra 6 to 20 minutes of sleep? You get side effects. At least 20 percent of sleeping pill users report adverse symptoms. The risk of having a driving accident while on these drugs increases; in fact, inserts for Belsomra and Ambien CR caution against driving at all during the day after use. Other side effects for prescription sleep medications and common OTC sleep aids include tolerance and dependence, daytime drowsiness, nervous tics, sexual impairment, and sleepwalking.

If you ultimately decide to use medications to help you sleep, treat them as a short-term fix, and talk with your doctor about the safest option for you. When taking sleep aids, make sure you have a 7- to 8-hour block for sleep, don't mix these medications with alcohol or other drugs, take the lowest possible dose, and be sure to read labels and follow directions. Better safe than sorry!

Sources: Consumer Reports, "The Problem with Sleeping Pills," February 2016, http://www.consumerreports.org/drugs/the-problem-with-sleeping-pills; Lester Holt, "Consumer Alert: Dangers of Over-the-Counter Sleep Aids," NBC News, January 2017, http://www.nbcnews.com/nightly-news/video/consumer-alert-dangers-of-over-the-counter-sleep-aids-867097667898; B. Duff-Brown, "Taking Painkillers with Sleeping Pills Is an Increasingly Risky Business," *SCOPE*, March 14, 2017, http://scopeblog.stanford.edu/2017/03/14/taking-painkillers-with-sleeping-pills-is-an-increasingly-risky-business; Consumer Reports, "Does Melatonin Really Help You Sleep?" January 5, 2016, http://www.consumerreports.org/vitamins-supplements/does-melatonin-really-help-you-sleep.

---

family or person living or sleeping with the sufferer is often the sleep-deprived person—and may not be tabulated in our overall sleep deficiency statistics!

LO 5 | GETTING A GOOD NIGHT'S SLEEP

Explore ways to improve your sleep through changing daily habits, modifying your environment, avoiding sleep disruptors, adopting mindfulness sleep strategies, and using other sound sleep hygiene approaches.

Many of us struggle with getting a good night's sleep on a regular basis. For problem sleepers, the good news is that there are many things you can do to improve sleep quality and duration. **Sleep hygiene** refers to the wide range of practices that can help you create and maintain normal, good-quality nighttime sleep and full daytime alertness.[84] The following sections provide proven strategies for improving your daily sleep patterns and getting the most out of the time you spend sleeping.

Create a Sleep-Promoting Environment

Where you sleep has much to do with how well you sleep. Making your bedroom into a calming, wind-down retreat is essential to setting the stage for restful and restorative sleep. Here are a few ways:

- **Chill.** Literally chill: Turn down the thermostat. The best sleep occurs in a cool bedroom—according to experts, one that is around 65 degrees. Normally, as you get sleepy, your body temperature starts to drop, and the body conserves energy through most of the sleeping hours, gradually increasing your temperature just before dawn. As light hits your room, your body temperature goes up along with your energy levels as part of normal circadian rhythms. In a room that is too hot or if you are sleeping in too many clothes or blankets or next to a person who exudes a lot of heat, the higher temperature may interfere with your natural body rhythms, making it harder to enter or remain in deep sleep, with resultant insomnia and other problems.[85] Everyone has an ideal sleep temperature based on percent body fat and other metabolic differences; finding out what seems to work best for you in different temperature and humidity situations is key to the environmental regulation of sleep. If you and your partner or roommate run hot and cold in ideal sleep temperatures, finding a good compromise temperature can help you both maintain sleep.

- **Create a Sleep "Cave."** As bedtime approaches, keep your bedroom quiet, calm, and dark with sensory stimuli at a minimum. Avoid exposure to bright light, particularly *blue light*, by turning off electronic devices or wearing an eye mask. Blue light is a key factor in our secretion of melatonin, a sleep hormone. If you get a lot of blue-light exposure from that glowing phone or tablet screen or from a computer monitor or TV in your room, your melatonin

> **sleep hygiene** The wide range of practices that can help you manage and create a systematic approach leading to normal, quality nighttime sleep and full daytime alertness.

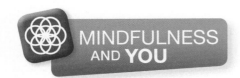

MINDFULNESS AND YOU

EVOKING THE RELAXATION RESPONSE

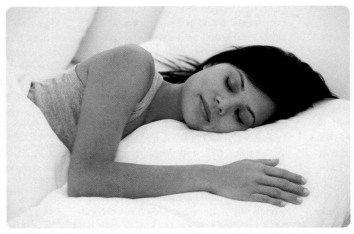

In one study, the use of mindfulness-based stress reduction helped 70 percent of participants experience significant relief from insomnia.

As scientists look for solutions to what appears to be an epidemic of sleeplessness, mindfulness-based interventions are receiving increasing clinical, community, individual, and research attention. In particular, research has focused on mindfulness-based stress reduction (MBSR), which is designed to help people focus on the moment in a calming, nonjudgmental way. MBSR is touted as a promising and effective program to help individuals learn to calm their mind and body as a means of helping them cope with challenges such as illness, pain, high stress, and anxiety. Key studies of the use of MBSR for insomnia over the course of an 8-week controlled intervention focused on sleep restrictions, stimulus control, and sleep hygiene along with mindfulness meditation have shown very promising results. Over 70 percent of participants in the treatment group experienced significant relief from insomnia up to 6 months after the intervention.

Together, MBSR, mindfulness meditation (a form of meditation that employs meditation using mindfulness calming techniques) and other mindfulness strategies have been shown to be effective in evoking the relaxation response—a shift in physiological activity that is the opposite of the stress response. A growing body of evidence indicates that taking simple actions to calm stressors may bring on a relaxation response that can help with insomnia and other sleep disturbances. Steps that you can take to evoke the relaxation response as you prepare yourself for sleep include the following:

■ **Choosing a calming focus**. Listening to your breathing and using positive words (such as *relax*, *listen to the quiet*, or *I am slowing down/relaxing*) are just some examples. Some people focus on a beautiful, peaceful setting, such as walking through the woods as snow gently falls on the trees or hearing loons over the lake at sunset. Allow yourself 10 minutes of calming focus several times a day.

■ **Letting go, feeling your body parts relax**. Slowly soften the muscles in your brow, face, neck, arms, and jaw, one by one until your body relaxes. Release tension, and let each part of your body sink into your mattress. Feel the coolness of your sheets against your skin or the cozy warmth of your comforter. If outside noises or thoughts intrude, take a deep breath and focus on how your body is beginning to drift. Some people find that meditative music or nature sounds can help to produce a peaceful, calming environment.

■ **Holding a nonjudgmental world view**. As you mindfully consider what you find around you and life in general, discard labeling thoughts, feelings, and sensations as being good or bad, right or wrong. Observe, but stop yourself from making judgments. Be open to things, experiences, people, and feelings.

■ **Non-striving**. Live in the moment and accept the moment as valuable. Instead of pushing ahead, take time out to just experience the now. Relax, observe, and feel.

■ **Letting be**. As you observe, don't try to change or fix people or things around you. Let things be as they are. Instead of viewing change as good or bad, try to observe, be more compassionate, and go with it.

■ **Having self–reliance**. Observe, trust yourself, and take actions that are based on truth and wisdom rather than emotions or spur-of-the moment decisions.

Sources: J. Corliss, "Mindfulness Meditation Helps Fight Insomnia, Improves Sleep," Harvard Health Publications, February 18, 2015, http://www.health.harvard.edu/blog/mindfulness-meditation-helps-fight-insomnia-improves-sleep-201502187726; S. Kim et al., "Effects of Mindfulness-Based Stress Reduction for Adults with Sleep Disturbance: A Protocol for an Update of a Systematic Review and Meta-analysis," *Systematic Reviews* 5, no. 1 (2016): 51; M. Bamber and J. Schneider, "Mindfulness-Based Meditation to Decrease Stress and Anxiety in College Students," *Educational Research Review* 18 (2016): 1–32; S. Garland et al., "The Quest for Mindful Sleep: A Critical Synthesis of the Impact of Mindfulness-Based Interventions for Insomnia," *Current Sleep Medicine Reports* 2, no. 3 (2016): 142–53; D. Black et al., "Mindfulness Meditation and Improvement in Sleep Quality and Daytime Impairments among Older Adults with Sleep Disturbances: A Randomized Clinical Trial," *JAMA Internal Medicine* 175, no. 4 (2015): 494–501; J. Ong et al., "A Randomized Controlled Trial of Mindfulness Meditation for Chronic Insomnia," *Sleep* 37, no. 9 (2014): 1553–63; M. Hafner et al, *Why Sleep Matters—The Economic Costs of Insufficient Sleep: A Cross-Country Comparative Analysis* (Santa Monica, CA: RAND Corporation, 2016).

production will drop, and you may find it hard to fall asleep or stay asleep.

- **Associate bed with sleep.** Make your bed a place for comfort and relaxation—a place for you to get the sleep you need to be productive and healthy; it shouldn't serve as your office or your social media center. You should spend a third of your time sleeping, so invest in a good mattress, and buy sheets that are smooth, cool, and relaxing and pillows that are right for you. Wash your bedding weekly or biweekly, and keep your bedroom clean and smelling fresh. Get rid of clutter, and keep things organized. Free yourself from intrusions by turning off the ringer on your phone, and charge your cell phone or tablet in a place that is out of reach so that you aren't tempted to look at it during sleep time. If you must have a TV in your bedroom, set it to turn off after an hour, and put the remote far from your bed so you aren't tempted to turn the TV back on.
- **Go to bed only when you are tired.** If you get in bed and can't sleep within 20 to 30 minutes, get up, keep the lights dim, and listen to relaxing music or meditate. Don't get into heavy studying on your computer or try to memorize complex details for an exam, and don't watch TV or grab your phone. This will keep you awake.
- **Establish bedtime and waking rituals.** Go to bed and get up at the same times each day. Establishing a bedtime ritual signals to your body that it's time for sleep. Listen to a quiet song, practice meditation and deep-breathing exercises, take a warm shower, or read something that lets you quietly wind down. Cool sheets and bedding and a lavender-scented room have been shown to be calming and promote more restful sleep. See the Mindfulness and You box for more on how mindfulness strategies can improve your sleep. On awakening, make your bed and air out your room.[86]

Adjust Your Daytime Habits

While we often focus on what happens in the bedroom as the key to sleep, what you do during the day can also have a significant impact on your sleep quality and duration.

Get Adequate Daytime Light Exposure
According to Kelly Brown, M.D., at the Vanderbilt Sleep Disorders Center, light is the best tool for controlling your internal clock. Light travels through the retina and regulates melatonin, slowing its production in daylight and encouraging it in darkness, helping to regulate the sleep-wake cycle.[87] If you want to stay awake in the daytime and sleep at night, get as much exposure to natural light outdoors during the day as you can. Open your blinds. Look for lamps and light bulbs that are recommended

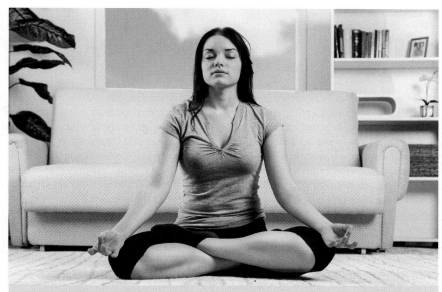
Try mindfulness meditation. Take steps to calm your thoughts and extinguish your stressors by focusing on your breathing, key words, or visualizations.

as therapy for seasonal ailments and to help with daytime alertness. These special lights increase your exposure to light and can help protect against other problems on dark winter days, in areas where daylight is in short supply, and if *seasonal affective disorder* (depression linked to the season of the year, typically winter) is a problem for you.

Exercise in the Morning or Afternoon
Have you ever noticed that after a day out hiking or a long swim or bike ride, you are tired when you get into bed? In fact, exercise may just be the great elixir when it comes to sleep.[88] You just need to make sure you exercise 3 to 4 hours before you go to bed. Why? Because exercise revs up your metabolism, makes you more alert, and depletes energy stores while raising body temperature. It takes hours to bring physiological changes down. Get in a workout in the morning or afternoon, and you will be awake for studying or writing that term paper. However, set a cutoff time for relaxing and cooling off the body for optimum sleep. Take time out for yourself. If you must walk the dog or want to go for a walk before bed or in the evening, keep it to a slow, mindful stroll, focusing on the things around you. Block negative thoughts and worries. Don't allow your mind to wander to problems you face or get worked up over assignments or upcoming tests. Focus on you and the moment and the sights and sounds around you.

Watch Your Diet, Particularly in the Hours before Bed
Avoid eating heavy meals within 2 to 3 hours of bedtime. Foods containing *tryptophan*, an amino acid (found in nut butters, bananas, tuna, eggs, chicken, turkey, yogurt, milk, and pork as well as in high-carbohydrate foods such as bread and pastries) may encourages sleepiness, particularly if you eat foods containing tryptophan on an empty stomach. However, foods that are high in protein and contain *tyramine* (such as sausage, eggplant, bacon, raspberries, chocolate, avocado, nuts, soy, and red wine) and greasy or spicy foods may keep you awake.[89]

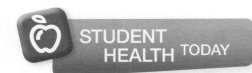

CAFFEINE, SLEEP, AND YOUR HEALTH

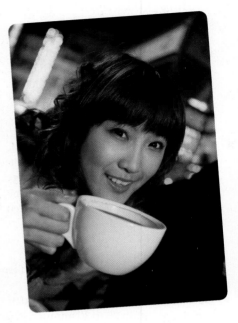

Caffeine has long been recognized for its ability to increase alertness and decrease sleepiness. Ingest too much caffeine, and you could end up wide awake when you want desperately to sleep.

A recent study indicated that effects of caffeine can last 5.5 to 7.7 hours or more—depending on how potent your coffee or energy drink really is. A double shot of espresso and a cup of your grandparents' drip coffee pot brew provide vastly different hits of caffeine with the potential for vastly different results. Many energy drinks are also high in calories and sugar. A nationally representative study of college students' caffeine consumption showed increasing trends in high caffeine consumption on campuses throughout the country and resulting problems with falling asleep and staying asleep. While it is clear that young adults are large consumers of caffeine, it is less clear whether they understand the health implications. Caffeine withdrawal, dependence, and addiction are all possible in addition to a significant drain on your finances. However, that's just the beginning. An ever-increasing body of research points to risk of cardiac irregularities, including,

but not limited to, arrhythmias, psychological problems such as depression and anxiety, and neurological side effects such as headaches and migraines. A growing concern about excess consumption of caffeine is that it can severely disrupt circadian cycles, leading to the inability to fall asleep and stay asleep. Consuming caffeinated beverages up to 8 hours before bedtime can have a significant effect on sleep! Think twice before ordering that large coffee or double shot espresso as you walk home from class. It may keep you up well past your bedtime, make you cranky and irritable, and add another layer of stress to an already stressful day.

Sources: N. Chaudhary et al., "Caffeine Consumption, Insomnia, and Sleep Duration: Results from a Nationally Representative Sample," *Nutrition* 32, no. 11 (2016): 1193–99; A. Haas et al., "Proportion as a Metric of Problematic Alcohol-Energy Drink Consumption in College Students," *Journal of Substance Use* (2017): 1–6; M.-D. Drici et al., "Cardiac Safety of So-Called 'Energy Drinks,'" *European Heart Journal* 35 (2014); H. Whiteman, "Rising Energy Drink Consumption May Pose a Threat to Public Health, Says WHO," *Medical News Today*, October 15, 2014, www.medicalnewstoday.com/articles/283929; J. J. Breda et al., "Energy Drink Consumption in Europe: A Review of the Risks, Adverse Health Effects and Policy Options," *Frontiers in Public Health* 2 (2014), doi:10.3389/fpubh.2014.00134.

Avoid Common Sleep Disruptors

Several factors play major roles in whether or not you can fall asleep and stay asleep. Some of the biggest sleep disruptors are common, and you'll recognize them right away. Other, lesser-known disruptors may be among the factors that hit you when you least expect them, leaving you staring at the ceiling when you should be catching z's. Avoid some of these behaviors and sleep on.

- **Go easy on the caffeine.** Long recognized for its ability to increase vigilance and alertness and decrease sleepiness when you need to stay awake, caffeine can be bad news for your sleep, particularly when consumed in the late afternoon or evening. See the Student Health Today box for more on caffeine and your health.
- **Avoid nicotine, alcohol, and liquids before bed.** Like caffeine, nicotine, alcohol, and liquids—even plain water—will increase the likelihood of sleep disturbances. Although

alcohol may make you sleepy initially, it disturbs other stages of sleep, keeping you from the restorative, deeper levels of sleep you need.[90] Alcohol, particularly binge drinking, has been shown to be a key sleep disruptor.[91] Heavy consumption of any liquids late in the day, even those without caffeine, can lead to **nocturia**, or overactive bladder, forcing you to get up several times during the night. (Pregnant women often suffer from nocturia, particularly in their first trimester.)

- **Turn off screens.** Watching TV, playing computer games, hanging out on Facebook or other social media sites, working on your latest paper on your laptop or tablet into the wee hours of the morning—all of these things can keep your mind alert and expose you to blue light, wrecking your chances for a good night's sleep.
- **Tune out conflict.** Avoid late-night phone calls, texts, or e-mails that can end up in arguments, disappointments, and other emotional stressors. If something does rile you up before bed, journal about it briefly, then promise yourself that you'll make time the next day to explore your thoughts and feelings more deeply.

nocturia Frequent urination at night caused by an overactive bladder.

LIVE IT! ASSESS YOURSELF

An interactive version of this assessment is available online on Mastering Health.

ASSESS | YOURSELF

Are You Sleeping Well?

Read each statement below, then circle True or False according to whether or not it applies to you in the current school term.

1. I sometimes doze off in my morning classes. True False

2. I sometimes doze off in my last class of the day. True False

3. I go through most of the day feeling tired. True False

4. I feel drowsy when I'm a passenger in a bus or car. True False

5. I often fall asleep while reading or studying. True False

6. I often fall asleep at the computer or watching TV. True False

7. It usually takes me a long time to fall asleep. True False

8. My roommate tells me I snore. True False

9. I wake up frequently throughout the night. True False

10. I have fallen asleep while driving. True False

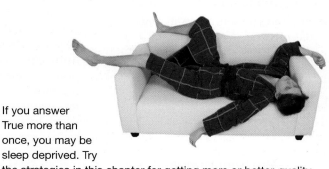

If you answer True more than once, you may be sleep deprived. Try the strategies in this chapter for getting more or better-quality sleep, but if you still experience sleepiness, see your health care provider.

YOUR PLAN FOR **CHANGE**

Here are some steps you can take to improve your sleep, starting tonight.

TODAY, YOU CAN:

☐ Identify things in your life that may prevent you from getting a good night's sleep. Develop a plan. What can you do differently starting today?

☐ Write a list of personal Do's and Don'ts. For instance: *Do* turn off your cell phone after 11 P.M. *Don't* drink anything containing caffeine after 3 P.M.

WITHIN THE NEXT TWO WEEKS, YOU CAN:

☐ Keep a sleep diary, noting not only how many hours of sleep you get each night, but also how you feel and function the next day.

☐ Arrange your room to promote restful sleep. Keep it quiet, cool, dark, and comfortable.

☐ Visit your campus health center for more information about getting a good night's sleep.

BY THE END OF THE SEMESTER, YOU CAN:

☐ Establish a regular sleep schedule. Get in the habit of going to bed and waking up at the same time, even on weekends.

☐ Create a ritual, such as stretching, meditation, reading something light, or listening to music, that you follow each night to help your body ease from the activity of the day into restful sleep.

☐ If you are still having difficulty sleeping, contact your health care provider.

STUDY **PLAN**

Visit the Study Area in Mastering Health to enhance your study plan with MP3 Tutor Sessions, Practice Quizzes, Flashcards, and more!

CHAPTER **REVIEW**

LO **1** | Sleepless in America

- Sleep deprivation, or insufficient sleep, is a major problem in the United States, affecting as many as 70 million adults overall and nearly 60 percent of students, resulting in major problems with excessive day-time sleepiness.

LO **2** | The Importance of Sleep

- Sleep serves as a mental and physical restorer, helps to conserve energy, reduces risks of cardiovascular disease and other chronic ailments, aids in having a healthy metabolism and good neurological functioning, improves motor tasks, and helps manage stress.

LO **3** | The Processes of Sleep

- The sleep cycle, known as the circadian rhythm, is regulated by a biological clock that coordinates the activity of nerve cells, proteins, and genes. Melatonin is the hormone that regulates the sleep cycle.
- REM and NREM sleep occur throughout the night. NREM sleep is slow-wave, restful sleep; REM sleep mimics waking states.
- How much sleep you need varies by age throughout the life span.

LO **4** | Sleep Disorders

- Sleep disorders, also known as somnipathy or dyssomnia, are any medical disorders that have a negative effect on sleep patterns. Although there are many sleep disorders, the most prevalent are insomnia, sleep apnea, restless legs syndrome, and narcolepsy, which have varying symptoms, causes, prevention, and treatment options.

LO **5** | Getting a Good Night's Sleep

- Staying active, paying attention to your sleep environment, improving your sleep hygiene, and avoiding emotional upset as well as food and drink before going to bed are all important to getting a good night's sleep. Practicing mindfulness meditation and other mindfulness strategies can help to ensure restful sleep.

POP **QUIZ**

LO **1** | Sleepless in America

1. Which of the following is NOT correct about sleeplessness in America?
   a. Women are more likely to suffer from insomnia than men.
   b. Men are more likely to snore and have sleep apnea than women.
   c. Hormonal changes or fluctuations have very little effect on restful sleep.
   d. Oversleeping on a regular basis may significantly increase your risk of premature dementia and/or Alzheimer's disease.

LO **2** | The Importance of Sleep

2. Which of the following age groups is reportedly most likely to fall asleep at the wheel?
   a. Over 60
   b. Over 45
   c. Under 26
   d. Under 18

LO **3** | The Processes of Sleep

3. Which of the following occurs when your body's circadian rhythm becomes out of sync with daylight hours?
   a. Jet lag
   b. REM sleep
   c. NREM sleep
   d. Somnolence

LO **4** | Sleep Disorders

4. Which sleep disorder involves difficulty falling asleep, waking up during the night, and/or difficulty falling back asleep?
   a. Obstructive sleep apnea
   b. Narcolepsy
   c. Restless legs syndrome
   d. Insomnia

LO 5 | Getting a Good Night's Sleep

5. Which of the following is *not* recommended if you want to get a good night's sleep?
   a. Getting adequate exposure to light, particularly sunlight during the day
   b. Exercising each day in the morning or afternoon
   c. Paying careful attention to your sleep environment, including lighting, clean scents, and cool temperatures
   d. Consume lots of fluids and foods that make you feel sleepy and full just prior to sleeping.

Answers to the Pop Quiz questions can be found on page A-1. If you answered a question incorrectly, review the section i dentified by the Learning Outcome. For even more study tools, visit **MasteringHealth**.

THINK ABOUT IT!

LO 1 | Sleepless in America

1. Why do you think the United States is one of the most sleep-deprived nations in the world? Although college students often do not get enough sleep-very few of them seek help. Why do you think this is the case? Do you think some people view their sleep-deprived status as an indicator of a positive work ethic?

LO 2 | The Importance of Sleep

2. Why is sleep so important to you while you are in college?

Do you notice changes in your health when you have longer periods of sleep deprivation? Does it affect your interactions with others?

LO 3 | The Processes of Sleep

3. What factors in your life are likely to disrupt your sleep cycles and cause sleep processes to be challenged? Are there things about these disruptions that you could change? Why does this matter?

LO 4 | Sleep Disorders

4. After reading this section, can you identify possible sleep disorders that you or a loved one might have? What behavior changes might you recommend for yourself or others to help with a specific disorder? Are there sleep specialists on campus or in your community?

LO 5 | Getting a Good Night's Sleep

5. What actions can you take to ensure that you get a good night's sleep at least 6 of the nights in every week? How might you use mindfulness strategies to help you? If either of your parents or friends are having sleep problems, what four things would you recommend they do to help them fall asleep and stay asleep each night?

ACCESS YOUR HEALTH ON THE INTERNET

Visit Mastering Health for links to the websites and RSS feeds.

If you are interested in finding out more about sleep topics or want to see how you could get a better nights sleep, the following websites might be of interest.

National Sleep Foundation. Information source for national and international sleep statistics, conducts a major national study on sleep each year, and provides a wealth of sleep information for consumers. **https ://sleepfoundation.org**

Harvard Health Publications. Mindfulness meditation helps fight insomnia, improves sleep, 2015. Overview of current research and options for those who have too many sleepless nights. Includes strategies for inducing sleep, tapes for mindfulness meditation, and other resources for gaining information about non-drug remedies for sleep. **https://www.health.harvard.edu /blog/mindfulness-meditation -helps-fight-insomnia-improves -sleep-201502187726**

CDC Sleep and Sleep Disorders. Provides national data/information about sleep, vetted by experts in the field. **www.cdc.gov/sleep/index.html**

5 Preventing Violence and Injury

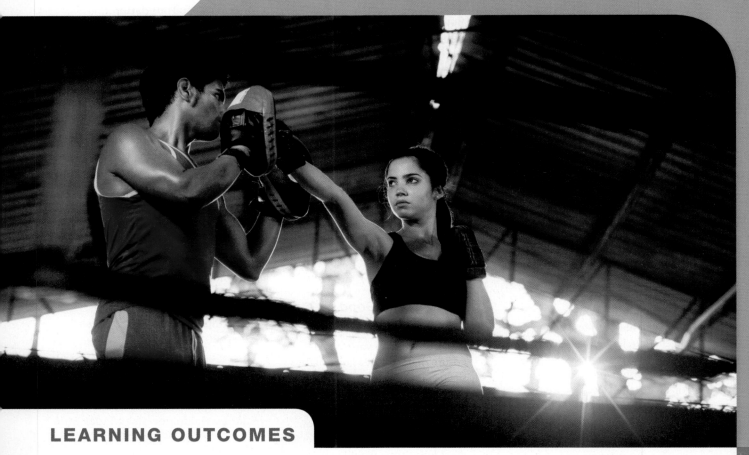

LEARNING OUTCOMES

LO **1** Differentiate between intentional and unintentional injuries, and discuss trends in violence in American society and on college campuses.

LO **2** List and explain factors that contribute to intentional acts of violence.

LO **3** Discuss the prevalence, common contributors to, and groups that are at risk for interpersonal and collective acts of violence, and describe intimate partner violence and the cycle of IPV.

LO **4** Describe various types of sexual victimization, environmental and social contributors, and the effectiveness of strategies to prevent and respond to sexual victimization.

LO **5** Discuss existing personal and community strategies for minimizing the risk of violence.

LO **6** Discuss key strategies that are likely to minimize the risk of unintentional injuries.

Violence seems to permeate many levels of our daily lives. We fear the threat of violence, and it touches us in subtle ways. We live our lives differently, distrust more, are taught to be wary of strangers, avoid certain areas where real or imagined danger may be lurking. We wonder what our futures may be like because of the uncertainty of events throughout the world. Imagine a world where the daily news was about good deeds, peaceful coexistence, caring about others, and working for the betterment of society—a world where everyone had the right and opportunity for the pursuit of health and happiness? In ways both large and small, we all have a part in creating that future.

Fear follows crime, and is its punishment.
—*Voltaire, 1694–1778*[1]

Nearly 25 years ago Deborah Prothrow-Stith, M.D., called violence in America *epidemic* and said that this epidemic was as potentially devastating to our society as any we had ever experienced.[2] She described what she saw as "an epidemic of meanness." Importantly, she believed its causes were human-made, including widespread availability of guns, rampant sale of illegal drugs, inadequate care for people with mental illness, and a divisive "have and have not society."

Today, we continue to have wars, homicides, rapes, domestic violence, child abuse, hate crimes, and many other serious problems. Protests, racial tensions, and civil unrest seem to be escalating. Terrorist threats, cyberthreats, and other threats to security seem to be spinning out of control. **Meanness** seems to be pervasive, as the media constantly tell us about some ugly event that has just played out. Even college campuses and public places such as shopping malls, churches, and nightclubs seem to be at risk, and people are increasingly fearful.

Put into perspective, violence has always been part of human existence. Throughout history, humans have sought to dominate others, achieve religious or political power, or acquire land and resources. They have fought for power, money, position in society, and sometimes basic survival. Today, we are much more aware of the violence occurring around us. We can now learn of violence in even the smallest towns of our nation and watch horrendous acts play out across the world from the safety of our own televisions, computers, and mobile devices, 24 hours a day. Violence touches us all. But is the world really as violent as it sometimes seems? To which kinds of violence are college students particularly vulnerable? Can individual, campus, and community policies and programs minimize violence in our communities?

LO 1 | WHAT IS VIOLENCE?

Differentiate between intentional and unintentional injuries, and discuss trends in violence in American society and on college campuses.

The World Health Organization defines **violence** as "the intentional use of physical force or power, threatened or actual, against oneself, another person, or a group or community that results in or has a high likelihood of resulting in injury, death, psychological harm, maldevelopment or deprivation."[3] Today, most experts realize that emotional and psychological forms of violence can be as devastating as physical blows to the body.

Historically, violence has been categorized as either *intentional* or *unintentional*, depending on whether there is intent to cause harm. Typically, **intentional injuries**—those committed with intent to harm—include assaults, homicides, self-inflicted injuries, and suicides. However, critics argue that people can get caught up in circumstances and emotional outbursts, making "intent" unclear. In contrast, **unintentional injuries** are those committed without apparent intent to harm, such as motor vehicle crashes or fires.

So why devote a chapter to violence and injury? Young adults are disproportionately affected by violence and injury. Unintentional injuries, particularly from motor vehicle crashes, are the number one cause of death among 15- to 44-year-olds in the United States today, and suicide and homicide are the second and third leading causes of death in 15- to 34-year-olds.[4]

Violence Overview

Although violence has long been part of the American landscape, it wasn't until the 1980s that the U.S. Public Health Service gave violence chronic disease status, indicating that it was a pervasive threat to society. Violent crimes involve force or threat of force and include four offenses: murder and non-negligent manslaughter, forcible rape, robbery, and aggravated assault. Statistics from the Federal Bureau of Investigation (FBI) have shown that, after increasing steadily from 1973 to 2006, the rates of overall crime and certain types of violent crime began a slow decline, falling by more than 10 percent between 2012 and 2014.[5] However, violent crime was up 1.7 percent in 2015 and increased 5.3 percent in the first half of 2016. In contrast, the Bureau of Justice Statistics reported little change in violent crime during those same periods.[6]

meanness Behaviors that demonstrate hatefulness, malevolence, cruelty, selfishness or viciousness and cause pain or suffering.

violence A set of behaviors that produces injuries, as well as the outcomes of these behaviors (the injuries themselves).

intentional injuries Injury, death, or psychological harm inflicted with the intent to harm.

unintentional injuries Injury, death, or psychological harm caused unintentionally or without premeditation.

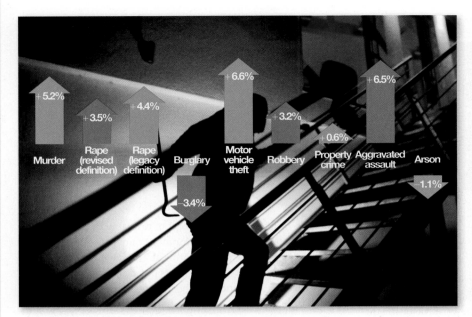

FIGURE 5.1 Changing Crime Rates FBI statistics show reported violent crimes increased by 6.2 percent in 2015 and 5.3 percent in 2016. Rates of crimes vary by type of crime, location, sex, and other variables; the most violent crimes are on the increase overall.

Source: FBI Crime in the United States, 2016 "Preliminary Semiannual Uniform Crime Report, January–June 2016," accessed March 2017, www.fbi.gov.

Which report was right? Actually, they both are! We use two measures for violence in the United States: the FBI's Uniform Crime Reporting (UCR) Program and the Bureau of Justice Statistics' National Crime Victimization Survey (NCVS). While the FBI's UCR collects data on violent crimes involving force or threat reported to law enforcement agencies, the Bureau of Justice Statistics collects detailed information on the frequency and nature of certain crimes twice a year through surveys of nearly 160,000 people in 90,000 homes.[7] The Bureau of Justice Statistics also does not track homicides or crimes against businesses, as the UCR Program does.

According to data from the first 6 months of 2016, all categories of violent crime were up except for property crime, burglary, larceny, and arson, which decreased. Murders were up 5.2 percent, and aggravated assaults were up 6.5 percent. Some regions of the United States reported dramatic increases. See **FIGURE 5.1** for the percent change of violent crimes reported in 2015 and **FIGURE 5.2** for the frequency of different types of crimes.

Whether total crime rates are up or down, there are huge disparities in crime rates based on race, sex, age, socioeconomic status, location, crime type, and other

WHAT DO YOU THINK?

Why do you think rates of violence in the United States are so much higher than those of other developed nations such as the United Kingdom and Japan? Can you think examples of pervasive meanness in society?

■ What factor do you think is the single greatest cause of violence?

■ What could be done to reduce risk from this factor?

factors. What's more, current numbers may not reflect actual offenses; over 54 percent of violent victimizations are not reported to the police.[8] Rates of nonreporting are even higher for some offenses such as rape. If those nonreports suddenly become reported, we might have a dramatically different profile. The good news is that, even though crime rates ebb and flow over the years, overall rates are considerably lower (nearly one third less) than they were in the early 1990s.[9]

Although you might never be a direct victim of crime, the people who live in fear of being victimized, are afraid to go out for a walk or run at night, won't let their children play outside because of violence in their neighborhoods, or avoid international travel or mass transit because of terrorist threats are already indirectly affected.

Violence on U.S. Campuses

The media frequently cover violence on campus, and gun violence has made headline news far too many times in recent years. Tragedies such as the one at Virginia Tech, where 32 people died in 2007 in the deadliest campus shooting in U.S. history, or at Marjory Stoneman Douglas High School in Parkland, Florida, where 17 people were gunned down in 2018, have sparked dialogue and action across the nation, prompting increases in campus security and safety measures. Today, it would be hard to find a campus without some form of safety plan in place to prevent

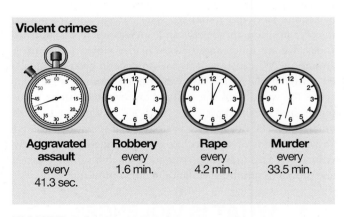

FIGURE 5.2 Crime Clock The crime clock represents the annual ratio of crime to fixed time intervals. The numbers are averages; the crime clock should not be taken to imply a regularity in the commission of crime.

Source: Adapted from Federal Bureau of Investigation, "Crime in the United States, 2015," Accessed March 2017, www.fbi.gov/about-us/cjis/ucr/crime-in-the-u.s/2014/crime-in-the-u.s.-2015/figs/crime-clock.jpg.

and respond to violent attacks. Knowing what actions will be taken in the event of a school shooting can help save lives and help avoid the inevitable anxiety and fear that occurs when lives are threatened.

While shootings make national news, many forms of campus violence continue to be hidden behind a veil of secrecy. Often, victims are reluctant to report assaults, and campuses are reluctant to have their images tarnished if violence is reported.

Relationship violence is one of the most prevalent problems on campus. In the most recent American College Health Association survey, 10.9 percent of women and 6.4 percent of men reported having been emotionally abused in the past 12 months in an intimate relationship.[10] Over 6.6 percent of women and 2.4 percent of men reported having been stalked, and 2 percent of women and 1.8 percent of men reported having been involved in a physically abusive relationship.[11] Nearly 1 percent of men and 2.7 percent of women reported having been in a sexually abusive relationship.[12]

However, statistics on reported campus violence represent only a glimpse of the big picture. Only 12.5 percent of rapes and 4.3 percent of sexual batteries are believed to have been reported to any authority.[13] Over 21 percent of undergraduate women and 7 percent of men have been sexually assaulted since entering college.[14]

Why do so few people report these assaults? Typical reasons include privacy concerns, fear of retaliation, embarrassment, lack of support, perception that the crime was too minor or that they were at fault, or uncertainty whether it was a crime.

LO 2 | FACTORS CONTRIBUTING TO VIOLENCE

List and explain factors that contribute to intentional acts of violence.

Several social, community, relationship, and individual factors increase the likelihood of violent acts. While no single criterion can explain what causes people to become violent offenders, key risk factors include the following:[15]

- **Community contexts.** Persistent poverty, particularly environments with unsafe housing, neighborhoods, schools, and workplaces increase risks of exposure to drugs, guns, and gangs. Inadequately staffed police and social services add to the risks.[16]
- **Societal factors.** Policies and programs that seek to remove inequality or disparity and discourage discrimination decrease risks. Social and cultural norms that support male dominance over women and violence as a means of settling problems increase risks.[17]
- **Religious beliefs and differences.** Extreme religious beliefs can lead people to think that violence against others is justified.
- **Political differences.** Civil unrest and differences in political party affiliations and beliefs have historically been triggers for violent acts.

- **Breakdowns in the criminal justice system.** Overcrowded prisons and inadequate availability of mental health services can precipitate repeat offenses and future violence.
- **Stress, depression, or other mental health issues.** People who are in crisis, are depressed, feel threatened, or are under stress are more apt to be highly reactive, striking out at others, displaying anger, or acting irrationally.[18]

What Makes Some Individuals Prone to Violence?

Personal factors can also increase risks for violence. Emerging evidence suggests that the family and home environment may be the greatest contributor to eventual violent behavior among family members.[19] Among key predictors of aggressive behavior are anger and substance abuse.[20]

Aggression and Anger
Aggressive behavior is often a key aspect of violent interactions. **Primary aggression** is goal-directed, hostile self-assertion that is destructive in nature. **Reactive aggression** is more often part of an emotional reaction brought about by frustrating life experiences. Whether aggression is reactive or primary, it is most likely to flare up in times of acute stress. See the **Mindfulness and You** box for tips on how to manage your own flare-ups.

Anger is a well-known catalyst for violence. Anger typically occurs when there is a *triggering event* or a person has learned that acting out in angry ways can get the person what he or she wants. Anger tends to be an active, attack-oriented emotion in which people feel powerful and in control for a short period.[21]

> **primary aggression** Goal-directed, hostile self-assertion that is destructive in nature.
>
> **reactive aggression** Hostile emotional reaction brought about by frustrating life experiences.

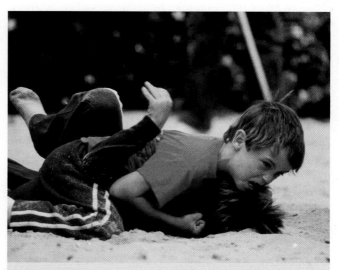

Most adults learn to control outbursts of anger in a rational manner. However, some people act out their aggressive tendencies in much the same way they did as children— with anger and violence that are a form of self-assertion or a response to frustration.

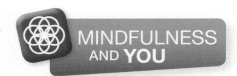

WHEN ANGER FLARES
Mindful Cooling Off Strategies

You know the feeling. You get home from classes, and someone has taken your parking place. Vaguely annoyed, you walk into your apartment to find a disaster: dishes piled high and smelly old leftovers on the counter. The food you had bought for your dinner is not in the fridge because someone else helped himself or herself to it. You're ready to explode in a screaming rant or fight. This lazy, inconsiderate slob has to go! Your blood pressure is up, and after a stressful day of exams, the relaxing evening at home you wanted is clearly history. Or is it?

You don't have to let anger control you. When frustration happens, try these mindfulness strategies to quell your anger:

1. Find a quiet place, and tune in to your physical anger sensations. Is your heart rate accelerated? Is your breathing increased? Is your mind racing? Is your face red? Are your muscles tight? Focus on what anger is doing to your body.

2. Close your eyes and breathe. Count out 10 slow, rhythmic breaths. Feel the warmth returning to your hands and arms. Soften your facial muscles, and feel your neck muscles relax.

3. Think of your anger as hot and burning. Focus on coolness—on the calming air that envelops you. Breathe.

4. Focus on your thoughts. Recognize that you may have been entitled to get mad, that it was probably what most people would do. But who is feeling the anger rippling through their body? And is it what you want to feel? Be compassionate with yourself. Cut yourself some slack. Accept the emotion and feel what anger just did to you, without judgment.

5. Step back. Observe your physical and emotional responses. Try to view the situation as a minor blip in your day. You can move through it. To change the dynamics, breathe slowly, soften your entire body, let

go. If you mind drifts toward ruminating on what made you angry, bring it back.

6. Once you are relaxed, take care of yourself. Let your roommate or partner know what bothered you, but be kind in your approach. Don't blast the person. Instead, tell him or her how you feel and what you would like to see happen. If you start to get frustrated, remember that you are in control of yourself. Feel the sensations in your body. If the heat starts rising, move back into your calm place emotionally or physical walk away.

7. Don't dwell. Relax. Do something that helps you remain calm. Work to change future dynamics through positive dialogue, consider your alternative options, or find a mediator to help resolve differences. Act kindly and compassionately. That will ultimately be best for you and others.

Physiological and genetic factors may influence people who have a short fuse. Increasing evidence suggests that people who act violently and unemotionally may have a genetic basis for increased anger and aggression; however, researchers acknowledge that there are several pathways by which a person may come to act violently.[22] Typically, anger-prone people come from families that are disruptive, chaotic, and unskilled in emotional expression and in which anger, domestic violence, and abuse occur regularly.[23] People who have been bullied in school may also be prone to react violently and suffer from PTSD as adults.[24]

2/3
of people in substance abuse treatment programs were **ABUSED AS CHILDREN**, as were 14% of men and 36% of women in U.S. prisons.

Substance Abuse Alcohol and drug abuse are often catalysts for violence at all levels of society, both nationally and internationally.[25]

- Forty percent of all violent crimes include alcohol as a factor; the Department of Justice reports that 37 percent of nearly 2 million convicted offenders in jail reported having been drinking when they were arrested.[26]
- An estimated 80 percent of offenses leading to prison, such as domestic violence, property offenses, and public-order offenses, include the involvement of alcohol and drugs.[27]
- Research suggests higher rates of alcohol use and violence in some athlete populations compared to nonathlete populations. Masculinity, antisocial norms, and violent social identity contribute to violence among athletes.[28]
- Numbers of suicide attempts and completions are highly correlated to drug and alcohol intake.[29]

How Much Impact Do the Media Have?

Although the media are often blamed for playing a role in the escalation of violence, this association has been challenged. Early studies seemed to support a link between excessive exposure to violent media and subsequent violent behavior, but much of this research has been criticized for methodological problems such as poor or inconsistent measures of violence, biased subject selection, and issues with sample size.[30]

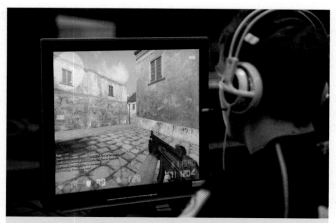

Arguably, Americans today, especially children, are exposed to more depictions of violence than ever before, but research has not shown a clear link between exposure to violent media and a propensity to engage in violent acts.

other groups and includes violent acts related to political, governmental, religious, cultural, or social clashes.[34] Gang violence and terrorism are two forms of collective violence that have become major threats in recent years.

▶ **SEE IT!** VIDEOS

How do we define a hate crime? Watch **Was North Carolina Killing a Hate Crime?** in the Study Area of Mastering Health.

1 IN 370

are the lifetime odds of dying in an assault by a firearm. For comparison, the odds are **1 IN 647** for dying as a passenger in a motor vehicle crash.

Do you think the media influence your behavior? If so, in what ways?

■ Could that influence lead to your becoming violent? Why or why not?

■ Are there instances in which restricting the nature and extent of violence and sex in the media is warranted? If so, under what circumstances?

A recent meta-analysis by the American Psychological Association indicates that playing violent games may increase risks of aggression and desensitize people when violence occurs. However, there is less evidence that watching violent videos increase risks for violent criminal activity. Other researchers continue to point out that exposure to violent videos has neither long-term nor short-term effects on either positive or negative behaviors.[31]

Critics of previous studies point out that today's young people are exposed to more media violence than any previous generation was, yet rates of violent crime among youth have fallen to 40-year lows.[32] Still, concerns have been raised about the effects of spending a disproportionate amount of time online instead of interacting in real-time, face-to-face communication.

LO 3 | INTERPERSONAL AND COLLECTIVE VIOLENCE

Discuss the prevalence, common contributors to, and groups that are at risk for interpersonal and collective acts of violence, and describe intimate partner violence and the cycle of IPV.

Interpersonal violence includes intentionally using "physical force or power, threatened or actual," to inflict violence against an individual that results in injury, death, or psychological harm.[33] Homicide, hate crimes, domestic violence, child abuse, elder abuse, and sexual victimization all fit into this category. **Collective violence** is violence perpetrated by groups against

Homicide

Homicide, defined as murder or nonnegligent manslaughter (killing another human), is the 13th leading cause of death in the United States. Overall, it is among the top five leading causes of death for people aged 1 to 44 years.[35] Nearly half of all homicides occur among people who know one another.[36] In two thirds of these cases, the perpetrator and the victim are friends or acquaintances; in one third, they are family members.[37]

Homicide rates reveal clear disparities across race, gender, and age. Homicides are the fifth leading cause of death for African American males, the sixth leading cause of death for Native Americans, and the ninth leading cause of death in Latino populations.[38] See the Health Headlines box for a discussion of guns and violence.

Hate Crimes and Bias-Motivated Crimes

A **hate crime** is a crime committed against a person, property, or group of people that is motivated by the offender's bias based on race, gender or gender identity, religion, disability, sexual orientation, or ethnicity.[39] Reports of hate crimes declined to 5,479 incidents in 2014, according to the FBI (FIGURE 5.3).[40] In sharp contrast, the anonymous Bureau of Justice Statistics National Crime Victimization Survey found that an estimated 294,000 violent and property hate crimes occurred in 2012.[41] Fear of retaliation keeps many hate crimes hidden. While 60 percent of hate crimes may never be reported, only about one fourth of those reported are reported by victims themselves.[42]

interpersonal violence Violence inflicted against one individual by another or by a small group of others.

collective violence Violence committed by groups of individuals.

homicide Death that results from intent to injure or kill.

hate crime Crime targeted against a particular societal group and motivated by bias against that group.

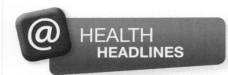

HEALTH HEADLINES

BRINGING THE GUN DEBATE TO CAMPUS

On average, each year in the United States 100,000 people are shot. Over 31,000 of them die, and of those who survive, many experience significant physical and emotional repercussions. Some facts about guns and gun violence include the following:

- Handguns are consistently responsible for more murders than any other type of weapon.
- Today, 35 percent of American homes have a gun on the premises, with nearly 300 million privately owned guns registered—and millions more that are unregistered and/or illegal.
- Firearms are the weapons most often used in attacks on American campuses. The most common reason for an incident is "related to an intimate relationship," followed by "retaliation for a specific action."
- The presence of a gun in the home triples the risk of a homicide in that location and increases suicide risk more than five times.

What factors contribute to gun deaths in the United States? Currently, this country has somewhere between 270 million and 350 million guns—meaning that, by some counts, there may be more guns than there are people. No other country on the planet even comes close in terms of civilian gun ownership. Advocates of background checks for weapons purchases and more strict gun control legislation argue that the uniquely large numbers of guns—particularly semiautomatic assault weapons with high-capacity magazines—in the United States as well as relatively easy access to powerful weapons are the main culprits. However, gun rights advocates say that the problem lies not with guns themselves, but with the people who own them.

High-profile shootings at schools and other public places have brought the gun debate to campuses. Over the last decade, numerous states have allowed concealed weapon carry, some of which allow them on campus. Critics argue that this is a dangerous situation in which alcohol and anger may converge to increase risks for faculty and students alike. Gun advocates argue that if people in mass-shooting situations had weapons, deaths and assaults would be prevented. What do you think?

Sources: C. Ingraham, "There Are Now More Guns Than People in the United States," *The Washington Post*, October 5, 2015, https://www.washingtonpost.com/news/wonk/wp/2015/10/05/guns-in-the-united-states-one-for-every-man-woman-and-child-and-then-some; J. Davidson and H. Jones, "The Orlando Shooting Is a Haunting Reminder of Just How Many Guns Are in America," *Time*, June 14, 2016, http://time.com/4188456/orlando-shooting-mass-shootings-gun-control; D. Drysdale, W. Modzeleski, and A. Simons, *Campus Attacks: Targeted Violence Affecting Institutions of Higher Learning* (Washington, DC: U.S. Secret Service, U.S. Department of Education, and Federal Bureau of Investigation, 2010); National Conference of State Legislatures, "Guns on Campus: Overview," 2015, http://www.ncsl.org/research/education/guns-on-campus-overview.aspx.

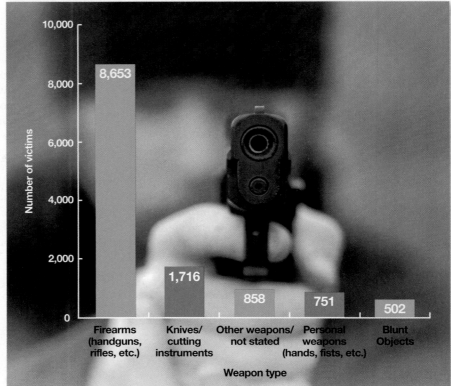

Homicide in the United States by Weapon Type, 2015. Sixty-seven percent of murders in the United States are committed by using firearms, far outweighing all other weapons combined.

Source: Data from U.S. Department of Justice, Federal Bureau of Investigation, "Crime in the United States, 2015, Expanded Homicide Data Table 8—Murder Victims by Weapon—2011–2015," 2015, https://ucr.fbi.gov/crime-in-the-u.s/2015/crime-in-the-u.s.-2015/tables/expanded_homicide_data_table_8_murder_victims_by_weapon_2011-2015.xls.

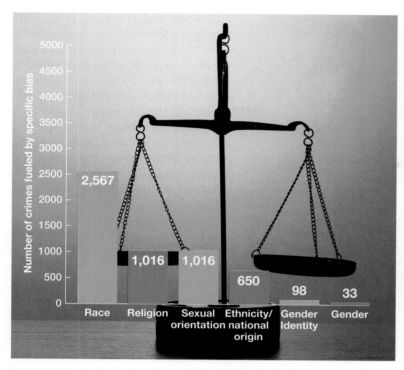

FIGURE 5.3 Bias-Motivated Crimes, Single-Bias Incidence, 2015

Source: Data from Federal Bureau of Investigation, "Hate Crime Statistics, 2015," Table 1, www.fbi.gov, November 2016.

Bias-motivated crime, sometimes referred to as **ethnoviolence**, describes violence based on prejudice and discrimination among ethnic groups in the larger society. **Prejudice** is an irrational attitude of hostility directed against an individual; a group; a race; or the supposed characteristics of an individual, group, or race. **Discrimination** constitutes actions that deny equal treatment or opportunities to a group of people, often based on prejudice.

Common reasons given to explain bias-motivated and hate crimes include (1) *thrill seeking* by multiple offenders through a group attack, (2) *feeling threatened* that others will take their jobs or property or beset them in some way, (3) *retaliating* for some real or perceived insult or slight, and (4) *fearing the unknown or differences*. For other people, hate crimes are a part of their mission in life because of religious zeal, lack of understanding, or distorted moral beliefs.

Campuses have responded to reports of hate crimes by offering courses that emphasize diversity, enforcing zero tolerance for violations, training faculty members to act appropriately, and developing policies that enforce punishment for hate crimes.

Gang Violence

Gang violence is increasing in many regions of the world; U.S. communities face escalating threats from gang networks engaged in drug trafficking, sex trafficking, shootings, beatings, thefts, carjackings, and the killing of innocent victims caught in the crossfire. There are over 33,000 gangs in the United States, with membership in excess of 1.4 million.[43] The vast majority are street gangs (88 percent), followed by prison gangs (9.5 percent) and outlaw motorcycle gangs (2.5 percent).[44] Gangs are believed to be responsible for 48 percent of U.S. violent crime overall and as much as 90 percent in some location.[45]

Why do young people join gangs? Often, gangs give members a sense of self-worth or belonging, companionship, security, and excitement. In some cases, gangs provide economic security through drug sales, prostitution, and other types of criminal activity. Friendships with delinquent peers, lack of parental monitoring, negative life events, and alcohol and drug use appear to increase risks for gang affiliation. Other risk factors include low self-esteem, academic problems, low socioeconomic status, alienation from family and society, a history of family violence, and living in a gang-controlled neighborhood.[46]

Cybercrime

Cyberattacks that attempt to disrupt infrastructure, influence elections, steal trade secrets, hijack and sell personal information and identities, exact payment for locking up sensitive information with ransomeware, and other threats are becoming more commonplace, more dangerous, and more sophisticated.[47] The FBI, which is the federal agency in charge of investigating cyberattacks, has prioritized personal and network security and ransomeware as national cyberthreats. To protect your own cybersecurity, the FBI recommends the following:[48]

■ **Keep your computer's firewall turned on.** Firewalls are important first lines of defense against potential cyberthreats.

The mass shooting at the Pulse Nightclub in Orlando, Florida in 2016 and other acts of violence based on gender identity exemplify growing threats to groups that are different.

ethnoviolence Violence directed at individuals affiliated with a particular ethnic group.

prejudice A negative evaluation of an entire group of people that is typically based on unfavorable and often wrong ideas about the group.

discrimination Actions that deny equal treatment or opportunities to a group, often based on prejudice.

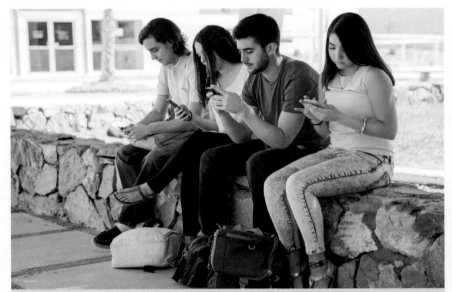

Staying safe from cybercrime requires vigilance and the use of the best available security on all your devices.

- **Choose antivirus and antispyware software from reputable sources.** Purchase high-quality programs from reputable sources, and look to independent sources for reviews.
- **Keep your operating system up to date.** Newer systems offer security patches and fixes to gaps in security. Buy newer systems, and keep them up to date on all of your devices.
- **Be careful what you download or open as attachments.** Don't open unknown attachments or items with subject lines meant to draw you in.
- **Turn off your computer when you aren't using it.** Constant connections allow malicious intruders to jump onto your account when nobody is watching.

Terrorism

Terrorist attacks around the world reveal the vulnerability of all nations to domestic and international threats. Effects on our economy, travel restrictions, additional security measures, and military buildups are but a few of the examples of how terrorist threats have affected our lives. As defined in the U.S. Code of Federal Regulations, **terrorism** is the "unlawful use of force or violence against persons or property to intimidate or coerce a government, the civilian population, or any segment thereof in furtherance of political or social objectives."[49] Increasingly, the Internet and social media are being used for

terrorism Unlawful use of force or violence against persons or property to intimidate or coerce a government, civilian population, or any segment thereof in furtherance of political or social objectives.

domestic violence The use of force to control and maintain power over another person in the home environment, including both actual harm and the threat of harm.

intimate partner violence (IPV) Physical, sexual, or psychological harm by a current or former partner or spouse.

recruitment and radicalization of youth throughout the world. Major groups in the United States and internationally are making efforts to counteract such activities.[50]

Over the past decade, the Centers for Disease Control and Prevention (CDC) established the Emergency Preparedness and Response Division. This group monitors potential public health problems, such as bioterrorism, chemical emergencies, radiation emergencies, mass casualties, national disaster, and severe weather; develops plans for mobilizing communities in case of emergency; and provides information about terrorist threats. In addition, the Department of Homeland Security works to prevent future attacks, and the FBI and other government agencies work to ensure citizens' health and safety. Increasing numbers of communities and individuals have enacted disaster and emergency preparedness plans. Check with your campus and community leaders to determine what plans are in force in your area and what you can do to stay safe.

Intimate Partner and Domestic Violence

Domestic violence has historically been described as the use of force to control and maintain power over another person in the home environment. It can occur between parent and child, between siblings or other family members, or, most commonly, between spouses or intimate partners. The violence may involve emotional abuse, verbal abuse, threats of physical harm, and physical violence ranging from slapping and shoving to beatings, rape, and homicide.

Intimate partner violence (IPV) includes physical, sexual, or psychological harm done by a current or former partner or spouse and doesn't have to occur within the home. On average, each minute, there are 20 new incidents of physical violence at the hands of an intimate partner in the United States.[51] This type of violence can occur among all types of couples and does not require sexual intimacy. Although we often think of violence as something perpetrated by a stranger, Americans are more likely to be victims of physical and psychological abuse, stalking, and other offenses by an intimate partner, often someone they know or who is living with them. Nearly 75 percent of all murder-suicides were perpetrated by an intimate partner and 96 percent of these deaths were women.[52] Homicide committed by a current or former intimate partner is the leading cause of death of pregnant women in the United States.[53]

Nearly half of all women and men in the United States have experienced psychological aggression by an intimate partner in their lifetime.[54] Women who are poor, less educated, living in high-poverty areas, socially isolated, and

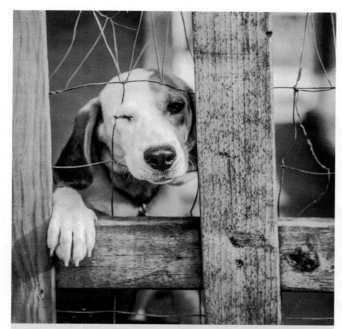

There is a strong relationship between animal abuse and family violence. Abusers batter family pets to exert power and control, to punish/hurt family members, for revenge and to keep family members fearful.

Source: M Newberg. "Pets in Danger: Exploring the Link Between Domestic Violence and Animal Abuse." *Aggression and Violent Behavior.* 2017. 34:273–281.

dependent on drugs and alcohol are at greatest risk of IPV.[55] This abuse can take the form of constant criticism, humiliation, verbal attacks, displays of explosive anger meant to intimidate, and controlling behavior. People who have experienced this violence are three times more likely to report mental health problems, such as depression, anxiety, high stress, gastrointestinal problems, insomnia, and other issues.[56]

The Cycle of IPV Have you ever heard of a woman repeatedly beaten by her partner and wondered, "Why doesn't she just leave him?" There are many reasons why some people find it difficult to break ties with abusers. Some, particularly women with small children, are financially dependent on their partners. Others fear retaliation. Some hope that the situation will change with time, and others stay because cultural or religious beliefs forbid divorce. Still others love the abusive partner and are concerned about what will happen if they leave.

In the 1970s, psychologist Lenore Walker developed a theory called the *cycle of violence* that explained predictable, repetitive patterns of psychological and/or physical abuse that seemed to occur in abusive relationships. The cycle consisted of three major phases:[57]

1. **Tension building.** Before the overtly abusive act, tension building includes breakdowns in communication, anger, psychological aggression, growing tension, and fear.

2. **Incident of acute abuse.** When the acute attack is over, the abuser may respond with shock and denial about his or her own behavior or blame the victim for making the abuser do it.

3. **Remorse/reconciliation.** During a "honeymoon" period, the abuser may be kind, loving, and apologetic, swearing to stop the abusive behavior.

After refining her work with the insights of other researchers, Walker expanded her research to focus on *battered woman syndrome*.[58] Today, battered woman syndrome is considered to be a subgroup of posttraumatic stress disorder (PTSD) and is often used to describe someone who has gone through the above cycle at least twice.

Child Abuse and Neglect

Child maltreatment is defined as any act or series of acts of commission or omission by a parent or caregiver that results in harm, potential for harm, or threat of harm to a child.[59] **Child abuse** refers to *acts of commission*, which are deliberate or intentional words or actions that cause harm, potential harm, or threat of harm to a child. The abuse may be sexual, psychological, physical, or a combination. **Neglect** is an *act of omission*, meaning a failure to provide for a child's basic physical, emotional, or education needs or failure to protect a child from harm or potential harm. Failure to provide food, shelter, clothing, medical care, or supervision or exposing a child to unnecessary environmental violence or threat are examples of neglect. Although reported cases may represent only a fraction of actual causes, **FIGURE 5.4** provides an overview of the most recent reported cases, representing over 3 million.[60] We lose four or five children a day, largely as a result of parental actions or lack thereof.[61]

Child abuse occurs at every socioeconomic level, across ethnic and cultural lines, within all religions, and at all levels of education. Not all violence against children is physical. Mental health can be severely affected by psychological violence—assaults on personality, character, competence, independence, or general dignity as a human being. The lifetime prevalence of PTSD, psychopathology, substance abuse, eating disorders, borderline personality disorders and emotional dysregulation are significantly higher in abuse/maltreatment survivors.[62] Victims of child abuse have a higher risk of depression, unintended pregnancy, sexually transmitted diseases (STIs), suicide, and drug and alcohol abuse and an overall lowered life expectancy, particularly among those who were repeatedly victimized.[63]

> **SEE IT! VIDEOS**
> Should strangers step in to prevent partner abuse? Watch **Will Anyone Confront Abusive Boyfriend?** available on Mastering Health.

child maltreatment Any act or series of acts of commission or omission by a parent or caregiver that results in harm, potential for harm, or threat of harm to a child.

child abuse Deliberate or intentional words or actions that cause harm, potential for harm, or threat of harm to a child.

neglect Failure to provide a child's basic needs such as food, clothing, shelter, and medical care.

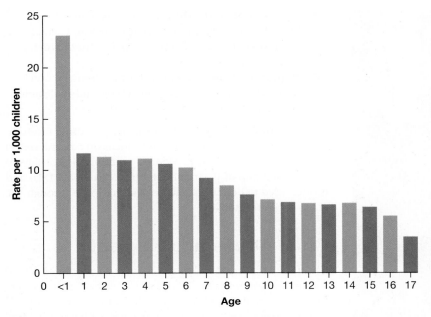

FIGURE 5.4 Child Abuse and Neglect Victims by Age, 2015

Source: U.S. Department of Health and Human Services, Administration for Children and Families 2015, Administration on Children, Youth and Families, Children's Bureau, 2015, Child Maltreatment, Exhibit 3-F, Victims by age. 2015, https://www.acf.hhs.gov/cb/resource/child-maltreatment-20.

Elder Abuse

By 2030, the number of people in the United States over the age of 65 will exceed 71 million—nearly double their number in 2000. Each year, hundreds of thousands of adults over the age of 60 are abused, neglected, or financially exploited as they enter the later years of life, and these statistics are likely an underestimate.[64] Many victims fail to report abuse because they are embarrassed or because they don't want the abuser to get in trouble or retaliate by putting them in a nursing home or escalating the abuse. A variety of social services focus on protecting our seniors, just as we endeavor to protect other vulnerable populations.

LO 4 | **SEXUAL** VICTIMIZATION

Describe various types of sexual victimization, environmental and social contributors, and the effectiveness of strategies to prevent and respond to sexual victimization.

The term *sexual victimization* refers to any situation in which an individual is coerced or forced to comply with or endure another person's sexual acts or overtures. It can run the gamut from harassment to stalking to assault and rape by perpetrators known or unknown to the victim. It can include sexual coercion and rape by spouses. Fear, sexual avoidance, sleeplessness, anxiety, and depression are just a few of the long-term consequences for victims.[65]

sexual assault Any act in which one person is sexually intimate with another without that person's consent.

rape Sexual penetration without the victim's consent.

aggravated rape Rape that involves one or multiple attackers, strangers, weapons, or physical beating.

simple rape Rape by one person, usually known to the victim, that does not involve physical beating or use of a weapon.

Sexual Assault and Rape

Sexual assault is any act in which one person is sexually intimate with another person without that person's consent. This may range from simple touching to forceful penetration and may include, for example, ignoring indications that intimacy is not wanted, threatening force or other negative consequences, and actually using force.

Considered the most extreme form of sexual assault, **rape** is defined as penetration without the victim's consent. However, a new, clarified definition of rape includes "[p]enetration, no matter how slight, of the vagina or anus with any body part or object, or oral penetration by a sex organ of another person, without the consent of the victim. This includes the offenses of rape, sodomy, and sexual assault with an object."[66]

Incidents of rape generally fall into one of two types: aggravated or simple. An **aggravated rape** is any rape involving one stranger or multiple attackers, use of weapons, or physical beatings. A **simple rape** is a rape perpetrated by one person whom the victim knows and does not involve a physical beating or use of a weapon. Most rapes are classified as simple rape, but that terminology should not be taken to mean that a simple rape is not violent or criminal.

Nearly 1 in 5 women and 1 in 59 men in the United States have been raped at some time in their lives; nearly 80 percent of female rape victims experience their first rape before the age of 25.[67] More than one fourth of male rape victims were raped before they were 10 years old.[68]

By most indicators, reported cases of rape appear to have declined in the United States since the early 1990s even as reports of other forms of sexual assault have increased. This decline is thought to be due to shifts in public awareness and attitudes about rape combined with tougher crime policies, major educational campaigns, and media attention. These changes enforce the idea that rape is a violent crime and should be treated as such. However, numerous sources indicate that rape is one of the most underreported crimes, particularly on college campuses.[69]

Acquaintance Rape The terms *date rape* and *acquaintance rape* were used interchangeably in the past. However, most experts now believe that the term *date rape* is inappropriate

OVER **20%** of undergraduate women have been **SEXUALLY ASSAULTED** one or more times during their undergraduate years.

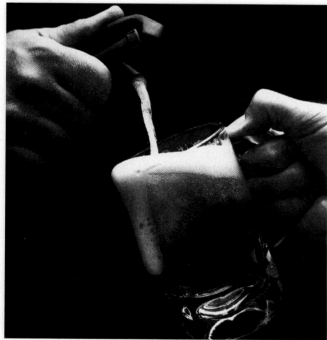

A lot of campus rapes start here.

Whenever there's drinking or drugs, things can get out of hand. So it's no surprise that many campus rapes involve alcohol.

But you should know that under any circumstances, sex without the other person's consent is considered rape. A felony, punishable by prison. And drinking is no excuse.

That's why, when you party, it's good to know what your limits are. You see, a little sobering thought now can save you from a big problem later.

Acquaintance rape is particularly common on college campuses, where alcohol and drug use can impair young people's judgment and self-control.

 Watch Video Tutor: Acquaintance Rape on Campus in Mastering Health.

because it implies a consensual interaction in an arranged setting and may minimize the criminality of the rape. Today, **acquaintance rape** refers to any rape in which the rapist is known to the victim. Acquaintance rape is more common when the offender and/or the victim has consumed drugs or alcohol; this makes the campus party environment a high-risk venue. Alcohol is frequently involved in acquaintance rape, as are a growing number of rape-facilitating drugs such as gamma-hydroxybutyrate (GHB), ketamine, and Rohypnol.

When you go out, be aware of your surroundings. If you have a drink, keep an eye on it at all times. Go with a group of people you know and trust, and be cautious if anyone offers you an unsealed beverage. If you feel incredibly tired or clumsy after drinking a relatively small amount, get to a safe place as soon as possible. The Skills for Behavior Change box identifies more practical tips for preventing dating violence.

▶ SEE IT! VIDEOS

What are the repercussions of sexual assault? Watch **Sexual Assaults on College Campuses: 95 Colleges under Federal Investigation** in the Study Area of Mastering Health.

Reducing Rape on Campus

As our awareness of the extent of the problem of rape on campus has increased, so has pressure to do something about it. Numerous campus activists, public health professionals and organizations, and key political figures have stepped forward with educational, policy, and legal actions designed to prevent rape, enforce penalties, and support victims.

acquaintance rape Any rape in which the rapist is known to the victim (replaces the formerly used term *date rape*).

In 1990, Congress passed the Clery Act, requiring institutions to collect and report data about sexual crimes on their campuses. As part of Clery Act, three main areas were to be addressed, or the institutions would lose federal aid: (1) victim's rights, (2) disciplinary procedures, and (3) educational programs.

Under further fire for failure to respond to student victimization on campus, Congress passed the Campus Sexual Assault Victim's Bill of Rights, known as the Ramstad Act, in 1992. The act gave victims the right to call in off-campus authorities to investigate serious campus crimes and required universities to develop educational programs and notify students of available counseling.

In 2013, under pressure from President Obama and in response to a detailed report from Senator Claire McCaskill about the existing risks to students on American campuses, the Campus Sexual Violence Elimination Act passed and was fully implemented by October 1, 2014.[70] As part of the act, intimate partner violence, dating violence, sexual assault, and stalking cases must be reported on annual campus crime reports. Notification procedures, options for victims and accused perpetrators, and consequences—including loss of federal support if schools don't conduct campus climate surveys and assess their prevention activities—are all part of the act's provisions.[71] Despite these changes, in 2014, many campuses that were not receiving federal funds did not report campus violence. In fact, as many as 500 of them reported no rapes or sexual assaults at all, prompting considerable national concern in the media.[72] As a result, several sources published rankings of the campuses

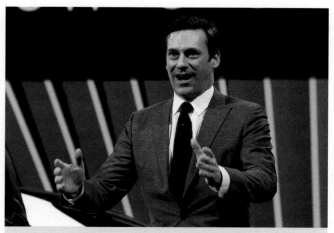

Well-known celebrities like Jon Hamm have helped raise awareness about sexual assault on campus through Joe Biden's "IT'S ON US" campaign.

with the highest numbers of rape occurrences—a scathing indictment of campus safety.

In 2014, California became the first state in the nation to implement a "yes means yes" law, changing the definition of sexual consent to require "an affirmative, conscious, and voluntary agreement to engage in sexual activity."[73] If one party is unable to give consent because of intoxication or other factors, the perpetrator could be prosecuted for sexual assault. The law also requires schools that receive funding from the state to develop policies for numerous situations related to sexual assault.[74] Additionally, President Obama and Vice President Joe Biden's "It's On Us" program was initiated between 2014 and 2017 to empower college men and women to work together to stop sexual assaults on campus through several action-oriented steps.

Marital Rape Although its legal definition varies within the United States, *marital rape* can be any unwanted intercourse or penetration (vaginal, anal, or oral) obtained by force or threat of force or when the spouse is unable to consent. This problem has undoubtedly existed since the origin of marriage as an institution, and it is noteworthy that marital rape was not a crime in all 50 states until 1993. Unfortunately, as many as 13 states still allow "marital exemptions" from prosecution, meaning that the judicial system may treat marital rape as a lesser crime.[75]

Decades of research have indicated that marital rape is not that uncommon, but exact percentages are difficult to assess because of differences in marital rape laws and different perceptions of whether rape within the confines of marriage is the same as rape by an acquaintance or a stranger. Internationally, women raised in cultures where male dominance is the norm and women are treated as property tend to have higher rates of forced sex within the confines of marriage. Women who are pregnant, ill, separated, or divorced have higher rates, as do women from homes where other forms of domestic violence are common and where there is a high rate of alcoholism or substance abuse.

Social Contributors to Sexual Violence Certain societal assumptions and traditions can promote sexual violence, including the following:

- **Trivialization.** Many people think that rape committed by a husband or intimate partner doesn't count as rape.
- **Blaming the victim.** In spite of efforts to combat this type of thinking, many believe that a scantily clad woman "asks" for sexual advances.
- **Pressure to be macho.** Males are taught from a young age that showing emotions is a sign of weakness. This often includes encouraging men to be aggressive and predatory to see females as passive targets.
- **Male socialization.** Many people still believe that behaviors implied in the phrases "sowing wild oats" and "boys will be boys" are merely a normal part of male development. Women are often objectified (treated as sexual objects) in the media, which contributes to the idea that it is natural for men to be predatory.

marital rape Unwanted sexual activity by a spouse or ex-spouse using force, threat of force, intimidation, or when a person is unable to consent.

Reducing Your Risk Of Dating Violence: Tips For Women And Men

Remember that if someone you are dating truly cares for and respects you, that person will respect your wishes and feelings. Here are some tips for dealing with sexual pressure or unwanted advances when dating and socializing:

- Before your date, think about your values, and set personal boundaries before you walk out the door. Have a plan for staying safe, and stick to it.

- Get consent for sexual activity. Educate yourself on what YES and NO really mean, and don't make assumptions, especially in situations involving drugs or alcohol. Ask yourself, "Is this worth my reputation, or is this worth having a sexual assault or rape charge and being prosecuted?" Ignorance is no excuse for illegal actions.

- Do not go off to a special room, car, or bedroom at a party where there is heavy drinking. Stay with friends. If you are getting intoxicated, don't let someone you don't know drive you home. There is safety in numbers, particularly if you stay in full view of others.

- Set limits. Practice what you will say to friends if they pressure you into actions that you would not normally engage in or if your date pressures you in an uncomfortable direction. If the situation feels as though it is getting out of control or someone is really coming on to you, change the dialogue. Say that you are uncomfortable. Say "no" directly, loudly, and firmly. Don't worry about hurting the other person's feelings.

- Don't accept drinks that you haven't had total control over from the moment of purchase. Don't leave drinks unattended.

- Remember that acts you might not consider serious could get you into a lot of trouble. Forced heavy kissing, touching, and pressing flesh are all grounds for charges of assault.

- Pay attention to your date's actions. If there is too much teasing, if there is encouragement to drink more and more, if there is a tendency to keep you from staying with your friends, or if you sense unusual pressure, it may mean trouble. Trust your intuition.

- Go out in groups when dating someone new. If you know the person, make sure he or she understands where you are coming from in terms of unwanted sexual advances.

- Stick with your friends. Agree to keep an eye out for one another at parties, and have a plan for leaving together and checking in with each other. Never leave a bar or party alone with a stranger. If you see someone being put into a compromising or dangerous situation, speak up. Try to steer the situation in another direction. You don't want your friends to be prosecuted for rape, and you don't want your friends to be victimized.

- **Male misperceptions.** Some men believe that when a woman says no, she is really being coy and inviting the man to seduce her. Later, these men may be surprised when the woman says she was raped.
- **Situational factors.** Dates during which one person makes all the decisions, pays for everything, and generally controls the entire situation are more likely to end in an aggressive sexual scenario. Use of alcohol and other drugs increases the risk and severity of assaults.

Sexual Harassment

Sexual harassment is defined as unwelcome sexual conduct that is related to any condition of employment or evaluation of student performance. Unwelcome sexual advances, requests for sexual favors, and other verbal or physical conduct of a sexual nature constitute sexual harassment in the following circumstances:

- Submission to such conduct is made either explicitly or implicitly a term or condition of an individual's employment or education.
- Submission to or rejection of such conduct by an individual is used as the basis for employment or education-related decisions affecting such an individual.
- Such conduct is sufficiently severe or pervasive that it has the effect, intended or unintended, of unreasonably interfering with an individual's work or academic performance because it has created an intimidating, hostile, or offensive environment and would have such an effect on a reasonable person of that individual's status.[76]

People often think of harassment as involving only faculty members or individuals in power who use sex to exhibit control of a situation. However, peers can harass one another too. Sexual harassment may include unwanted touching; unwarranted sex-related comments or subtle pressure for sexual favors; deliberate or repeated humiliation or intimidation based on sex; and gratuitous comments, jokes, questions, or remarks about clothing or body, sexuality, or past sexual relationships.

Most schools and companies have sexual harassment policies in place, as well as procedures for dealing with harassment problems. Faculty, students, and employees on U.S. campuses are protected from sexual harassment and other sexual offenses under Title IX of the Education Amendment of 1972, which prohibits discrimination based on sex in all education programs or activities that receive federal funds.

If you believe you are being harassed, the most important thing you can do is be assertive:

- **Tell the harasser to stop.** Be clear and direct. Tell the person that if it continues, you will report it. If the harassing is via phone or Internet, block the person.
- **Document the harassment.** Make a record of each incident. If the harassment becomes intolerable, a record of exactly what occurred (and when and where) will help make your case. Save copies of all communication from the harasser.

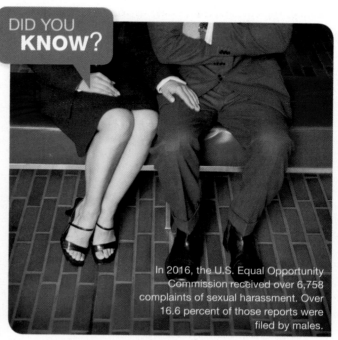

DID YOU KNOW?

In 2016, the U.S. Equal Opportunity Commission received over 6,758 complaints of sexual harassment. Over 16.6 percent of those reports were filed by males.

Source: Data are from U.S. Equal Employment Opportunity Commission, "Charges Alleging Sexual Harassment, FY 2010–2016," 2017, www.eeoc.gov.

- **Try to make sure you aren't alone in the harasser's presence.** Witnesses to harassment can ensure appropriate validation of the event.
- **Complain to a higher authority.** Talk to legal authorities or your instructor, adviser, or counseling center psychologist about what happened.
- **Remember that you have not done anything wrong.** You will likely feel awful after being harassed (especially if you have to complain to superiors). However, feel proud that you are not keeping silent.

Traditional and Tech-Facilitated Stalking

Stalking can be defined as a course of conduct directed at a specific person that would cause a reasonable person to feel fear. Often, the victim is a former or current intimate partner. Traditionally, stalking meant someone following you, showing up where you were, contacting you, sending gifts, or peering into your windows in the night—forms of personal unwanted space invasion that are fairly easy to spt.[77] Online intrusions and monitoring are called **cyberstalking**. Today's stalkers often use *technology-facilitated methods* that are even more insidious. By using technology, the perpetrator tries to create a sense of omnipresence and to isolate and humiliate victims, by exploiting shared sexual content, photos, or messages and making the victim feel that he or she is continually being surveilled. Security cameras, tracking and GPS devices that can provide

sexual harassment Any form of unwanted sexual attention related to any condition of employment, education, or performance evaluation.

stalking Willful, repeated, and malicious following, harassing, or threatening of another person.

cyberstalking Stalking that occurs online.

location, spyware, and inexpensive devices can instill fear and cause people to modify normal behavior.[78]

College students are more likely to be stalked than the general public by 200 percent, and 18-24 year olds are the most likely to be stalked overall.[79] College students are also more vulnerable to a form of *coercive control*—a situation in which a person is dominated by an intimate partner through isolation, manipulation, micromanagement, and veiled and direct threats. Stalking is often one of the most pervasive forms of coercive control, as victims begin to feel trapped—as though everywhere they go, everyone is part of a surveillance plot. Although men are often the perpetrators, people of all genders and sexual orientations can be victims or victimizers.[80]

Over 15 percent of women and nearly 6 percent of men have been victims of stalking during their lifetimes.[81] Fewer than 10 percent of stalkers are strangers to their victims.[82] Like sexual harassment, stalking is an underreported crime. Often, students do not think a stalking incident is serious enough to report, or they worry that the police will not take it seriously.

Child Sexual Abuse

Sexual abuse of children by adults or older children includes sexually suggestive conversations; inappropriate kissing; touching; petting; oral, anal, or vaginal intercourse; and other kinds of sexual interaction. In 2015, there were 315,000 reported cases of child sexual abuse in the United States.[83] Recent studies indicate that the rates of sexual abuse in children range from 1 to 35 percent of all children, one in four girls and one in six boys being sexually abused before the age of 18.[84]

The shroud of secrecy surrounding this problem makes it likely that the number of actual cases is grossly underestimated both in the United States and globally. Unfortunately, the programs taught in schools today, often with an emphasis on "stranger danger," may give children the false impression that they are more likely to be assaulted by a stranger. In reality, 90 percent of child sexual abuse victims know their perpetrator; nearly 70 percent of children are abused by family members, usually an adult male.[85]

People who were abused as children bear spiritual, psychological, and/or physical scars. Studies have shown that child sexual abuse has an impact on later life. Children who experience sexual abuse are at increased risk for anxiety disorders, depression, eating disorders, PTSD, and suicide attempts.[86] Youth who have been sexually abused are 25 percent more likely to experience teen pregnancy, 30 percent more likely to abuse their own children, and much more likely to have problems with alcohol abuse or drug addiction.[87]

LO 5 | PREVENTING VIOLENCE

Discuss existing personal and community strategies for minimizing the risk of violence.

It is far better to prevent a violent act than to have to recover from it. Both individuals and communities can play important roles in preventing violence and intentional injuries.

Self-Defense against Personal Assault and Rape

Assault can occur no matter what preventive actions you take, but commonsense self-defense tactics can lower the risk. Self-defense is a process that includes increasing your awareness, developing self-protective skills, taking reasonable precautions, and having the judgment necessary to respond quickly to changing situations. It is important to know ways to avoid and extract yourself from potentially dangerous situations.

Most attacks by unknown assailants are planned in advance. Many rapists use certain ploys to initiate their attacks. Examples include asking for help, offering help, staging a deliberate "accident" such as bumping into you, or posing as a police officer or other authority figure. Sexual assault frequently begins with a casual, friendly conversation.

The Skills for Behavior Change box describes some steps you can take to reduce your risk of being assaulted. In addition, trust your intuition. Be assertive and direct with someone who is getting out of line or becoming threatening. This may convince a would-be attacker to back off. Don't try to be nice, and don't fear making a scene. Use the following tips to

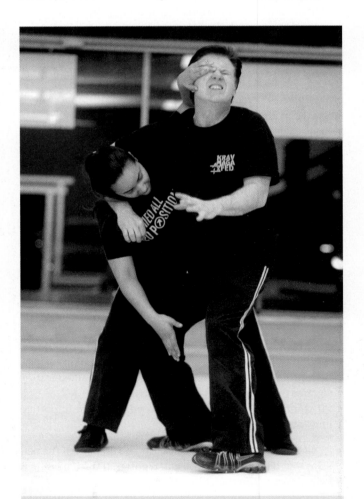

College campuses often offer safety workshops and self-defense classes to provide students with physical and mental skills that may help them repel or deter an assailant.

SKILLS FOR
BEHAVIOR CHANGE

Stay Safe On All Fronts

Follow these tips to protect yourself from assault.

Outside Alone

◉ Carry a cell phone and keep it turned on, but stay off it. Be aware of what is happening around you.

◎ If you are being followed, don't go home. Head for a location where there are other people. If you decide to run, run fast and scream loudly to attract attention.

◎ Vary your routes. Stay close to other people.

◎ Walk or park in lighted areas; avoid dark areas where someone could hide.

◎ Carry pepper spray or other deterrents. Consider using your campus escort service.

◎ Tell other people where you are going and when you expect to be back.

In Your Car

◎ Lock your car doors. Do not open your doors or windows to strangers.

◎ If someone hits your car, drive to the nearest gas station or other public place if you can. Call the police or road service for help, and stay in your car until help arrives.

◎ If a car appears to be following you, do not drive home. Drive to the nearest police station.

In Your Home

◎ Install dead bolts on all doors, and locks on all windows. Make sure the locks work, and don't leave a spare key outside.

◎ Lock doors when at home, even during the day. Close blinds and drapes whenever you are away and in the evening when you are home.

◎ Rent apartments that require a security code or clearance to gain entry, and avoid easily accessible apartments, such as first-floor units. When you move into a new residence, pay a locksmith to change the keys and locks (making sure that you have permission from the landlord if you are renting).

◎ Don't let repair people in without asking for identification, and have someone else with you when repairs are being made.

◎ Keep a cell phone near your bed, and call 9-1-1 in emergencies. Buy phones that have E911 locators so that emergency personnel can find you even if you can't respond or don't know where you are.

◎ If you return home to find your residence has been broken into, don't enter. Call the police. If you encounter an intruder, it is better to give up money or valuables than to resist.

let a potential assailant know that you are prepared to defend yourself:

- **Speak in a strong voice.** State, "Leave me alone!" rather than "Will you please leave me alone?" Sound like you mean it.
- **Maintain eye contact.** This keeps you aware of the person's movements and conveys an aura of strength and confidence.
- **Stand up straight, act confident, and remain alert.** Walk as though you own the sidewalk.

If you are attacked, act immediately. Draw attention to yourself and your assailant. Scream "Fire!" as loudly as you can. Passersby are much more likely to help if they hear the word *fire* rather than just a scream.

What to Do If Rape Occurs
If you are a rape victim, report the attack. Follow these steps:

- Call 9-1-1.
- Do not bathe, shower, douche, clean up, or touch anything the attacker may have touched.
- Save the clothes you were wearing at the time of the rape, and do not launder them. They will be needed as evidence. Bring a clean change of clothes to the clinic or hospital.
- Contact the rape assistance hotline in your area, and ask for advice on counseling if you need additional help.

If someone you know is assaulted, here's how you can help:

- Believe the rape victim. Don't ask questions that might seem to imply that the person is at a fault in any way for the assault.
- Encourage the person to see a doctor immediately, because she or he may have medical needs but feel too embarrassed to seek help. Offer to go along with your friend.
- Encourage the person to report the crime to the police.
- Be understanding, and let the person know you will be there if she or he needs help or to talk.
- Recognize that this is an emotional situation and it may take time for the person to bounce back.
- Encourage the person to seek counseling.

Campus-Wide Responses to Violence

Many college administrators have been proactive in establishing violence prevention policies, programs, and services. Campuses are conducting emergency response drills and reviewing the effectiveness of emergency messaging systems, including mobile phone alert systems. The Reverse 9-1-1 system uses database and geographic information system (GIS) mapping technologies to notify campus police and community members in the event of problems, and other systems allow administrators to send out alerts in text, voice, e-mail, or instant message format. Some schools program the phone numbers, photographs, and basic student information for all incoming first-year students into a university security system so that in the event of a threat, students need only hit a button on their phones, whereupon campus police will be notified, and tracking devices will pinpoint the students' location.

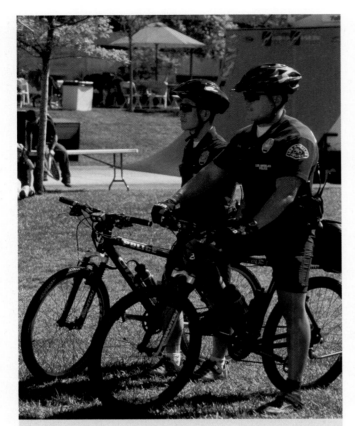

The presence and visibility of campus law enforcement have increased in recent years.

impaired driving Driving under the influence of alcohol or other drugs.

There are many changes that can be made to the campus environment to improve safety. More and better campus lighting, parking lot security, emergency call boxes, removal of overgrown shrubbery, safe ride programs, and stepped-up security are increasingly on the radar of campus safety personnel. Buildings can be designed with better lighting and enhanced security features, and security cameras can be installed in hallways, classrooms, and public places.

Campus law enforcement has changed over the years by increasing both its numbers and its authority to prosecute student offenders. Campus police are responsible for emergency responses, and they have the power to enforce laws with students in the same way they are handled in the general community. In fact, many campuses now hire state troopers or local law enforcement officers to deal with campus issues rather than maintaining a separate police staff.

Community Strategies for Preventing Violence

There are many steps you can take to ensure your personal safety; however, it is also necessary to address the issues of violence and safety at a community level. Strategies recommended by the CDC's injury response initiatives include the following:

- Inoculate children against violence in the home. Teaching young people principles of respect and responsibility are fundamental to the health and well-being of future generations.
- Develop policies and laws that prevent violence. Enforce laws so that offenders know you mean business in your settings.
- Develop skills-based educational programs that teach the basics of interpersonal communication, elements of healthy relationships, anger management, conflict resolution, appropriate assertiveness, stress management, and other health-based behaviors.
- Involve families, schools, community programs, athletics, music, faith-based organizations, and other community groups in providing experiences that help young people to develop self-esteem and self-efficacy.
- Promote tolerance and acceptance, and establish and enforce policies that forbid discrimination. Offer diversity training and mandate involvement.
- Improve community services that focus on family planning, mental health services, day care and respite care, and alcohol and substance abuse prevention.
- Make sure walking trails, parking lots, and other public areas are well lit, unobstructed, and patrolled regularly.
- Improve community-based support and treatment for victims, and ensure that individuals have choices available when they are trying to stop violence in their lives.

LO 6 | UNINTENTIONAL INJURIES

Discuss key strategies that are likely to minimize the risk of unintentional injuries.

Unintentional injuries occur without planning or intention to harm. They are the leading cause of death for Americans age 1 through 44, and the fourth leading cause of death overall.[88] Over 136,00 Americans are killed by unintentional injuries each year.[89]

Recently, unintentional poisonings, the great majority of which are due to drug overdose, overtook motor vehicle crashes (MVCs) as the number one cause of unintentional death.[90] Among young adults, other common causes of significant unintentional mortalities each year include falls, drownings, and fires.

Motor Vehicle Safety

In 2016, over 40,200 Americans died of injuries sustained in MVCs, a 6 percent increase over the previous year.[91] What caused the increase? Several factors probably contributed. Cheaper gas and a strong economy mean more miles driven. An aging highway infrastructure may increase risk, and budget cuts to police patrols may be factors. Aggressive driving and failure to use seatbelts add to increasing numbers of deaths. Impaired and distracted drivers are on the increase and are major factors in injury and deaths on the roads.[92]

Impaired Driving: Alcohol In 2014, nearly one third of all motor vehicle fatalities involved an alcohol-impaired driver,

▶ **SEE IT!** VIDEOS

Are you at risk of falling asleep at the wheel? Watch **Dozing and Driving: 1 in 24 Asleep at Wheel**, available on Mastering Health.

making alcohol the primary cause of **impaired driving**.[93] Of alcohol-impaired drivers involved in fatalities, 7 percent had a previous conviction for driving while impaired (DWI) and another 24 percent had a history of license suspension or revocation.[94] The age group with the highest percentage of alcohol-impaired drivers involved in fatal crashes is people aged 21 to 24 years.[95]

After alcohol, marijuana is the drug most often linked to impaired driving.[96] Marijuana use reduces attention, increases weaving in and out of traffic, and slows reaction time.[97] A recent study in Colorado shows increases in the number of fatal crashes since the legalization of marijuana.[98] Prescription drugs, mainly opioids and sedatives, are also common factors in MVC fatalities.[99]

Impaired Driving: Drowsiness

Drowsiness is a form of impairment that plays a major role in fatal crashes. Many researchers contend that driving while sleep-deprived is as dangerous as driving drunk. Drowsy driving is estimated to cause up to 6,000 fatal MVCs each year.[100]

Impaired Driving: Distractions

Three types of activities constitute **distracted driving**: taking your eyes off the road, taking your hands off the steering wheel, and taking your mind off driving.[101] Examples include using a cell phone, eating and drinking, talking with passengers, adjusting your music or navigation system, reading, doing personal grooming, playing with pets, changing clothes, picking up things that you've dropped, and daydreaming. Distracted driving kills at least 4,000 people per year and injures over 400,000 more, and these statistics may be underestimates.[102]

Recent research indicated that distracted driving was a factor increasing percentages of crashes, including 76 percent of rear-end crashes and 89 percent of road-departure crashes.[103] Texting is one of the most dangerous forms of distracted driving—over 600 percent more dangerous than drunk driving.[104] Despite clear statistics to the contrary, a recent study indicated that 20 percent of drivers age 18 to 20 years and nearly 30 percent of drivers aged 21 to 34 said that texting does not affect their driving![105] Highway safety experts estimate that the average text takes the driver's eyes off the road for long enough, traveling 55 miles per hour, to cross a football field.[106] Currently, 46 states ban texting while driving, and 14 states ban all handheld cell phone use of any kind while driving.[107]

> **distracted driving** Driving while performing any nondriving activity that has the potential to distract the driver from the primary task of driving and increase the risk of crashing.

Vehicle Safety Issues

Wearing a safety belt cuts the risk of death or serious injury in a crash by almost half.[108] Although about 87 percent of Americans report wearing a safety belt, 49 percent of people killed in MVCs in 2014 were not wearing one at the time of the crash.[109] Each year, safety belt use is estimated to save more than 12,000 lives.[110] So buckle up, and insist that any passengers do the same. If you're transporting an infant or child in your vehicle, follow state laws governing use and location of age-appropriate safety seats.

In addition, it makes good sense to buy vehicles with the highest crash safety ratings, side and knee airbags, antilock brakes, traction and stability controls, impact-absorbing crumple zones, strong compartment and roof supports, and automatic braking for impending frontal crashes and blind spot assistance if you are trying to keep yourself and loved ones safe on the road. Unfortunately, people who don't have the financial resources to drive vehicles with all of these safety features—and that group often includes college students—are at increased risk during MVCs.

Improve Your Driving Skills

Even the most careful drivers may find themselves having to avoid a crash at some time in their lives. Although you can't control what other drivers are doing, you can

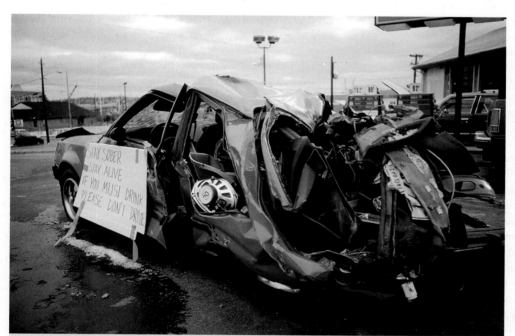

Driving under the influence of alcohol greatly increases the risk of being involved in a motor vehicle crash. Of all drivers between the ages of 21 and 24 years involved in fatal crashes, nearly one of three was legally drunk.

Source: National Highway and Traffic Safety Administration, "Traffic Safety Facts 2012 Data: Alcohol-Impaired Driving," DOT HS 811 870, December 2013, www-nrd.nhtsa.dot.gov/Pubs/811870.pdf.

WHAT DO YOU THINK?

How often are you distracted by incoming messages in texts, e-mails, or tweets when driving? Have you ever felt uneasy while riding with other people who are using distracted by devices? What are your own state's laws regarding cell phone use?

- How would you feel if someone you cared about were killed or injured by a distracted driver?
- How would you feel if the auto industry or cell phone providers installed software that would not allow incoming messages while you were on Bluetooth in your car?

reduce your risk of injury in an MVC by practicing risk management driving techniques. These include the following:

- Don't use electronic devices while driving. Avoid talking on a cell phone while driving, even if the phone is hands free. Never ever text while driving.
- Don't drink and drive. Take a taxi or arrange for someone to be the designated driver.
- Keep your eyes on the road. Scan the road ahead of you and to both sides.
- Keep your mind on the road. Don't drive when tired, highly stressed, worried, or emotional.

- Avoid aggressive driving. This includes speeding, unnecessary lane changes, passing where prohibited, running red lights, and failing to yield the right of way. It also includes tailgating: The rear bumper of the car ahead of you should be at least 3 seconds' worth of distance away, making stopping safely possible. Increase the distance when visibility is reduced, speed is increased, or roads are slick.
- Drive with your low-beam headlights on, *day and night*, to make your car more visible to other drivers.
- Drive defensively. Be on the alert for unsignaled lane changes, sudden braking, or other unexpected maneuvers.
- Obey all traffic laws.
- Always wear a safety belt, whether you're the driver or the passenger.

Cycling Safety

The National Highway and Traffic Safety Administration reports that in 2014, 726 bicyclists died in traffic collisions, and 50,000 were injured.[111] Most fatal collisions involving bicycles occur at nonintersections (60 percent) between the hours of 4:00 P.M. and midnight. Alcohol also plays a significant role in bicycle deaths and injuries: In about one third of all fatal crashes involving both motor vehicles and bicycles, either the driver or the cyclist was drunk.[112]

All cyclists should wear a properly fitted bicycle helmet every time they ride. Wearing a properly fitted bicycle helmet has been estimated to reduce the risk of head injury by half.[113] In addition to wearing a helmet approved by the American

personal flotation device (PFD) A device worn to provide buoyancy and keep the wearer, conscious or unconscious, afloat with the nose and mouth out of the water; the most commonly used PFD is a life jacket.

National Standards Institute or the Snell Memorial Foundation, cyclists should consider the following suggestions:

- Watch the road and listen for traffic sounds! Never listen to music with headphones or talk on a cell phone while cycling.
- Don't drink and ride.
- Follow all traffic laws, signs, and signals.
- Ride with the flow of traffic.
- Wear light or brightly colored reflective clothing that is easily seen at dawn, at dusk, and during full daylight.
- Avoid riding after dark. If you must ride at night, use a front light and a red reflector or a flashing rear light, as well as reflective tape or other markings on your bike and clothing.
- Use proper hand signals.
- Keep your bicycle in good condition.
- Use bike paths whenever possible.
- Stop at stop signs and traffic lights.

Stay Safe in the Water

According to the latest statistics, 3,406 Americans die each year in the United States by drowning, making it the fifth leading cause of unintentional injury death among Americans of all ages.[114] Children aged 1 to 4 years have the highest rate of drowning, but young Americans aged 15 to 24 years experience the most drownings: 507 per year.[115] People who survive near-drownings may experience severe brain damage.[116]

Drowning Risk Factors Lack of swimming ability, lack of barriers around unsupervised swimming areas, lack of skilled supervision around water locations, failure to wear a **personal flotation device (PFD)** such as a life jacket, temperature extremes that cause hypothermia, riptides and other hazardous conditions, seizure disorders, and excess alcohol use all increase the risk for drowning. In fact, the vast majority of adults who drown are not wearing PFDs (88 percent) and are under the influence of alcohol (70 percent).[117]

Most drownings occur during water recreation, either in backyard pools or in natural water locations where people congregate to have fun. Often, parents or lifeguards are not present, and people unexpectedly find themselves in dangerous situations. Many victims are strong swimmers but can't get out of dangerous waters quickly enough. To be safe, take the following precautions around water:

- Learn how to swim. It is never too late.
- Learn CPR. When seconds can mean the difference between life and death, you want to be ready and able to save a loved one's life.
- Don't drink alcohol or take other drugs before or while swimming.
- Never swim alone, even if you are a skilled swimmer. Tell other people where you are going.
- Pay attention to water temperature. Hypothermia can cause you to become disoriented and weak very quickly.

- Never leave a child unattended, even in extremely shallow water. Keep gates and barriers to backyard pools locked at all times.
- Before entering the water, check the depth. Most neck and back injuries result from diving into water that is too shallow.
- Never swim in a river with currents that are too swift for easy, relaxed swimming.
- Watch riptide warnings and beach conditions. If you are caught in a rip current, swim parallel to the shore. Once you are free of the current, swim toward the shore.

Boating In 2015, the U.S. Coast Guard received reports of 2,613 injured boaters and 626 deaths.[118] About 76 percent of these boating fatalities were drownings, and 85 percent of those who drowned were not wearing a PFD.[119]

Although operator inattention, inexperience, excessive speed, and mechanical failure also contributed to these deaths, alcohol consumption was the leading factor.[120] The U.S. Coast Guard and every state have "boating under the influence" (BUI) laws that carry stringent penalties for violation, including fines, license revocation, and even jail time.[121]

To stay safe when boating, the American Boating Association recommends sharing your plans for your outing, checking the weather ahead of time, making sure your boat is in good condition and has the proper safety equipment, and carrying an emergency radio and cell phone.[122] In addition, make sure you have enough PFDs for all who are on board, put on your life jacket before setting out, and wear it at all times while on the water or at a boat dock. If you run into problems, there is unlikely to be time to put the life jacket on.

If you are going on a snorkeling, diving, sailing, parasailing, or other water-related venture, check the qualifications and safety record of the company you are using. Don't sign up for trips on which boat operators party with their passengers.

Drowning is not the only hazard to be aware of when swimming or boating. Remember that water reflects UV rays, so wear sun-protective clothing, sunscreen on exposed skin, a hat, and sunglasses with UV protection.

Safety at Home

Common unintentional injuries in the home include poisonings, falls, and burns. Although older adults are particularly vulnerable, thousands of young adults, teens, and children are brought to emergency rooms for treatment of such injuries.

Prevent Poisoning A **poison** is any substance that is harmful to the body when ingested, inhaled, injected, or absorbed through the skin. In 2015, of the substance abuse disorders in more than 20 million Americans, roughly 10 percent involved prescription pain relievers, around 5 percent involved heroin.[123] Drug overdose is the leading cause of accidental death in the United States, with 52,404 lethal drug overdoses in 2015.[124] Addiction to opioids is a significant player in this epidemic, causing 20,101 prescription pain reliever overdose deaths and 12,990 heroin overdose deaths in 2015.[125]

Over-the-counter drugs are also commonly implicated in overdose incidents. These include cough syrup and sleep medications as well as aspirin and other pain relievers.

In 2015, 55 poison control centers in the United States logged more than 2.1 million calls for poisonings of humans, 50,000 for dogs, and 5,000 for cats.[126] For comprehensive drug and chemical safety precautions, talk with your doctor or pharmacist, and read labels. If you have questions, call the poison control center.[127]

Avoid Falls Falls are the third most common cause of death from unintentional injury in the United States, leading to 31,959 deaths in 2014.[128] About 20 percent of people who fall suffer serious injury, such as a hip fracture or a head injury. In fact, falls are the most common cause of both these injuries.[129] Observe the following measures to reduce your risk of falls:

- Keep floors and stairs clear of all objects.
- Avoid using small scatter rugs and mats, which can slide out from under your feet. Use rubberized liners or strips to secure large rugs to the floor.
- Train your pets to stay away from your feet.
- Install slip-proof mats, treads, or decals in showers and tubs and on the stairs.
- If you need to reach something in a high cupboard or closet or change a ceiling light, use an appropriate step stool or short ladder.

Reduce Your Risk of Fire In 2014, nearly 3,500 Americans died in a fire.[130] Although fire-related deaths are not common on college campuses in the United States, a total of 85 fatal campus fires occurred between January 2000 and May 2015, claiming 118 lives.[131]

Smoke alarms were missing or disconnected in 58 percent of these fatal fires. Alcohol was a factor in 76 percent; specifically, at least one of the students involved was legally drunk.[132] Intoxication increases the risk for not only a fire, but also for injury and death once a fire begins, in part because of less effective responses and evacuations. The primary causes of fires in campus housing are cooking, use of candles, smoking, faulty wiring, and arson.[133]

Tips to prevent fires include the following:

- Extinguish all cigarettes in ashtrays before bed, and never smoke in bed.
- Set lamps and candles away from curtains, linens, paper, and other combustibles. Never leave candles unattended or burning while you sleep.
- In the kitchen, keep hot pads, kitchen cloths, and paper towels away from stove burners. Avoid reaching over hot pans. Use caution when lighting barbecue grills.
- Avoid overloading electrical circuits with appliances and cords.
- Have the proper fire extinguishers ready in case of fire, and replace batteries in smoke alarms and test them periodically.

> **poison** Any substance harmful to the body when ingested, inhaled, injected, or absorbed through the skin.

ASSESS YOURSELF

Are You at Risk for Violence or Injury?

LIVE IT! ASSESS YOURSELF

An interactive version of this assessment is available online on Mastering Health.

How often are you at risk for sustaining an intentional or unintentional injury? Answer the questions below to find out.

1 Relationship Risk

How often does your partner:

	Never	Sometimes	Often
1. Criticize you for your appearance (weight, dress, hair, etc.)?	○	○	○
2. Embarrass you in front of others by putting you down?	○	○	○
3. Blame you or others for his or her mistakes?	○	○	○
4. Curse at you, shout at you, say mean things, insult, or mock you?	○	○	○
5. Demonstrate uncontrollable anger?	○	○	○
6. Criticize your friends, family, or others who are close to you?	○	○	○
7. Threaten to leave you if you don't behave in a certain way?	○	○	○
8. Manipulate you to prevent you from spending time with friends or family?	○	○	○
9. Express jealousy, distrust, and anger when you spend time with other people?	○	○	○
10. Make threats to harm others you care about, including pets?	○	○	○
11. Control your telephone calls, monitor your messages and where you go, or read your e-mail without permission?	○	○	○
12. Punch, hit, slap, or kick you?	○	○	○
13. Force you to perform sexual acts that make you uncomfortable or embarrassed?	○	○	○
14. Threaten to kill himself or herself if you leave?	○	○	○

2 Risk for Assault or Rape

How often do you:

	Never	Sometimes	Often
1. Leave your drink unattended when you get up to dance or go to the restroom?	○	○	○
2. Accept drinks from strangers while out at a bar or party?	○	○	○
3. Leave parties with people you barely know or just met?	○	○	○
4. Walk alone in poorly lit or unfamiliar places?	○	○	○
5. Open the door to strangers?	○	○	○
6. Leave your car or home door unlocked?	○	○	○
7. Talk on your cell phone, oblivious to your surroundings?	○	○	○

3 Risk for Vehicular Injuries

How often do you:

	Never	Sometimes	Often
1. Drive after you have had one or two drinks?	○	○	○
2. Drive after you have had three or more drinks?	○	○	○
3. Drive when you are sleepy or extremely tired?	○	○	○
4. Drive while you are extremely upset?	○	○	○
5. Drive while using and holding your cell phone?	○	○	○
6. Drive or ride in a car while not wearing a seatbelt?	○	○	○
7. Drive faster than the speed limit?	○	○	○
8. Accept rides from friends who have been drinking?	○	○	○

4 Online Safety

How often do you:

	Never	Sometimes	Often
1. Use the same password on multiple sites for long periods of time?	○	○	○
2. Use the same firewall, security software, or anti-spyware program that came with your computer or laptop?	○	○	○
3. Put personal information on your social networking pages, such as personal pictures, travel or vacation plans, and other private material?	○	○	○
4. Date people you meet online?	○	○	○
5. Use a shared or public computer to check e-mail without clearing the browser cache?	○	○	○

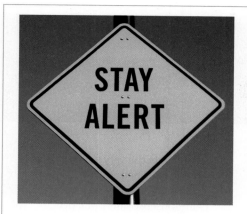

Analyzing Your Responses

Look at your responses to the list of questions in each of these sections. Part 1 focused on relationships. If you answered "sometimes" or "often" to several of these questions, you may need to evaluate your situation. In Parts 2 through 4, if you answered "often" to any question, you may need to take action to ensure that you stay safe.

YOUR PLAN FOR **CHANGE**

The **ASSESS YOURSELF** activity gave you the chance to consider symptoms of abuse in your relationships and signs of unsafe behavior in other realms of your life. Now that you are aware of these signs and symptoms, you can work on changing behaviors to reduce your risk.

TODAY, YOU CAN:

☐ Pay attention as you walk your normal route around campus, and think about whether you are taking the safest route. Is it well lit? Do you walk in areas that receive little foot traffic? Are there any emergency phone boxes along your route? Does campus security patrol the area? If part of your route seems unsafe, look around for alternative routes. Vary your route when possible.

☐ Look at your residence's safety features. Is there a secure lock, dead bolt, or keycard entry system on all outer doors? Can windows be shut and locked? Is there a working smoke alarm in every room and hallway? Are the outside areas well lit? If you live in a dorm or apartment building, is there a security guard at the main entrance? If you notice any potential safety hazards, report them to your landlord or campus residential life administrator right away.

WITHIN THE NEXT TWO WEEKS, YOU CAN:

☐ If you are worried about potentially abusive behavior in a partner or a friend's partner, visit the campus counseling center and ask about resources on campus or in your community to help you deal with potential relationship abuse. Consider talking to a counselor about your concerns or sitting in on a support group.

☐ Next time you go out to a bar or a party, set limits for yourself to avoid putting yourself in a dangerous or compromising position. Decide ahead of time on the number of drinks you will have, arrange with a friend to look out for each other during the party, and be sure you have a reliable, safe way of getting home.

BY THE END OF THE SEMESTER, YOU CAN:

☐ Sign up for a self-defense or violence prevention class or workshop.

☐ Get involved in an on-campus or community group dedicated to promoting safety. You might want to attend a meeting of an antiviolence group, join in a Take Back the Night rally, or volunteer at a local rape crisis center or battered women's shelter.

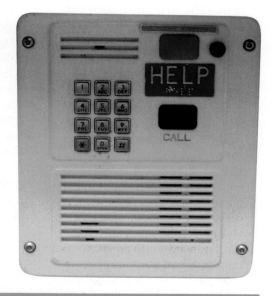

STUDY **PLAN**

Visit the Study Area in Mastering Health to enhance your study plan with MP3 Tutor Sessions, Practice Quizzes, Flashcards, and more!

CHAPTER **REVIEW**

LO **1** | What Is Violence?

- Violence continues to be a major problem in the United States today. Intentional injuries result from actions committed with the intent to do harm; unintentional injuries are committed without the intent to harm. Violence affects everyone in society—from the direct victims to children and families who witness it to the people who modify their behaviors because they are fearful.

LO **2** | Factors Contributing to Violence

- Factors that lead to violence include poverty or economic difficulties, unemployment, parental and family influences, cultural beliefs, discrimination or oppression, religious or political differences, breakdowns in the criminal justice system, and stress. Anger and substance abuse can contribute to violence and aggression.

LO **3** | Interpersonal and Collective Violence

- Interpersonal violence includes homicide, hate crimes, intimate partner violence, and elder abuse. Victims of these crimes often suffer long-term emotional, social, and physical consequences. Forms of collective violence, including gang violence, cybercrimes, and terrorism, are increasing in prevalence and cause increased fear and anxiety in society.

LO **4** | Sexual Victimization

- Most sexual victimization crimes are committed by someone the victim already knows. Key forms of sexual victimization includes unwanted touching, stalking, harassment, rape, unwanted sexual advances, and child sexual abuse.

LO **5** | Preventing Violence

- To reduce the risk of becoming a victim of violence, recognize how to protect yourself and your friends; know where to turn for help; and have honest, straightforward conversations about sexual matters in dating situations. Moderation in alcohol consumption is another key factor in reducing your risks. Campuses have stepped up educational programs, increased support for victims, increased surveillance, used technologies to improve their response, and provided clear messages about victim rights and consequences for offenders. They have also mandated campus climate surveys so that they can better understand what is happening on campus before problems arise. With increasing reports of violence on campus, national attention has sharply focused what we can do to change a culture of violence. Preventing violence on a community level means prioritizing mental and emotional health, providing services to people in trouble, alcohol and drug abuse prevention, and providing behavioral skills training.

LO **6** | Unintentional Injuries

- Unintentional injuries, particularly motor vehicle injuries, continue to be a leading cause of death for people aged 1 to 44 years. Impaired driving, drowsy driving, and distracted driving are key contributors to vehicular deaths and injuries. To avoid unintentional injuries, focus on personal protection, reduce your risks, and pay attention to threats.
- Injuries from bicycles, drownings, poisonings, falls, and fires pose threats for people of all ages, particularly the very young and old Americans. They also affect young adults who are impaired or not using commonsense safety practices. Young males are at significantly greater risk of unintentional injury than young females.

POP **QUIZ**

LO **1** | What Is Violence?

1. _____ is an example of an intentional injury.
   a. A car accident
   b. Murder
   c. Accidental drowning
   d. A cycling collision

LO **2** | Factors Contributing to Violence

2. An emotional reaction brought about by frustrating life experience is called
   a. reactive aggression.
   b. primary aggression.
   c. secondary aggression.
   d. tertiary aggression.

LO **3** | Interpersonal and Collective Violence

3. Which of the following is *not* a common explanation for bias-motivated crimes?
   a. Fear of the unknown
   b. Self-defense
   c. Thrill seeking
   d. Retaliation for a perceived slight

4. Which of the following is an example of collective violence?
   a. Sexual assault
   b. Homicide
   c. Domestic violence
   d. Terrorism

5. Psychologist Lenore Walker developed a theory known as the

a. aggression cycle.

b. sexual harassment cycle.

c. cycle of child abuse.

d. cycle of violence.

LO 4 | Sexual Victimization

6. When Jane began a new job with all male coworkers, her supervisor told her that he enjoyed having an attractive woman in the workplace, and he winked at her. His comment constitutes
   a. poor judgment but not a problem if Jane likes compliments.
   b. sexual assault.
   c. sexual harassment.
   d. sexual battering.

7. Rape by a person known to the victim that does not involve a physical beating or use of a weapon is called
   a. simple rape.
   b. sexual assault.
   c. simple assault.
   d. aggravated rape.

8. Which of the following is *not* an example of stalking?
   a. Making sexually charged comments to another person
   b. Doing "drive-bys" to see whether a person is home or has visitors.
   c. Showing up at places where you know the other person is going to be.
   d. Sending texts and messages to someone you like even though they ignore you.

LO 5 | Preventing Violence

9. Which of the following is a tip to protect yourself from assault?
   a. If a car is following you, drive home, go in, and lock your doors.
   b. If you get home and find that your residence has been broken into, go inside, assess damages, and call the police.
   c. Talk or text on your phone when you're outside alone to look busy.
   d. If you're going somewhere alone, tell others where you are going and when you expect to be back.

LO 6 | Unintentional Injuries

10. What is the leading cause of death for persons aged 15 to 44 years in the United States?
    a. Homicide
    b. Heart disease/CVD
    c. Unintentional injury
    d. Suicide

Answers to the Pop Quiz can be found on page A-1. If you answered a question incorrectly, review the section identified by the Learning Outcome. For even more study tools, visit **MasteringHealth***.*

THINK ABOUT IT!

LO 1 | What Is Violence?

1. What forms of violence do you think are most significant or prevalent in the United States today? Why?

2. What type of violence is most common on your campus? How do you think campus violence affects students at your school? Are there differences in how men and women respond to news that there has been a rape or violent assault on campus? If so, why?

LO 2 | Factors Contributing to Violence

3. Why do some people develop into violent or abusive adults and others become pacifists or peaceful adults? What key factors influence violent offenders to be violent?

LO 3 | Interpersonal and Collective Violence

4. Have you been affected by acts of terrorism or gang violence? If so, how were you affected? What strategies can you take to discourage collective violence, as an individual and as a community?

LO 4 | Sexual Victimization

5. Have you known anyone personally who has been sexually assaulted on campus? What actions were taken to help the person cope with the assault? What campus services, if any, were used?

LO 5 | Preventing Violence

6. What are some everyday decisions you can make to minimize your risk of becoming a victim of violence? How can you be a good friend to someone who has become a victim of violence?

7. Is your campus safe? What steps has your campus administration and community taken to reduce levels of campuswide violence?

LO 6 | Unintentional Injuries

8. Think about an unintentional injury that affected you. What led up to it? What could have been done to prevent it? How much control did you have over the situation, and how much was it affected by other people?

ACCESS YOUR HEALTH ON THE INTERNET

Visit Mastering Health for links to the websites and RSS feeds.

The following websites explore further topics and issues related to violence and injury.

Not Alone. This site houses the report of the White House Task Force to Protect Students from Sexual Assault and recommendations for reporting, responding to, and preventing future assaults. Detailed recommendations and action plans are presented. www.whitehouse.gov/sites/default/files/docs/report_0.pdf

Men Can Stop Rape. Practical suggestions for men who are interested in helping to protect women from sexual predators and assault are provided on this site. www.mencanstoprape.org

National Center for Injury Prevention and Control. The Web-based Injury Statistics Query and Reporting System (WISQARS) database of this CDC section provides statistics and information on fatal and nonfatal injuries, both intentional and unintentional. www.cdc.gov/injury

National Sexual Violence Resource Center. This is an excellent resource for victims of sexual violence. www.nsvrc.org

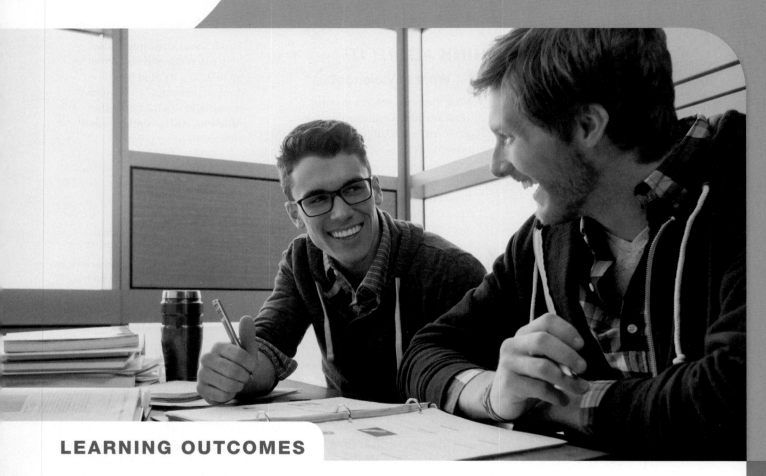

6

Connecting and Communicating in the Modern World

LEARNING OUTCOMES

LO **1** Describe the types of social support that are available and the impact of social networks on health status.

LO **2** Discuss the purpose and common forms of intimate relationships.

LO **3** Discuss ways to improve communication skills and interpersonal interactions, particularly in the digital environment.

LO **4** Identify the characteristics of successful relationships, including how to overcome common conflicts, and discuss how to cope when a relationship ends.

LO **5** Compare and contrast the types of committed relationships and singlehood.

Humans are social beings. We have a basic need to belong and to feel loved, accepted, and wanted. We can't thrive without relating to and interacting with others. Strong connections to other people reduce depression, build our immune systems, improve sleep, and strengthen our resolve.[1] In fact, people who have positive, fulfilling relationships with spouses, family members, friends, and coworkers are 30 percent more likely to survive over time than people who are socially isolated.[2] However, having a healthy social life is not a given, even for people who regularly interact with many others. A person can feel lonely, even in a crowd, because loneliness does not result from being physically alone; it is caused by feeling disconnected from others.[3] In this chapter, we examine the vital role relationships play in our lives and the communication skills necessary to create and maintain them.

LO 1 | THE VALUE OF RELATIONSHIPS

Discuss the types of social support that are available and the impact of social networks on health status.

Historically, research examining the benefits of intimate relationships has focused on marriage; however, recent studies report that all types of close relationships are good for our health.[4] The benefits range from a decreased likelihood of catching a cold to a faster recovery from stressful tasks to a longer life span. On the flip side, people with poor social connections have decreased immune function, higher blood pressure, and higher rates of depression, pain, and fatigue.[5] One recent study analyzing data from more than 14,000 people over multiple decades revealed that the effects of social isolation are long lasting, raising future risks for increased blood pressure, body mass index, waist circumference, and inflammation (a risk factor for heart disease and cancer).[6]

Why do relationships make us healthier? First, they affect our choices. For example, we eat healthier when our friends eat healthy foods.[7] Second, friends often provide us with **social support**—the type of help we receive from our contact with others. Social support is delivered in four forms: emotional, instrumental, informational, and belonging.[8] For a college student who breaks her leg playing basketball, social support might be as follows:

- **Emotional support.** Displays of caring, love, trust, and empathy, as when close friends and family members provide a listening ear about frustrations and pain.

- **Instrumental support.** Concrete help and service, such as a roommate carrying the student's backpack to class as she learns to use her crutches and keeping the apartment tidy so she doesn't trip.

- **Informational support.** Advice, suggestions, and information, as when an aunt shows her some tricks to better navigate on crutches.

- **Belonging support.** Sharing activities or a sense of belonging, as when her teammates encourage her to still come to basketball practice while her leg heals.

Third, having friends can change your perspective on how challenging a task is. In one clever study, a group of students were taken to the foot of a steep hill, and each was fitted with a heavy backpack. The students were then told to estimate how steep the hill was. Students standing with friends estimated the hill to be less steep than students standing alone. The hill appeared even less steep the longer the friends had known each other. Evidence suggests that with support, challenges look easier to us, thus reducing our stress.[9]

That the length of the friendship affected the students' estimate of the difficulty of the climb should come as no surprise. Research shows that it is the quality of our friendships, not the quantity, that matters when it comes to health. There's a lot of wisdom in the quip often attributed to Al Capone: "I'd rather have 4 quarters than 100 pennies." He was right. A few close friends are worth far more to our health than 100 acquaintances—or 500 Facebook friends. The good news is that the average number of confidants reported by Americans is on the rise, averaging a little over two per person. Sadly, 9 percent of Americans report that they have no one to whom they can turn for discussing important matters.[10]

Besides our closest relationships, we all have a constellation of neighbors, relatives, classmates, coworkers, and friends of friends that make up our **social network**. The collective value of all the people in your social network—and the likelihood of those people providing social support when you need it—determines your **social capital**. The more social capital we have, the happier and healthier we are.[11]

To build social capital, we can both strengthen our existing ties and widen our network. John Cacioppo, a leading researcher on loneliness, describes these actions as building *relational connectedness* and *collective connectedness*.[12]

social support Help that you receive from people in your social network in the form of emotional, instrumental, informational, and appraisal support.

social network People you know who can provide social support when needed.

social capital Collective value of all the people in your social network and the likelihood of those people providing social support when you need it.

Relational connectedness comes from mutually rewarding face-to-face contact. We deepen our relational connectedness each time we interact positively with people in our social network, strengthening our ties and increasing the likelihood of someone coming to our aid when asked. So helping a friend move or celebrating your sister's birthday is more than just being nice or socializing; these acts are important steps in building relational connectedness.

Collective connectedness comes from the feeling that you are part of a group beyond yourself. It manifests itself in feelings such as trust and having a sense of community, as well as in actions like voting and volunteering. The groups you belong to deepen your collective connectedness and can expand your social network. People find collective connectedness in many ways: cheering for the same sports team, volunteering together, or worshipping at the same temple. The important thing is feeling that you are a part of a larger whole, even when you might not have intimate ties to individuals in the group.

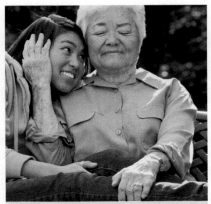

We may be accustomed to the term *intimacy* being used to describe romantic or sexual relationships, but intimate relationships can take many forms. The emotional bonds that characterize intimate relationships often span generations and help individuals gain insight into and understanding of each other's worlds.

- **Intimacy.** Someone with whom we can share our feelings freely.
- **Social integration.** Someone with whom we can share worries and concerns.
- **Nurturance.** Someone we can take care of and who will take care of us.
- **Assistance.** Someone to help us in times of need.
- **Affirmation.** Someone who will reassure us of our own worth.

In mutually rewarding intimate relationships, partners and friends meet each other's needs. They disclose feelings, share confidences, and provide support and reassurance. Each person comes away feeling better for the interaction and validated by the other person.

In addition to behavioral interdependence and need fulfillment, intimate relationships involve strong bonds of *emotional attachment*, or feelings of love. When we hear the word *intimate*, we often think of a sexual relationship. Although sex can play an important role in emotional attachment to a romantic partner, relationships can be intimate without being sexual. For example, two people can be emotionally intimate (share feelings) or spiritually intimate (share spiritual beliefs and practices) without being sexually intimate.

Emotional availability, the ability to give emotionally to and receive emotionally from others without fear of being hurt or rejected, is the fourth characteristic of intimate relationships. For this to be possible, people need to be in touch with their own emotions and be mindfully aware of the emotional cues of others. At times, it is healthy to limit our emotional availability. For example, after a painful breakup, we may decide not to jump into another relationship immediately, or we may decide to talk about it only with close friends. Holding back can offer time for introspection, healing, and considering lessons learned. Some people who have experienced intense trauma find it difficult to ever be fully available emotionally, which can limit their ability to experience intimate relationships.[14]

LO 2 | **INTIMATE** RELATIONSHIPS: WHEN CONNECTING GETS PERSONAL

Discuss the purpose and common forms of intimate relationships.

We all need people in our lives who affirm who we are and provide **intimate connectedness**.[13] These **intimate relationships** often include four characteristics: *behavioral interdependence*, *need fulfillment*, *emotional attachment*, and *emotional availability*. Each of these characteristics may be related to interactions with family, close friends, and romantic partners.

Behavioral interdependence refers to the mutual impact that people have on each other as their lives intertwine. What one person does influences what the other person wants to do and can do. Behavioral interdependence usually becomes stronger over time, to the point at which each person would feel a great void if the other were gone.

Intimate relationships are also a means of *need fulfillment*. Through relationships with others, we fulfill our needs for the following:

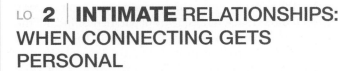

relational connectedness Mutually rewarding face-to-face contacts.

collective connectedness Feeling that you are part of a community or group.

intimate connectedness A relationship that makes you feel that who you are is affirmed.

intimate relationships Relationships with family members, friends, and romantic partners, characterized by behavioral interdependence, need fulfillment, emotional attachment, and emotional availability.

Caring for Yourself

You have probably heard the old saying that you must love yourself before you can love someone else. What does this mean exactly? Learning how you function emotionally and how to nurture yourself through all life's situations is a lifelong task. You should certainly not postpone intimate connections with other people until you achieve this state. However, a certain level of individual maturity will help you maintain relationships.

Two personal qualities that are especially important to any good relationship are *accountability* and *self-nurturance*.

Accountability means that you recognize responsibility for your own choices and actions. You don't hold other people responsible for positive or negative experiences. **Self-nurturance** means developing individual potential through a balanced and realistic appreciation of self-worth and ability. To make good choices in life, a person must balance many physical and emotional needs: sleeping, eating, exercising, working, relaxing, and socializing. When the balance is disrupted, self-nurturing people are patient with themselves as they put things back on course. Learning to live in a balanced and healthy way is a lifelong process. Individuals who are on a path of accountability and self-nurturance have a much better chance of achieving this balance and maintaining satisfying relationships with others.

Important factors that affect your ability to nurture yourself and maintain healthy relationships with others include the way you define yourself (*self-concept*) and the way you evaluate yourself (*self-esteem*). Your self-concept is like a mental mirror that reflects how you view your physical features, emotional states, talents, likes and dislikes, values, and roles. A person might define herself as an activist, a mother, an honor student, an athlete, or a musician. As we discuss in other chapters, how you feel about yourself or evaluate yourself constitutes your self-esteem.

Family Relationships

A family is a recognizable group of people with roles, tasks, boundaries, and personalities whose central focus is to protect, care for, love, and socialize with one another. Because the family is a dynamic institution that changes as society changes, the definition of *family* changes over time. Historically, most families have been made up of people related by blood, marriage or long-term committed relationships or adoption. Today, however, many groups of people are recognized and function as family units. Although there is no "best" family type, we do know that a healthy family's key roles and tasks include nurturance and support. Healthy families foster a sense of security and feelings of belonging that are central to growth and development.

Families provide our most significant relationships during our childhood years. It is from our **family of origin**, the people present in our household during our first years of life, that we initially learn about feelings, problem solving, love, intimacy, and gender roles. We learn to negotiate relationships and have opportunities to communicate effectively, develop attitudes and values, and explore spiritual belief systems. It is not uncommon when we establish relationships outside the family to rely on these initial experiences and on skills modeled by our family of origin.

Friendships

Friendships are often the first relationships we form outside our immediate families. Establishing and maintaining strong friendships may be a good predictor of your success in establishing romantic relationships, as both require shared interests and values, mutual acceptance, trust, understanding, respect, and self-confidence.

Developing meaningful friendships is more than merely "friending" someone on Facebook. Getting to know someone well requires time, effort, and commitment. But the effort is worth it. A good friend can be a trustworthy companion, someone who respects your strengths and accepts your weaknesses, someone who can share your joys and your sorrows, and someone you can count on for support.

> **accountability** Accepting responsibility for personal decisions, choices, and actions.
> **self-nurturance** Developing individual potential through a balanced and realistic appreciation of self-worth and ability.
> **family of origin** People who are present in the household during a child's first years of life, usually parents and siblings.

Romantic Relationships

At some point, most people choose to enter an intimate romantic and sexual relationship with another person. Beyond the characteristics of friendship, romantic relationships typically include the following characteristics related to passion and caring:

- **Fascination.** Lovers tend to pay attention to the other person even when they should be involved in other activities. They are preoccupied with the other and want to think about, talk to, and be with the other.
- **Exclusivity.** Lovers have a special relationship that usually precludes having the same kind of relationship with a third party. The love relationship often takes priority over all others.
- **Sexual desire.** Lovers desire physical intimacy and want to touch, hold, and engage in sexual activities with the other.
- **Giving the utmost.** Lovers care enough to give the utmost when the other is in need, sometimes to the point of extreme sacrifice.
- **Being a champion or advocate.** Lovers actively champion each other's interests and attempt to ensure that the other succeeds.

Theories of Love There is no single definition of *love*, and the word may mean different things to different people, depending on cultural values, age, gender, and situation. Although we may not always know how to put our feelings into words, we know it when the "lightning bolt" of love strikes.

Several theories related to how and why love develops have been proposed. In his classic triangular theory of love, psychologist Robert Sternberg proposed the following three key components to loving relationships (**FIGURE 6.1**):[15]

- **Intimacy.** The emotional component, which involves closeness, sharing, and mutual support
- **Passion.** The motivational component, which includes lust, attraction, and sexual arousal
- **Commitment.** The cognitive component, which includes the decision to be open to love in the short term and commitment to the relationship in the long term. (See the Student Health Today box for a discussion of the shortest type of relationship, hooking up.)

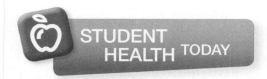

HOOKING UP *The New Norm or Nothing New?*

Hooking up is a vague term often used to describe sexual encounters, from kissing to intercourse, without the expectation of commitment. While the media often report about the new "hookup culture" on campus, research tells a different story. Longitudinal data indicate that young adults' sexual behavior hasn't changed much in the past few decades. College students are not having more sex or a greater number of partners than their counterparts 20 or 30 years ago. Today's college students are more likely to describe their sex partner as a "friend" than in the past, but today's college students are still twice as likely to have sex with a romantic partner than with a hookup.

While hookup behavior may not be as pervasive as some think, college students should understand the risks involved:

- **Recognize the role of emotions in sex.** Sternberg's triangular theory of love would place hooking up in the infatuation category, passion with no commitment or intimacy, far from Sternberg's picture of "ideal." Additionally, according to Fisher, attraction and sex create a chemical reaction in the brain that fosters an emotional response even if we say, "It's just about the sex."

- **Recognize the role of alcohol in hooking up.** In a recent study of college hookups, students reported that they were more likely to hook up if they had been drinking alcohol. Among participants who consumed alcohol before their last hookup, 31 percent of females and 28 percent of males indicated that they would likely not have hooked up with their partners had alcohol not been involved.

- **Recognize the risk of unintended pregnancy and STIs.** In one study, only 70 percent of students reported condom use during their last hookup. Reduced inhibitions due to alcohol plus a lack of communication with a new partner increase the risk of unprotected sex and thus the risk for unintended pregnancy and STIs.

Sources: M.A. Monto and A.G. Carey, "A New Standard of Sexual Behavior? Are Claims Associated with the "Hookup Culture" Supported by General Social Survey Data?," *Journal of Sex Research* 56, no. 6 (2014): 605–15; P.N.E. Roberson et al., "Hooking Up During College Years: Is There a Pattern?," *Culture, Health & Sexuality* 17, no. 5 (2015): 576–91; J.M. Bearak, "Casual Contraception in Casual Sex: Life-Cycle Change in Undergraduates' Sexual Behavior in Hookups," *Social Forces* 93, no. 2 (2014): 483–513.

According to Sternberg, the quality of a love relationship is related to the level of intimacy, passion, and commitment each person brings to the relationship over time. He suggests that relationships that include two or more of those components are more likely to endure than those that include only one. He uses the term **consummate love** to describe a combination of intimacy, passion, and commitment—an ideal and deep form of love that is, unfortunately, all too rare.[16]

Quite different from Sternberg's approach are theories of love and attraction based on brain circuitry and chemistry. Anthropologist Helen Fisher, among others, hypothesizes that attraction and falling in love follow a fairly predictable pattern based on (1) *imprinting*, in which our evolutionary patterns, genetic predispositions, and past experiences trigger a romantic reaction; (2) *attraction*, in

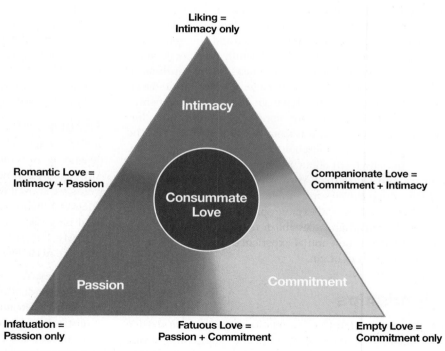

FIGURE 6.1 Sternberg's Triangular Theory of Love According to Sternberg's model, three elements—intimacy, passion, and commitment—existing alone or in combination, form different types of love. The most complete, ideal type of love in the model is consummate love, which combines balanced amounts of all three elements.

consummate love A relationship that combines intimacy, compassion, and commitment.

WHAT DO **YOU** THINK?

What factors do you consider most important in a potential partner?

- Are any of these factors absolute musts?
- Does what you believe to be important in a relationship differ from what your parents might think is important?

which neurochemicals produce feelings of euphoria and elation; (3) *attachment*, in which endorphins (natural opiates) cause lovers to feel peaceful, secure, and calm; and (4) *production of a cuddle chemical*; that is, the brain secretes the hormone oxytocin, which stimulates sensations during lovemaking and elicits feelings of satisfaction and attachment.[17]

According to Fisher's theory, lovers who claim to be swept away by passion may not be far from the truth. A love-smitten person's endocrine system secretes chemical substances such as dopamine and norepinephrine.[18] Attraction may in fact be a "natural high"; however, this passion "buzz" lessens over time as the body builds up a tolerance. Fisher speculates that some people become attraction junkies, seeking out the intoxication of new love much as a drug user seeks a chemical high.

Choosing a Romantic Partner Attraction theory suggests that more than just chemical and psychological processes influence who a person falls in love with. This theory suggests proximity, similarities, reciprocity, and physical attraction also play strong roles.[19] *Proximity* is being in the same place at the same time. When you are out and about in the community, you are more likely to cross paths with a potential partner than you are if you stay at home. And if you meet a person while you are at work, at the dog park, or at a religious event, it is likely that you will share interests. While

73%

of Americans list "similar ideas about having and raising children" as the **MOST IMPORTANT TRAIT** when choosing a partner, followed by "a steady job" (63%).

physical proximity is important, with the growth of Internet dating sites, it has become easier to meet people outside your geographic proximity.

You also choose a partner based on *similarities* (in attitudes, values, intellect, interests, education, and socioeconomic status); the old adage that "opposites attract" usually isn't true, at least not in the long run. If a potential partner expresses interest, you may react with mutual regard—*reciprocity*. The more you express interest, the safer it is for someone else to reciprocate, continuing the cycle and strengthening the connection.

A final factor that plays a significant role in selecting a partner is *physical attraction*. Attraction is a complex notion, influenced by social, biological, and cultural factors.[20] People seem to seek out similarly attractive partners, meaning more attractive people seek out more attractive partners and vice versa; however, as relationships evolve, status and personality become more important and the importance of personal appearance diminishes.[21]

LO 3 | BUILDING COMMUNICATION SKILLS

Discuss ways to improve communication skills and interpersonal interactions, particularly in the digital environment.

From the moment of birth, we struggle to be understood. We flail our arms, cry, scream, smile, frown, and make sounds and gestures to attract attention or to communicate our wants or needs. By adulthood, each of us has developed a unique way of communicating through gestures, words, expressions, and body language. No two people communicate in exactly the same way or have the same need for connecting with others, yet we all need to connect.

Different cultures have different ways of expressing feelings and using body language. Members of some cultures gesture broadly; others maintain a closed body posture. Some are offended by direct eye contact; others welcome a steady gaze. Men and women also tend to differ in communication styles (**FIGURE 6.2**)—though it is important to note that there may be significant variation within groups of men and women, and that communication patterns vary based on numerous contextual factors, such as culture, age, geography, and method of communication (e.g.face-to-face vs online social media.)

Although people differ in how they communicate, this doesn't mean that one gender, culture, or group is better at communication than another. We have to be willing to accept differences and work to keep lines of communication open and fluid. Remaining interested, actively engaging in interaction, and being open and willing to exchange ideas and thoughts are all things we can typically learn with practice. By understanding how to deliver and interpret information, we can enhance our relationships.

Learning Appropriate Self-Disclosure

Sharing personal information with others is called **self-disclosure**. If you are willing to share personal information with other people, they will likely share personal information with you. Likewise, if you want to learn more about someone, you have to be willing to share some of your personal background and interests with that person. Self-disclosure is not only storytelling or sharing secrets; it is also sharing emotions about what you are currently experiencing in life and providing any information about the past that is relevant to the other person's understanding of your current reactions.

self-disclosure Sharing feelings or personal information with others.

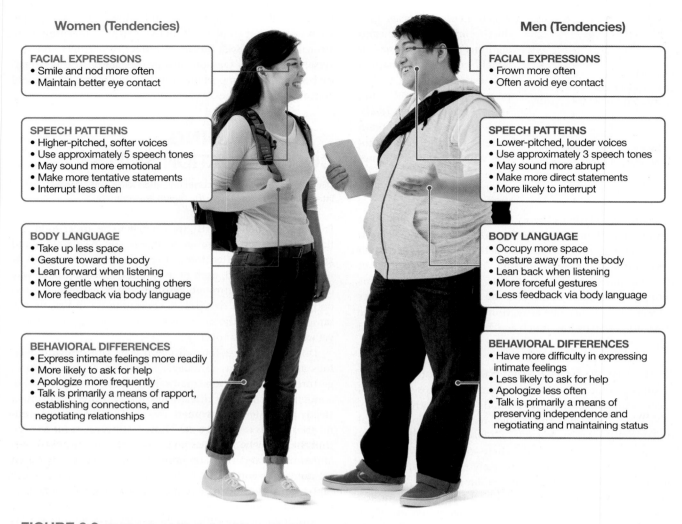

Women (Tendencies)

FACIAL EXPRESSIONS
• Smile and nod more often
• Maintain better eye contact

SPEECH PATTERNS
• Higher-pitched, softer voices
• Use approximately 5 speech tones
• May sound more emotional
• Make more tentative statements
• Interrupt less often

BODY LANGUAGE
• Take up less space
• Gesture toward the body
• Lean forward when listening
• More gentle when touching others
• More feedback via body language

BEHAVIORAL DIFFERENCES
• Express intimate feelings more readily
• More likely to ask for help
• Apologize more frequently
• Talk is primarily a means of rapport, establishing connections, and negotiating relationships

Men (Tendencies)

FACIAL EXPRESSIONS
• Frown more often
• Often avoid eye contact

SPEECH PATTERNS
• Lower-pitched, louder voices
• Use approximately 3 speech tones
• May sound more abrupt
• Make more direct statements
• More likely to interrupt

BODY LANGUAGE
• Occupy more space
• Gesture away from the body
• Lean back when listening
• More forceful gestures
• Less feedback via body language

BEHAVIORAL DIFFERENCES
• Have more difficulty in expressing intimate feelings
• Less likely to ask for help
• Apologize less often
• Talk is primarily a means of preserving independence and negotiating and maintaining status

FIGURE 6.2 Tendencies in Verbal and Nonverbal Communication by Gender

* Note that styles of communication can vary widely within groups of men and women. Sources: Tannen, D. (2007). *You just don't understand: Women and men in conversation*. New York: Harper Collins; Torppa, C.B. (2010). *Gender issues: Communication differences in interpersonal relationships*. Retrieved from https://ohioline.osu.edu/factsheet/FLM-FS-4-02-R10; Wood, J. and Fixmer-Oraiz, N. (2017). *Gendered lives*. Boston: Cengage.

Self-disclosure can be a double-edged sword because there is risk in divulging personal insights and feelings. If you sense that sharing feelings and personal thoughts will result in a closer relationship, you will likely take such a risk. But if you believe that the disclosure may result in rejection or alienation, you might not open up so easily. If the confidentiality of previously shared information has been violated, you might hesitate to be as open in the future. However, the risk in not disclosing yourself to others is a lack of intimacy in relationships.[22]

If self-disclosure is a key element in creating healthy communication but fear is a barrier to that process, what can be done? The following suggestions can help:

■ **Get to know yourself.** Remember that your *self* includes your feelings, beliefs, thoughts, and concerns. The more you know about yourself, the more likely you will be able to share yourself with others.

■ **Become more accepting of yourself.** No one is perfect or has to be.

■ **Be willing to talk about sex.** Mainstream culture in the United States puts many taboos on discussions of sex, so it's no wonder we find it hard to disclose our sexual past to those with whom we are sexually intimate. However, the threats of unintended pregnancy and sexually transmitted infections make it important for partners to discuss sexual history.

■ **Choose a safe context for self-disclosure.** When and where you make such disclosures and to whom may greatly influence the response you receive. Choose a setting where you feel safe to let yourself be heard.

Becoming a Better Listener

Listening is a vital part of interpersonal communication. Good listening skills enhance our relationships, improve our grasp of information, and allow us to more effectively interpret what

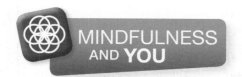

MINDFUL LISTENING

Good communication starts with good listening. When we listen mindfully, we focus on the speaker's words and on the speaker's tone of voice, facial expressions, and body language. We are aware, fully listening, and receptive to the person's message. We avoid interrupting except possibly to encourage or ask for clarification. This allows us to hear the meta-message—the message underlying the words that tells the whole story the speaker is trying to convey. It takes discipline to listen without judging or arguing or being defensive, but mindful listening helps to avoid conflict and allows the speaker to feel fully heard, improving our relationships and connections with others.

To listen more mindfully, practice these listening skills on a daily basis:

- To avoid distractions, turn off the TV, shut your laptop lid, and put your phone away.
- Be present in the moment. Good listeners participate and acknowledge what the other person is saying through nonverbal cues such as nodding or smiling and asking questions at appropriate times.
- Ask for clarification. If you aren't sure what the speaker means, say that you don't completely understand, or paraphrase what you think you heard.
- Control the desire to interrupt. Try taking a deep breath for 2 seconds, then hold your breath for another second, and really listen to what is being said as you slowly exhale.

Sources: F. Hennessey, "The Skill of Mindfully Listening," Psych Central, July 2016, https://psychcentral.com/lib/the-skill-of-mindful-listening; M. Hartwell-Walker, "Meta-communication: What I Said Isn't What I Meant," Psych Central, February 2017, https://psychcentral.com/lib/ meta -communication-what-i-said-isnt-what-i-meant.

---

others say. We listen best when (1) we believe that the message is somehow important and relevant to us; (2) the speaker holds our attention through humor, dramatic effect, or other techniques; and (3) we are in the mood to listen (free of distractions and worries). Listening to someone is a choice—a gift—that communicates to the other person that he or she is valuable and the person's ideas are worth hearing. See the **Mindfulness and You** box for information on how mindfully listening can improve your relationships.

The Three Basic Listening Modes
There are three main ways in which we listen:

- *Passive listening* occurs when we are listening but not providing either verbal or nonverbal feedback to the speaker. The speaker may feel unsure whether the message is being received, and without feedback, it is easy for the listener to be distracted or lose a train of thought.[23]
- *Selective listening* occurs when we are engaged but listening only for information that supports what we already believe; otherwise, we are tuned out while thinking of our rebuttal or waiting for a chance to break into the conversation.[24]
- *Active listening* occurs when we not only hear the words, but also are trying to understand what is really being said. The listener confirms understanding by restating or paraphrasing the speaker's message before responding. By actively listening, we show genuine interest in and an open mind to what the other person is thinking and feeling.[25]

Using Nonverbal Communication

Understanding what someone is saying usually involves more than listening and speaking. Often, what is not said speaks more loudly than any words could. Rolling the eyes, looking at the floor or ceiling rather than maintaining eye contact, body movements, and hand gestures—all these nonverbal clues influence the way we interpret messages. **Nonverbal communication** includes all unwritten and unspoken messages, both intentional and unintentional, including touch, gestures, interpersonal space, body language, tone of voice, and facial expressions.[26] Ideally, our nonverbal communication matches and supports our verbal communication, but this is not always the case. Research shows that when verbal communication and nonverbal communication don't match, we are more likely to believe the nonverbal cues.[27] This is one reason it is important to be aware of the nonverbal cues we use regularly and to understand how others might interpret them.

While facial expressions such as smiling are believed to have near universal meaning, other facial expressions and most body language is culturally specific.[28] A gesture of agreement or approval in one culture can be offensive in another. To communicate as effectively as possible, it is important to recognize and use appropriate nonverbal cues that support and help clarify your verbal messages. Awareness and practice of your verbal and nonverbal communication will help you better understand other people.

Connecting Digitally

You may have noticed that, in the definition of *relational connectedness*, Dr. Cacioppo specifically describes the contact as "face-to-face." Did you wonder whether Facetime counts as face-to-face? Were you curious about whether *oxytocin*—the hormone that make us feel happy when we interact with

> **nonverbal communication**
> Unwritten and unspoken messages, both intentional and unintentional.

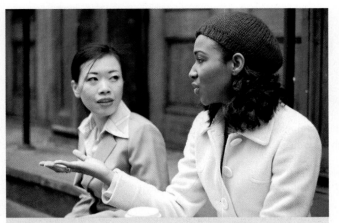

One way to communicate better is to pay attention to your body language. Much of your message is conveyed by nonverbal cues. Laughing, smiling, and gesturing all help to convey meaning and assure your partner that you are actively engaged in the conversation.

friends in person—is released when we receive a Snap or when we comment on a friend's Facebook post? The research on technology's impact on health is far from definitive. At this point, it appears there can be both benefit and harm, depending on who the user is and how the technology is used.

On one hand, digital communication allows us to have a diverse social network and easily keep in touch over long distances.[29] According to some reports, Americans spend more time on social networking sites (SNSs) than on any other online activity.[30] These connections seem to strengthen our social networks; frequent Facebook users report 9 percent more close core ties than other Internet users.[31] Frequent Facebook users also report feeling significantly more social support, specifically emotional and instrumental support.[32]

On the other hand, research shows that some SNS users feel more depressed, stressed, and disconnected. When people spend more time on Facebook, they report higher levels of depression.[33] Researchers first thought the depression was related to envy of the activities and lifestyles of their friends, but newer research shows that social comparison (paying attention to how one does things compared with how other people do things) may be what mediates the depressive symptoms. No matter whether the comparison is upward, downward, or neutral and whether the user is male or female, constant comparison fuels depression.[34]

Another concern is stress caused by reading Snaps or Facebook posts. When social media makes users aware of stressful events in other people's lives about which they otherwise would not know, their stress levels can increase. Because social media allows wide dissemination of news about illness, death, car crashes, or just bad days, we now have details about other people's lives that, in the past, we would have known only about our closest friends. This phenomenon has been dubbed "the cost of caring" and has been found only in females; males do not report increased stress in similar circumstances.[35]

Another group that reports technology-related stress is what the American Psychological Association refers to as the "constant checker"—the 43 percent of Americans who are always checking their e-mails, texts, and/or social media accounts. Constant checkers feel more stress than non–constant checkers related to political and cultural discussions on social media and work-related email. Constant checkers report feeling disconnected from family even if they're in the same place (44 percent of constant checkers compared to 25 percent of non–constant checkers). Even among non–constant-checkers, disconnection is an issue. Almost half of millennials (45 percent) report feeling disconnected from family even when they are together.[36]

A final concern about SNS use relates to the lack of nonverbal communication in text-based digital communication, which can lead to confusion and misunderstanding.[37] Some experts are concerned that, over time, reduced exposure to nonverbal communication may reduce people's ability to read facial expressions, affecting their in-person communication skills and making relationship building more difficult.[38] See the Skills for Behavior Change box for information on how to deal with social media meanness.

Thus, while social media can improve our lives, it may be wise to limit the time spent on social media and monitor our

SKILLS FOR
BEHAVIOR CHANGE

Social Media Meanness

Why does technology seem to bring out the worst in people? Psychologists often identify anonymity and invisibility as the culprits for this lack of restraint. When people feel anonymous, they are more willing to say things they normally wouldn't. Even when people aren't anonymous, impulse control is reduced because it's so easy to respond or vent immediately. What can you do when people are rude or are trolling you?

- Try not to respond emotionally. Don't type anything you wouldn't say to the person's face.

- When you are angry, press "pause," not "send." Take time to think about your response.

- Watch your words. Reread your response, and think about how your words could be interpreted without the benefit of tone of voice or other nonverbal cues.

- End the conversation. If you want to respond without continuing the rudeness, you can thank the person for giving you their thoughts, ask to meet to talk about it in person, or "agree to disagree."

Sources: A.G. Zimmerman and G.J. Ybarra, "Online Aggression: The Influences of Anonymity and Social Modeling," *Psychology of Popular Media Culture* 5, no. 2 (2016): 181–93; C.P. Barlett, "Anonymously Hurting Others Online: The Effect of Anonymity on Cyberbullying Frequency," *Psychology of Popular Media Culture* 4, no. 2 (2015): 70.

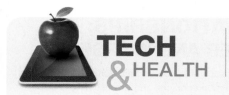

TECH & HEALTH | LOVE IN THE TIME OF TWITTER

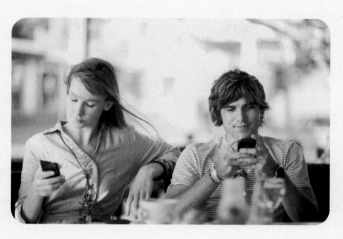

Technology has revolutionized our access to information and how we communicate. Couples can meet on Tinder, keep in constant contact via texting, and tell the world about their relationship highs and lows via Facebook, Twitter, Instagram, and Snapchat. Nancy Baym, author of *Personal Connections in the Digital Age*, suggests that we currently lack standard etiquette for the use of new media in relationships. At its best, social media can bring people closer together. At its worst, it can be used intentionally or unintentionally to embarrass or hurt. Consider the following suggestions to safeguard yourself:

When Meeting

- If you join a dating site, be honest about yourself. State your own interests and characteristics fairly, including things that you think might be less attractive than stereotypes and cultural norms dictate.
- If you meet someone online and want to meet in person, put safety first. Plan something brief, preferably during daylight hours. Meet in a public place, such as a coffee shop. Tell a friend or family member the details of when and where you are meeting and any information you have on the person you are meeting.

While Dating

- Discuss with your partner limits on the type of information each of you wants shared online. Agree to share only within those limits.
- Recognize that constant electronic updates throughout the day can leave little to share when you are together. Save some information for face-to-face talks.
- Sober up before you click "submit." Things that seem funny under the influence might not seem funny the next morning—and could possibly get you in trouble.
- Remember that the Internet is forever. Once a picture or a post has been sent, it can never be completely erased.
- Never post anything that would embarrass someone if it were seen by a family member or potential employer. "Social media screening," the practice of searching out all possible information on a prospective employee, is done by about a third of employers.

- Respect your partner's privacy. Logging onto his or her e-mail or Facebook account to look at private messages is a breach of trust.
- Know that a phone's GPS can be used to track your location, and cell phone spyware can allow e-mail and texts to be read from another device. If you think you may be a victim of cyberstalking, get a new phone or ask the service provider to reinstall the phone's operating system to wipe out the software.

If Breaking up

- Do not break up with someone via text, e-mail, tweet, Facebook, or chat. People deserve the respect of a face-to-face breakup.
- When you break up, be sure to change any passwords you may have confided to your partner. The temptation to use those for ill might be too strong to resist.

Source: K. Stolz, *Unfriending My Ex: Confessions of a Social Media Addict* (New York: Scribner, 2015); N. Baym, *Personal Connections in the Digital Age* (Cambridge, UK: Polity, 2015); CareerBuilder.com, "Number of Employers Using Social Media to Screen Candidates Has Increased 500 Percent over the Last Decade," April 28, 2016, http://www.careerbuilder.com/share/aboutus/pressreleasesdetail.aspx?ed=12%2F31%2F2016&id=pr945&sd=4%2F28%2F2016.

emotions related to its use. When using social media, remember that people often show the most flattering image of themselves possible; it is not always an accurate representation of their lives. Furthermore, the number of likes or followers you have is not a reflection of your worth as a person.

▶ SEE IT! VIDEOS

Meet Elise and learn about her project: 100 Dates of Summer. Watch **One Woman's Journey Through 100 Dates** in the Study Area of Mastering Health.

The bottom line is that real hugs and kisses cannot be replaced by typing XOXO, and the lack of accompanying nonverbal communication with most digital communication can create confusion or conflict due to a lack of clarity. While technology allows us to be more connected than during any other time in history, we must be sure to use digital communication as a complement to other ways of communicating, not a replacement. See the **Tech & Health** box for more on social media and relationships.

27%

of 18- to 24-year-olds have used **ONLINE DATING**—triple the rates of just 2 years ago.

Managing Conflict through Communication

A **conflict** is an emotional state that arises when the behavior of one person interferes with that of another. Conflict is inevitable whenever people live or work together. Not all conflict is bad; in fact, airing feelings and coming to resolution over differences can sometimes strengthen relationships. **Conflict resolution** and successful conflict management form a systematic approach to resolving differences fairly and constructively rather than allowing them to fester. The goal of conflict resolution is to solve differences peacefully and creatively.

Here are some strategies for conflict resolution:

1. **Identify the problem or issue.** Talk with each other to clarify exactly what the conflict is. Try to understand both sides. In this first stage, you must say what you want and listen to what the other person wants. Focus on using "I" messages, and avoid "you" messages. Be an active listener: Repeat what the other person has said, and ask questions for clarification.

2. **Generate several possible solutions.** Base your search for solutions on the goals and interests identified in the first step. Come up with several different alternatives, and avoid evaluating any of them until you have finished brainstorming.

3. **Evaluate the alternative solutions.** Narrow solutions to one or two that seem to work for both parties. Be honest with each other about a solution that feels unsatisfactory, but also be open to compromise.

4. **Decide on the best solution.** Choose a solution that is acceptable to both parties. You both need to be committed to the decision for it to be effective.

5. **Implement the solution.** Discuss how the decision will be carried out. Establish who is responsible to do what and when. The solution stands a better chance of working if you agree on how it will be implemented.

6. **Follow up.** Evaluate whether the solution is working. Check in with the other person to see how he or she feels about it. Are you satisfied with the way the solution is working out? If something is not working as planned or if circumstances have changed, discuss revising the plan. Remember that both parties must agree to any changes to the plan, as they did with the original idea.

conflict Emotional state that arises when opinions differ or the behavior of one person interferes with the behavior of another.

conflict resolution Concerted effort by all parties to constructively resolve differences or points of contention.

LO **4** | **RELATIONSHIPS:** FOR BETTER AND WORSE

Identify the characteristics of successful relationships, including how to overcome common conflicts, and discuss how to cope when a relationship ends.

Success in a relationship is often defined by whether a couple stays together and remains close over the years. Learning to communicate, respecting each other, and sharing a genuine fondness are crucial. Many social scientists agree that the happiest committed relationships are flexible enough to allow partners to grow throughout their lives.

Characteristics of Healthy and Unhealthy Relationships

Satisfying and stable relationships are based on good communication, intimacy, friendship, and other factors. A key ingredient is *trust*, the degree to which each partner feels that he or she can rely on the integrity of the other. Without trust, intimacy will not develop, and the relationship will likely fail. Trust includes three fundamental elements:

- **Predictability** The ability to predict your partner's behavior based on past actions.
- **Dependability** The ability to rely on your partner's emotional support in all situations, particularly those in which you feel threatened or hurt.
- **Faith** Belief that your partner has positive intentions and behavior.

What does a healthy relationship look and feel like? Healthy and unhealthy relationships are contrasted in **FIGURE 6.3**. Answering some basic questions can also help you determine whether a relationship is working.

- Do you love and care for yourself to the same extent that you did before the relationship? Can you be yourself in the relationship?
- Are there genuine caring and goodwill? Do you share interests, values, and opinions? Is there mutual respect for differences?
- Is there mutual encouragement? Do you support each other unconditionally?
- Do you trust each other? Are you honest with each other? Can you comfortably express your feelings, opinions, and needs?
- Is there room in your relationship for growth as you both evolve and mature?

Relationships are nourished by consistent communication, actions, and self-reflection. Poor communication can weaken bonds and create mistrust. We all need to reflect periodically on how we typically relate to others through our words and actions. Have we been honest, direct, and fair in our conversations? Have we listened to other people's thoughts, wants, and needs? Have we behaved in ways that are consistent with our words, values, and beliefs?

In an unhealthy relationship...	In a healthy relationship...
You care for and focus on another person only and neglect yourself, or you focus only on yourself and neglect the other person.	You both love and take care of yourselves before and while in a relationship.
One or both of you feels pressure to change to meet the other person's standards and is afraid to disagree or voice ideas.	You respect each other's individuality, embrace your differences, and allow each other to "be yourselves."
One or both of you has to justify what you do, where you go, and people you see.	You both do things with friends and family and have activities independent of each other.
One of you makes all the decisions and controls everything without listening to the other's input.	You discuss things with each other, allow for differences of opinion, and compromise equally.
One or both of you feels unheard and is unable to communicate what you want.	You express and listen to each other's feelings, needs, and desires.
You lie to each other and find yourself making excuses for the other person.	You both trust and are honest with yourselves and with each other.
You don't have any personal space and have to share everything with the other person.	You respect each other's need for privacy.
Your partner keeps his or her sexual history a secret or hides a sexually transmitted infection from you, or you do not disclose your history to your partner.	You share sexual histories and information about sexual health with each other.
One of you is scared of asking the other to use protection or has refused the other's requests for safer sex.	You both practice safer sex methods.
One or both of you has forced or coerced the other to have sex.	You both respect sexual boundaries and are able to say no to sex.
One or both of you yells and hits, shoves, or throws things at the other in an argument.	You resolve conflicts in a rational, peaceful, and mutually agreed upon way.
You feel stifled, trapped, and stagnant. You are unable to escape the pressures of the relationship.	You both have room for positive growth, and you both learn more about each other as you develop and mature.

FIGURE 6.3 Healthy versus Unhealthy Relationships

Source: Advocates for Youth, Washington, DC, 2006, www.advocatesforyouth.org. Copyright © 2000. Used with permission.

Breakdowns in relationships often begin with a change in communication, however subtle. Either partner may stop listening and cease to be emotionally present for the other. In turn, the other feels ignored, unappreciated, or unwanted. Unresolved conflicts increase, and unresolved anger can cause problems in sexual relations, which can further increase communication difficulties. Using technology to communicate adds a whole new dimension to communication between partners (see the Student Health Today box for more on digital communication).

College students, particularly those who are socially isolated and far from family and hometown friends, may be particularly vulnerable to staying in unhealthy relationships. They may become emotionally dependent on a partner. Mutual obligations, such as shared rental, financial, or transportation arrangements and sometimes childcare, can complicate a decision to end an unhealthy relationship. It's also easy to mistake sexual advances for physical attraction or love. Without a strong social network to validate their feelings or share concerns, students can feel stuck in an unhealthy relationship.

Honesty and verbal affection are usually positive aspects of a relationship. In a troubled relationship, however, they can be used to cover up irresponsible or hurtful behavior. Saying "at least I was honest" is not an acceptable substitute for acting in a trustworthy way, and claiming "but I really do love you" is not a license for being inconsiderate or hurtful.

Confronting Couples Issues

Couples who seek a long-term relationship must confront a number of issues that can either enhance or diminish their chances of success. These issues can involve jealousy, sharing power and responsibility, and communication about unmet expectations.

Technology such as dating websites can help couples meet, and texting can help people get to know each other better, but what about after a relationship begins? Does technology help or hurt? Two University of Nevada–Las Vegas researchers attempted to find out by interviewing 410 college students about the good and bad of technology in relationships.

■ **The Good:** Not surprisingly, text messaging was highly praised for its ability to keep couples in constant contact. People also reported using the Internet to search for information to improve their relationship, on topics from relationship building to sexual positions. Couples appreciated that they could make their relationship public, both by setting a status to "in a relationship" and by posting pictures that their friends could see. Using technology as a way to manage conflict

was also a common theme. People reported that it was easier to use text messaging to apologize, to test the waters after a fight, and to argue slowly and more clearly.

■ **The Bad:** Texting sometimes seemed impersonal and detached, especially sexting. The presence of phones made people feel that they did not always have their partner's full attention. People were concerned with who else their partner might be in contact with—that a phone is "another outlet for infidelity." Finally, the lack of nonverbal cues made it harder to interpret messages, creating opportunities for misunderstanding and for information to be taken out of context.

■ **Consider:** How has technology improved or injured your relationships? How can people set boundaries on phone use to improve relationships?

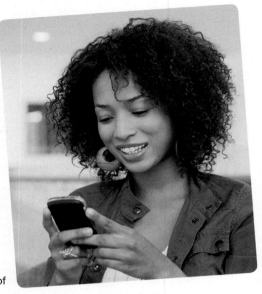

Source: K. Herlein and K. Ancheta, "Advantages and Disadvantages of Technology in Relationships: Findings from an Open-Ended Survey," *Qualitative Report* 19, no. 22 (2014): 1–11, Available at www.nova.edu/ssss/QR/QR19/hertlein22.pdf.

WHAT DO YOU THINK?

Have you ever been jealous in a relationship?

■ Can you identify what actions or events caused you to feel jealous?

■ Did you have actual facts to support your feelings, or was your response based on suspicions?

Jealousy Jealousy is a negative reaction evoked by a real or imagined relationship between one's partner and another person. Contrary to what many people believe, jealousy is not a sign of intense devotion. Instead, jealousy often indicates underlying problems, such as insecurity or possessiveness—significant barriers to a healthy relationship. Often, jealousy is rooted in past experiences of deception or loss. Other causes of jealousy typically include:

■ **Overdependence on the relationship.** People who have few social ties and rely exclusively on their partners tend to be overly fearful of losing them.

■ **Severity of the threat.** People may feel uneasy if someone with good looks or a great personality appears to be interested in their partner.

■ **High value on sexual exclusivity.** People who believe that sexual exclusivity is a crucial indicator of love are more likely to become jealous.

■ **Low self-esteem.** People who think poorly of themselves are more likely to fear that someone else will gain their partner's affection.

■ **Fear of losing control.** Some people need to feel in control of every situation. Feeling that they may be losing control over a partner can cause jealousy.

In both men and women, jealousy is also related to believing that it would be difficult to find another relationship if the current one ends. Although a certain amount of jealousy can occur in any loving relationship, it doesn't have to threaten the relationship as long as partners communicate openly about it.[39]

Sharing Power and Responsibilities

Power can be defined as the ability to make and implement decisions. Historically, men have been the primary wage earners and, consequently, had decision-making power. Women exerted much influence, but most women needed a man's income and often a man's physical protection for survival. As increasing numbers of women have entered the workforce and generated their own financial resources, the power dynamics between women and men have shifted considerably. The increase in the divorce rate in the past century was partly due to working

jealousy Aversive reaction evoked by a real or imagined relationship involving a person's partner and a third person.

power Ability to make and implement decisions.

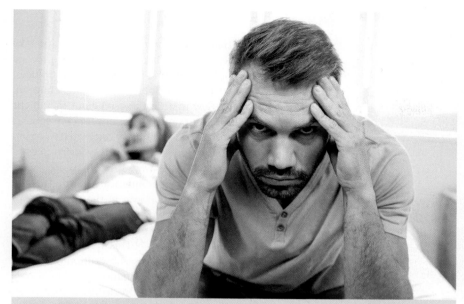

All couples have conflicts. Learning to handle them maturely is vital to relationship success.

personality conflicts. Many people enter a relationship with certain expectations about how they and their partner will behave. Failure to communicate these beliefs can lead to resentment and disappointment. Differences in sexual needs may also contribute to the demise of a relationship. Under stress, communication and cooperation between partners can break down. Conflict, negative interactions, and a general lack of respect between partners can erode even the most loving relationship.

What behaviors signal trouble? On the basis of 35 years of research and couples therapy, therapist John Gottman has identified four behavior patterns in couples that predict future divorce with better than 90 percent accuracy:[41]

- **Criticism.** Phrasing complaints in terms of a partner's defect; for example, "You never talk about anyone but yourself. You are self-centered."
- **Defensiveness.** Righteous indignation as a form of self-protection; for example, "It's not my fault we missed the flight. You always make us late."
- **Stonewalling.** Withdrawing emotionally from a given interaction; for example, the listener seems to ignore the speaker, giving no indication that the speaker was heard.
- **Contempt.** Talking down to a person; for example, "How could you be so stupid?"[42]

Of these, contempt is the biggest predictor of divorce. While these behaviors do not guarantee that an individual couple will divorce, they are "red flags" that the relationship is at high risk for failure.

women gaining the ability to support themselves rather than having to stay in a difficult or abusive relationship solely for financial reasons.

Whereas gender roles and tasks were rigid in the past, modern society has very few gender-specific roles. Both women and men work outside the home, care for children, drive, run businesses, manage family finances, and perform equally well in the tasks of daily living. Rather than taking on traditional female and male roles, many couples find that it makes more sense to divide tasks on the basis of schedule, convenience, and preference. However, while many women work as many hours outside the home as men, the division of labor at home is rarely equal. The Bureau of Labor Statistics estimates that on a typical day, 50 percent of women do household chores such as cleaning or laundry, while the same is true of only 22 percent of men; 70 percent of women prepare food or clean up afterward, but only 43 percent of men share those tasks.[40] Over time, if couples can't communicate how they feel about sharing power and responsibility and arrive at an equitable solution, the relationship is likely to suffer.

Unmet Expectations
We all have expectations of ourselves and our partners: how we will spend our time and our money, how we will express love and intimacy, and how we will grow together as a couple. Expectations are an extension of our values, beliefs, hopes, and dreams for the future. When communicated and agreed upon, these expectations help relationships thrive. If we are unable to communicate our expectations, we set ourselves up for disappointment and hurt. Partners in healthy relationships can communicate wants and needs and have honest discussions when things aren't going as expected.

When and Why Relationships End
Relationships end for many reasons, including illness, financial concerns, career problems, geographical separation, and

Coping with Failed Relationships
No relationship comes with a guarantee. Losing love is as much a part of life as falling in love. Nevertheless, uncoupling can be very painful. Whenever we get close to another person, we risk getting hurt if things don't work out. Consider the following tips for coping with a failed relationship:[43]

- **Acknowledge that you have gone through a rough experience.** You may feel grief, loneliness, rejection, anger, guilt, relief, sadness, or all of these. Seek out trusted friends and, if needed, professional help.
- **Let go of negative thought patterns and habits.** Engage in activities that make you happy. Take a walk, read, listen to music, go to the movies or a concert, spend time with friends you enjoy, volunteer with a community organization, write in a journal. Seek out joy!
- **Make a promise to yourself: no new relationships until you have moved past the last one.** You need time

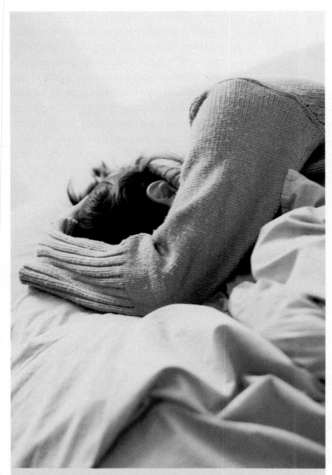

It might feel as if there is no end to the sorrow, anger, and guilt that often accompany a difficult breakup, but time is a miraculous healer. Acknowledging your feelings and finding healthful ways to express them will help you deal with the end of a romantic relationship.

to resolve your experience rather than escaping from it by getting involved with someone new. It can be difficult to be trusting and intimate in a new relationship if you are still working on getting over a past relationship. Heal first before looking for love again.

LO 5 | PARTNERING AND SINGLEHOOD

Compare and contrast the types of committed relationships and singlehood.

Commitment in a relationship means that one intends to act over time in a way that perpetuates the well-being of the other person, oneself, and the relationship. Polls show that the majority of Americans strive to develop a committed relationship, whether in the form of marriage, cohabitation, or partnerships, but an increasing number of young Americans remain single by choice.[44]

Marriage

In many societies, traditional committed relationships take the form of marriage. In the United States, marriage means entering into a legal agreement that includes shared finances, property, and often the responsibility for raising children. Many Americans also view marriage as a religious sacrament that emphasizes certain rights and obligations for each spouse. Marriage is socially sanctioned and highly celebrated in American culture, so there are numerous incentives for couples to formalize their relationship in this way.

Historically, close to 90 percent of Americans married at least once during their lifetime: today, however, the percentage of Americans who are married is at its lowest point since 1920. Only half of people aged 18 and over were married in 2015, compared with 72 percent in 1960 (FIGURE 6.4).[45] This decrease is due to a combination of delay of first marriages, substitution of cohabitation for marriage, and concerns over finances.[46] When people do marry, they do so later than ever before. In 1960, the median age for first marriage was 22.8 years for men and 20.3 years for women; today, the median age for first marriage has risen to 29.5 years for men and 27.4 years for women.[47] Although marriage rates seem to be declining, remarriage rates are increasing. Men are more likely to remarry (67 percent) than are women (52 percent), but most people do opt to give marriage another go.

Divorce rates in the United States have been high for decades. Some estimates indicate that approximately 50 percent of first marriages end in divorce with even higher divorce rates for second and third marriages.[48] However, other studies

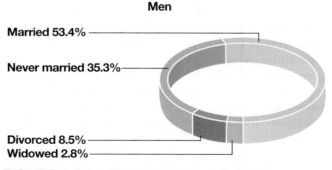

Women

Married 50.8%
Never married 29.4%
Divorced 11.2%
Widowed 8.6%

Men

Married 53.4%
Never married 35.3%
Divorced 8.5%
Widowed 2.8%

FIGURE 6.4 Marital Status of the U.S. Population by Sex

Note: The figure combines the percentages of people who are married, separated, and married with a spouse absent.

Source: U.S. Census Bureau, "Table MS-1, Marital Status of People 15 Years and Over, by Sex, Race, and Hispanic Origin: 1950 to Present," America's Families and Living Arrangements, 2016, www.census.gov.

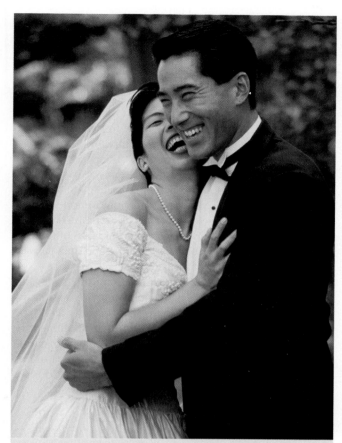

For many people, weddings or commitment ceremonies serve as the ultimate symbol of a long-term, exclusive relationship between two people.

benefits of marriage, indicating that friendship is the critical element of these benefits.[54]

Couples in healthy marriages have less stress, which in turn contributes to better overall health.[55] A healthy marriage contributes to lower stress levels in three important ways: less risky personal behaviors, expanded support networks, and financial stability.[56] Risky personal behaviors, including smoking and heavy alcohol use, are lower in married adults, who are about half as likely to be smokers as are cohabitating, divorced, separated, or widowed adults.[57] They are also less likely to be heavy drinkers, more likely to get enough sleep, and more likely to use preventive health care than are divorced adults.[58] While it may be that marriage causes the improved behaviors, it may also be that people who engage in healthier behaviors are just more likely to get married. Marriage also provides the possibility for integration into an existing social network of family and friends to provide assistance and help couples cope when stressors inevitably arise. Finally, marriage is strongly related to economic well-being, which can alter people's health status and stress levels.

Cohabitation

Cohabitation is a relationship in which two unmarried people with an intimate connection live together in the same household. For a variety of reasons, more Americans—now more than 9 million couples, about 7 percent of adults 18 and older—are choosing cohabitation.[59] In some states, cohabitation that lasts a designated number of years (usually 7) legally constitutes a **common-law marriage** for purposes of purchasing real estate and sharing other financial obligations.

Cohabitation can offer many of the same benefits as marriage: love, sex, companionship, and the opportunity to get to know a partner better over time. In addition to emotional and physical benefits, some people may live together for practical reasons, such as the opportunity to share bills and housing costs. Most young couples now live together before marriage; in fact, it is common for cohabitation to be the first living arrangement for young adults after leaving home.[60] On average, the first cohabitation before marriage for people over age 20 lasts about 18 months, and about 40 percent of couples transition into marriage within 3 years.[61]

Cohabitation before marriage has been a controversial issue for decades. While some voiced moral objections, other concerns were related to higher divorce rates among couples who cohabited before marriage. However, according to recent research based on more than 7,000 respondents to the National Survey of Family Growth, cohabitation before marriage is no longer a predictor of divorce.[62] In fact, avoiding divorce may be part of the motivation for cohabiting, as 60 percent of female respondents and 67 percent of male respondents to that same

suggest that the divorce rate for new marriages is only 30 percent and that it has been declining since the early 1980s.[49] This decrease is related to an increase in the number of couples who cohabit instead of marrying, an increase in the age at which people first marry, and a higher level of education among those who do marry.[50] The risk of divorce is lower for college-educated people marrying for the first time; it is lower still for people who wait to marry until their mid-twenties and who haven't cohabited with multiple partners before marriage.[51]

Many Americans believe that marriage involves **monogamy**, or exclusive sexual involvement with one partner. However, the lifetime pattern for an increasing number of young Americans appears to be **serial monogamy**, in which a person has a monogamous sexual relationship with one partner before moving on to another monogamous relationship.[52] A small number of couples choose an **open relationship** (or open marriage), in which the partners agree that there may be sexual involvement outside their relationship.

A healthy marriage provides emotional support by combining the benefits of friendship with a loving, committed relationship. It also provides stability both for the couple and for the people who are involved in their lives. Considerable research indicates that married people live longer, feel happier, remain mentally alert longer, and suffer fewer physical and mental health problems.[53] A new study by the National Bureau of Economic Research confirms the long-lasting

monogamy Exclusive sexual involvement with one partner.

serial monogamy A nonoverlapping series of monogamous sexual relationships.

open relationship A relationship in which partners agree that sexual involvement can occur outside the relationship.

cohabitation Intimate partners living together without being married.

common-law marriage Cohabitation lasting a designated period of time (usually 7 years) that is considered legally binding in some states.

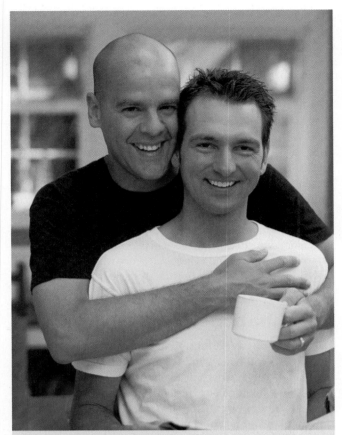

Most adults want to form committed, lasting relationships, regardless of their sexual orientation.

survey agreed with the statement "Living together before marriage may help prevent divorce."[63]

While cohabitation can serve as a prelude to marriage for some people, for others it is a permanent alternative to marriage. The most likely to cohabit include people of lower socioeconomic status, those who are less religious, those who have been divorced, and those who have experienced parental divorce or high levels of parental conflict during childhood.[64] Although cohabitation has advantages, it also has drawbacks. Perhaps the greatest disadvantage is the lack of societal validation for the relationship, especially if the couple subsequently has children. Many cohabitants must deal with pressure to marry from parents and friends, difficulties in obtaining insurance and tax benefits, and legal issues over property and health care decision-making powers.

Gay and Lesbian Marriage and Partnerships

The U.S. Census Bureau reports that in 2014, there were 783,100 same-sex couples in the United States, 25 percent of whom were legally married.[65] Whatever their gender or sexual orientation, most adults want intimate, committed relationships that include love, passion, friendship, communication, validation, companionship, and a sense of stability.

In addition to facing the same challenges to successful relationships as heterosexual couples do, lesbian and gay couples often face discrimination and difficulties dealing with social, religious, and legal issues. For lesbian and gay couples, obtaining the same level of marriage benefits such as tax deductions, power-of-attorney rights, partner health insurance, and child custody rights has been a longstanding challenge. However, in 2015, the Supreme Court's ruling in *Obergefell v. Hodges* made same-sex marriage is legal in all 50 states.[66]

This was a long hoped-for decision for many same-sex couples across the country, especially those in the 13 states that had yet to legalize same-sex marriage. Supreme Court Justice Anthony Kennedy, the justice who cast the deciding vote in the decision, said that the Court's decision was based on the acknowledgement of four fundamental principles: that marriage is inherent to the concept of individual autonomy, that marriage is of unparalleled importance to committed couples, that marriage is crucial for safeguarding the rights of the children of couples in committed relationships, and that marriage has long been a keystone of social order.[67]

In explaining his opinion, Justice Kennedy stated, "It would misunderstand these men and women to say they disrespect the idea of marriage. Their plea is that they do respect it, respect it so deeply that they seek to find its fulfillment for themselves. Their hope is not to be condemned to live in loneliness, excluded from one of civilization's oldest institutions. They ask for equal dignity in the eyes of the law. The Constitution grants them that right."[68]

Staying Single

Increasing numbers of adults of all ages are electing to marry later in life or to remain single. According to data from the most recent U.S. Census, 57 percent of women and 67 percent of men aged 20 to 34 are single.[69] Over a lifetime, 29 percent of females and 35 percent of males remain single, having never married.[70]

Being single allows for rich and productive lives. Single people volunteer more, have larger social circles, and go out more than their married peers. They are more likely to stay frequently in touch with, provide help to, and receive help from family members, neighbors, and friends than are married people. Additionally, many single people report enjoying the solitude, self-sufficiency, and the time to pursue what is personally meaningful that singlehood allows.[71]

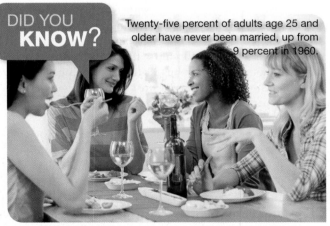

DID YOU KNOW?

Twenty-five percent of adults age 25 and older have never been married, up from 9 percent in 1960.

Source: K. Parker, W. Wang, and M. Rohol, "Record Share of Americans Have Never Married," Pew Research (2014), www.pewsocialtrends.org /files/2014/09/2014-09-24_Never-Married-Americans.pdf.

LIVE IT! ASSESS YOURSELF

An interactive version of this assessment is available online on Mastering Health.

ASSESS YOURSELF

How Well Do You Communicate?

How do you think you rate as a communicator? How do you think others might rate you? Are you generally someone who expresses his or her thoughts easily, or are you more apt to say nothing for fear of saying the wrong thing? Read the following scenarios, and indicate how each describes you, according to the following rating scale.

5 = Would describe me *all* or *nearly all* of the time

3 = Would describe me *sometimes*, but it would be a struggle for me

1 = Would describe me *never* or *almost never*

1. In a roomful of mostly strangers, you find it easy to mingle and strike up conversations with just about anyone in the room.

2. Someone you respect is very critical or hateful about someone you like a lot. You are comfortable speaking up and saying that you disagree and why you feel this way.

3. Someone in your class is not doing her part on a group project, and her work is substandard. You can be direct and tell her the work isn't acceptable.

4. One of your friends asks you to let him look at your class assignment because he hasn't had time to do his. You know that he skips class regularly and seems never to do his own work, so you politely tell him no.

5. You realize that the person you are dating is not right for you, and you are probably not right for him or her. When the person blurts out, "I love you," you say, "I'm sorry, but I don't have those same feelings for you."

6. Your instructor asks you to give a speech at a state conference, discussing health problems faced by students on campus. You tell the instructor that you would love to do it and begin planning what you will say.

7. You don't want to go to a party on Friday night, even though all of your good friends are going to go. When asked what time they should pick you up, you tell them that you appreciate the offer, but you really don't want to go.

8. Your best friend is in an abusive relationship. You tell your friend that you think he or she might benefit by visiting the campus counseling center.

9. Students in your class have done poorly on a recent exam and believe that the test was unfair. You volunteer to be the spokesperson and talk with the instructor, telling her what the class thinks of the exam.

10. You see someone you are really attracted to. You walk up to the person and strike up a conversation with the intention of asking him or her out for a cup of coffee.

How Did You Do?

The higher your score on the above scenarios (that is, the more 5s you have), the more likely it is that you are a direct and clear communicator. Are there areas that you rated as 3 or as 1? Why do you think you would have difficulties in these situations? How might you best communicate in these situations to achieve the results you want? Any time you have to communicate with others about difficult topics, it is best to speak and listen carefully, keep the other person's feelings in mind, and show respect for the individual. Try to think ahead of time about what you might say so that you will be prepared to speak.

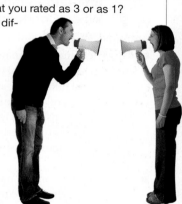

YOUR PLAN FOR CHANGE

The **ASSESS YOURSELF** activity gave you the chance to look at how you communicate. Now that you have considered your responses, you can take steps toward becoming a better communicator and improving your relationships.

TODAY, YOU CAN:

☐ Call a friend you haven't talked to in a while or arrange to meet a new acquaintance for coffee to get to know each other better.

☐ Start a journal for keeping track of communication and relationship issues that arise. Look for trends and think about ways in which you can change your behavior to address them.

WITHIN THE NEXT TWO WEEKS, YOU CAN:

☐ Spend some time letting the people you care about know how important they are to you and how you appreciate the social support they provide.

☐ If there is someone with whom you have a conflict, arrange a time to talk about the issues. Be sure to meet in a neutral setting away from distractions.

BY THE END OF THE SEMESTER, YOU CAN:

☐ Practice being an active listener, and notice when your mind wanders while you are listening to someone.

☐ Think about the ways in which you communicate with a sexual partner. Consider removing yourself from an unhappy relationship or improving communication with a partner to reach a satisfying relationship.

STUDY **PLAN**

CHAPTER **REVIEW**

LO 1 | The Value of Relationships

■ All types of relationships can bolster our health. Social support, in the form of emotional, instrumental, informational, and belonging support, helps to reduce our stress and strengthen our resolve.

■ In addition to our need for feeling close to family and friends, collective connectedness, the feeling of being part of a group, widens our social network and increases our social capital.

LO 2 | Intimate Relationships: When Connecting Gets Personal

■ Characteristics of intimate relationships include behavioral interdependence, need fulfillment, emotional attachment, and emotional availability. Relationships help us fulfill our needs for intimacy, social integration, nurturance, assistance, and affirmation.

■ Family, friends, and romantic partners provide the most common opportunities for intimacy. Each relationship may include healthy and unhealthy characteristics that can affect daily functioning.

LO 3 | Building Communication Skills

■ To improve our communication with others, we need to develop our skills related to self-disclosure, listening effectively, conveying and interpreting nonverbal communication, and managing and resolving conflicts.

■ Digital communication allows us to keep in contact like at no other time in history, but there are concerns about its relationship to depression, envy, and a lack of nonverbal cues.

LO 4 | Relationships: For Better and Worse

■ There are many strategies for building better relationships. Examining one's own behaviors to determine what to change and how to change is an important ingredient of success. Characteristics of successful relationships include good communication, intimacy, friendship, and trust.

■ Factors that can cause problems in romantic relationships include breakdowns in communication, erosion of mutual respect, jealousy, difficulty sharing power and responsibilities, and unmet expectations. Before relationships fail, warning signs often appear. By recognizing these signs and taking action to change behaviors, partners may save and enhance their relationship.

LO 5 | Partnering and Singlehood

■ For most people, commitment is an important part of a successful relationship. Types of committed relationships include marriage, partnership, and cohabitation. Success in committed relationships requires understanding the elements of a good relationship.

■ Remaining single is more common than ever before. Most single people lead healthy, happy, and well-adjusted lives, although they may feel pressure from others to partner.

POP **QUIZ**

LO 1 | The Value of Relationships

1. When Neil had a D in his chemistry course on his midterm report, Mariah told him about the tutors who are available. This is an example of
   a. appraisal support.
   b. emotional support.
   c. informational support.
   d. instrumental support.

2. The power of all the people who could come to your aid with their resources is your
   a. social support.
   b. social potential.
   c. social network.
   d. social capital.

LO 2 | Intimate Relationships: When Connecting Gets Personal

3. Intimate relationships fulfill our psychological need for someone to listen to our worries and concerns. This is known as our need for
   a. dependence.
   b. social integration.
   c. enjoyment.
   d. spontaneity.

4. According to anthropologist Helen Fisher, attraction and falling in love follow a pattern based on
   a. lust, attraction, and attachment.
   b. intimacy, passion, and commitment.
   c. imprinting, attraction, attachment, and the production of a cuddle chemical.
   d. fascination, exclusiveness, sexual desire, giving the utmost, and being a champion.

LO 3 | Building Communication Skills

5. Sharika sits quietly while listening to her sister, not providing any

nonverbal feedback. This is an example of:

    a. competitive listening.

    b. passive listening.

    c. active listening.

    d. reflective listening.

6. The goal of conflict resolution is to

    a. constructively resolve points of contention.

    b. declare a winner and a loser.

    c. ensure that couples argue as little as possible.

    d. set a time limit on discussion of difficult issues.

LO 4 | Relationships: For Better and Worse

7. Predictability, dependability, and faith are three fundamental elements of

    a. trust.

    b. friendship.

    c. attraction.

    d. attachment.

8. All of the following are typical causes of jealousy *except*

    a. overdependence on the relationship.

    b. low self-esteem.

    c. a past relationship that involved deception.

    d. belief that relationships can easily be replaced.

LO 5 | Partnering and Singlehood

9. A relationship in which two unmarried people with an intimate connection share the same household is known as

    a. monogamy.

    b. cohabitation.

    c. a common-law household.

    d. a civil union.

10. Sofia is 30 years old, and she decides to stay single rather than getting married. Which of the following is *true* about Sofia's decision?

    a. Sofia needs to seek out sexual intimacy to stay content throughout life.

    b. Sofia is unusual, as staying single is becoming less common.

    c. Sofia is in the minority of women ages 20 to 34, as most are married.

    d. Sofia can obtain intimacy through relationships with family and friends.

Answers can be found on page A-1. If you answered a question incorrectly, review the section identified by the Learning Outcome. For even more study tools, visit **Mastering Health**.

THINK ABOUT IT!

LO 1 | The Value of Relationships

1. What are the four types of social support? What are examples of social support you give and receive in your life?

2. How can people increase the social capital in their lives? How does social capital affect health status?

LO 2 | Intimate Relationships: When Connecting Gets Personal

3. What are the characteristics of intimate relationships? What are behavioral interdependence, need fulfillment, emotional attachment, and emotional availability, and why is each important in relationship development?

4. What problems can form barriers to intimacy? What actions can you take to reduce or remove these barriers?

LO 3 | Building Communication Skills

5. What is nonverbal communication, and why is it important to develop skills in this area? Give examples of some things you do to communicate without words.

6. Why might Facebook users report more social support in their lives? How can Facebook affect social capital?

LO 4 | Relationships: for Better and Worse

7. What are common elements of good relationships? What are some warning signs of trouble? What actions can you take to improve your own interpersonal relationships?

8. How can you tell the difference between a love relationship and one that is based primarily on attraction? What characteristics do love relationships share?

9. What are some of the common warning signs that a relationship is going to fail? What are some actions people can take to change behaviors to save or even enhance a troubled relationship?

LO 5 | Partnering and Singlehood

10. What are the different types of committed relationships? How do they differ? What does it take for any kind of committed relationship to succeed?

11. Name some common misconceptions about people who choose to remain single. Why might people hold those opinions?

ACCESS YOUR HEALTH ON THE INTERNET

Visit Mastering Health for links to the websites and RSS feeds.

The following websites explore further topics and issues related to communicating in the modern world.

National Center for Health Statistics. This division of the Centers for Disease Control and Prevention has up-to-date statistics on trends in marriage, divorce, and cohabitation. **www.cdc.gov/nchs**

The Gottman Institute. This organization helps couples directly and provides training to therapists. The website includes research information, self-help tips for relationship building, and a relationship quiz. **www.gottman.com**

The National Gay and Lesbian Task Force. This organization works toward lesbian, gay, bisexual, and transgender (LGBT) equality and provides research and policy analysis to create social change. **www.thetaskforce.org**

National Healthy Marriage Resource Center. This website provides a clearinghouse for news and research related to healthy marriages. **www .healthymarriageinfo.org**

Pew Research Center. This organization is a nonpartisan think tank that researches trends shaping America. **www.pewresearch.org**

The Hotline. This site provides information about domestic violence, including how to recognize abuse and how to get help in your local area. Phone support is available 24/7 at 1-800-799-SAFE (7233). **www .thehotline.org**

FOCUS ON Understanding Your Sexuality

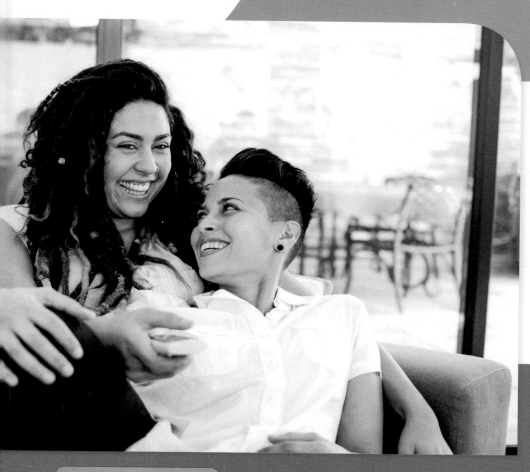

LEARNING OUTCOMES

LO **1** Define *sexual identity*, and discuss its major components, including biology, gender identity, gender roles, and sexual orientation.

LO **2** Identify the primary structures of male and female sexual and reproductive anatomy, and explain the functions of each.

LO **3** List and describe the stages of the human sexual response, and classify types of sexual dysfunctions.

LO **4** Discuss the variety of sexual expression and their implications for sexual health and safety.

WHY SHOULD I CARE?

It is more difficult to please a partner sexually and to describe to a partner how to please you if you don't understand basic sexual anatomy. For example, the clitoris in females is very responsive to touch, and stimulation of the clitoris often leads to orgasm. The urethral opening located nearby is not.

Human sexuality is complex and involves physical health, personal values, and interpersonal relationships as well as cultural traditions, social norms, new technologies, and changing political agendas. **Sexuality** is much more than sexual feelings or intercourse.

It includes all the thoughts, feelings, and behaviors associated with being male or female, experiencing attraction, being in love, and being in relationships that include sexual intimacy. Having a comprehensive understanding of your sexuality will help you make responsible and satisfying decisions about

your behaviors and your interpersonal relationships.

sexuality Thoughts, feelings, and behaviors associated with being male or female, experiencing attraction, being in love, and being in relationships that include sexual intimacy.

163

LO 1 | YOUR SEXUAL IDENTITY

Define sexual identity, and discuss its major components, including biology, gender identity, gender roles, and sexual orientation.

Sexual identity is a combination of the sex assigned at birth, the gender the person identifies as, and who the person is attracted to, both physically and emotionally. The beginning of sexual identity occurs at conception with the combining of chromosomes that

---

sexual identity Recognition of oneself as a sexual being; a composite of biological sex characteristics, gender identity, gender roles, and sexual orientation.

gonads The reproductive organs that produce germ cells and sex hormones in a man (testes) or woman (ovaries).

intersexuality Not exhibiting exclusively male or female sex characteristics.

disorders of sexual development (DSDs) A more descriptive way of describing intersexuality that may be used interchangeably or alone.

puberty The period of sexual maturation.

pituitary gland The endocrine gland in the brain controlling the release of hormones from the gonads.

secondary sex characteristics Characteristics associated with sex but not directly related to reproduction, such as vocal pitch, amount of body hair, breast enlargement, and location of fat deposits.

gender The characteristics and actions associated with being feminine or masculine as defined by the society or culture in which one lives.

gender roles Expressions of maleness or femaleness in everyday life that conform to society's expectations.

socialization The process by which a society communicates behavioral expectations to its members.

gender role stereotypes Generalizations about how men and women should express themselves and the characteristics each possess.

androgyny The combination of traditional masculine and feminine traits in a single person.

gender identity A personal sense or awareness of being masculine or feminine, a male or a female.

transgender Having a gender identity that does not match one's assigned biological sex.

cisgender Having a gender identity that matches the biological sex an individual is assigned at birth.

sexual orientation A person's enduring emotional, romantic, sexual, or affectionate attraction to other persons.

---

determine sex. All normal eggs carry an X sex chromosome; normal sperm may carry either an X or a Y chromosome. If a sperm carrying an X chromosome fertilizes an egg, the resulting combination of sex chromosomes (XX) provides the blueprint to produce a female. If a sperm carrying a Y chromosome fertilizes an egg, the XY combination produces a male.

The genetic instructions included in the sex chromosomes lead to the differential development of male and female **gonads** (reproductive organs) at about the eighth week of fetal life. Once the male gonads (testes) and the female gonads (ovaries) develop, they play a key role in all future sexual development through the production of sex hormones. The primary female sex hormones are estrogen and progesterone. The primary male sex hormone is testosterone. The release of testosterone in a maturing fetus stimulates the development of a penis and other male genitals. If no testosterone is produced, female genitals form.

On rare occasions, chromosomes are added, lost, or rearranged in this process, and the sex of the offspring is not clear. For example, a baby girl may have a large clitoris but not have a vaginal opening, making the question "Is the baby a boy or a girl?" not always easy to answer. This condition is known as **intersexuality**. Today, many professional groups are using the term **disorders of sexual development (DSDs)**, a less confusing term, to describe intersex conditions, which occur in an estimated 1 in 1,500 births.[1]

At the time of **puberty**, sex hormones again play major roles in development. Hormones released by the **pituitary gland**, called *gonadotropins*, stimulate the testes and ovaries to make appropriate sex hormones. The increase of estrogen production in females and testosterone production in males leads to the development of **secondary sex characteristics**. Male secondary sex characteristics include deepening of the voice, development of facial and body hair, and growth of the skeleton and musculature. Female secondary sex characteristics include growth of the breasts, widening of the hips, and development of pubic and underarm hair.[2]

In addition to a person's biological status as a male or female, an important component of sexual identity is gender. **Gender** refers to characteristics and actions typically associated with men or women (masculine or feminine) as defined by the culture in which one lives. **Gender roles**, then, are socially constructed behavioral norms that we use to express masculinity or femininity in ways that conform to society's expectations. Our sense of masculine and feminine traits is largely a result of **socialization** during our childhood. For example, your parents may have influenced your perception of gender roles by the toys they gave you (trucks or dolls), your clothing (pink or blue) or chores they assigned you (doing dishes or yard work).[3]

Gender roles can be confining when they lead to stereotyping. Boundaries established by **gender role stereotypes** can make it difficult to express one's true gender identity. In the United States, common masculine gender role stereotypes include being independent, aggressive, logical, and in control of emotions; common feminine gender role stereotypes include being passive, nurturing, intuitive, sensitive, and emotional.[4] **Androgyny** refers to the combination of traditional masculine and feminine traits in a single person. Androgynous people do not always follow traditional gender roles but instead choose behaviors on the basis of a given situation.

While gender roles are an expression of cultural expectations for behavior, **gender identity** is a person's perception of their being male/masculine or female/feminine, including the choice of gender pronouns (e.g., *he* or *she*).[5] When the sex assigned at birth (male or female) does not match a person's gender identity, based on cultural expectations of gender, the person is **transgender**. When a person's gender identity matches the sex assigned at birth, the person is **cisgender**.[6]

Sexual Orientation

Sexual orientation refers to a person's enduring emotional, romantic, or sexual attraction to others. You may be primarily attracted to members of the opposite sex (**heterosexual**), the same sex (**homosexual**), or both sexes (**bisexual**). Many prefer the term **gay**, queer, or **lesbian** to describe their sexual orientation. *Gay* and *queer* can apply to both men and women, but *lesbian* refers specifically to women.[7]

Most researchers today agree that sexual orientation is best understood by using a model that incorporates biological, psychological, and socioenvironmental factors. Biological explanations focus on research into genetics, hormones, and differences in brain anatomy. Psychological and socioenvironmental explanations examine parent-child interactions, sex roles, and early sexual and interpersonal interactions. Collectively, this growing body of research suggests that the origins of homosexuality, like those of heterosexuality, are complex.[8] To diminish the complexity of sexual orientation to "a choice" is a clear misrepresentation of current research.

While support for gay rights and marriage equality continues to increase each year in the United States,[9] lesbian, gay, bisexual, and transgender people are still often targets of **sexual prejudice**. Sexual prejudice involves negative attitudes and hostile actions directed at people on the basis of their sexual orientation. Hate crimes, discrimination, and hostility toward sexual minorities are evidence of ongoing sexual prejudice.[10] Recent data from the U.S. Department of Justice indicates that prejudice related to sexual orientation is the motivation for 19 percent of all hate crimes in the United States.[11]

LO 2 | SEXUAL AND REPRODUCTIVE ANATOMY AND PHYSIOLOGY

Identify the primary structures of male and female sexual and reproductive anatomy, and explain the functions of each.

Understanding the functions of the female and male reproductive systems will help you derive pleasure and satisfaction from your sexual relationships,

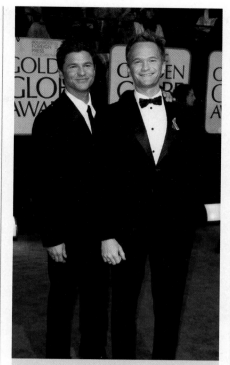

The presence of gay and lesbian celebrities in the media, such as actor Neil Patrick Harris and his husband David Burtka, has contributed to the increasing acceptance of gay relationships in everyday life.

be sensitive to your partner's wants and needs, and make responsible choices about your own sexual health.

Female Sexual and Reproductive Anatomy and Physiology

The female reproductive system includes two major groups of structures: the external genitals and the internal organs (**FIGURE 1**). The external female genitals are collectively known as the **vulva** and include all structures that are outwardly visible: the mons pubis, the labia minora and labia majora, the clitoris, the urethral and vaginal openings, and the vestibule of the vagina and its glands. The **mons pubis** is a pad of fatty tissue covering and protecting the pubic bone; after the onset of puberty, it becomes covered with coarse hair. The **labia majora** are folds of skin and erectile tissue that enclose the urethral and vaginal openings; the **labia minora**, or

▶ **SEE IT!** VIDEOS

Is being gay in the spotlight no big deal? Watch **Celebrities Coming Out, Casually**, available on Mastering Health.

inner lips, are folds of mucous membrane found just inside the labia majora.

The **clitoris** is located at the upper end of the labia minora and beneath the mons pubis; its only known function is to provide sexual pleasure. Directly below the clitoris is the **urethral opening** through which urine is expelled from the body. Below the urethral opening is the vaginal opening. In some women, the vaginal opening is covered by a thin membrane called the **hymen**. It is a myth that an intact hymen is proof of virginity; the hymen is not present in all women and, if present, is sometimes stretched or torn by physical activity.

The **perineum** is the area of smooth tissue found between the vulva and the anus. Although it is not technically part of the external genitalia, the tissue in this area has many nerve endings and is sensitive to touch; it can play a part in sexual excitement.

heterosexual Experiencing primary attraction to and preference for sexual activity with people of the other sex.

homosexual Experiencing primary attraction to and preference for sexual activity with people of the same sex.

bisexual Experiencing attraction to and desire for sexual activity with people of both sexes.

gay Sexual orientation involving primary attraction to people of the same sex; usually applies to men attracted to men.

lesbian Sexual orientation involving attraction of women to other women.

sexual prejudice Negative attitudes and hostile actions directed at those with a different sexual orientation.

vulva The region that consists of the female's external genitalia.

mons pubis Fatty tissue covering the pubic bone in females; in physically mature women, the mons is covered with coarse hair.

labia majora The "outer lips," or folds of tissue covering the female sexual organs.

labia minora The "inner lips," or folds of tissue just inside the labia majora.

clitoris A pea-sized nodule of tissue located at the top of the labia minora; central to sexual arousal and pleasure in women.

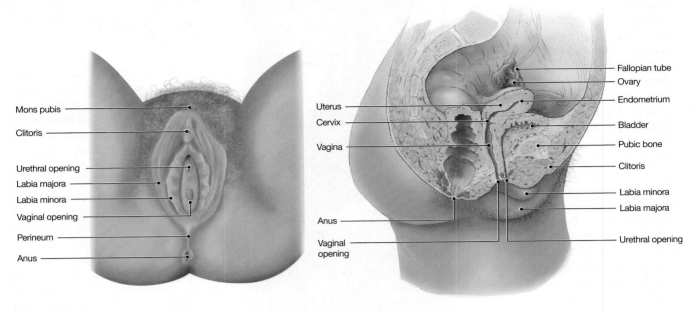

External Anatomy

Mons pubis
Clitoris
Urethral opening
Labia majora
Labia minora
Vaginal opening
Perineum
Anus

Internal Organs

Uterus
Cervix
Vagina
Anus
Vaginal opening

Fallopian tube
Ovary
Endometrium
Bladder
Pubic bone
Clitoris
Labia minora
Labia majora
Urethral opening

FIGURE 1 The Female Reproductive System

The internal female genitals include the vagina, uterus, fallopian tubes, and ovaries. The **vagina** is a muscular, tubular organ that serves as a passageway from the uterus to the outside of the body. It allows menstrual flow to exit the uterus during a woman's monthly cycle, receives the penis during intercourse, and serves as the birth canal during childbirth. The **uterus (womb)** is a hollow, muscular, pear-shaped organ. Hormones acting on the inner lining of the uterus (the **endometrium**) either prepare the uterus for the implantation and development of a fertilized egg or signal that no fertilization has taken place by deteriorating and becoming menstrual flow.

The lower end of the uterus, the **cervix**, extends down into the vagina. The **ovaries**, almond-sized organs suspended on either side of the uterus, have two main functions: producing hormones (estrogen, progesterone, and small amounts of testosterone) and serving as the reservoir for immature eggs. All the eggs a woman will ever have are present in her ovaries at birth. Eggs mature and are released from the ovaries in response to hormone levels. Extending from the upper end of the uterus are two thin, flexible tubes called the **fallopian tubes**. The fallopian tubes, which do not actually touch the ovaries, capture eggs as they are released from the ovaries during ovulation and are the site where sperm and egg meet and fertilization normally takes place. The fallopian tubes then serve as the passageway to the uterus, where the fertilized egg becomes implanted and development continues.

The Onset of Puberty and the Menstrual Cycle

With the onset of puberty, the female reproductive system matures, and the development of secondary sex characteristics transforms young girls into young women. The first sign of puberty is the beginning of breast development, which generally occurs around age 10.[12] Around age 9½ to 11½ the **hypothalamus** receives the message to begin secreting *gonadotropin-releasing hormone (GnRH)*. The release of GnRH in turn signals the pituitary gland to release two hormones, *follicle-stimulating hormone (FSH)* and *luteinizing hormone (LH)*, which signal the ovaries to start producing **estrogens** and **progesterone**. Estrogen regulates the menstrual cycle, and increased estrogen levels assist in the development of female secondary sex characteristics. Progesterone helps the endometrium to develop in preparation for nourishing a fertilized egg and helps to maintain pregnancy.

urethral opening The opening through which urine is expelled.

hymen A piece of thin tissue that covers the vaginal opening in some women.

perineum The region between the vulva and the anus.

vagina The passage in females leading from the vulva into the uterus.

uterus (womb) A hollow, muscular, pear-shaped organ whose function is to contain the developing fetus.

endometrium The soft, spongy matter that makes up the uterine lining.

cervix The lower end of the uterus that opens into the vagina.

ovaries The almond-size organs that house developing eggs and produce hormones.

fallopian tubes The tubes that extend from near the ovaries to the uterus; site of fertilization and passageway for fertilized eggs.

hypothalamus An area of the brain located near the pituitary gland; works in conjunction with the pituitary gland to control reproductive functions.

estrogens Hormones secreted by the ovaries that control the menstrual cycle and assists in the development of female secondary sex characteristics.

progesterone A hormone secreted by the ovaries that helps the endometrium develop and helps to maintain pregnancy.

The normal age range for the onset of the first menstrual period, termed **menarche**, is 10 to 18 years; the average age falls between 12 and 13 years.[13] The average menstrual cycle lasts 28 days and consists of three phases: the proliferative phase, the secretory phase, and the menstrual phase (**FIGURE 2**).

The *proliferative phase* begins with the end of menstruation, when the hypothalamus senses very low blood levels of estrogen and progesterone. In response, the hypothalamus increases secretion of GnRH, which in turn triggers the pituitary gland to release FSH. FSH signals several **ovarian follicles** to begin maturing. While the follicles mature, they begin producing estrogen, which in turn signals the endometrium to proliferate or build up. High estrogen levels signal the pituitary gland to slow down FSH production and increase release of LH. Under the influence of LH, the mature ovarian follicle (known as a **Graafian follicle**) ruptures and releases a mature **ovum** (plural: *ova*), a single mature egg cell, near a fallopian tube (around day 14). This is the process of **ovulation**.

The phase following ovulation is called the *secretory phase*. The ruptured Graafian follicle, which remains in the ovary, is transformed into the **corpus luteum** and begins secreting large amounts of estrogen and progesterone.

These hormone secretions peak around day 20 or 21 of the average cycle and cause the endometrium to thicken. If fertilization and implantation take place, cells surrounding the developing embryo release a hormone called *human chorionic gonadotropin (HCG)*, increasing estrogen and progesterone secretions that maintain the endometrium and signal the pituitary gland not to start a new menstrual cycle.

If no implantation occurs, the hypothalamus responds by signaling the pituitary gland to stop producing FSH and LH, thus causing the levels of progesterone in the blood to peak. The corpus luteum begins to decompose, leading to rapid declines in estrogen and progesterone levels. Without these hormones, the endometrium is sloughed off in the menstrual flow, and this begins the *menstrual phase*. The low estrogen levels of the menstrual phase signal the hypothalamus to release GnRH, which acts on the pituitary gland to secrete FSH, and the cycle begins again.

Menstrual Problems

Premenstrual syndrome (PMS) is a term used for a collection of physical, emotional, and behavioral symptoms that many women experience 7 to 14 days before the beginning of their menstrual period. The most common symptoms are tender breasts, bloating, food cravings, fatigue, irritability, and depression. It is estimated that 85 percent of menstruating women experience at least one symptom of PMS each month.[14] For the majority of women, these disappear as their period begins, but for a small subset of women (5 to 8 percent), symptoms are severe enough to affect their daily routines and activities to the point of being disabling. This severe form of PMS has its own diagnostic category in the fifth edition of the *Diagnostic and Statistical Manual of Mental Disorders* (*DSM-5*), **premenstrual dysphoric disorder (PMDD)**, with symptoms that include severe depression, hopelessness, anger, anxiety, low self-esteem, difficulty concentrating, irritability, and tension.[15]

There are several natural approaches to managing PMS that can also help PMDD. These strategies include eating a diet that is rich in whole grains, fruits, and vegetables; reducing caffeine and salt intake; exercising regularly; and taking measures to reduce stress.[16] Recent research on methods of controlling the severe emotional swings has led to the use of antidepressants for treating PMDD.[17]

Dysmenorrhea is a medical term for menstrual cramps, the pain or discomfort in the lower abdomen that many women experience just before or during

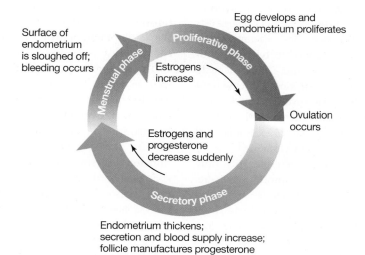

FIGURE 2 The Three Phases of the Menstrual Cycle

Source: S.A. Rathus et al., Human Sexuality in a World of Diversity, 10th ed., © 2017. Figure "The Three Phases of the Menstrual Cycle," © 2005 Allyn & Bacon. Reproduced with permission of Pearson Education, Inc.

menarche The first menstrual period.

ovarian follicles The areas within the ovary in which individual eggs develop.

Graafian follicle A mature ovarian follicle that contains a fully developed ovum (egg).

ovum A single mature egg cell.

ovulation The point of the menstrual cycle at which a mature egg ruptures through the ovarian wall.

corpus luteum A body of cells that forms from the remains of the Graafian follicle following ovulation; it secretes estrogen and progesterone during the second half of the menstrual cycle.

premenstrual syndrome (PMS) The set of mood changes and physical symptoms that occur in some women during the 1 or 2 weeks prior to menstruation.

premenstrual dysphoric disorder (PMDD) The collective name for a group of negative symptoms similar to but more severe than PMS.

dysmenorrhea A condition of pain or discomfort in the lower abdomen just before or during menstruation.

menstruation. Along with cramps, some women can experience nausea and vomiting, loose stools, sweating, and dizziness. Menstrual cramps can be classified as primary or secondary dysmenorrhea. Primary dysmenorrhea doesn't involve any physical abnormality and usually begins 6 months to 1 year after a woman's first period; secondary dysmenorrhea has an underlying physical cause such as endometriosis or uterine fibroids.[18] The discomfort of primary dysmenorrhea can be reduced by using over-the-counter nonsteroidal anti-inflammatory drugs (NSAIDs) such as aspirin or ibuprofen. Other self-care strategies such as soaking in a hot bath or using a heating pad on the abdomen may ease cramps. For severe cramping, your health care provider may recommend a low-dose oral contraceptive to prevent ovulation. Without ovulation, there are fewer **prostaglandins** to trigger muscle contractions, thus reducing the severity of the cramps caused by the muscle contractions. Managing secondary dysmenorrhea involves treating the underlying cause.

Toxic shock syndrome (TSS) is a rare but life-threatening complication caused by toxins produced by a bacterial infection.

---

prostaglandin A hormone-like substance associated with muscle contractions and inflammation.

menopause The permanent cessation of menstruation, generally occurring between the ages of 40 and 60 years.

hormone replacement therapy (HRT) The use of synthetic or animal estrogens and progesterone to compensate for decreases in estrogens in a woman's body during menopause.

penis The male sexual organ that releases sperm into the vagina.

ejaculation The propulsion of semen from the penis.

scrotum The external sac of tissue that encloses the testes.

testes The male sex organs that manufacture sperm and produce hormones.

testosterone The male sex hormone manufactured in the testes.

sperm The cell manufactured by male sex organs that combines with the female's ovum in fertilization.

epididymis The duct system where sperm mature and are stored.

vas deferens A tube that transports sperm from the epididymis to the ejaculatory duct.

It usually follows skin wounds, injury, or the use of a superabsorbent tampon, diaphragm, cervical cap, or contraceptive sponge during a woman's period (see Chapter 7 for more on these contraceptive methods). TSS symptoms include a sudden high fever, vomiting, diarrhea, dizziness, muscle aches, or a rash that looks like sunburn. If you have symptoms such as a high fever and vomiting and have been using a tampon or one of the previously mentioned contraceptive devices, remove it immediately and contact a health care provider. Proper treatment usually ensures recovery in 2 to 3 weeks.[19]

Menopause

Just as menarche signals the beginning of a woman's reproductive years, **menopause**—the permanent cessation of menstruation—signals the end. *Perimenopause* refers to the 4 to 6 years preceding menopause when hormonal changes take place and menstrual cycles and flow can become irregular. Menopause generally occurs after age 45 among U.S. women.[20] Menopausal changes result in decreased estrogen levels, which may produce troublesome symptoms in some women, such as hot flashes, night sweats, decreased vaginal lubrication, headaches, dizziness, and joint pain.[21]

From the 1970s to the 2000s, women commonly relieved these symptoms with synthetic forms of estrogen and progesterone known as **hormone replacement therapy (HRT)**, also called menopausal hormone therapy. This therapy was believed to relieve menopausal symptoms and simultaneously reduce the risk of heart disease and osteoporosis. However, research later revealed that HRT increased the risk for heart disease, stroke, blood clots, and breast cancer in some women.[22]

Today, doctors prescribe HRT only when menopause symptoms are severe; the woman is under age 60 years; and she is free of heart disease, diabetes, high cholesterol, high blood pressure, and a history of breast, ovarian, or uterine cancer.[23] Women are now encouraged to manage mild symptoms by using lifestyle techniques such as exercising regularly, sleeping in a cooler room, and limiting caffeine and alcohol intake.[24]

Male Sexual and Reproductive Anatomy and Physiology

The structures of the male reproductive system are divided into external and internal genitals (**FIGURE 3**). The external genitals are the penis and the scrotum. The internal male genitals include the testes, epididymides, vasa deferentia, ejaculatory ducts, urethra, and other structures—the seminal vesicles, the prostate gland, and the Cowper's glands—that secrete components that, with sperm, make up semen.

The **penis** is the male organ through which urine and semen are expelled from the body. The urethra, a tube that passes through the center of the penis, acts as the passageway for both semen and urine to exit the body. During sexual arousal, the spongy tissue in the penis fills with blood, making the organ stiff (erect). Further sexual excitement leads to **ejaculation**, a series of rapid, spasmodic contractions that propel semen out of the penis.

Situated outside the body behind the penis is a sac called the **scrotum**, containing the testes. The scrotum not only protects the testes, but also maintains them at an ideal temperature—vital to sperm production—by raising them closer to the body or lowering them. The **testes** (singular: *testis*) manufacture sperm and **testosterone**, the hormone responsible for the development of male secondary sex characteristics.

The development of **sperm** is called *spermatogenesis*. Like the maturation of eggs in the female, this process is governed by the pituitary gland. FSH is secreted into the bloodstream to stimulate the testes to manufacture sperm. Immature sperm are released into a comma-shaped structure on the back of each testis called the **epididymis** (plural: *epididymides*), where they ripen and reach full maturity.

Each epididymis contains coiled tubules that gradually straighten out to become the **vas deferens** (plural: *vasa deferentia*). These make up the tubular transportation system whose sole function is to store and move sperm. Along

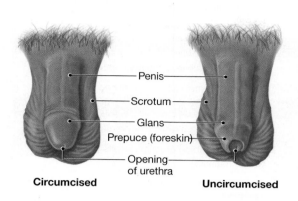

External Anatomy

Penis
Scrotum
Glans
Prepuce (foreskin)
Opening of urethra

Circumcised   **Uncircumcised**

Internal Organs

Rectum
Seminal vesicle
Prostate gland
Ejaculatory duct
Anus
Cowper's gland
Epididymis
Testis
Scrotum

Bladder
Pubic bone
Vas deferens
Urethra
Spongy bodies of erectile tissue
Penis
Glans

FIGURE 3 The Male Reproductive System

the way, the **seminal vesicles** provide sperm with nutrients and other fluids that compose **semen**.

The vasa deferentia eventually connect each epididymis to the **ejaculatory ducts**, which pass through the prostate gland and empty into the urethra. The **prostate gland** contributes more fluids to the semen, including chemicals that help the sperm fertilize an ovum and neutralize the acidic environment of the vagina to make it more conducive to sperm motility (ability to move) and potency (potential for fertilizing an ovum). Just below the prostate gland are two pea-shaped nodules called the **Cowper's glands**. The Cowper's glands secrete a preejaculate fluid that lubricates the urethra and neutralizes any acid that may remain in the urethra after urination. Urine and semen do not come into contact with each other; during ejaculation, a small valve closes off the tube to the urinary bladder.

Debate continues over the practice of *circumcision*, the surgical removal of the fold of skin, known as the *foreskin*, covering the **glans**. While circumcision was nearly universal in the United States in the past, only about 60 percent of baby boys are now circumcised,[25] mostly for religious or cultural reasons or because of hygiene concerns. Research supports

the claim that circumcision yields medical benefits, including decreased risk of urinary tract infections in the first year, decreased risk of penile cancer (although cancer of the penis is very rare), and decreased risk of sexual transmission of human papillomavirus (HPV) and human immunodeficiency virus (HIV).[26] Strong arguments against circumcision include a lack of medical necessity; a possible reduction in sexual sensitivity; and the possibility of bleeding, infection, and surgical complications. The American Academy of Pediatrics and the Centers for Disease Control and Prevention counsel that the benefits of newborn male circumcision outweigh the risks but that the benefits are not great enough for routine circumcision to be recommended in infants, thus leaving the decision to families.[27]

LO **3** | **HUMAN SEXUAL RESPONSE**

List and describe the stages of the human sexual response, and classify types of sexual dysfunctions.

Sexual response is a physiological process that can be roughly divided into four stages: excitement/arousal, plateau,

orgasm, and resolution. Regardless of the type of sexual activity (stimulation by a partner or self-stimulation), the response stages are the same; however, researchers agree that each individual has a personal response pattern that may or may not exactly conform to these phases.

During the first stage, *excitement/arousal*, **vasocongestion** (increased blood flow that causes swelling in the genitals) stimulates male and female genital responses. The vagina begins to lubricate, and the penis becomes partially erect. Both sexes may exhibit a "sex

seminal vesicles The glandular ducts that secrete nutrients for the semen.

semen Fluid containing sperm and nutrients that increases sperm viability and neutralizes vaginal acid.

ejaculatory duct The tube formed by the junction of the seminal vesicle and the vas deferens that carries semen to the urethra.

prostate gland The gland that secretes chemicals that helps sperm fertilize an ovum and provides neutralizing fluids into the semen.

Cowper's glands Glands in the male reproductive system that secrete a fluid that lubricates the urethra and neutralizes any acid remaining in the urethra after urination.

glans The head of the penis.

vasocongestion The engorgement of the genital organs with blood.

flush," or light blush all over their bodies. This happens in people of all skin tones, although it is less apparent in those with darker skin tones. Excitement/arousal can be generated through fantasy or by touching parts of the body, kissing, viewing pornography, or reading erotic literature.

During the *plateau phase*, the initial responses intensify. Voluntary and involuntary muscle tensions increase. A woman's nipples become fully erect, as does a man's penis. The penis secretes a few drops of preejaculatory fluid, which may contain sperm.

During the *orgasmic phase*, vasocongestion and muscle tensions reach their peak, and rhythmic contractions occur through the genital regions. In women, these contractions are centered in the uterus, outer vagina, and anal sphincter. In men, the contractions occur in two stages. First, contractions within the prostate gland begin propelling semen through the urethra. In the second stage, the muscles of the pelvic floor, urethra, and anal sphincter contract. Semen usually, but not always, is ejaculated from the penis. In both sexes, spasms in other major muscle groups also occur, particularly in the buttocks and abdomen. Feet and hands may also contract, and facial features often contort.

Muscle tension and congested blood subside in the *resolution phase* as the genital organs return to their prearousal states. Both sexes usually experience deep feelings of well-being and profound relaxation. Many women can experience multiple orgasms during the orgasmic phase. Most men experience a refractory period, during which their systems are incapable of subsequent arousal. This refractory period may last from a few minutes to several hours and tends to lengthen with age.

Men and women experience the same stages in the sexual response cycle; however, the length of time spent in any one stage varies. Thus, one partner may be in the plateau phase while the other is in the excitement or orgasmic phase. Sexual pleasure and satisfaction are also possible without orgasm or intercourse. Expressing sexual feelings for another person involves many pleasurable activities, of which intercourse and orgasm are only a part.

TABLE 1 | Types of Sexual Dysfunction

Disorder	Description
Desire Disorders	
Inhibited sexual desire	Lack of interest in sexual activity
Sexual aversion disorder	Phobias (fears) or anxiety about sexual contact
Arousal Disorders	
Erectile dysfunction	Inability to achieve or maintain an erection
Female sexual arousal disorder	Inability to remain sexually aroused
Orgasmic Disorders	
Premature ejaculation	Reaching orgasm rapidly or prematurely
Delayed ejaculation	Difficulty reaching orgasm despite normal desire and stimulation
Female orgasmic disorder	Inability to have an orgasm or difficulty or delay in reaching orgasm
Pain Disorders	
Dyspareunia	Pain during or after sex
Vaginismus	Forceful contraction of the vaginal muscles that prevents penetration from occurring

Sexual Dysfunction

Research indicates that *sexual dysfunction*, the term used to describe problems that can hinder sexual functioning, is quite common. Sexual dysfunction can be divided into four major categories: desire disorders, arousal disorders, orgasmic disorders, and pain disorders (see **TABLE 1**), all of which can be treated successfully.

People should not feel embarrassed about sexual dysfunction. The reproductive system can malfunction just as any other body system can. If you experience repeated problems with sexual

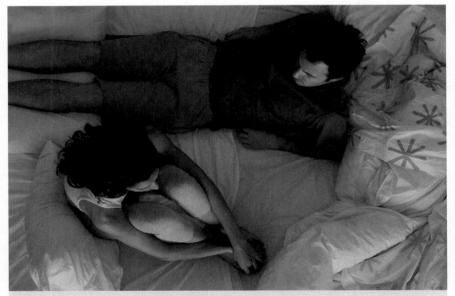

Sexual disorders can have both physical and psychological roots and can occur as a result of stress, fatigue, depression, or anxiety. They frequently have a physiological origin, such as overall poor health, chronic disease, or the use of alcohol or drugs.

 Watch Video Tutor: **Male and Female Sexual Response** in Mastering Health.

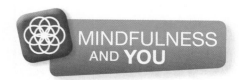

MEDITATION BEFORE MEDICATION

What better time is there to be mindful, to pay close attention on purpose, than during sex? Yet 1 in 10 people admit to having taken a look at their phones while having sex! Distraction, whether from phones or thoughts or nerves, can easily get in the way of sexual pleasure.

Giving pleasure our full focus is good advice for all of us, but it may be especially important for people who are struggling with sexual dysfunction. Mindfulness has

been shown to improve sexual response, desire, lubrication, and sexual satisfaction in women with low sexual desire. In males, mindfulness has led to improvement in erectile dysfunction, premature ejaculation, and sex-related pain.

If you are experiencing sexual dysfunction, it is important to talk to a health care provider rather than suffering silently. But before you take medication, ask how mindfulness-based therapies could help.

Sources: K. Kushlev et al., "Silence Your Phones: Smartphone Notifications Increase Inattention and Hyperactivity Symptoms," *Proceedings of the 2016 CHI Conference on Human Factors in Computing Systems*, Association for Computing Machinery, (2016); L.A. Brotto and R. Basson, "Group Mindfulness-based Therapy Significantly Improves Sexual Desire in Women," *Behaviour Research and Therapy* 57, (2014): 43–54; L.A. Brotto and D. Goldmeier, "Mindfulness Interventions for Treating Sexual Dysfunctions: The Gentle Science of Finding Focus in a Multitask World," *The Journal of Sexual Medicine* 12, no. 8 (2015): 1687–89.

function, an important first step is to investigate the possible causes with a qualified health care provider. Causes can be varied and overlapping and commonly include biological or medical factors; substance-induced factors (recreational, over-the-counter, or prescription drug use); psychological factors (stress, performance pressure); and factors related to social context (relationship tensions, poor communication).[28] See the **Mindfulness and You** box for information on mindfulness and sexual dysfunction.

LO 4 | SEXUAL EXPRESSION AND BEHAVIOR

Discuss the variety of sexual expression and their implications for sexual health and safety.

Finding healthy ways to express your sexuality is an important part of developing sexual maturity. How do we know which sexual behaviors are considered appropriate or normal? Every society

sets standards and attempts to normalize sexual behavior. Boundaries arise that distinguish good from bad or acceptable from unacceptable and result in what is viewed as normal or abnormal. These may change over time. The common standards for sexual behavior in Western culture today include the following:[29]

- **The coital standard.** Penile-vaginal intercourse (coitus) is viewed as the ultimate sex act.
- **The orgasmic standard.** Sexual interaction should lead to orgasm.
- **The two-person standard.** Sex is an activity to be experienced by two people.
- **The romantic standard.** Sex should be related to love.
- **The safer-sex standard.** A person who chooses to be sexually active should act to prevent disease transmission and unintended pregnancy.

These are not laws or rules, but rather social scripts that have been adopted to fit the current culture. Sexual standards often shift through the years, and some people choose to ignore them altogether. The standards can feel limiting, as they do not fit everyone; for example, a lesbian couple cannot participate in penile-vaginal intercourse, and people who enjoy hooking up may disagree with the romantic standard. Rather than accepting societal standards, we might consider the CERTS Model for Healthy Sexuality. The acronym CERTS stands for:[30]

- **Consent.** You freely chooses to engage in the sexual activity and can stop the activity at any time.
- **Equality.** Neither partner is dominant; both feel equal power in the relationship.
- **Respect.** You accept and respect your partner and yourself.
- **Trust.** You trust your partner with your body physically and emotionally. You can be vulnerable together.
- **Safety.** You feel safe from sexually transmitted infections, unintended pregnancy, and violence, and you feel comfortable with where, when, and what sexual activity takes place. You are not making decisions under the power of drugs and alcohol.

By using the CERTS model, rather than societal standards for "normal," all behaviors can be evaluated as either healthy or unhealthy for an individual. As you read about the options for sexual expression in the section ahead, use the CERTS model to explore your feelings about what is right for you.

Options for Sexual Expression

The range of human sexual expression is virtually infinite. What you find enjoyable may not be an option for someone else. The ways you choose to meet your sexual needs today may be very different from what they were 2 weeks ago or will be 2 years from now. Accepting yourself as a sexual person with individual desires and preferences is the first step in achieving sexual satisfaction.

Celibacy and Abstinence

While celibacy and abstinence are related terms, they aren't synonymous. **Celibacy** can refer to abstention from all sexual activities whatsoever, including masturbation (complete celibacy), or abstention from sexual activities with another person (partial celibacy).[31] Some individuals choose celibacy for religious or moral reasons. Others may be celibate for a period of time because of illness, a breakup, or lack of an acceptable partner. For some, celibacy is a lonely, agonizing state; others find it an opportunity for introspection, values assessment, and personal growth.

Abstinence usually refers to refraining from intercourse: oral, vaginal, or anal. People who are abstinent may engage in other sexual behaviors, such as kissing, touching, or masturbation. While no good estimates of celibacy exist, 32.8 percent of college students report being abstinent (no oral, vaginal, or anal sex) for the past 12 months.[32]

Autoerotic Behaviors

Autoerotic behaviors involve sexual self-stimulation. The two most common are sexual fantasy and masturbation.

Sexual fantasies are sexually arousing thoughts and dreams. Fantasies may reflect real-life experiences, forbidden desires, or the opportunity to practice new or anticipated sexual experiences. The fact that you may fantasize about a particular sexual experience does not

---

celibacy Avoidance of any sexual activities (complete) or sexual activities with others (partial).

abstinence Avoidance of intercourse.

autoerotic behaviors Sexual self-stimulation.

sexual fantasies Sexually arousing thoughts and dreams.

masturbation Self-stimulation of genitals.

erogenous zones Areas of the body of both men and women that, when touched, lead to sexual arousal.

cunnilingus Oral stimulation of a woman's genitals.

fellatio Oral stimulation of a man's genitals.

vaginal intercourse The insertion of the penis into the vagina.

---

mean that you want to, or have to, act out that experience. Sexual fantasies are just that—fantasy.

Masturbation is self-stimulation of the genitals. Although many people are uncomfortable discussing masturbation, it is a common sexual practice across the life span. Masturbation is a natural pleasure-seeking behavior that begins in infancy. It is a valuable and important means for adolescents, as well as adults, to explore their sexual feelings and responsiveness. Masturbation does not have to be a solitary activity. Some couples masturbate together, and when separated physically, many couples use technology to connect sexually (see the **Tech & Health** box).

Kissing and Erotic Touching

Kissing and erotic touching are two very common forms of nonverbal sexual communication. Both men and women have **erogenous zones**, areas of the body that when touched lead to sexual arousal. Erogenous zones may include genital as well as nongenital areas, such as the earlobes, mouth, nipples, and inner thighs. Almost any area of the body can be conditioned to respond erotically to touch. Spending time with your partner to explore and learn about his or her erogenous areas is another pleasurable, safe, and satisfying means of sexual expression.

Manual Stimulation

Both men and women can be sexually aroused and achieve orgasm through manual stimulation of the genitals by a partner. For many women, orgasm is more likely to be achieved through manual stimulation than through intercourse. *Sex toys* include a wide variety of objects that can be used for sexual stimulation alone or with a partner. They can be used both to enhance the sexual experience and as therapeutic devices to help with issues such as orgasmic difficulty and erectile dysfunction.

Oral-Genital Stimulation

Cunnilingus is oral stimulation of a woman's genitals; **fellatio** is oral stimulation of a man's genitals. Many partners find oral-genital stimulation

---

38%

of sexually active college students report having had **MORE THAN ONE** sex partner in the past 12 months.

intensely pleasurable. In the most recent National College Health Assessment (NCHA), 43.9 percent of all college students reported having had oral sex in the past month.[33] Remember, HIV (human immunodeficiency virus) and other sexually transmitted infections (STIs) can be transmitted via unprotected oral-genital sex, just as they can through intercourse. Use of an appropriate barrier device (a dental dam for cunnilingus and a condom for fellatio) is strongly recommended if either partner's disease status is positive or unknown.

Vaginal Intercourse

The term *intercourse* generally refers to **vaginal intercourse** (coitus, or insertion of the penis into the vagina), which is the most frequently practiced form of sexual expression. In the latest NCHA survey, 47.1 percent of college students reported having had vaginal intercourse in the past month.[34] Coitus can involve a variety of positions, including the missionary position (the man on top facing the woman), the woman on top, side by side, or the man behind (rear entry). It is essential to protect yourself from unintended pregnancy and STIs during vaginal intercourse. (See Chapter 7 for information on contraceptives and Chapter 14 for information on safer sex.)

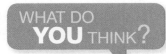

WHAT DO YOU THINK?

Why do we place so much importance on orgasm?

- Can sexual pleasure and satisfaction be achieved without orgasm?
- What is the role of desire in sexual response?

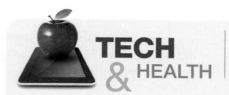

TECH & HEALTH | CONSENSUAL TEXTS

Actress Jennifer Lawrence was livid. "I can't even describe to anybody what it feels like to have my naked body shoot across the world like a news flash against my will. It just makes me feel like a piece of meat." Photos on her phone, in various states of nudity, were hacked from the cloud and posted online. "I didn't tell you that you could look at my naked body," she said. She worried it would affect her career. She was mad that her friends looked at the pictures. She said she would rather give back the money from *The Hunger Games* than tell her dad about the pictures.

But wait, this wasn't a case of paparazzi stalking her and secretly taking a picture. She willingly shot those selfies and sent them to her boyfriend. What she didn't consent to was the pictures being shared with the world.

What can we take from Ms. Lawrence's story? First, once a photo has been taken, we have limited control over its future. Second, "consent," a concept that we usually associate with sexual activity, may apply to sexting, too. According to popular video blogger and sex educator Laci Green, there are three times when consent can never be truly given: when the person is underage, when the person is drunk, or when the

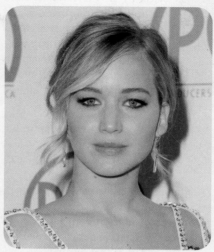

Once a photo of us has been taken, we may have limited control over what happens to it.

person is under pressure from someone is power. Perhaps we need to consider similar rules for texting.

- Never take or send a sexy image of a person under 18 years of age. It is illegal.
- When you are under the influence, you may post pictures that you will later regret. Wait to sober up before posting.

- If you feel pressured to send a picture to someone, don't send it. While the vast majority of people report no negative outcomes of sexting, people who felt pressured to send the sext were more likely to have a negative outcome.

Perhaps the same rule we use for sex, "Yes means yes," could be applied to sharing photos too. Did the person who willingly sent you this photo say that you could share it? Yes? Then, go ahead. No? Then it was meant for you only, so keep it that way.

Consider: Do you engage in any sexting activity that could cause you future hurt or embarrassment? Do males and females face the same threat of embarrassment from shared photos or videos? Why or why not? If you receive a sexy photo from a person you barely know, what is your responsibility to protect this person's privacy?

Sources: S. Kashner, "Both Huntress and Prey," *Vanity Fair* 56, no. 11, November 2014, Available at www.vanityfair.com/hollywood/2014/10/jennifer-lawrence-photo-hacking-privacy; L. Green, "Wanna Have Sex: Consent 101," Video, www.youtube.com/watch?v=TD2EooMhqRl, March 2014; E. Englander, "Coerced Sexting and Revenge Porn among Teens," *Bullying, Teen Aggression and Social Media* 1, no. 2 (2015): 19–21.

Anal Intercourse

The anal area is highly sensitive to touch, and some couples find pleasure in stimulating it. **Anal intercourse** is the insertion of the penis into the anus. Research indicates that 5.3 percent of college students have had anal sex in the past month.[35] Note that condom use is especially important with anal intercourse, as the delicate tissues of the anus are more likely to tear than are vaginal tissues, significantly increasing the risk of transmission of HIV and other STIs. Also, anything inserted into the anus (fingers, penis, or toys) should not then be inserted directly into the vagina without being cleaned, as bacteria commonly found in the anus can cause vaginal infections.

Variant Sexual Behavior

Although attitudes toward sexuality have changed radically over time, some behaviors are still considered to be outside the norm. People who study sexuality prefer the neutral term **variant sexual behavior** to describe less common sexual activities, such as group sex, swinging (partner swapping), fetishism (using inanimate objects to heighten sexual arousal), and BDSM (a catch-all term for bondage, discipline, domination, submission, sadism, and masochism). These activities are all legal in the United States when they involve consenting adults.

Some variant sexual behaviors can be harmful and are illegal in most

circumstances. These include exhibitionism (exposing one's genitals to strangers in public places), voyeurism (observing other people for sexual gratification without their consent), and pedophilia (any sexual activity involving a minor).

Drugs and Sex

Because psychoactive drugs affect the body's entire physiological functioning, it is logical that they also affect sexual behavior. Promises of increased pleasure make drugs very tempting to people who

anal intercourse The insertion of the penis into the anus.

variant sexual behavior A sexual behavior that most people do not engage in.

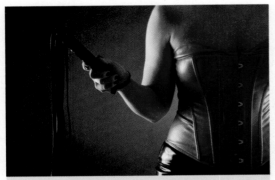

As with any other human behavior, the idea of "normal" sexual behavior varies from person to person and from society to society, usually along a spectrum of perceived acceptability or appropriateness.

are seeking greater sexual satisfaction. But if drugs are necessary to increase sexual feelings, it is likely that partners are being dishonest about their feelings for each other. Good sex should not depend on chemical substances. Alcohol is notorious for reducing inhibitions and promoting feelings of well-being and desirability. At the same time, alcohol inhibits sexual response; the mind may be willing, but the body may not be.

Recreational Use of Erectile Dysfunction Medications

An emerging issue is the recreational use of drugs intended to treat erectile dysfunction (e.g., Viagra). Young men who take this type of medication report that they hope to increase their sexual stamina or counteract performance anxiety or the effects of alcohol or other drugs.[36] However, these drugs probably have only a placebo effect in men with normal erections, and combining them with other drugs, such as ketamine, amyl nitrate (poppers), or methamphetamine, can lead to potentially fatal drug interactions.[37]

Date Rape Drugs

"Date rape drugs" such as Rohypnol or gamma-hydroxybutyrate (GHB) are used to interfere with an individual's ability to consent to sexual activity. Most often ingested by an unsuspecting person in alcoholic drinks, these drugs make it easier for a perpetrator to commit sexual assault because the victim is less able to resist. Victims often wake with little or no memory of what occurred.[38] See more detail on these drugs in chapters covering drugs (Chapter 8) and violence (Chapter 5).

Responsible and Satisfying Sexual Behavior

Healthy sexuality results from assimilating information and building skills, exploring values and beliefs, and making responsible and informed choices. In addition to CERTS, healthy and responsible sexuality should include the following:[39]

- **Good communication as the foundation.** Open and honest communication with your partner is the basis for establishing respect, trust, and intimacy. Can you share your thoughts and emotions freely with your partner? Do you talk about being sexually active and what that means? Can you comfortably share your sexual history with your partner? Do you discuss contraception and disease prevention? Are you able to communicate what you like and don't like?
- **Acknowledging that you are a sexual person.** People who can see and accept themselves as sexual beings are more likely to make informed decisions and take responsible actions. If you see yourself as a potentially sexual person, you will plan ahead for contraception and disease prevention. If you are comfortable being a sexually active person, you will not need or want your sexual experiences clouded by alcohol or other drug use. If you choose not to be sexually active, you will do so consciously, as a personal decision.
- **Understanding sexual functions and safety.** If you understand how the human body works, sexual pleasure and response will not be mysterious events. You will be better able to pleasure yourself and communicate to your partner how best to pleasure you. You will understand how pregnancy and STIs can be prevented. You will be able to recognize sexual dysfunction and take responsible actions to address the problem.
- **Accepting and embracing your gender identity and your sexual orientation.** "Be comfortable in your own skin" is an old saying that is particularly relevant when it comes to sexuality. It is difficult to feel sexually satisfied if you are conflicted about your gender identity or sexual orientation. You should explore and address questions and feelings you may have.

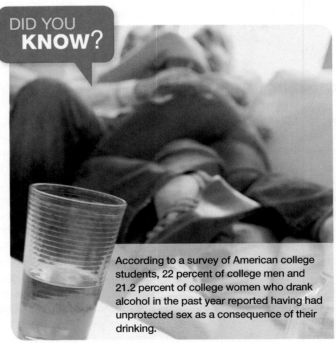

DID YOU **KNOW**?

According to a survey of American college students, 22 percent of college men and 21.2 percent of college women who drank alcohol in the past year reported having had unprotected sex as a consequence of their drinking.

Source: Data from American College Health Association, *American College Health Association—National College Health Assessment II (ACHA-NCHA II) Reference Group Data Report, Fall 2016* (Baltimore: American College Health Association, 2017).

ASSESS YOURSELF

LIVE IT! ASSESS YOURSELF
An interactive version of this assessment is available online in Mastering Health.

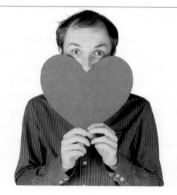

What Are Your Attitudes about Sexual Differences?

Sexuality and sexual differences can be uncomfortable or difficult topics for many people. To complete this assessment, think about your attitudes regarding sexual differences, and indicate how comfortable you would be in the following situations.

	Completely Comfortable				Not at All Comfortable
1. Your close friend, who is of the same sex as you, reveals to you his or her preference for same-sex partners.	1	2	3	4	5
2. Your roommate tells you that he or she likes sexual encounters that involve three or more partners at one time.	1	2	3	4	5
3. Your sister tells you that she would like to have a sex-change operation.	1	2	3	4	5
4. Your 85-year-old grandfather reveals that he is sexually active with his 85-year-old girlfriend.	1	2	3	4	5
5. A male friend reveals that, although he is primarily heterosexual, he occasionally has sex with men.	1	2	3	4	5
6. Your lab partner, who looks and acts like a man, reveals that he is transgender.	1	2	3	4	5
7. Your blind date tells you that he or she occasionally likes to engage in BDSM sexual play.	1	2	3	4	5
8. Two women from your health class invite you to attend their commitment ceremony.	1	2	3	4	5
9. Your cousin reveals that he or she has made a personal commitment not to engage in sexual activity until marriage.	1	2	3	4	5
10. The person with whom you are romantically involved asks you to tell him or her your sexual fantasies.	1	2	3	4	5
11. Your divorced mother reveals that she is dating a man who is 20 years younger than she is.	1	2	3	4	5
12. Your partner says that he or she would like to try anal sex.	1	2	3	4	5
13. Your roommate believes that it is important to be a virgin until marriage but engages in oral sex with his or her partner.	1	2	3	4	5
14. Two of your classmates invite you over for "porn" night.	1	2	3	4	5
15. Your close friend confides in you that he couldn't get an erection the last time he wanted to have intercourse.	1	2	3	4	5
16. You walk in on your partner as he is trying on a dress and high heels.	1	2	3	4	5
17. You go out dancing with friends at a gay bar and run into two men from your residence hall.	1	2	3	4	5
18. Your sister and her husband share with you that their first child was born with a DSD.	1	2	3	4	5
19. A same-sex acquaintance hits on you at a party.	1	2	3	4	5
20. Your housemate asks how often you masturbate.	1	2	3	4	5

YOUR PLAN FOR CHANGE

If you were surprised or unhappy with any of your responses to the ASSESS YOURSELF activity, consider ways to change the attitudes you want to work on.

TODAY, YOU CAN:

☐ Review your responses to the questionnaire, and think about attitudes you would like to change. Evaluate your behavior, and identify patterns and specific things you are doing. What can you change now? What can you change in the near future?

☐ Think about the level of sexual prejudice on campus. Consider joining or starting a group such as the Gay-Straight Alliance that works against sexual prejudice.

WITHIN THE NEXT TWO WEEKS, YOU CAN:

☐ Establish a time to sit down with the person with whom you are having a sexual relationship, and have an honest and open discussion about sex. Before the discussion, think about what you would like to talk about and how you will bring it up. Are there sexual issues between you that need to be addressed? Are you and your partner both satisfied with the nature of your sexual relationship?

☐ Take steps to be more responsible about your sexuality. If you have had unprotected sex, make an appointment to be tested for STIs. If you have found yourself without protection, stop by a drugstore and purchase several packages of condoms.

BY THE END OF THE SEMESTER, YOU CAN:

☐ Develop a greater understanding of and tolerance for people with different sexual values and lifestyles. Learn about different viewpoints by doing research, attending meetings on campus, or getting to know sexually diverse people.

☐ Expand your sense of gender identity. Consider taking a class or workshop in an activity or subject area that you traditionally associate with the opposite gender.

☐ If you are concerned that your sexual decision making is sometimes impaired by drugs or alcohol, set goals to limit and control your use of these substances.

STUDY **PLAN**

Visit the Study Area in Mastering Health to enhance your study plan with MP3 Tutor Sessions, Practice Quizzes, Flashcards, and more!

CHAPTER **REVIEW**

LO **1** | Your Sexual Identity

- Sexual identity is determined by a complex interaction of genetic, physiological, environmental, and social factors. Biological sex, gender identity, gender roles, and sexual orientation all are blended into our sexual identity. Sexual orientation refers to a person's enduring emotional, romantic, sexual, or affectionate attraction to others.

LO **2** | Sexual and Reproductive Anatomy and Physiology

- The major structures of female reproductive anatomy include the mons pubis, labia minora and majora, clitoris, vagina, uterus cervix, fallopian tubes, and ovaries. The major structures of male reproductive anatomy are the penis, scrotum, testes, epididymides, vasa deferentia, ejaculatory ducts, urethra, seminal vesicles, prostate gland, and Cowper's glands.

LO **3** | Human Sexual Response

- Physiologically, both males and females experience four stages of sexual response: excitement/arousal, plateau, orgasm, and resolution.
- Sexual dysfunctions can be categorized into four classes: desire disorders, arousal disorders, orgasmic disorders, and pain disorders. Stress, relationship issues, lack of exercise, smoking, alcohol and drug use, and other lifestyle choices can lead to sexual dysfunction.

LO **4** | Sexual Expression and Behavior

- People can express themselves sexually in a variety of ways, including celibacy, autoerotic behaviors, kissing and erotic touch, manual stimulation, oral-genital stimulation, vaginal intercourse, and anal intercourse. Variant sexual behaviors are those that are less common.
- Alcohol and other psychoactive drugs can affect sexual behavior. Alcohol and drug use can decrease inhibitions and lead people to engage in undesired or unsafe sexual activity.
- Responsible and satisfying sexuality involves good communication, acknowledging yourself as a sexual being, understanding sexual structures and functions, and accepting your gender identity and sexual orientation.

POP **QUIZ**

LO **1** | Your Sexual Identity

1. Your personal inner sense of masculinity or femininity is known as your
   a. sexual identity.
   b. sexual orientation.
   c. gender identity.
   d. gender.

LO **2** | Sexual and Reproductive Anatomy and Physiology

2. The most sensitive or erotic spot in the female genital region is the
   a. mons pubis.
   b. clitoris.
   c. vagina.
   d. labia.

LO **3** | Human Sexual Response

3. Which of the following is *true* about the first stage of the human sexual response?
   a. In men, testes become completely engorged.
   b. In men and women, the rectal sphincter contracts.
   c. In men, the Cowper's gland may release fluid containing sperm.
   d. In men and women, vasocongestion occurs.

LO **4** | Sexual Expression and Behavior

4. What is the effect of alcohol on sex?
   a. It promotes feelings of aversion.
   b. It promotes greater sexual satisfaction.
   c. It inhibits sexual response.
   d. It inhibits pregnancy.

*Answers to the Pop Quiz questions can be found on page A-1. If you answered a question incorrectly, review the section identified by the Learning Outcome. For even more study tools, visit **Mastering Health**.*

7 Considering Your Reproductive Choices

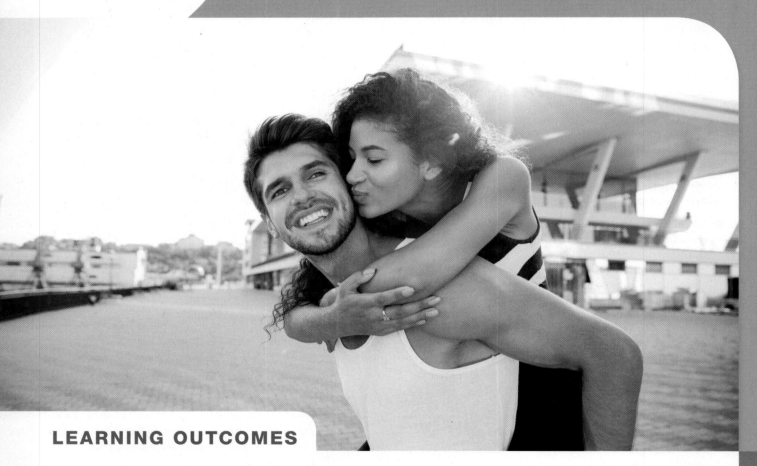

LEARNING OUTCOMES

LO **1** Explain the process of conception, and describe how the effectiveness of contraception is measured.

LO **2** Compare and contrast the advantages, disadvantages, and effectiveness of different types of contraception in preventing pregnancy and sexually transmitted infections, and describe emergency contraception and its use.

LO **3** List and explain factors that you should consider when choosing a method of contraception.

LO **4** Summarize the political issues surrounding abortion and the various types of abortion procedures.

LO **5** Discuss key issues to consider in planning a pregnancy, describe the process of pregnancy and fetal development, and explain the importance of prenatal care.

LO **6** Explain the basic stages of childbirth and complications that can arise during pregnancy, childbirth, and the postpartum.

LO **7** Review primary causes of and possible solutions for infertility.

Do you feel ready to care for another human being for the next 18 years? Do you have the financial and emotional resources? If not, there is a wide range of options to postpone parenthood until you're ready! If you are ready, there are many actions you can take now to prepare for a healthy pregnancy.

Today, we not only understand the intimate details of reproduction, but also possess technologies that can control or enhance our **fertility**, that is, our ability to reproduce. Along with information and technological advances comes choice, which goes hand in hand with responsibility. Choosing whether and when to have children is one of our greatest responsibilities. Children transform people's lives. They require a lifelong personal commitment of love and nurturing. Before having children, a person should ask, "Am I mature enough physically and emotionally, and do I have the resources to care for another human being for the next 18 years?"

One measure of maturity is the ability to discuss reproduction and birth control with your sexual partner before engaging in sexual activity. Men often assume that their partners are taking care of birth control. Women sometimes feel that broaching the topic implies promiscuity. Both may feel that bringing up the subject interferes with romance and spontaneity.

Too often, neither partner brings up the topic, resulting in unprotected sex. In a recent national survey, only 78 percent of sexually active college women and 73 percent of sexually active college men reported having used a method of contraception the last time they had vaginal intercourse.[1] Ambivalence toward contraception has serious consequences: 45 percent of all pregnancies in the United States—nearly 3 million a year—are unintended, and the highest rates are among women ages 18 to 24.[2]

Discussing this topic with your health care provider or your sexual partner will be easier if you understand human reproduction and contraception and honestly consider your attitudes toward these matters. Here, we discuss information to consider as you contemplate your own sexual and reproductive choices.

LO 1 | BASIC PRINCIPLES OF CONTRACEPTION

Explain the process of conception, and describe how the effectiveness of contraception is measured.

The term **contraception** refers to methods of preventing conception. **Conception** occurs when a sperm fertilizes an egg (ovum). This usually takes place in a woman's fallopian tube. The following conditions are necessary for conception:

- **A viable egg.** A sexually mature woman will release one egg (sometimes more) from one of her two ovaries every 28 days on average. Eggs remain viable for 24 to 36 hours after their release into the fallopian tube.

- **A viable sperm.** Each ejaculation contains between 200 and 500 million sperm cells. Once sperm reach the fallopian tubes, they survive an average of 48 to 72 hours—and can survive up to a week.

- **Access to the egg by the sperm.** To reach the egg, sperm must travel up the vagina, through the cervical opening into the uterus, and from there to the fallopian tubes.

Contraceptive methods prevent conception by interfering with one of these three conditions.

Although the terms *contraceptives* and **birth control** are commonly used interchangeably, contraceptives are devices, behaviors, or drugs that prevent conception, while birth control includes any method that reduces the likelihood of pregnancy or childbirth, including contraceptives, contragestion (e.g., the morning-after pill), abortion, or government policies that discourage childbearing.

Without contraceptives, 85 percent of sexually active women would become pregnant within 1 year.[3] Societies have searched for a simple, infallible, and risk-free way to prevent pregnancy since people first associated sexual activity with pregnancy. Outside of abstinence, we have not yet found one.

To evaluate the effectiveness of a particular contraceptive method, you must be familiar with two concepts: perfect-use failure rate and typical-use failure rate. The **perfect-use failure rate** is the number of pregnancies that are likely to occur in the first year of use per 100 users of the method if the method is used absolutely perfectly—without any error. The **typical-use failure rate** is the number of pregnancies per 100 users of the method that are likely to occur in the first year of typical use—that is, with the normal number of errors, memory lapses, and incorrect or incomplete use. The typical-use failure rate is always higher. Because it reflects how people actually use the method, it is more practical in helping to make informed decisions about contraceptive methods.

fertility A person's ability to reproduce.

contraception Methods of preventing conception.

conception Fertilization of an ovum by a sperm.

birth control Any method that reduces the likelihood of conception or childbirth.

perfect-use failure rate The number of pregnancies per 100 users that are likely to occur in the first year of use of a particular birth control method if the method is used consistently and correctly.

typical-use failure rate The number of pregnancies per 100 users that are likely to occur in the first year of use of a particular birth control method if the method's use is not consistent or always correct.

LO 2 | CONTRACEPTIVE METHODS

Compare and contrast the advantages, disadvantages, and effectiveness of different types of contraception in preventing pregnancy and sexually transmitted infections, and describe emergency contraception and its use.

Present methods of contraception fall into several categories. **Barrier methods** block the egg and sperm from joining. **Hormonal methods** prevent ovulation, thicken cervical mucus, or prevent a fertilized egg from implanting. **Intrauterine methods** interfere with sperm movement and egg fertilization. **Behavioral methods** can involve temporary or permanent abstinence, planning intercourse around fertility patterns, or reducing exposure of the egg to semen. **Permanent methods** surgically block the sperm's ability to fertilize the egg. Contraceptive methods could also be categorized whether they are available with or without a visit to a health care provider, the length of time it takes fertility to return after ending use, their cost, or their ability to protect against **sexually transmitted infections (STIs)**. **TABLE 7.1** summarizes the effectiveness, STI protection, frequency of use, and cost of various contraceptive methods.

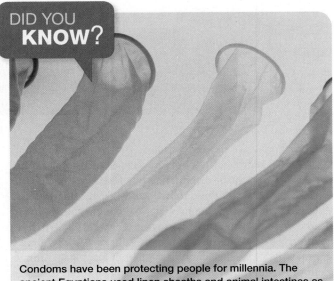
76%

of college students report using a **CONTRACEPTIVE METHOD** the last time they had intercourse.

barrier method Contraceptive methods that block the meeting of egg and sperm by means of a physical barrier (such as a condom), a chemical barrier (such as a spermicide), or both.

hormonal methods Contraceptive methods that introduce synthetic hormones into a woman's system to prevent ovulation, thicken cervical mucus, or prevent a fertilized egg from implanting.

intrauterine methods Contraceptive methods in which a device is inserted into the uterus to either introduce synthetic hormones or interfere with sperm movement or egg fertilization.

behavioral methods Temporary or permanent abstinence or planning intercourse in accordance with fertility patterns.

permanent methods Surgically altering a man's or woman's reproductive system to permanently prevent pregnancy.

sexually transmitted infections (STIs) Infectious diseases caused by pathogens transmitted through some form of sexual contact.

spermicide A substance that kills sperm.

male condom A single-use sheath of thin latex or other material designed to fit over an erect penis and to catch semen on ejaculation.

Barrier Methods

Barrier methods work on the simple principle of preventing sperm from ever reaching the egg by use of a physical or chemical barrier. Some barrier methods prevent semen from coming into contact with the woman's body. Others prevent sperm from getting past the cervix. Many barrier methods contain or are used in combination with **spermicide**, a substance that kills sperm.

Male Condom The **male condom** is a thin sheath designed to cover the erect penis and prevent semen from entering the vagina. Used consistently and correctly, male condoms can both prevent pregnancy and help to prevent the spread of HIV and other STIs. Most male condoms are made of latex, although condoms made of polyurethane, polyisoprene, or lambskin are available. While lambskin condoms can prevent pregnancy, they are not effective protection against HIV and STIs. Condoms come in a wide variety of styles and may be purchased in pharmacies, supermarkets, some public restrooms, and many health clinics. A new condom must be used for each act of vaginal, oral, or anal intercourse.

A condom must be rolled onto the penis before the penis touches the vagina, and it must be held in place when the penis is removed from the vagina after ejaculation to prevent slippage (see **FIGURE 7.1**). Uncircumcised males should retract the foreskin slightly before putting on a condom. In condoms without a reservoir tip, a half-inch space should be left to catch the ejaculate. To do so, the user can pinch the tip to remove air while unrolling the condom down the shaft of the penis.

Condoms come with or without lubrication. If desired, users can lubricate their own condoms with contraceptive foams, creams, and jellies or other

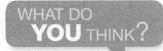

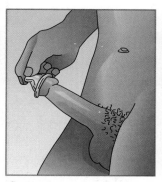
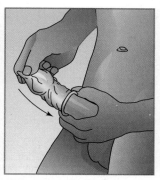
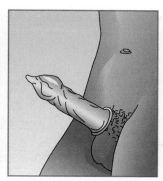
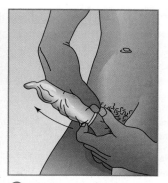

1 Pinch the air out of the top half-inch of the condom to allow room for semen.

2 Holding the tip of the condom with one hand, use the other hand to unroll it onto the penis.

3 Unroll the condom all the way to the base of the penis, smoothing out any air bubbles.

4 After ejaculation, hold the condom around the base until the penis is totally withdrawn to avoid spilling any semen.

FIGURE 7.1 How to Use a Male Condom

 Watch Video Tutor: **Choosing Contraception** in Mastering Health.

water-based lubricants. Never use products such as baby oil, cooking oils, petroleum jelly, vaginal yeast infection medications, or body lotion with a condom. These products contain substances that will cause the latex to disintegrate.

Condoms are available with or without spermicide. Recent research indicates that the most commonly used spermicide, nonoxynol-9 (N-9), can cause irritation and increase the likelihood of infection, including HIV infection, when used multiple times per day. However, N-9 can be used safely by women who are at low risk for HIV and STIs and who do not use N-9 more than once a day.[4] The current recommendation is that users purchase condoms without spermicide and lubricate the condom themselves with water-based lubricants. Of course, the use of condoms with N-9 is safer than using no condom at all.

Condom options are seemingly endless. If partners are unhappy with one type, they should try another. They should also be aware that not all condoms are labeled for contraceptive and STI prevention purposes. Some novelty condoms, such as flavored, glow-in-the-dark, or ticklers, may be designed only for pleasure enhancement, so be sure check the label.

Condoms are less effective and more likely to break during intercourse if they are old or improperly stored. To maintain effectiveness, store them in a cool place (not in a wallet or glove compartment). Lightly squeeze the package before opening to feel that air is trapped inside and the package has not been punctured. Discard all condoms that don't pass this test and condoms that have passed their expiration date.

Many people choose condoms because they are inexpensive and readily available without a prescription, and their use is limited to times of sexual activity with no negative health effects. However, there is considerable potential for user error with the condom; as a result, the effectiveness rate of condoms is only 82 percent.[5] Improper use of a condom can lead to breakage, leakage, or slippage, potentially exposing users to STI transmission or unintended pregnancy. For example, if the penis is not removed from the vagina before it becomes flaccid (soft), semen may leak out of the condom. Even when used perfectly, a condom doesn't protect against STIs that may have external areas of infection (e.g., herpes).

Female Condom The **female condom** is a single-use, soft, lubricated, loose-fitting sheath meant for internal vaginal use. The

> **female condom** A single-use nitrile sheath for internal use during vaginal intercourse to catch semen on ejaculation.

new and improved version, called FC2, is made from nitrile rather than polyurethane. The sheath has a flexible ring at each end. One ring lies inside the sheath to serve as an insertion mechanism and hold the condom in place over the cervix. The other ring remains outside the vagina and protects the labia and the base of the penis from exposure to STIs. **FIGURE 7.2** shows the proper use of the female condom.

Used consistently and correctly, female condoms can help to prevent the spread of HIV and other STIs, including those transmitted by external genital contact (e.g., herpes). The female condom can be inserted in advance, so its use doesn't have to interrupt lovemaking. Some women choose the female condom because it gives them more personal control over pregnancy prevention and STI protection or because they cannot rely on their partner to use a male condom. Because the nitrile material is thin and pliable, there is less loss of sensation with the female condom than there is with the latex male condom. The female condom is relatively inexpensive, is readily available without a prescription, and causes no negative health effects.

As with the male condom, there is potential for user error with the female condom, including possible slipping or leaking, both of which could lead to STI transmission or an unintended pregnancy. Because of the potential problems, the typical-use effectiveness rate of the female condom is 79 percent.[6] As with the male condom, a new condom is required for each act of intercourse, so users must always have them on hand. Male and female condoms should never be used simultaneously; the friction will cause breakage.

Jellies, Creams, Foams, Suppositories, and Film Like condoms, some other barrier methods—jellies, creams, foams, suppositories, sponges, and film—do not

TABLE 7.1 | Contraceptive Effectiveness, STI Protection, Frequency of Use, and Cost

Method	Effectiveness		STI/HIV Protection	Frequency of Use	Cost
	Typical Use	Perfect Use			
Continuous abstinence	100	100	Yes	N/A	None
Nexplanon/ Implanon	99.95	99.95	No	Inserted every 3 years	$0–$800 for exam, device, and insertion; $0–$300 for removal
Male sterilization (Vasectomy)	99.85	99.9	No	Done once	$0–$1,000 for interview, counseling, examination, operation, and follow-up sperm count
Female sterilization (tubal ligation)	99.5	99.5	No	Done once	$0–$6,000 for interview, counseling, examination, operation, and follow-up
IUD (intrauterine device)					
Mirena/Skyla/Kyleena/ Liletta	99.8	99.8	No	Inserted every 3–5 years	$0–$1,000 for exam, insertion, and follow-up visit
ParaGard (copper T)	99.2	99.4	No	Inserted every 12 years	$0–$1,000 for exam, insertion, and follow-up visit
Depo-Provera	94	99.8	No	Injected every 12 weeks	$0–$100 per 3-month injection; $0–$250 for initial exam
Oral contraceptives (combined pill and progestin-only pill)	91	99.7	No	Take daily	$0–$50 monthly pill pack at drugstores, often less at clinics; check for family planning programs in your student health center, $0–$250 for initial exam
Xulane patch	91	99.7	No	Applied weekly	$0–$80 per month at drugstores; often less at clinics, $0–$250 for initial exam
NuvaRing	91	99.7	No	Inserted every 4 weeks	$0–$80/month at drugstores, often less at clinics; $0–$250 for initial exam
Diaphragm (with spermicidal cream or jelly)	88	94	No	Used every time	$0–$75 for diaphragm; $0–$250 for initial exam; $0–$17 for supplies of spermicide jelly or cream
Today Sponge					
Women who have never given birth	88	91	No	Used every time	$0–$15 per package of three sponges. Available at family planning centers, drugstores, online, and in some supermarkets
Women who have given birth	76	80	No	Used every time	
Cervical cap (FemCap) (with spermicidal cream or jelly)					
Women who have never given birth	86	96	No	Used every time	$0–$75 for cap; $0–$250 for initial exam; $0–$17 for supplies of spermicide jelly or cream
Women who have given birth	68	No data	No	Used every time	
Male condom (without spermicides)	82	98	Some	Used every time	$0–1.00 and up per condom. Some family planning or student health centers give them away or charge very little. Available in drugstores, family planning clinics, some supermarkets, and from vending machines
Female condom (without spermicides)	79	95	Some	Used every time	$2–$4 per condom. Available at family planning centers, drugstores, and in some supermarkets
Withdrawal	78	96	No	Used every time	None
Fertility awareness–based methods	76	95-99	No	Followed every month	$10–$12 for temperature kits. Charts and classes often free in health centers and churches
Spermicides (foams, creams, gels, vaginal suppositories, and vaginal film)	72	82	No	Used every time	$8 for an applicator kit of foam and gel ($4–$8 for refills). Film and suppositories are priced similarly. Available at family planning clinics, drugstores, and some supermarkets
No method	15	15	No	N/A	None
Emergency contraceptive pill	Treatment initiated within 72–120 hours after unprotected intercourse reduces the risk of pregnancy by 75–89% (with no protection against STIs). Costs depend on what services are needed: $25–$65 for over-the-counter pills. Not meant for frequent use. Many women report nausea and vomiting.				

Note: "Effectiveness" refers to the number of women not experiencing unintended pregnancies during the first year of use per 100 users. "Typical use" refers to failure rates for those whose use is not consistent or always correct. "Perfect use" refers to failure rates for those whose use is consistent and always correct.
Some family planning clinics charge for services and supplies on a sliding scale according to income. Cost varies based on insurance coverage; many forms of contraception are supplied at no cost.

Advantages	Disadvantages
Women who abstain until their 20s have fewer partners in their lifetimes and are less likely to get STIs, become infertile, or develop cervical cancer.	Can be difficult to maintain. Partners must decide together on a definition of abstinence.
3 years of continuous protection. The ability to get pregnant returns quickly. Nothing to remember to take or use. For most women, periods become fewer and lighter. May be used while breastfeeding.	Minor surgery is required for insertion. Pain during insertion and removal. Irregular bleeding is common in the first 6 to 12 months.
Permanent. No long-term side effects. Allows for privacy. Allows men to be actively involved in their fertility.	Difficult to reverse if the man changes his mind in the future.
Permanent. No long-term side effects. Allows for privacy.	Difficult to reverse if the woman changes her mind in the future.
Continuous protection for 3 to 5 years. Ability to get pregnant returns quickly. Nothing to remember to take or use. Reduces cramps and menstrual flow by 90%. Many women report no period after first few months. May be used while breastfeeding.	Minor surgery is required for insertion. Pain during insertion and removal.
Continuous protection for 12 years. Ability to get pregnant returns quickly. No hormones. May be used while breastfeeding.	Some women report heavier periods and more cramping. Minor surgery is required for insertion. Pain during insertion and removal. Not a good choice for women with multiple partners.
Nothing to remember daily. Private, no evidence of use. Can help to prevent endometrial cancer. Most women stop having periods in the first year of use. May be used while breastfeeding.	Prescription is required. Irregular bleeding in first months. Some women have longer, heavier periods. No way to stop side effects until shot wears off. May cause some weight change, moodiness, or headaches. May reduce bone density over time.
Nothing to remember right before sex. Reduces PMS symptoms, makes periods lighter. Protects against bone thinning and PID. Lowers risks of ovarian and endometrial cancer.	Prescription is required. In first months, there can be breast tenderness and nausea. Some brands have high risks for blood clots. Not good for women over 35 who smoke. Must be taken at the same time each day. May delay return of fertility for a few months after taking.
Nothing to remember daily. Lighter, shorter periods. Like the pill, some benefits against cramps, PID, and PMS.	Prescription is required. Similar to the pill, but must remember weekly, not daily. Higher risks for blood clots, heart attacks and strokes than with pills.
Nothing to remember daily. Lighter, shorter periods. Like the pill, some benefits against cramps, PID, and PMS.	Prescription is required. Similar to the pill, but must remember monthly. Higher risks for blood clots, heart attacks, and strokes than with pills.
No hormones. Immediately effective and reversible. Can be inserted hours in advance of sex.	Doctor visit is required. Takes practice to insert correctly. Must be used every time. Can be dislodged with deep thrusting during sex. Cannot be used with silicone or spermicide sensitivity/allergy.
Similar benefits as diaphragm. No doctor visit required.	Cannot be used during period. Do not leave in more than 30 hours or risk for TSS. Must be used every time. Can be difficult for beginners to insert and remove. Cannot be used with spermicide sensitivity or allergy.
Similar benefits as diaphragm. Good for people with a latex allergy.	Doctor visit is required. Cannot be used during menstruation or risk for TSS. Must be used every time. Can be difficult for beginners to insert and remove. Cannot be used with silicone or spermicide sensitivity or allergy. Can be dislodged with deep thrusting during sex.
No doctor visit required. Easily reversible. Helps to protect against STIs and HIV. Can be used in conjunction with other forms of birth control. No side effects. No effect on hormones. Safe with water-based lubricants. This is the only temporary option for men.	Have to use every time. Have to have on hand. Can be disruptive to sex. Can reduce sensitivity during intercourse. Rare allergies to latex require use of condoms made from materials other than latex.
No doctor visit required. Easily reversible. Helps protect against STIs and HIV. Can be used in conjunction with other forms of birth control. No side effects. No effect on hormones. Safe with oil or water-based lubricants. Latex-free, so no allergy issues. Can be inserted in advance of sex.	Have to use every time. Have to have on hand. Can cause irritation. Can reduce sensitivity during intercourse. Takes practice to insert.
No side effects. Easily reversible. No effect on hormones. Can be used when no other method is available. Can improve the effectiveness of other methods.	Requires strong self-control and trust. Not good for sexually inexperienced or premature ejaculators.
No side effects. Easily reversible. Consistent with teachings of the Roman Catholic Church. Actively involves males.	Both partners must be willing to abstain for 10 days per month. Requires a regular cycle.
No doctor visit required. Easily reversible. No side effects. Easily reversible. No effect on hormones. Can improve the effectiveness of other methods.	Can be messy or leak. Some risk related to frequent use of nonoxynol-9. Must be applied shortly before sex.
No hormones, no prescription.	N/A

Sources: Adapted from R. Hatcher et al., Contraceptive Technology, 20th rev. ed. (New York: Ardent Media, 2011); Planned Parenthood, "Birth Control," Accessed March 2017, www.plannedparenthood.org.

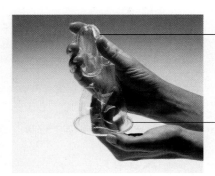

Inner ring is used for insertion and to help hold the sheath in place during intercourse.

Outer ring covers the area around the opening of the vagina.

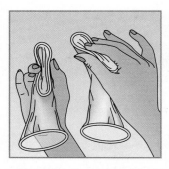

❶ Grasp the flexible inner ring at the closed end of the condom, and squeeze it between your thumb and second or middle finger so it becomes long and narrow.

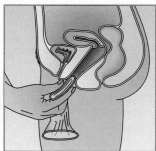

❷ Choose a comfortable position for insertion: squatting, with one leg raised, or sitting or lying down. While squeezing the ring, insert the closed end of the condom into your vagina.

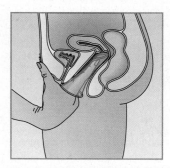

❸ Placing your index finger inside of the condom, gently push the inner ring up as far as it will go. Be sure the sheath is not twisted. The outer ring should remain outside of the vagina.

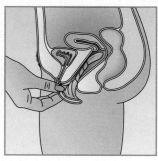

❹ During intercourse, be sure that the penis is not entering on the side, between the sheath and the vaginal wall. When removing the condom, twist the outer ring so that no semen leaks out.

FIGURE 7.2 How to Use a Female Condom

require a prescription. They are referred to as spermicides. The active ingredient in most of them is N-9.

Jellies and creams are packaged in tubes, and *foams* are available in aerosol cans. All have applicators designed for insertion into the vagina. They must be inserted far enough for the substance to cover the cervix, thus providing both a chemical barrier that kills sperm and a physical barrier that keeps sperm from an egg. Jellies and creams usually need to be inserted at least 10 minutes before intercourse. They remain effective for about 1 hour after insertion.

Suppositories are waxy capsules inserted deep into the vagina, where they melt. They must be inserted 10 to 20 minutes before intercourse; they should be inserted no more than 1 hour before intercourse, or they lose their effectiveness. An additional suppository or other spermicide must be inserted for each act of intercourse.

Vaginal contraceptive film is another method of spermicide delivery. A thin film infused with spermicidal gel is inserted into the vagina 15 minutes before intercourse so that it covers the cervix. The film dissolves into a spermicidal gel that is effective for up to 3 hours. A new film must be inserted for each act of intercourse.

Like condoms, spermicides are inexpensive, do not require a prescription or pelvic examination by a health care provider, and are readily available. They are simple to use, and their use is limited to the time of sexual activity. The most effective way to use spermicides is in conjunction with another barrier method; used alone, they have a typical-use effectiveness rate of 72 percent.[7] Spermicides can be messy and must be reapplied for each act of intercourse. Some people experience irritation or allergic reactions to spermicides, and recent studies indicate that while spermicides containing N-9 are effective at preventing pregnancy, they are not effective in preventing transmission of HIV, chlamydia, or gonorrhea.[8] Frequent use of N-9 spermicides (i.e., multiple times a day) has been shown to cause irritation and breaks in the mucous layer or skin of the genital tract, creating a point of entry for viruses and bacteria that cause disease. Spermicides containing N-9 have also been associated with increased risk of urinary tract infection.[9] Contragel, popular in Europe, and Amphora, currently undergoing testing in the United States, are spermicides that use lactic acid to create an environment that is hostile to sperm. These and others will, it is hoped, provide future N-9 alternatives.

Diaphragm with Spermicidal Jelly or Cream

Invented in the mid-nineteenth century, the **diaphragm** was the first widely used birth control method for women. The device is a soft, shallow cup made of thin latex rubber. Its flexible, rubber-coated metal ring is designed to fit

vaginal contraceptive film A thin film infused with spermicidal gel that is inserted into the vagina so that it covers the cervix.

diaphragm A cup-shaped latex device that is designed to cover the cervix and block access to the uterus; should always be used with spermicide.

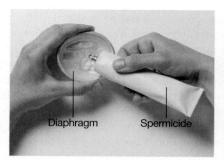
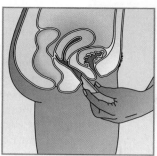
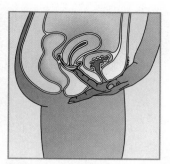

① Place spermicidal jelly or cream inside the diaphragm and all around the rim.

② Fold the diaphragm in half and insert dome-side down (spermicide-side up) into the vagina, pushing it along the back wall as far as it will go.

③ Position the diaphragm with the cervix completely covered and the front rim tucked up against your pubic bone; you should be able to feel your cervix through the rubber dome.

FIGURE 7.3 Proper Use and Placement of a Diaphragm

snugly behind the pubic bone in front of the cervix and over the back of the cervix on the other side so that it blocks access to the uterus. Because diaphragms come in different sizes, they must be fitted by a trained health care provider.

Spermicidal cream or jelly must be applied to the inside of the diaphragm before it is inserted, up to 6 hours before intercourse. The diaphragm holds the spermicide in place, creating a physical and chemical barrier against sperm; without spermicide, the diaphragm is ineffective (**FIGURE 7.3**). Although the diaphragm can be left in place for multiple acts of intercourse, additional spermicide must be applied each time. The diaphragm must then stay in place for 6 to 8 hours after intercourse. After removal, the diaphragm should be cleaned, inspected for damage, and stored safely.

Because the diaphragm can be inserted up to 6 hours in advance, some users find it less disruptive than other barrier methods. Diaphragms have a higher typical-use effectiveness rate (88 percent) than other barrier methods.[10] The U.S. Food and Drug Administration (FDA) has recently approved a new one-size-fits-most diaphragm, Caya. It is not yet widely available, but your health care provider or pharmacy can order it. The term *one-size-fits-most* means that women for whom a conventional diaphragm 65 to 80 mm in diameter is effective will not have to be fitted to use a Caya or be refitted for a different size if they gain or lose weight.[11]

Some women find inserting a diaphragm awkward at first. When inserted incorrectly, diaphragms are much less effective. It is also possible for a diaphragm to slip out of place as a result of heavy thrusting during sex. As with other barrier methods, supplies must be kept on hand, as additional spermicide is required for each act of intercourse. The device cannot be used during the woman's menstrual period or for longer than 48 hours because of the risk of **toxic shock syndrome (TSS)**, a potentially life-threatening disease that results when certain bacteria multiply in environments such as tampons and diaphragms and their toxins spread to the bloodstream.

Cervical Cap with Spermicidal Jelly or Cream

Early **cervical caps** were made from beeswax, silver, or copper. These were among the oldest methods used to prevent pregnancy. The only cervical cap available in the United States, the FemCap, is a clear silicone cup that fits snugly over the entire cervix and has a ring on the back to assist with removal. It comes in three sizes and must be fitted by a health care provider. The FemCap is designed for use with spermicidal jelly or cream. It is held in place by suction created during application and works by blocking sperm from the uterus. The FemCap can be inserted up to 6 hours before intercourse. The device must be left in place for 6 to 8 hours after sex, and additional spermicide must

toxic shock syndrome (TSS) A rare, potentially life-threatening disease that occurs when specific bacterial toxins multiply and spread to the bloodstream, most commonly through improper use of tampons, diaphragms, or cervical caps.

cervical cap A small cup made of silicone that is designed to fit snugly over the entire cervix; should always be used with spermicide.

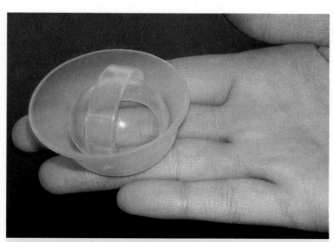

FemCap is used in conjunction with spermicide and is positioned to cover the cervix. It is shaped like a sailor's cap and has a loop to aid in removal.

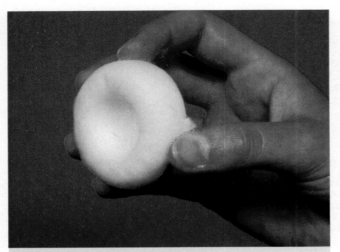

The Today Sponge is a barrier method infused with spermicide. It is a round pillow of polyurethane foam with a loop to assist with removal.

be used for any additional intercourse during this time. After removal, the cervical cap should be cleaned, inspected for damage, and stored safely.

With a typical-use effectiveness rate of 86 percent,[12] cervical caps are reasonably effective. They are relatively inexpensive, as the only ongoing cost is the spermicide, and they last for 2 years.[13] Some users find the FemCap less disruptive than other barrier methods because, like the diaphragm, it can be inserted up to 6 hours before intercourse and may be used for multiple acts of intercourse.

The FemCap is somewhat more difficult to insert than a diaphragm because of its smaller size. Like a diaphragm, it requires an initial fitting by a physician and may require subsequent refitting if a woman's cervix size changes (e.g., after giving birth). Because the FemCap can become dislodged during intercourse, placement must be checked periodically. The device cannot be used during the menstrual period or for longer than 48 hours because of the risk of TSS. Some women report unpleasant vaginal odors after use. As with other barrier methods, users must keep a supply of spermicidal cream or jelly on hand.

Contraceptive Sponge

The **contraceptive sponge** (sold in the United States as the Today Sponge) is a small, round pillow of polyurethane foam with a loop on the back to assist with removal and a dimple on the front to help it fit closely to the cervix. Before insertion, the sponge must be moistened with water to activate the infused spermicide. It is then folded and inserted deep into the vagina, where it fits over the cervix and creates a barrier against sperm. Protection begins immediately on insertion and lasts for up to 24 hours. There is no need to reapply spermicide or insert a new sponge for any subsequent acts of intercourse within the same 24-hour period;

contraceptive sponge A contraceptive device containing nonoxynol-9 and made of polyurethane foam that fits over the cervix to create a barrier against sperm.

oral contraceptives Pills containing synthetic hormones that prevent ovulation by regulating hormones.

the sponge must be left in place for at least 6 hours after the last intercourse. After one use, it is thrown away.

The main advantage of the sponge is convenience, because it does not require a trip to a health care provider for fitting. The sponge allows for more spontaneity than some other barrier methods because protection begins immediately on insertion and lasts for 24 hours without reapplication of spermicide for additional intercourse.

The effectiveness of the sponge is similar to that of the diaphragm for women who have never given birth (88 percent typical-use effectiveness rate) but less effective for women who have previously given birth (76 percent typical-use effectiveness rate).[14] Allergic reactions are more common with the sponge than with other barrier methods. If the vaginal lining becomes irritated, the risk of yeast infections and other STIs may increase. The sponge should not be used during menstruation. Some cases of TSS have been reported in women using the sponge; therefore, the same precautions should be taken as with the diaphragm and cervical cap. Finally, the sponge is infused with nonoxynol-9, so users should be aware of risks related to this chemical.

Hormonal Methods

The term *hormonal contraception* refers to birth control that contains synthetic estrogen, progestin (synthetic progesterone), or both—similar to the hormones estrogen and progesterone that a woman's ovaries produce naturally for the process of ovulation and the menstrual cycle. Synthetic estrogen works to prevent the ovaries from releasing an egg. If no egg is released, there is nothing to be fertilized by the sperm, and pregnancy cannot occur. Progestin thickens the cervical mucus, which hinders the movement of the sperm, inhibits the egg's ability to travel, and suppresses the sperm's ability to unite with the egg. Progestin also thins the uterine lining, making it unlikely for a fertilized egg to implant in the uterine wall. Most errors are due to user error, not method failure, so it is easier for a motivated user to approach perfect use with hormonal methods than with barrier contraceptives.

Oral Contraceptives

Oral contraceptive pills were first marketed in the United States in 1960. Today, oral contraceptives are a commonly used birth control method among college women (58 percent of sexually active women report using pills, second only to condoms at 61 percent).[15] Birth control pills are highly effective at preventing pregnancy (91 percent effective with typical use).[16] Much of the pill's popularity is due to its convenience and ability to be used discreetly. Users tend to like the fact that the pill doesn't interrupt lovemaking.

The greatest disadvantage of oral contraceptives is that they must be taken every day at the same time, without fail. If a woman misses a pill, she should use a backup method of contraception for the remainder of that cycle. After discontinuing use of the pill, return of fertility may be delayed, but the pill is not known to cause infertility. Other drawbacks are that the pill does not protect against HIV and STIs and that its effectiveness may be affected by certain medications, including St. John's wort and the antibiotic rifampin, and by some treatments for seizures, HIV, and yeast infections.

More than 40 brands of oral contraceptives exist, fitting into two categories: combination pills and progestin-only pills. *Combination pills* work through the combined effects of synthetic estrogen and progestin and are taken in a cycle. At the end of each 3-week cycle, the user stops taking pills or takes placebo pills for 1 week. The resultant drop in hormone level causes the uterine lining to be shed, and the user will have a menstrual period, usually within 1 to 3 days. Menstrual flow is generally lighter than it is for women who don't use the pill, because the hormones in the pill prevent thick endometrial buildup.

Several brands of combination pills have *extended cycles*, such as the 91-day Seasonale and Seasonique. A woman using this regimen takes active pills for 12 weeks, followed by 1 week of placebos. On this cycle, women can expect a menstrual period every 3 months. Lybrel, another extended-cycle pill, supplies an active dose of hormones every day for 365 days, eliminating menstruation completely during use. While the idea of not having a period for a year may be unsettling, there is no known physiological need for a woman to have a monthly period, and no known risks are associated with avoidance.

In addition to effectively preventing pregnancy, the combination pill may lessen menstrual difficulties, such as cramps and premenstrual syndrome (PMS), and lower the risk of several health conditions, including endometrial and ovarian cancers, noncancerous breast disease, osteoporosis, ovarian cysts, pelvic inflammatory disease, and iron-deficiency anemia.[17] Many different brands of combination pills are on the market, some of which contain progestins that offer additional benefits, such as reducing acne, minimizing fluid retention, or relieving cramps.

Although the estrogen in combination pills is associated with increased risk of several serious health problems among older women, the risk is low for most healthy, nonsmoking women under age 35. Problems include increased risk for blood clots and higher risk for increased blood pressure, thrombotic stroke, and myocardial infarction. These risks increase with age and cigarette smoking. Early warning signs of complications associated with oral contraceptives include severe abdominal, chest, or leg pain; severe headache; and/or eye problems.[18]

Different brands of contraceptive pills have varying minor side effects. Some of the most common are spotting between periods, breast tenderness, moodiness, and nausea. With most pills, side effects clear up within a few months. Other, less common side effects include acne, hair loss or growth, and a change in sexual desire. With so many brands available, most women who wish to use the pill are able to find one without unpleasant side effects.

Progestin-only pills (or minipills) contain small doses of progestin and no estrogen. These pills are available in 28-day packs of active pills (menstruation usually occurs during the fourth week even though the active dose continues through the entire month). Ovulation may occur, but the progestin prevents pregnancy by thickening cervical mucus and interfering with implantation of a fertilized egg. Progestin-only pills are a good choice for women who are at high risk for estrogen-related side effects or who cannot take estrogen-containing

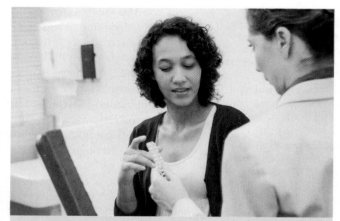

Studies show that college-age women are most familiar with the birth control pill and the male condom; talk to your health care provider about other options that are available to you and your partner.

pills because of diabetes, high blood pressure, or other cardiovascular conditions. They also can be used safely by women who are older than age 35 and by women who are currently breastfeeding.

Like combination pills, progestin-only pills are highly effective at preventing pregnancy: 91 percent with typical use.[19] Progestin-only pills share many of the health benefits of combination pills, but unlike combination pills, they carry no estrogen-related cardiovascular risks. Also, some of the typical side effects of combination pills, including nausea and breast tenderness, usually do not occur with progestin-only pills. With progestin-only pills, women's menstrual periods generally become lighter or stop altogether.

Because of the lower dose of hormones in progestin-only pills, it is especially important to take them at the same time each day. If a woman takes a pill 3 or more hours later than usual, she will need to use a backup method of contraception for the next 48 hours.[20] The most common side effect of progestin-only pills is irregular menstrual bleeding or spotting. Less common side effects include mood changes, changes in sex drive, and headaches.

Contraceptive Skin Patch Xulane (a generic form of Ortho Evra, which has been removed from the market) is a square transdermal (i.e., the substance is absorbed through the skin) adhesive patch less than 2 inches wide, as thin as a plastic bandage. It is worn for 1 week and replaced on the same day of the week for 3 consecutive weeks; during the fourth week, no patch is worn. Xulane works by delivering continuous levels of estrogen and progestin into the bloodstream. The patch can be worn on the buttocks, abdomen, upper torso (front or back, excluding the breasts), or upper outer arm. It should not be used by women over age 35 who smoke cigarettes and is less effective in women who weigh more than 198 pounds.[21]

Xulane is anticipated to have the same level of effectiveness with typical use (91 percent) as the brand-name patch Ortho Evra.[22] Women who choose

Xulane A patch that releases hormones similar to those in oral contraceptives; each patch is worn for 1 week.

to use the patch often do so because they find it easier to remember to replace it weekly than to take a daily pill. Xulane has not yet been shown to offer health benefits similar to those of combination pills (reduction in risk of certain cancers and diseases, lessening of PMS symptoms, etc.), though it is likely that it does. Like other hormonal methods, the patch regulates a woman's menstrual cycle. Because the user has to think about her birth control only once a week, it may increase convenience and spontaneity.

Like other hormonal birth control methods, the patch offers no protection against HIV or other STIs. Some women experience minor side effects like those associated with combination pills. Rarely, women report the patch falling off or irritation at the site of application. The estrogen in the patch is associated with cardiovascular risks, particularly in women who smoke and women over the age of 35.[23] Amid evidence that the patch may increase the risk of life-threatening blood clots, the FDA mandated an additional warning label explaining that patch use exposes women to about 60 percent more estrogen than a typical combination pill.[24] There may be some delay in return of fertility with the patch, especially if a woman had irregular menstrual cycles before beginning use. As with oral contraceptives, some medications can make Xulane less effective.

Vaginal Contraceptive Ring

NuvaRing is a soft, flexible plastic hormonal contraceptive ring about 2 inches in diameter. The user inserts the ring into the vagina, leaves it in place for 3 weeks, then removes it for 1 week, during which she will have a menstrual period. Once the ring has been inserted, it releases a steady flow of estrogen and progestin.

The ring is 91 percent effective with typical use.[25] Advantages of NuvaRing include lower risk of user error, as there is no pill to take daily or patch to change weekly, no need to be fitted by a health care provider, and rapid return of fertility when use is stopped. It also exposes the user to a lower dosage of estrogen than do the patch and some combination pills, and it may have fewer estrogen-related side effects. It likely offers some of the same potential health benefits as combination pills, and it regulates the menstrual cycle.

Like other hormonal methods, the ring provides no protection against STIs or HIV. Like combination pills, the ring poses rare but potentially serious

health risks for some women. Possible side effects that are unique to the ring include increased vaginal discharge and vaginal irritation or infection.

Contraceptive Injections

Depo-Provera (injected intramuscularly) and the newer **Depo-subQ Provera** (injected just beneath the skin in a lower dose) are long-acting progestins that are injected every 3 months by a health care provider. Both prevent ovulation, thicken cervical mucus, and thin the uterine lining, all of which prevent pregnancy.

Depo-Provera and Depo-subQ Provera take effect within 24 hours of the first shot, so there is usually no need for a backup method. There is little room for user error, as a health care provider administers the injection every 3 months. With typical use, Depo-Provera and Depo-subQ Provera are 94 percent effective.[26] With continued use, a woman's menstrual periods become lighter and may eventually cease. There are no estrogen-related health risks associated with Depo-Provera and Depo-subQ Provera, and they offer the same potential health benefits as progestin-only pills. Unlike estrogen-containing hormonal methods, this method can be used by women who are breastfeeding.

The main disadvantage of this method is irregular bleeding, which can be troublesome at first, but within a year, most women are amenorrheic (have no menstrual periods). Also, this method offers no protection against STIs or HIV. Prolonged use of Depo-Provera has been linked to loss of bone density, and some medications can make contraceptive injections less effective.[27] A disadvantage for women who want to get pregnant is that fertility may not return for up to 1 year after the final injection.

Contraceptive Implants

A single-rod implantable contraceptive, **Nexplanon** (formerly called **Implanon**) is a small, soft plastic capsule (about the size of a matchstick) that is inserted just beneath the skin on the inner side of a woman's upper underarm by a health care provider. Nexplanon continually releases a low, steady dose of progestin for 3 years, suppressing ovulation during that time.

After insertion, Nexplanon is generally not visible, so it is a discreet method of birth control. It is highly effective, allowing no user error, and has a more than 99 percent typical-use effectiveness rate.[28] It has benefits similar to those of other progestin-only forms of contraception, including lighter or no menstrual periods, the lack of estrogen-related side effects, and safety for use by breastfeeding women.

Xulane is an adhesive patch that delivers estrogen and progestin through the skin for 1 week. Patches are changed weekly and worn for 3 out of 4 weeks.

Implants are fully reversible; that is, after removal, there is usually no delay in return of fertility. Although implants are effective for 3 years, a health care provider can remove the implant at any time if a woman wants to become pregnant.

Potential minor side effects of Nexplanon include irritation, allergic reaction, and swelling or scarring around the area of insertion, and a possibility of infection or complications with removal. Like all other hormonal methods, Nexplanon offers no protection against STIs or HIV.[29]

Intrauterine Contraceptives

The **intrauterine device (IUD)** is a small, flexible plastic device with a nylon string attached. It is placed in the uterus through the cervix and provides protection from pregnancy for 3 to 12 years. The exact mechanism by which it works is not clearly understood, but researchers believe that IUDs affect the way sperm and eggs move, thereby preventing fertilization, and/or affect the lining of the uterus to prevent a fertilized ovum from implanting.

IUDs were once extremely popular in the United States. However, in the 1970s, most brands were removed from the market because of serious complications such as pelvic inflammatory disease and infertility. Redesigned for safe use, IUDs are again very popular with women around the world and are experiencing a resurgence of popularity among U.S. women.[30]

Five IUDs are currently available in the United States. Para-Gard is a T-shaped plastic device with copper around the shaft. It does not contain any hormones and can be left in place for

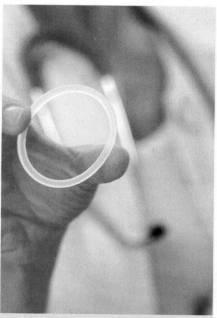

NuvaRing is inserted into the vagina, where it releases estrogen and progestin for 3 weeks.

12 years. Mirena is effective for 5 years and releases small amounts of progestin. Skyla and Kyleena are smaller versions of Mirena, specifically designed for women who have not yet had a baby. Skyla is effective for 3 years, and Kyleena is effective for 5 years. Liletta, also smaller and effective for 3 years, was designed to be a more affordable choice.

An IUD must be inserted by a health care provider. One or two strings extend from the IUD into the vagina so the user can periodically check to make sure that the device is in place. Although IUDs were initially not recommended for women who had never had a baby, the American Congress of Obstetricians and Gynecologists now supports their use for women of all ages, whether they have borne children or not.[31]

The IUD is a safe, discreet, and highly effective method that is more than 99 percent effective.[32] ParaGard has the benefit of containing no hormones and so has none of the potential negative health effects of hormonal contraceptives. Skyla, Mirena, Kyleena, and Liletta, by contrast, likely offer some of the same potential health benefits as other progestin-only methods. IUDs are fully reversible; that is, after removal, there is usually no delay in return of fertility. Although IUDs are effective for 3 to 12 years, a health care provider can remove the IUD at any time if the woman decides to become pregnant.

Some disadvantages of IUDs include possible discomfort during insertion and removal and potential complications, such as expulsion. Also, IUDs do not protect against HIV and STIs. In some women, Paraguard can cause heavy menstrual flow and severe cramps for the first few months; other negative side effects of Paraguard include acne, headaches, mood changes, uterine cramps, and backache, which seem to occur most often in women who have never been pregnant and go away after the first few months.

Behavioral Methods

Some methods of contraception rely on one or both partners altering their sexual behavior. In general, these methods require more self-control, diligence, and commitment, making them more prone to user error than hormonal and barrier methods.

Withdrawal Withdrawal, also called *coitus interruptus*, involves removing the penis from the vagina just before ejaculation. In the American College Health Association's 2015 National College Health Assessment (ACHA-NCHA), 32 percent of respondents reported that withdrawal was the method of birth control (or one of the

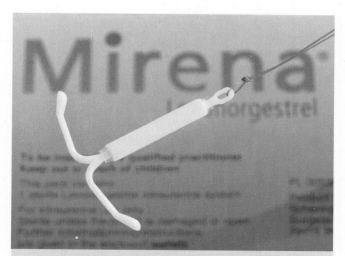

The Mirena IUD is a flexible plastic device inserted by a health care provider into a woman's uterus, where it releases progestin for up to 5 years.

intrauterine device (IUD) A device, often T-shaped, that is implanted in the uterus to prevent pregnancy.

withdrawal A contraceptive method that involves withdrawing the penis from the vagina before ejaculation; also called *coitus interruptus.*

methods) they used the last time they had sexual intercourse.[33] This statistic is startlingly high, considering the high risk of both STI transmission and pregnancy (only 78 percent effective with typical use) associated with this method of birth control.[34]

Even with "perfect" use, withdrawal is unreliable because there are a half-million sperm in just the drops of preejaculate fluid that are released *before* ejaculation. Timing withdrawal is also difficult, and males who are concentrating on accurate timing might not be able to relax and enjoy intercourse. Withdrawal offers no protection against STIs and requires a high degree of self-control, experience, and trust.

Abstinence and "Outercourse"

Strictly defined, *abstinence* means avoiding oral, vaginal, and anal sex. This definition would allow one to engage in forms of sexual intimacy such as fondling, kissing, and masturbation. Couples who go beyond fondling and kissing to activities such as oral sex and mutual masturbation, but not vaginal or anal sex, are sometimes said to be engaging in "outercourse."

Abstinence is the only method of avoiding pregnancy that is 100 percent effective. It is also the only method that is 100 percent effective against transmitting and contracting STIs. Like abstinence, outercourse can be 100 percent effective for birth control as long as the male does not ejaculate near the vaginal opening. Unlike abstinence, however, outercourse is not 100 percent effective against STIs. Oral–genital contact can transmit disease, although the practice can be made safer by using a condom on the penis or a latex barrier, such as a **dental dam**, over the vulva. Both abstinence and outercourse require discipline and commitment for couples to sustain over long periods of time. Thirty-four percent of college students report having been abstinent for the past 12 months. Thirty-five percent report never having engaged in vaginal sex, 32 percent never in oral sex, and 76 percent never in anal sex.[35]

Fertility Awareness Methods

Fertility awareness methods (FAMs) of birth control, sometimes referred to as periodic abstinence, natural family planning, or the "rhythm" method, rely on altering sexual behavior during certain times of the month (**FIGURE 7.4**).

Fertility awareness methods are rooted in an understanding of basic physiology. A released ovum can survive about 36 hours after ovulation, and sperm can live for about 7 days in the reproductive tract. These techniques require observing female fertile periods and abstaining from sexual intercourse (or any penis–vagina contact) during the times when a sperm and egg could meet. Some of the more common forms are the following:

dental dam A square of latex that is used as a barrier between the mouth and a woman's genitals to protect from vaginal fluids.

fertility awareness methods (FAMs) Several types of birth control that require alteration of sexual behavior rather than chemical or physical intervention in the reproductive process.

- **Cervical mucus method.** This method requires the woman to examine the consistency and color of her normal vaginal secretions. Before ovulation, vaginal mucus becomes slippery, thin, and stretchy, and normal vaginal secretions may increase. To prevent pregnancy, partners must avoid sexual activity involving penis–vagina contact while this mucus is present and for several days afterward.
- **Body temperature method.** This method relies on the fact that a woman's basal (resting) body temperature rises between 0.4 and 0.8 degrees after ovulation has occurred. For this method to be effective, a woman must chart her temperature for several months to learn to recognize her body's temperature fluctuations. To prevent pregnancy, partners must abstain from penis–vagina contact before the temperature rise until several days after the temperature rise is observed.
- **Calendar method.** This method requires the woman to record the exact number of days in her menstrual cycle. Because few women menstruate with complete regularity, this method involves keeping a record of the menstrual cycle for 12 months, during which time some

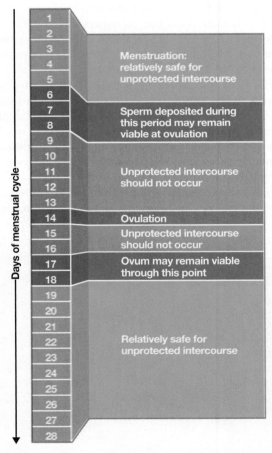

FIGURE 7.4 The Fertility Cycle Fertility awareness methods (FAMs) can combine the use of a calendar, the cervical mucus method, and body temperature measurements to identify the fertile period. It is important to remember that most women do not have a consistent 28-day cycle.

other method of birth control must be used. This method assumes that ovulation occurs during the midpoint of the cycle. To prevent pregnancy, the couple must abstain from penis–vagina contact during the fertile time.

Fertility awareness methods are the only forms of birth control that comply with certain religious teachings, including those of the Roman Catholic Church. The effectiveness of FAMs depends on diligence, commitment, and self-discipline; they have a 76 percent effectiveness rate with typical use.[36] Women who attempt to use these methods without proper training run a high risk of unintended pregnancy. Anyone interested in using them is advised to take a class, often offered for free by health centers and churches. These methods offer no STI protection, and they may not work for women with irregular menstrual cycles.

Emergency Contraception

Emergency contraception is the use of a contraceptive to prevent pregnancy after unprotected intercourse, a sexual assault, or the failure of another birth control method. Combination estrogen-progestin pills and progestin-only pills are two common types of **emergency contraceptive pills (ECPs)**, sometimes referred to as "morning-after pills." ECPs contain the same type of hormones as regular birth control pills and are used after unprotected intercourse but before a woman misses her period. A woman takes ECPs to prevent pregnancy; the method will not work if she is already pregnant, nor will it harm an existing pregnancy.

Multiple types of ECPs are available in the United States with no prescription. They must be taken within 72 hours (3 days) of intercourse. The FDA has more recently approved *ella*, which is available only by prescription and can prevent pregnancy when taken up to 120 hours (5 days) after unprotected intercourse. ECPs use the same hormones that other hormonal contraceptives do and prevent pregnancy in the same way: by delaying or inhibiting ovulation, inhibiting fertilization, or blocking implantation of a fertilized egg, depending on the phase of the woman's menstrual cycle. When taken within 24 hours, ECPs reduce the risk of pregnancy by up to 95 percent; when taken 2 to 5 days later, ECPs reduce the risk of pregnancy by 88 percent.[37]

Today, anyone of any age can purchase ECPs, and they are kept on the regular store shelves, usually near other family planning supplies. According to a recent national survey, about 1 in 11 sexually active college students reported using (or their partner using) emergency contraception within the past year.[38] Although ECPs are no substitute for taking proper precautions before having sex (such as using a condom), widespread availability of emergency contraception has the potential to significantly reduce the rates of unintended pregnancies and abortions, particularly among young women.

Permanent Methods of Birth Control

In the United States, **sterilization** has become the second leading method of contraception for women of all ages and the leading method of contraception among women over age 35.[39] Because sterilization is permanent, anyone considering it should think through possibilities such as divorce and remarriage or a future improvement in financial status that might make pregnancy realistic or desirable.

Female Sterilization One method of sterilization for women is **tubal ligation**, a surgical procedure in which the fallopian tubes are cut or tied shut to block the sperm's access to released eggs (see **FIGURE 7.5**). The operation is usually done laparoscopically (via a half-inch incision in the abdomen) on an outpatient basis. The procedure usually takes less than an hour and is performed under local or general anesthesia; the patient is usually allowed to return home within a short time after the procedure. A tubal ligation does not affect ovarian and uterine function. The woman's menstrual cycle continues; released eggs simply disintegrate and are absorbed by the lymphatic system.

A newer sterilization procedure, *Essure*, involves the placement of small microcoils into the fallopian tubes via the vagina. The entire procedure takes about 35 minutes and can be performed in a physician's office, usually under local anesthetic, not general anesthesia. Once in place, the metallic microcoils expand to the shape of the fallopian tubes. The coils promote the growth of scar tissue around the coils and lead to a blockage in the fallopian tubes. Like traditional forms of tubal ligation, Essure is permanent. It is recommended for women who cannot have tubal ligation because of chronic health conditions such as obesity or heart disease. However, Essure has been under review by the FDA because of concerns about its safety and effectiveness, so if a woman is interested in this method, it is important to be informed of potential risks.[40]

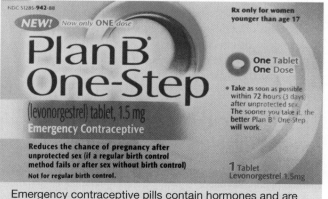

Emergency contraceptive pills contain hormones and are used after an act of unprotected intercourse. When taken within 24 hours of unprotected intercourse, ECPs reduce the risk of pregnancy by up to 95 percent.

emergency contraceptive pills (ECPs) Drugs taken within 3 to 5 days after unprotected intercourse to prevent pregnancy.

sterilization Permanent fertility control achieved through surgical procedures.

tubal ligation Sterilization of a woman that involves cutting and tying off or cauterizing the fallopian tubes.

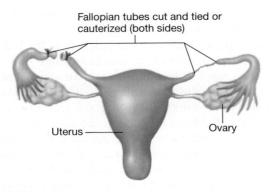

FIGURE 7.5 Female Sterilization: Tubal Ligation In a tubal ligation, both fallopian tubes are cut and tied or sealed shut.

A **hysterectomy**, or removal of the uterus, is a method of sterilization requiring major surgery. It is usually done only when a woman's uterus is diseased or damaged, not as a primary means of female sterilization.

The main advantage to female sterilization is that it is highly effective (less than a 1 percent failure rate) and permanent.[41] After the one-time expense of the procedure, no other cost or ongoing action is required. Sterilization has no negative effect on a woman's sex drive. These methods require no use of hormones, are discreet, and require no ongoing purchase of supplies or remembering to use them, thus allowing sex with full spontaneity.

As with any surgery, there are risks involved with a tubal ligation. Although rare, possible complications include infection, pulmonary embolism, hemorrhage, anesthesia complications, and ectopic pregnancy. Of course, sterilization offers no protection against STIs and is not effective immediately. A backup method of birth control is needed for 3 months. While the permanent nature of this method is considered an advantage, the woman and her partner (if she is in a long-term relationship) need to seriously consider whether they may want children later; reversal is possible in some instances, but the procedure should be considered permanent.

Male Sterilization Sterilization in men is less complicated than it is in women. A **vasectomy** is frequently done on an outpatient basis, using a local anesthetic (see **FIGURE 7.6**). This procedure involves making a small incision in the side of the scrotum to expose a vas deferens, cutting the vas deferens and either tying off or cauterizing the ends, then repeating the procedure on the other side.

Many men are reluctant to consider sterilization because they fear that the operation will affect their sexual performance or sex drive. However, a vasectomy in no way affects sexual response. The testes continue to produce sperm, but the sperm can no longer enter the ejaculatory duct via the vas deferens. Any sperm that are manufactured disintegrate and are absorbed into the lymphatic system. Because sperm constitute

hysterectomy Surgical removal of the uterus.

vasectomy A male sterilization procedure that involves cutting and tying off the vasa deferentia.

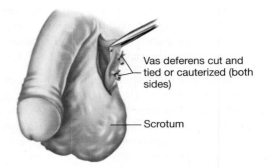

FIGURE 7.6 Male Sterilization: Vasectomy In a vasectomy, the surgeon makes an incision in the scrotum, then locates and cuts the vasa deferentia, either sealing or tying both sides shut.

only a small part of the semen (about 2 percent), the amount and consistency of ejaculate are not noticeably changed.

A vasectomy is a highly effective and permanent means of preventing pregnancy; typical effectiveness rates are more than 99 percent.[42] A vasectomy is a fairly simple outpatient procedure requiring minimal recovery time, and after the one-time expense, no other cost or ongoing action is required. It is discreet, uses no hormones, allows for spontaneity, and is one of the few methods that allow men to be in charge of fertility. Of course, men don't necessarily have to make permanent body alterations to be more involved with birth control choices. See Student Health Today for more information.

Male sterilization offers no protection against STI transmission. Also, a vasectomy is not immediately effective in preventing pregnancy. Because sperm are stored in other areas of the reproductive system besides the vasa deferentia, couples must use alternative birth control methods for at least 1 month after the vasectomy. A physician will do a semen analysis to determine when unprotected intercourse can take place. As with any surgery, there are some risks involved with a vasectomy. In a small percentage of cases, serious complications occur, such as formation of a blood clot in the scrotum, infection, or inflammatory reactions. Very infrequently, the vasa deferentia may create a new path, canceling out the procedure. A vasectomy is initially expensive if not covered by the man's insurance plan. While the permanent nature of this method is considered an advantage, the man and his partner (if he is in a long-term relationship) need to seriously consider whether they may want children later if their circumstances change. While vasectomies can be reversed in some instances, the procedure is costly and not guaranteed to work.

LO 3 | CHOOSING A METHOD OF CONTRACEPTION

List and explain factors that you should consider when choosing a method of contraception.

With all the options available, how does a person or a couple decide what method of contraception is best? Take some time to research the various methods, ask questions of your

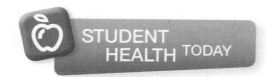

HOW CAN MEN BE MORE INVOLVED IN BIRTH CONTROL?

The sexual health needs of young men have been largely overlooked in the field of reproductive health. Most of the research and outreach related to preventing unintended pregnancy is focused on women, leading to missed opportunities to emphasize the importance of shared responsibility for reproductive health.

There are many reasons for the disparity: Men seek health care less often; it is sometimes incorrectly assumed that men are not interested in reproductive health issues; and because women carry the baby, they are often seen as having a bigger stake in pregnancy prevention. Male contraceptive methods are also more medically challenging, as they need to suppress millions of sperm per ejaculation, only one of which is needed for fertilization—in contrast to one egg per month in women.

However, healthy sexual relationships and ongoing good reproductive health require that both partners be stakeholders. So how can men be more involved in responsible sexual decision making?

- Initiate discussions with your partner about contraception and your sexual health histories.
- Take an active role in discussing and deciding what type of contraception is best for you and your partner.
- Buy and use condoms every time you have sex.
- Help pay for contraceptive costs.
- If an unintended pregnancy occurs, share in the responsibility and decision making about the best way to handle the situation.

---

health care provider, and be honest with yourself about your own preferences. **TABLE 7.2** lists the most popular forms of contraception among sexually active college students. Questions to ask yourself and discuss with your partner include the following:

- **How comfortable would I be using this particular method?** If you aren't at ease with a method, you might not use it consistently, and it probably will not be a reliable choice for you. Consider your own comfort level with touching your body or whether the method may cause discomfort for you or your partner.
- **Will this method be convenient for me and my partner?** Some methods require more effort than others. Be honest with yourself about how likely you are to use the method consistently. Are you willing to interrupt lovemaking, to abstain from sex during certain times of the month, or to take a pill at the same time every day?
- **Am I at risk for the transmission of STIs?** If you have multiple sex partners or are uncertain about the sexual history or disease status of your current sex partner, then you are at risk of contracting HIV or other STIs. Besides abstinence, condoms (male and female) are the only contraceptive methods that provide some protection against STIs and HIV.
- **Do I want to have a biological child in the future?** If you are unsure about your plans for future childbearing, you should use a temporary birth control method rather than a permanent one such as sterilization. If you know you want to have children in the future, consider how soon that will be, since some methods, such as Depo-Provera, will cause a delay in return to fertility.
- **How would an unplanned pregnancy affect my life?** If an unplanned pregnancy would be a potentially devastating event for you or would have a serious impact on your plans for the future, then you should choose a highly

effective birth control method. However, if, you are in a stable relationship, have a reliable source of income, are planning to have children in the future, and would embrace a pregnancy if it occurred now, then you may be comfortable with a less reliable method.

- **What are my religious and moral values?** If your beliefs prevent you from considering other birth control methods,

TABLE **7.2** | Contraception Methods Used by College Students or Their Partners the Last Time They Had Sex

Method	Male	Female	Total
Male condom	69%	61%	64%
Birth control pills (monthly or extended cycle)	62%	58%	59%
Withdrawal	29%	39%	32%
Intrauterine device	8%	9%	9%
Nexplanon/implant	7%	6%	7%
Depo-Provera/shots	5%	4%	4%
Spermicide (foam, jelly, cream)	5%	3%	3%
Sterilization	2%	2%	2%
Xulane/patch	2%	1%	1%
Female condom	1%	0%	1%
Diaphragm/cervical cap	0%	0%	0.3%
Sponge	0%	0%	0.2%

Note: Survey respondents could select more than one method.

Source: Data from American College Health Association, *American College Health Association—National College Health Assessment II: Reference Group Data, Spring 2016* (Hanover, MD: American College Health Association, 2016).

FAMs are a good option. When both partners are motivated to use these methods, they can be successful at preventing unintended pregnancy. If you are considering this option, sign up for a class to get specific training for using the method effectively.

■ **How much will the birth control method cost?** Some contraceptive methods involve an initial outlay of money and few continuing costs (e.g., sterilization, IUD), whereas others are fairly inexpensive but must be purchased repeatedly (e.g., condoms, spermicides, monthly pills). You should consider whether a method will be cost-effective for you in the long run. Remember that prescription methods require routine checkups, which may involve some cost to you, depending on your health insurance coverage. Because health insurance coverage varies, consider your local family planning clinic or campus health center for affordable care.

■ **Do I have any health factors that could limit my choice?** Hormonal birth control methods can pose potential health risks to women with certain preexisting conditions, such as high blood pressure, a history of stroke or blood clots, liver disease, migraines, or diabetes. In addition, women who smoke or are over age 35 are at risk for complications of combination hormonal contraceptives. Breastfeeding women can use progestin-only methods but should avoid methods containing estrogen. Men and women with latex allergies can use barrier methods made of polyurethane, polyisoprene, silicone, or other materials rather than latex condoms.

■ **Are there any additional benefits I would like from my contraceptive?** Hormonal birth control methods may have desirable secondary effects, such as the reduction of acne or the lessening of premenstrual symptoms. Some hormonal birth control methods have been associated with reduced risks of certain cancers. Extended-cycle pills and some progestin-only methods cause menstrual periods to be less frequent or to stop altogether, which some women find desirable. Condoms have the added health benefit of protecting against STIs.

LO 4 | ABORTION

Summarize the political issues surrounding abortion and the various types of abortion procedures.

An **abortion** is the termination of a pregnancy by expulsion or removal of an embryo or fetus from the uterus. The vast majority of abortions occur because of unintended pregnancies, as even the best birth control methods can fail.[43] In addition, some pregnancies are terminated because they are a consequence of rape or incest or because of health risks to the mother. Other commonly cited reasons include not being ready financially or emotionally to care for a child.[44] When an unintended pregnancy does occur, a woman must decide whether to terminate the pregnancy, carry to

abortion Termination of a pregnancy by expulsion or removal of an embryo or fetus from the uterus.

term and keep the baby, or carry to term and give the baby up for adoption. This is a personal decision that each woman must make on the basis of her personal beliefs, values, and resources and after carefully considering all alternatives.

In 1973, the landmark U.S. Supreme Court decision in *Roe v. Wade* stated that the "right to privacy . . . founded on the Fourteenth Amendment's concept of personal liberty . . . is broad enough to encompass a woman's decision whether or not to terminate her pregnancy."[45] The decision maintained that during the first trimester of pregnancy, a woman and her health care provider have the right to terminate the pregnancy through abortion without legal restrictions. It allowed individual states to set conditions for second-trimester abortions. Third-trimester abortions were ruled illegal unless the mother's life or health was in danger. Before this decision legalized abortions, women who wanted to terminate a pregnancy had to travel to a country where the procedure was legal, consult an illegal abortionist, or perform their own abortions. These procedures sometimes led to infertility from internal scarring or death from hemorrhage or infection.

The Abortion Debate

Abortion is a highly charged and politically thorny issue in American society. In a recent national poll, 47 percent of Americans described themselves as pro-choice, while 46 percent described themselves as pro-life.[46] Pro-choice individuals believe that it is a woman's right to make decisions about her own body and health, including the decision to continue or terminate a pregnancy. On the other side of the issue, pro-life individuals believe that the embryo or fetus is a human being with rights that must be protected.

In the more than 40 years since *Roe v. Wade* legalized abortion nationwide, hundreds of laws have been passed at the state and federal level to narrow or expand its limits. In 2016 alone, more than 60 new abortion-related laws were passed in the United States, most of which focused on regulation of abortion providers or facilities or limitations on the provision of abortions.[47] These types of laws make abortions more difficult and costly to provide, consequently reducing the number of clinics and providers willing and able to provide abortion services. Thus, although abortion remains legal in all 50 states, its availability is severely limited for many women as a result of difficulty accessing abortion services. Abortion services are especially constrained for low-income women who are less able to travel long distances to a clinic, visit a clinic multiple times, or pay out of pocket for an abortion.

Emotional Aspects of Abortion

The best scientific evidence available indicates that among adult women who have an unplanned pregnancy, the risk of mental health problems is no greater if they have an abortion than if they deliver a baby. Although a variety of feelings such as regret, guilt, sadness, relief, and happiness are normal, evidence does not show that having an abortion causes an increase in anxiety, depression, or suicidal ideation.[48] Researchers have

21%

of Americans will only vote for a **POLITICAL CANDIDATE** with their same views on abortion.

found that the best predictor of a woman's emotional well-being after an abortion was her emotional well-being before the procedure.[49] The factors that place a woman at higher risk for negative psychological responses after an abortion include perception of stigma, need for secrecy, low levels of social support for the abortion decision, prior history of mental health issues, low self-esteem, and avoidance and denial coping strategies.[50]

Methods of Abortion

The choice of abortion procedure is determined by how many weeks the woman has been pregnant. Length of pregnancy is calculated from the first day of her last menstrual period.

Surgical Abortions The majority of abortions performed in the United States today are surgical. If performed during the first trimester, abortion presents a relatively low health risk to the mother. About 89 percent of abortions occur during the first 12 weeks of pregnancy (see **FIGURE 7.7**).[51] The most commonly used method of first-trimester abortion is **suction curettage**, also called vacuum aspiration or dilation and curettage (D&C), which is usually performed under local anesthesia (**FIGURE 7.8**). The cervix is dilated with instruments or by placing laminaria, a sterile seaweed product, in the cervical canal. The laminaria is left in place for a few hours or overnight and slowly dilates the cervix. After the laminaria is removed, a long tube is inserted through the cervix and into the uterus,

and gentle suction removes fetal tissue from the uterine walls.

Pregnancies that progress into the second trimester (after week 12) are usually terminated through **dilation and evacuation (D&E)**. For this procedure, the cervix is dilated for 1 to 2 days, and a combination of instruments and vacuum aspiration is used to scrape and suck fetal tissue from the uterus. The D&E can be performed on an outpatient basis (usually in a physician's office), usually under general anesthesia. This procedure may cause moderate to severe uterine cramping and blood loss. After a D&E, a follow-up visit to the clinic is necessary and important.

Abortions during the third trimester are very rare (fewer than 2 percent of abortions in the United States).[52] When they are performed, a D&E is the most commonly used procedure. The much debated, **intact dilation and extraction (D&X)**, often referred to as "partial birth abortion," is illegal in the United States. However, several states do not enforce the law and allow the procedure when the mother's life or health is at risk.[53]

The risks associated with surgical abortion include infection, incomplete abortion (when parts of the placenta remain in the uterus), excessive bleeding, and cervical and uterine trauma. Follow-up and attention to danger signs decrease the chances of long-term problems.

The mortality rate for women undergoing first-trimester abortions in the United States averages 3 deaths for every 1 million

suction curettage An abortion technique that uses gentle suction to remove fetal tissue from the uterus; also called vacuum aspiration or dilation and curettage (D&C).

dilation and evacuation (D&E) An abortion technique that uses a combination of instruments and vacuum aspiration.

intact dilation and extraction (D&X) A late-term abortion procedure in which the body of the fetus is extracted up to the head and then the contents of the cranium are aspirated.

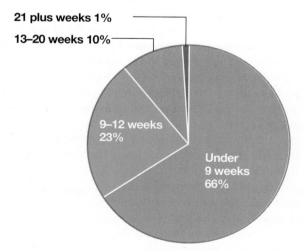

FIGURE 7.7 When Women Have Abortions (in weeks from the last menstrual period)

Source: T.C. Jatlaoi et al., "Abortion Surveillance—United States 2013," *Morbidity and Mortality Weekly Report* 65, no. SS12 (2016), 1–44.

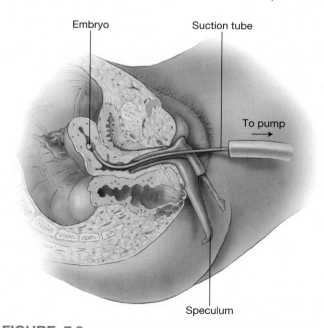

FIGURE 7.8 Suction Curettage Abortion This procedure, in which a long tube and gentle suction are used to remove fetal tissue from the uterine walls, can be performed until the twelfth week of pregnancy.

procedures at 8 or fewer weeks.[54] The risk of death increases with the length of pregnancy. At 18 weeks or later, the mortality rate is 7 per 100,000.[55] This higher rate later in the pregnancy is due to the increased risk of uterine perforation, bleeding, infection, and incomplete abortion; these complications occur because the uterine wall becomes thinner as the pregnancy progresses. As a point of comparison, for every 100,000 live births, nearly 24 women die of childbirth-related causes.[56]

Medical Abortions Unlike surgical abortions, a **medical abortion** (also called medication abortion) is performed without inserting an instrument into the uterus. Mifepristone, formerly known as RU-486 and currently sold in the United States under the brand name Mifeprex, is a steroid hormone that induces abortion by blocking the action of progesterone, the hormone produced by the ovaries and placenta that maintains the uterine lining. As a result, the lining and embryo are expelled from the uterus, terminating the pregnancy. Medical abortions must be performed early in the pregnancy, no later than 9 weeks after a woman's last menstrual period.

Mifepristone's nickname, "the abortion pill," may imply an easy process; however, this treatment actually involves more steps than a suction curettage abortion, which takes approximately 15 minutes followed by a physical recovery of about 1 day. With mifepristone, an initial visit to the clinic involves a physical examination and a dose of mifepristone and antibiotics, which may cause minor side effects such as nausea, headaches, weakness, and fatigue. The patient returns 2 to 3 days later for a dose of prostaglandins (misoprostol), which causes uterine contractions that expel the fertilized egg. The patient is required to stay under observation at the clinic for 4 hours and to make a follow-up visit within 2 weeks.[57]

More than 99 percent of women who use mifepristone early in pregnancy will experience a complete abortion.[58] The side effects are similar to those reported during heavy menstruation and include cramping, minor pain, and nausea. Fewer than 1 percent of women have more serious outcomes requiring a blood transfusion because of severe bleeding or the administration of intravenous antibiotics.[59]

LO 5 | PREGNANCY

Discuss key issues to consider in planning a pregnancy, describe the process of pregnancy and fetal development, and explain the importance of prenatal care.

Pregnancy is an important event in a woman's life and the life of her partner. The actions taken before pregnancy as well as behaviors engaged in during pregnancy can significantly affect the health of both infant and mother.

Planning for Pregnancy and Parenthood

Today, sexually active people are able to choose whether and when they want to have children. As you approach the decision of whether or not to have children or when to do so, take the time to evaluate your emotions, finances, and physical health. If you decide not to have children, you will be part of a growing number of Americans remaining childless. See the **Health in a Diverse World** box for more information.

Emotional Health First and foremost, consider why you may want to have a child. To fulfill an inner need to carry on the family? To share love? To give your parents grandchildren? To have a close tie or friendship? Then consider the responsibilities involved with becoming a parent. Are you ready to make all the sacrifices necessary to bear and raise a child? Can you care for this new human being in a loving and nurturing manner? Do you have a strong social support system? This emotional preparation for parenthood can be as important as the physical preparation.

Financial Evaluation Finances are another important consideration. Can you afford to give your child the life you would like him or her to enjoy? The U.S. Department of Agriculture estimates that it will cost an average of $233,610 to raise a child born today to age 18, not including college tuition.[60]

It is important to check whether your medical insurance provides maternity benefits. If not, you can expect to pay, on average, $8,775 for a normal delivery and $11,525 for a cesarean section, not including prenatal care.[61] Both partners should investigate their employers' policies on parental leave, including length of leave available and conditions for returning to work.

Maternal Age The average age at which a woman has her first child has been creeping up (from 21 in 1970 to almost 26 today), so a woman who becomes pregnant in her 30s has plenty of company.[62] In fact, births to women in their 20s are declining, while the rate of first births to women between the ages of 30 and 39 is the highest reported in four decades. Births to women over age 39 have continued to increase slightly over the years.[63]

Statistically, the chances of having a baby with birth defects rise after the age of 35. Researchers believe that this is due to a decline in the quality of eggs after this age. Two specific age-related risks are **Down syndrome** and miscarriage. The risk of miscarriage nearly doubles for women 35 to 45 compared to women under 35.[64] Another concern is that a woman's fertility begins to decline as she ages. A gradual decline in fertility begins around age 32 and fertility decreases

medical abortion Termination of a pregnancy during the first 9 weeks using hormonal medications that cause the embryo to be expelled from the uterus.

Down syndrome A genetic disorder caused by the presence of an extra chromosome that results in mental disabilities and distinctive physical characteristics.

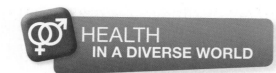

HEALTH IN A DIVERSE WORLD

CHILDLESS BY CHOICE

After carefully considering whether or not to have children, an increasing number of Americans are choosing to remain child-free. While, only around one in 10 women were childless (defined as no children by age 44) in the 1970s, today the number is closer to one in seven.

Certainly, not all people who are currently childless are so by choice. Estimates indicate that about 40 percent of people who are childless are voluntarily childless, about 30 percent want to conceive but haven't been successful, and 30 percent expect to have children in the future but have not yet. Those that are postponing parenthood until their late 30s and beyond report they are waiting for the right partner, financial stability, or the desire to have children to "kick in."

Who is choosing to remain child-free? More research on the topic is being done in European countries than the United States. There, people who value their freedom and independence highly, have negative or ambivalent feelings toward children, grew up in large cities, have well-educated parents, have no siblings, or have poor opinions of their own parents are more likely to choose childlessness. Being highly educated is related to childlessness for women but not for men.

The decision to be childless is not always easy. There can be pressure from family, friends, and even partners to have a child. People sometimes even question their own decision, concerned that at some point in the future, they might regret not having children.

Hollywood star Cameron Diaz, herself childless by choice, summed it up well: "It's so much more work to have children. To have lives besides your own that you are responsible for . . . . Not having a baby might really make things easier, but that doesn't make it an easy decision."

Sources: G. Livingston, "Childlessness Falls, Family Size Grows among Highly Educated Women," Pew Research Center, May 7, 2015, http://www.pewsocialtrends.org/2015/05/07/childlessness-falls-family-size-grows-among-highly-educated-women; A. Furnham, "Choosing to be Child-free," *Psychology Today*, April 21, 2015, https://www.psychologytoday.com/blog/sideways-view/201504/choosing-be-child-free; S. Kanazawa, "Intelligence and Childlessness," *Social Science Research* 48 (2014): 157–70; K. Schlosser, "Cameron Diaz's Naked Truth: No Kids Makes Things Much Easier," *Today: Pop Culture*, July 1, 2014, http://www.today.com/popculture/cameron-diazs-naked-truth-no-kids-makes-things-easier-1D79872076.

---

more rapidly after age 37 because of the reduction in the number and quality of eggs in the ovaries.[65] While some risks increase with age, many doctors note that older mothers bring some advantages to their pregnancies: They tend to follow medical advice during pregnancy more thoroughly and are more mature psychologically, better prepared financially, and generally more ready to care for an infant than are some younger women.

Physical Health: Maternal Health

The birth of a healthy baby depends in part on the mother's **preconception care** (the medical care she receives before becoming pregnant). The fetus is most susceptible to developing certain problems in the first 4 to 10 weeks after conception, before prenatal care is normally initiated. Because many women don't realize that they are pregnant until later, they often can't reduce health risks unless intervention begins before conception.[66] Maternal factors that can affect a fetus or infant include drug use (illicit, prescription, or over-the-counter), alcohol consumption, tobacco use, or obesity. To promote good preconception health, a woman should get the best medical care she can, practice healthy behaviors, build a strong support network, and encourage safe environments at home and at work.[67]

Nutrition counseling is an important part of preconception care. Among the many important nutrition issues is intake of folic acid (folate). When consumed the month before conception and during early pregnancy, folate reduces the risk of spina bifida, a congenital birth defect resulting from failure of the spinal column to close. A woman also needs to make sure her immunizations are up to date before

she becomes pregnant. For example, if she has never had rubella (German measles), a woman needs to be immunized before becoming pregnant. A rubella infection can cause miscarriage or intellectual, visual, or hearing impairments in the infant.

Physical Health: Paternal Health

Fathers-to-be are encouraged to practice the same healthy habits as mothers-to-be because, by one route or another, dozens of chemicals studied so far (from occupational exposures to by-products of cigarette smoke to hormones) appear to harm sperm.[68] A fathers' age may also play a role; research shows a relationship between older fathers and autism, ADHD, bipolar disorder, and schizophrenia.[69]

The Process of Pregnancy

The process of pregnancy begins the moment a sperm fertilizes an ovum in the fallopian tubes. From there, the single fertilized cell, now called a *zygote*, multiplies and becomes a sphere-shaped cluster of cells called a *blastocyst* that travels toward the uterus, a journey that may take 3 to 4 days. On arrival, the embryo burrows into the thick, spongy endometrium (implantation) and is nourished from this carefully prepared lining.

Pregnancy Testing

A positive test is based on the secretion of **human chorionic**

> **preconception care** Medical care received before becoming pregnant that helps a woman assess and address potential health issues.
>
> **human chorionic gonadotropin (HCG)** A hormone that is detectable in blood or urine samples of a mother within the first few weeks of pregnancy.

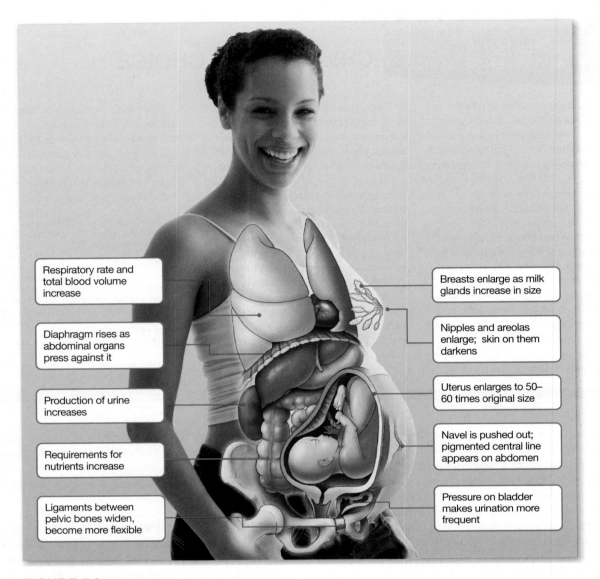

FIGURE 7.9 Changes in a Woman's Body during Pregnancy

Respiratory rate and total blood volume increase

Diaphragm rises as abdominal organs press against it

Production of urine increases

Requirements for nutrients increase

Ligaments between pelvic bones widen, become more flexible

Breasts enlarge as milk glands increase in size

Nipples and areolas enlarge; skin on them darkens

Uterus enlarges to 50–60 times original size

Navel is pushed out; pigmented central line appears on abdomen

Pressure on bladder makes urination more frequent

gonadotropin (HCG), which is found in the woman's urine or blood. Some home pregnancy test kits, sold over the counter in drugstores, can be used as early as a week after conception and many are 99 percent reliable.[70] If the test is done too early in the pregnancy, it may show a false negative. Other causes of false negatives are unclean testing devices, ingestion of certain drugs, and vaginal or urinary tract infections. A blood test administered and analyzed by the health care provider at the woman's first prenatal appointment will officially confirm a pregnancy.

Early Signs of Pregnancy

A woman's body undergoes substantial changes during a pregnancy (**FIGURE 7.9**). The first sign of pregnancy is usually a missed menstrual period (although some women "spot"

in early pregnancy, which may be mistaken for a period). Other signs include breast tenderness, emotional upset, extreme fatigue, sleeplessness, nausea, and vomiting (especially in the morning).

Pregnancy typically lasts 40 weeks and is divided into three phases, or **trimesters**, of approximately 3 months each. The due date is calculated from the expectant mother's last menstrual period.

The First Trimester

During the first trimester, few noticeable changes occur in the mother's body. She may urinate more frequently and experience morning sickness, swollen breasts, or undue fatigue. These symptoms may not be frequent or severe, so women often do not realize they are pregnant right away. During the first 8 weeks after conception, the **embryo** differentiates and develops its various organ systems, beginning with the nervous and circulatory systems. At the start of the third month, the embryo is called a **fetus**,

trimester A 3-month phase of pregnancy.

embryo The fertilized egg from conception through the eighth week of development.

fetus The developing human from the ninth week until birth.

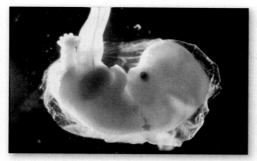

(a) A human embryo during the first trimester. The embryonic period lasts from the third to the eighth week of development. By the end of the embryonic period, all organs have formed.

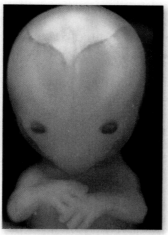

(b) A human fetus during the second trimester. Growth during the fetal period is very rapid.

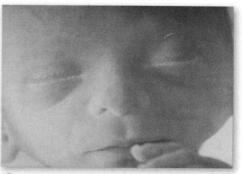

(c) A human fetus during the third trimester. By the end of the fetal period, the growth rate of the head has slowed relative to the growth rate of the rest of the body.

FIGURE 7.10 Fetoscopic Photographs Showing Development in the First, Second, and Third Trimesters of Pregnancy

indicating that all organ systems are in place. For the rest of the pregnancy, growth and refinement occur in each body system so that at birth they can function independently yet in coordination with each other. The photos in **FIGURE 7.10** illustrate physical changes during fetal development.

The Second Trimester At the beginning of the second trimester, the fourth through sixth months of pregnancy, physical changes in the mother become more visible. Her breasts swell and her waistline thickens. During this time, the fetus makes greater demands on the mother's body. In particular, the **placenta**, the network of blood vessels that carries nutrients and oxygen to the fetus and fetal waste products to the mother, becomes well established.

The Third Trimester The end of the sixth month through the ninth month comprise the third trimester. This is the period of greatest fetal growth. The growing fetus depends entirely on the mother for nutrition and must receive large amounts of calcium, iron, and protein from the mother's diet. Although the fetus may survive if born during the seventh month, it needs the layer of fat it acquires during the eighth month and time for the organs (especially the respiratory and digestive organs) to develop fully. Infants who are born prematurely usually require intensive medical care.

A doctor-approved exercise program during pregnancy can help to control weight, make delivery easier, and have a healthy effect on the fetus.

Prenatal Care

A successful pregnancy depends on a mother who takes good care of herself and her fetus. Good nutrition and exercise; avoiding drugs, alcohol, and other harmful substances; and regular medical checkups from the beginning of pregnancy are all essential. Early detection of fetal abnormalities, identification of high-risk mothers and infants, and screening for possible complications are the major purposes of prenatal care.

Ideally, a woman should begin prenatal appointments in the first trimester. On the first visit, the health care practitioner should obtain a complete medical history of the mother and her family and note any hereditary conditions that could put the woman or her fetus at risk. Regular checkups to measure weight gain and blood pressure and to monitor the fetus's size and position should continue throughout the pregnancy.

placenta A network of blood vessels connected to the umbilical cord that transports oxygen and nutrients to a developing fetus and carries away fetal wastes.

Nutrition and Exercise Despite "eating for two," pregnant women need only about 300 additional calories a day. Special attention should be paid to getting enough folic acid (found in dark leafy greens, citrus fruits, and beans), iron (dried fruits, meats, legumes, liver, egg yolks), calcium (nonfat or low-fat dairy products and some canned fish), and fluids.

While vitamin supplements can correct some deficiencies, there is no substitute for a well-balanced diet. Babies born to poorly nourished mothers run high risks of substandard mental and physical development.

Weight gain during pregnancy helps to nourish a growing baby. For a woman of normal weight before pregnancy, the recommended gain during pregnancy is 25 to 35 pounds.[71] For overweight women, weight gain of 15 to 25 pounds is recommended, and for obese women, 11 to 20 pounds is recommended.[72] Underweight women should gain 28 to 40 pounds, and women carrying twins should gain about 35 to 45 pounds.[73] Gaining too much or too little weight can lead to complications. With higher weight gains, women may develop gestational diabetes, hypertension, or increased risk of delivery complications. Gaining too little increases the chance of a low birth weight baby.

As in all other stages of life, exercise is an important factor in overall health during pregnancy. Regular exercise is recommended for pregnant women; however, they should consult with their health care provider before starting any exercise program. Exercise can help to control weight, make labor easier, and help with a faster recovery by contributing to increased strength and endurance. Women can usually maintain their customary level of activity during most of the pregnancy, although there are some cautions: Pregnant women should avoid exercise that puts them at risk of falling or having an abdominal injury, and exercise that involves lying on the back should be avoided in the third trimester, as it can restrict blood flow to the uterus.

Avoiding Drugs, Alcohol, Tobacco, and Other Teratogens

A woman should consult with a health care provider about the safety of any drugs she might use during pregnancy. Even too much of common over-the-counter medications such as aspirin can damage a developing fetus. During the first 3 months of pregnancy, the fetus is especially subject to the **teratogenic** (birth defect–causing) effects of drugs, environmental chemicals, X-rays, or diseases. The fetus can also develop an addiction to or tolerance for drugs that the mother is using.

Maternal consumption of alcohol is detrimental to a growing fetus. Birth defects associated with **fetal alcohol syndrome (FAS)** include developmental disabilities, neural and cardiac impairments, and cranial and facial deformities. The exact amount of alcohol that causes FAS is not known; therefore, the American Congress of Obstetricians and Gynecologists recommends completely avoiding alcohol during pregnancy.[74]

Women who smoke during pregnancy have a greater chance of miscarriage, complications, premature births, low birth weight infants, stillbirth, and infant mortality specifically due to sudden infant death syndrome.[75] Smoking restricts the blood supply to the developing fetus and thus limits oxygen and nutrition delivery and waste removal. Tobacco use also appears to be a significant factor in the development of cleft lip and palate.[76]

A pregnant woman should avoid exposure to X-rays, toxic chemicals, heavy metals, pesticides, gases, and other hazardous compounds. She should also avoid cleaning litter boxes, if possible, because cat feces can contain organisms that cause **toxoplasmosis**. If a pregnant woman contracts this disease, the baby may be stillborn or suffer intellectual disabilities or other birth defects.

Prenatal Testing and Screening

Modern technology enables medical practitioners to detect health defects in a fetus as early as the tenth week of pregnancy. One common test is **ultrasonography** or **ultrasound**, which uses high-frequency sound waves to create a *sonogram*, or visual image, of the fetus in the uterus. The sonogram is used to determine the fetus's size and position, which can help to safely deliver the infant. Sonograms can also detect birth defects in the nervous and digestive systems.

Chorionic villus sampling (CVS) involves snipping tissue from the developing fetal sac. Chorionic villus sampling can be used at 10 to 13 weeks of pregnancy. This is an attractive option for couples who are at high risk for having a baby with Down syndrome or a debilitating hereditary disease.

The **triple marker screen** (often called the TMS or AFT [alpha-fetoprotein] test) is a commonly used maternal blood test that is optimally conducted between the sixteenth and eighteenth weeks of pregnancy. The TMS is a screening test, not a diagnostic tool; it can detect susceptibility for a birth defect or genetic abnormality, but it is not meant to confirm a diagnosis of any condition. A *quad screen test* (or AFP-plus test), which screens for an additional protein in maternal blood, is more accurate than the triple marker screen.

Amniocentesis is a common testing procedure that is strongly recommended for women over age 35. This test involves inserting a long needle through the mother's abdominal and uterine walls into the **amniotic sac**, the protective pouch surrounding the fetus. The needle draws out 3 to 4 teaspoons of fluid, which is analyzed for genetic information about the baby. Amniocentesis can be performed between weeks 15 and 20.

If any of these tests reveals a serious birth defect, the parents are advised to undergo counseling. In the case of a chromosomal abnormality such as Down syndrome, the parents are usually offered the option of a therapeutic abortion. Some parents choose this option; others research the condition and decide to continue the pregnancy.

teratogenic Causing birth defects; may refer to drugs, environmental chemicals, radiation, or diseases.

fetal alcohol syndrome (FAS) A pattern of birth defects, developmental disabilities, and behavioral problems in a child caused by the mother's alcohol consumption during pregnancy.

toxoplasmosis A disease caused by an organism found in cat feces that, when contracted by a pregnant woman, may result in stillbirth or birth defects.

ultrasonography (ultrasound) A common prenatal test that uses sound waves to create a visual image of a developing fetus.

chorionic villus sampling (CVS) A prenatal test that involves snipping tissue from the fetal sac to be analyzed for genetic defects.

triple marker screen (TMS) A common maternal blood test that can be used to identify certain birth defects and genetic abnormalities in a fetus.

amniocentesis A medical test in which a small amount of fluid is drawn from the amniotic sac to test for Down syndrome and other genetic abnormalities.

amniotic sac The protective pouch surrounding the fetus.

LO 6 | CHILDBIRTH

Explain the basic stages of childbirth and complications that can arise during pregnancy, childbirth, and the postpartum.

Prospective parents need to make several key decisions before the baby is born. These include where to have the baby, whether to use pain medication during labor and delivery, which childbirth method to choose, and whether to breast-feed or use formula. Answering these questions in advance will help to smooth the passage into parenthood.

Labor and Delivery

During the final weeks before delivery, the baby normally shifts to a head-down position, and the cervix begins to dilate (widen). The junction of the pubic bones loosens to permit expansion of the pelvic girdle during birth. The exact mechanisms that initiate labor are unknown. A change in the hormones in the fetus and mother cause strong uterine contractions to occur, signaling the beginning of labor. Another early signal can be the breaking of the amniotic sac, which causes a rush of fluid from the vagina (commonly referred to as "water breaking"), but this happens in only 10 to 15 percent of pregnancies.

The birth process has three stages, shown in **FIGURE 7.11**, which can last from several hours to more than a day. In some cases, toward the end of the second stage, the attending health care provider may perform an *episiotomy*, a straight incision in the mother's perineum (the area between the vulva and the anus) to prevent the baby's head from tearing vaginal tissues and to speed the baby's exit from the vagina. After delivery, the attending provider assesses the baby's overall condition, clears the baby's mucus-filled breathing passages, and ties and severs the umbilical cord. The mother's uterus continues to contract in the third stage of labor until the placenta is expelled.

Managing Labor Pain medication given to the mother during labor can cause sluggish responses in the newborn and other complications. For this reason, some women choose a drug-free labor and delivery. However, it is important to keep a flexible attitude about pain relief, because each labor is different. One person is not a "success" for delivering without medication or another a "failure" for using medical measures.

The Lamaze method is the most popular technique of childbirth preparation in the United States. It discourages the use of pain medication. Prelabor classes teach the mother to control her pain through special breathing patterns, focusing exercises, and relaxation. The partner (or labor coach) assists by giving emotional support, physical comfort, and coaching for proper breath control during contractions.

Cesarean Section (C-Section) If labor lasts too long or if the baby is in physiological distress or is about to exit the uterus any way but headfirst, a **cesarean section (C-section)** may be necessary. This surgical procedure involves making an incision across the mother's abdomen and through the uterus to remove the baby. A C-section may also be performed

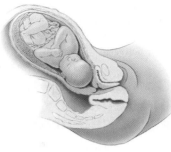
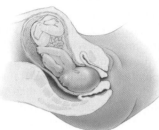
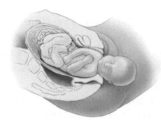
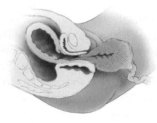
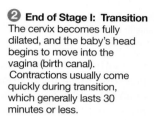

❶ **Stage I: Dilation of the cervix** Contractions in the abdomen and lower back push the baby downward, putting pressure on the cervix and dilating it. The first stage of labor may last from a couple of hours to more than a day for a first birth, but it is usually much shorter during subsequent births.

❷ **End of Stage I: Transition** The cervix becomes fully dilated, and the baby's head begins to move into the vagina (birth canal). Contractions usually come quickly during transition, which generally lasts 30 minutes or less.

❸ **Stage II: Expulsion** Once the cervix has become fully dilated, contractions become rhythmic, strong, and more intense as the uterus pushes the baby headfirst through the birth canal. The expulsion stage lasts 1 to 4 hours and concludes when the infant is finally pushed out of the mother's body.

❹ **Stage III: Delivery of the placenta** In the third stage, the placenta detaches from the uterus and is expelled through the birth canal. This stage is usually completed within 30 minutes after delivery.

FIGURE 7.11 The Birth Process The entire process of labor and delivery usually takes from 2 to 36 hours. Labor is generally longer for a woman's first delivery and shorter for subsequent births.

if labor is extremely difficult, maternal blood pressure falls rapidly, the placenta separates from the uterus too soon, the mother has diabetes, or other problems occur. Risks are the same as for any major abdominal surgery, and recovery from birth takes considerably longer after a C-section.

The rate of delivery by C-section in the United States has increased from 5 percent in the mid-1960s to nearly one-third of all births today.[77] Although this procedure is necessary in certain cases, some doctors and critics, including the Centers for Disease Control and Prevention, think that C-sections are performed too often in this country. Advocates of natural birth suggest that hospitals, driven by profits and worried about malpractice, are too quick to intervene in the birth process. Some

cesarean section (C-section) A surgical birthing procedure in which the baby is removed through an incision made in the mother's abdominal wall and uterus.

doctors say that the increase is due to maternal demand because busy mothers want to schedule their deliveries.[78]

Complications of Pregnancy and Childbirth

Pregnancy carries the risk for potential complications and problems that can interfere with the proper development of the fetus or threaten the health of the mother and child. Some complications may result from a preexisting health condition of the mother, such as diabetes or an STI, and others can develop during pregnancy and may result from physiological problems, genetic abnormalities, or exposure to teratogens.

Preeclampsia and Eclampsia

Preeclampsia is a condition characterized by high blood pressure, protein in the urine, and edema (fluid retention), which usually causes swelling of the hands and face. Symptoms may include sudden weight gain, headache, nausea or vomiting, changes in vision, racing pulse, mental confusion, and stomach or right shoulder pain. If preeclampsia is not treated, it can cause strokes and seizures, a condition called *eclampsia*. Potential problems can include liver and kidney damage, internal bleeding, poor fetal growth, and fetal and maternal death.

Preeclampsia tends to occur in the late second or third trimester. The cause is unknown; however, the incidence is higher in first-time mothers; women over 40 or under 18 years of age; women carrying multiple fetuses; and women with a history of chronic hypertension, diabetes, or kidney disorder or a previous history of preeclampsia.[79] A family history of preeclampsia is also a risk factor. Treatment for preeclampsia ranges from bed rest and monitoring for mild cases to hospitalization and close monitoring for more severe cases.

Miscarriage

Even when a woman does everything "right," not every pregnancy ends in delivery. In fact, in the United States, between 10 and 15 percent of known pregnancies end in **miscarriage** (also referred to as *spontaneous abortion*).[80] Most miscarriages occur during the first trimester.

Reasons for miscarriage vary. In some cases, the fertilized egg has failed to divide correctly. In others, genetic abnormalities, maternal illness, or infections are responsible. Maternal hormonal imbalance may also cause a miscarriage, as may a weak cervix, toxic chemicals in the environment, or physical trauma to the mother. In most cases, the cause is not known.

Ectopic Pregnancy

The implantation of a fertilized egg outside the uterus, usually in the fallopian tube or occasionally in the pelvic cavity, is called an **ectopic pregnancy**. Because these structures are not capable of expanding and nourishing a developing fetus, the pregnancy must be terminated surgically, or a miscarriage will occur. If an ectopic pregnancy progresses undiagnosed and untreated, the fallopian tube will rupture, which puts the woman at great risk of hemorrhage, peritonitis (infection in the abdomen), and even death. Ectopic pregnancy occurs in about 2 percent of pregnancies in North America and is a leading cause of maternal mortality in the first trimester.[81]

Stillbirth

Stillbirth is the death of a fetus after the twentieth week of pregnancy but before delivery. A stillborn baby is born dead, often for no apparent reason. Each year in the United States, there is about 1 stillbirth in every 160 births.[82] Birth defects, placental problems, poor fetal growth, infections, and umbilical cord accidents are known contributing factors.

The Postpartum Period

The postpartum period lasts 6 weeks after delivery. During this period, many women experience fluctuating emotions. Many new mothers experience what is called the "baby blues," characterized by periods of sadness, anxiety, headache, sleep disturbances, and irritability. About 1 in 7 new mothers experience

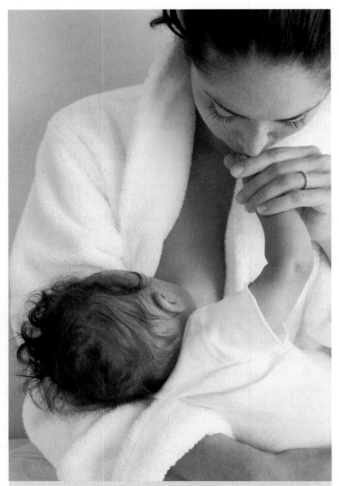

In addition to its numerous health benefits, breastfeeding enhances the development of intimate bonds between mother and child.

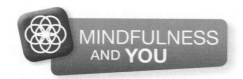
postpartum depression, a more disabling syndrome characterized by mood swings, lack of energy, crying, guilt, and depression any time within the first year after childbirth.[83] Women who experience postpartum depression should seek professional treatment. Counseling is the most common type of treatment, but sometimes medication is recommended.[84] See the **Mindfulness and You** box for discussion of depression during pregnancy.

Breastfeeding

Although the new mother's milk will not begin to flow for 2 or more days after delivery, her breasts secrete a yellow fluid called *colostrum* beginning immediately after birth. Because colostrum contains vital antibodies to help fight infection and boost the baby's immune system, all newborns should be allowed to suckle.

The American Academy of Pediatrics strongly recommends that infants be exclusively breast-fed for 6 months and breast-fed as a supplement until 12 months of age.[85] Scientific findings indicate there are many advantages to breastfeeding. Breast milk is perfectly matched to babies' nutritional needs as they grow. Breast-fed babies have fewer illnesses and much lower hospitalization rates because breast milk contains maternal antibodies and immunological cells that stimulate the infant's immune system. When breast-fed babies do get sick, they recover more quickly. They are also less likely to be obese later in life than are babies who are fed formula, and breast-fed babies tend to have fewer allergies. They may even be more intelligent: A recent study found that the longer a baby was breast-fed, the higher the IQ in adulthood.[86] Breastfeeding also has the added benefit of helping mothers lose weight after birth because the production of milk burns hundreds of calories a day. Breastfeeding also causes the hormone oxytocin to be released, which makes the uterus return to its normal size faster.

Breast milk is not the only way to nourish a baby. Some women are unable or unwilling to breast-feed; women who have certain medical conditions or who are taking certain medications are advised not to breast-feed. Prepared formulas can provide nourishment that allows a baby to grow and thrive. Both feeding methods can supply the physical and emotional closeness essential to the parent–child relationship.

Infant Mortality

After birth, infant death can be caused by birth defects, low birth weight, injuries, or unknown causes. In the United States, the unexpected death of a child under 1 year of age for no apparent reason is called **sudden infant death syndrome (SIDS)**. SIDS is responsible for about 1,500 deaths a year.[87] It is the leading cause of death for children age 1 month to 1 year and most commonly occurs in babies less than 6 months old.[88] It is not a specific disease; rather, it is ruled a cause of death after all other possibilities are ruled out. A SIDS death is sudden and silent; death occurs quickly, often during sleep, with no signs of suffering. The exact cause of SIDS is unknown, but a few risk factors are known. For example, babies who are placed to sleep on their stomachs are more likely to die from SIDS than those placed on their backs, as are babies who are placed on or covered by soft bedding. Breastfeeding and avoiding exposure to tobacco smoke are known protective factors.[89]

postpartum depression A mood disorder experienced by women who have given birth; involves depression, fatigue, and other symptoms and may last for weeks or months.

sudden infant death syndrome (SIDS) Sudden death of an infant under 1 year of age for no apparent reason.

LO 7 | INFERTILITY

Review primary causes of and possible solutions for infertility.

An estimated 1 in 10 American couples experiences **infertility**, usually defined as the inability to conceive after trying for a year or more.[90] Although the focus is often on women, in about one third of cases, infertility is due to a cause involving only the male partner, and in another third of cases, infertility is due to causes involving both partners or an unknown origin.[91] Because of this, it is important for both partners to be medically evaluated.

Causes in Women

The most common cause for female infertility is *polycystic ovary syndrome (PCOS)*. A woman's ovaries have follicles, which are tiny, fluid-filled sacs that hold the eggs. When an egg is mature, the follicle breaks open to release the egg so that it can travel to the fallopian tubes for fertilization. In women with PCOS, immature follicles bunch together to form large cysts or lumps. The eggs mature within the bunched follicles, but the follicles don't break open to release them. As a result, women with PCOS often don't have menstrual periods, or they have periods infrequently. Researchers estimate that 5 to 10 percent of women of childbearing age—as many as 5 million women in the United States—have PCOS.[92] Although obesity doesn't cause infertility, it is a risk factor for PCOS. It also increases the level of estrogen in the body and can cause ovulatory disorders, both of which interfere with getting pregnant.[93] In some women, the ovaries stop functioning before natural menopause, a condition called *premature ovarian failure*. Another cause of infertility is **endometriosis**. In this very painful disorder, parts of the lining of the uterus implant outside the uterus, blocking the fallopian tubes.

Pelvic inflammatory disease (PID) is a serious infection that scars the fallopian tubes and blocks sperm migration. Infection-causing bacteria (chlamydia or gonorrhea) can invade the fallopian tubes, causing normal tissue to turn into scar tissue. This scar tissue blocks or interrupts the normal movement of eggs into the uterus. About 1 in 10 women with PID becomes infertile, and if a woman has multiple episodes of PID, her chance of becoming infertile increases.[94]

Causes in Men

Among men, the single largest fertility problem is **low sperm count**.[95] Although only one viable sperm is needed for fertilization, research has shown that all the other sperm in the ejaculate aid in the fertilization process. There are normally at least 40 million sperm per milliliter of semen. When the count drops below 20 million, fertility declines.[96]

Low sperm count may be attributable to environmental factors (such as exposure of the scrotum to intense heat or cold, radiation, certain chemicals, or altitude), being overweight, or wearing excessively tight underwear or clothing. Other factors, such as the mumps virus, can damage the cells that make sperm. Varicocele (enlarged veins on a man's testicle) can heat the testicles and damage the sperm.[97]

Infertility Treatments

Medical procedures can identify the cause of infertility in about 90 percent of cases.[98] Once the cause has been determined and an appropriate treatment has been instituted, the chances of pregnancy range from 30 to 70 percent, depending on the reason for infertility.[99]

Fertility Drugs Fertility drugs stimulate ovulation in women who are not ovulating. Of women who use these drugs, 60 to 80 percent will begin to ovulate; of those who ovulate, about half will conceive.[100] Fertility drugs can have many side effects, including headaches, depression, fatigue, fluid retention, and abnormal uterine bleeding. Women using fertility drugs are also at increased risk of developing multiple ovarian cysts and liver damage. The drugs sometimes trigger the release of more than one egg. As many as 1 in 3 women treated with fertility drugs will become pregnant with more than one child.[101]

Alternative Insemination and Assisted Reproductive Technology Another treatment option is **alternative insemination** (also known as *artificial insemination*) of a woman with her partner's sperm. The couple may also choose insemination by an anonymous donor through a sperm bank. At a properly managed sperm bank, donated sperm are medically screened, classified according to the donor's physical characteristics (such as hair and eye color), and then frozen for future use.

There are many different assisted reproductive technologies (ART) available. The most common is **in vitro fertilization (IVF)**. During IVF, eggs and sperm are mixed in a laboratory dish to fertilize, and some of the fertilized eggs (zygotes) are then transferred to the woman's uterus. Another option is nonsurgical embryo transfer, in which a donor egg is fertilized by the man's sperm and then implanted in the woman's uterus. Infertile couples could also participate in an embryo adoption program. Fertility treatments such as IVF often produce excess fertilized eggs that couples may choose to donate for other infertile couples to adopt. In addition to helping infertile couples, ART can help young women who are not yet ready to have a baby but who are concerned

infertility The inability to conceive after trying for a year or more.

endometriosis A disorder in which endometrial tissue establishes itself outside the uterus.

pelvic inflammatory disease (PID) Inflammation of the female genital tract that may cause scarring or blockage of the fallopian tubes, resulting in infertility.

low sperm count A sperm count below 20 million sperm per milliliter of semen.

alternative insemination A fertilization procedure in which semen from a partner or donor is deposited into a woman's uterus via a thin tube.

in vitro fertilization (IVF) Fertilization of an egg in a nutrient medium and subsequent transfer back into the mother's body.

⏵ **SEE IT!** VIDEOS

Looking for a new breakthrough in infertility treatment? Watch **New Pill to Help Women Get Pregnant Soon to Be Available Over the Counter** in the Study Area of Mastering Health.

about future infertility. A woman can have her eggs frozen to be fertilized in the future when she is ready for a child.

There are many ethical and moral questions surrounding infertility treatments. Before deciding on a treatment, you must ask yourself important questions: Has infertility been confirmed? Have all alternatives and potential risks been considered? Have you examined your attitudes, values, and beliefs about conceiving a child in this manner? Finally, will you tell your child about the method of conception and, if so, how?

Surrogate Motherhood

Infertile couples who still cannot conceive after treatment may choose to live without children, or

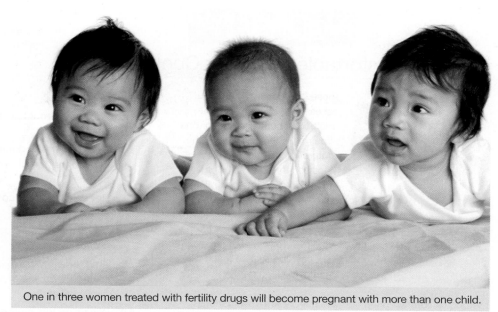

One in three women treated with fertility drugs will become pregnant with more than one child.

Source: American Society for Reproductive Medicine, "Fertility Drugs and the Risk for Multiple Births," Accessed March 2015, www.asrm.org/uploadedFiles/ASRM_Content/Resources/Patient_Resources/Fact_Sheets_and_Info_Booklets/fertilitydrugs_multiplebirths.pdf.

they may decide to pursue surrogate motherhood or adoption. With surrogacy, a woman is hired to carry another person's pregnancy to term, at which point the intended parents gain custody. In traditional surrogacy, the gestational carrier is also the biological mother of the child. In gestational surrogacy, the surrogate is not the biological mother; instead, an embryo is created via IVF using the couple's own (or donor) egg and sperm. In the United States, an estimated 750 children a year are born via surrogates.[102]

Adoption

Adoption provides a way for individuals and couples who may not be able or do not wish to have a biological child to form a legal parental relationship with a child who needs a home. Adoption benefits children whose birth parents are unable or unwilling to raise them and provides adults who are unable to conceive or carry a pregnancy to term a means to create a family. Approximately 2 percent of U.S. children are adopted.[103]

There are two types of adoption: *confidential* and *open*. In confidential adoption, the birth parents and the adoptive parents never know each other. Adoptive parents are given only basic information about the birth parents, such as medical information that they need to care for the child. In open adoption, birth parents and adoptive parents know some information about each other. There are different levels of openness, from information exchange to the birth parents being involved in the child's life. Both parties must agree to this plan, and open adoption is not available in every state.

Some couples choose to adopt children from other countries. Each year, U.S. families adopt more than 5,000 foreign-born children.[104] The cost of international adoption varies widely, but it can cost more than $20,000, including agency fees, dossier and immigration-processing fees, travel, and court costs.[105] In some cases, the adoptive parents must travel to the child's country at least once and remain there for a time that may vary from a few days to several weeks. Some families find it beneficial to serve as foster parents before deciding to adopt. Others choose to adopt older children from the foster system in the United States rather than waiting for an infant placed through international adoption.

ASSESS YOURSELF

LIVE IT! ASSESS YOURSELF
An interactive version of this assessment is available online in Mastering Health.

Are You Comfortable with Your Contraception?

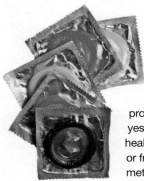

These questions will help you assess whether your current method of contraception or one you may consider using in the future will be effective for you. Answering yes to any of these questions predicts potential problems. If you have more than a few yes responses, consider talking to a health care provider, counselor, partner, or friend to decide whether to use this method or how to use it so that it will really be effective.

Method of contraception you use now or are considering:

	Yes	No
1. Have I or my partner ever become pregnant while using this method?	Y	N
2. Am I afraid of using this method?	Y	N
3. Would I really rather not use this method?	Y	N
4. Will I have trouble remembering to use this method?	Y	N
5. Will I have trouble using this method correctly?	Y	N
6. Does this method make menstrual periods longer or more painful for me or my partner?	Y	N
7. Does this method cost more than I can afford?	Y	N
8. Could this method cause serious complications?	Y	N
9. Am I, or is my partner, opposed to this method because of any religious or moral beliefs?	Y	N
10. Will using this method embarrass me or my partner?	Y	N
11. Will I enjoy intercourse less because of this method?	Y	N
12. Am I at risk of being exposed to HIV or other sexually transmitted infections if I use this method?	Y	N

Total number of yes answers: ___

Based on Robert Hatcher and Anita Nelson, *Contraceptive Technology*, 19th edition, New York: Ardent Media, 2009.

YOUR PLAN FOR CHANGE

The **ASSESS YOURSELF** activity gave you the chance to assess your comfort and confidence with a contraceptive method you are using now if you are sexually active or may use in the future. Depending on the results of the assessment, you might decide to consider changing your birth control method.

TODAY, YOU CAN:

☐ Visit your local drugstore, and study the forms of contraception that are available without a prescription. Think about those you would consider using and why.

☐ If you are not currently using any contraception or are not in a sexual relationship now but might be in the future, purchase a package of condoms (or pick up free samples from your campus health center) to keep on hand just in case.

WITHIN THE NEXT TWO WEEKS, YOU CAN:

☐ Make an appointment for a checkup with your health care provider. Be sure to ask him or her any questions you have about contraception.

☐ Sit down with your partner and discuss contraception. Talk about how your current method is working for both of you, whether the effectiveness level of the method you are using is high enough, and, if you aren't using birth control consistently, what you can do together to improve.

BY THE END OF THE SEMESTER, YOU CAN:

☐ Periodically reevaluate whether your new or continued contraception is still effective for you. Review your experiences, and take note of any consistent problems you may have encountered.

☐ Always keep a backup form of contraception on hand. Check this supply periodically, and throw out and replace any supplies that have expired.

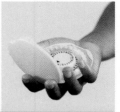

STUDY **PLAN**

Visit the Study Area in Mastering Health to enhance your study plan with MP3 Tutor Sessions, Practice Quizzes, Flashcards, and more!

CHAPTER **REVIEW**

LO **1** | Basic Principles of Contraception

- Contraception, commonly called birth control, prevents conception, the fertilization of an egg by sperm. Types of contraception include barrier, hormonal, intrauterine, behavioral, and permanent methods.

LO **2** | Contraceptive Methods

- Male and female condoms, when used correctly are most effective at preventing sexually transmitted infections (STIs). Other barrier methods include spermicides, the diaphragm, the cervical cap, and the contraceptive sponge.
- Hormonal contraceptives contain synthetic estrogen and/or progestin.
- Intrauterine devices are small devices that can be placed in the uterus and provide contraception for 3 to 12 years.
- Fertility awareness methods rely on altering sexual practices to avoid pregnancy, as do abstinence, outercourse, and withdrawal.
- Emergency contraception may be used up to 5 days after unprotected intercourse or the failure of another contraceptive method.
- While most methods of contraception are reversible, sterilization should be considered permanent.

LO **3** | Choosing a Method of Contraception

- Choosing a method of contraception involves researching the various options, asking questions of your health care provider, being honest with yourself, and having open conversations with potential partners.

LO **4** | Abortion

- Abortion is legal in the United States but strongly opposed by many Americans. Abortion methods include suction curettage, dilation and evacuation (D&E), and medical abortions.

LO **5** | Pregnancy

- Prospective parents must consider emotional health, maternal and paternal health, and financial resources. Full-term pregnancy has three trimesters. Prenatal care includes a complete physical examination within the first trimester, checkups throughout the pregnancy, healthy nutrition and exercise, and avoidance of all teratogenic substances. Prenatal tests, can be used to detect birth defects.

LO **6** | Childbirth

- Childbirth occurs in three stages. Partners should jointly choose a labor method early in the pregnancy to be better prepared when labor occurs. Possible complications of pregnancy and childbirth include preeclampsia and eclampsia, miscarriage, ectopic pregnancy, and stillbirth.

LO **7** | Infertility

- Infertility in women may be caused by polycystic ovary syndrome (PCOS), pelvic inflammatory disease (PID), or endometriosis. In men, infertility is most often caused by low sperm count. Treatments may include fertility drugs, alternative insemination, in vitro fertilization (IVF), assisted reproductive technology (ART), embryo transfer, and embryo adoption programs. Surrogate motherhood and adoption are also options.

POP **QUIZ**

LO **1** | Basic Principles of Contraception

1. What is meant by the *failure rate* of contraceptive use?
   a. The number of times a woman fails to get pregnant when she wanted to
   b. The number of times a woman gets pregnant when she did not want to
   c. The number of pregnancies that occur in women using a particular method of birth control
   d. The number of times a couple fails to use birth control

LO **2** | Contraception Methods

2. Which type of lubricant could you safely use with a latex condom?
   a. Coconut oil
   b. Water-based lubricant
   c. Body lotion
   d. Petroleum jelly

3. Mariana and David want to practice a method of avoiding pregnancy that is 100 percent effective. What method would you recommend?
   a. abstinence
   b. calendar method
   c. NuvaRing
   d. condoms

4. Emergency contraception is up to 88 percent effective when used within how many days of unprotected intercourse?
   a. 1
   b. 2 to 5
   c. 5 to 7
   d. 7 to 14

5. Benjamin wants to be sterilized. The male sterilization process his health care provider will perform is called
   a. suction curettage.
   b. tubal ligation.
   c. hysterectomy.
   d. vasectomy.

LO **3** | Choosing a Method of Contraception

6. Emily wants to use a contraception method that also protects against STIs. Her best option is

a. Xulane.
b. condoms.
c. a contraceptive sponge.
d. an IUD.

LO 4 | Abortion

7. What is the most commonly used method of first-trimester abortion?
a. Suction curettage
b. Dilation and evacuation (D&E)
c. Medical abortion
d. Induction abortion

LO 5 | Pregnancy

8. What is the recommended pregnancy weight gain for a woman who is at a healthy weight before pregnancy?
a. 15 to 20 pounds
b. 20 to 30 pounds
c. 25 to 35 pounds
d. 30 to 45 pounds

LO 6 | Childbirth

9. In an ectopic pregnancy, the fertilized egg implants in the woman's
a. fallopian tube.
b. uterus.
c. vagina.
d. ovaries.

LO 7 | Infertility

10. The number of American couples who experience infertility is
a. 1 in 10.
b. 1 in 25.
c. 1 in 50.
d. 1 in 100.

Answers to the Pop Quiz can be found on page A-1. If you answered a question incorrectly, review the section identified by the Learning Outcome. For even more study tools, visit **Mastering Health**.

THINK ABOUT IT!

LO 1 | Basic Principles of Contraception

1. How, in general, do contraceptives work? What is the difference between perfect-use and typical-use failure rates? Which do you think is a better predictor of effectiveness? Why?

LO 2 | Contraceptive Methods

2. What are the options for birth control methods? What are their major advantages and disadvantages?

3. Do your religious views affect your sexual behavior or choice of birth control methods? If so, how do your religious views affect your family planning decisions?

LO 3 | Choosing a Method of Contraception

4. List the most effective contraceptive methods. What are their drawbacks? What medical conditions would keep a person from using each one? Which methods do you think would be most effective for you? Why?

LO 4 | Abortion

5. What are the various methods of abortion? What are the two opposing viewpoints concerning abortion? What is *Roe v. Wade*, and what impact has it had on the abortion debate in the United States?

LO 5 | Pregnancy

6. Discuss the growth of the fetus through the three trimesters. What medical checkups or tests should be done during each trimester?

LO 6 | Childbirth

7. What are some of the complications that can occur during pregnancy and childbirth? What actions can we take to prevent these complications?

LO 7 | Infertility

8. If you and your partner are unable to have children, what alternative methods of conception would you consider? Would you consider adoption?

ACCESS YOUR HEALTH ON THE INTERNET

Use the following websites to further explore topics and issues related to reproductive health. For links to the websites below, visit Mastering Health.

Guttmacher Institute. This is a nonprofit organization focused on sexual and reproductive health research, policy analysis, and public education. www.guttmacher.org

Association of Reproductive Health Professionals. This independent organization provides education for health care professionals and the general public. The *Patient Resources* portion of the website includes information on birth control and an interactive tool to help you choose a method that will work for you. www.arhp.org

Planned Parenthood. This site offers a range of up-to-date information on sexual health issues, such as birth control, the decision of when and whether to have a child, sexually transmitted infections, abortion, and safer sex. www.plannedparenthood.org

Bedsider. This easy to read and humorous website offers up-to-date and thorough information on contraceptives. www.bedsider.org

The American Pregnancy Association. This is a national organization that offers a wealth of resources to promote reproductive and pregnancy wellness. The website includes educational materials and information on the latest research. www.americanpregnancy.org

Sexuality Information and Education Council of the United States. Information, guidelines, and materials for the advancement of sexuality education are all found here. The site advocates the right of individuals to make responsible sexual choices. www.siecus.org

International Council on Infertility Information Dissemination. This site includes current research and information on infertility. www.inciid.org

8 Recognizing and Avoiding Addiction and Drug Abuse

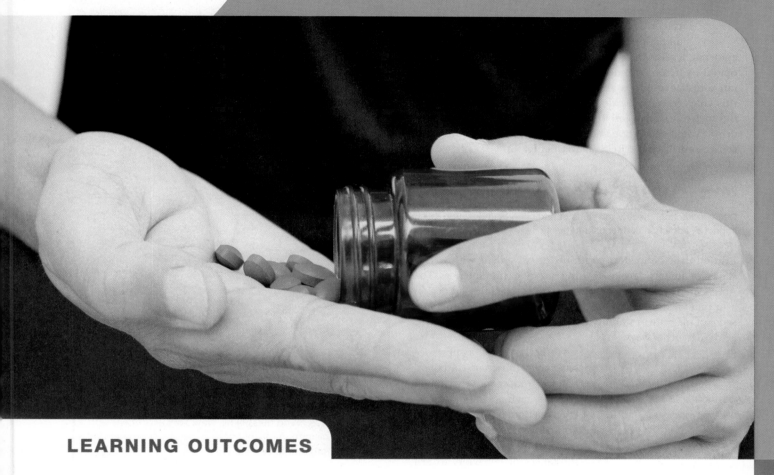

LEARNING OUTCOMES

LO **1** Define addiction, identify the signs of addiction, and describe the impact of addiction on friends and family.

LO **2** Describe types of process addictions, such as gambling disorder, exercise addiction, technology addictions, and compulsive buying disorder.

LO **3** Identify the six categories of drugs and their routes of administration.

LO **4** Review problems relating to the misuse and abuse of prescription drugs, including the use of illicit drugs among college students.

LO **5** Discuss the use and abuse of controlled substances, including stimulants, marijuana and other cannabinoids, depressants, opioids (narcotics), hallucinogens, inhalants, and anabolic steroids.

LO **6** Discuss treatment and recovery options for addicts, as well as public health approaches to preventing drug abuse and reducing the impact of addiction on our society.

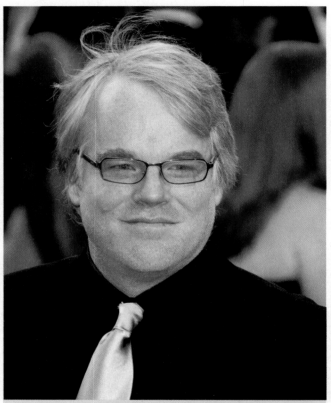

WHY SHOULD I CARE?

You might think drugs are helping you relax, improving your concentration, or enhancing your social enjoyment, but those effects are transient—and often illusory—and they are nothing compared to the many negative effects those same drugs can have on your life and health. Sooner or later, drug misuse and abuse is likely to catch up with you and cause problems, be they academic, social, career, legal, financial, or health related. Are a few moments of excitement really worth a lifetime of trouble?

These days, it's easy to find high-profile cases of compulsive and destructive behavior. Stories of celebrities, athletes, and politicians struggling with addiction are common. Heroin deaths have reached epidemic levels. An American dies every 19 minutes from an opioid or heroin overdose.[1] Millions of people from a wide range of backgrounds are waging battles with addiction. In this chapter, we will examine addictions to common activities such as eating, gambling, and shopping, as well as specific drugs that are addictive and commonly abused. (Alcohol and tobacco are discussed in detail in Chapter 9.)

LO 1 | WHAT IS ADDICTION?

Define addiction, identify the signs of addiction, and describe the impact of addiction on friends and family.

Addiction is defined as continued involvement with a substance or activity despite ongoing negative consequences. The American Psychiatric Association (APA) classifies addiction as a mental disorder. Addictive behaviors initially provide a sense of pleasure or stability that is difficult for some people to achieve in other ways.

Addiction affects all kinds of people. Academy Award–winning actor Philip Seymour Hoffman, widely respected for his work, was found dead in his New York apartment with a needle in his arm. A mix of cocaine, heroin, and other drugs ultimately proved fatal.

addiction Continued involvement with a substance or activity despite ongoing negative consequences.

physiological dependence The adaptive state of brain and body processes that occurs with regular addictive behavior and results in withdrawal if the addictive behavior stops.

tolerance A phenomenon in which progressively larger doses of a drug or more intense involvement in a behavior are needed to produce the desired effects.

withdrawal A series of temporary physical and psychological symptoms that occur when an addict abruptly abstains from an addictive chemical or behavior.

psychological dependence Dependency of the mind on a substance or behavior, which can lead to psychological withdrawal symptoms such as anxiety, irritability, or cravings.

To be addictive, a substance or behavior must have the potential to produce positive mood changes, such as euphoria, anxiety reduction, or pain reduction. The danger develops when the person comes to depend on these substances or behaviors to feel normal or function on a daily basis. Signs of addiction become apparent when people continue to use the substance despite knowing the harm that it causes to themselves and others.

People with **physiological dependence** on a substance, such as an addictive drug, experience **tolerance** when they require increased amounts of the drug to achieve the desired effect. They also experience **withdrawal**, a series of temporary physical and psychological symptoms that occurs when substance use stops. Tolerance and withdrawal are important criteria for determining whether or not someone is addicted.

Psychological dependence can also play an important role in addiction. Behaviors unrelated to the use of drugs, such as gambling, working, and sex, can create changes at the cellular level along with positive mood changes.[2] A person with an intense, uncontrollable urge to continue engaging in a particular activity is said to have developed a psychological dependence. In fact, psychological and physiological dependence are so intertwined that it is not really possible to separate them. Although the mechanism is not well understood, all forms of addiction probably reflect dysfunction of certain biochemical systems in the brain.[3]

Common Characteristics of Addiction

Our brains are wired to ensure that we will repeat life-sustaining activities by associating those activities with reward or pleasure. We all engage in potentially addictive behaviors because some behaviors that are essential to our survival are also highly reinforcing, such as eating, drinking, and sex. At some point, however, some individuals are not able to engage in these behaviors moderately, and these individuals become addicted.

Addiction has five common characteristics: (1) **compulsion**, which is characterized by **obsession** (excessive preoccupation) with the behavior and an overwhelming need to perform it; (2) **loss of control**, or the inability to predict reliably whether any isolated occurrence of the behavior will be healthy or damaging; (3) **negative consequences**, such as physical damage, legal trouble, financial problems, academic failure, or family dissolution; (4) **denial**, the inability to perceive that the behavior is self-destructive; and (5) **inability to abstain**. These five components are present in all addictions, whether chemical or behavioral.[4]

Addiction is a process that evolves over time (**FIGURE 8.1**). It begins when a person repeatedly seeks the illusion of relief to avoid unpleasant feelings or situations. This pattern, known as *nurturing through avoidance*, is a maladaptive way of taking care of emotional needs. As a person increasingly depends on the addictive behavior, there is a corresponding deterioration in relationships as well as personal and professional life. Eventually, addicts do not find the addictive behavior pleasurable but consider it preferable to the unhappy realities they seek to escape.

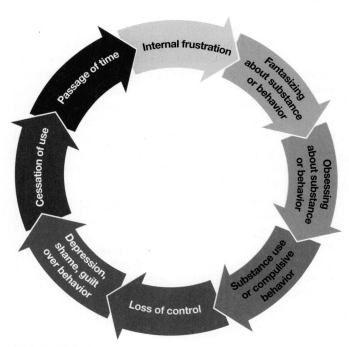

FIGURE 8.1 The Cycle of Psychological Addiction

Source: Adapted from Recovery Connection, Cycle of Addiction, 2016, www.recoveryconnection.org/cycle-of-addiction.

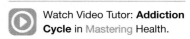 Watch Video Tutor: **Addiction Cycle** in Mastering Health.

Addiction Affects Family and Friends

The family and friends of an addicted person also suffer many negative consequences. Often, they struggle with **codependence**, a self-defeating relationship pattern in which a person is controlled by an addict's addictive behavior. A codependent person will often put his or her needs aside to take care of the addict. They find it hard to set healthy boundaries and often live in a chaotic, crisis-oriented mode. Although the word *codependent* is used less frequently today, treatment professionals still recognize the importance of helping addicts see how their behavior affects those around them and of working with family and friends to establish healthier relationships.

Family and friends can play an important role in getting an addict to seek treatment, particularly when they refuse to be **enablers**, that is, people who knowingly or unknowingly protect addicts from the natural consequences of their behavior. If addicts don't have to deal with the consequences, they cannot see the self-destructive nature of their behavior and will continue it. Enabling is rarely conscious or intentional.

LO 2 | ADDICTIVE BEHAVIORS

Describe types of process addictions, such as gambling disorder, exercise addiction, technology addictions, compulsive buying disorder, and compulsive sexual behavior.

Drugs are not the only source of addiction. New knowledge about the brain's reward system suggests that, for the brain, a reward is a reward, whether brought on by a chemical or a behavior.[5] **Process addictions** are behaviors that are known to be addictive because they are mood altering. Examples include disordered gambling, compulsive buying, compulsive Internet or technology use, work addiction, compulsive exercise, and sexual addiction.

Gambling Disorder

Gambling is a form of recreation and entertainment for millions of Americans. Most people who gamble do so casually and moderately

compulsion Preoccupation with a behavior and an overwhelming need to perform it.

obsession Excessive preoccupation with an addictive substance or behavior.

loss of control Inability to predict reliably whether a particular instance of involvement with an addictive substance or behavior will be healthy or damaging.

negative consequences Physical damage, legal trouble, financial ruin, academic failure, family dissolution, and other severe problems that do not occur with healthy involvement in any behavior.

denial Inability to perceive or accurately interpret the self-destructive effects of an addictive behavior.

inability to abstain Failure to avoid drug use over a sustained period of time.

codependence A self-defeating relationship pattern in which a person helps or encourages addictive behavior in another.

enabler A person who knowingly or unknowingly protects an addict from the consequences of the addict's behavior.

process addiction A condition in which a person is dependent on (addicted to) some mood-altering behavior or process, such as gambling, buying, or exercise.

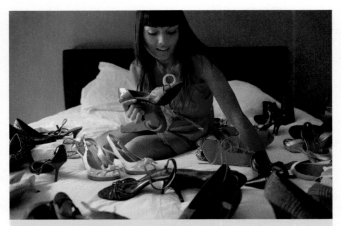

Once a person recognizes a habit and decides to change it, the habit can usually be broken. With addiction, however, the sense of compulsion is so strong that a behavior can't be controlled. For example, you might like to shop or spend time online hunting for bargains, but it isn't considered an addiction unless you have lost control over where and when you shop and how much you spend.

to experience the excitement of anticipating a win. However, more than 5 million people in the United States meet the criteria for having a gambling addiction, and many others are directly or indirectly affected by the gambling behavior of friends or relatives.[6] The APA recognizes **gambling disorder** as an addictive disorder. According to the fifth edition of the APA's *Diagnostic and Statistical Manual of Mental Disorders* (DSM-5), characteristic behaviors include a preoccupation with gambling, unsuccessful efforts to cut back or quit, gambling when feeling distressed, and lying to family members to conceal the extent of gambling.[7]

A gambling addiction typically progresses through four phases:[8]

- The winning phase often begins with a large win, which reinforces the excitement and reward associated with gambling. The gambler begins to feel as though he or she cannot lose.
- In the losing phase, gamblers become preoccupied with gambling, trying to win back what they have lost. This often interferes with work and family life.
- In the desperate phase, gamblers lose the ability to control their gambling. They feel ashamed and guilty but cannot stop. They may resort to stealing or cheating to continue their gambling.
- In the hopeless phase, gamblers give up the hope of quitting. They don't believe that anyone cares or that help is possible.

gambling disorder A set of behaviors including preoccupation with gambling, unsuccessful efforts to cut back or quit, using gambling to escape problems, and lying to family members to conceal the extent of involvement with gambling.

compulsive buying disorder A preoccupation with shopping and spending accompanied by little control over the impulse to buy.

exercise addict A person who always works out alone, following the same rigid pattern; exercises for more than 2 hours daily, repeatedly, and when sick or injured; focuses on weight loss or calories burned; exercises to the point of pain and beyond; and skips work, class, or social activities for workouts.

Strong evidence suggests that disordered gambling has a biological component. Gambling addiction has come to be viewed as a disorder of the dopamine neurotransmitter system coupled with decreased blood flow to a key section of the brain's reward system. Individuals with gambling disorder may compensate for this reward deficiency by overdoing it and getting hooked.[9] Like drug abusers, gambling addicts show tolerance—needing to increase the amount of their bets—and have withdrawal symptoms, including sleep disturbance, sweating, irritability, and craving.[10]

Although gambling is illegal for anyone under the age of 21, college students have easier access to gambling opportunities than ever before. The percentage of college students who gamble—close to 75 percent—is consistent with these growing opportunities.[11] Nearly 18 percent of those students reported gambling once a week or more.[12] It is estimated that 6 percent of college students in the United States have a serious gambling problem, which can result in psychological difficulties, debt, and failing grades.[13]

Compulsive Buying Disorder

In the United States, many people shop to make themselves feel better. But people who engage in "retail therapy" in excess, running their credit cards to the limit, may have **compulsive buying disorder**. Compulsive buyers are preoccupied with shopping and spending, and they exercise little control over their impulses. Compulsive buying is estimated to afflict up to 6 percent of adults.[14] Most compulsive buyers are women.[15]

Symptoms that a person has crossed the line into compulsive buying include preoccupation with shopping and spending, buying more than one of the same item, shopping for longer than intended, repeatedly buying much more than the person needs or can afford, and buying that interferes with social activities or work and creates financial problems. Compulsive buying frequently results in psychological distress as well as conflict with friends and between couples.[16]

The Internet provides instant access to millions of tempting purchases, information about the newest fashions, and continual alerts about new products. These features enable a compulsive buyer to be alone with his or her addiction, shopping with little or no direct interaction, either verbal or face to face. Compulsive buyers often do not want others (including family members) to know what, how frequently, and how much they buy.[17] It is not uncommon for the goods they buy to be useless or left unused.[18]

> ▶ **SEE IT! VIDEOS**
> How do you battle compulsive shopping? Watch **Woman's Shopping Addiction Revealed**, available on Mastering Health.

Exercise Addiction

Generally speaking, most Americans get too little physical activity, not too much. However, when taken to extremes, exercise can become addictive as a result of its powerful mood-enhancing effects. **Exercise addicts** use exercise compulsively

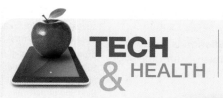

TECH & HEALTH | MOBILE DEVICES, MEDIA, AND THE INTERNET *Could You Unplug?*

If someone asked you to unplug for 24 hours, how hard would it be? Judging from the results of a study with participants from 37 countries on six continents, it would be extremely hard! All students followed the same assignment: Give up Internet, newspapers, magazines, TV, radio, phones, iPods/MP3 players, movies, video games, and any other form of electronic or social media for 24 hours.

Students around the world repeatedly used the term *addiction* to speak about their media dependence and likened their reactions to feelings of withdrawal. "Media is my drug; without it I was lost," said one student from the United Kingdom. A student from the United States noted: "I was itching, like a crackhead, because I could not use my phone." A student from Slovakia simply said, "I felt sad, lonely, and depressed."

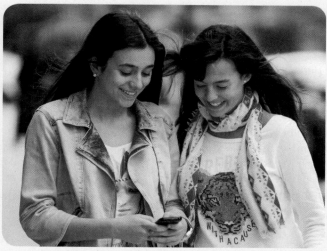

As the world goes wireless, many of us are increasingly attached to our cell phones, laptops, and tablet computers.

Students also reported that media—especially mobile phones—have become virtual extensions of themselves. Going without made it seem as though they had lost part of themselves.

Despite the withdrawal symptoms, many students found that there were definite benefits to being unplugged for 24 hours. Some students found that they had more time to talk, listen, and share with others. Students also reported feeling liberated. They took time to do things they normally would not do, such as visiting relatives and having face-to-face conversations.

How do you "unplug" without the anxiety of ignoring your friends online? Apps can actually help! Some apps can post automatic status updates to Facebook and Twitter, send you reminders about scheduled technology breaks, or temporarily lock out your access to the Internet. Here are a few:

- **Off time.** http://Offtime.co//
- **Unplug and Reconnect.** (Free: Android) www.unplugreconnect.com
- **Unplug** www.weareunplugged.com

Source: Adapted from The World Unplugged, "Going 24 Hours without Media," 2011, http://theworldunplugged.wordpress.com.

---

to try to meet needs—for nurturance, intimacy, self-esteem, and self-competency—that an object or activity cannot truly meet. Addictive or compulsive exercise results in negative consequences similar to those of other addictions: alienation of family and friends, injuries from overdoing it, and a craving for more. Warning signs of exercise addiction include injuring and reinjuring the body through excess or lack of proper rest; difficulty concentrating; feeling restless; adhering to a rigid workout plan; becoming fixated on burning calories or losing weight; canceling social plans, skipping work, or missing class to exercise; or working out beyond the point of pain.[19]

Technology Addictions

Are you or your friends more concerned with texting or tweeting than with eating, studying, or having a face-to-face conversation? These attitudes and behaviors are not unusual; many experts suggest that technology addiction is real and can present serious problems. An estimated one in eight Internet users will likely experience **Internet addiction**.[20] Younger people are more likely to be addicted to the Internet than are middle-aged users.[21] Approximately 9 percent of college students report that Internet use and computer games have interfered with their academic performance.[22] To read about students taking part in an "unplug from technology day," see the **Tech & Health** box.

Some online activities, such as gaming and cybersex, seem to be more compelling and potentially addictive than others. Internet addicts typically exhibit symptoms such as general disregard for their health, sleep deprivation, neglecting family and friends, lack of physical activity, euphoria when online, low grades, and poor job performance. Internet addicts may feel moody or uncomfortable when offline. They may use their behavior to compensate for loneliness, marital or work problems, an unsatisfying social life, or financial problems.

Work Addiction

Work addiction is the compulsive use of work and the work persona to fulfill needs of intimacy, power, and success. The disorder is characterized by

> **Internet addiction** Compulsive use of the computer, PDA, cell phone, or other form of technology to access the Internet for activities such as e-mail, games, shopping, and blogging.
>
> **work addiction** The compulsive use of work and the work persona to fulfill needs for intimacy, power, and success.

excessive time spent working, difficulty disengaging from work, going above and beyond what the job calls for, a compulsive work style, high levels of stress, low life satisfaction, marital conflict, and work burnout.[23] Work addicts may feel too busy to take care of their health, and there is some evidence that work addiction can cause physical symptoms such as sleep problems and exhaustion, high blood pressure, anxiety and depression, weight gain, ulcers and chest pain, or more chronic health conditions such as heart disease and asthmatic attacks.[24] **FIGURE 8.2** identifies other signs of work addiction.

Work addiction is found among all age, racial, and socioeconomic groups but typically develops in people in their 40s and 50s. Male work addicts outnumber female work addicts, but this is changing as women gain equality in the workforce.[25] Most work addicts come from homes in which one or more parents were work addicts, rigid, violent, or otherwise dysfunctional.[26] While work addiction can bring admiration, as the addicts often excel in their professions, the negative effects on individuals and those around them may be far-reaching.[27]

Compulsive Sexual Behavior

Everyone needs love and intimacy, but the sexual practices of people addicted to sex involve neither. **Sexual addiction** is compulsive involvement in sexual activity.

Compulsive sexual behavior may involve a normally enjoyable sexual experience that becomes an obsession, or it may involve fantasies or activities outside the bounds of culturally, legally, or morally acceptable behavior.[28] People with compulsive sexual behavior may participate in a wide range of sexual activities, including affairs, sex with strangers, prostitution, voyeurism, exhibitionism, rape, incest, or pedophilia. They frequently experience crushing episodes of depression and anxiety, fueled by the fear of discovery. Compulsive sexual behavior can lead to loss of intimacy with loved ones, family disintegration, and other related problems.

While compulsive sexual behavior is most common in men, it can affect anyone, regardless of sexual preference. Many sex addicts have a history of physical, emotional, and/or sexual abuse, or trauma.[29]

Although process addictions are becoming more commonly recognized in society, drug addiction still garners most public attention.

LO **3** | **WHAT** IS A DRUG?

Identify the six categories of drugs and their routes of administration.

Drugs are substances other than food that are intended to affect the structure or function of the mind or the body

through chemical action. Many drugs have important benefits. However, the potential for addiction is great for even the most therapeutic substances, owing to their potent effects on the brain.

Scientists divide drugs into six categories: prescription, over-the-counter (OTC), recreational, herbal preparations, illicit, and commercial. Each category includes some drugs that stimulate the body, some that depress body functions, and some that produce hallucinations (sounds, images, or other sensations that are perceived but are not real). Each category also includes psychoactive drugs.

> **sexual addiction** Compulsive involvement in sexual activity.
>
> **drugs** Nonnutritional nonfood substances that are intended to affect the structure or function of the mind or body through chemical action.

- **Prescription drugs.** Prescription drugs can be obtained only with a prescription from a licensed health practitioner. Approximately 49 percent of Americans have reported using at least one prescription medication in the past month.[30] The percentage of people taking five or more prescription drugs is 11 percent.[31] Close to 75 percent of physician office visits involve receiving some drug therapy.[32]
- **Over-the-counter drugs.** OTC drugs, used to treat everything from headaches to athlete's foot, are available without a prescription. They create substantial savings for the health care system through decreased visits to health care providers and decreased use of prescription medications.[33] However, they can be misused.[34]
- **Recreational drugs.** Generally, people use recreational drugs to relax or socialize. Most of them are legal even though they are psychoactive. Alcohol, tobacco, and caffeine products are included in this category.
- **Herbal preparations.** Herbal preparations encompass approximately 750 substances, including teas and other

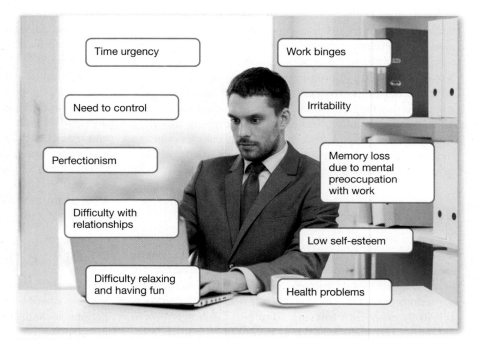

FIGURE 8.2 Signs of Work Addiction

- Time urgency
- Work binges
- Need to control
- Irritability
- Perfectionism
- Memory loss due to mental preoccupation with work
- Difficulty with relationships
- Low self-esteem
- Difficulty relaxing and having fun
- Health problems

products of botanical (plant) origin, that are believed to have medicinal properties.

- **Illicit (illegal) drugs.** Illicit drugs are the most notorious type of drug. Although laws governing their use, possession, cultivation, manufacture, and sale differ from state to state, illicit drugs are generally recognized as harmful. All are psychoactive.

- **Commercial drugs.** Commercial drugs are those found in commercially sold products. More than 1,000 exist, including those used in seemingly benign items such as perfumes, cosmetics, household cleaners, paints, glues, inks, dyes, and pesticides.

How Drugs Affect the Brain

Pleasure, which scientists call *reward*, is a powerful biological force for survival. The brain is wired such that you tend to want to repeat pleasurable experiences. Life-sustaining activities, such as eating, activate a circuit of specialized nerve cells devoted to producing and regulating pleasure. One important set of nerve cells, which uses a chemical **neurotransmitter** called *dopamine*, sits at the very top of the brain stem. These dopamine-containing neurons relay messages about pleasure through their nerve fibers to nerve cells in the limbic system,

structures in the brain that regulate emotions. Still other fibers connect to a related part of the frontal region of the cerebral cortex, the area of the brain that plays a key role in memory, perception, thought, and consciousness. Thus, this "pleasure circuit," known as the *mesolimbic dopamine system*, spans the survival-oriented brain stem, the emotional limbic system, and the thinking frontal cerebral cortex.

All addictive substances and behaviors can activate the brain's pleasure circuit. Drug addiction is a biological, pathological process that alters the way in which the pleasure center, as well as other parts of the brain, functions. Almost all **psychoactive drugs** (those that change the way the brain works) affect chemical neurotransmission by enhancing it, suppressing it, or interfering with it. While some drugs mimic the effects of natural neurotransmitters, others block receptors and thereby prevent neuronal messages from getting through. Still other drugs block the *reuptake* of neurotransmitters by neurons, thus increasing the concentration of the neurotransmitters in the synaptic gap, the space between individual neurons (**FIGURE 8.3**). Finally, some drugs cause neurotransmitters to be released in greater amounts than is normal.

neurotransmitter A chemical that relays messages between nerve cells or from nerve cells to other body cells.

psychoactive drugs Drugs that affect brain chemistry and have the potential to alter mood or behavior.

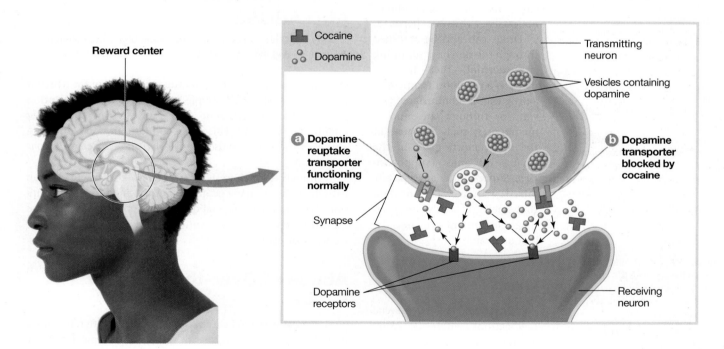

FIGURE 8.3 **The Action of Cocaine at Dopamine Receptors in the Brain** (a) In normal neural communication, dopamine is released into the synapse between neurons. It binds temporarily to dopamine receptors on the receiving neuron and then is recycled back into the transmitting neuron by a transporter. (b) When cocaine molecules are present, they attach to the dopamine transporter and block the recycling process. Excess dopamine remains active in the synaptic gaps between neurons, creating feelings of excitement and euphoria.

Watch Video Tutor: **Psychoactive Drugs Acting on the Brain** in Mastering Health.

Source: Adapted from NIDA "Cocaine—How the Brain Responds to Cocaine," February 2016, Available at http://www.drugabuse.gov/videos/reward-circuit-how-brain-responds-to-cocaine.

Routes of Drug Administration

Route of administration refers to the way a given drug is taken into the body. The most common method is by swallowing a tablet, capsule, or liquid (**oral ingestion**). Drugs taken orally may not reach the bloodstream for as long as 30 minutes.

Drugs can also enter the body through the respiratory tract via sniffing, smoking, or inhaling (**inhalation**). Drugs that are inhaled and absorbed by the lungs travel the most rapidly of all the routes of drug administration.

Another rapid form of drug administration is by **injection** directly into the bloodstream (intravenously), into a muscle (intramuscularly), or just under the skin (subcutaneously). Intravenous injection, which involves inserting a hypodermic needle directly into a vein, is the most common method of injection for drug users, owing to the rapid speed (within seconds in most cases) with which a drug's effect is felt. It is also the most dangerous method because of the risk of damaging blood vessels and contracting HIV (human immunodeficiency virus) and hepatitis.

Drugs can also be absorbed through the skin or tissue lining (**transdermal**)—the nicotine patch is a common example of a drug that is administered this way—or through the mucous membranes, such as those in the nose (snorting) or in the vagina or anus (**suppositories**). Suppositories are typically mixed with a waxy medium that melts at body temperature, releasing the drug into the bloodstream.

Using a needle to inject drugs poses health threats beyond the effects of the drug.

Drug Interactions

Polydrug use—taking several medications, vitamins, recreational drugs, or illegal drugs simultaneously—can be dangerous. Alcohol in particular frequently has dangerous interactions with other drugs. Hazardous interactions include synergism, inhibition, antagonism, intolerance, and cross-tolerance.

Synergism, also called *potentiation*, is an interaction of two or more drugs in which the effects of the individual drugs are multiplied beyond what would normally be expected if they were taken alone. You might think of synergism as $2 + 2 = 10$. A synergistic reaction can be very dangerous—even deadly.

Antagonism, although usually less serious than synergism, can also produce unwanted and unpleasant effects. In an antagonistic reaction, drugs work at the same receptor site, and one drug blocks the action of the other. The blocking drug occupies the receptor site and prevents the other drug from attaching, thus altering its absorption and action.

With **inhibition**, the effects of one drug are eliminated or reduced by the presence of another drug at the receptor site. **Intolerance** occurs when drugs combine in the body to produce extremely uncomfortable reactions. The drug Antabuse, which is used to help alcoholics give up alcohol, works by producing this type of interaction.

Cross-tolerance occurs when a person develops a physiological tolerance to one drug that also increases the body's tolerance to other substances that act similarly on the body.

LO 4 | DRUG MISUSE AND ABUSE

Review problems relating to the misuse and abuse of prescription drugs, including the use of illicit drugs among college students.

Drug misuse involves using a drug for a purpose for which it was not intended. For example, taking a friend's prescription painkiller for your headache is misuse. So is using Adderall or Ritalin as a study aid. This is not too far removed from **drug abuse**, or the excessive use of any drug, and may cause serious harm.

Although drug abuse is usually referred to in connection with illicit drugs, many people also abuse and misuse prescription, OTC, and recreational drugs. In this section, we discuss these drug-related behaviors and focus in particular on college students' drug use.

Abuse of Over-the-Counter Drugs

Over-the-counter medications come in many different forms, including pills, liquids, nasal sprays, and topical creams. Although many people assume that no harm can come from legal nonprescription drugs, OTC medications can be abused, with resultant health complications and potential addiction. Teenagers, young adults, and people over the age of 65 appear to be most vulnerable to abusing OTC drugs.

OTC drug abuse can involve taking more than the recommended dosage, combining the drug with other drugs, or taking a drug over a longer period of time than is recommended.

oral ingestion Intake of drugs through the mouth.

inhalation The introduction of drugs into the body through the respiratory tract.

injection The introduction of drugs into the body via a hypodermic needle.

transdermal The introduction of drugs into the body through the skin.

suppositories Mixtures of drugs and a waxy medium designed to melt at body temperature after being inserted into the anus or vagina.

polydrug use Use of multiple medications, vitamins, recreational drugs, or illicit drugs simultaneously.

synergism Interaction of two or more drugs that produces more profound effects than would be expected if the drugs were taken separately; also called *potentiation*.

antagonism A type of interaction in which two or more drugs work at the same receptor site so that one blocks the action of the other.

inhibition A drug interaction in which the effects of one drug are eliminated or reduced by the presence of another drug at the same receptor site.

intolerance A type of interaction in which two or more drugs produce extremely uncomfortable reactions.

cross-tolerance Development of a tolerance to one drug that reduces the effects of another, similar drug.

drug misuse Use of a drug for a purpose for which it was not intended.

drug abuse Excessive use of a drug.

Abuse of and addiction to OTC drugs can be accidental. A person may develop tolerance from continued use, creating an unintended dependence. However, teenagers and young adults sometimes intentionally abuse OTC medications in search of a cheap high—by drinking large amounts of cough medicine, for instance. The following are a few types of OTC drugs that are subject to misuse and abuse.

- **Caffeine pills and energy drinks.** Energy drinks, OTC caffeine pills, and pain relievers containing caffeine are commonly abused for the energy boost they provide. Caffeine in large doses can result in tremors/shaking, restlessness and edginess, insomnia, dehydration, panic attacks, heart irregularities, and other symptoms.

- **Cold medicines (cough syrups and tablets).** Of particular concern, one ingredient that is present in many cough and cold medicines is dextromethorphan (DXM). As many as 5 percent of high school seniors report taking drugs containing DXM to get high.[35] Large doses of products containing DXM can cause hallucinations, loss of motor control, and "out-of-body" (dissociative) sensations. In combination with alcohol or other drugs, large doses of DXM can be deadly. Some states have passed laws limiting the amount of products containing DXM a person can purchase or prohibiting sale to individuals under age 18.[36]

- **Diet pills.** Although diet pills are intended to help people lose weight, some teens use them as a way of getting high. Diet pills often contain a stimulant such as caffeine or an herbal ingredient that is claimed to promote weight loss, such as *Hoodia gordonii*. Although they can sometimes cause serious side effects, many diet pills are marketed as dietary supplements and so are regulated by the Food and Drug Administration (FDA) as food, not as drugs. This means that their manufacturers may make unsubstantiated claims of effectiveness or can use untested and unsafe ingredients.

- **Sleep aids.** Using sleep aids in excess may be harmful, as they can cause problems with the sleep cycle, weaken areas of the body, or induce narcolepsy (a condition of excessive, intrusive sleepiness). Continued use can lead to tolerance and dependence.

Nonmedical Use or Abuse of Prescription Drugs

In the United States today, the abuse of prescription medications is at an all-time high. Only marijuana is more widely abused.[37] Individuals abuse prescription medications because they are an easily accessible and inexpensive means of altering a user's mental and physical state. The latest available data

Over-the-counter cough syrup is frequently abused by young people seeking a high from the ingredient DXM.

indicate that approximately 6.4 million Americans aged 12 years and older used prescription drugs for nonmedical reasons in the past month.[38]

Prescription drug abuse is particularly common among teenagers and young adults. In 2015, 2 percent of teenagers age 12 to 17 years and 5 percent of people 18 to 25 years reported abusing prescription drugs in the past month.[39] Often, these drugs are taken surreptitiously from friends or family members who have prescriptions or are given freely or sold by the person with the prescription. The problem may be getting worse, with approximately 13 percent of twelfth-graders reporting abuse of prescription drugs by the time they graduate from high school.[40]

College Students and Prescription Drug Abuse Prescription drug abuse among college students has increased dramatically over the past decade. Because drugs are prescribed by doctors and approved by the FDA, many college students perceive prescription drugs as being safer and more socially acceptable than illicit drugs, or they believe that prescription drugs will enhance their well-being or performance. However, nothing could be farther from the truth when these drugs are misused.

According to the 2016 *American College Health Association–National College Health Assessment*, approximately 12 percent of surveyed students reported having illegally used prescription drugs in the last year.[41] The most commonly abused prescription drugs on college campuses are stimulants—drugs that are intended to treat attention deficit/hyperactivity

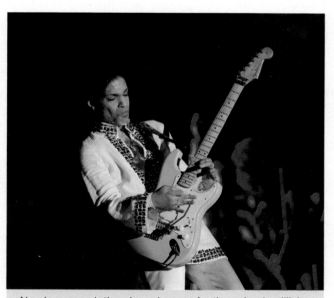

Abusing prescription drugs is no safer than abusing illicit drugs, as was tragically demonstrated by the 2016 death of pop star Prince from an overdose of fentanyl, a narcotic that is prescribed to treat pain.

disorder (ADHD) such as Ritalin or Adderall—followed by painkillers (e.g., OxyContin and Vicodin).[42] Approximately 7 percent of students reported having used stimulants not prescribed to them in the past 12 months, while 5 percent of students reported having used painkillers that were not prescribed to them in the past 12 months.[43]

Students who misuse prescription stimulants such as Adderall primarily report using them for academic gain.[44] According to a recent study, students indicate that it is easy or very easy to get prescription medications, and friends with prescriptions were the most commonly reported source.[45] Users generally believed that the drugs were beneficial, despite frequent reports of adverse reactions. The most commonly reported adverse effects were sleeping difficulties, irritability, and reduced appetite.

Use and Abuse of Illicit Drugs

The problem of illicit (illegal) drug use touches us all. We may use illicit substances ourselves, watch someone we love struggle with drug abuse, or become the victim of a drug-related crime. At the very least, we pay increasing taxes for law enforcement and drug rehabilitation. When our coworkers use drugs, the effectiveness of our own work may be diminished.

Illicit drug use spans all age groups, genders, ethnicities, occupations, and socioeconomic groups. Illicit drug use peaked around 25 million users between 1979 and 1986, declined until 1992, rose up to around 27 million users per year, and has remained stable over the past several decades.[46] Among youth, however, illicit drug use, notably of marijuana and heroin, has been rising in recent years.[47]

Illicit Drug Use on Campus Close to 50 percent of college-aged students nationwide have tried an illicit drug at some point; the vast majority of them reported having used marijuana (see **TABLE 8.1**).[48] The most startling trend is how many students smoke marijuana daily or almost daily; one in

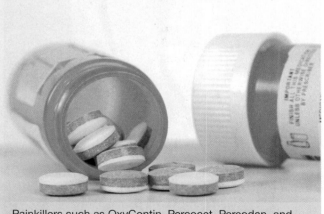

Painkillers such as OxyContin, Percocet, Percodan, and Vicodin are highly addictive. If they are taken daily for several weeks, that is enough time for addiction to develop. OxyContin in particular can be a highly addictive and dangerous narcotic when abused.

5.3%

of college students report having abused prescription **PAINKILLERS** such as codeine, vicodin, and oxycontin in the past year.

17 college students smokes pot at least 20 times a month.[49] While 28 states have legalized marijuana for medicinal and/or recreational use, the drug remains illegal in much of the U.S.

TABLE **8.1** | 30-Day Drug Use Prevalence, Full-Time College Students vs. Respondents 1 to 4 Years beyond High School

	Full-Time College (%)	Others (%)
Any illicit drug	23.4	28.2
Any illicit drug other than marijuana	9.2	9.2
Marijuana	21.1	25.4
Inhalants	0.2	*
Hallucinogens	1.4	1.6
LSD	0.7	1.2
Hallucinogens other than LSD	0.9	0.4
Ecstasy (methylene-dioxymethamphetamine, MDMA)	0.7	1.5
Cocaine	1.5	1.2
Crack	*	0.2
Other cocaine	1.4	1.3
Heroin	*	0.2
Narcotics other than heroin	1.3	2.1
Amphetamines, adjusted	4.2	3.3
Crystal methamphetamine	*	0.6
Sedatives (barbiturates)	1.0	1.7
Tranquilizers	1.6	2.0
Alcohol	63.2	51.1
Been drunk	38.4	24.9
Flavored alcoholic beverage	30.5	26.3
Cigarettes	11.3	23.4
Approximate weighted N =	1,020	570

*Indicates prevalence less than 0.05 percent.

Source: L. D. Johnston et al., *Monitoring the Future National Survey Results on Drug Use, 1975–2013,* Volume 2: *College Students and Adults Ages 19–55* (Ann Arbor, MI: Institute for Social Research, University of Michigan, 2016), Available at http://monitoringthefuture.org/new.html.

College administrators, staff, and faculty are concerned about the link between substance abuse and poor academic performance, depression, anxiety, suicide, property damage, vandalism, fights, serious medical problems, and death. Students who use marijuana and/or other illicit drugs are at increased risk for disruptions in college attendance.[50] A longer-term consequence of illicit drug use among college students is a significantly increased chance of unemployment after college. The most recent research shows that 10 percent of people who were persistent drug users during college experienced unemployment after college compared with 1.7 percent of students who did not use drugs and 4.8 percent of those who used drugs sporadically.[51]

Why Do Some College Students Use Drugs?

Research has identified the following factors in a student's life that increase the risk of substance abuse; the more factors, the greater the risk.

- **Positive expectations.** Some students take drugs such as Adderall and Ritalin in hopes of improving their ability to study. But the vast majority of students say they take drugs to relax, reduce stress, and forget problems.[52]
- **Genetics and family history.** Genetics and family history play a significant role in the risk for developing an addiction.
- **Substance use in high school.** Two thirds of college students who use illicit drugs began in high school.[53]
- **Curiosity.** College students are learning a lot about themselves. Sometimes, that self-discovery includes experimenting with different mind-altering substances.
- **Social norms.** College students often overestimate the amount of drug use on campus. Surveys conducted on college campuses found that students perceived that 85.5 percent of their peers used marijuana within the last 30 days, when actually 18.4 percent had used the drug.[54]
- **Sorority and fraternity membership.** Being a member of a sorority or fraternity increases the likelihood of abusing alcohol and drugs.[55] A few factors that may contribute to more drinking and use of drugs in sororities and fraternities include group living, hazing or initiation rituals, lack of supervision, and social pressure.[56]

To prepare yourself for a possible offer of drugs, see the Skills for Behavior Change box.

LO 5 | COMMON DRUGS OF ABUSE

Discuss the use and abuse of controlled substances, including stimulants, marijuana and other cannabinoids, depressants, opioids (narcotics), hallucinogens, inhalants, and anabolic steroids.

Hundreds of drugs are subject to abuse. For general purposes, drugs can be divided into the following categories: *stimulants, cannabis products (cannabinoids) including marijuana, depressants, opioids (narcotics), hallucinogens, inhalants,* and *anabolic*

steroids. **TABLE 8.2** summarizes the categorization, uses, and effects of various drugs of abuse, both legal and illicit.

> **stimulant** A drug that increases activity of the central nervous system.

Stimulants

A **stimulant** is a drug that increases activity of the central nervous system. Its effects usually involve increased activity, anxiety, and agitation; users often seem jittery or nervous while high. Commonly used illegal stimulants include cocaine, amphetamines, and methamphetamine. Legal stimulants include caffeine and nicotine. (See Chapter 9 for a discussion of nicotine.)

Cocaine A white crystalline powder derived from the leaves of the South American coca shrub (not related to cocoa plants),

TABLE 8.2 | Drugs of Abuse: Uses and Effects

Category	Drugs	Trade or Street Names	Dependence	Usual Method	Possible Effects	Overdose Effects	Withdrawal Syndrome
Stimulants	Cocaine	Coke, flake, snow, crack, *coca*, *blanca*, *perico*,	*Physical:* Possible *Psychological:* High *Tolerance:* Yes	Snorted, smoked, injected	Increased alertness, excitation, euphoria, increased pulse rate and blood pressure, insomnia, loss of appetite	Agitation, increased body temperature, hallucinations, convulsions, possible death	Apathy, long periods of sleep, irritability, depression, disorientation
	Amphetamine, methamphetamine	Crank, ice, cristal, crystal meth, speed, Adderall, Dexedrine	*Physical:* Possible *Psychological:* High *Tolerance:* Yes	Oral, injected, smoked			
	Methylphenidate	Ritalin, Concerta, Focalin, Metadate	*Physical:* Possible *Psychological:* High *Tolerance:* Yes	Oral, injected, snorted, smoked			
Cannabis	Marijuana	Pot, grass, sinsemilla, blunts, *mota*, *yerba*	*Physical:* Possible *Psychological:* High *Tolerance:* Yes	Oral, smoked	Euphoria, relaxed inhibitions, increased appetite, disorientation	Fatigue, paranoia, possible psychosis	Hyperactivity, decreased appetite, insomnia
	Hashish, hashish oil	Hash, hash oil	*Physical:* Unknown *Psychological:* Moderate *Tolerance:* Yes	Smoked, oral			
Narcotics	Heroin	Diamorphine, horse, smack, black tar, *chiva*	*Physical:* High *Psychological:* High *Tolerance:* Yes	Injected, snorted, smoked	Euphoria, drowsiness, respiratory depression, constricted pupils, nausea	Slow and shallow breathing, clammy skin, convulsions, coma, possible death	Watery eyes, runny nose, yawning, loss of appetite, irritability, tremors, panic, cramps, nausea, chills and sweating
	Morphine	MS-Contin, Roxanol	*Physical:* High *Psychological:* High *Tolerance:* Yes	Oral, injected			
	Hydrocodone, oxycodone	Vicodin, Oxy-Contin, Percocet, Percodan	*Physical:* High *Psychological:* High *Tolerance:* Yes	Oral			
	Codeine	Acetaminophen with codeine, Tylenol with codeine	*Physical:* Moderate *Psychological:* Moderate *Tolerance:* Yes	Oral, injected			
Depressants	Gamma-hydroxybutyrate	GHB, liquid Ecstasy, liquid X	*Physical:* Moderate *Psychological:* Moderate *Tolerance:* Yes	Oral	Slurred speech, disorientation, drunken behavior without odor of alcohol, impaired memory of events, interacts with alcohol	Shallow respiration, clammy skin, dilated pupils, weak and rapid pulse, coma, possible death	Anxiety, insomnia, tremors, delirium, convulsions, possible death

Continued on next page

TABLE **8.2** | Drugs of Abuse: Uses and Effects (Continued)

Category	Drugs	Trade or Street Names	Dependence	Usual Method	Possible Effects	Overdose Effects	Withdrawal Syndrome
	Benzodiaz-epines	Valium, Xanax, Halcion, Ativan, Rohypnol (roofies, R-2), Klonopin	*Physical:* Moderate *Psychological:* Moderate *Tolerance:* Yes	Oral, injected			
	Other depressants	Ambien, Sonata, barbiturates, methaqualone (Quaalude)	*Physical:* Moderate *Psychological:* Moderate *Tolerance:* Yes	Oral			
Hallucino-gens	Methylene-dioxymeth-amphetamine (MDMA), analogs	Ecstasy, XTC, Adam, MDA (love drug), MDEA (Eve)	*Physical:* None *Psychological:* Moderate *Tolerance:* Yes	Oral, snorted, smoked	Heightened senses, teeth grinding, dehydration	Increased body temperature, electrolyte imbalance, cardiac arrest	Muscle aches, drowsiness, depression, acne
	LSD	Acid, micro-dot, Sunshine, Boomers	*Physical:* None *Psychological:* Unknown *Tolerance:* Yes	Oral	Hallucinations, altered perception of time and distance	Longer, more intense "trips"	None
	Phencycli-dine, analogs	PCP, angel dust, hog, ketamine (special K)	*Physical:* Possible *Psychological:* High *Tolerance:* Yes	Smoked, oral, injected, snorted		Unable to direct movement, feel pain, or remember	Drug-seeking behavior
	Other hallucinogens	*Psilocybe* mushrooms, mescaline, peyote, dextromethorphan	*Physical:* None *Psychological:* None *Tolerance:* Possible	Oral			
Inhalants	Amyl and butyl nitrite	Pearls, poppers, Rush, Locker Room	*Physical:* Unknown *Psychological:* Unknown *Tolerance:* No	Inhaled	Flushing, hypotension, headache	Methemo-globinemia	Agitation
	Nitrous oxide	Laughing gas, balloons, whippets	*Physical:* Unknown *Psychological:* Low *Tolerance:* No	Inhaled	Impaired memory, slurred speech, drunken behavior, slow-onset vitamin deficiency, organ damage	Vomiting, respiratory depression, loss of consciousness, possible death	Trembling, anxiety, insomnia, vitamin deficiency, confusion, hallucinations, convulsions
	Other inhalants	Adhesives, spray paint, hairspray, lighter fluid	*Physical:* Unknown *Psychological:* High *Tolerance:* No	Inhaled			
Anabolic Steroids	Testosterone	Depo testosterone, Sustanon, Sten, Cypt	*Physical:* Unknown *Psychological:* Unknown *Tolerance:* Unknown	Injected	Virilization, edema, testicular atrophy, gynecomastia, acne, aggressive behavior	Unknown	Possible depression
	Other anabolic steroids	Parabolan, Winstrol, Equipose, Anadrol, Dianabol	*Physical:* Unknown *Psychological:* Yes *Tolerance:* Unknown	Oral, injected			

Source: Adapted from U.S. Department of Justice Drug Enforcement Administration, "DEA Drug Fact Sheets," 2011, www.justice.gov.

cocaine ("coke") has been described as one of the most powerful naturally occurring stimulants. Cocaine can be taken in several ways, including snorting, smoking, and injecting. The powdered form is snorted through the nose, which can damage mucous membranes and cause sinusitis. It can destroy the user's sense of smell and occasionally even eat a hole through the septum. When snorted, the drug enters the bloodstream through the lungs in less than 1 minute and reaches the brain in less than 3 minutes. It binds at receptor sites in the central nervous system, producing an intense high that disappears quickly, leaving a powerful craving for more.

Cocaine alkaloid, or *freebase*, is obtained from removing the hydrochloride salt from cocaine powder. *Freebasing* refers to smoking freebase by placing it at the end of a pipe and holding a flame near it to produce a vapor, which is then inhaled. *Crack* is identical pharmacologically to freebase, but the hydrochloride salt is still present and is processed with baking soda and water. It is a cheap, widely available drug that is very potent. Crack is commonly smoked in the same manner as freebase. Because crack takes little time to achieve the desired high, a crack user can become addicted quickly.

Some cocaine users occasionally inject the drug intravenously, which introduces large amounts into the body rapidly, creating a brief, intense high and a subsequent crash. Injecting users place themselves at risk not only for contracting HIV and hepatitis through shared needles, but also for skin infections, vein damage, inflamed arteries, and infection of the heart lining.

Cocaine is both an anesthetic and a central nervous system stimulant. In tiny doses, it can slow the heart rate. In larger doses, the physical effects are dramatic: increased heart rate and blood pressure, loss of appetite that can lead to dramatic weight loss, convulsions, muscle twitching, irregular heartbeat, and even death from overdose. Other effects include temporary relief of depression, decreased fatigue, talkativeness, increased alertness, and heightened self-confidence. However, as the dose increases, users become irritable and apprehensive, and their behavior may turn paranoid or violent.

Amphetamines

The **amphetamines** include a large and varied group of synthetic agents that stimulate the central nervous system. Small doses improve alertness, lessen fatigue, and generally elevate mood. With repeated use, however, physical and psychological dependence develops. Sleep patterns are affected (insomnia); heart rate, breathing rate, and blood pressure increase; and restlessness, anxiety, appetite suppression, and vision problems are common. High doses over long periods can produce hallucinations, delusions, and disorganized behavior.

Certain types of amphetamines or amphetamine-like drugs are used for medicinal purposes. Drugs prescribed to treat ADHD are stimulants and are increasingly abused on campus.

An increasingly common form of amphetamine, *methamphetamine* (commonly called "meth") is a potent, long-acting, inexpensive drug that is highly addictive. In the short term, methamphetamine produces increased physical activity, alertness, euphoria, rapid breathing, increased body temperature, insomnia, tremors, anxiety, confusion, and decreased appetite. Over 897,000 Americans are regular users. The largest proportion of people using methamphetamine are people over the age of 18 years.[57] In 2015, about 1 percent of high school seniors reported having used methamphetamine in their lifetime.[58] The rate of methamphetamine use may be increasing because the drug is relatively easy to make. Recipes often include common OTC ingredients such as ephedrine and pseudoephedrine.

Methamphetamine can be snorted, smoked, injected, or ingested orally. When it is snorted, the effects can be felt in 3 to 5 minutes; when it is ingested orally, effects occur within 15 to 20 minutes. The pleasurable effects of methamphetamine typically last only a few minutes when it is snorted; in contrast, smoking the drug can produce a high that lasts more than 8 hours. Users often experience tolerance after the first use, making methamphetamine highly addictive.

Methamphetamine increases the release of and blocks the reuptake of the neurotransmitter dopamine, leading to high levels of the chemical in the brain. This action occurs rapidly and produces the intense euphoria, or "rush," that many users feel. Over time, meth destroys dopamine receptors, making it impossible to feel pleasure. Researchers have now established that because of the destruction of dopamine receptors, people who abuse methamphetamine (or cocaine) are at increased risk for developing Parkinson's disease later in life.[59]

Other long-term effects of methamphetamine use can include severe weight loss, cardiovascular damage, increased risk of heart attack and stroke, hallucinations, extensive tooth decay and tooth loss ("meth mouth"), violence, paranoia,

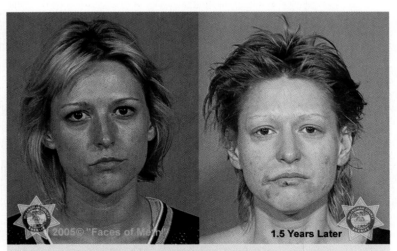

1.5 Years Later

The physical consequences of methamphetamine use are often dramatic. The photo at left shows a person before she began using methamphetamine. The photo at right shows the same person after just a year and a half of methamphetamine use.

psychotic behavior, and even death. Chronic methamphetamine abusers often demonstrate severe structural and functional changes in areas of the brain associated with emotion and memory, which may account for many of the emotional and cognitive problems that are observed in chronic methamphetamine abusers. Some of these changes persist after the methamphetamine abuse has stopped. Other changes reverse after sustained periods of abstinence from methamphetamine, lasting typically longer than a year, but problems can remain even after a long period of abstinence.[60]

Meth users are at increased risk for transmission of HIV, hepatitis B and C, and other sexually transmitted diseases. Meth can alter judgment, increase libido, and lessen inhibitions, leading users to engage in unsafe behaviors, including risky sexual behavior. HIV and other infectious diseases can be spread through sharing of contaminated needles, syringes, and other injection equipment.

Bath Salts *Bath salts* are synthetic (human-made) cathinones—drugs that are chemically related to the stimulant cathinone, which occurs naturally in the khat plant.[61] Although banned for use by humans in 2012, bath salts are often sold in online or in smoke shops or drug paraphernalia stores under a variety of names and are labeled "not for human consumption" to reduce risks of legal prosecution. These packages contain various amphetamine-like or cocaine-like substances, such as methylene-dioxypyrovalerone (MPDV), which act much like cocaine does but are at least 10 times stronger.[62] The powder can be smoked, snorted, injected, and wrapped in pieces of paper and ingested ("bombed"). These chemicals cannot be detected by routine drug screening, making them attractive for misuse.[63]

Effects include intense stimulation, alertness, euphoria, elevated mood, and a pleasurable rush. Users may describe feelings of closeness, sociability, and moderate sexual arousal. Other symptoms can include tremor, shortness of breath, and loss of appetite. Changes in body temperature regulation are accompanied by hot flashes and sweating, and the drug may cause bleeding from the nose and throat from ulcerations when it is snorted.[64]

This drug also can have significant effects on the cardiovascular system, resulting in rapid heart rate, increased blood pressure, and chest pain. Psychiatric effects at higher doses consist of anxiety, agitation, hallucinations, paranoia, and erratic behavior. Depression and suicide have also been reported as a result of use. Although withdrawal symptoms are reported as minimal, users often describe a strong craving.[65]

Caffeine Unlike cocaine and methamphetamine, **caffeine** is a legal stimulant. More than 85 percent of Americans drink at least one caffeinated beverage per day.[66] Ninety-six percent of beverage caffeine

consumed is from coffee, soft drinks, and tea.[67] Beverages such as energy drinks, chocolate drinks, and energy shots represent only a small portion of overall caffeine intakes.[68] One of the many reasons caffeine-containing products are loved is for their wake-up effects. Caffeine is so commonplace that it may seem entirely benign, but excessive consumption of caffeine is associated with addiction and certain health problems.

> **caffeine** A stimulant drug that is legal in the United States and found in many coffees, teas, chocolates, energy drinks, and certain medications.

Caffeine is derived from the chemical family called *xanthines*, which are found in plant products such as coffee, tea, and chocolate. The xanthines are mild central nervous system stimulants that enhance mental alertness, reduce feelings of fatigue, and increase heart muscle contractions, oxygen consumption, metabolism, and urinary output. A person feels these effects within 15 to 45 minutes of ingesting a caffeinated product. It takes 4 to 6 hours for the body to metabolize half of the caffeine ingested, so depending on the amount of caffeine taken in, it may continue to exert effects for a day or longer. **FIGURE 8.4** compares the caffeine content of various products.

As the effects of caffeine wear off, frequent users may feel let down—mentally or physically depressed, tired, and weak. To counteract this, they may choose to drink another cup of coffee or tea or another soda. Habitually engaging in this practice leads to tolerance and psychological dependence. Symptoms of excessive caffeine consumption include chronic insomnia, jitters, irritability, nervousness, anxiety, and involuntary muscle twitches. Withdrawing from caffeine may compound the effects and produce severe headaches, fatigue, and nausea. Because caffeine meets the requirements for addiction—tolerance, psychological dependence, and withdrawal symptoms—it can be classified as addictive.

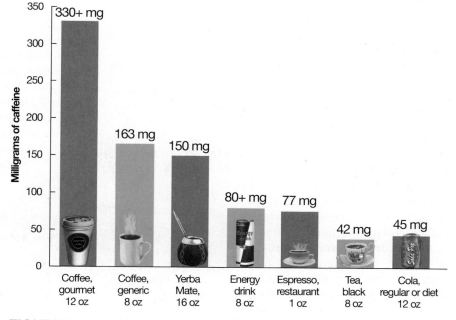

FIGURE 8.4 Caffeine Content Comparison

Source: Caffeine Informer, "Caffeine Content of Drinks," Accessed June 2016, http://www.caffeineinformer.com/the-caffeine-database.

marijuana Chopped leaves and flowers of *Cannabis indica* or *Cannabis sativa* plants (hemp); a psychoactive stimulant.

tetrahydrocannabinol (THC) The chemical name for the active ingredient in marijuana.

Heavy levels of caffeine use have been suspected of being linked to several serious health problems such as high blood pressure, and arrhythmias increased risk of heart attacks among young adults, and increased anxiety and depression.[69] However, no strong evidence exists to suggest that moderate caffeine use (less than 300 mg daily, or approximately three cups of regular coffee) produces harmful effects in healthy, nonpregnant people. For most people, caffeine poses few health risks and may actually have some benefits, such as improved memory, faster reaction time, reduction of chronic inflammation, and possibly prevention of skin cancer.[70]

Marijuana and Other Cannabinoids

Although archaeological evidence documents the use of **marijuana** ("grass," "weed," or "pot") as far back as 6,000 years ago, the drug did not become popular in the United States until the 1960s. Today, marijuana is the most commonly used illicit drug in the United States.[71] In 2015, some 33 million Americans reported having used marijuana in the past year, and more than 22 million reported having used marijuana within the past month.[72] Marijuana use is also on the rise on college campuses; approximately 36 percent of students reportedly used marijuana in the past year, following the trends of increased use in the general population as well as legalization for recreational use in a number of states.[73]

Methods of Use and Short-Term Physical Effects
Marijuana is derived from either the *Cannabis sativa* or *Cannabis indica* (hemp) plant. When marijuana is smoked, it is usually rolled into cigarettes (joints) or placed in a pipe or water pipe (bong).

Consumption of marijuana in edibles is becoming an increasingly popular alternative to smoking. Infusing food items with marijuana provides a more convenient and discreet way to consume cannabis. However, there are challenges with consuming edibles. The effects are hard to predict and can differ between individuals. It also takes longer to feel the effects—sometimes 30 to 60 minutes—and the effects can last longer.[74] The potency of edibles can also be quite a bit stronger; a marijuana-infused chocolate bar, for example, may contain as much as 100 milligrams of THC, far too much for consumption at one time.[75]

Tetrahydrocannabinol (THC) is the principal psychoactive substance in marijuana and the key to determining how powerful a high it will produce. More potent forms of the drug can contain up to 27 percent THC, but most average 15 percent.[76] *Hashish*, a potent cannabis preparation derived mainly

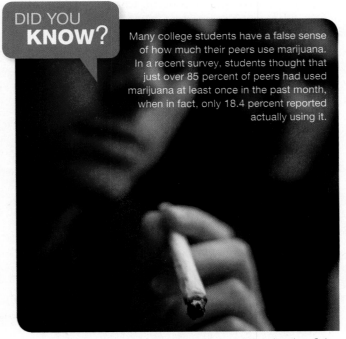

Source: Data are from American College Health Association, *American College Health Association—National College Health Assessment II: Reference Executive Summary, Fall 2016* (Hanover, MD: American College Health Association, 2017).

DID YOU **KNOW?**

Many college students have a false sense of how much their peers use marijuana. In a recent survey, students thought that just over 85 percent of peers had used marijuana at least once in the past month, when in fact, only 18.4 percent reported actually using it.

from the plant's thick, sticky resin, contains high THC concentrations. Smoking THC-rich resin extracts, called *dabbing*, is becoming much more common among marijuana users. These extracts contain high levels of THC, and people who have smoked them have ended up in the emergency room. Another danger is the extraction process, which involves butane lighter fluid; people have suffered burns and explosions or fires in their homes resulting from extracting resin extracts.[77]

The effects of smoking marijuana are generally felt within 30 minutes and usually wear off within 3 hours. The most noticeable effect of THC is the dilation of the eyes' blood vessels, which gives the smoker bloodshot eyes. Marijuana smokers also exhibit coughing, dry mouth and throat ("cotton mouth"), impaired body movement, increased heart rate, and changes in mood. Users can also experience severe anxiety, panic, paranoia, and psychosis and may have intensified reactions to various stimuli. Colors, sounds, and the speed at which things move may seem altered.[78]

One common way of smoking marijuana is to use a pipe.

Marijuana and Driving
Marijuana use presents clear hazards for drivers of motor vehicles and others on the road with them. The drug substantially reduces a driver's ability to react and make quick decisions. Perceptual and other performance deficits resulting from marijuana use may persist for some time after the high subsides. Users who attempt to drive, fly, or operate heavy machinery often fail to recognize their impairment. In the state of

10 MILLION

people reported **DRIVING** under the influence of illicit drugs in the past year.

Washington, where recreational use of marijuana is legal, one in six drivers involved in fatal car crashes had recently used marijuana.[79] Recent research indicates that a person is two and a half times more likely to be involved in a motor vehicle accident if driving under the influence of marijuana.[80] Combining even a low dose of marijuana and alcohol enhances the impairing effects of both drugs.

Effects of Chronic Marijuana Use Smoke from marijuana has been shown to contain many of the same toxins, irritants, and carcinogens as tobacco smoke.[81] Because marijuana smokers typically inhale more deeply and hold the smoke in their lungs longer than do tobacco smokers, the lungs are exposed to more tar per breath. Furthermore, effects from irritation similar to those experienced by tobacco smokers can occur.[82] Lung conditions such as chronic bronchitis, emphysema, and other lung disorders are also associated with smoking marijuana.

Some marijuana users believe that "vaping" marijuana poses fewer health risks than smoking. Vaporizers heat marijuana to a temperature that releases THC without creating smoke. While a small percentage of recreational marijuana users (7.6 percent) report vaping as a way to use marijuana, the majority still smoke.[83] Studies report very minimal difference between vaping and smoking in the effects on the lungs.[84]

Frequent and/or long-term marijuana use may significantly increase a man's risk of developing testicular cancer. The risk was particularly elevated (about twice the risk for those who never smoked marijuana) for men who used marijuana at least weekly or who had long-term exposure to the substance beginning in adolescence.[85]

The link between marijuana use and common mental health disorders is somewhat conflicting. A recent study found that using marijuana as an adult is not associated with a variety of mood and anxiety disorders, including depression and bipolar disorder, challenging some previous research.[86] However, use of marijuana is associated with a higher likelihood of drug dependence.[87]

The American Academy of Pediatrics has stated that marijuana is harmful to adolescent health and development.[88] For adolescents, marijuana use can disrupt concentration and memory. It can also cause problems with learning and is linked to lower rates of high school and college completion.[89] It can also affect motor control, coordination, and judgment, which increase the risk of unintentional deaths and injuries.[90]

Other risks associated with marijuana use include suppression of the immune system, blood pressure changes, and impaired memory function. Recent studies suggest that pregnant women who smoke marijuana may have children who have subtle brain changes that can cause difficulties with problem-solving skills, memory, and attention.[91]

Legalization of Marijuana and Medicinal Uses Although classified as a dangerous drug by the U.S. government, marijuana is known to have several medical purposes and has been legalized for medicinal uses in 28 states and the District of Columbia. It helps to control the severe nausea and vomiting that are often side effects of chemotherapy, the chemical treatment for cancer. It improves appetite and forestalls the loss of lean muscle mass associated with AIDS-wasting syndrome. Marijuana reduces the muscle pain and spasticity caused by diseases such as multiple sclerosis. Opponents of medical marijuana argue that there are FDA-approved drugs that are just as effective in treating the same conditions and that the potential side effects of marijuana make it inappropriate for FDA approval. Although several states have legalized marijuana for medicinal and/or recreational purposes, its legal status continues to be hotly debated (see the **Points of View** box).

Synthetic Marijuana Also known as K2 or "Spice," synthetic marijuana comprises a diverse family of herbal blends marketed under many names, including K2, fake marijuana, Yucatan Fire, Skunk, and Moon Rocks. These products contain dried, shredded plant material and one or more synthetic cannabinoids, with results that mimic marijuana intoxication but with longer duration and poor detectability in urine drug screens. K2 is sold legally as herbal blend incense. However, Spice is smoked by people to gain effects similar to marijuana, hashish, and other forms of cannabis.[92]

Spice is used by nearly one in seven college students, most commonly by males and first- and second-year college students.[93] Students who reported using Spice were more likely to have smoked cigarettes, marijuana, and hookahs.[94] Spice is also gaining attention among high school seniors, with reports that one in every nine, or 11.3 percent, of high school seniors are using this drug.[95]

The most common way of smoking Spice is by rolling it in papers (as with marijuana or handmade tobacco cigarettes).[96] Sometimes it is mixed with marijuana. Some users also make it into herbal tea for drinking.[97] People who smoke Spice may experience several adverse health effects such as hallucinations, severe agitation, extremely elevated heart rate and blood pressure, coma, suicide attempts, and drug dependence, which is not common among cannabis users.[98] Emergency departments are also reporting a significant increase in the numbers of people being treated for Spice use.[99]

Depressants

Whereas central nervous system stimulants increase muscular and nervous system activity, **depressants** have the opposite effect. These drugs slow down neuromuscular activity and

> **depressants** Drugs that slow down the activity of the central nervous and muscular systems and cause sleepiness or calmness.

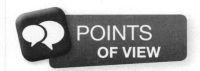
MARIJUANA

Currently, 28 states and the District of Columbia have chosen to legalize marijuana for medicinal use, and eight of these states—Washington, Colorado, Oregon, Alaska, California, Nevada, Maine, and Massachusetts—have legalized marijuana for recreational use. The arguments for and against the legalization of marijuana have been very strong over the past few decades. Following are some of the major points from both sides.

Arguments for Legalization

- There are medical benefits for individuals dealing with cancer and other chronic diseases.
- Legalizing marijuana and taxing its sale would bring in revenue for the government.
- Legal government and U.S. Food and Drug Administration (FDA) oversight would allow for standardization of marijuana growth and production and could promote more responsible cultivation methods.
- Legalizing marijuana would result in more effective law enforcement and criminal justice, since police officers would have more time and money to pursue the perpetrators of more serious crimes.
- Having legal outlets for drugs such as marijuana may reduce illegal drug trafficking from off-shore criminal elements and reduce the risk of harmful drug additives.

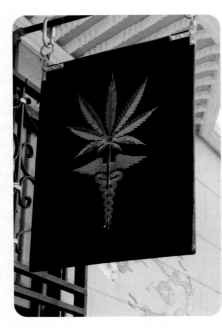

Arguments against Legalization

- Some individuals believe that it is morally wrong to consume marijuana.
- Research indicates that marijuana use affects young users the most in the long term.
- Research has found that people who used marijuana heavily as teenagers lose an average of 8 IQ points that are not recovered with quitting or aging.
- Marijuana use can cause or worsen respiratory symptoms or conditions such as bronchitis, alter mood and judgment, damage the immune system, and impair short-term memory and motor coordination. These side effects make it inappropriate for FDA approval.
- Marijuana is known to be addictive; approximately 9 percent of people who experiment with marijuana become addicted.
- Legalization could make marijuana more available to children and teenagers.

WHERE DO YOU STAND?

- Do you think marijuana should be legalized by the federal government? What potential problems do you think this would create or solve?
- What criteria do you think should be used to determine the legality of a particular substance? Who should make those determinations?
- What are your feelings on drug laws in general? Do you think they should be more or less prohibitive? What sort of policies would you propose to protect individuals and their rights?

Sources: National Institute on Drug Abuse, "DrugFacts: Is Marijuana Medicine?," July 2015, www.drugabuse.gov; DrugRehab.us, "Pros and Cons of Legalizing Recreational Marijuana," 2016, www.drugrehab.us/news/pros-cons-legalizing-recreational-marijuana; N. Volkow et al., "Adverse Health Effects of Marijuana Use," *New England Journal of Medicine* 370 (2014): 2219–27.

---

benzodiazepines A class of central nervous system depressant drugs with sedative, hypnotic, and muscle relaxant effects; also called *tranquilizers*.

barbiturates Drugs that depress the central nervous system, have sedative and hypnotic effects, and are less safe than benzodiazepines.

cause sleepiness or calmness. If the dose is high enough, brain function can stop, causing death. Alcohol is the most widely used central nervous system depressant. (For details on alcohol's effect on the body, see Chapter 9.) Other depressants are benzodiazepines, barbiturates, and GHB.

Benzodiazepines and Barbiturates A *sedative* drug promotes mental calmness and reduces anxiety, whereas a *hypnotic* drug promotes sleep or drowsiness. The most common sedative-hypnotic drugs are **benzodiazepines**, more commonly known as *tranquilizers*.[100] These include prescription drugs such as Valium, Ativan, and Xanax. Benzodiazepines are most commonly prescribed for tension, muscle strain, sleep problems, anxiety, panic attacks, and alcohol withdrawal.[101] **Barbiturates** are sedative-hypnotic drugs such as Amytal and Seconal. Today, benzodiazepines have largely replaced barbiturates, which were used medically in the past for relieving tension and inducing relaxation and sleep.

Sedative-hypnotic drugs have a synergistic effect when combined with alcohol, another central nervous system depressant. Taken together, these drugs can lead to respiratory failure and death. All sedative or hypnotic drugs can produce physical and psychological dependence in several weeks. A complication specific to sedatives is cross-tolerance, which occurs when users develop tolerance for one sedative or become dependent on it and develop tolerance for others as well. Withdrawal from sedative or hypnotic drugs may range from mild discomfort to severe symptoms, depending on the degree of dependence.[102]

One benzodiazepine of concern is Rohypnol, a potent tranquilizer that is similar to Valium but many times stronger. The drug produces a sedative effect, amnesia, muscle relaxation, and slowed psychomotor responses. Rohypnol, the most publicized "date rape" drug, has gained notoriety as a growing problem on college campuses. The drug has been added to punch and other drinks at parties, where it is reportedly given to a woman in hopes of incapacitating her so that she is unable to resist sexual assault. (See Chapter 5 for more on drug-facilitated rape.)

GHB

Gamma-hydroxybutyrate (GHB) is a central nervous system depressant known to have euphoric, sedative, and anabolic (bodybuilding) effects. It was originally sold over the counter to bodybuilders to help reduce body fat and build muscle. Concerns about GHB led the FDA to ban OTC sales in 1992, and GHB is now a Schedule I drug. (Schedule I drugs are classified as having a high potential for abuse, with no currently accepted medical use in the United States.)[103] GHB is an odorless, tasteless fluid. Like Rohypnol, GHB has been slipped into drinks without being detected, resulting in loss of memory, unconsciousness, amnesia, and even death. Other dangerous side effects include nausea, vomiting, seizures, hallucinations, coma, and respiratory distress.

Opioids (Narcotics)

Opioids cause drowsiness, relieve pain, and produce euphoria. Also called *narcotics*, opioids are derived from the parent drug **opium**, a dark, resinous substance made from the milky juice of the opium poppy seedpod, and they are all highly addictive. Opium and heroin are both illegal in the United States, but some opioids are available by prescription for medical purposes: Morphine is sometimes prescribed for severe pain, and codeine is found in prescription cough syrups and other painkillers. Several prescription drugs, including Vicodin, Percodan, OxyContin, Demerol, and Dilaudid, contain synthetic opioids.

Opium is extracted from opium poppy seedpods like this one.

Physical Effects of Opioids

Opioids are powerful depressants of the central nervous system. Opioid drugs are derived naturally from the opium plant or created synthetically. Side effects include drowsiness, mental confusion, nausea, and constipation.[104]

The human body's physiology could be said to encourage opioid addiction. Opioid-like hormones called **endorphins** are manufactured in the body and have multiple receptor sites, particularly in the central nervous system. When endorphins attach themselves at these points, they create feelings of painless well-being; medical researchers refer to them as "the body's own opioids." When their endorphin levels are high, people feel euphoric. The same euphoria occurs when opioids or related chemicals are active at the endorphin receptor sites.

Of all the opioids, heroin has the greatest notoriety as an addictive drug. *Heroin* is a white powder derived from morphine. *Black tar heroin* is a sticky, dark brown, foul-smelling form of heroin that is relatively pure and inexpensive. Once considered a cure for morphine dependence, heroin was later discovered to be even more addictive and potent than morphine. Today, heroin has no medical use.

Heroin is a depressant that produces drowsiness and a dreamy, mentally slow feeling. It can cause drastic mood swings, with euphoric highs followed by depressive lows. Chronic heroin users may develop a number of complications, including liver and kidney diseases, collapsed veins, abscesses, constipation, and infection of the heart lining. Symptoms of tolerance and withdrawal can appear within 3 weeks of first use.[105]

In 2015, 591,000 Americans reported having used heroin in the past year, a considerable increase since 2002.[106] Once predominantly found in urban areas, heroin use is becoming increasingly common in suburban and rural communities, particularly among white men and women.[107] Deaths from heroin overdoses have skyrocketed in recent years, rising from just over 1,800 deaths in 2000 to nearly 12,990 in 2015, particularly among those who are finding that heroin is a cheaper high than prescription opiates such as the oxycodone and hydrocodone to which they have become addicted.[108] This trend appears to be driven largely by 18- to 25-year-olds. Young and older adults hooked on painkillers are finding that heroin is cheaper and easier to obtain than prescription opioids.[109]

Although heroin is usually injected intravenously ("mainlined"), the contemporary version of heroin is so potent that users can get high by snorting or smoking the drug. This has attracted a more affluent group of users who

opioids Drugs that induce sleep, relieve pain, and produce euphoria; include derivatives of opium and synthetics with similar chemical properties; also called *narcotics*.

opium The parent drug of the opioids; made from the seedpod resin of the opium poppy.

endorphins Opioid-like hormones that are manufactured in the human body and contribute to natural feelings of well-being.

may not want to inject, for reasons such as the increased risk of contracting diseases like HIV.

Many users describe the rush they feel when injecting themselves as intensely pleasurable; others report unpredictable and unpleasant side effects. The temporary nature of the rush contributes to the drug's high potential for addiction; many addicts shoot up four or five times a day. Mainlining can cause veins to scar and eventually collapse. Once a vein has collapsed, it can no longer be used to introduce heroin into the bloodstream. Addicts become expert at locating new veins to use: in the feet, in the legs, in the temples, under the tongue, or in the groin.

Heroin addicts experience a distinct pattern of withdrawal. Symptoms of withdrawal include intense desire for the drug, sleep disturbance, dilated pupils, loss of appetite, irritability, goose bumps, and muscle tremors. The most difficult time in the withdrawal process occurs 24 to 72 hours after last use. All of the preceding symptoms continue, along with nausea, abdominal cramps, restlessness, insomnia, vomiting, diarrhea, extreme anxiety, hot and cold flashes, elevated blood pressure, and rapid heartbeat and respiration. Once the peak of withdrawal has passed, all these symptoms begin to subside.[110]

Hallucinogens

Hallucinogens, or *psychedelics*, are substances that are capable of creating auditory or visual hallucinations and unusual changes in mood, thoughts, and feelings. The major receptor sites for most of these drugs are in the reticular formation (located in the brain stem at the upper end of the spinal cord), which is responsible for interpreting outside stimuli before allowing these signals to travel to other parts of the brain. When a hallucinogen is present at a reticular formation site, sensory input becomes scrambled, and the user may see wavy walls instead of straight ones or may "smell" colors and "hear" tastes. This mixing of sensory messages is known as *synesthesia*. Users may also become less inhibited or may recall events long buried in the subconscious mind. The most widely recognized hallucinogens are LSD, Ecstasy, PCP, mescaline, psilocybin, and ketamine. All are illegal and carry severe penalties for manufacture, possession, transportation, or sale.

LSD First synthesized in the late 1930s by Swiss chemist Albert Hoffman, *lysergic acid diethylamide (LSD)* received media attention in the 1960s when

young people used the drug to "turn on, tune in, drop out." In 1970, federal authorities placed LSD on the list of controlled substances (Schedule I). Today, this dangerous psychedelic drug, known alternatively as "acid," has been making a comeback. It is estimated that 9.5 percent of Americans aged 12 or older have used LSD at least once in their lifetime.[111] A national survey of college students showed that fewer than 4.5 percent had used the drug in their lives.[112]

LSD is one of the most potent hallucinogenic drugs. An odorless, water-soluble substance, it is synthesized from lysergic acid, a compound found in rye fungus. A common method for taking LSD is by using blotter acid—small squares of blotter-like paper that have been impregnated with a liquid LSD mixture. The blotter is swallowed or chewed briefly. LSD also comes in tiny thin squares of gelatin called *windowpane* and in tablets called *microdots*, which are less than an eighth of an inch across (it would take ten or more to equal the size of an aspirin tablet).[113]

The psychological effects of LSD vary. LSD also distorts ordinary perceptions, such as the movement of stationary objects, as well as auditory or visual hallucinations. In addition, the drug shortens attention span, causing the mind to wander. Thoughts may be interposed and juxtaposed, so the user experiences several different thoughts simultaneously. Users become introspective, and suppressed memories may surface, often taking on bizarre symbolism. Many more effects are possible, including decreased aggressiveness and enhanced sensory experiences.[114]

In addition to its psychedelic effects, LSD produces several physical effects, including increased heart rate, elevated blood pressure and temperature, goose bumps, increased reflex speeds, muscle tremors and twitches,

> **hallucinogens** Substances capable of creating auditory or visual distortions and unusual changes in mood, thoughts, and feelings.

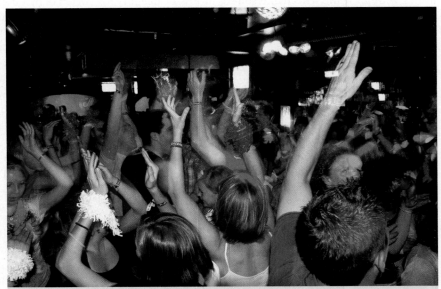

Although users may think so-called club drugs (such as Ecstasy, GHB, and ketamine) are harmless, research has shown that they can produce hallucinations, paranoia, amnesia, dangerous increases in heart rate and blood pressure, coma, and in some cases death.

perspiration, increased salivation, chills, headaches, and mild nausea. Because the drug also stimulates uterine muscle contractions, it can lead to premature labor and miscarriage in pregnant women.

Although there is no evidence that LSD is addictive, it does produce tolerance, so users may need to take more of the drug to get the same effect. This is a dangerous practice, as the drug is unpredictable.[115]

Ecstasy *Ecstasy* is a common street name for the drug *methylene-dioxymethamphetamine (MDMA)*, a synthetic compound with both stimulant and mildly hallucinogenic effects. It is one of the best-known **club drugs** or "designer drugs," a term applied to synthetic analogs of existing illicit drugs popular at nightclubs and all-night parties. Ecstasy creates feelings of extreme euphoria, openness and warmth; an increased willingness to communicate; feelings of love and empathy; increased awareness; and heightened appreciation for music. Young people may use Ecstasy initially to improve their mood or get energized. Ecstasy can enhance the sensory experience and distort perceptions, but it does not create visual hallucinations. Effects can last for 3 to 6 hours.[116]

Some of the risks associated with Ecstasy use are similar to those of other stimulants. Because of the nature of the drug, Ecstasy users are at risk of inappropriate or unintended emotional bonding and have a tendency to say things they might feel uncomfortable about later. Physical consequences of Ecstasy use may include mild to extreme jaw clenching, tongue and cheek chewing, short-term memory loss or confusion, increased body temperature, and increased heart rate and blood pressure. Combined with alcohol, Ecstasy can be extremely dangerous and sometimes fatal. As the effects of the drug wear off, the user can experience mild depression, fatigue, and a hangover that can last from days to weeks. Chronic use appears to damage the brain's ability to think and to regulate emotion, memory, sleep, and pain. Some studies indicate that Ecstasy may cause long-lasting neurotoxic effects by damaging brain cells that produce serotonin.[117]

MDMA in powder or crystal form—called "Molly," short for molecule—has become a popular festival drug. Unlike Ecstasy, which tends to be laced with ingredients such as caffeine or methamphetamine, Molly is considered pure MDMA. Still, many powders that are sold as Molly contain no actual MDMA. Some typical side effects of using Molly include grinding ones teeth, becoming dehydrated, feeling anxious, having trouble sleeping, fever, and losing one's appetite, as well as uncontrollable seizures, elevated blood pressure, high body temperature, and depression.[118]

PCP The synthetic substance *phencyclidine (PCP)* was originally developed as a dissociative anesthetic; patients who were given this drug could keep their eyes open, apparently remain conscious, and feel no pain during a medical procedure. Afterward, they would experience amnesia for the time that the drug was in their system. Such a drug had obvious advantages as an anesthetic, but its unpredictability and drastic effects (postoperative delirium, confusion, and agitation) caused it to be withdrawn from the legal market.[119]

> **club drugs** Synthetic analogs that produce effects similar to those of existing drugs.

On the illegal market, PCP is a white, crystalline powder that users often sprinkle onto marijuana cigarettes. It is dangerous and unpredictable, regardless of the method of administration. The effects of PCP depend on the dose. A small dose can produce effects similar to those of strong central nervous system depressants: slurred speech, impaired coordination, reduced sensitivity to pain, and reduced heart and respiratory rate. Large doses can cause fever, salivation, nausea, vomiting, and total loss of sensitivity to pain. PCP can also cause a rise in blood pressure, seizures, violent outbursts, coma and possibly death.[120]

Psychologically, PCP may produce either euphoria or dysphoria. It also is known to produce hallucinations as well as delusions and overall delirium. Some users experience a prolonged state of "nothingness." The long-term effects of PCP use are unknown.

Mescaline *Mescaline* is one of hundreds of chemicals derived from the peyote cactus, a small, button-like plant that grows in the southwestern United States and in Latin America. Natives of these regions have long used the dried peyote buttons for religious purposes. It is both a powerful hallucinogen and a central nervous system stimulant.

Users typically either swallow pieces of the cactus, called buttons, or soak them in water, creating an intoxicating liquid that can then be ingested. The effects of mescaline include visual hallucinations, altered states of consciousness, and occasionally feelings of anxiety or revulsion. Side effects of mescaline may include vomiting, dizziness, diarrhea, and headache. Effects may persist for up to 12 hours.[121]

Products sold on the street as mescaline are likely to be synthetic chemical relatives of the true drug. Street names of these products include DOM, STP, TMA, and MMDA. Any of these can be toxic in small quantities.

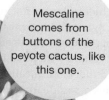

Mescaline comes from buttons of the peyote cactus, like this one.

Psilocybin *Psilocybin* and *psilocin* are the active chemicals in a group of mushrooms that are sometimes called "magic mushrooms." *Psilocybe* mushrooms, which grow throughout the world, can be cultivated from spores or harvested wild. When consumed, these mushrooms can cause hallucinations. Because many mushrooms resemble the *Psilocybe* variety, people who harvest wild mushrooms for any purpose should be certain of what they are doing.

Mushroom varieties can be easily misidentified, and mistakes can be fatal. Psilocybin is similar to LSD in its physical effects, which generally wear off in 6 to 12 hours.[122]

Ketamine The liquid form of *ketamine* ("Special K") is used as an anesthetic in some hospitals and veterinary clinics. After stealing it from hospitals or medical suppliers, dealers typically dry the liquid (usually by cooking it) and grind the residue into powder. Special K causes hallucinations because it inhibits the relay of sensory input; the brain fills the resulting void with visions, dreams, memories, and sensory distortions. The effects of ketamine are similar to those of PCP—confusion, agitation, aggression, and lack of coordination—but are even less predictable. Aftereffects of ketamine are less severe than those of Ecstasy, so it has grown in popularity as a club drug.[123]

Psilocybe mushrooms produce hallucinogenic effects when ingested.

Salvia Native to Southern Mexico, salvia is an herb from the mint family.[124] Its main active ingredient, salvinorin A, causes hallucinations by changing brain chemistry.[125] Although associated hallucinatory episodes have been described as intense, they are relatively short lasting, typically beginning after a minute and fading after 30 minutes.[126] These brief but extreme hallucinations often include changes in mood, body sensations, changes to visual perception, emotional swings, feeling detached, and an altered sense of self and reality.[127] Salvia's long-term effects have not been studied.

Inhalants

Inhalants are chemicals whose vapors, when inhaled, can cause hallucinations and create intoxicating and euphoric effects. Not commonly recognized as drugs, inhalants are legal to purchase and widely available but dangerous. They generally appeal to young people who can't afford or obtain illicit substances. Some misused products include rubber cement, model glue, paint thinner, aerosol sprays, lighter fluid, varnish, wax, spot removers, and gasoline. Most of these substances are sniffed or "huffed" by users in search of a quick, cheap high. Amyl nitrite, a vasodilator, and nitrous oxide ("laughing gas"), an anesthetic, are also sometimes abused.

Because they are inhaled, the volatile chemicals in these products reach the bloodstream within seconds. This characteristic, along with the fact that

inhalants Chemical vapors that are sniffed or inhaled to produce highs.

anabolic steroids Artificial forms of the hormone testosterone that promote muscle growth and strength.

ergogenic drugs Substances that are believed to enhance athletic performance.

dosages are extremely difficult to control because everyone has unique lung and breathing capacities, makes inhalants particularly dangerous. The effects of inhalants resemble those of central nervous system depressants: dizziness, disorientation, impaired coordination, reduced judgment, and slowed reaction times.[128]

An overdose of fumes from inhalants can cause unconsciousness and even death. Because the effect lasts only a few minutes, users may continue to inhale over several hours; this can lead to loss of consciousness and death.[129]

Anabolic Steroids

Anabolic steroids are artificial forms of the male hormone testosterone that promote muscle growth and strength. Steroids are available in two forms: injectable solutions and pills. **Ergogenic drugs** are used primarily by people who believe that the drugs will increase their strength, power, bulk (weight), speed, and athletic performance.

It was once estimated that up to 20 percent of college athletes used steroids.[130] Now that the National Collegiate Athletic Association (NCAA) has instituted stricter drug-testing policies, reported use of anabolic steroids among intercollegiate athletes has decreased. In 2014, fewer than half of 1 percent of college athletes surveyed reported use of anabolic steroids within the past 12 months.[131] Those who reported using anabolic steroids used them less than once per week. Of those, half reported that their first experience with anabolic steroids occurred after the age of 18.[132] The perceived use of anabolic steroid on college campuses is much higher than reality.[133] In a 2014 survey, fewer than 1 percent of students reported using them within the past 30 days.[134]

Physical Effects of Steroids Although their primary effects are not psychotropic, anabolic steroids can produce a state of euphoria and diminished fatigue in addition to increased bulk and power in both sexes. These qualities give steroids an addictive quality. When users stop, they can experience psychological withdrawal and sometimes severe depression, in some cases leading to suicide attempts.[135]

Men and women who use steroids experience a variety of adverse effects, including mood swings (aggression and violence, sometimes known as "roid rage"), acne, liver damage, elevated cholesterol levels, kidney damage, and immune system disturbances.[136] There is also a danger of transmitting HIV and hepatitis through shared needles. In women, large doses of anabolic steroids may trigger the development of masculine attributes such as lowered voice, increased facial and body hair, and male-pattern baldness; large doses may also result in an enlarged clitoris, smaller breasts, and changes in or absence of menstruation. When taken by healthy men, anabolic steroids shut down the body's production of testosterone, causing men's breasts to grow and their testicles to atrophy.

Steroid Use and Society The Anabolic Steroids Control Act (ASCA) of 1990 makes it a crime to possess, prescribe, or distribute anabolic steroids for any use other than the treatment of specific diseases. Penalties for their illegal use include up to 1 year of imprisonment and/or a fine of $1,000 for the first offense, mandatory imprisonment of 15 days to 2 years and a $2,500 fine for a second offense, and mandatory imprisonment of 90 days to 3 years and a fine of $2,500 or more for a third offense. Federal punishment for intent to distribute steroids is not more than 5 years of imprisonment, with 2 years of parole and a $250,000 fine for the first offense and 10 years of imprisonment with a minimum 4 years of parole and/or higher fines for a second offense. The statutory maximum punishment may be doubled if the person is convicted of selling steroids to a minor or near schools and colleges.[137]

In recent years, high-profile athletes in sports such as cycling, track and field, swimming, and baseball have been in the media spotlight for suspected use of steroids or other banned performance-enhancing drugs. Over 100 Russian track and field athletes were barred from the 2016 Summer Olympic Games for illegal drug use.

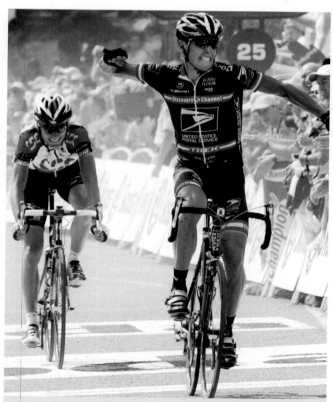

After being stripped of seven Tour de France titles in 2012 and an Olympic medal in 2013, cyclist Lance Armstrong publicly ended his years of denial and admitted to doping. He was banned from cycling for life and has been sued by the U.S. federal government and others for fraud.

LO 6 | TREATING AND REDUCING DRUG ABUSE

Discuss treatment and recovery options for addicts, as well as public health approaches to preventing drug abuse and reducing the impact of addiction on our society.

An estimated 20.8 million (one in seven) Americans aged 12 years or older needed treatment for an illicit drug or alcohol use problem in 2015.[138] Only 10 percent of those addicted will receive treatment.[139] Recovery from drug addiction or addiction to a behavior is a long-term process and frequently requires multiple episodes of treatment. The first step generally begins with abstinence—refraining from the behavior. **Detoxification** refers to an early abstinence period during which an addict adjusts physically and cognitively to being free from the addiction's influence. It occurs in virtually every recovering addict, and it is uncomfortable for most addicts and can be dangerous for some. This is true primarily for those addicted to chemicals, especially alcohol and heroin, and painkillers such as OxyContin. For these people, early abstinence may involve profound withdrawals that require medical supervision. Because of this, most inpatient treatment programs provide a pretreatment component of supervised detoxification to achieve abstinence safely before treatment begins. In this section, we will discuss some common approaches to treating substance abuse problems.

Over the years, scientific research has shown that treatment can help addicts recover from their addiction. The Surgeon General's Report on Alcohol, Drugs and Health (2016) identified key findings that support the effectiveness of treatment interventions, therapies, services and medications for substance abuse disorders. Some of these findings are as follows:

- Substance abuse disorders can be treated effectively, with reoccurrence rates no higher than those for other chronic diseases such as diabetes, asthma, and hypertension.
- Substance abuse disorders can be easily identified through brief screenings in clinical settings that include brief conversations with a health care provider and other brief interventions.
- Treatment for substance abuse disorders is less costly in the long run than no treatment.

detoxification The process, which involves abstinence, of freeing a drug user from an intoxicating or addictive substance in the body or from dependence on such a substance.

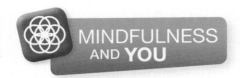

MINDFULNESS-BASED RELAPSE PREVENTION FOR ADDICTION RECOVERY

Mindfulness is becoming recognized as an effective way to prevent relapse in addiction recovery. Similar to mindfulness-based cognitive therapy used to help treat depression, Mindfulness-Based Relapse Prevention (MBRP) focuses on two major predictors of relapse: negative emotions and cravings. MBRP is a group-based program that typically meets for eight sessions. It was originally created for people coming out of treatment who needed an aftercare program, but it has since evolved to provide continued support throughout the recovery process. The theoretical framework for the integration of mindfulness and cognitive-behavioral relapse prevention is that mindfulness may help people become less attached to emotions, helping them prevent spiraling thoughts that might lead to relapse. By increasing emotional awareness, redefining how one responds to triggers for relapse such as boredom, and developing coping skills, the person in recovery learns how to interrupt the familiar cycle of substance abuse behavior. If a lapse does occur, mindfulness can help to reduce the feelings of guilt and shame that increase the risk of relapse. To focus on bringing awareness to your own triggers and cravings, try the following activity:

Over the next week, pay attention to the way your body responds to pleasant events. Be aware of detailed body sensations, thoughts and emotions occurring with the pleasant event. Use the following chart to record your experiences in as much detail as you can. Do your best to pay attention to at least one pleasant occurrence each day.

Pleasant Events

	What was the experience?	Were you aware of the pleasant feelings while the event was happening?	How did your body feel in detail during the experience?	What moods, feelings, and thoughts accompanied this event?	What thoughts are in your mind now as you write about this event?
Monday					
Tuesday					
Wednesday					
Thursday					
Friday					
Saturday					
Sunday					

Sources: C. Gregoire, "Mindfulness-Based Relapse Prevention Holds Promise for Treating Addiction," *Science,* 11/18/2015, http://www.huffingtonpost.com/entry/mindfulness-based-relapse-prevention-interview_us_5645fd24e4b08cda3488638b; S. Weerasinghe and S. Barotine, "Mindfulness for Addiction Recovery: A Cognitive Disciplinary Preventive Approach to Avoid Relapse in Substance Abuse," *Journal of Basic & Applied Sciences* 12 (2016): 81–91; Wired for Compassion, "Mindfulness Based Relapse Prevention: 8 Week Programme Course Handbook, http://www.wiredforcompassion.org.uk/wp-content/uploads/2012/02/Mindfulness-relapse-prevention-workbook.pdf.

- Behavioral therapies can be effective in treating substance abuse disorders.
- Medications can be effective in treating serious substance abuse disorders but are often underutilized.

Treatment Approaches

Outpatient behavioral treatment encompasses a variety of programs for people with substance abuse problems who visit a clinic at regular intervals. Most of the programs involve individual or group drug counseling. *Residential treatment programs* can also be very effective, especially for people with more severe problems. Therapeutic communities are highly structured programs in which addicts remain at a residence, typically for 6 to 12 months, with a focus on resocializing the addict to a drug-free lifestyle.

After a serious substance abuse disorder goes into remission, it can take as long as 4 to 5 years for the person's risk of relapse to drop below 15 percent, the risk of the general population of developing a substance use disorder.[140] As for others with chronic diseases, support systems that provide monitoring and management to help maintain remission and prevent relapse are recommended. Such support systems can help individuals focus on more self awareness and *self-compassion*, allowing those who slip in their path to recovery to cut themselves some slack; acknowledge the difficulties of their addiction and reasons for the slip; and provide support for getting back on track with positive self-talk and behaviors. Some of these recovery support systems can include housing, education, and support groups.[141] See **Mindfulness and You** for more on mindfulness-based relapse prevention.

WHAT DO YOU THINK?

Do you believe that an athlete's admission of steroid use invalidates his or her athletic achievements?

- How do you think professional athletes who have used steroids or other performance enhancers should be disciplined?
- If you are an athlete, have you ever considered using some type of ergogenic aid to improve your performance?

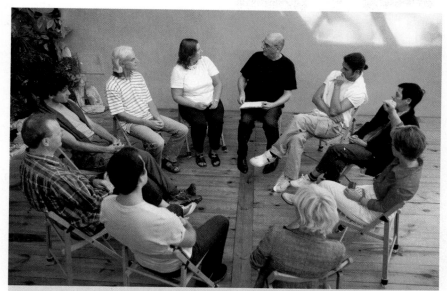

For most addicts, recovery is a long, difficult process; for some people it can be a lifelong journey. Therapy often takes the form of group meetings, such as those held by Alcoholics Anonymous, Narcotics Anonymous, and other 12-step programs.

12-Step Programs The first 12-step program was Alcoholics Anonymous (AA), begun in 1935 in Akron, Ohio. The 12-step program has since become the most widely used approach to dealing not only with alcoholism, but also with drug abuse and various other addictive or dysfunctional behaviors. There are more than 130 different recovery programs based on the program, including Narcotics Anonymous, Cocaine Anonymous, Crystal Meth Anonymous, Gamblers Anonymous, and Pills Anonymous.[142]

The 12-step program is nonjudgmental and based on the idea that a program's only purpose is to work on personal recovery. Working the 12 steps includes admitting to having a serious problem, recognizing there is an outside power that could help, consciously relying on that power, admitting and listing character defects, seeking deliverance from defects, apologizing to the individuals one has harmed in the past, and helping other people who have the same problem. There is no membership cost, and the meetings are open to anyone who wishes to attend.

Recovery Coaching Recovery coaching is relatively new to the addiction field. Recovery coaches are not treatment providers but help people who are being discharged from treatment to connect with community resources. The responsibility of recovery coaches is to provide four types of support: emotional support, informational support, help in accessing health and social services, and help in finding healthy social connections and recreational activities.[143]

Social, Recreational, and Social Media Support Systems An increasing number of social and recreational programs provide support for people in recovery. These programs make it easier to maintain sobriety in an environment that does not involve alcohol or other drugs.

Programs or businesses such as recovery cafes, clubhouses, sports leagues, musician's organizations, and arts and theater groups are just a few examples of alternatives available.

Social media, mobile health apps, and specific online recovery programs can provide social support to people in recovery. The ability to connect with others for social interaction, support, and friendship helps to reduce the isolation that those in recovery can experience. Studies are beginning to show that these emerging tools have positive benefits for preventing relapse and support those in recovery.[144]

Vaccines against Addictive Drugs Vaccines have the potential to offer people who have kicked their habit a way to stay clean by making the body immune to the effects of the drug, thereby decreasing the motivation to use.

To help manage the opioid and heroin epidemic, two vaccines are advancing toward human clinical trials. The first stimulates the immune system to attack the heroin and eliminate it from the body. The second keeps heroin from reaching the brain and also prevents HIV infection.[145]

A promising new cocaine vaccine that keeps the user from getting high by stimulating the immune system to attack the drug when it is taken is in development. Clinical human trials are expected to begin soon. Vaccines against nicotine and methamphetamine are also in development.[146]

Other Pharmacological Treatments Methadone maintenance is one treatment available for people addicted to heroin or other opioids. Methadone, a synthetic narcotic, is chemically similar enough to opioids to control the tremors, chills, vomiting, diarrhea, and severe abdominal pains of withdrawal. Methadone dosage is decreased over a period of time until the addict is weaned off it.

Methadone maintenance is controversial because of the drug's own potential for addiction. Critics contend that the program merely substitutes one addiction for another. Proponents argue that people on methadone maintenance are less likely to engage in criminal activities to support their habits than heroin addicts are. For this reason, many methadone maintenance programs are financed by state or federal government and are available free of charge or at reduced cost.

Naltrexone (Trexan), an opioid antagonist, has been approved as a treatment. It is used to treat opioid use disorders and alcohol use disorders. While on naltrexone, recovering addicts do not have the compulsion to use heroin, and if they do use it, they don't get high, so there is no point in using the drug.[147]

A number of new drug therapies for opioid dependence are emerging. Another new drug therapy, buprenorphine

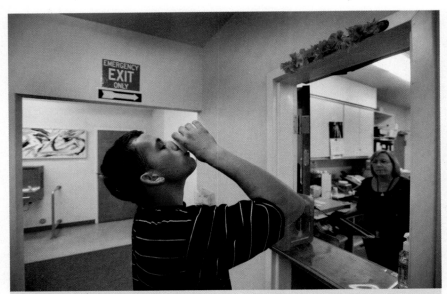

Methadone is a synthetic narcotic that blocks the effects of heroin withdrawal. Although it is a narcotic and must be administered under the supervision of clinic or pharmacy staff, methadone allows many heroin addicts to lead somewhat normal lives.

(Temgesic), is a mild, nonaddicting synthetic opioid; it works a lot like methadone by blocking withdrawal symptoms and heroin cravings. One of the advantages of buprenorphine is that it does not require addicts to go to a clinic or pharmacy to get their medication; rather, it can be taken at home.

Drug Treatment and Recovery for College Students

A growing number of college campuses provide collegiate recovery programs for students. While these programs vary from campus to campus, most provide some combination of recovery residence halls or recovery-specific wings, counseling services and on-campus meetings, and other educational and social supports. Many students who participate in collegiate recovery programs may have mental health problems, such as depression or an eating disorder, in addition to their substance use disorder, which can complicate recovery.[148]

Early intervention increases the likelihood of successful treatment. Depending on the severity of abuse or dependence, college students undergoing drug treatment may be required to spend time away from school in a residential drug rehabilitation inpatient facility. The needs of college students seeking drug treatment in rehab do not differ greatly from those of other adult recovering addicts, but for best results, the community of addicts should include people of a similar age and educational background. Private therapy, group therapy, cognitive training, nutrition counseling, and health therapies can all be used to help with recovery.

Addressing Drug Misuse and Abuse in the United States

Illegal drug use in the United States costs about $193 billion per year.[149] This estimate includes $11 billion in the cost of health care, $120 billion in lost productivity, and $61 billion in the cost of criminal investigation, prosecution, incarceration, and other associated criminal justice costs.[150] Americans are alarmed by the persistent problem of illegal drug use. Respondents in public opinion polls think that the government should focus on treatment for people who use illegal drugs such as heroin or cocaine. There is increased support for moving away from mandatory sentences for nonviolent drug crimes. Many strategies include prevention strategies that focus on helping individuals develop the knowledge, attitudes, and skills to make good decisions. Other approaches encourage use of community prevention strategies to make it easier to act in healthy ways. These strategies involve community leaders, parents, and local officials working together to shift individual attitudes and community norms.[151] To address safety concerns, many employers have instituted mandatory drug testing. Despite controversies over the accuracy of urinalysis tests, this practice is becoming more common.

All of these approaches will probably help up to a point, but they do not offer a total solution to the problem. Drug abuse has been a part of human behavior for thousands of years, and it is not likely to disappear in the near future. For this reason, it is necessary to educate ourselves and to develop the self-discipline necessary to avoid dangerous drug dependence.

In general, researchers in the field of drug education agree that a multimodal approach is best. Young people should be taught the difference between drug use, misuse, and abuse. Factual information that is free of scare tactics must be presented; lecturing and moralizing have proven not to work.

ASSESS YOURSELF

Do You Have a Problem with Drugs?

LIVE IT! ASSESS YOURSELF

An interactive version of this assessment is available online in Mastering Health.

Answering the following questions will help you determine whether you have developed a drug problem:

Yes   **No**

___   ___ **1.** In the past year, have you found it significantly difficult to pay attention in class, at work, or at home?

___   ___ **2.** Have you ever thought that you should cut down on your drug use?

___   ___ **3.** Have you had blackouts or flashbacks as a result of your drug use?

___   ___ **4.** Have people annoyed (irritated, angered, etc.) you by criticizing your drug use?

___   ___ **5.** Have you ever been arrested or in trouble with the law because of your drug use?

___   ___ **6.** Have you lost friends because of your drug use?

___   ___ **7.** Have you ever felt bad or guilty about your drug use?

___   ___ **8.** Have you ever thought you might have a drug problem?

If you answered "yes" to *any* of the questions, you should consider talking to a counselor or health care provider either on campus at your health or counseling center or your family health care provider.

Source: Hazelden Betty Ford Foundation, "Do You Need to Talk to Someone about a Drug, Alcohol or Mental Health Problem?," 2016, http://www.hazelden.org/web/public/talk_about_drug_alcohol_mental_health.page.

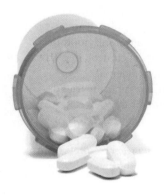

YOUR PLAN FOR **CHANGE**

The **ASSESS YOURSELF** activity describes signs of being controlled by drugs or having a drug problem. Depending on your results, you may need to change certain behaviors that may be detrimental to your health.

TODAY, YOU CAN:

☐ Imagine a situation in which someone offers you a drug and think of several different ways of refusing. Rehearse these scenarios in your head.

☐ Think about the drug use patterns among your social group. Are you ever uncomfortable with these people because of their drug use? Is it difficult to avoid using drugs when you are with them? If the answers are yes, begin exploring ways to expand your social circle.

WITHIN THE NEXT TWO WEEKS, YOU CAN:

☐ Stop by your campus health center to find out about drug treatment programs or support groups they may have.

☐ If you are concerned about your own drug use or the drug use of a close friend, make an appointment with a counselor to talk about the issue.

BY THE END OF THE SEMESTER, YOU CAN:

☐ Participate in clubs, activities, and social groups that do not rely on substance abuse for their amusement.

☐ If you have a drug problem, make a commitment to enter a treatment program. Acknowledge that you have a problem and that you need the assistance of others to help you overcome it.

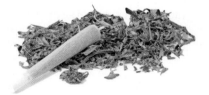

STUDY **PLAN**

Visit the Study Area in Mastering Health to enhance your study plan with MP3 Tutor Sessions, Practice Quizzes, Flashcards, and more!

CHAPTER **REVIEW**

LO 1 | What Is Addiction?

- Addiction is the continued involvement with a substance or activity despite ongoing negative consequences of that involvement; without the behavior, the addict experiences withdrawal. All addictions have four common symptoms: compulsion, loss of control, negative consequences, and denial.
- Codependents are typically friends or family members who are controlled by an addict's behavior. Enablers are people who knowingly or unknowingly protect addicts from the consequences of their behavior.

LO 2 | Addictive Behaviors

- Addictive behaviors include disordered gambling, compulsive buying, exercise addiction, technology addiction, work addiction, and compulsive sexual behavior.

LO 3 | What Is a Drug?

- Drugs are substances other than food that are intended to affect the structure or function of the mind or the body through chemical action. Almost all psychoactive drugs affect neurotransmission in the brain.
- The six categories of drugs are prescription drugs, OTC drugs, recreational drugs, herbal preparations, illicit (illegal) drugs, and commercial drugs. Routes of administration include oral ingestion, inhalation, injection (intravenous, intramuscular, and subcutaneous), transdermal, and suppositories.

LO 4 | Drug Misuse and Abuse

- OTC medications are drugs that do not require a prescription. Some

OTC medications, including sleep aids, cold medicines, and diet pills, can be addictive.
- Prescription drug abuse is at an all-time high, particularly among college students. Only marijuana is more commonly abused. The most commonly abused prescription drugs are opioids/narcotics, depressants, and stimulants.
- People from all walks of life use illicit drugs. Drug use declined from the mid-1980s to the early 1990s but has remained steady since then. However, among young people, use of drugs has been rising in recent years.

LO 5 | Common Drugs of Abuse

- Drugs of abuse (both legal and illegal) include stimulants; cannabis products, including marijuana; narcotics/depressants; hallucinogens; inhalants; and anabolic steroids. Each has its own set of risks and effects.

LO 6 | Treating and Reducing Drug Abuse

- Treatment begins with abstinence from the drug or addictive behavior. Treatment programs may be outpatient or residential and may include individual, group, or family therapy, as well as 12-step programs.
- The drug problem affects everyone through crime and elevated health care costs. Researchers agree that a multimodal approach to drug misuse and abuse is best.

POP **QUIZ**

LO 1 | What Is Addiction?

1. Which of the following is not a characteristic of addiction?

a. Denial
b. Acknowledgment of self-destructive behavior
c. Loss of control
d. Obsession with a substance or behavior

LO 2 | Addictive Behaviors

2. An example of a process addiction is
a. a cocaine addiction.
b. a gambling addiction.
c. a marijuana addiction.
d. a caffeine addiction.

LO 3 | What Is a Drug?

3. Rebecca takes a number of medications for various conditions, including Prinivil (an antihypertensive drug), insulin (a medication for diabetes), and Claritin (an antihistamine). This is an example of
a. synergism.
b. illegal drug use.
c. polydrug use.
d. antagonism.

4. Cross-tolerance occurs when
a. drugs work at the same receptor site so that one blocks the action of the other.
b. the effects of one drug are eliminated or reduced by the presence of another drug at the receptor site.
c. a person develops a physiological tolerance to one drug and shows a similar tolerance to certain other drugs as a result.
d. two or more drugs interact and the effects of the individual drugs are multiplied beyond what normally would be expected if they were taken alone.

LO 4 | Drug Misuse and Abuse

5. The excessive use of any drug is called
   a. drug misuse.
   b. drug addiction.
   c. drug tolerance.
   d. drug abuse.

6. Which of the following is *not* an example of drug misuse?
   a. Developing tolerance to a drug
   b. Taking a friend's prescription medicine
   c. Taking medicine more often than is recommended
   d. Not following the instructions when taking a medicine

LO 5 | Common Drugs of Abuse

7. Which of the following is classified as a stimulant?
   a. Methamphetamine
   b. Alcohol
   c. Marijuana
   d. LSD

8. The psychoactive drug mescaline is found in what plant?
   a. Mushrooms
   b. Peyote cactus
   c. Marijuana
   d. Belladonna

LO 6 | Treating and Reducing Drug Abuse

9. Generally, the first step in a drug treatment program is
   a. cognitive therapy.
   b. behavioral therapy.
   c. resocialization.
   d. detoxification.

10. Which of the following statements is *false*?
    a. Only one in ten people with a substance abuse disorder receive treatment.
    b. Treatment for substance abuse disorders are less costly in the long run than no treatment.
    c. Identification of a substance abuse disorder requires a set of complex screenings on admission to a treatment center.
    d. Medications can be effective in treating serious substance abuse disorders.

*Answers to the Pop Quiz can be found on page A-1. If you answered a question incorrectly, review the section identified by the Learning Outcome. For even more study tools, visit **Mastering Health**.*

THINK ABOUT IT!

LO 1 | What Is Addiction?

1. Discuss how addiction affects family and friends. What role do family and friends play in helping the addict get help and maintain recovery?

LO 2 | Addictive Behaviors

2. What differentiates a process (behavioral) addiction from a substance abuse addiction?

LO 3 | What Is a Drug?

3. Explain the terms *synergism* and *antagonism*.

4. Why and how to drugs work? What are some of the different ways in which different types of drugs interact with brain chemistry?

LO 4 | Drug Misuse and Abuse

5. Do you think there is such a thing as responsible use of illicit drugs? Would you change any of the current laws governing drugs? How would you determine what is legitimate and illegitimate use?

6. Why do you think so many young people today are abusing prescription drugs? Do you perceive prescription drug abuse as being less dangerous or illegal than illicit drug use? Why? Do you think this is an accurate or biased perception?

LO 5 | Common Drugs of Abuse

7. Why do you think many people today think that marijuana use is not dangerous? What are the arguments in favor of legalizing marijuana? What are the arguments against legalization?

8. What accounts for the fact that some drugs are more addictive than others, chemically, culturally, and psychologically?

LO 6 | Treating and Reducing Drug Abuse

9. What types of programs do you think would be effective in preventing drug abuse among high school and college students? How would programs for high school students differ from those for college students?

ACCESS YOUR HEALTH ON THE INTERNET

For links to the websites below, visit the Study Area in Mastering Health.

The following websites explore further topics and issues related to drug addiction and alcohol abuse.

Club Drugs. The website provides science-based information about club drugs. **www.drugabuse.gov/ drugs-abuse/club-drugs**

Join Together. An excellent site for the most current information related to substance abuse. Also includes information on alcohol and drug policy and provides advice on organizing and taking political action. **www.drugfree. org/join-together**

National Institute on Drug Abuse (NIDA). The home page of this U.S. government agency has information on the latest statistics and findings in drug research. **www.nida.nih.gov**

Substance Abuse and Mental Health Services Administration (SAMHSA). Outstanding resource for information about national surveys, ongoing research, and national drug interventions. **www.samhsa.gov**

National Center for Responsible Gambling. A resource for gambling information pertinent to college campuses. **www. collegegambling.org**

9 Drinking Alcohol Responsibly and Ending Tobacco Use

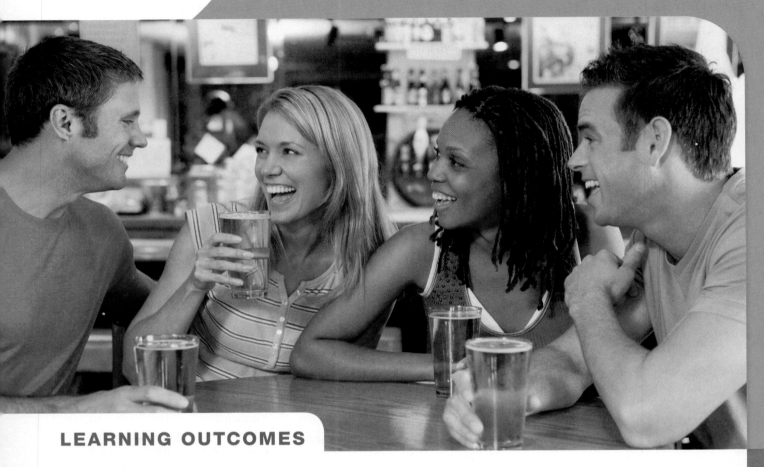

LEARNING OUTCOMES

LO **1** Explain the physiological and behavioral effects of alcohol, including absorption, metabolism, and blood alcohol concentration.

LO **2** Identify short-term and long-term effects of alcohol consumption.

LO **3** Describe alcohol use patterns of college students, practical strategies for drinking responsibly, and ways to cope with campus and societal pressures to drink.

LO **4** Describe alcohol use disorder and its risk factors, causes, and costs to society, and discuss options for treatment.

LO **5** Discuss the rate of tobacco use in the United States in general and among college students in particular, and explain the social and political issues involved in tobacco use and prevention.

LO **6** Identify different types of tobacco products and the chemicals they contain, and explain their effects on the body.

LO **7** Describe the health risks and physical impact associated with using tobacco products and with environmental tobacco smoke.

LO **8** Describe methods and benefits of smoking cessation.

Alcohol is not just a beverage. It's a drug that can interact with other drugs you may be using. When alcohol and prescription drugs are taken together, severe medical problems can result, including alcohol poisoning, unconsciousness, respiratory depression, and death. And if the life-threatening health consequences aren't enough to make you give up smoking, consider the negative impact smoking can have on your social (and romantic!) life. Popular media may make smoking seem glamorous and sexy, but in reality, smoking makes your breath, hair, and clothing smell bad; it causes your skin to age prematurely; it yellows your teeth; and it can interfere with a man's ability to achieve and maintain an erection.

When many of us think of dangerous drugs, we automatically think of illegal substances such as heroin or cocaine. But in reality, two socially accepted drugs—alcohol and tobacco—kill far more people. Annually, excessive use of alcohol is responsible for about 88,000 deaths—twice as many as illicit drugs[1]—and tobacco use is the single largest preventable cause of death in the United States, claiming nearly 480,000 lives a year.[2]

LO 1 | ALCOHOL: AN OVERVIEW

Explain the physiological and behavioral effects of alcohol, including absorption, metabolism, and blood alcohol concentration.

Throughout history, humans have used alcohol for everything from social gatherings to religious ceremonies. The consumption of alcoholic beverages is interwoven with many traditions, and moderate use of alcohol can enhance celebrations or special times. Research shows that very low levels of alcohol consumption, particularly wine, may actually lower some health risks in older adults.[3] Although alcohol may play a positive role in some people's lives, it is first and foremost a chemical substance that affects physical and mental behavior. Alcohol is a drug; if not used responsibly, it can be dangerous.

86%

of people age 18 or older report drinking ALCOHOL at some point in their life.

More than half of Americans consume alcoholic beverages regularly, and about 21 percent abstain from drinking alcohol altogether.[4] Among those who drink, consumption patterns vary. More men are regular drinkers, and men typically drink more than women. White drinkers are more likely to drink daily or nearly daily than nonwhites. Abstainers are more likely to be women, Asian American or African American, and employed. Adults in poor families are more than twice as likely to be lifetime abstainers as are adults in nonpoor families.[5]

The Chemistry and Potency of Alcohol

The intoxicating substance in beer, wine, liquor, and liqueurs is **ethyl alcohol**, or **ethanol**. It is produced during a process called **fermentation**, in which yeast organisms break down plant sugars, yielding ethanol and carbon dioxide. For beer and wine, the process ends with fermentation. Hard liquor is produced through **distillation**, a process during which alcohol vapors are condensed and mixed with water to make the final product.

The **proof** of an alcoholic drink is a measure of the percentage of alcohol in the beverage and therefore its strength. The alcohol percentage is half of the given proof. For example, 80 proof whiskey is 40 percent alcohol by volume, and 100 proof vodka is 50 percent alcohol by volume. Lower-proof drinks will produce fewer alcohol effects than the same amount of higher-proof drinks. Most wines are between 12 and 15 percent alcohol, and most beers are between 2 and 8 percent alcohol, depending on state laws and type of beer.

When discussing alcohol consumption, researchers usually talk in terms of standard drinks. As defined by the National Institute on Alcohol Abuse and Alcoholism (NIAAA), a **standard drink** is any drink that contains about 14 grams of pure alcohol (about 0.6 fluid ounce or 1.2 tablespoons; see **FIGURE 9.1**). The actual size of a standard drink depends on the proof: A 12-ounce can of beer and a 1.5-ounce shot of vodka are both considered one standard drink because they contain the same amount of alcohol—about 0.6 fluid ounce. If you are estimating your blood alcohol concentration using standard drinks as a measure, keep in mind the size of your drinks as well as their proof. For example, you may have bought only one beer at the ballpark last weekend, but if it came in a 22-ounce cup, you actually consumed two standard drinks.

ethyl alcohol (ethanol) Addictive drug produced by fermentation that is the intoxicating substance in alcoholic beverages.

fermentation The process in which yeast organisms break down plant sugars to yield ethanol.

distillation The process in which alcohol vapors are condensed and mixed with water to make hard liquor.

proof The measure of the percentage of alcohol in a beverage; the proof is double the percentage of alcohol in the drink.

standard drink The amount of any beverage that contains about 14 grams of pure alcohol.

Standard drink equivalent (and % alcohol)	Approximate number of standard drinks in:
Beer = 12 oz (~5% alcohol)	12 oz = 1 16 oz = 1.3 22 oz = 2 40 oz = 3.3
Malt liquor = 8.5 oz (~7% alcohol)	12 oz = 1.5 16 oz = 2 22 oz = 2.5 40 oz = 4.5
Table wine = 5 oz (~12% alcohol)	750-mL (25-oz) bottle = 5
80 proof spirits (gin, vodka, etc.) = 1.5 oz (~40% alcohol)	mixed drink = 1 or more* pint (16 oz) = 11 fifth (25 oz) = 17 1.75 L (59 oz) = 39

FIGURE 9.1 **What Is a Standard Drink?**

*Note: It can be difficult to estimate the number of standard drinks in a single mixed drink made with hard liquor. Depending on factors such as the type of spirits and the recipe, a mixed drink can contain from one to three or more standard drinks.

Source: Adapted from National Institute on Alcohol Abuse and Alcoholism, *Rethinking Drinking: Alcohol and Your Health*, NIH Publication No. 15-3770 (Bethesda, MD: National Institutes of Health, Revised 2016).

Absorption and Metabolism

Whereas the compounds found in most foods and drugs have to be broken down via digestion before they can be absorbed into the bloodstream, alcohol molecules are small enough to be absorbed. Approximately 20 percent of ingested alcohol diffuses through the stomach lining into the bloodstream, and nearly 80 percent passes through the lining of the upper third of the small intestine. A negligible amount of alcohol is absorbed through the lining of the mouth.

Several factors influence how quickly your body will absorb alcohol: the alcohol concentration in your drink, the amount of alcohol you consume, the amount of food in your stomach, your metabolism, your weight, and your mood. The higher the concentration of alcohol in your drink, the more rapidly it will be absorbed. As a rule, wine and beer are absorbed more slowly than distilled beverages.

"Fizzy" alcoholic beverages, such as champagne and carbonated wines, are absorbed more rapidly than those containing no carbonation. Carbonated beverages and drinks served with mixers cause the pyloric valve—which controls passage of stomach contents into the small intestine—to relax, thereby emptying the stomach contents more rapidly into the small intestine. Because the greatest absorption of alcohol occurs in the small intestine, carbonated beverages increase the rate of absorption. In drinkers of high concentrations of alcohol, the pyloric valve can become stuck in the closed position—a condition called pylorospasm. During pylorospasm, alcohol becomes trapped in the stomach, causing irritation and often inducing vomiting. The Student Health Today box discusses the effects of mixing energy drinks with alcohol.

The more alcohol you consume, the longer absorption takes. Absorption of alcohol also takes longer if there is food in your stomach, because the surface area exposed to alcohol is smaller and because a full stomach retards the emptying of alcoholic beverages into the small intestine.

Mood is another factor in absorption. In fact, powerful moods such as those that occur during stress and tension are likely to cause the stomach to dump its contents into the small intestine rapidly, meaning that alcohol is absorbed much faster when people are tense than when they are relaxed.

Once absorbed into the bloodstream, alcohol circulates throughout the body and is metabolized in the liver, where it is converted to *acetaldehyde*—a toxic chemical that can cause nausea and vomiting as well as long-term effects such as liver damage—by the enzyme *alcohol dehydrogenase*. It is then rapidly oxidized to *acetate*, converted to carbon dioxide and water, and eventually excreted from the body. A very small portion of alcohol is excreted unchanged by the kidneys, lungs, and skin.

Alcohol contains 7 calories (kcal) per gram. This means that the average beer contains about 150 calories. Mixed drinks may contain more calories if the alcohol is combined with sugary soda or fruit juice. The body uses the calories in alcohol in the same way as those found in carbohydrates: for immediate energy or for storage as fat if the calories are not immediately needed.

Alcohol breakdown occurs at a fairly constant rate of 0.5 ounce per hour (slightly less than one standard drink)—approximately equivalent to 12 ounces of 5 percent beer, 5 ounces

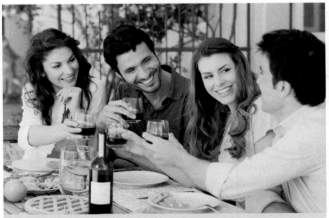

Eating while drinking slows the absorption of alcohol into the bloodstream. Other factors that influence how rapidly a person's body absorbs alcohol include gender, body weight, body composition, and mood.

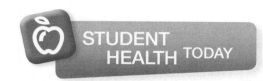
ALCOHOL AND ENERGY DRINKS
A Dangerous Mix

Energy drinks are aggressively marketed on college campuses. Manufacturers often give away samples to promote them. The success of these products is based on claims that they provide a burst of energy from caffeine and other plant-based stimulants and vitamins. Thirty-four percent of 18- to 24-year-olds are regular consumers of energy drinks.

Alcohol energy drink products such as Rockstar 21 and Sparks are almost impossible to find these days since, for the most part, they have been forced off the market by the FDA and other governing bodies. They originally became popular in the second half of the last decade, but by 2010 warning letters were sent out by the FDA and these alcohol and caffeine beverages began to disappear. In the United States, you will not find these products on the shelves. However, there are many independent websites that still promote mixing alcohol and energy drinks.

Students often mix energy drinks with alcohol, and these combinations can be particularly dangerous. College men who use alcohol-mixed energy drinks score more highly on risk-taking measures. In a recent study, most college students had neutral or negative views of alcohol-mixed drinks. Those who most frequently consume alcohol-mixed energy drinks had positive expectations, such as being able to party longer. Other reasons for alcohol-mixed energy drinks include "liking the taste" and wanting to drink something else.

Students who are involved in intercollegiate or intramural sports, fraternities, and sororities are more likely to use alcohol-mixed energy drinks than other students. Living off campus also appears to increase consumption of alcohol-mixed energy drinks, as does pregaming. Students who drink alcohol-mixed energy drinks while pregaming are more likely to drink heavily throughout the night, because caffeine counters alcohol's sedative effect, which would normally cause them to stop drinking. Students also report not noticing the signs of intoxication (dizziness, fatigue, headache, or lack of coordination) when they had consumed alcohol-mixed energy drinks.

Studies indicate that students who report drinking alcohol-mixed energy drinks are more likely to consume large amounts of alcohol, have unprotected sex or sex under the influence of alcohol or drugs, be hurt or injured, and meet criteria for alcohol dependency.

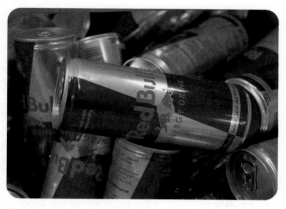

Mixing alcohol with energy drinks, such as Red Bull, can have serious consequences.

Sources: Centers for Disease Control and Prevention, "Alcohol and Public Health: Fact Sheets—Caffeine and Alcohol," 2015, https://www.cdc.gov/alcohol/fact-sheets/caffeine-and-alcohol.htm; M. Patrick et al., "Who Uses Alcohol Mixed with Energy Drinks? Characteristics of College Student Users," *Journal American College Health*, 64, no. 1 (2016): 74–7; A. Haas et al., "Proportion as a Metric of Problematic Alcohol-Energy Drink Consumption in College Students," *Journal of Substance Abuse*, doi:10.1080/14659891.2016.1271037; Verster et al., "Motives for Mixing Alcohol with Energy Drinks and Other Nonalcoholic Beverages and Consequences for Overall Alcohol Consumption," *International Journal of Internal Medicine* 7 (2014): 285–93.

---

of 12 percent wine, or 1.5 ounces of 40 percent (80 proof) liquor. Unmetabolized alcohol circulates in the bloodstream until enough time passes for the body to break it down.

Blood Alcohol Concentration

Blood alcohol concentration (BAC) is the ratio of alcohol to total blood volume. It is the factor used to measure the physiological and behavioral effects of alcohol. Despite individual differences, alcohol produces some general behavioral effects, depending on BAC (see **FIGURE 9.2**).

At a BAC of 0.02 percent, a person feels slightly relaxed and in a good mood. At 0.05 percent, relaxation increases, there is some motor impairment, and the person becomes more talkative. At 0.08, the person feels euphoric, and there is further motor impairment. The legal limit for driving a motor vehicle is 0.08 percent BAC in all states and the District of Columbia. At 0.10 percent, the depressant effects of alcohol become apparent, drowsiness sets in, and motor skills are further impaired, followed by a loss of judgment. Thus, a driver may

not be able to estimate distance or speed, and some drinkers may do things they wouldn't do when sober. As BAC increases, the drinker suffers increasingly negative physiological and psychological effects.

A drinker's BAC depends on weight and percentage of body fat, the water content in body tissues, the concentration of alcohol in the beverage consumed, the rate of consumption, and the volume of alcohol consumed. Heavier people have larger body surfaces through which to diffuse alcohol; therefore, they have lower concentrations of alcohol in their blood than do thin people after drinking the same amount. Alcohol does not diffuse as rapidly into body fat as into water; therefore, alcohol concentration is higher in a person with more body fat. Because women tend to have more body fat and less water in their tissues than men of the same weight, women become more intoxicated after drinking the same amount of alcohol.

Body fat is not the only contributor to the differences

blood alcohol concentration (BAC) The ratio of alcohol to total blood volume; the factor used to measure the physiological and behavioral effects of alcohol.

Blood Alcohol Concentration (BAC)	Psychological and Physical Effects
Not Impaired	
<0.01%	Negligible
Sometimes Impaired	
0.01–0.04%	Slight muscle relaxation, mild euphoria, slight body warmth, increased sociability and talkativeness
Usually Impaired	
0.05–0.07%	Lowered alertness, impaired judgment, lowered inhibitions, exaggerated behavior, loss of small muscle control
Always Impaired	
0.08–0.14%	Slowed reaction time, poor muscle coordination, short-term memory loss, judgment impaired, inability to focus
0.15–0.24%	Blurred vision, lack of motor skills, sedation, slowed reactions, difficulty standing and walking, passing out
0.25–0.34%	Impaired consciousness, disorientation, loss of motor function, severely impaired or no reflexes, impaired circulation and respiration, uncontrolled urination, slurred speech, possible death
0.35% and up	Unconsciousness, coma, extremely slow heartbeat and respiration, unresponsiveness, probable death

FIGURE 9.2 The Psychological and Physical Effects of Alcohol

in alcohol's effects on men and women. Compared to men, women have a less active form of alcohol dehydrogenase in the stomach. Recall that this enzyme helps break down alcohol. So if a man and a woman drink the same amount of alcohol, the woman's BAC will be approximately 30 percent higher than the man's. Hormonal differences can also play a role; certain points in the menstrual cycle and the use of hormonal contraceptives likely contribute to longer periods of intoxication. **FIGURE 9.3** compares blood alcohol levels in men and women by weight and number of drinks consumed.

learned behavioral tolerance The ability of heavy drinkers to modify their behavior so that they appear to be sober even when they have high BAC levels.

Both breath analysis (breathalyzer tests) and urinalysis are used to determine whether an individual is legally intoxicated, but blood tests are more accurate measures of BAC. An increasing number of states require blood tests for people who are suspected of driving while intoxicated. In some states, refusal to take the breath, urine, or blood test results in immediate suspension of a person's driver's license.

People can develop physical and psychological tolerance to the effects of alcohol through regular use. Over time, the nervous system adapts, requiring greater amounts of alcohol to produce the same physiological and psychological effects. Though their BAC may be quite high, some individuals learn to modify their behavior to appear sober. This ability is called **learned behavioral tolerance**.

LO 2 | ALCOHOL AND YOUR HEALTH

Identify short-term and long-term effects of alcohol consumption.

The immediate and long-term effects of alcohol consumption can vary greatly (**FIGURE 9.4**). Whether or not you experience any immediate or long-term consequences depends on you as an individual, the amount of alcohol you consume, and your circumstances.

Short-Term Effects of Alcohol Use

Ethanol's most dramatic effects occur in the central nervous system (CNS). Alcohol depresses CNS functions, decreasing

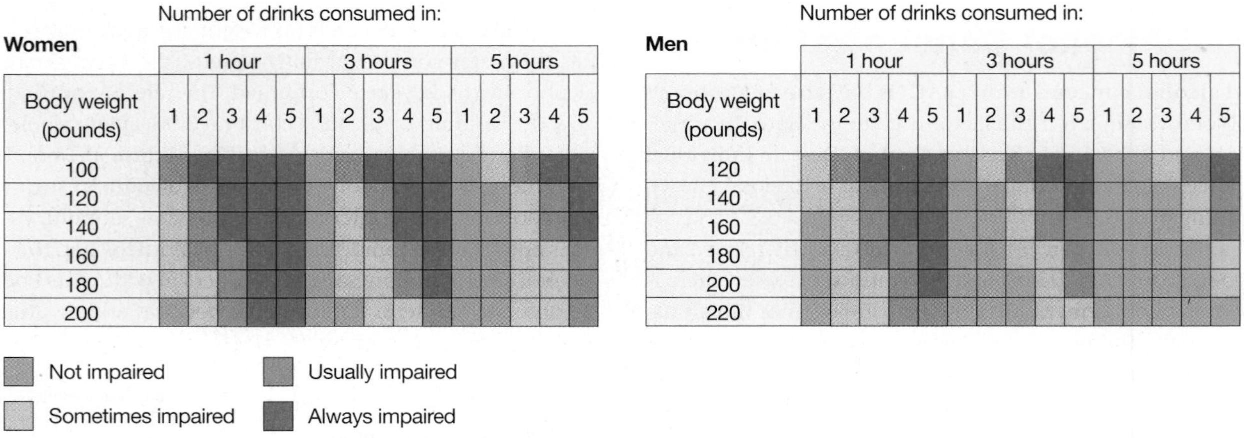

Number of drinks consumed in:

Women

Body weight (pounds)	1 hour					3 hours					5 hours				
	1	2	3	4	5	1	2	3	4	5	1	2	3	4	5
100															
120															
140															
160															
180															
200															

Number of drinks consumed in:

Men

Body weight (pounds)	1 hour					3 hours					5 hours				
	1	2	3	4	5	1	2	3	4	5	1	2	3	4	5
120															
140															
160															
180															
200															
220															

Not impaired   Usually impaired
Sometimes impaired   Always impaired

FIGURE 9.3 Approximate Blood Alcohol Concentration (BAC) and the Physiological and Behavioral Effects
Remember that there are many variables that can affect BAC, so this is only an estimate of what your BAC would be.

respiratory rate, pulse rate, and blood pressure. As CNS depression deepens, vital functions become noticeably affected. In extreme cases, coma and death can result.

Alcohol is a diuretic; that is, it increases urinary output. Although this effect might be expected to lead to **dehydration**, the body actually retains water, most of it in the muscles or cerebral tissues. Because water is usually pulled out of the *cerebrospinal fluid* (fluid within the brain and spinal cord), drinkers may suffer symptoms that include "morning-after" headaches.

Alcohol irritates the gastrointestinal system and may cause indigestion and heartburn if consumed on an empty stomach. In addition, both binge drinking and long-term drinking may increase the risk of experiencing an irregular heartbeat.[6] Drinking too much even on a single occasion may increase the risk of stroke, high blood pressure, or damage to the heart muscle.[7]

Hangover A **hangover** is often experienced the morning after heavy drinking. Its symptoms include: headache, muscle aches, upset stomach, anxiety, depression, diarrhea, and thirst. **Congeners**, forms of alcohol that metabolize more slowly than ethanol and are more toxic, are thought to play a role in hangover development. The body metabolizes the congeners after the ethanol is gone from the system, and their toxic by-products may contribute to the hangover. Alcohol also upsets the water balance in the body, and the result may be excess urination, dehydration, and thirst the next day. Increased production of hydrochloric acid can irritate the stomach lining and cause nausea. Recovery from a

> **dehydration** Loss of water from body tissues.
>
> **hangover** Physiological reactions to excessive drinking, including headache, upset stomach, anxiety, depression, diarrhea, and thirst.
>
> **congeners** Forms of alcohol that are metabolized more slowly than ethanol and produce toxic by-products.

Short-Term Health Effects

NERVOUS SYSTEM
- Slowed reaction time, slurred speech
- Impaired judgment and motor coordination
- High BACs can lead to coma and death

SENSES
- Dulled senses of taste and smell
- Less acute vision and hearing

SKIN
- Broken capillaries
- Flushing, sweating, heat loss

HEART AND LUNGS
- Decreased pulse and respiratory rate
- Lowered blood pressure

STOMACH
- Nausea
- Irritation and inflammation

URINARY SYSTEM
- Increased urination

SEXUAL RESPONSE
- **Women:** decreased vaginal lubrication
- **Men:** erectile dysfunction

Long-Term Health Effects

BRAIN
- Memory impairment
- Damaged/destroyed brain cells

IMMUNE SYSTEM
- Lowered disease resistance

HEART
- Weakened heart muscle
- Elevated blood pressure

LIVER
- Increased risk of liver cancer
- Fatty liver and cirrhosis

DIGESTIVE SYSTEM
- Chronic inflammation of the stomach and pancreas
- Increased risk of cancers of the mouth, esophagus, stomach, pancreas, and colon

BONES
- Increased risk of osteoporosis

REPRODUCTIVE SYSTEM
- **Women:** menstrual irregularities and increased risk of birth defects
- **Men:** impotence and testicular atrophy
- **Both sexes:** increased risk of breast cancer

FIGURE 9.4 Effects of Alcohol on the Body and Health

Watch Video Tutor: **Long- and Short-Term Effects of Alcohol** in Mastering Health.

hangover usually takes 12 hours. Bedrest, solid food, plenty of water, and aspirin or ibuprofen may help to relieve a hangover's discomforts, but the only sure way to avoid one is to abstain from excessive alcohol use in the first place.

There is good news for people suffering from a hangover. The U.S. Food and Drug Administration (FDA) has approved Blowfish, the only over-the-counter hangover drug. The tablet is a combination of aspirin, an antacid, and caffeine, and it is intended to fight headache, fatigue, and upset stomach after a night of drinking.[8]

Alcohol and Injuries

Alcohol use plays a significant role in the types of injuries people experience. The relationship between alcohol and a variety of accidents, such as automobile crashes, falls, and fires, has long been established. Approximately 70 percent of fatal injuries during activities such as swimming and boating involve alcohol.[9] Drinking affects psychomotor skills and cognitive skills; in other words, drinking can have an adverse effect on a person's reaction time as well as judgment, meaning that people under the influence of alcohol often set themselves up for injury.[10]

Alcohol use is also a key risk factor for suicide, playing a role in approximately 20 percent of suicides in the United States.[11] Alcohol may increase the risk for suicide by intensifying depressive thoughts or feelings of hopelessness, lowering inhibitions to hurt oneself, and interfering with the ability to assess future consequences of one's actions.[12]

Alcohol and Sexual Decision Making

Because it lowers inhibitions, alcohol has a clear influence on one's ability to make good decisions about sex. Intoxicated people are less likely to use safer sex practices and more likely to engage in high-risk sexual activity.[13] Over 21 percent of college students report engaging in sexual activity after drinking, including having sex with someone they just met and having unprotected sex.[14] The chance of acquiring a sexually transmitted infection or experiencing unplanned pregnancy also increases as students drink more heavily.[15]

Alcohol and Rape, Sexual Assault, and Dating Violence

In a recent survey, almost 20 percent of undergraduate women and 5 percent of undergraduate men reported having been sexually assaulted by physical force or while incapacitated while in college.[16] Among the women who experienced a sexual assault or unwanted sexual contact, 61 percent had been drinking alcohol, and 88 percent reported not taking or using any drug other than alcohol before the incident.[17] Alcohol use by women makes them more vulnerable to sexual assault.[18] While men, when drinking, are also at increased risk of victimization, they are also more likely to engage in coercive sexual behaviors, including sexual assault.[19] Alcohol is sometimes used as an excuse for unacceptable behavior. When a man sexually assaults an acquaintance, he is often viewed as bearing less responsibility for his actions if he was drunk. The double standard in our society often places blame for the assault on the victim if she was intoxicated. No one deserves to be raped. Rape is a violent crime. Choosing to imbibe alcohol is not volunteering to be sexually assaulted.

alcohol poisoning (acute alcohol intoxication) Potentially lethal BAC that inhibits the brain's ability to control consciousness, respiration, and heart rate; usually occurs as a result of drinking a large amount of alcohol in a short period of time.

Alcohol Poisoning

Alcohol poisoning (also known as **acute alcohol intoxication**) occurs frequently and can be fatal.

The amount of alcohol that causes a person to lose consciousness—0.35 percent BAC for most (see Figure 9.4)—is dangerously close to the lethal dose. Death from alcohol poisoning can be caused by CNS and respiratory system depression or by inhaling vomit or fluid into the lungs. Alcohol depresses the nerves that control involuntary actions such as breathing and the gag reflex (which prevents choking). As BAC levels reach higher concentrations, these functions can eventually be completely suppressed. If a drinker becomes unconscious and vomits, there is a danger of asphyxiation through choking to death on the person's own vomit.

Blood alcohol concentration can continue rising even after a drinker becomes unconscious because alcohol in the stomach and intestine continues to be absorbed into the bloodstream. Signs of alcohol poisoning include inability to be roused; a weak, rapid pulse; an unusual or irregular breathing pattern; and cool (possibly damp), pale, or bluish skin. If you are with someone who has been drinking heavily and exhibits these symptoms or if you are unsure about the person's condition, call your local emergency number (9-1-1 in most areas) for immediate assistance.

Drinking and Driving

Traffic accidents are the leading cause of accidental death for all age groups from 1 to 25 years old.[20] In the United States, adults drink too much and get behind the wheel approximately 121 million times (based on self-reports) in a year.[21] Alcohol-impaired drivers are involved in about 1 in 3 crash deaths, resulting in nearly 10,000 deaths a year—roughly one traffic fatality every 53 minutes.[22] College students are overrepresented in alcohol-related crashes. A recent survey reported over 20 percent of college students have driven after drinking, and about 1.6 percent said they had driven after drinking five or more drinks in the past 30 days.[23]

Over the past 20 years, the percentage of intoxicated drivers involved in fatal crashes decreased for all age groups (FIGURE 9.5). Several factors probably contributed: laws that raised the drinking age to 21 years, stricter law enforcement, laws prohibiting anyone under 21 from driving with any detectable BAC, increased automobile safety, and educational programs designed to discourage drinking and driving. Furthermore, all states have zero-tolerance laws for driving while intoxicated, and the penalty is usually suspension of the driver's license.

Despite these measures, the risk of being involved in an alcohol-related automobile crash remains substantial.

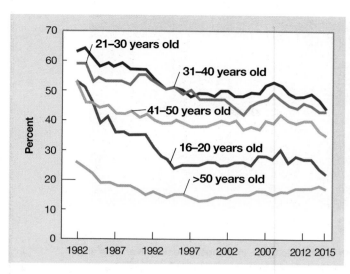

FIGURE 9.5 Percentage of Fatally Injured Drivers with BACs Greater Than 0.08 Percent, by Driver Age, 1982–2015

Source: Insurance Institute for Highway Safety, "Alcohol Impaired Driving 2015: Alcohol," Copyright 2017. Reprinted with permission.

Laboratory and test track research shows that the vast majority of drivers are impaired even at 0.08 BAC with regard to critical driving tasks. The likelihood of a driver being involved in a fatal crash rises significantly with a BAC of 0.05 percent and even more rapidly after 0.08 percent.[24]

Alcohol-related fatal crashes occur more often at night than during the day, and the hours between 9:00 P.M. and 6:00 A.M. are the most dangerous.[25] Fifty-three percent of fatally injured drivers involved in nighttime single-vehicle crashes had BACs at or above 0.08 percent.[26] The risk of being involved in an alcohol-related crash increases not only with the time of day, but also with the day of the week; 23 percent of all fatal crashes during the week were alcohol related, compared with 42 percent on weekends.[27]

Long-Term Effects of Alcohol

Alcohol is distributed throughout most of the body and may affect many organs and tissues. Problems associated with long-term, habitual use of alcohol include diseases of the nervous system, cardiovascular system, and liver as well as some cancers.

Effects on the Nervous System

The CNS is especially sensitive to alcohol. Even people who drink moderately experience shrinkage in brain size and weight and a loss of some degree of intellectual ability. Research suggests that adolescents' developing brains are much more prone to damage than was previously thought. Alcohol appears to damage the frontal areas of the adolescent brain, which are crucial for controlling impulses and thinking through consequences of intended actions.[28] In addition, researchers suggest that people who begin drinking at an early age are at much higher risk of experiencing alcohol abuse or dependence, drinking five or more drinks per drinking occasion, and driving under the influence of alcohol at least weekly.[29]

Alcohol and Weight Gain

Alcohol contains 7 calories per gram—nearly as much as fat (9 calories per gram) and more than carbohydrates or protein (4 calories per gram)—and the calories from alcohol provide few nutrients. A standard drink contains 12 to 15 grams of alcohol, so a single drink can add about 100 empty calories to your daily intake. By drinking an extra 150 calories a day more than you need, you can gain 1 pound a month and up to 12 pounds a year.[30]

Cardiovascular Effects

Several studies have associated light to moderate consumption of red wine (no more than two drinks a day) with a reduced risk of coronary artery disease.[31] How? The strongest evidence points to an increase in high-density lipoprotein (HDL) cholesterol—"good" cholesterol—among moderate drinkers.[32] Alcohol's effects on blood clotting, insulin sensitivity, and inflammation are also thought to play a role in protecting against heart disease. However, alcohol consumption is not a preventive measure against heart disease; it causes many more hazards than benefits. Regular or heavy drinking is a major cause of *cardiomyopathy*, a degenerative disease of the heart muscle, and of *heart arrhythmias* (irregular heartbeats).[33] Drinking too much alcohol also contributes to high blood pressure, increasing the risk of a stroke and heart attack in some people.[34] Combining the use of alcohol with tobacco and other drugs increases the likelihood of damage to the heart.[35]

Liver Disease

One result of heavy drinking is that the liver begins to store fat—a condition known as *fatty liver*. If there is insufficient time between drinking episodes, this fat cannot be transported to storage sites, and the fat-filled liver cells stop functioning. Continued drinking can cause a further stage of liver deterioration called *fibrosis*, in which the damaged area of the liver develops fibrous scar tissue. Cell function can be partially restored at this stage with proper nutrition and abstinence from alcohol. However, if the person continues to drink, **cirrhosis** of the liver results (**FIGURE 9.6**). A common cause of death in the United States, cirrhosis occurs as liver cells die and damage becomes permanent. **Alcoholic hepatitis** is another serious condition resulting from prolonged use of alcohol. A chronic inflammation of the liver develops, which may be fatal in itself or progress to cirrhosis.

> **cirrhosis** The last stage of liver disease associated with chronic heavy use of alcohol, during which liver cells die and damage becomes permanent.
>
> **alcoholic hepatitis** A condition resulting from prolonged use of alcohol, in which the liver is inflamed; can be fatal.

Alcohol-related **LIVER DISEASE** is the primary cause of almost

1 IN 3

liver transplants in the United States.

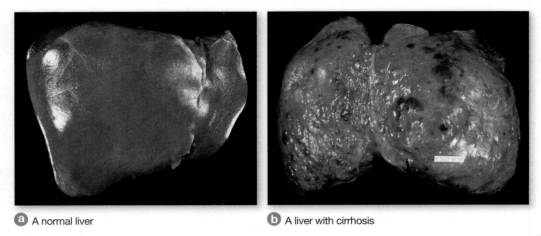

(a) A normal liver   (b) A liver with cirrhosis

FIGURE 9.6 **Comparison of a Healthy Liver with a Cirrhotic Liver** In cirrhosis, healthy liver cells are replaced with scar tissue that interferes with the liver's ability to perform its many vital functions.

Cancer In its *Report on Carcinogens*, the U.S. Department of Health and Human Services lists alcoholic beverages as known carcinogens.[36] Two recent studies have indicated that alcohol use is strongly associated with the risk of cancer in both women and men.[37] For women, the increased cancer risk appears at lower levels of alcohol consumption then in men, and the total amount of alcohol consumption rather than the regularity of drinking or binge drinking seem to have greatest effect.[38] Alcohol use has been linked to cancers of the esophagus, colon, rectum, breast, stomach, oral cavity, and liver. The leading alcohol-related cancer in women is breast cancer; the leading cancer for men is colorectal cancer.[39]

There is substantial evidence to suggest that women who consume even low levels of alcohol have a higher risk of breast cancer than those who abstain. A recent study found that women who consumed 0.5 to 1.5 drinks per day had a 6 percent increased risk of breast cancer compared to those who drank up to half a drink a day.[40] The risk was elevated for women who have a family history of breast cancer.[41]

Other Effects Alcohol abuse is a major cause of chronic inflammation of the pancreas, the organ that produces digestive enzymes and insulin. Chronic alcohol abuse inhibits enzyme production, which further inhibits the absorption of nutrients. Drinking alcohol can block the absorption of calcium, a nutrient that strengthens the bones. This should be of particular concern to women because of their risk for osteoporosis.

Alcohol and Pregnancy

Teratogenic substances cause birth defects. Of the 30 known teratogens in the environment, alcohol is one of the most dangerous. If a woman ingests alcohol while pregnant, it will pass through the placenta and enter the growing fetus's bloodstream. In the United States, more than 1 in 5 pregnant women report alcohol use during early pregnancy.[42] Fetal development can be disrupted by alcohol at any point during a woman's pregnancy, even before she is aware that she is pregnant. When a woman is pregnant, no amount of alcohol is known to be safe to drink.[43] Alcohol consumed during the first trimester poses the greatest threat to organ development; exposure during the last trimester, when the brain is developing rapidly, is most likely to affect CNS development.[44]

A disorder called **fetal alcohol syndrome (FAS)** is associated with alcohol consumption during pregnancy. FAS is the third most common birth defect and the second leading cause of mental retardation in the United States, with an estimated incidence of 0.2 to 1.5 cases per 1,000 live births.[45] FAS is the most common preventable cause of mental impairment in the Western world.[46]

Among the symptoms of FAS are mental retardation; small head size; tremors; and abnormalities of the face, limbs, heart, and brain. Children with FAS may experience problems such

fetal alcohol syndrome (FAS) A birth defect involving physical and mental impairment that results from the mother's alcohol consumption during pregnancy.

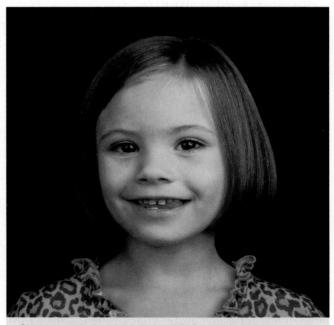

Characteristic facial features of FAS include a small, upturned nose with a low bridge and a thin upper lip.

binge drinking A pattern of drinking alcohol that brings BAC to 0.08 gram-percent or above; corresponds to consuming five or more drinks (adult male) or four or more drinks (adult female) in 2 hours.

as poor memory and impaired learning, reduced attention span, impulsive behavior, and poor problem-solving abilities, among others.

Some children may have fewer than the full physical or behavioral symptoms of FAS and may be diagnosed with disorders such as partial fetal alcohol syndrome (PFAS) or alcohol-related neurodevelopmental disorder (ARND); all of these disorders, including FAS, fall under the umbrella term *fetal alcohol spectrum disorders (FASD)*. An estimated 1 in 20 U.S. schoolchildren may be affected by FASD.[47] Infants whose mothers binge-drink when pregnant are at higher risk for FASD.[48] Risk levels for babies whose mothers consume smaller amounts are uncertain.[49] To avoid any chance of harming her fetus, any woman of childbearing age who is pregnant or may become pregnant is advised to refrain from consuming any amount of alcohol.

LO 3 | ALCOHOL USE IN COLLEGE

Describe alcohol use patterns of college students, practical strategies for drinking responsibly, and ways to cope with campus and societal pressures to drink.

Alcohol is the most popular drug on college campuses; over 64 percent of students report having consumed alcoholic beverages in the past 30 days (**FIGURE 9.7**).[50] Approximately 38 percent of all college students engage in **binge drinking**.[51] For a typical adult, this means consuming five or more drinks (men) or four or more drinks (women) in about 2 hours.[52] Students who drink only once a week are considered binge drinkers if they consume these amounts within 2 hours. Binge drinking is especially dangerous because it can lead to extreme intoxication, unconsciousness, alcohol poisoning, and even death.

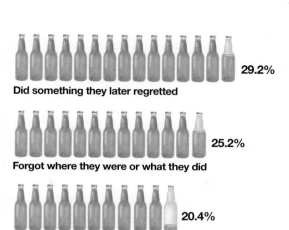

29.2%
Did something they later regretted

25.2%
Forgot where they were or what they did

20.4%
Had unprotected sex

11.7%
Physically injured self

2.1%
Got in trouble with the police

1.3%
Physically injured another person

FIGURE 9.8 Prevalence of Negative Consequences of Drinking among College Students, Past Year

Source: Data from American College Health Association, *American College Health Association—National College Health Assessment II (ACHA-NCHA II) Reference Group Data Report Spring 2016* (Linthicum, MD: American College Health Association, 2016).

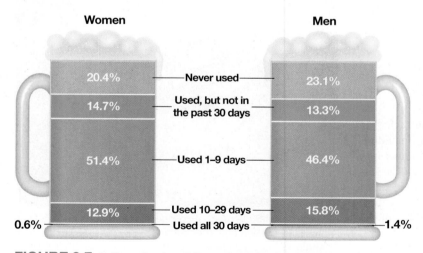

Women

20.4%	Never used	23.1%
14.7%	Used, but not in the past 30 days	13.3%
51.4%	Used 1–9 days	46.4%
12.9%	Used 10–29 days	15.8%
0.6%	Used all 30 days	1.4%

Men

FIGURE 9.7 College Students' Patterns of Alcohol Use in the Past 30 Days

Source: Data from American College Health Association, *American College Health Association—National College Health Assessment II: Reference Group Executive Summary, Fall 2016* (Hanover, MD: American College Health Association, 2017).

Drinking competitions, celebrations, or games and hazing rituals encourage this type of drinking.

College is a critical time to become aware of and responsible for one's drinking. Many students are away from home, often for the first time, and are excited by their newfound independence. For some students, this rite of passage into college culture is symbolized by alcohol use. Many students say they drink to have fun. "Having fun," which often means drinking simply to get drunk, may really be a way of coping with stress, boredom, anxiety, or pressures created by academic and social demands.

A significant number of students experience negative consequences as a result of their alcohol consumption (**FIGURE 9.8**). Nearly 2 percent reported having had sex with someone without giving consent, and 0.3 percent reported having had sex with someone without getting consent.[53] A recent study found that students who played intramural sports, were in abusive relationships, had high stress levels, belonged to a

pregaming Drinking heavily at home before going out to an event or other location.

fraternity or sorority, or were depressed reported higher levels of drinking and negative alcohol-related effects.[54]

Alcohol use among college students also has consequences related to academic performance.[55] Alcohol consumption tends to disrupt sleep and decreases REM sleep. Alcohol use is associated with shorter sleep duration, greater sleep irregularity, bedtime delay, weekend oversleeping, and sleep-related impairment.[56] These disruptive effects increase daytime sleepiness and decrease alertness, which can also negatively affect students' academic performance.[57]

Fortunately, many college students report practicing protective behaviors when consuming alcohol to reduce the risk of negative consequences as a result of their alcohol use. The Skills for Behavior Change box provides some strategies for drinking responsibly.

High-Risk Drinking and College Students

According to one study, 1,825 college students die each year because of alcohol-related unintentional injuries, including car accidents.[58] Consumption of alcohol is the number one cause of preventable death among undergraduate college students in the United States today.[59]

Although everyone who drinks is at some risk for alcohol-related problems, college students seem particularly vulnerable for the following reasons:

- Alcohol exacerbates their already high risk for suicide, automobile crashes, and falls.
- Many college and university students' customs and celebrations encourage certain dangerous practices and patterns of alcohol use.

- The alcoholic beverage industry heavily targets university campuses.
- Drink specials enable students to consume large amounts of alcohol cheaply.
- College students are particularly vulnerable to peer influence.
- College administrators often deny that alcohol problems exist on their campuses.

Pregaming, Binge Drinking, and Calorie "Saving"

Pregaming (also called preloading or front-loading) involves planned heavy drinking in a compressed time frame, usually in someone's home, apartment, or residence hall, before going out to a bar, party, or sporting event. In a recent study, 92 percent of students reported pregaming during the academic year.[60] Students who pregame consume more drinks and have higher BACs. They are also more likely to drink in the extreme—consuming 8 drinks at a time for women, 10 for men—and reach an estimated BAC of 0.16 percent.[61] Additional negative consequences of pregaming include passing out, drunk driving, aggression, alcohol poisoning, and violent acts.[62]

Competitive drinking is also common on college campuses, where students often play drinking games such as beer pong, quarters, and flip cup.[63] Some of the games involve some type of cognitive and physical task that specify how much and when participants should drink. Others involve chugging—as with keg stands—and encourage extreme consumption of alcohol.[64] People who play drinking games are less likely to monitor or regulate how much they drink and are at risk for extreme intoxication and negative related outcomes.[65] Drinking games have been associated with blacking out, regrettable sexual experiences, and alcohol-related injuries and deaths from alcohol poisoning.[66]

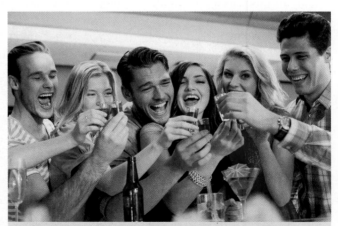

While about 63 percent of college students drink only occasionally and 20.2 percent don't drink at all, college students have high rates of binge drinking. Take control of when you drink and how much.

Source: American College Health Association, *American College Health Association—National College Health Assessment II (ACHA-NCHA II) Reference Group Data Report Spring 2016* (Linthicum, MD: American College Health Association, 2016).

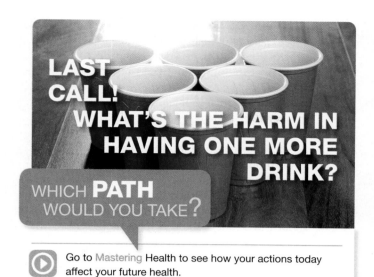

LAST CALL! WHAT'S THE HARM IN HAVING ONE MORE DRINK?

WHICH PATH WOULD YOU TAKE?

Go to Mastering Health to see how your actions today affect your future health.

Some people use extreme measures to control their eating and/or exercise excessively so that they can save calories, consume more alcohol, and become intoxicated faster.[67] **Drunkorexia** is a colloquialism used to describe the combination of two dangerous behaviors: disordered eating and heavy drinking. Early studies have found that college students who restrict the number of calories they consume before drinking are more likely to drink heavily.[68] One study found that 28 percent of women and 8 percent of men surveyed said that they "saved" calories for drinking by restricting normal caloric intake.[69] The same study found that 29 percent of those surveyed had engaged in drunkorexia before all drinking occasions and that highly physically active college students are more likely to binge-drink than their nonactive peers.[70] Motivations for drunkorexia include preventing weight gain, getting drunk faster, and saving money that would be spent on food to buy alcohol. Potential risks of drunkorexia include blackouts, forced sexual activity, unintended sexual activity, and alcohol poisoning.

A Dangerous Alternative: Alcohol Inhalation

Motivated by wanting to get drunk faster or to get drunk without the calories, some students have begun "vaping" alcohol by using nebulizers or by dropping carbon dioxide pills into a container of alcohol or pouring alcohol over dry ice and inhaling with a straw. While a very small number of students actually participate in vaping alcohol, the risks for those who do are very high.[71] When alcohol is inhaled, it goes directly from the lungs to the brain and bloodstream, getting the drinker drunk very quickly. Bypassing the stomach and liver, inhaled alcohol isn't metabolized, so it doesn't lose any potency. When alcohol is absorbed into the bloodstream that quickly, the body's natural defense against alcohol overdose, the gag reflex, is bypassed, and the body cannot expel the alcohol.[72] Risks include liver and brain damage.

▶ SEE IT! VIDEOS

Heavy drinking during spring break can lead to bad decisions or worse. Watch **Sloppy Spring Breaker**, available on Mastering Health.

Efforts to Reduce Student Drinking

What are colleges doing to address the problem of drinking on campus? Programs that have proven particularly effective use cognitive–behavioral skills training with *motivational interviewing*, a nonjudgmental approach to working with students to change behavior. The NIAAA has recognized Brief Alcohol Screening and Intervention for College Students (BASICS) as an effective program for students who drink heavily and have experienced or are at risk for alcohol-related problems.[73] E-interventions—electronically based alcohol education interventions using Web-based interventions such as the Alcohol EDU® and e-Check Up to Go (e-Chug)—have also shown to be highly effective in reducing alcohol-related problems among students.[74]

Web-based education for first-year students has become an increasingly important intervention. Because first-year students are at increased risk for alcohol-related problems, schools must ensure that students are made aware of risks and effects of alcohol as well as educating them about campus resources available for dealing with issues with alcohol use.

WHAT DO YOU THINK?

Why do some college students drink excessive amounts of alcohol?

■ Are there particular traditions or norms related to when and why students drink on your campus?

■ Have you ever had your sleep or studies interrupted or had to babysit a friend because he or she had been drinking?

LO 4 | ALCOHOL ABUSE AND DEPENDENCE

Describe alcohol use disorder and its risk factors, causes, and costs to society, and discuss options for treatment.

The fifth edition of the *Diagnostic and Statistical Manual of Mental Disorders* (DSM-5) has integrated alcohol abuse and alcohol dependence into a single disorder: **alcohol use disorder (AUD)**. Any person who meets two or more of the new criteria would receive a diagnosis of AUD. Severity of AUD falls along a spectrum from mild to moderate to severe, according to the number of criteria a person meets (**FIGURE 9.9**). For example a student who shares having a strong desire or craving to use alcohol and a high tolerance for alcohol with a counselor or clinician would meet the criteria for mild AUD.

Identifying an Alcoholic

As with other addictions, craving, loss of control, tolerance, psychological dependence, and withdrawal symptoms must be

drunkorexia A colloquial term to describe the combination of disordered eating, excessive physical activity, and heavy alcohol consumption.

alcohol use disorder Problem drinking so severe that at least two or more alcohol-related issues are present, such as engaging in risky behaviors, having problems at work or school, or issues with relationships.

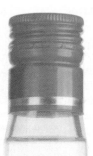

Answer each of these questions for the past year:

Do you ever drink more or for longer periods of time than you'd planned?

Do you have a strong desire to cut down, or are you unable to control your alcohol use?

At times, are you unable to think of anything other than your next drink?

Do you spend considerable time in activities related to drinking or recovering from drinking?

Have you reduced your involvement in pleasurable social, occupational, or recreational activities?

Have you neglected responsibilities at work, school, and/or at home?

Do you continue drinking despite knowing that physical/psychological problems are caused or exacerbated by your drinking? Or after a memory blackout?

Have you more than once physically endangered yourself during or after drinking?

Have you continued to use alcohol despite social or interpersonal problems caused or aggravated by use?

Do you meet the definition of having developed tolerance based on these criteria?
1) You need increasingly greater amounts of alcohol to get the same desired effect.
2) Over time, you experience fewer effects from alcohol when you drink the same amount.

Do you experience characteristic signs of alcohol withdrawal when you stop drinking or do you use another substance to relieve or avoid withdrawal?

If you answered yes to two or more of the questions, you are considered someone with an alcohol use disorder (AUD). The level of AUD is defined as: **mild**: 2–3 items; **moderate**: 4–5 items; and **severe**: 6 or more items.

FIGURE 9.9 Alcohol Use Disorder Criteria

Source: National Institutes of Health, *Alcohol Use Disorder: A Comparison between DSM-IV and DSM-5*, National Institute on Alcohol Abuse and Alcoholism NIH Publication No. 13-7999, July 2015, http://pubs.niaaa.nih.gov/publications/dsmfactsheet/dsmfact.htm.

present to qualify a drinker as an addict. Irresponsible and problem drinkers, such as people who get into fights or embarrass themselves or others when they drink, are not necessarily alcoholics. Alcoholics can be found at all socioeconomic levels and in all professions, ethnic groups, geographical locations, religions, and races. Data indicate that about 15 percent of people

in the United States are problem drinkers, and about 5 to 10 percent of male drinkers and 3 to 5 percent of females would be diagnosed as alcohol dependent.[75]

Recognizing and admitting the existence of an alcohol problem can be extremely difficult. Alcoholics often deny their problem, claiming that they can stop any time. The fear of being labeled a "problem drinker" often prevents people from seeking help. People who recognize alcoholic behaviors in themselves should seriously consider seeking professional help. (The Skills for Behavior Change box gives tips for cutting down on drinking.)

AUD is not uncommon among college students; about 1 in 5 college students meet the criteria.[76] In a recent study, the progression to alcohol dependency based on college students' drinking patterns when they entered college indicated that 1.9 percent of nondrinkers, 4.3 percent of light drinkers, 12.8 percent of moderate drinkers, and 19 percent of heavy drinkers developed alcohol dependency.[77]

Functional Alcoholics Most of us picture an alcoholic as someone who drinks too much too often, with obviously negative impact on the person's life. However, not all alcoholics fit that stereotype. Functional alcoholics are typically educated, have a steady job, have a family, and have made it to middle age.[78] By all outward appearances, functional alcoholics seem to have their personal and professional lives in order. Functional alcoholics also suffer from denial. Having a job, being able to pay bills, and having a lot of friends might keep functional alcoholics from thinking they have a problem. However, no one can drink heavily and maintain major responsibilities. Over time, the drinking catches up with them.

The Causes of Alcohol Use Disorder

We know that alcoholism is a disease with biological and social/environmental components, but we do not know what role each component plays.

Biological and Family Factors Research into the hereditary and environmental causes of alcoholism has found higher rates of alcoholism among children of alcoholics than in the general population. Alcoholism among individuals with a family history of alcoholism is about four to eight times more common than it is among individuals with no such family history.[79]

Despite evidence of heredity's role, scientists do not yet understand the precise role of genes in increased risk for alcoholism, nor have they identified a specific "alcoholism" gene. Alcohol use disorders are approximately 60 percent heritable.[80] Adoption studies demonstrate a strong link between biological parents' substance use and their children's risk for addiction.[81] Research has found that alcohol stimulates the production of dopamine, which activates the pleasure center of the brain. In alcoholics, the dopamine response to alcohol is diminished, leading them to drink more alcohol to feel the same pleasurable effects.[82] Alcohol gives individuals with the gene a stronger sense of reward from alcohol, making it more likely for them to be heavy drinkers. However, there is nothing deterministic about the genetic basis for addiction. Although no single gene causes addiction, multiple genes can affect the ability to develop addiction.

Social and Cultural Factors

Some people begin drinking as a way to dull the pain of an acute loss or an emotional or social problem. Unfortunately, they become even sadder as the depressant effect of the drug begins to take its toll, sometimes causing them to antagonize friends and other social supports. Eventually, the drinker becomes physically dependent on the drug.

Family attitudes toward alcohol also seem to influence whether a person will develop a drinking problem. People who are raised in cultures in which drinking is a part of religious or ceremonial activities or part of the family meal are less prone to alcohol dependence. In contrast, societies in which alcohol purchase is carefully controlled and drinking is regarded as a rite of passage to adulthood appear to have greater tendency for abuse. The Health in a Diverse World box discusses some of the patterns of alcohol use and abuse around the world.

The amount of alcohol a person consumes seems to be directly related to the drinking habits of that individual's social group. People whose friends and relatives drink heavily are more likely to drink heavily themselves. The opposite is also true: people with abstinent friends or family members are less likely to drink themselves. This finding has increased importance for individuals in treatment or who have been in treatment and their need to sever ties with heavy drinkers to maintain abstinence.

Alcohol Use Disorder in Women

Women tend to become alcoholics at later ages and after fewer years of heavy drinking than do men. Women also get addicted faster with less alcohol use, with greater risks for cirrhosis; excessive memory loss and shrinkage of the brain; heart disease; and cancers of the mouth, throat, esophagus, liver, and colon than male alcoholics. The risk of breast cancer increases with alcohol use.[83] Also, women suffer the consequences of alcoholism more profoundly, with alcoholism death rates that are 50 to 100 percent higher than those of alcoholic men.[84]

The highest risks for alcoholism occur among women who are unmarried but living with a partner, are in their twenties or early thirties, or have a husband or partner who drinks heavily. Other risk factors for women include a family history of drinking problems, pressure to drink from a peer or spouse, depression, and stress.

Alcohol and Prescription Drug Abuse

When alcohol and prescription drugs are taken together, severe medical problems can result, including alcohol poisoning, unconsciousness, respiratory depression, and death. The greatest risks from drug mixing occur when alcohol is mixed with prescription painkillers. Both drugs slow breathing rates in unique ways and inhibit the coughing reflex; when combined, they can stop breathing altogether. Alcohol also interacts with antianxiety medications, antipsychotics, antidepressants, sleep medications, and muscle relaxants, causing dizziness and drowsiness and making falls and unintentional injuries more likely. The prescription drugs that are most commonly combined with alcohol include opioids (e.g., Vicodin, OxyContin, Percocet), stimulants (e.g., Ritalin, Adderall, Concerta), sedative/anxiety medications (e.g., Ativan, Xanax), and sleeping medications (e.g., Ambien, Halcion).

Costs to Society

Alcohol-related costs to society are estimated to be well over $249 billion per year when health insurance, criminal justice

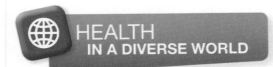
Alcohol consumption comes with many serious social and developmental issues, including violence, child neglect and abuse, and absenteeism in the workplace. Throughout the world, alcohol is a factor in 60 types of diseases and injuries and a component cause in 200 others. Almost 4 percent of all deaths worldwide are attributed to alcohol, more than deaths caused by HIV/AIDS, violence, or tuberculosis. Worldwide, the impact of alcohol use is as follows:

■ Alcohol use results in 3.3 million deaths each year.

■ 7.6 percent of male deaths and 4.0 percent of female deaths worldwide are attributable to alcohol consumption.

■ Early alcohol use (before the age of 14) is positively correlated with harmful behaviors later in life, including alcohol addiction and drunk driving.

■ At the same level of alcohol consumption, men are more likely to become injured and women are more likely to experience negative health outcomes such as cancer (particularly breast cancer), cardiovascular disease, and gastrointestinal problems.

A large variation exists in adult per capita alcohol consumption. The highest consumption levels can be found in the developed world, including Europe and the Americas. Intermediate consumption levels can be found in regions of the Western Pacific and Africa. Low consumption levels can be found in Southeast Asia and the Eastern Mediterranean regions. Many factors, including culture, religion, economic development, and socioeconomic status, contribute to these differences.

Source: World Health Organization, "Global Status Report on Alcohol and Health," 2014, www.who.int/substance_abuse/publications/global_alcohol_report/en.

---

costs, treatment costs, and lost productivity are considered.[85] These costs break down to a 72 percent loss in workplace productivity, 11 percent related to health care expenses for treating problems caused by excessive drinking, 10 percent related to criminal justice costs, and 5 percent related to losses from motor vehicle crashes.[86] Binge drinking alone accounts for the majority (77 percent) of the economic cost. Excessive drinking cost $807 per person, or $2.05 for each drink consumed.[87] Alcoholism is directly or indirectly responsible for more than 25 percent of the nation's medical expenses and lost earnings.[88] Emotional, mental, and physical costs are impossible to measure; however, the toll that alcohol takes in terms of loss of loved ones in drunk-driving accidents, alcohol-related violence and abuse in homes, and the damage to families and relationships are likely to be huge.

Treatment and Recovery

Only a very small percentage of alcoholics ever receive care in special treatment facilities. Numerous factors contribute to this low treatment utilization, including an inability or unwillingness to admit to an alcohol problem, the social stigma, the fact that seeking treatment would require abstinence, and the desire to deal with alcohol problems on one's own.[89] Most problem drinkers who seek help have experienced a turning point when the person recognizes that alcohol controls his or her life.

Alcoholics who decide to quit drinking will experience *detoxification*, the process by which their bodies are purged of the addictive substance. Withdrawal symptoms include hyperexcitability, confusion, agitation, sleep disorders, convulsions, tremors, depression, headache, and seizures.

delirium tremens (DTs) A state of confusion, delusions, and agitation brought on by withdrawal from alcohol.

For a small percentage of people, alcohol withdrawal results in a severe syndrome known as **delirium tremens (DTs)**, characterized by confusion, delusions, agitated behavior, and hallucinations.

The alcoholic who is ready for help has several avenues of treatment: psychologists and psychiatrists who specialize

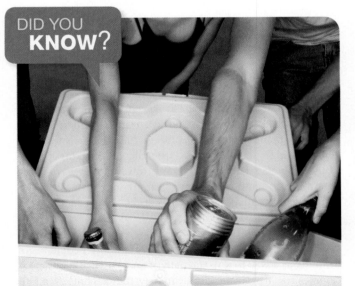

DID YOU KNOW?

The average college student spends about $1,800 per year on alcohol—compared to spending an average of about $1,250 a year on books.

Source: Data from College Board, Trends in Higher Education, https://trends.collegeboard.org/college-pricing/figures-tables/average-estimated-undergraduate-budgets-2016-17; Spread the Health, "Party Foul: Spending Too Much on Booze," Accessed March 17, 2017, https://spreadthehealthbu.com/2013/10/22/party-foul-spending-too-much-on-booze.

in addiction treatment, private treatment centers, hospitals specifically designed to treat alcoholics, community mental health facilities, and support groups such as **Alcoholics Anonymous (AA)**.

Private Treatment Facilities

On admission to a private treatment facility, the patient receives a complete physical examination to determine whether underlying medical problems will interfere with treatment. Shortly after detoxification, alcoholics begin their treatment for psychological addiction. Most treatment facilities keep their patients from 3 to 6 weeks. Treatment at private centers can cost several thousand dollars, but some insurance programs or employers will assume most of this expense.

Therapy

Several types of therapy are commonly used in alcoholism recovery programs. In family therapy, the person and family members examine the psychological reasons underlying the addiction and the environmental factors that have enabled it. In individual and group therapy, alcoholics learn positive coping skills for situations that have regularly caused them to turn to alcohol.

The high prevalence of alcohol and other drug use on college campuses makes attending college a threat to sobriety. While there are many recovery management strategies for adults, understanding an appropriate recovery support system for college students has received less attention. In particular, there has been a lack of campus-based services for recovering students. However, many campuses recognize the need to create recovery-friendly space and supportive environments for students engaged in recovery. Common features of such programs include a designated campus meeting space, drug-free housing options, individual or group counseling, relapse prevention, and sober leisure activities. Peer support and 12-step tenets are typically emphasized.[90]

Relapse

Success in recovery varies with the individual. Treating an addiction requires more than getting the addict to stop using a substance; it also requires getting the person to break a pattern of behavior that has dominated his or her life. Many alcoholics refer to themselves as "recovering" throughout their lifetime rather than "cured." In fact, only about one-third of people who are abstinent less than a year will remain abstinent.[91]

People seeking to regain a healthy lifestyle must not only confront their addiction, but also guard against the tendency to relapse. For alcoholics, it is important to identify situations that could trigger a relapse, such as becoming angry or frustrated and being around other people who drink. During the initial recovery period, it can help to join a support group, maintain stability (resisting the urge to move, travel, assume a new job, or make other drastic life changes), set aside time each day for reflection, and maintain a pattern of assuming responsibility for their own actions. To be effective, recovery programs must offer alcoholics ways to increase self-esteem and resume personal growth.

LO 5 | TOBACCO USE IN THE UNITED STATES

Discuss the rate of tobacco use in the United States in general and among college students in particular, and explain the social and political issues involved in tobacco use and prevention.

In the United States, tobacco use is the single most preventable cause of death. Close to a half a million Americans die each year of tobacco-related diseases.[92] Moreover, another 16 million people suffer from health disorders caused by tobacco. To date, tobacco is known to cause about 20 diseases, and about half of all regular smokers die of smoking-related diseases.[93]

Approximately 36 million Americans age 18 and older report using tobacco products (cigarettes, cigars, smokeless tobacco, and pipe tobacco) at least once in the past month.[94] Declines in cigarette smoking over the past two decades have slowed in comparison with earlier periods. In 2015, 16.7 percent of men and 13.6 percent of women were current cigarette smokers. Nearly 13 percent of adults age 18 to 24 years are cigarette smokers, yet adults age 25 to 44 years had the highest

Alcoholics Anonymous (AA) An organization whose goal is to help alcoholics stop drinking; includes auxiliary branches such as Al-Anon and Alateen.

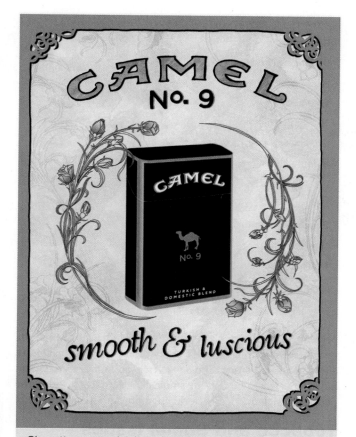

Cigarette companies have become adept at marketing to women using "glamorous" packaging and ad campaigns borrowed from cosmetics, perfume (such as the famous Chanel scents evoked by this Camel No. 9 brand), and the fashion industry.

TABLE 9.1 | Percentage of Population That Smokes (Age 18 and Older) among Selected Groups in the United States

	Percentage
United States overall	15.1
Race	
Asian	7.0
Black, non-Hispanic	16.7
Hispanic	10.1
Native American	21.9
White, non-Hispanic	16.6
Multiple race	20.2
Age (years)	
18–24	13.0
25–44	17.7
45–64	17.0
65+	8.4
Gender	
Male	16.7
Female	13.6
Education	
Undergraduate degree	7.4
High School diploma	19.8
GED diploma	34.1
12th grade, (no diploma)	26.3
Graduate degree	3.6
Income Level	
Below poverty level	26.1
At or above poverty level	13.9
Sexual Orientation	
Straight	14.9
Lesbian/gay/bisexual	20.6

Source: Centers for Disease Control and Prevention, "Current Cigarette Smoking among Adults—United States, 2005–2015," *Morbidity and Mortality Weekly* 65, no. 44 (2016): 1205–1211.

percentage of current cigarette smoking (18 percent); then the percentage continues to decrease with age, with 17 percent of adults age 45 to 64 years and 8 percent of adults age 65 years and older reported to be current smokers.[95] **TABLE 9.1** shows the percentages of Americans, by demographic group, who smoke.

Tobacco and Social Issues

The production and distribution of tobacco products involve many political and economic issues. Tobacco-growing states derive substantial income from tobacco production, and federal, state, and local governments benefit enormously from cigarette taxes.

Advertising The tobacco industry spends an estimated $26 million per day on advertising and promotional material.[96] With the number of smokers declining by about 1 million each year, the industry must actively recruit new smokers.[97] Studies have found that kids are three times as susceptible to advertising run by tobacco companies as are adults, are more likely to actually smoke as a result of cigarette marketing than of peer pressure, and that tobacco company advertising and promotion can be cited as the culprit for one-third of underage experimentation with smoking.[98]

Tobacco products are heavily advertised to specific populations. In women's magazines, the advertising implies that smoking is the key to financial success, desirability, beauty, weight control, independence, social acceptance, and being "cool." These ads have apparently been working. From the mid-1970s through the early 2000s, cigarette sales to women increased dramatically. Not coincidentally, by 1987, cigarette-induced lung cancer had surpassed breast cancer as the leading cancer killer among women and has remained the leading cancer killer in every year since.[99]

Women are not the only targets of gender-based cigarette advertisements. Men are depicted in locker rooms, charging over rugged terrain in off-road vehicles, or riding stallions into the sunset in blatant appeals to a need to feel and appear masculine. Minorities are also often the targets of heavy marketing. Tobacco advertising, particularly of menthol cigarettes, is much more common in magazines aimed at African Americans, such as *Jet* and *Ebony*, than in similar magazines aimed at broader audiences, such as *Time* and *People*. Billboards and posters spreading the cigarette message have dotted the landscape in Hispanic communities for many years, especially in

WHAT DO **YOU** THINK?

Nicotine is highly addictive, so should it be regulated as a controlled substance?

- How could tobacco be regulated effectively?
- Should more resources be used for research into nicotine addiction? Why or why not?

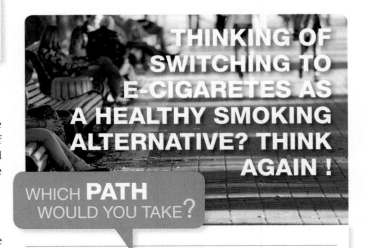

WHICH **PATH** WOULD YOU TAKE?

Go to Mastering Health to see how your actions today affect your future health.

low-income areas. Tobacco companies also sponsor community-based events such as festivals and annual fairs.

Financial Costs to Society
Annual costs attributed to smoking in the United States are estimated to be between $289 and $333 billion.[100] The economic burden of tobacco use totals more than $170 billion in direct medical expenditures and more than $150 billion in lost productivity.[101] It is estimated that smoking-related health costs and productivity losses are $19.16 per pack of cigarettes sold.[102]

College Students and Tobacco Use

College students are the targets of heavy tobacco marketing and advertising campaigns. The tobacco industry has set up aggressive marketing promotions at bars, music festivals, and other events specifically targeted at the 18- to 24-year-old age group. On top of targeted advertising, peer influence can prompt students to start smoking, and many colleges and universities still sell tobacco products in campus stores. However, cigarette smoking among U.S. college students has decreased in recent years (**FIGURE 9.10**). In a 2016 survey, over 10 percent of college students reported having smoked cigarettes in the past 30 days.[103] College men have slightly higher rates of smoking (13 percent) compared to women (8 percent).[104] Men also use more cigars and smokeless tobacco.[105]

See the **Points of View** box for a discussion of banning smoking on campuses.

Why Do College Students Smoke?
Among the reasons students smoke are to relax and to reduce stress. Smokers are more likely to have high levels of perceived stress than nonsmokers. Students also smoke to fit in or because they are addicted to tobacco. For some students, weight control is an important motivator, and fear of weight gain is a common reason for smoking relapse among those who quit. Students who have been diagnosed or treated for depression are much more likely to use tobacco compared to students who have not.

Social Smoking
Many college-age smokers identify themselves as "social smokers," that is, they smoke only with other people rather than alone. Social smokers typically smoke on weekends, at night, at social events, or when just hanging out with friends. Often, social smokers smoke to fit in with groups and to help social interactions.[106] Even occasional smoking is not without risks of damaging health effects. Smoking less than a pack of cigarettes a week has been shown to damage blood vessels and to increase the risk of heart disease and cancer.[107] In women who take birth control pills, even a few cigarettes a week can increase the likelihood of heart disease, blood clots, stroke, liver cancer, and gallbladder disease.[108]

Tobacco Use and Prevention Policies

It has been more than 40 years since the U.S. government began warning that tobacco use was hazardous to health. Despite all the education on the health hazards of tobacco use,

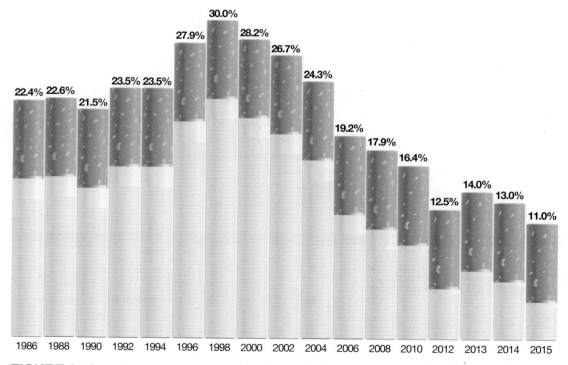

FIGURE 9.10 Trends in Prevalence of Cigarette Smoking in the Past Month among College Students

Source: Data from L. D. Johnston et al., *Monitoring the Future National Survey Results on Drug Use, 1975–2015, Volume II: College Students and Adults Ages 19–50* (Ann Arbor, MI: Institute for Social Research, University of Michigan, 2016).

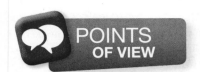

SMOKING ON COLLEGE AND UNIVERSITY CAMPUSES *Should Smoking Be Banned?*

In recent years, hundreds of campuses have implemented all-out prohibitions or significant restrictions on tobacco use, with many more campuses pursuing becoming smoke-free. Currently, there are an estimated 1,757 smoke-free campuses. Of these, 1,468 are completely free of tobacco, 1,331 ban e-cigarettes use, and 652 prohibit hookah use anywhere on campus. The debate regarding tobacco-free campuses (including the ban of e-cigarettes) is contentious at many schools. Following are some of the major points on both sides of the question.

Arguments for Banning Tobacco on Campuses

- The majority of college students— 4 out of 5—do not smoke.
- Two-thirds of students and most employees prefer to attend classes held on a smoke-free campus.
- One in five students say that they have experienced some immediate health impact from exposure to environmental tobacco smoke.
- Nonsmokers are 40 percent less likely to become smokers if they live in smoke-free dorms.
- Very little is known about the harmful effects caused by exposure to e-cigarettes.
- Secondhand e-cigarette vapor contains nicotine, low levels of carcinogens, and ultrafine particles.

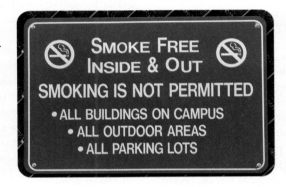

Arguments against Banning Tobacco on Campuses

- There are so many other causes of potentially harmful fumes on campus—from diesel trucks, for example—that banning smoking wouldn't really affect the overall health and air quality on campus.
- The policy would be difficult if not impossible to enforce.
- Smokers who are forced outside to light up are possibly being put in danger at night or in other situations when they would have to leave residence halls.
- Smoking bans in public and private places violate the rights of smokers and encourage discriminatory treatment of people who are addicted to nicotine.

WHERE DO YOU STAND?

- Is smoking on a college campus a threat to public health?
- Do you think that smokers have the right to smoke in dorms, in campus buildings, in adjacent parks, or in other public places on campus? Why or why not?
- How do you feel when you are walking across campus and someone is smoking close to you? Do you feel as though you could or should ask smokers to put out their cigarettes?
- Would banning smoking be discriminatory? Would it be a violation of individual rights? Should student smokers be singled out for exclusion on college campuses?

Sources: American Nonsmokers' Rights Foundation, Smoke-Free and Tobacco-Free U.S. and Tribal Colleges and Universities, January 2, 2017; American Nonsmokers' Rights Foundation, Colleges and Universities, February 15, 2017, http://no-smoke.org/goingsmokefree.php?id=447; University of Michigan, National Tobacco Free Campus Initiative, http://sph.umich.edu.

health care and lost productivity associated with smoking cost between $289 billion and $333 billion each year.[109]

In 1998, the tobacco industry reached the Master Settlement Agreement with 46 states. The agreement requires tobacco companies to pay out more than $206 billion over 25 years. The agreement includes a variety of measures to support antismoking education and advertising and to fund research to determine effective smoking-cessation strategies. The agreement also curbs certain advertising and promotions directed at youth.

Unfortunately, most of the money designated for tobacco control and prevention at the state level has not been used for this purpose. Facing budget woes, many states have drastically cut spending on antismoking programs. In the few states that have spent the settlement money on smoking-cessation programs, there has been some reported success in decreasing cigarette use.[110] The Family Smoking Prevention and Tobacco Control Act of 2009 allows the FDA to forbid tobacco advertising geared toward children, to lower the amount of nicotine in tobacco products, to ban sweetened cigarettes that appeal to young people, and to prohibit labels such as "light" and "low tar."[111] One of the most significant impacts of the law is that it requires more prominent health warnings on advertising of tobacco products. Smokeless tobacco ads now must contain a warning that fills 20 percent of the advertising space. The FDA attempted to require cigarette packages and advertising to have larger, graphical warnings depicting the negative consequences of smoking, but a federal judge declared the requirement unconstitutional in 2012.

LO 6 | TOBACCO AND ITS EFFECTS

Identify different types of tobacco products and the chemicals they contain, and explain their effects on the body.

Smoking, the most common form of tobacco use, delivers a strong dose of nicotine as well as 7,000 other chemical substances, including arsenic, formaldehyde, and ammonia, directly to the lungs. Among these chemicals are more than 70 known or suspected carcinogens.[112] Inhaling hot toxic gases exposes sensitive mucous membranes to irritating chemicals that weaken the tissues and contribute to cancers of the mouth, larynx, and throat. The heat from tobacco smoke is also harmful to tissues.

Nicotine

The highly addictive chemical stimulant **nicotine** is the major psychoactive substance in all tobacco products. In its natural form, nicotine is a colorless liquid that turns brown on exposure to air. When tobacco leaves are burned in a cigarette, pipe, or cigar, nicotine is released and inhaled into the lungs. Sucking or chewing tobacco releases nicotine into the saliva, and the nicotine is then absorbed through mucous membranes in the mouth. In e-cigarettes, nicotine is released when a mixture of nicotine, glycol, glycerin, and flavorings is vaporized into an aerosol that the smoker inhales.

Nicotine is a powerful CNS stimulant producing a variety of physiological effects. In the cerebral cortex, it produces an aroused, alert mental state. Nicotine stimulates the adrenal glands, which increases the production of adrenaline. It also increases heart and respiratory rates, constricts blood vessels, and, in turn, increases blood pressure because the heart must work harder to pump blood through the narrowed vessels.

Beginning smokers usually feel the effects of nicotine with their first puff. These symptoms, called **nicotine poisoning**, can include dizziness, lightheadedness, rapid and erratic pulse, clammy skin, nausea and vomiting, and diarrhea. These unpleasant effects cease as tolerance develops, which happens almost immediately in new users, perhaps after the second or third cigarette. In contrast, tolerance to most other drugs, such as alcohol, develops over a period of months or years. Regular smokers generally do not experience a "buzz" from smoking. They continue to smoke simply because quitting is so difficult.

nicotine The primary stimulant chemical in tobacco products; nicotine is highly addictive.

nicotine poisoning Symptoms often experienced by beginning smokers, including dizziness, diarrhea, light-headedness, rapid and erratic pulse, clammy skin, nausea, and vomiting.

tar Thick, brownish sludge condensed from particulate matter in smoked tobacco.

Tar and Carbon Monoxide

Cigarette smoke is a complex mixture of chemicals and gases produced by the burning of tobacco and its additives. Particulate matter condenses in the lungs to form a thick, brownish sludge called **tar**, which contains various carcinogenic agents such as benzopyrene and chemical irritants such as phenol. Phenol has the potential to combine with other chemicals that contribute to developing lung cancer.

In healthy lungs, millions of tiny hairlike projections (*cilia*) on the surfaces lining the upper respiratory passages sweep away foreign matter, which is expelled from the lungs by coughing. However, the cilia's cleansing function is impaired in smokers' lungs by nicotine, which paralyzes the cilia for up to 1 hour after a single cigarette. This allows tars and other solids in tobacco smoke to accumulate and irritate sensitive lung tissue. **FIGURE 9.11** illustrates how tobacco smoke damages the lungs.

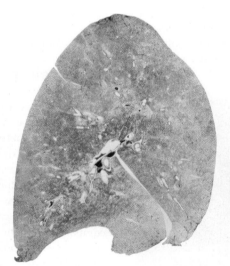

 A healthy lung

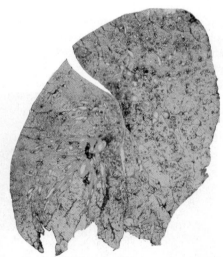

ⓑ A smoker's lung permeated with deposits of tar

FIGURE 9.11 Lung Damage from Chemicals in Tobacco Smoke Smoke particles irritate lung pathways, causing extra mucus production, and nicotine paralyzes the cilia that normally function to keep the lungs clear of excess mucus. The result is difficulty breathing, "smoker's cough," and chronic bronchitis. At the same time, tar collects within the alveoli (air sacs), ultimately causing their walls to break, leading to emphysema. Tar and other carcinogens in tobacco smoke also cause cellular mutations that lead to cancer.

carbon monoxide A gas found in tobacco smoke that reduces the ability of blood to carry oxygen.

Cigarette smoke also contains poisonous gases, the most dangerous of which is **carbon monoxide**, the deadly gas that is emitted in car exhaust. Carbon monoxide reduces the oxygen-carrying capacity of red blood cells by binding with the receptor sites for oxygen, causing oxygen deprivation in many body tissues. It is at least partly responsible for increased risk of heart attacks and strokes in smokers.

Tobacco Use Disorder

The American Psychiatric Association defines tobacco use disorder as a "problematic pattern of tobacco use leading to clinically significant impairment or distress"[113] that is characterized by at least two of the following signs and symptoms in a 12-month period: (1) use of tobacco in larger amounts or over a longer period of time than intended; (2) persistent desire and unsuccessful efforts to cut down or quit; (3) spending a large amount of time getting or using tobacco; (4) craving tobacco; (5) tobacco use interfering with work, school, or social obligations; (6) reoccurring social or personal relationship issues caused by smoking; (7) giving up or reducing important activities; (8) persistent tobacco use in physically hazardous situations, such as smoking in bed; (9) continued tobacco use despite a persistent or reoccurring physical or psychological problem resulting from tobacco use; (10) increasing tolerance, such as smoking an increasing number of cigarettes to obtain the desired effect; and (11) withdrawal symptoms related to reducing or quitting tobacco use.[114]

Tobacco Products

Tobacco comes in several forms. Cigarettes, cigars, pipes, and bidis are used for burning and inhaling tobacco. Smokeless tobacco is sniffed or placed in the mouth. Electronic cigarettes are an increasingly popular vehicle for nicotine, with their own health risks.

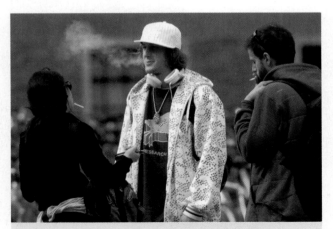

There is no safe amount of tobacco use. Any exposure to smoke increases your risks for negative health effects. Even if you consider yourself "only" a social smoker, chances are you're on the road to dependence and a more frequent smoking habit.

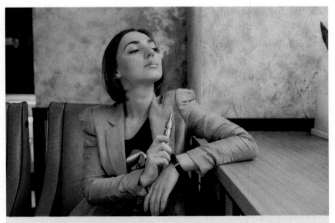

Electronic cigarette, or e-cigarette.

Cigarettes *Filtered cigarettes* are the most common form of tobacco available today. Almost all manufactured cigarettes have filters designed to reduce levels of gases such as hydrogen cyanide and carbon monoxide, but these products may actually deliver more hazardous gases to the user than do non-filtered brands. Some smokers use low-tar and low-nicotine products as an excuse to smoke more cigarettes, thus exposing themselves to more harmful substances than they would with regular-strength cigarettes.

Clove cigarettes contain about 40 percent ground cloves (a spice) and about 60 percent tobacco. Many users mistakenly believe that these products are made entirely of ground cloves and that smoking them eliminates the risks associated with tobacco. In fact, clove cigarettes contain higher levels of tar and carbon monoxide than do regular cigarettes, and the numbing effect of eugenol, the active ingredient in cloves, allows smokers to inhale the smoke more deeply. The same effect is true of *menthol cigarettes*; the throat-numbing effect of the menthol allows for deeper inhalation.

E-Cigarettes Electronic cigarettes (also called *e-cigarettes*, *electronic nicotine delivery systems*, *vape pens*, or simply *vapes*) typically deliver nicotine, flavorings (e.g., mint, chocolate), and other additives as vapor instead of smoke. When a user draws air through one of these devices, an airflow sensor activates the battery and heats the atomizer to vaporize propylene glycol and nicotine. On inhalation, the aerosol vapor delivers a dose of nicotine into the lungs, after which residual aerosol is exhaled into the environment. Beyond exposing users to chemicals such as nicotine, carbonyl compounds, and volatile organic compounds, the health effects and harmful doses of heated and aerosolized constituents of e-cigarette fluids, including solvents, flavorings, and toxicants are not fully understood.[115]

In a recent survey, about 11 percent of college students reported using e-cigarettes in the past, with 4.3 percent reporting usage in the past 30 days.[116] Students who use e-cigarettes are more likely to be heavy drinkers. While many campuses and many student apartments

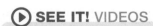

SEE IT! VIDEOS

What are the dangers of e-cigarettes for children? Watch **GMA Investigates Liquid Nicotine** in the Study Area of Mastering Health.

and rental houses have become tobacco or smoke free, the availability of e-cigarettes—and their barely detectable odor—may allow students to work around those bans and more easily use nicotine along with alcohol.[117]

Cigars As cigarette use has declined, sales of large cigars have more than tripled.[118] Many people believe that cigars are safer than cigarettes when the opposite is true. Cigars have higher levels of cancer-causing substances, more tar per gram of tobacco smoked, and higher levels of toxins than do cigarettes.[119] In addition, smoking cigars causes many of the same diseases as cigarette smoking and smokeless tobacco. Regular cigar smokers are at risk for developing cancers of the lung, oral cavity, larynx, esophagus, and possibly pancreas. Cigar smokers have 4 to 10 times the risk of dying from lung, laryngeal, oral, or esophageal cancer compared to people who have never smoked.[120] Most cigars contain as much nicotine as several cigarettes, and when cigar smokers inhale, nicotine is absorbed as rapidly as it is with cigarettes. Smokers who don't inhale still expose the lips, tongue, throat, and larynx to a number of toxic chemicals contained in tobacco smoke, and high levels of nicotine are still absorbed through the mouth's mucous membranes. A single cigar can potentially provide as much nicotine as a pack of cigarettes.[121]

Bidis Generally made in India or Southeast Asia, **bidis** are small, hand-rolled cigarettes that come in a variety of flavors, such as vanilla, chocolate, and cherry. They have become increasingly popular with college students because they are viewed as safer and cheaper than cigarettes. However, they are far more toxic than cigarettes. Smoke from a bidi contains three to five times as much nicotine as is found in cigarettes.[122] The leaf wrappers are nonporous, which means that smokers must suck harder to inhale and inhale more to keep the bidi lit. This results in much more exposure to higher amounts of tar, nicotine, and carbon monoxide.

Pipes and Hookahs Pipes have had a long history of use throughout the world, including ritualistic and ceremonial use in many cultures. According to the National Cancer Institute and the American Cancer Society, pipe smoking carries risks similar to those of cigar smoking.

Hookahs, a type of water pipe with a long hose for inhaling, originated in the Middle East but have become particularly popular among young adults in the United States. Many students believe that smoking a hookah is safer than smoking cigarettes. However, many of the same harmful toxins and chemicals found in cigarettes—those associated with lung cancer, respiratory disease, low birth weight babies, and periodontal disease—are also found in hookah smoke.[123] Health risks associated with hookah use also include the possibility of infectious disease transmission by sharing a pipe.

Smokeless Tobacco There are two types of smokeless tobacco: chewing tobacco and snuff.

Chewing tobacco comes in three forms—loose leaf, plug, or in a pouch—and contains tobacco leaves treated with molasses and other flavorings. The user "dips" the tobacco by placing a small amount between the lower lip and teeth to stimulate the flow of saliva and release the nicotine. **Dipping** releases nicotine rapidly into the bloodstream. While cigarette smoking has been on the decline in the United States among youth, use of smokeless tobacco by youth has held steady since 1999.[124]

Snuff is a finely ground form of tobacco that can be inhaled, chewed, or placed against the gums. It comes in dry or moist powdered form or sachets (pouches that resemble tea bags). In 2009, *snus* became the latest form of smokeless tobacco to hit the market in the United States. Popular for more than 100 years in Sweden, these small sachets of tobacco are placed inside the cheek and sucked. Some people prefer snus to chewing tobacco because snus doesn't require the user to spit frequently.

Smokeless tobacco is just as addictive as cigarettes and actually contains more nicotine; holding an average-sized dip or chew in the mouth for 30 minutes delivers as much nicotine as smoking four cigarettes. A two-can-a-week snuff user gets as much nicotine as a ten-pack-a-week smoker.

bidis Hand-rolled flavored cigarettes.

chewing tobacco A stringy form of tobacco that is placed in the mouth and then sucked or chewed.

dipping Placing a small amount of chewing tobacco between the lower lip and teeth for rapid nicotine absorption.

snuff A powdered form of tobacco that is sniffed and absorbed through the mucous membranes in the nose or placed inside the cheek and sucked.

LO 7 | **HEALTH** HAZARDS OF TOBACCO PRODUCTS

Describe the health risks and physical impact associated with using tobacco products and with environmental tobacco smoke.

Each day, tobacco contributes to approximately 1,200 deaths from cancer, cardiovascular disease, and respiratory disorders.[125] In addition, tobacco use can negatively affect the health of almost every system in your body. **FIGURE 9.12** summarizes some physiological and health effects of smoking.

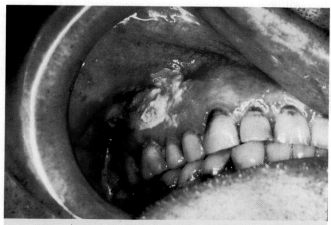

Leukoplakia can appear on the tongue or gums, as shown here.

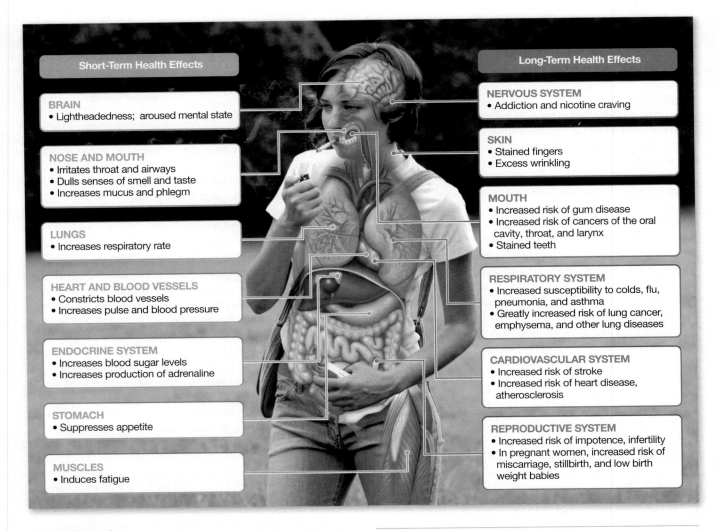

Short-Term Health Effects

BRAIN
• Lightheadedness; aroused mental state

NOSE AND MOUTH
• Irritates throat and airways
• Dulls senses of smell and taste
• Increases mucus and phlegm

LUNGS
• Increases respiratory rate

HEART AND BLOOD VESSELS
• Constricts blood vessels
• Increases pulse and blood pressure

ENDOCRINE SYSTEM
• Increases blood sugar levels
• Increases production of adrenaline

STOMACH
• Suppresses appetite

MUSCLES
• Induces fatigue

Long-Term Health Effects

NERVOUS SYSTEM
• Addiction and nicotine craving

SKIN
• Stained fingers
• Excess wrinkling

MOUTH
• Increased risk of gum disease
• Increased risk of cancers of the oral cavity, throat, and larynx
• Stained teeth

RESPIRATORY SYSTEM
• Increased susceptibility to colds, flu, pneumonia, and asthma
• Greatly increased risk of lung cancer, emphysema, and other lung diseases

CARDIOVASCULAR SYSTEM
• Increased risk of stroke
• Increased risk of heart disease, atherosclerosis

REPRODUCTIVE SYSTEM
• Increased risk of impotence, infertility
• In pregnant women, increased risk of miscarriage, stillbirth, and low birth weight babies

FIGURE 9.12 Effects of Smoking on the Body and Health

Watch Video Tutor: **Long- and Short-Term Effects of Tobacco** in Mastering Health.

Cancer

Lung cancer is the leading cause of cancer deaths in the United States. The American Cancer Society estimates that tobacco smoking causes 90 percent of all cases of lung cancer in men and 78 percent in women.[126] There were an estimated 222,500 new cases of lung cancer in the United States in 2017 alone, and an estimated 155,870 Americans died from the disease in 2017.[127]

If you are a smoker, your risk of developing lung cancer depends on several factors. First, the amount you smoke per day is important. The more you smoke, the more likely you are to develop lung cancer. A second factor is the age at which you started smoking; if you started in your teens, you have a greater chance of developing lung cancer than do people who start later. A third factor is whether you inhale deeply when you smoke, which increases your risk. Smokers are also more susceptible to the cancer-causing effects of exposure to other irritants, such as asbestos and radon, than are nonsmokers.

A major risk of chewing tobacco is **leukoplakia**, a condition characterized by leathery white patches inside the mouth, produced by contact with irritants in tobacco juice. While the majority of leukoplakia cases do not develop into cancer, some are precancerous and can eventually progress to cancer without proper treatment or are already cancerous on initial sighting.[128]

Over 49,670 cases of oral cancer were diagnosed in 2017, the vast majority of which were caused by smokeless tobacco or cigarettes.[129] Smokeless tobacco users have significantly higher rates of oral cancer than do nonusers. Warning signs include lumps in the jaw or neck; color changes or lumps inside the lips; white, smooth, or scaly patches in the mouth or on the neck, lips, or tongue; a red spot or sore on the lips or gums or inside the mouth that does not heal in 2 weeks; repeated bleeding in the mouth; and difficulty or abnormality in speaking or swallowing.

leukoplakia A condition characterized by leathery white patches inside the mouth; produced by contact with irritants in tobacco juice.

The lag time between first use and contracting cancer is shorter for smokeless tobacco users than for smokers because absorption through the gums is the most efficient route of nicotine administration. Many smokeless tobacco users eventually "graduate" to cigarettes and increase their risk for developing additional problems.

Tobacco use is linked to other cancers as well. The rate of pancreatic cancer is more than twice as high for smokers as for nonsmokers. Typically, the prognosis for people with pancreatic cancer is not good; the 5-year survival rate is 7 percent.[130] Smokers are at increased risk to develop cancers of the lip, tongue, salivary glands, and esophagus. A growing body of evidence suggests that long-term use of smokeless tobacco increases the risk of cancers of the larynx, esophagus, nasal cavity, pancreas, colon, kidney, and bladder.

Cardiovascular Disease

Smoking tobacco is a major risk factor for cardiovascular disease and stroke.[131] Smoking poses as great a risk for developing heart disease as high blood pressure and high cholesterol do.

Smoking contributes to heart disease by aging the arteries.[132] This occurs because smoking and exposure to environmental tobacco smoke (ETS) encourage and accelerate the buildup of fatty deposits (plaque) in the heart and major blood vessels (*atherosclerosis*). Smokers can experience a 50 percent increase in plaque accumulation in the arteries, compared with former smokers. Nonsmokers who are regularly exposed to ETS can have a 20 to 25 percent increase in plaque buildup.[133] For unknown reasons, smoking decreases blood levels of HDLs, the "good cholesterol" that helps to protect against heart attacks.

Smoking also contributes to **platelet adhesiveness**, the sticking together of red blood cells associated with blood clots. The oxygen deprivation associated with smoking decreases the oxygen supplied to the heart and can weaken tissues. Smoking also contributes to irregular heart rhythms, which can trigger a heart attack. Both carbon monoxide and nicotine can precipitate angina attacks (chest pain due to the heart muscle not getting the blood supply it needs).

Smokers are two to four times as likely to suffer strokes as nonsmokers.[134] A stroke occurs when a small blood vessel in the brain bursts or is blocked by a blood clot, denying oxygen and nourishment to vital portions of the brain. Depending on the area of the brain affected, stroke can result in paralysis, loss of mental functioning, or death. Smoking contributes to strokes by raising blood pressure, which increases the stress on vessel walls, and platelet adhesiveness contributes to blood clot formation.

Respiratory Disorders

Smoking quickly impairs the respiratory system in the form of breathlessness, chronic cough, and excess phlegm production. Over time, cumulative lung damage can lead to chronic obstructive pulmonary disease, including chronic bronchitis and emphysema. Ultimately, smokers are up to 25 times more likely to die of lung disease than are nonsmokers.[135]

Chronic bronchitis may develop in smokers because their inflamed lungs produce more mucus, which they constantly try to expel along with foreign particles. This results in the persistent cough known as "smoker's hack." Smokers are also more prone than nonsmokers to respiratory ailments such as influenza, pneumonia, and colds.

Emphysema is a chronic disease in which the alveoli (the tiny air sacs in the lungs) are destroyed, impairing the lungs' ability to obtain oxygen and remove carbon dioxide. As a result, breathing becomes difficult. Whereas healthy people expend only about 5 percent of their energy in breathing, people with advanced emphysema expend nearly 80 percent. Because the heart has to work harder to do even the simplest tasks, it may become enlarged, and death from heart damage may result. There is no known cure for emphysema, and the damage is irreversible. Approximately 80 to 90 percent of all cases of emphysema are related to cigarette smoking.[136]

Sexual Dysfunction and Fertility Problems

Despite attempts by tobacco advertisers to make smoking appear sexy, research shows that it can cause impotence in men. Studies have found that male smokers are much more likely to experience erectile dysfunction than are nonsmokers.[137] Toxins in cigarette smoke damage blood vessels, reducing blood flow to the penis and leading to an inadequate erection. Impotence may indicate oncoming cardiovascular disease.

In women, smoking can lead to infertility and problems with pregnancy. Women who smoke increase their risk for infertility, ectopic pregnancy, miscarriage, and stillbirth. Smoking also increases the risk of sudden infant death syndrome and the chances of a baby being born with a cleft lip or cleft palate.[138] Smoking during pregnancy increases the chance of premature birth and the risk of low birth weight (less than 5.5 pounds), which in turn increases the likelihood of illness or death of an infant.[139]

Other Health Effects

Studies have shown tobacco use to be a serious risk factor in the development of gum disease.[140] In addition, smoking increases risk of macular degeneration, one of the most common causes of blindness in older adults. It also causes premature skin wrinkling, staining of the teeth, yellowing of the fingernails, and bad breath. Nicotine speeds up the process by which the body uses and eliminates drugs, making medications less effective. In addition, recent research suggests smoking significantly increases the risk for Alzheimer's disease.[141]

Environmental Tobacco Smoke

Although fewer Americans smoke than was the case in the past, air pollution from smoking in public places continues to be a problem. **Environmental tobacco smoke (ETS)** is divided into two categories: mainstream and sidestream

platelet adhesiveness Stickiness of red blood cells associated with blood clots.

emphysema Chronic lung disease in which the tiny air sacs in the lungs are destroyed, making breathing difficult.

environmental tobacco smoke (ETS) Smoke from tobacco products, including secondhand and mainstream smoke.

mainstream smoke Smoke that is drawn through tobacco while inhaling.

sidestream smoke Smoke from the burning end of a cigarette, pipe, or cigar or exhaled by nonsmokers; commonly called *secondhand smoke*.

smoke. **Mainstream smoke** refers to smoke drawn through tobacco while inhaling; **sidestream smoke** (commonly called *secondhand smoke*) refers to smoke from the burning end of a cigarette or smoke exhaled by a smoker. People who breathe smoke from someone else's smoking product are said to be *involuntary* or *passive* smokers.

Between 1988 and 2008, detectable levels of nicotine exposure in nonsmoking Americans decreased from 87.9 percent to 25.3 percent.[142] The decrease in exposure to secondhand smoke is due to the growing number of laws that ban smoking in workplaces and other public areas. As of 2016, 41 states and the District of Columbia had laws requiring workplaces, restaurants, and bars to be 100 percent smoke-free.[143] There are 22,578 municipalities—home to 82 percent of the U.S. population—that are covered by either state, commonwealth, territorial, or local law.[144] Groups such as Action on Smoking and Health and Americans for Nonsmokers' Rights continue to push for policies and laws in support of smoke-free public places.[145]

Risks from Environmental Tobacco Smoke

Although involuntary smokers breathe less tobacco than active smokers do, they still face risks from exposure. According to the American Lung Association, secondhand smoke contains hundreds of chemicals that are known to be toxic or carcinogenic, including formaldehyde, benzene, vinyl chloride, arsenic ammonia, and hydrogen cyanide.[146] Every year, ETS is estimated to be responsible for approximately 3,400 lung cancer deaths in nonsmoking adults, 46,000 coronary and heart disease deaths in nonsmoking adults who live with smokers, and higher risk of death in newborns from sudden infant death syndrome.[147]

The Environmental Protection Agency has designated secondhand smoke as a known carcinogen. More than 70 cancer-causing agents are found in secondhand smoke.[148] There is also strong evidence that secondhand smoke interferes with normal functioning of the heart, blood, and vascular systems, significantly increasing the risk for heart disease. Studies indicate that nonsmokers who had been exposed to secondhand smoke were far more likely to have coronary heart disease and stroke than were nonsmokers who had not been exposed to smoke.[149]

LO 8 | QUITTING SMOKING

Describe methods and benefits of smoking cessation.

Approximately 70 percent of U.S. adult smokers want to quit smoking, and up to 55 percent make a serious attempt to quit each year.[150] Quitting is often a lengthy process involving several unsuccessful attempts before success is finally achieved. Even successful quitters suffer occasional slips. Smokers who are unable to quit can expect to lose at least one decade of life compared to people who do not smoke.

Benefits of Quitting

Many body tissues damaged by smoking can repair themselves. As soon as the person stops smoking, the body begins the repair process. Within 12 hours, carbon monoxide levels return to normal, and "smoker's breath" disappears.[151] Often, within a month of quitting, the mucus that clogs airways is broken up and eliminated. Circulation and the senses of taste and smell improve within weeks. Many former smokers say that they have more energy, sleep better, and feel more alert.

After 1 year, the risk for heart disease decreases,[152] and women are less likely to bear babies of low birth weight.[153] After 10 smoke-free years, the risk of developing cancer of the lung, larynx, pancreas, kidney, bladder, or cervix is considerably reduced.[154] See **FIGURE 9.13** for a timeline of how the body recuperates after a smoker quits.

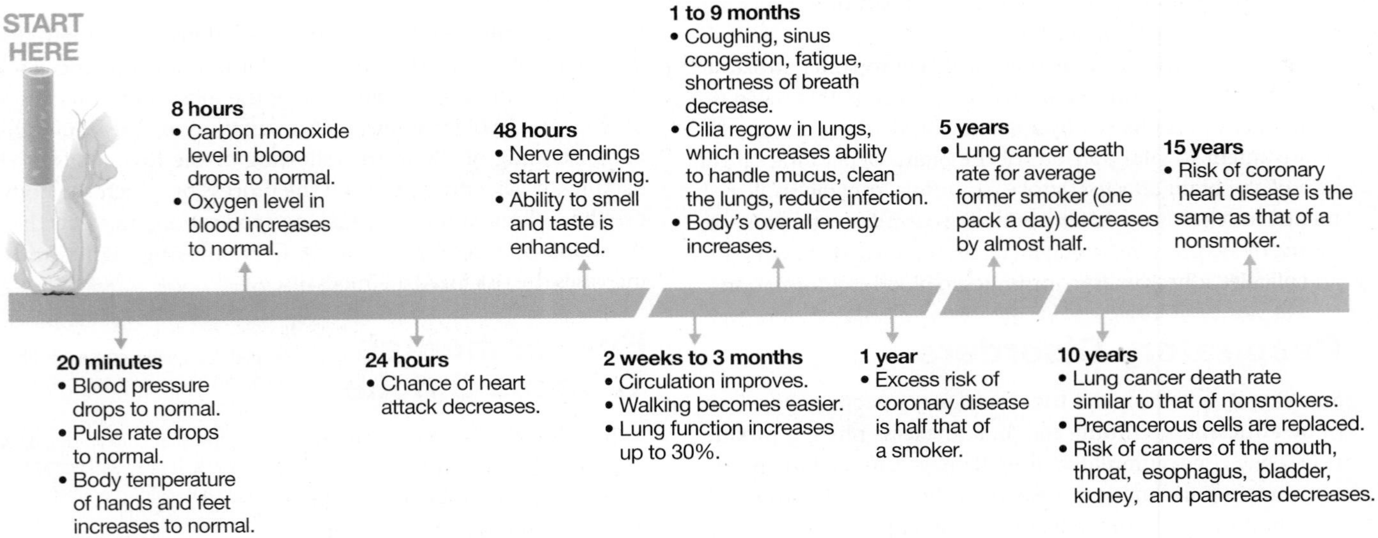

START HERE

8 hours
- Carbon monoxide level in blood drops to normal.
- Oxygen level in blood increases to normal.

48 hours
- Nerve endings start regrowing.
- Ability to smell and taste is enhanced.

1 to 9 months
- Coughing, sinus congestion, fatigue, shortness of breath decrease.
- Cilia regrow in lungs, which increases ability to handle mucus, clean the lungs, reduce infection.
- Body's overall energy increases.

5 years
- Lung cancer death rate for average former smoker (one pack a day) decreases by almost half.

15 years
- Risk of coronary heart disease is the same as that of a nonsmoker.

20 minutes
- Blood pressure drops to normal.
- Pulse rate drops to normal.
- Body temperature of hands and feet increases to normal.

24 hours
- Chance of heart attack decreases.

2 weeks to 3 months
- Circulation improves.
- Walking becomes easier.
- Lung function increases up to 30%.

1 year
- Excess risk of coronary disease is half that of a smoker.

10 years
- Lung cancer death rate similar to that of nonsmokers.
- Precancerous cells are replaced.
- Risk of cancers of the mouth, throat, esophagus, bladder, kidney, and pancreas decreases.

FIGURE 9.13 When Smokers Quit Within 20 minutes of smoking that final cigarette, the body begins to undergo a series of changes that continues for years. However, by smoking just one cigarette a day, the smoker loses all these benefits, according to the American Cancer Society.

Another significant benefit of quitting smoking is the money saved. The cost of a single pack of cigarettes, including taxes, ranges from about $5.19 to as much as $12.60 in the most expensive state, so a pack-a-day smoker who lives in an area where cigarettes cost $8.00 per pack spends $56.00 per week, or $2,912 per year.[155]

How Can You Quit?

Smokers who want to quit have several options. Most people who succeed quit "cold turkey," that is, they decide simply not to smoke again, and they don't. Others focus on gradual reduction in smoking levels, which can reduce risks over time. Some rely on short-term programs based on behavior modification and a system of self-rewards. Still others turn to treatment centers, community outreach programs, or a telephone helpline. Finally, some people work privately with their physicians to reach their goal. Programs that combine several approaches have shown the most promise.

Breaking the Nicotine Addiction

Nicotine addiction may be one of the toughest addictions to overcome. Symptoms of **nicotine withdrawal** include irritability, restlessness, nausea, vomiting, and intense cravings for tobacco (see **TABLE 9.2**). The evidence is strong that consistent pharmacological treatments can double a smoker's chances of quitting. The FDA has approved seven medications to help with smoking cessation. Three of these are over-the-counter medications: nicotine gum, patches, and lozenges. There are four prescription options: nicotine inhalers, nicotine nasal sprays, Zyban (bupropion, an antidepressant), and Chantix (varenicline, a drug that blocks the effects of nicotine in the brain).[156]

The **Skills for Behavior Change** box presents one of the American Cancer Society's approaches for quitting smoking. The **Mindfulness and You** box talks about how mindfulness may help break the habit.

Nicotine Replacement Products Nontobacco products that replace depleted levels of nicotine in the bloodstream have helped some people stop using tobacco. The two most common

nicotine withdrawal Symptoms, including nausea, headaches, irritability, and intense tobacco cravings, suffered by nicotine-addicted individuals who stop using tobacco.

SKILLS FOR
BEHAVIOR CHANGE

Tips for Quitting Smoking

Are you ready to quit tobacco? These strategies can help:

- Ask smokers who live with you to keep cigarettes out of sight and not offer you any.
- Use the four Ds: deep breaths, drink water, do something else, and delay (tell yourself you'll smoke in 10 minutes when the urge hits).
- Keep "mouth toys" handy: hard candy, chewing gum, toothpicks or coffee stirrers, or carrot or celery sticks can help.
- Ask your doctor about nicotine gum, patches, nasal sprays, inhalers, or lozenges.
- Make an appointment with your dental hygienist to have your teeth cleaned.
- Examine the associations that trigger your urge to smoke.
- Spend your time in places that don't allow smoking.
- Take up a new sport, exercise program, hobby, or organizational commitment. This will help to shake up your routine and distract you from smoking.

TABLE **9.2** | Coping Strategies for Common Smoking Withdrawal Problems

Withdrawal Challenge	Estimated Length of Symptoms	Coping Strategies*
Anger, frustration, and irritability	Peaks in first week after quitting but can last 2–4 weeks	Avoid caffeine, which can amp up an already agitated mood. Get a massage; try deep breathing or exercise.
Anxiety	Builds over the first 3 days and may last up to 2 weeks	Same strategies as above. Also remind yourself that the symptoms usually pass by themselves over time.
Mild depression	One month or less	Be with supportive friends, increase physical activity, make a list of things that are upsetting you, and write down possible solutions. If depression lasts longer than a month, seek medical advice.
Weight gain	Usually begins in the early weeks and continues through the first year after quitting	Studies show that nicotine replacement products such as gum and lozenges can help to counter weight gain. You may also ask your doctor about the drug bupropion (brand name: Zyban), which has also been shown to counter weight gain.

*Asking your doctor for nicotine-replacement products or other medications is a valid coping strategy for any of the withdrawal challenges listed here.

Source: Adapted from National Cancer Institute, "Handling Withdrawal Symptoms When You Decide to Quit," National Cancer Institute Fact Sheet, accessed March 2017, www.cancer.gov.

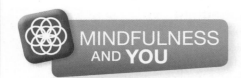

MINDFULNESS FOR SMOKING CESSATION

More people are addicted to nicotine than to any other drug in the United States. Research suggests that nicotine maybe as addictive as heroin, cocaine, or alcohol. Successfully quitting smoking is a challenge that often requires more than one attempt. About 70 percent of adult smokers report wanting to quit smoking completely. Fifty-five percent tried to stop smoking for more than one day in the past year.

Recently, mindfulness-based therapies have been found to offer greater chances of success for those attempting to quit smoking. Mindfulness interventions have also been shown to decrease negative affect and craving in smokers.

Dr. Judson Brewer, the Director of Research at the Center for Mindfulness at the University of Massachusetts, has found that people who use mindfulness training may have better outcomes than those who use standard methods of quitting. Dr. Brewer uses the acronym RAIN to help people manage their nicotine cravings.

- **R**ecognize the craving that is occurring, and relax with it.
- **A**ccept the moment. Pay attention to how your body is feeling.
- **I**nvestigate the experience. Ask yourself what is happening to your body in this moment.
- **N**ote what is happening. As you acknowledge anxiousness, irritability, and other feelings, realize that they are nothing more than body sensations that will pass.

Using mindfulness techniques in this way will help the body become familiar with the cravings and learn that it can adapt.

Cravings usually last from 90 seconds to 3 minutes. Simply using the acronym above helps many smokers to acknowledge and get through the craving, which should then become weaker over time.

Sources: J. Brewer, "A Randomized Controlled Trial of Smartphone-Based Mindfulness Training for Smoking Cessation: A Study Protocol," *BMC Psychiatry* 15, no. 83 (2015): 2–7; J. Brewer, "A Simple Way to Break A Habit," TED TalkMED, November, 2015; Centers for Disease Control and Prevention, "Smoking & Tobacco Use: Quitting Smoking," February 1, 2017, https://www.cdc.gov/tobacco/data_statistics/fact_sheets/cessation/quitting; L. Peltz, "Practicing Mindfulness to Help You Break the Habit of Smoking," Expert Beacon, 2016, https://expertbeacon.com/practicing-mindfulness-help-you-break-habit-smoking/#.WM2YbhAfSPV; A. Ruscio et al., "Effect of Brief Mindfulness Practice on Self-Reported Affect, Craving and Smoking: A Pilot Randomized Controlled Trial Using Ecological Momentary Assessment," *Nicotine Tobacco Research* 18, no. 1 (2016): 64–73.

are nicotine chewing gum and the nicotine patch, both available over the counter. The FDA has also approved a nicotine nasal spray, a nicotine inhaler, and nicotine lozenges.

Nicotine gum delivers about as much nicotine as a cigarette does. Users experience no withdrawal symptoms and fewer cravings for nicotine as the dosage is reduced until they are completely weaned. Users chew up to 20 pieces of gum a day for 1 to 3 months. Nicotine-containing lozenges are available in two strengths, and a 12-week program of use is recommended to allow users to taper off the drug.

The nicotine patch is generally used in conjunction with a comprehensive smoking-behavior-cessation program. A small, thin patch delivers a continuous flow of nicotine through the skin, helping to relieve cravings. Patches can be bought with or without a prescription and are available in different dosages. It is recommended that people who use the patch as a part of their smoking-cessation program use it for 9 to 10 weeks.[157] During this time, the dose of nicotine is gradually reduced until the smoker is fully weaned from the drug. The patch costs less than a pack of cigarettes—about $4—and some insurance plans will pay for it.[158]

The nasal spray, which requires a prescription, is much more powerful and delivers nicotine to the bloodstream faster than gum, lozenges, or the patch. Patients are warned to be careful not to overdose; as little as 40 mg of nicotine taken at one time could be lethal. The FDA has advised that the nasal spray should be used for no more than 3 months and never for more than 6 months, so that smokers don't become dependent. The FDA also advises that no one who experiences nasal or sinus problems, allergies, or asthma should use it.

The nicotine inhaler, which also requires a prescription, consists of a mouthpiece and a cartridge. By puffing on the mouthpiece, the smoker inhales air saturated with nicotine, which is absorbed through the lining of the mouth, entering the body much more slowly than does the nicotine in cigarettes. Using the inhaler mimics the hand-to-mouth actions used in smoking and causes the back of the throat to feel as it would when inhaling tobacco smoke.

Smoking-Cessation Medications
Bupropion (brand name: Zyban), an antidepressant, is FDA approved as a smoking-cessation aid. Varinicline (brand name: Chantix) reduces nicotine cravings and the urge to smoke and blocks the effects of nicotine at nicotine receptor sites in the brain. Both drugs may cause changes in behavior such as agitation, depression, hostility, and suicidal thoughts or actions. People taking one of these drugs who experience any unusual changes in mood are advised to stop taking the drug immediately and contact their health care professional.[159]

LIVE IT! ASSESS YOURSELF

An interactive version of this assessment is available online in Mastering Health.

ASSESS | YOURSELF

Alcohol and Tobacco: Are Your Habits Placing You at Risk?

1 What's Your Risk of Alcohol Abuse?

Many college students engage in potentially dangerous drinking behaviors. Do you have a problem with alcohol use? Take the following quiz to see.

1. How often do you have a drink containing alcohol?
- ⓪ Never
- ① Monthly or less
- ② 2 to 4 times a month
- ③ 2 to 3 times a week
- ④ 4 or more times a week

2. How many alcoholic drinks do you have on a typical day when you are drinking?
- ⓪ 1 or 2
- ① 3 or 4
- ② 5 or 6
- ③ 7 to 9
- ④ 10 or more

3. How often do you have six drinks or more on one occasion?
- ⓪ Never
- ① Less than monthly
- ② Monthly
- ③ Weekly
- ④ Daily or almost daily

4. How often during the past year have you been unable to stop drinking once you had started?
- ⓪ Never
- ① Less than monthly
- ② Monthly
- ③ Weekly
- ④ Daily or almost daily

5. How often during the past year have you failed to do what was normally expected of you because of drinking?
- ⓪ Never
- ① Less than monthly
- ② Monthly
- ③ Weekly
- ④ Daily or almost daily

6. How often during the past year have you needed a first drink in the morning to get yourself going after a heavy drinking session?
- ⓪ Never
- ① Less than monthly
- ② Monthly
- ③ Weekly
- ④ Daily or almost daily

7. How often during the past year have you had a feeling of guilt or remorse after drinking?
- ⓪ Never
- ① Less than monthly
- ② Monthly
- ③ Weekly
- ④ Daily or almost daily

8. How often during the past year have you been unable to remember what happened the night before because you had been drinking?
- ⓪ Never
- ① Less than monthly
- ② Monthly
- ③ Weekly
- ④ Daily or almost daily

9. Have you or someone else been injured as a result of your drinking?
- ⓪ No
- ① Yes, but not in the past year
- ② Yes, during the past year

10. Has a relative, friend, or a doctor or other health care professional been concerned about your drinking or suggested you cut down?
- ⓪ No
- ① Yes, but not in the past year
- ② Yes, during the past year

Interpreting Part 1

Scores above 8: Your drinking patterns are putting you at high risk for illness, unsafe sexual situations, or alcohol-related injuries, and may even affect your academic performance.

Source: T. Babor et al., "The Alcohol Use Disorders Identification Test: Interview Version," *Audit: The Alcohol Use Disorders Identification Test*, 2nd Edition. Copyright © 2001.

YOUR PLAN FOR **CHANGE**

This **ASSESS YOURSELF** activity gave you the chance to evaluate your alcohol consumption. If some of your answers surprised you or if you were unsure how to answer some of the questions, consider taking steps to change your behavior.

TODAY, YOU CAN:

☐ Start a journal of your drinking habits to track how much alcohol you consume and what you spend on it.

☐ If you have a family history of alcohol abuse or addiction, consider whether your current use is healthy or is likely to create problems for you in the future.

WITHIN THE NEXT TWO WEEKS, YOU CAN:

☐ Make your first drink at a party something nonalcoholic.

☐ Intersperse alcoholic drinks with nonalcoholic beverages to help you pace yourself.

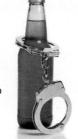

BY THE END OF THE SEMESTER, YOU CAN:

☐ Commit yourself to limiting your alcohol intake at every social function.

☐ Cultivate friendships and explore activities that do not center on alcohol. If your friends drink heavily, you may need to step back from the group for a while or make an effort to meet people who do not make drinking a major focus of their social activity.

2 Why Do You Smoke?

Identifying why you smoke can help you develop a plan to quit. Answer the following questions and evaluate your reasons for smoking.

1. I smoke to keep from slowing down.
   ❑ Often ❑ Sometimes ❑ Never

2. I feel more comfortable with a ciga-rette in my hand.
   ❑ Often ❑ Sometimes ❑ Never

3. Smoking is pleasant and enjoyable.
   ❑ Often ❑ Sometimes ❑ Never

4. I light up a cigarette when some-thing makes me angry.
   ❑ Often ❑ Sometimes ❑ Never

5. When I run out of cigarettes, it's almost unbearable until I get more.
   ❑ Often ❑ Sometimes ❑ Never

6. I smoke cigarettes automatically without even being aware of it.
   ❑ Often ❑ Sometimes ❑ Never

7. I reach for a cigarette when I need a boost.
   ❑ Often ❑ Sometimes ❑ Never

8. Smoking relaxes me in a stressful situation.
   ❑ Often ❑ Sometimes ❑ Never

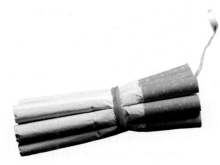

Interpreting Part 2

Use your answers to identify some of the key reasons why you smoke, then use the tips presented in this chapter to develop a plan for quitting.

Source: Abridged and adapted from National Institutes of Health, *Why Do You Smoke?* , NIH Publication No. 93-1822 (Washington, DC: U.S. Department of Health and Human Services, 1990).

YOUR PLAN FOR CHANGE

This **ASSESS YOURSELF** activity gave you the chance to evaluate your current smoking habits. Regardless of your current level of nicotine addiction, if you smoke at all, now is the time to take steps toward kicking the habit.

TODAY, YOU CAN:

☐ Develop a plan to kick the tobacco habit. The first step in quitting smok-ing is to identify why you want to quit. Write your reasons down, and carry a copy of your list with you. Every time you are tempted to smoke, go over your reasons for stopping.

☐ Think about the times and places you usually smoke. What could you do instead of smoking at those times? Make a list of positive tobacco alternatives.

WITHIN THE NEXT TWO WEEKS, YOU CAN:

☐ Pick a day to stop smoking, and tell a family member or friend your plan to gain support and accountability.

☐ Throw away all your cigarettes, light-ers, and ashtrays.

BY THE END OF THE SEMESTER, YOU CAN:

☐ Focus on the positives. Now that you have stopped smoking, your mind and body will begin to feel better. Make a list of the good things about not smoking. Carry a copy with you, and look at it whenever you have the urge to smoke.

☐ Reward yourself for stopping. Go to a movie, go out to dinner, or buy yourself a gift.

☐ If you are having difficulty quitting, consult with your campus health center or your doctor to discuss medications or other therapies that may help you quit.

STUDY PLAN

Visit the Study Area in Mastering Health to enhance your study plan with MP3 Tutor Sessions, Practice Quizzes, Flashcards, and more!

CHAPTER REVIEW

LO 1 | Alcohol: An Overview

- Alcohol is a central nervous system depressant used by about half of all Americans. Alcohol's effect on the body is measured by the blood alcohol concentration (BAC). The higher the BAC, the greater the drowsiness and impaired judgment and motor function.

LO 2 | Alcohol and Your Health

- Excessive alcohol consumption can cause long-term damage to the nervous system and cardiovascular system, liver disease, and increased risk for cancer. Alcohol-impaired drivers are responsible for about one in three car crash deaths. College students have high rates of alcohol-related crashes. Drinking during pregnancy can cause fetal alcohol spectrum disorders.

LO 3 | Alcohol Use in College

- Large numbers of college students report drinking in the past 30 days. Negative consequences associated with alcohol use among college students include academic problems, traffic accidents, unplanned sex and sexually transmitted infections, hangovers, alcohol poisoning, injury to self or others, relationship problems, and dropping out of school.

LO 4 | Alcohol Abuse and Dependence

- Alcohol use becomes alcoholism when it interferes with school, work, or social and family relationships or entails violations of the law. Causes of alcoholism include biological, family, social, and cultural factors. Treatment options include detoxification at private medical facilities, therapy (family, individual, or group), and self-help programs. Most recovering alcoholics relapse (over half within 3 months) because alcoholism is a behavioral addiction as well as a chemical addiction.

LO 5 | Tobacco Use in the United States

- Tobacco use involves many social and political issues, including advertising targeted at youth and women, the fastest-growing populations of smokers. Costs attributed to smoking in the United States are estimated to be between $289 and $333 billion per year.
- College students are heavily targeted by tobacco marketing and advertising campaigns. College students smoke to reduce stress, to fit in socially, and because they are addicted. The FDA requires prominent health warnings on tobacco products and enacts other policies to prevent young people from using tobacco products.

LO 6 | Tobacco and Its Effects

- Smoking delivers over 7,000 chemicals to the lungs of smokers. Tobacco comes in smoking and smokeless forms; both contain nicotine, an addictive psychoactive substance.

LO 7 | Health Hazards of Tobacco Products

- Health hazards of smoking include markedly higher rates of cancer, heart and circulatory disorders, respiratory diseases, sexual dysfunction, fertility problems, low birth weight babies, and gum diseases. Smokeless tobacco increases risks for oral cancer and other oral problems. Environmental tobacco smoke puts nonsmokers at greater risk for cancer and heart disease.

LO 8 | Quitting Smoking

- To quit, smokers must kick both a chemical addiction and a behavioral habit. Nicotine-replacement products or drugs such as Zyban and Chantix can help to wean smokers off nicotine. Therapy methods can also help.

POP QUIZ

LO 1 | Alcohol: An Overview

1. If a man and a woman drink the same amount of alcohol, the woman's blood alcohol concentration (BAC) will be approximately
   a. the same as the man's BAC.
   b. 60 percent higher than the man's BAC.
   c. 30 percent higher than the man's BAC.
   d. 30 percent lower than the man's BAC.

LO 2 | Alcohol and Your Health

2. Which of the following is *not* a potential long-term effect of alcohol use?
   a. Increased risk of some cancers
   b. Increased risk of liver damage
   c. Increased risk of eye disorders
   d. Increased risk of nervous system damage

LO 3 | Alcohol Use in College

3. Which of the following statements is *false*?
   a. College students drink in an effort to deal with stress and boredom.
   b. College students tend to underestimate the amount that their peers drink.
   c. Rape is linked to binge drinking.
   d. Consumption of alcohol is the number one cause of preventable death among undergraduates.

4. When Amanda goes out on the weekends, she usually has four or five beers in a row. This type of high-risk drinking is called
   a. tolerance.
   b. alcoholic addiction.
   c. alcohol overconsumption.
   d. binge drinking.

LO 4 | Alcohol Abuse and Dependence

5. The alcohol withdrawal syndrome that results in confusion, delusion, agitated behavior, and hallucination is known as
   a. automatic detoxification.
   b. delirium tremens.
   c. acute withdrawal.
   d. transient hyperirritability.

LO 5 | Tobacco Use in the United States

6. Which of the following does *not* contribute to college students' vulnerability to tobacco?
   a. Targeting by tobacco marketers
   b. The new, stressful environment of college
   c. Presence of tobacco products on campus
   d. Lack of information about the dangers of smoking

LO 6 | Tobacco and Its Effects

7. What does nicotine do to cilia in the lungs?

   a. Instantly destroys them
   b. Thickens them
   c. Paralyzes them
   d. Accumulates on them

8. What effect does carbon monoxide have on a smoker's body?
   a. It accumulates on the alveoli in the lungs, making breathing difficult.
   b. It increases heart rate.
   c. It interferes with the ability of red blood cells in the blood to carry oxygen.
   d. It dulls taste and smell.

LO 7 | Health Hazards of Tobacco Products

9. A major health risk of chewing tobacco is
   a. lung cancer.
   b. leukoplakia.
   c. heart disease.
   d. emphysema.

LO 8 | Quitting Smoking

10. How quickly will an individual begin to see health benefits after quitting smoking?
    a. Within 8 hours
    b. Within a month
    c. Within a year
    d. Never

Answers to the Pop Quiz can be found on page A-1. If you answered a question incorrectly, review the section identified by the Learning Outcome. For even more study tools, visit **Mastering Health**.

THINK ABOUT IT!

LO 1 | Alcohol: An Overview

1. Would a person be more intoxicated after having four gin and tonics instead of four beers? Why or why not?

LO 2 | Alcohol and Your Health

2. At what point in your life should you start worrying about the long-term effects of alcohol abuse?

LO 3 | Alcohol Use in College

3. When it comes to drinking alcohol, how much is too much? How can you avoid drinking amounts that will affect your judgment? If you see a friend having too many drinks at a party, what actions could you take?

4. What are some of the most common negative consequences college students experience as a result of drinking? What negative impacts do students experience as a result of other students' excessive drinking?

LO 4 | Alcohol Abuse and Dependence

5. Describe the difference between a problem drinker and an alcoholic. What factors can cause someone to become an alcoholic?

LO 5 | Tobacco Use in the United States

6. What tactics do tobacco companies use to target different groups of people?

7. What are some of the main reasons college students choose to use tobacco?

LO 6 | Tobacco and Its Effects

8. Discuss the various ways in which tobacco is used. Is any method less addictive or less hazardous to health than another?

LO 7 | Health Hazards of Tobacco Products

9. Discuss health hazards associated with tobacco. Who should be responsible for the medical expenses of smokers? Insurance companies? Smokers themselves?

LO 8 | Quitting Smoking

10. Describe the various methods of tobacco cessation. Which would be most effective for you? Why?

ACCESS YOUR HEALTH ON THE INTERNET

Visit Mastering Health for links to the websites and RSS feeds.

Use the following websites to explore further topics and issues related to smoking and tobacco use.

Alcoholics Anonymous. This website provides general information about AA and the 12-step program. **www.aa.org**

American Lung Association. This site offers a wealth of information about smoking trends, environmental smoke, and advice on smoking cessation. **www.lungusa.org**

ASH (Action on Smoking and Health). The nation's oldest and largest antismoking organization, ASH fights smoking and protects nonsmokers' rights. **www.ash.org**

College Drinking: Changing the Culture. This resource center targets three audiences: the student population as a whole, the college and its surrounding environment, and the individual at risk or alcohol-dependent drinker. **www.collegedrinkingprevention .gov**

Students against Destructive Decisions. SADD is an organization of students dedicated to raising awareness about the dangers of underage drinking, drug use, and impaired driving, among other destructive decisions. **www.sadd.org**

10 Nutrition: Eating for a Healthier You

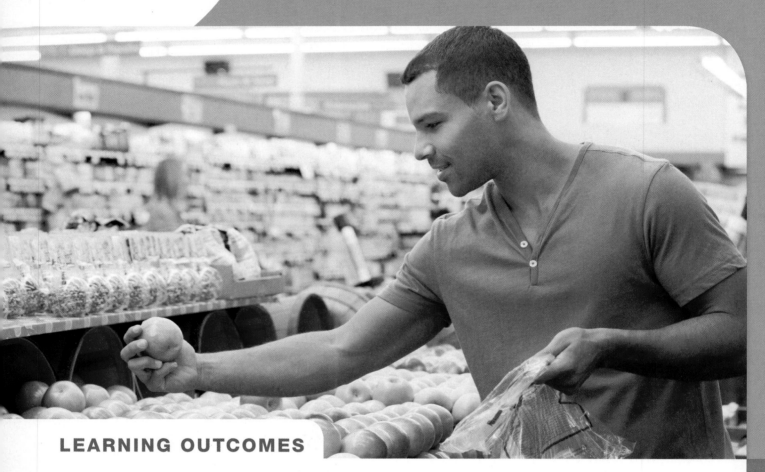

LEARNING OUTCOMES

LO **1** List the six classes of nutrients, and explain the primary functions of each.

LO **2** Explain how the Dietary Guidelines for Americans and the MyPlate food guidance system can help you follow a healthful eating pattern.

LO **3** Discuss strategies for healthful eating, including how to read food labels, the role of vegetarian diets and dietary supplements, how to eat mindfully, and how to choose healthful foods on and off campus.

LO **4** Explain food safety concerns facing Americans and people in other regions of the world.

When was the last time you ate because you felt truly hungry? True **hunger** occurs when our brains initiate a physiological response that prompts us to seek food for the energy and **nutrients** that our bodies require to maintain proper functioning. Often, people in wealthy nations don't eat in response to hunger; instead, we eat because of **appetite**, a learned psychological desire to consume food. The sight and smell of food, food advertising, cultural factors, our social interactions, emotions, finances, and even the time of day can influence the choices we make to satisfy our appetites. Given all these influences, how can we make more healthful choices more often?

Nutrition is the science that investigates the relationship between physiological function and the essential elements of the foods we eat. With an understanding of nutrition, you will be able to make more informed choices about your diet. Your health depends largely on what you eat, how much you eat, and the amount of exercise you get throughout your life. This chapter focuses on fundamental principles of nutrition—how you can eat for a healthier you.

LO 1 | ESSENTIAL NUTRIENTS FOR HEALTH

List the six classes of nutrients, and explain the primary functions of each.

Foods and beverages provide the chemicals needed to maintain the body's tissues and perform its functions. *Essential nutrients* are those the body cannot synthesize (or cannot synthesize in adequate amounts); we must obtain them from our diet. Of the six groups of essential nutrients, the four we need in the largest amounts—water, proteins, carbohydrates, and fats—are called *macronutrients*. The other two groups—vitamins and minerals—are needed in smaller amounts, so they are called *micronutrients*.

Before the body can use food, the digestive system must break down larger food particles into smaller, more usable forms. The **digestive process** is the sequence of functions by which the body breaks down foods into molecules small enough to be absorbed, absorbs nutrients, and excretes waste.

▶ SEE IT! VIDEOS

How accurate are restaurant calorie counts? Watch **Menu Calorie Counts**, available on Mastering Health.

Recommended Intakes for Nutrients

In the next sections, we discuss each nutrient group and identify how much of each group you need. These recommended amounts, known as the **Dietary Reference Intakes (DRIs)**, are published by the Food and Nutrition Board of the Institute of Medicine.[1] The DRIs establish the amount of each nutrient needed to prevent deficiencies or reduce the risk of chronic disease and identify maximum safe intake levels for healthy people. The DRIs are umbrella guidelines and include the following categories:

- **Recommended Dietary Allowances (RDAs).** RDAs are daily nutrient intake levels that meet the nutritional needs of 97 to 98 percent of healthy individuals.
- **Adequate Intakes (AIs).** AIs are daily intake levels that are assumed to be adequate for most healthy people. AIs are used when there isn't enough research to support establishing an RDA.
- **Tolerable Upper Intake Levels (ULs).** ULs are the highest amounts of a nutrient that an individual can consume daily without risking adverse health effects.
- **Acceptable Macronutrient Distribution Ranges (AMDRs).** AMDRs are ranges of protein, carbohydrate, and fat intake that provide adequate nutrition and are associated with a reduced risk for chronic disease.

Whereas the RDAs, AIs, and ULs are expressed as amounts—usually milligrams (mg) or micrograms (μg)—AMDRs are expressed as percentages. The AMDR for protein, for example, is 10 to 35 percent, meaning that no less than 10 percent and no more than 35 percent of the calories you consume should come from proteins. But that raises a new question: What are calories?

Calories

A *kilocalorie* is a unit of measure used to quantify the amount of energy in food. On nutrition labels and in consumer publications, the term is shortened to

hunger The physiological impulse to seek food.

nutrients The constituents of food that sustain humans physiologically: water, proteins, carbohydrates, fats, vitamins, and minerals.

appetite The learned desire to eat; normally accompanies hunger but is more psychological than physiological.

nutrition The science that investigates the relationship between physiological function and the essential elements of foods eaten.

digestive process The process by which the body breaks down foods into smaller components and either absorbs or excretes them.

Dietary Reference Intakes (DRIs) A set of recommended intakes for each nutrient published by the Institute of Medicine.

TABLE 10.1 | Estimated Daily Calorie Needs

	Calorie Range		
	Sedentary[a]		Active[b]
Children			
2 to 3 years old	1,000	→	1,400
Females			
4 to 13 years old	1,200–1,600	→	1,400–2,200
14 to 18	1,800	→	2,400
19 to 25	2,000	→	2,400
26 to 50	1,800	→	2,200–2,400
51 to 55	1,600	→	2,000–2,200
Males			
4 to 12 years old	1,200–1,800	→	1,600–2,400
13 to 18	2,000–2,400	→	2,600–3,200
19 to 20	2,600	→	3,000
21 to 40	2,400	→	2,800–3,000
41 to 60	2,200	→	2,800
61+	2,000	→	2,400–2,600

[a] A lifestyle that includes only the light physical activity associated with typical day-to-day life.
[b] A lifestyle that includes physical activity equivalent to walking more than 3 miles per day at 3 to 4 miles per hour in addition to the light physical activity associated with typical day-to-day life.

Source: U.S. Department of Agriculture and U.S. Department of Health and Human Services, *2015–2020 Dietary Guidelines for Americans*, 8th ed., Appendix 2, Table A2-1. (Washington, DC: U.S. Government Printing Office).

calorie. *Energy* is defined as the capacity to do work. We derive energy from the energy-containing nutrients in the foods we eat. These energy-containing nutrients—proteins, carbohydrates, and fats—provide calories. Vitamins, minerals, and water do not. **TABLE 10.1** shows the caloric needs for various individuals.

calorie A unit of measure that indicates the amount of energy obtained from a particular food.

dehydration Abnormal depletion of body fluids, typically a result of lack of water.

proteins Large molecules made up of chains of amino acids; essential constituents of all body cells.

amino acids The nitrogen-containing building blocks of protein.

essential amino acids The nine basic nitrogen-containing building blocks of human proteins that must be obtained from foods.

complete proteins Proteins that contain all nine of the essential amino acids.

Water: A Crucial Nutrient

The human body consists of 50 to 70 percent water by weight. The water in our system bathes cells; aids in fluid, electrolyte, and acid–base balance; and helps to regulate body temperature. Water is the major component of our blood, which carries oxygen, nutrients, and hormones and other substances to body cells and removes metabolic wastes. Humans can survive for several weeks without food but only several days without water.

Individual needs for water vary drastically according to dietary factors, age, size, overall health, environmental temperature and humidity levels, and exercise. The general recommendations are approximately 9 cups of total water from all beverages and foods each day for women and an average of 13 cups for men.[2] However, critics have questioned whether we really need to consume this much additional water, as the average healthy person gets considerable water in the foods they eat.[3] In fact, fruits and vegetables are 80 to 95 percent water, meats are more than 50 percent water, and even dry bread and cheese are about 35 percent water!

Contrary to popular opinion, caffeinated drinks, including coffee, tea, and soda, also count toward total fluid intake. Consumed in moderation, caffeinated beverages have not been found to dehydrate people whose bodies are used to caffeine.[4]

There are situations in which a person needs additional fluids to avoid **dehydration**, a state of abnormal depletion of body fluids. Dehydration can develop within a single day, especially when you engage in strenuous physical activity in a hot climate. Dehydration is also a risk when you have a fever or an illness involving vomiting or diarrhea and in people with kidney disease, diabetes, or cystic fibrosis. Older adults and the very young are at increased risk for dehydration.

Excessive water intake can also pose a serious health risk if it prompts *hyponatremia*, a condition characterized by low blood levels of the mineral sodium. If you are an athlete and wonder about water consumption, visit the American College of Sports Medicine's website (www.acsm.org) to download its brochure "Selecting and Effectively Using Hydration for Fitness."[5]

▶ DO IT! NUTRITOOLS

Ever wondered how your favorite meal stacks up, nutrition-wise? Complete the **Build a Meal, Build a Salad, Build a Pizza,** and **Build a Sandwich** activities, available on Mastering Health.

Proteins

Next to water, **proteins** are the most abundant compounds in the human body. In fact, proteins are major components of all living cells. They are called the "body builders" because of their role in developing and repairing bone, muscle, skin, and blood cells. They are the key elements of antibodies that protect us from disease, enzymes that control chemical activities in the body, and many hormones that regulate body functions. Proteins also supply an alternative source of energy to cells when fats and carbohydrates are not available. Specifically, every gram of protein you eat provides 4 calories. (There are about 28 grams in an ounce by weight.) Adequate protein in the diet is vital to many body functions and ultimately to survival.

The body breaks down proteins into smaller nitrogen-containing molecules known as **amino acids**, the building blocks of protein. Nine of the 20 different amino acids needed by the body are termed **essential amino acids**, which means the body must obtain them from the diet; the other 11 amino acids are considered nonessential because the body can make them. Dietary protein that supplies all the essential amino acids is called **complete protein**. Typically, protein from

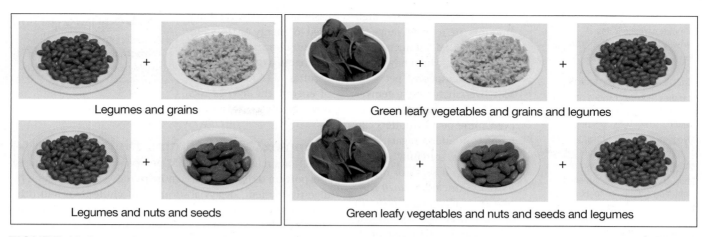

FIGURE 10.1 **Foods Providing Complementary Amino Acids** Complementary combinations of plant-based foods can provide all essential amino acids. In some cases, you might need to combine three sources of protein to supply all nine; however, the foods do not necessarily have to be eaten in the same meal. Two of the limited amino acids in leafy green vegetables are supplied by either grains or nuts and seeds, and the third is found in legumes.

animal products is complete, and quinoa and soy are complete plant proteins.

Other proteins from plant sources are **incomplete proteins** because they lack one or more of the essential amino acids. However, it is easy to combine plant foods to produce a complete protein meal (**FIGURE 10.1**). Plant foods that are rich in incomplete proteins include *legumes* (beans, lentils, peas, peanuts, and soy products); *grains* (e.g., wheat, corn, rice, and oats); and *nuts and seeds*. Certain vegetables, such as leafy green vegetables and broccoli, also contribute valuable plant proteins. Consuming a variety of foods from these categories will provide all the essential amino acids.

Although protein deficiency poses a threat to the global population, few Americans suffer from protein deficiencies. In fact, the average American age 20 years and over consumes 83 grams of protein daily, much of it from high-fat animal flesh and dairy products.[6] The AMDR for protein is 10 to 35 percent of calories. The RDA is 0.8 gram (g) per kilogram (kg) of body weight.[7] To calculate your protein needs, divide your body weight in pounds by 2.2 to get your weight in kilograms, then multiply by 0.8. The result is your recommended protein intake per day. For example, a woman who weighs 130 pounds should consume about 47 grams of protein each day. A 6-ounce steak provides 53 grams of protein—more than she needs!

People who need to eat extra protein include pregnant women and patients who are fighting a serious infection, recovering from surgery or blood loss, or recovering from burns. In these instances, proteins that are lost to cellular repair and development need to be replaced. Athletes also require more protein to build and repair muscle fibers.[8]

⊙ DO IT! NUTRITOOLS

Complete the **Know Your Protein Sources** activity, available on Mastering Health.

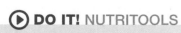

protein takes longer to digest than carbohydrates. Protein also releases certain satiety hormones that contribute to feeling full longer.

Carbohydrates

Carbohydrates supply much of the energy we need to sustain normal daily activity. In comparison to proteins or fats, carbohydrates are broken down more quickly and efficiently, yielding a fuel called glucose. All body cells can burn glucose for fuel; moreover, glucose is the only fuel that red blood cells can use and is the primary fuel for the brain. Carbohydrates are the best fuel for moderate to intense exercise because they can be readily broken down to glucose even when we're breathing hard and our muscle cells are getting less oxygen.

Like proteins, carbohydrates provide 4 calories per gram. The RDA for adults is 130 grams of carbohydrate per day.[9] There are two major types of carbohydrates: simple and complex.

Simple Carbohydrates **Simple carbohydrates** or *simple sugars* are found naturally in fruits, many vegetables, and dairy foods. The most common form of simple carbohydrates is *glucose*. Fruits and berries contain *fructose* (commonly called *fruit sugar*). Glucose and fructose are **monosaccharides**. **Disaccharides** are combinations of two monosaccharides. Perhaps the best-known example is *sucrose* (granulated table sugar). *Lactose* (milk sugar), found in milk and milk products, and *maltose* (malt sugar) are other examples of common disaccharides. Eventually, the human body converts all types of simple sugars to glucose to provide energy to cells.

In addition, a sedentary person may find it easier to stay in energy balance when consuming a high-protein, low-carbohydrate diet because

incomplete proteins Proteins that lack one or more of the essential amino acids.

carbohydrates Basic nutrients that supply the body with glucose, the energy form most commonly used to sustain normal activity.

simple carbohydrates A carbohydrate made up of only one sugar molecule or of two sugar molecules bonded together; also called simple sugars.

monosaccharides A sugar that is not broken down further during digestion, including fructose and glucose.

disaccharides Combinations of two monosaccharides such as lactose, maltose, and sucrose.

complex carbohydrates A carbohydrate that can be broken down during digestion into monosaccharides or disaccharides; also called a polysaccharide.

starches Polysaccharides that are the storage forms of glucose in plants.

glycogen The polysaccharide form in which glucose is stored in the liver and, to a lesser extent, in muscles.

fiber The indigestible portion of plant foods that helps to move food through the digestive system and softens stools by absorbing water.

whole grains Grains that are milled in their complete form and therefore include the bran, germ, and endosperm, with only the husk removed.

Sugar is found in high amounts in a wide range of processed food products such as soft drinks, which have more than 10 teaspoons per can. Moreover, such diverse items as breakfast cereals, yogurts, and even some peanut butters can be high in added sugars. Read food labels carefully before purchasing. If sugar or one of its aliases (including *high fructose corn syrup* and *cornstarch*) appears near the top of the ingredients list, then that product contains a lot of sugar and is probably not your best nutritional bet.

Complex Carbohydrates: Starches and Glycogen

Complex carbohydrates are found in grains, cereals, legumes, and other vegetables. Also called *polysaccharides*, they are formed by long chains of monosaccharides. *Starches*, *glycogen*, and *fiber* are the main types of complex carbohydrates.

Starches make up the majority of the complex carbohydrate group and come from cereals, breads, pasta, rice, corn, oats, barley, potatoes, and related foods. The body breaks down these complex carbohydrates into glucose, which can be easily absorbed by cells and used as energy or stored in the muscles and the liver as **glycogen**. When the body requires a sudden burst of energy, the liver breaks down glycogen into glucose.

Complex Carbohydrates: Dietary Fiber

Fiber, sometimes referred to as "bulk" or "roughage," is the indigestible portion of plant foods that helps move foods through the digestive system, delays absorption of cholesterol and other nutrients, and softens stools by absorbing water. Dietary fiber is found only in plant foods, such as fruits, vegetables, nuts, and grains.

Fiber is either *soluble* or *insoluble*. Soluble fibers, such as pectins, gums, and mucilages, dissolve in water, form gel-like substances, and can be digested easily by bacteria in the colon. Major food sources of soluble fiber include citrus fruits, berries, oat bran, dried beans, and some vegetables. Insoluble fibers, such as lignins and cellulose, typically do not dissolve in water and cannot be fermented by bacteria in the colon. They are found in most fruits and vegetables and in **whole grains**, such as brown rice, whole wheat, wheat or oat bran, and whole-grain breads and cereals (**FIGURE 10.2**). The AMDR for carbohydrates is 45 to 65 percent of total calories, and health experts recommend that the majority of this intake be fiber-rich carbohydrates.

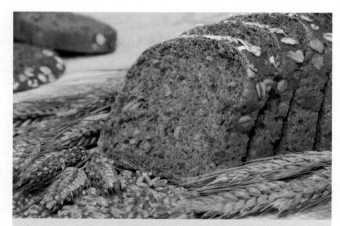

A recent study that followed more than 367,000 participants over 14 years found that the higher the consumption of whole grains, the lower the risk for death from cardiovascular disease, diabetes, and cancer. The risk of death was reduced by an average of 17%. Unfortunately, nearly 100% of Americans fail to meet their recommended intakes for whole grains.

Sources: T. Huang et al., "Consumption of Whole Grains and Cereal Fiber and Total and Cause-Specific Mortality: Prospective Analysis of 367,442 Individuals," *BMC Medicine* 13, no. 1 (2015): 59; 2015 Dietary Guidelines Advisory Committee, "Advisory Report to the Secretary of Health and Human Services and the Secretary of Agriculture," 2015, Available at http://health .gov/dietaryguidelines/2015-scientific-report.

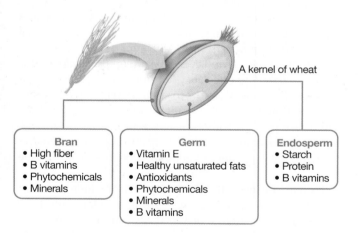

A kernel of wheat

Bran	Germ	Endosperm
• High fiber	• Vitamin E	• Starch
• B vitamins	• Healthy unsaturated fats	• Protein
• Phytochemicals	• Antioxidants	• B vitamins
• Minerals	• Phytochemicals	
	• Minerals	
	• B vitamins	

FIGURE 10.2 Anatomy of a Whole Grain Whole grains are more nutritious than refined grains because whole grains contain the bran, germ, and endosperm of the seed, sources of fiber, vitamins, minerals, and beneficial phytochemicals (chemical compounds that occur naturally in plants).

Source: Adapted from Joan Salge Blake, Kathy D. Munoz, and Stella Volpe, *Nutrition: From Science to You*, 3rd ed. © 2015, page 132. Printed and electronically reproduced by permission of Pearson Education, Inc., Upper Saddle River, New Jersey.

Fiber is associated with a reduced risk for obesity, heart disease, constipation, and possibly even type 2 diabetes and colon and rectal cancers. The DRI for dietary fiber is 25 grams per day for women and 38 grams per day for men.[10] What's the best way to increase your intake? Eat fewer refined carbohydrates in favor of more fiber-rich carbohydrates, including whole-grain breads and cereals, fresh fruits, legumes and other vegetables, nuts, and seeds. As with most nutritional advice, however, too much of a good thing can pose problems. A sudden increase in dietary fiber may cause flatulence (intestinal gas), cramping, or bloating. Consume plenty of water or other (sugar-free) liquids to reduce such side effects. Find out more about the benefits of fiber in the Skills for Behavior Change box.

Fats

Cholesterol and triglycerides (commonly called fats) are two forms of a large group of biological compounds known as *lipids*, which are not soluble in water. The term *dietary fats* technically refers to **triglycerides**—the majority of our body fat. And at 9 calories per gram, they are our most significant source of fuel for low to moderate levels of activity and during rest and sleep. They also play a vital role in insulating body organs against cold and shock, as well as maintaining healthy skin and hair. When we consume too many calories from any source, the liver converts the excess into triglycerides, which are stored in fat cells throughout our bodies. Dietary fats are also broken down into components that contribute to cell structures and many important body chemicals. Finally, we need to consume dietary fat in order for the body to absorb the fat-soluble vitamins A, D, E, and K.

The remaining fat in our bodies is composed of substances such as **cholesterol**—which are technically *sterols*. The ratio of total cholesterol to a group of compounds called **high-density lipoproteins (HDLs)** is important in determining risk for heart disease. Lipoproteins facilitate the transport of cholesterol in the blood. High-density lipoproteins are capable of transporting more cholesterol than are **low-density lipoproteins (LDLs)**. Whereas LDLs transport cholesterol to the body's cells, HDLs transport circulating cholesterol to the liver for metabolism and elimination from the body. For this reason, a high level of HDL cholesterol in the blood is desirable, as is a low level of LDL cholesterol.

triglycerides The most common form of fat in our food supply and in the body; made up of glycerol and three fatty acid chains.

fats Basic nutrients composed of carbon and hydrogen atoms; needed for the proper functioning of cells, insulation of body organs against shock, maintenance of body temperature, and healthy skin and hair.

cholesterol A substance that, like fats, is not soluble in water. It is found in animal-based foods and is synthesized by the body. Although essential to functioning, cholesterol circulating in the blood can accumulate on the inner walls of blood vessels.

high-density lipoproteins (HDLs) Compounds that facilitate the transport of cholesterol in the blood to the liver for metabolism and elimination from the body.

low-density lipoproteins (LDLs) Compounds that facilitate the transport cholesterol in the blood to the body's cells.

saturated fats Fats that are unable to hold any more hydrogen in their chemical structure; derived mostly from animal sources; solid at room temperature.

unsaturated fats Fats that have room for more hydrogen in their chemical structure; derived mostly from plants; liquid at room temperature.

Types of Dietary Fats Triglycerides contain *fatty acid* chains of oxygen, carbon, and hydrogen atoms. Fatty acid chains that cannot hold any more hydrogen in their chemical structure are called **saturated fats**. They generally come from animal sources, such as meat, dairy, and poultry products, and are solid at room temperature. **Unsaturated fats** have room for additional hydrogen atoms in their chemical structure and are liquid at room temperature. They generally come from plants and include most vegetable oils.

The terms *monounsaturated fatty acids* and *polyunsaturated fatty acids* refer to the relative number of hydrogen atoms that are missing in a fatty acid chain. Peanut, canola, and olive oils are high in monounsaturated fats, which appear to lower LDL levels and increase HDL levels. Corn, sunflower, and safflower oils are high in polyunsaturated fats. For a breakdown of the types of fats in common vegetable oils, see **FIGURE 10.3**.

Two specific types of polyunsaturated fatty acids essential to a healthful diet are *omega-3 fatty acids* (found in many types of fatty fish, leafy dark green vegetables, walnuts, and flaxseeds) and *omega-6 fatty acids* (found in corn, soybean, peanut, sunflower, and cottonseed oils). Both are classified as *essential fatty acids*—that is, those we must receive from our diets because the body requires them for functioning but cannot synthesize

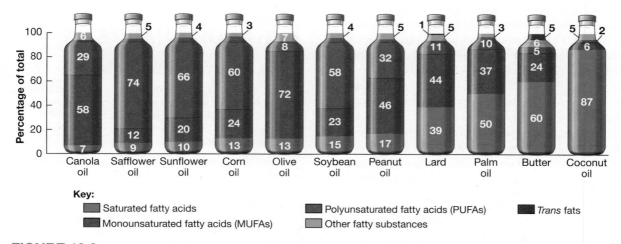

FIGURE 10.3 Percentages of Saturated, Polyunsaturated, Monounsaturated, and *Trans* Fats in Common Vegetable Oils

Key:

- Saturated fatty acids
- Monounsaturated fatty acids (MUFAs)
- Polyunsaturated fatty acids (PUFAs)
- Other fatty substances
- *Trans* fats

---

trans fatty acids Fatty acids that are produced when polyunsaturated oils are hydrogenated to make them more solid.

them. The most important fats in these groups are *linoleic acid*, an omega-6 fatty acid, and *alpha-linolenic acid*, an omega-3 fatty acid. The body needs these to make hormone-like compounds that control immune function, pain perception, and inflammation, to name a few key benefits. You may also have heard of EPA (eicosapentaenoic) and DHA (docosahexaenoic acid). These are derivatives of alpha-linolenic acid that are found abundantly in oily fish such as salmon and tuna and are associated with a reduced risk for heart disease.[11]

Avoiding *Trans* Fatty Acids

For decades, Americans shunned butter, cream, and other foods high in saturated fats. What they didn't know is that fats called *trans* **fatty acids** increase the risk for cardiovascular disease even more than saturated fats do. Research shows that consuming *trans* fats decreases levels of HDL-cholesterol and increases levels of LDL-cholesterol. For every 2 percent increase in intake of *trans* fats, the risk for cardiovascular disease increases 23 percent.[12]

Although a small amount of *trans* fatty acids do occur in some animal products, the great majority are in processed foods made with partially hydrogenated oils (PHOs).[13] PHOs are produced when food manufacturers add hydrogen to a plant oil, solidifying it, helping it to resist rancidity, and giving the food in which it is used a longer shelf life. The hydrogenation process straightens out the fatty acid chain so that it is more like a saturated fatty acid, and it has similar harmful effects, lowering HDLs and raising LDLs. *Trans* fats have been used in margarines, many commercial baked goods, and restaurant deep-fried foods.

In 2015, the U.S. Food and Drug Administration (FDA) ruled that PHOs are no longer "generally recognized as safe" for consumption. Food companies have until July 2018 to remove PHOs from their products.[14] In the meantime, *trans* fats are being removed from most foods. The FDA allows foods with less than 0.5 grams

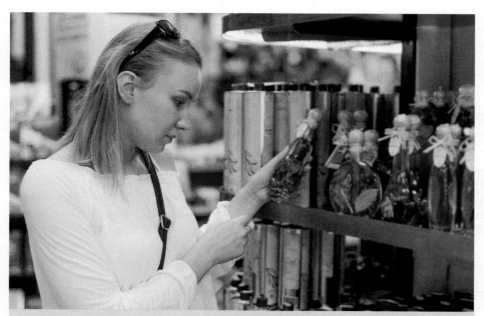

Not all fats are the same, and your body needs some fat to function. Try to reduce saturated fats, which are in meat, full-fat dairy, and poultry products, and avoid *trans* fats, which typically come in stick margarines, commercially baked goods, and deep-fried foods. Replace these with unsaturated fats, such as those in plant oils, fatty fish, and nuts and seeds.

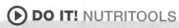

DO IT! NUTRITOOLS

Complete the **Know Your Fat Sources** activity, available on Mastering Health.

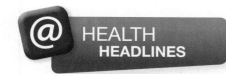

COCONUT OIL *Friend or Foe?*

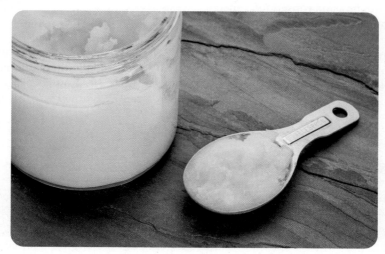

If you're a label reader, you have probably noticed coconut oil on the ingredients list of milk, spreads, and yogurt. Or maybe you've seen jars filled with this semi-solid milky-white fat on the grocery store shelves. Once thought of as unhealthy, coconut oil consumption is now being touted for several beneficial effects, including a reduced risk for cardiovascular disease. Let's see what the science says.

Whereas most plant oils are about 7 to 17 percent saturated fat, 87 percent of the fatty acids in coconut oil are saturated. Coconut oil also doesn't contain any essential fatty acids, and it is known to raise levels of LDL cholesterol. Still, it also raises levels of HDL cholesterol, and it is rich in vitamin E and a variety of phytochemicals.

The original study that sparked interest in coconut oil was observational. It found that Polynesian people, who have a low prevalence of cardiovascular disease, ingest mostly fat from coconuts. This association between consumption of coconut oil and reduced rates of cardiovascular disease does not, of course, prove cause and effect. More recently, however, some clinical studies have demonstrated mechanisms—such as reductions in blood pressure and metabolic stress—by which coconut oil does appear to exert a cardioprotective effect.

Health professionals are therefore divided over whether to recommend replacing heart-healthy polyunsaturated vegetable oils with coconut oil. There is a larger body of research in humans that monounsaturated and polyunsaturated fatty acids lower LDL cholesterol levels and reduce the risk of cardiovascular disease, but only a few studies support coconut oil as beneficial for heart health. At this point, the American Heart Association advises against adding coconut oil to your diet.

Source: F. Hamam, "Specialty Lipids in Health and Disease," *Food and Nutrition Sciences* 4 (2013): 63–70; A. S. Babu et al., "Virgin Coconut Oil and Its Potential Cardioprotective Effects," *Postgraduate Medicine* 126, no. 7 (2014): 76–83; Y. Kamisah et al., "Cardioprotective Effect of Virgin Coconut Oil in Heated Palm Oil Diet-Induced Hypertensive Rats," *Pharmaceutical Biology* 53, no. 9 (2015): 1243–49; American Heart Association, "Fats and Oils: AHA Recommendations," Accessed April 2015, Available at www.heart.org.

of *trans* fat per serving to be labeled as *trans*-fat free. However, if you see the words *partially hydrogenated oils, fractionated oils, shortening, lard,* or *hydrogenation* on a food label, then *trans* fats are present, even if the amount listed on the label is zero.

Fat Intake Recommendations
The AMDR for fats is 20 to 35 percent of total calories. Saturated fat should make up less than 10 percent of your total calories, and you should keep *trans* fat intake to an absolute minimum.[15] Instead of trying to eat a low-fat diet, replace the saturated and *trans* fats you eat with healthful unsaturated fats from plants and fish. Many studies have shown that balanced higher-fat diets such as the Mediterranean diet, which is rich in plant oils and fish, produce significant improvements in body weight and cardiovascular risk factors.[16]

Follow these guidelines to add more healthful fats to your diet:

- Eat fatty fish (herring, mackerel, salmon, sardines, or tuna) at least twice weekly.
- Use olive, peanut, soy, and canola oils instead of butter or lard. See Health Headlines for more information on coconut oil.

- Add leafy green vegetables, walnuts, walnut oil, and ground flaxseed to your diet.

Follow these guidelines to reduce your intake of saturated and *trans* fats:

- Read the Nutrition Facts panel on food labels to find out how much saturated fat is in a product.
- Chill meat-based soups and stews, remove any fat that hardens on top, and then reheat the soup or stew to serve.
- Fill up on fruits and vegetables.
- Hold the creams and sauces.
- Avoid all products with *trans* fatty acids. Use *trans* fat–free margarines, vegetable spreads, bean spreads, nut butters, low-fat cream cheese, and the like.
- Choose lean meats, fish, or skinless poultry. Broil or bake whenever possible. Drain off fat after cooking.
- Choose fewer cold cuts, bacon, sausages, hot dogs, and organ meats.
- Select nonfat and low-fat dairy products.

Vitamins

Vitamins are organic compounds that promote growth and are essential to life and health. Every minute of every day, vitamins help to maintain nerves and skin, produce blood cells, build bones and teeth, heal wounds, and convert food energy to body energy, and they do all this without adding any calories to your diet.

Vitamins are classified as either *fat soluble*, which means that they are absorbed through the intestinal tract with the help of fats, or *water soluble*, which means that they dissolve easily in water. Vitamins A, D, E, and K are fat soluble; B-complex vitamins and vitamin C are water soluble. Fat-soluble vitamins tend to be stored in the body, and toxic levels can accumulate in a person who regularly consumes more than the UL. Excesses of water-soluble vitamins generally are excreted in the urine and rarely cause toxicity problems. See **TABLE 10.2** for functions, recommended intake amounts, and food sources of specific vitamins.

Vitamin D Vitamin D, the "sunshine vitamin," is formed from a compound in the skin when it is exposed to the sun's ultraviolet rays. In most people, an adequate amount of vitamin D can be synthesized with 5 to 30 minutes of sun on

TABLE 10.2 | A Guide to Vitamins

Vitamin Name	Primary Functions	Recommended Intake	Reliable Food Sources
Thiamin	Carbohydrate and protein metabolism	Men: 1.2 mg/day Women: 1.1 mg/day	Pork, fortified cereals, enriched rice and pasta, peas, tuna, legumes
Riboflavin	Carbohydrate and fat metabolism	Men: 1.3 mg/day Women: 1.1 mg/day	Beef liver, shrimp, dairy foods, fortified cereals, enriched breads and grains
Niacin	Carbohydrate and fat metabolism	Men: 16 mg/day Women: 14 mg/day	Meat/fish/poultry, fortified cereals, enriched breads and grains, canned tomato products
Vitamin B_6	Carbohydrate and amino acid metabolism	Men and women aged 19–50: 1.3 mg/day	Garbanzo beans, meat/fish/poultry, fortified cereals, white potatoes
Folate	Amino acid metabolism and DNA synthesis	Men: 400 µg/day Women: 400 µg/day	Fortified cereals, enriched breads and grains, spinach, legumes, liver
Vitamin B_{12}	Formation of blood cells and nervous system	Men: 2.4 µg/day Women: 2.4 µg/day	Shellfish, all cuts of meat/fish/poultry, dairy foods, fortified cereals
Pantothenic acid	Fat metabolism	Men: 5 mg/day Women: 5 mg/day	Meat/fish/poultry, shiitake mushrooms, fortified cereals, egg yolks
Biotin	Carbohydrate, fat, and protein metabolism	Men: 30 µg/day Women: 30 µg/day	Nuts, egg yolks
Vitamin C	Collagen synthesis, iron absorption, and promotes healing	Men: 90 mg/day Women: 75 mg/day Smokers: 35 mg more per day than RDA	Sweet peppers, citrus fruits and juices, broccoli, strawberries, kiwi
Vitamin A	Immune function, maintains epithelial cells, healthy bones and vision	Men: 900 µg Women: 700 µg	Beef and chicken liver, egg yolks, milk Carotenoids found in spinach, carrots, mango, apricots, cantaloupe, pumpkin, yams
Vitamin D	Promotes calcium absorption and healthy bones	Adults aged 19–70: 15 µg/day (600 IU/day)	Canned salmon and mackerel, milk, fortified cereals
Vitamin E	Protects cell membranes and acts as a powerful antioxidant	Men: 15 mg/day Women: 15 mg/day	Sunflower seeds, almonds, vegetable oils, fortified cereals
Vitamin K	Blood coagulation and bone metabolism	Men: 120 µg/day Women: 90 µg/day	Kale, spinach, turnip greens, Brussels sprouts

Note: Values are for all adults aged 19 and older, except as noted. Values increase among women who are pregnant or lactating.

Source: Data from Food and Nutrition Board, Institute of Medicine, National Academies, "Dietary Reference Intakes (DRIs): Estimated Average Requirements," Accessed February 2016, Available at https://iom.nationalacademies.org/~/media/Files/Activity%20Files/Nutrition/DRIs/5_Summary%20Table%20Tables%20 1-4.pdf.

the face, neck, hands, arms, and legs twice a week without sunscreen.[17] However, the sun is not high enough in the sky during late fall to early spring in northern climates to allow for vitamin D synthesis. For people who cannot rely on the sun to meet their daily vitamin D needs, consuming vitamin D–fortified milk, yogurt, soy milk, cereals, and fatty fish such as salmon can also supply this vitamin.

Vitamin D promotes the body's absorption of calcium, the primary mineral component of bone. It also assists in the processes of bone growth, repair, and remodeling. For these reasons, a deficiency of vitamin D can promote loss of bone density and strength, a condition called *osteoporosis*. Two other bone disorders, *rickets* in children and its adult version, *osteomalacia*, both of which cause softening and distortion of the bones, can also be prevented with adequate intake of vitamin D.[18] An adequate level of vitamin D may also reduce the risk for cardiovascular disease, diabetes, and some forms of cancer.

More is not always better, however.[19] Vitamin D is stored in the body's fat tissues, and an excessive intake can be toxic.

Folate
Folate, one of the B vitamins, is needed for the production of compounds necessary for DNA synthesis in body cells. It is particularly important for proper cell division during embryonic development; folate deficiencies during the first few weeks of pregnancy, typically before a woman even realizes she is pregnant, can prompt a neural tube defect such as spina bifida, in which the primitive tube that eventually forms the brain and spinal cord fails to close properly. The FDA requires that all bread, cereal, rice, and pasta products sold in the United States be fortified with folic acid, the synthetic form of folate, to reduce the incidence of neural tube defects.

Minerals

Minerals are indestructible inorganic elements that build body tissues and assist body processes. They are readily absorbed and excreted. *Major minerals* are the minerals that the body needs in fairly large amounts: sodium, calcium, phosphorus, magnesium, potassium, sulfur, and chloride. *Trace minerals* include iron, zinc, manganese, copper, fluoride, selenium, chromium, and iodine. Only very small amounts of trace minerals are needed, and serious problems may result if excesses or deficiencies occur (see **TABLE 10.3**).

Sodium Sodium is necessary for the regulation of blood volume and blood pressure, fluid balance, transmission of nerve impulses, heart activity, and certain metabolic functions. It enhances flavors, acts as a preservative, and tenderizes meats,

> **vitamins** Essential organic compounds that promote metabolism, growth, and reproduction and help to maintain life and health.
>
> **minerals** Inorganic, indestructible elements that aid physiological processes.

TABLE 10.3 | A Guide to Minerals

Mineral Name	Primary Functions	Recommended Intake	Reliable Food Sources
Sodium	Fluid and acid–base balance; nerve impulses and muscle contraction	Adults: 1.5 g/day (1,500 mg/day)	Table salt, pickles, most canned soups, snack foods, luncheon meats, canned tomato products
Potassium	Fluid balance; nerve impulses and muscle contraction	Adults: 4.7 g/day (4,700 mg/day)	Most fresh fruits and vegetables: potato, banana, tomato juice, orange juice, melon
Phosphorus	ATP, fluid balance and bone formation	Adults: 700 mg/day	Milk/cheese/yogurt, soy milk and tofu, legumes, nuts, poultry
Selenium	Regulates thyroid hormones and reduces oxidative stress	Adults: 55 μg/day	Seafood, milk, whole grains, and eggs
Calcium	Part of bone; muscle contraction, acid–base balance, and nerve transmission	Adults: 1,000 mg/day	Milk/yogurt/cheese, sardines, collard greens and spinach, calcium-fortified juices
Magnesium	Part of bone; muscle contraction	Men: 400 mg/day Women: 310 mg/day	Spinach, kale, collard greens, whole grains, seeds, nuts, legumes
Iodine	Synthesis of thyroid hormones	Adults: 150 μg/day	Iodized salt, saltwater seafood
Iron	Part of hemoglobin and myoglobin	Men: 8 mg/day Women: 18 mg/day	Meat/fish/poultry, fortified cereals, legumes
Zinc	Immune system function; growth and sexual maturation	Men: 11 mg/day Women: 8 mg/day	Meat/fish/poultry, fortified cereals, legumes

Note: Values are for all adults aged 19 and older.

Source: Data from Food and Nutrition Board, Institute of Medicine, National Academies, "Dietary Reference Intakes (DRIs): Estimated Average Requirements," Accessed February 2016, Available at https://iom.nationalacademies.org/~/media/Files/Activity%20Files/Nutrition/DRIs/5_Summary%20Table%20Tables%201-4.pdf.

so it is often present in high quantities in the foods we eat. A common misconception is that table salt and sodium are the same thing: Table salt is a compound containing both sodium and chloride. It accounts for only 15 percent of our sodium intake. The majority of sodium in our diet comes from processed foods that are infused with sodium to enhance flavor and for preservation. Pickles, fast foods, salty snacks, processed cheeses, canned and dehydrated soups, frozen dinners, many breads and bakery products, and smoked meats and sausages often contain several hundred milligrams of sodium per serving.

The AI for sodium is just 1,500 milligrams, which is about 0.65 of a teaspoon.[20] The *2015–2020 Dietary Guidelines for Americans* suggest keeping your sodium intake below 2,300 mg/day. Unfortunately, 89 percent of Americans exceed this limit.[21]

Why is high sodium intake a concern? Salt-sensitive individuals respond to a high-sodium diet with an increase in blood pressure (hypertension), which contributes to heart disease and stroke. Although the cause of the majority of cases of hypertension is unknown, lowering sodium intake can reduce the risk.

Calcium Calcium is the primary mineral component of bones and teeth. It is also essential for muscle contraction, nerve impulse transmission, blood clotting, and acid–base balance. The issue of calcium consumption has gained national attention with the rising incidence of osteoporosis among older adults. Calcium is an underconsumed "nutrient of public health concern"; that is, most Americans do not consume the recommended 1,000–1,300 milligrams of calcium per day.[22]

Milk is one of the richest sources of dietary calcium. Calcium-fortified soy milk is an excellent vegetarian alternative. Many leafy green vegetables are good sources of calcium, but some contain oxalic acid, which makes their calcium harder to absorb. Spinach, chard, and beet greens are not particularly good sources of calcium, whereas broccoli, cauliflower, and many peas and beans offer good supplies.

It is generally best to take calcium throughout the day, consuming it with foods that also contain protein, vitamin D, and vitamin C for optimal absorption. Many dairy products are both excellent sources of calcium and fortified with vitamin D, which is known to improve calcium absorption.

Do you consume carbonated soft drinks? Be aware that the added phosphoric acid (phosphate) in these drinks can cause you to excrete extra calcium, which may result in calcium loss from your bones. One study of 2,500 men and women found that in women who consumed at least three cans of cola per week, even diet cola, bone density of the hip was 4 to 5 percent lower than in women who drank fewer than one cola per month. Colas did not seem to have the same effect on

anemia A condition that results from the body's inability to produce adequate hemoglobin.

Even if you never use table salt, you still may be getting excess sodium in your diet.

men.[23] There may also be a "milk displacement" effect, meaning that people who drank soda were not drinking milk, thereby decreasing their calcium intake.

Iron Worldwide, iron deficiency is the most common nutrient deficiency, affecting more than 2 billion people, nearly 30 percent of the world's population.[24] In the United States, iron deficiency is less prevalent; however, because iron is a key component of red blood cells, deficiency can develop with blood loss and in menstruating women who fail to maintain a balanced diet. Women aged 19 to 50 years need about 18 milligrams of iron per day, and men aged 19 to 50 years need about 8 milligrams.[25]

Iron deficiency can lead to *iron-deficiency anemia.* **Anemia** results from the body's inability to produce adequate amounts of hemoglobin (the oxygen-carrying component of the blood). When iron-deficiency anemia occurs, body cells receive less oxygen. As a result, the person feels tired. Iron is also important for energy metabolism, DNA synthesis, and other body functions.

Iron overload or iron toxicity due to ingesting too many iron-containing supplements is the leading cause of accidental poisoning in small children in the United States. Symptoms of iron toxicity include nausea, vomiting, diarrhea, rapid heartbeat, weak pulse, dizziness, shock, and confusion. Excess iron intake from high meat consumption, iron fortification, and supplementation is also associated with problems such as cardiovascular disease and cancer.[26]

Beneficial Non-Nutrient Components of Foods

Increasingly, nutrition research is focusing on components of foods that are not nutrients themselves but interact with

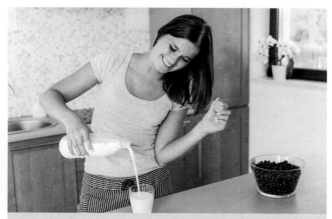
Milk is a great source of calcium and other nutrients. If you don't like milk or can't drink it, make sure to get enough calcium—at least 1,000 milligrams a day—from other sources.

nutrients to promote human health.[27] Foods that may confer health benefits beyond the nutrients they contribute to the diet—whole foods, fortified foods, enriched foods, or enhanced foods—are called **functional foods**. As part of a varied diet, functional foods have the potential to have positive effects on health.[28]

Some of the most popular functional foods today are those containing **antioxidants**. These substances appear to protect against oxidative stress, a complex process in which *free radicals* (atoms with unpaired electrons) destabilize other atoms and molecules, prompting a chain reaction that can damage cells, cell proteins, or genetic material in the cells. Free radical formation occurs as a result of normal cell metabolism. Antioxidants combat it by donating their electrons to stabilize free radicals; activating enzymes that convert free radicals to less-damaging substances; or reducing or repairing the damage they cause. Free radical damage is associated with many chronic diseases, including cardiovascular disease, cancer, age-related vision loss, and other diseases of aging.

Some antioxidants are nutrients. These include vitamins C and E as well as the minerals copper, iron, manganese, selenium, and zinc. Other potent antioxidants are **phytochemicals**, compounds that occur naturally in plants and are thought to protect them against ultraviolet radiation, pests, and other threats. Common examples include carotenoids and polyphenols.

Carotenoids are pigments found in red, orange, and dark green fruits and vegetables. Beta-carotene, the most researched carotenoid, is a precursor of vitamin A, meaning that vitamin A can be produced in the body from beta-carotene. Along with beta-carotene, other carotenoids, such as lutein, lycopene, and zeaxanthin, are associated in numerous studies with a reduced risk for chronic disease.[29]

Polyphenols, which include a group known as flavonoids, are the largest class of phytochemicals. They are found in an array of fruits and vegetables as well as soy products, tea, and chocolate. Like carotenoids, they are thought to have potent antioxidant properties.[30]

Although research supporting the health benefits of antioxidant nutrients and phytochemicals is not conclusive, studies do show that individuals who are deficient in antioxidant vitamins and minerals have an increased risk for age-related diseases and that antioxidants consumed in whole foods, mostly fruits and vegetables, may reduce these individuals' risks.[31] In contrast, antioxidants that are consumed as supplements do not necessarily confer such a benefit, and some studies suggest that they may be harmful, acting as "pro-oxidants" and increasing the risk of certain cancers and overall mortality in some populations, such as smokers.[32]

Foods that are rich in nutrients and phytochemicals are increasingly being referred to as "superfoods." Do they live up to their name? See the Health Headlines box.

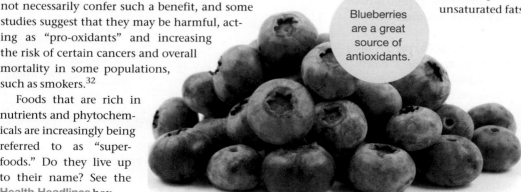

Blueberries are a great source of antioxidants.

Explain how the Dietary Guidelines for Americans and the MyPlate food guidance system can help you follow a healthful eating pattern.

Americans consume about 900 more calories per day than they did 50 years ago (see **FIGURE 10.4**).[33] When this trend combines with our increasingly sedentary lifestyle, it is not surprising that we have seen a dramatic rise in obesity.

The U.S. Department of Health and Human Services and the U.S. Department of Agriculture (USDA) publish two tools for consumers to make healthy eating easy: the Dietary Guidelines for Americans and the MyPlate food guidance system.

Dietary Guidelines for Americans

The Dietary Guidelines for Americans (DGAs) are recommendations for eating a healthy, nutritionally adequate diet. They are revised every 5 years. The most recent, the *2015–2020 Dietary Guidelines for Americans*, include the following five key guidelines:[34]

1. **Follow a healthy eating pattern across the lifespan.** Recognize that every food and beverage choice you make throughout the day can positively influence your health, providing you nutrients and fiber at an appropriate calorie level to help you achieve and maintain a healthy body weight, and reduce your risk for chronic disease. The DGAs identify the following components of a healthful eating pattern:
   - A variety of vegetables of different types and colors, plus legumes
   - Fruits, especially whole fruits
   - Grains, at least half of which are whole grains
   - Fat-free or low-fat dairy choices
   - A variety of lean-protein foods, including seafood, lean meats and poultry, eggs, legumes, soy products, and nuts and seeds
   - Oils.

2. **Focus on variety, nutrient density, and amount.** Choose the densest versions of foods within all food groups. Nutrient-dense foods provide a relatively high level of nutrients and fiber for a relatively low number of calories. For example, a slice of whole-grain toast with peanut butter provides healthful unsaturated fats, protein, and fiber-rich

functional foods Foods that are believed to have specific health benefits beyond their basic nutrients.

antioxidants Substances that are believed to protect against oxidative stress and resultant tissue damage.

phytochemicals Naturally occurring non-nutrient plant chemicals that are believed to have beneficial health effects.

HEALTH CLAIMS OF SUPERFOODS

Functional foods contain both nutrients and other active compounds that may improve overall health, reduce the risk for certain diseases, or delay aging. These foods are increasingly being referred to as "superfoods." But do they live up to their name? Let's look at a few.

Salmon is a rich source of the omega-3 fatty acids EPA and DHA, which combat inflammation, improve HDL/LDL blood profiles, and reduce the risk for cardiovascular disease. These essential fatty acids may also promote a healthy nervous system, reducing the risk for mood disorders and age-related dementia.

Yogurt makes it onto most superfood lists because it contains living, beneficial bacteria called probiotics. You will see their genus name—for example, *Lactobacillus* or *Bifidobacterium*—in the list of ingredients on the product's label. Probiotics colonize the large intestine, where they help to complete digestion and produce certain vitamins, and may reduce the risk of diarrhea and other bowel disorders, boost immunity, and help to regulate body weight.

Yogurt and kefir (a fermented milk drink) are dairy products that contain beneficial bacteria called *probiotics*.

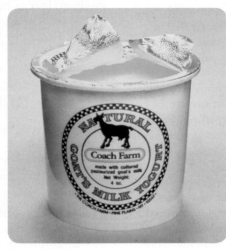

Cocoa is particularly rich in phytochemicals called flavonols that have been shown in many studies to reduce the risk for cardiovascular disease, diabetes, and even arthritis. Dark chocolate has a higher level of flavonols than milk chocolate does.

Given such claims, it's easy to get carried away by the idea that superfoods, like superheros, have superpowers. But eating a square of dark chocolate won't rescue you from the ill effects of a fast-food burger and fries. What matters is your whole diet. Focus on including superfoods as components of a varied diet that is rich in fresh fruits, legumes and other vegetables, whole grains, lean sources of protein, and nuts and seeds. These are the "everyday heroes" of a super-healthful diet.

Source: Academy of Nutrition and Dietetics, "Position of the Academy of Nutrition and Dietetics: Functional Foods," *Journal of the Academy of Nutrition and Dietetics* 113 (2013): 1096–1103; S. C. Dyall, "Long-Chain Omega-3 Fatty Acids and the Brain: A Review of the Independent and Shared Effects of EPA, DPA, and DHA," *Frontiers in Aging Neuroscience* 7 (2015): 52; A P.S. Hungin et al., "Systematic Review: Probiotics in the Management of Lower Gastrointestinal Symptoms in Clinical Practice—An Evidence-Based International Guide," *Alimentary Pharmacology and Therapeutics* 38, no. 8 (2013): 864–86; N. Khan et al., "Cocoa Polyphenols and Inflammatory Markers of Cardiovascular Disease," *Nutrients* 6, no. 2 (2014): 844–80.

---

carbohydrates as well as vitamins and minerals, for about 300 calories, whereas a plain waffle with butter and maple syrup provides little more than refined carbohydrates, saturated fats, and added sugars, for about 400 calories. The toast with peanut butter is also more satiating, so you won't be as likely to feel hungry as quickly.

3. **Limit calories from added sugars and saturated fats, and reduce sodium intake.** Specifically, the DGAs advise you to do the following:

   ▪ Consume less than 10 percent of calories per day from added sugars. Avoid sugary drinks, and make sweet desserts occasional treats.

   ▪ Consume less than 10 percent of calories per day from saturated fats. Limiting your intake of animal-based foods will help you meet this goal.

   ▪ Consume less than 2,300 mg per day of sodium.

   ▪ If alcohol is consumed, it should be consumed in moderation—up to one drink per day for adult women and two drinks per day for adult men.

4. **Shift to healthier food and beverage choices.** The DGAs recommend that you shift your intake of vegetables, fruits, dairy, and healthful fish and plant oils upward by replacing snack foods such as chips with raw

vegetables, meat-based entrées with fish and legumes, sugary drinks with milk or soy milk, and desserts high in added sugars with whole fruits.

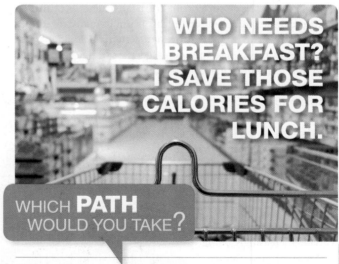

WHO NEEDS BREAKFAST? I SAVE THOSE CALORIES FOR LUNCH.

WHICH **PATH** WOULD YOU TAKE?

Go to Mastering Health to see how your actions today affect your future health.

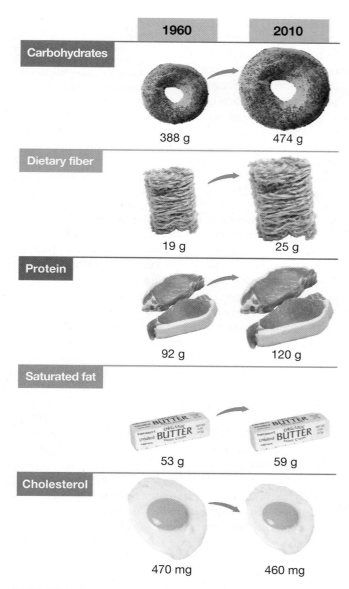

	1960	2010
Carbohydrates	388 g	474 g
Dietary fiber	19 g	25 g
Protein	92 g	120 g
Saturated fat	53 g	59 g
Cholesterol	470 mg	460 mg

FIGURE 10.4 Trends in Per Capita Nutrient Consumption Since 1960, Americans have increased their caloric intake from 3,100 to 4,000 and their daily consumption of carbohydrates, protein, and saturated fat.

Source: Data are from the USDA Center for Nutrition Policy and Promotion, February 1, 2015, www.ers.usda.gov/data-products/food-availability-(per-capita)-data-system/.aspx#26715.

5. **Support healthy eating patterns for all.** Citing the socioecological model of health, the DGAs point out that each of your choices—while shopping, eating out, standing in line at your campus dining hall, or cooking for friends—can promote the availability of healthy foods aligned with the Dietary Guidelines. You can also encourage others to join you in physical activity.

MyPlate Food Guidance System

To help consumers understand and implement the Dietary Guidelines, the USDA has developed an easy-to-follow graphic and guidance system called MyPlate, which can be found at www.choosemyplate.gov and is illustrated in **FIGURE 10.5**. The MyPlate food guidance system takes into consideration the dietary and caloric needs for a wide variety of individuals, such as pregnant or breastfeeding women, those trying to lose weight, and adults with different activity levels. The interactive website can create personalized dietary and exercise recommendations based on the individual information you enter.

MyPlate's key messages, which support the Dietary Guidelines, include the following:

- **Eat nutrient-dense foods.** While eating the recommended number of servings from MyPlate, make the most nutrient-dense choices within a given food group.
- **Eat seafood twice a week.** Replace red meat or poultry with grilled, broiled, or baked seafood twice a week. In addition to salmon, tuna, and other fatty finfish, clams, mussels, oysters, and calamari are all high in omega-3 fatty acids.
- **Avoid empty calories.** MyPlate refers to calories from added sugars and saturated fats as *empty calories*. Here are some examples of empty-calorie foods:[35]
  - Sausages, hot dogs, bacon, and ribs. Adding a sausage link to your breakfast adds 96 empty calories.
  - Cheese. Switching from whole-milk mozzarella cheese to nonfat mozzarella cheese saves you 76 empty calories per ounce.
  - Refined grains, including crackers, bagels, and white rice. Switching to whole-grain versions can save you 25 or more empty calories per serving.

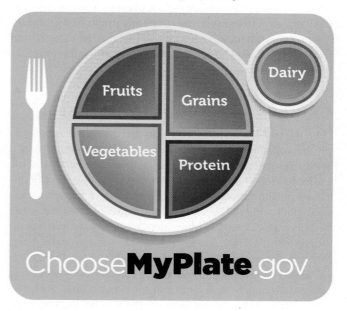

FIGURE 10.5 The MyPlate System The USDA MyPlate food guidance system takes a new approach to dietary and exercise recommendations. Each colored section of the plate represents a food group. An interactive tool at the MyPlate website helps you analyze and track your foods and physical activity and provides helpful tips to personalize your plans.

Source: U.S. Department of Agriculture, 2013, www.choosemyplate.gov.

6 OR MORE

teaspoons of **SUGAR** are present in most national brands of fruit yogurt per serving!

- Cakes, cookies, pastries, and ice cream. Approximately 75 percent of the calories in a slice of chocolate cake or a serving of ice cream are empty calories.
- Wine, beer, and all alcoholic beverages. A whopping 155 empty calories are consumed with each 12 fluid ounces of beer.
- **Engage in physical activity**. Any activity that gets your heart pumping counts, including walking on campus, playing basketball, and dancing. MyPlate offers personalized recommendations for weekly physical activity.

LO 3 | HOW CAN I EAT MORE MINDFULLY AND HEALTHFULLY?

Discuss strategies for healthful eating, including how to read food labels, the role of vegetarian diets and dietary supplements, how to eat mindfully, and how to choose healthful foods on and off campus.

Whether you follow a vegetarian diet, eat only organic foods, take dietary supplements, or choose to eat locally grown foods, there are ways to improve the nutrient content of your meals. Let's begin with how to read a food label. The information contained in a food label can be useful when it comes to planning a healthy meal plan.

Read Food Labels

How do you know what nutrients the packaged foods you eat are contributing to your diet? To help consumers evaluate the nutritional values of packaged foods, the FDA and the USDA developed the Nutrition Facts label that is typically displayed on the side or back of cans, cartons, or boxes of packaged foods. One of the most helpful items on the label is the **% daily values (%DVs)** list, which tells you how much of an average adult's allowance for a particular substance (fat, fiber, calcium, etc.) is provided by a serving of the food. The %DV is calculated based on a diet containing 2,000 calories per day, so your values may be different from those listed on a label. The label also includes information on the serving size and calories. In 2016, the FDA published a new label that is more helpful for consumers. It identifies the calories per serving in much larger type and uses a serving size that better reflects the amount of the food that people

% daily values (%DVs) Items on food and supplement labels that identify how much of each listed nutrient or other substance a serving of food contributes to a 2,000 calorie/day diet.

typically eat. **FIGURE 10.6** walks you through the old and new Nutrition Facts labels. For the latest information on the new label, go to www.fda.gov and search "Nutrition Facts label."

Food labels contain other information as well, such as the name and manufacturer of the product, an ingredients list, and sometimes claims about the product's contents or effects. The FDA allows three types of claims on the packages of foods and dietary supplements:[36]

- Health claims describe a relationship between a food product and health promotion, but no food label is allowed to claim that a food can treat or cure a disease. FDA-approved health claims are supported by current scientific evidence and meet the standard for *significant scientific agreement (SSA)* among experts. If there is agreement that a food may reduce the risk of a disease and experts are confident that their opinion won't change with more scientific study, the health claim is approved. For example, an approved health claim on a package of whole-grain bread may state, "In a low-fat diet, whole-grain foods like this bread may reduce the risk of heart disease."
- Nutrient content claims indicate a specific nutrient is present at a certain level. For example, a product label might say "High in fiber" or "Low in fat" or "This product contains 100 calories per serving." Nutrient content claims can use the following words: *more, less, fewer, good source of, free, light, lean, extra lean, high, low,* and *reduced*.
- Structure and function claims describe the effect that a component in the food product has on the body. For example, the label of a carton of milk is allowed to state, "Calcium builds strong bones." Be aware that the FDA does not regulate structure and function claims.

In addition to food labels, shoppers are increasingly being guided in their food choices by nutritional rating systems. What are these systems, and can they help you make smarter choices? See the Student Health Today box for answers.

Front of Package Labeling The FDA requires several types of information on the front of food labels. These include the name of the food, the manufacturer or distributor, the ingredients, and the net weight of the food. Other aspects of the labeling on the front of packages are unregulated and may cause confusion for consumers.

The *Facts Up Front* initiative is a voluntary labeling system that manufacturers can use to provide quick, accurate information for the consumer. The most important information from the Nutrition Facts label is placed on the front of the package. As shown in **FIGURE 10.7**, Facts Up Front illustrates the kilocalories, saturated fat, sodium, and added sugars per serving. It also lists the amount and %DV of other "encouraged" micronutrients, such as potassium, that are underconsumed by Americans if a serving of the food contains more than 10 percent of the %DV.

▶ **SEE IT!** VIDEOS

Cut back on sugar while satisfying your sweet tooth! Watch **Ditching Sugar**, available on Mastering Health.

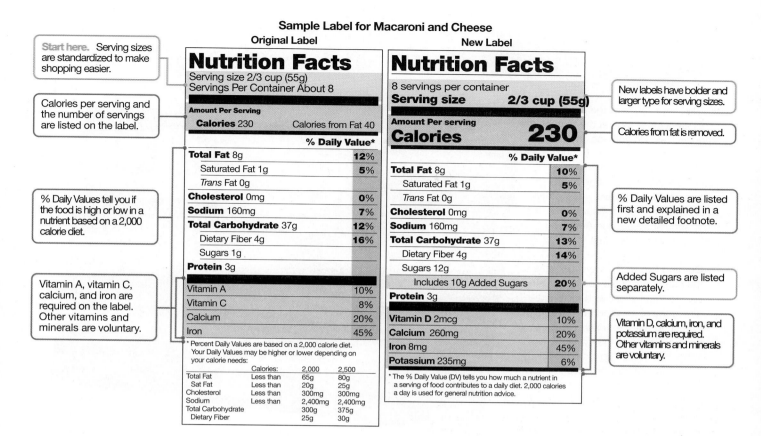

FIGURE 10.6 Reading a Food Label

Sources: U.S. Food and Drug Administration, "How to Understand and Use the Nutrition Facts Panel," April 2015, www.fda.gov/Food/IngredientsPackagingLabeling/LabelingNutrition/ucm274593.htm; U.S. Food and Drug Administration, "Changes to the Nutrition Facts Label," August 2016, http://www.fda.gov/Food/GuidanceRegulation/GuidanceDocumentsRegulatoryInformation/LabelingNutrition/ucm385663.htm.

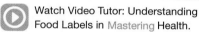 Watch Video Tutor: Understanding Food Labels in Mastering Health.

Understand Serving Sizes

MyPlate presents personalized dietary recommendations based on servings of particular nutrients. But how much is one serving? Is it different from a portion? Although these two terms are often used interchangeably, they actually mean very different things. A *serving* is the recommended amount you should consume; a *portion* is the amount you choose to eat at any one time. See FIGURE 10.8 for a handy pocket guide with tips on recognizing serving sizes.

Even when we read the label, we don't always get a clear idea of what a serving of the product really is. Consider a bottle of chocolate milk: The food label may list one serving size as 8 fluid ounces and 150 calories. However, note the size of the bottle. If it holds 16 ounces, drinking the entire contents will get you 300 calories.

Vegetarianism: A Healthy Diet?

The word **vegetarian** means different things to different people. Strict vegetarians, or *vegans*, avoid all foods of animal origin, including dairy products and eggs. Their diet is based on vegetables, grains, fruits, nuts, seeds, and legumes. Far more common are *lacto-vegetarians*, who eat dairy products but avoid flesh foods and eggs. *Ovo-vegetarians* add eggs to a vegan diet, and *lacto-ovo-vegetarians* eat both dairy products and eggs. *Pesco-vegetarians* eat fish, dairy products, and eggs; and *semivegetarians* eat chicken, fish, dairy products, and eggs. Some people in the semivegetarian category prefer to call themselves "non–red meat eaters."

According to a poll conducted by the Vegetarian Resource Group, 3.4 percent of U.S. adults, approximately 8 million adults, are vegetarians or vegans.[37] Among young adults (ages 18 to 34), 6 percent are vegetarian.[38]

vegetarian A person who follows a diet that excludes some or all animal products.

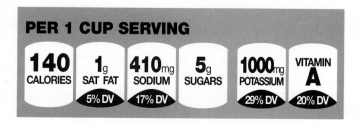

FIGURE 10.7 Facts Up Front Information is placed on the front of the package for a quick, accurate picture of the nutritional content of a serving of the food.

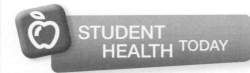

NUTRITION RATING SYSTEMS

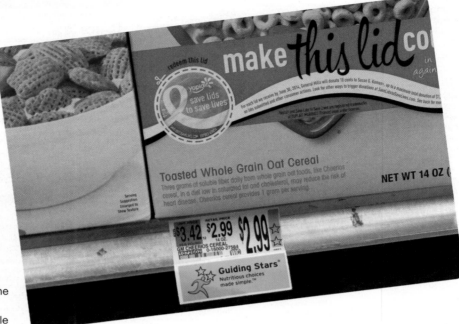

Next time you're at the grocery store, take a close look at the tags on the store shelves. Do you see anything different—stars, perhaps, or numbers inside blue hexagons? If so, you're looking at a nutrition rating system designed to help you quickly locate healthful foods. Four of the most popular systems in American markets are the following:

- **Guiding Stars.** This system rates the nutritional quality of foods using zero to three stars, with three indicating the highest nutritional quality. A fresh tomato, for example, gets three stars. What the system lacks in subtlety it makes up for in simplicity. Even consumers who haven't been introduced to it can quickly understand the basic message behind it: The product with the most stars "wins."

- **NuVal.** The NuVal System uses a scale of 1 to 100. The higher the number, the higher the nutritional quality. In rating each food, the system considers more than 30 dietary components—not just nutrients, but fiber and phytochemicals, too. In this system, a tomato gets a top score of 100 points. The 100-point rating scale allows consumers to make more subtle distinctions between very similar foods. For example, if two brands of whole-grain bread get scores of 48 and 29, the bread with the higher score is lower in calories and sodium and higher in fiber.

- **American Heart Association Heart Check.** The AHA Heart Check identifies foods that promote good heart health. To receive a Heart Check rating, the food must meet specific criteria for levels of saturated fat, sodium, and other nutrients. For example, to receive a Heart Check rating, a serving of food cannot contain more than 20 milligrams of cholesterol and cannot contain any partially hydrogenated oils. Each serving must also contain 10 percent or more of the daily value for dietary fiber or at least one of the following nutrients: protein, vitamin A, vitamin C, iron, or calcium.

- **Aggregate Nutrient Density Index (ANDI).** This index ranks foods according to the number of micronutrients per calorie and takes into account as many known beneficial phytochemicals as possible. However, it does not consider macronutrient density, such as the amount of high-quality protein or essential fatty acids in the food. A top score is 1,000. How does this system rate our tomato? It gets just 164 points! In contrast, kale gets a top score of 1,000. Here's why: A medium-sized tomato and two-thirds of a cup of kale have about the same number of calories, but the kale has more vitamin C, calcium, and beta-carotene.

Do these ranking systems prompt shoppers to choose more healthful foods? Research suggests that they might.

A recent study that followed shoppers in 150 supermarkets for 2 years found that the systems may be most effective in discouraging unhealthful choices. Sales of less nutritious foods fell by as much as 31 percent, resulting in an average purchase of more nutritious foods overall. Moreover, an evaluation of the AHA Heart Check system found that people who purchase the AHA-approved foods have a higher diet quality and a lower risk of cardiovascular disease and diabetes.

Source: J. Cawley et al., "The Impact of a Supermarket Nutrition Rating System on Purchases of Nutritious and Less Nutritious Foods," *Public Health Nutrition* 18, no. 1 (2015): 8–14; A.H. Lichtenstein et al., "Food-Intake Patterns Assessed by Using Front-of-Pack Labeling Program Criteria Associated with Better Diet Quality and Lower Cardiometabolic Risk," *American Journal of Clinical Nutrition* 99, no. 3 (2014): 454–62.

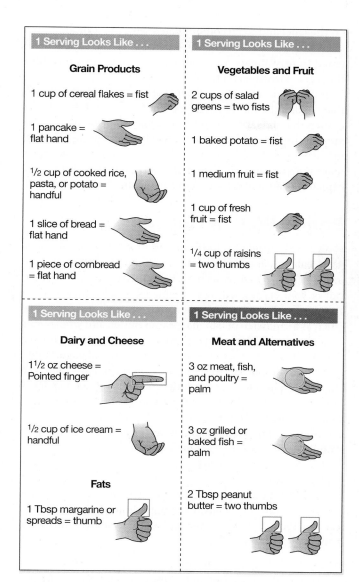

1 Serving Looks Like . . .	1 Serving Looks Like . . .
Grain Products	**Vegetables and Fruit**
1 cup of cereal flakes = fist	2 cups of salad greens = two fists
1 pancake = flat hand	1 baked potato = fist
1/2 cup of cooked rice, pasta, or potato = handful	1 medium fruit = fist
1 slice of bread = flat hand	1 cup of fresh fruit = fist
1 piece of cornbread = flat hand	1/4 cup of raisins = two thumbs

1 Serving Looks Like . . .	1 Serving Looks Like . . .
Dairy and Cheese	**Meat and Alternatives**
1 1/2 oz cheese = Pointed finger	3 oz meat, fish, and poultry = palm
1/2 cup of ice cream = handful	3 oz grilled or baked fish = palm
Fats	
1 Tbsp margarine or spreads = thumb	2 Tbsp peanut butter = two thumbs

FIGURE 10.8 Serving Size Card One of the challenges of following a healthy diet is judging how big a portion size should be and how many servings you are really eating. The comparisons on this card can help you recall what a standard food serving looks like. For easy reference, photocopy or cut out this card, fold on the dotted lines, and keep it in your wallet. You can even laminate it for long-term use.

Sources: National Heart, Lung and Blood Institute, "Serving Size Card," Accessed March 2017, http://hp2010.nhlbihin.net/portion/servingcard7.pdf; National Dairy Council, "Serving Size Comparison Chart," Accessed March 2017, www.healthyeating.org/Portals/0/Documents/Schools/Parent%20Ed/Portion_Sizes_Serving_Chart.pdf.

Common reasons for choosing a vegetarian lifestyle include concern for animal welfare, the environmental costs of meat production, food safety, personal health, weight loss, and weight maintenance. Generally, people who follow a balanced vegetarian diet weigh less and have better cholesterol levels, fewer problems with irregular bowel movements (constipation and diarrhea), and a lower risk of heart disease than do non-vegetarians. A recent analysis of 29 studies involving a total of more than 20,000 participants found that people who follow

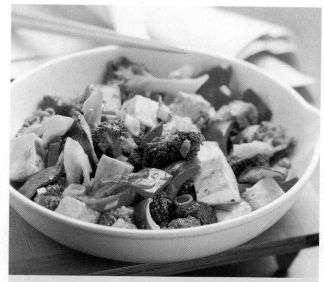

A vegetarian diet can be a very healthy way to eat. Make sure you get complementary essential amino acids throughout the day. Adding a whole grain, such as brown rice, can further enhance a tofu and vegetable stir-fry.

a vegetarian diet have an average blood pressure several points lower than that of nonvegetarians.[39] Some studies suggest that vegetarianism may also reduce the risk of some cancers, particularly colon cancer.[40]

With proper meal planning, vegetarianism provides a healthful alternative to a meat-based diet. Eating a variety of healthful foods throughout the day helps to ensure proper nutrient intake. Vegan diets are of greater concern than diets that include dairy products and eggs. Vegans may be deficient in vitamins B_2 (riboflavin), B_{12}, and D as well as calcium, iron, zinc, and other minerals; however, many foods are fortified with these nutrients, or vegans can obtain them from supplements. Vegans also have to pay more attention to the amino acid content of their foods, but eating a variety of types of plant foods throughout the day will provide adequate amounts of protein. Pregnant women, older adults, sick people, and families with young children who are vegans need to take special care to ensure that their diets are adequate. In all cases, seek advice from a health care professional if you have questions.

WHAT DO **YOU** THINK?

Why are so many people becoming vegetarians?

■ How easy is it to be a vegetarian on your campus?

■ What concerns about vegetarianism do you have, if any?

Supplements: Research on the Daily Dose

Dietary supplements are products that contain one or more dietary ingredients taken by mouth and intended to supplement existing diets. Ingredients

dietary supplements Products taken by mouth and containing dietary ingredients such as vitamins and minerals that are intended to supplement existing diets.

ONLY 5.4%

of college students eat the recommended five or more servings of **FRUITS AND VEGETABLES** a day.

mindful eating Eating with an awareness of how enjoyable eating can be and how food affects your body, feelings, and mind.

range from vitamins, minerals, and herbs to enzymes, amino acids, fatty acids, and organ tissues. They can come in tablet, capsule, liquid, powder, and other forms. A majority of Americans—68 percent—take at least one dietary supplement.[41] Among supplements users, 98 percent take vitamin–mineral supplements.[42]

It is important to note that dietary supplements are not regulated the way foods or drugs are. The FDA does not evaluate the safety and efficacy of supplements before they are put on the market, and it can take action to remove a supplement from the market only after the product has been proven harmful. Currently, the United States has no formal guidelines for supplement marketing and safety, and supplement manufacturers are responsible for self-monitoring their products.

Do you really need to take dietary supplements? The Office of Dietary Supplements, part of the National Institutes of Health, states that some supplements may help to ensure that you get adequate amounts of essential nutrients but warns that supplements cannot take the place of a varied, healthful diet. They are also not intended to prevent or treat disease, and the U.S. Preventive Services Task Force concluded that there is insufficient evidence to recommend that healthy people take multivitamin–mineral supplements to prevent cardiovascular disease or cancer.[43] The individuals who may benefit from using multivitamin–mineral supplements include pregnant and breastfeeding women, older adults, vegans, people on a very low-calorie weight-loss diet, individuals dependent on alcohol, and patients with malabsorption problems or other significant health problems. On the other hand, the efficacy of many dietary supplements is unproven. The benefit of fish consumption in reducing the risk for cardiovascular disease is well established, for example, but studies of fish-oil supplements have yielded conflicting results.[44]

Taking high-dose supplements of the fat-soluble vitamins A, D, and E can be harmful or even fatal. You should also be aware that supplements can interact with certain medications, including aspirin, diuretics, and steroids, potentially resulting in problems. Moreover, supplements often do not contain the ingredients listed on the label; in 2015, the New York State Office of the Attorney General required several national supplements retailers to cease selling a variety of herbal supplements that had been found to entirely lack the ingredients indicated

on the label and to be contaminated with plant products not identified on the label. Only 4 percent of the supplements tested from Walmart stores, for example, had DNA matching the plants identified on the ingredients list.[45]

If you do decide to take dietary supplements, choose brands that contain the U.S. Pharmacopeia or Consumer Lab seal. This ensures that the supplement is free of toxic ingredients and contains the ingredients stated on the label. Store your supplements in a dark, dry place (not the bathroom or other damp spots), make sure they are out of reach of small children, and check the expiration date and discard supplements that have passed it.

Eating Well in College

College students, in particular, find it hard to fit a well-balanced meal into the day. It is important to eat breakfast and lunch if you are to keep energy levels up and get the most out of your classes. Eating a complete breakfast that includes fiber-rich carbohydrates, protein, and healthy unsaturated fat (such as a sandwich of banana, peanut butter, and whole-grain bread or a bowl of oatmeal topped with dried fruit and nuts) is key. If you are short on time, bring a container of yogurt and a handful of almonds to your morning class. For many of us, eating can be a mindless, consuming, and guilt-ridden practice. A slower, more thoughtful and focused way of consuming food, known as **mindful eating**, can help you to avoid processed foods and unhealthy food and beverage choices. For more on mindful eating, see the **Mindfulness and You** box.

If your campus is like many others, your lunchtime options include a variety of fast-food restaurants. Generally speaking, you can eat more healthfully and for less money if you bring food from home or eat at your campus dining hall. If you must eat fast food, follow the tips below to get more nutritional bang for your buck:

- Ask for nutritional analyses of menu items. The FDA requires that most restaurants provide calorie and other nutritional information on menus or menu boards.
- Order salads, but be careful about what you add to them. Taco salads and Cobb salads are often high in fat, calories, and sodium. Ask for low-fat dressing on the side, and use it sparingly. Stay away from high-fat add-ons such as bacon bits, croutons, and crispy noodles.
- If you crave french fries, try baked "fries," which may be lower in fat.
- Avoid giant sizes, and refrain from ordering extra sauce, bacon, cheese, and other toppings that add calories, sodium, and fat.
- Limit sodas and other beverages that are high in added sugars.
- At least once per week, swap a vegetable-based meat substitute into your fast-food choices. Most places now offer veggie burgers and similar products, which provide excellent sources of protein and often have less fat and fewer calories.

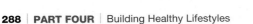

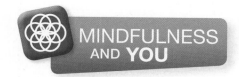

MINDFUL EATING

Do you ever eat meals standing at the counter, sitting in front of your computer or TV, or in your car? Some research has suggested that a slower, more thoughtful way of eating, may reduce body weight and processed, unhealthy food choices. Eating on autopilot or using food as a reward interferes with the body's ability to feel hunger, stop when full, or enjoy food. Eating this way makes it easy to overeat and gain weight. The key is to slow down and enjoy food, free of distractions. This is called *mindful eating*. Mindful eating is eating intentionally, with the understanding and awareness that what you're putting in your mouth has an effect on your body. That eating isn't just filling up the gas tank—something to do as quickly as possible. It's an opportunity to get to know yourself, what you enjoy, and what your body is telling you.

Once you have developed a healthy relationship with food, you're less likely to use food as a coping mechanism for stress, social rejection, anxiety, depression, or even anger. This is the goal of mindful eating. Mindfulness applied to eating may be achieved by following these simple steps:

- **Eat at the table.** Food eaten at the table is often eaten more slowly. When you eat food in the car or between classes, you tend to eat quickly and often simply to satisfy hunger. Foods eaten at the table tend to be healthier options.
- **Make food the main focus.** Notice the colors, smells, flavors, and textures of your food. Get rid of distractions such as smartphones, tablets, or television while eating.
- **Slow eating down.** Take small bites, and slow your eating. When you sit down to eat, set a timer for 20 minutes. Serve foods that take longer to eat, such as soups or salads, and chew slowly.
- **Choose food you enjoy.** Plan meals that are colorful, satisfying, and also nourishing to the body
- **Eating should nourish your soul.** Learn to use all your senses to eat foods that are both satisfying to your soul as well as nourish your body.
- **Eat until you are satisfied and then stop.** Become aware of your own cues for when to begin eating and when to stop.

Start slowly to begin the practice of mindful eating and self-compassion. Begin with just one meal a day or one per week to eat in a more attentive manner, as old eating habits may be difficult to change.

Sources: E. Forman et al., "Mindful Decision Making and Inhibitory Control Training as Complementary Means to Decrease Snack Consumption," *Appetite* 103 (2016): 176–83; M. Mantzios and J.C. Wilson, "Mindfulness, Eating Behaviours, and Obesity: A Review and Reflection on Current Findings," *Current Obesity Reports* 4, no. 1 (2015): 141–46; S. Katteman et al., "Mindfulness Meditation as an Intervention for Binge Eating, Emotional Eating, and Weight Loss: A Systematic Review," *Eating Behaviors* 15, no. 2 (2014): 197–204; C. Dawn et al., "Impact of Non-Diet Approaches on Attitudes, Behaviors, and Health Outcomes: A Systematic Review," *Journal of Nutrition Education and Behavior* 47, no. 2 (2015): 143–55; M. Mantzios and J.C. Wilson, "Making Concrete Construals Mindful: A Novel Approach for Developing Mindfulness and Self-Compassion to Assist Weight Loss," *Psychology and Health* 29, no. 4 (2014): 422–41. doi:10.1080/08870446.2013.863883.

In the dining hall, try these ideas:

- Choose lean meats, grilled chicken, fish, or vegetable dishes. Avoid fried chicken, fatty cuts of red meat, and meat dishes smothered in creamy or oily sauce.
- Hit the salad bar, and load up on leafy greens, beans, tuna, or tofu. Choose items such as avocado or nuts for "good" fat. Go easy on the dressing, or substitute vinaigrette or low-fat dressings.
- When choosing items from a made-to-order food station, ask the preparer to hold the butter or oil, mayonnaise, sour cream, and cheese- or cream-based sauces.
- Avoid going back for seconds and consuming large portions.
- If there are healthy foods you would like but don't see in your dining hall, speak to your food service manager and provide suggestions.
- Pass up high-calorie, low-nutrient foods such as sugary cereals, ice cream, and other sweet treats. Choose fruit or low-fat yogurt to satisfy your sweet tooth.

Between classes, avoid vending machines. Reach into your backpack for an apple, banana, some dried fruit and nuts, a single serving of unsweetened applesauce, or whole-grain crackers spread with peanut butter. Energy bars can be a nutritious option if you choose well. Check the Nutrition Facts label for bars that are below 200 calories and provide at least 3 grams of dietary fiber. Cereal bars usually provide less protein than energy bars; however, they also tend to be much lower in calories and sugar and high in fiber.

Maintaining a nutritious diet within the confines of a typical college student's budget can be challenging. The **Money & Health** box identifies ways to include fruits and vegetables in your diet without breaking the bank.

LO 4 | FOOD SAFETY: A GROWING CONCERN

Explain food safety concerns facing Americans and people in other regions of the world.

Eating unhealthy food is one thing. Eating food that has been contaminated with a pathogen, toxin, or other harmful substance is quite another. As outbreaks of foodborne illness

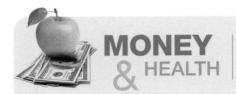

MONEY & HEALTH | ARE FRUITS AND VEGGIES BEYOND YOUR BUDGET?

Many people who are on tight budgets, including college students, think that they can't afford fruits and vegetables. If that sounds like you, it's time for some facts. In 2015, the Economic Research Service of the USDA published data showing that substituting any of several common fruits or vegetables—such as bananas, grapes, applesauce, carrots, or celery—for more typical snack items—such as chips, crackers, cookies, muffins, or candy—costs less. Contrary to popular opinion, people on a tight budget can eat healthfully, including plenty of fruits and vegetables, and spend less on food.

So how can you do it? Here are some tips:

- **Celebrate the season.** From apples to zucchini, when fruits and vegetables are in season, they cost less. If you can freeze them, stock up. If not, enjoy them fresh while you can.
- **Buy small amounts frequently.** Most fresh produce keeps only a few days, so buy amounts that you know you'll be able to eat or freeze.
- **Do it yourself.** Avoid prewashed, precut fruits and vegetables, including salad greens. They cost more and often spoil faster. Also choose frozen 100 percent juice concentrate, and add the water yourself.
- **Buy canned or frozen on sale, in bulk.** Canned and frozen produce, especially when it's on sale, may be much less expensive than fresh. Most frozen items are just as nutritious as fresh and can be even more so, depending on how long ago the fresh food was harvested. For canned items, choose fruits without added sugars and vegetables without added salt or sauces. Bear in mind that beans are legumes and count as a vegetable choice. Low-sodium canned beans are one of the most affordable, convenient, and nutritious foods you can buy. If you can't find low-sodium beans, just rinse them before heating.
- **Don't pay full price.** Use coupons, watch for sales, or shop at larger supermarkets or discount warehouses.
- **Fix and freeze.** Make large batches of homemade soups, vegetable stews, and pasta sauce, and store them in single-serving containers in your freezer.
- **Grow your own.** All it takes is one sunny window, a pot, soil, and a packet of seeds. Lettuce, spinach, and fresh herbs are particularly easy to grow indoors in small spaces.

Sources: U.S. Department of Agriculture, Economic Research Service, "Snacks: Impact on Food Costs of Substituting Fruits and Vegetables for Other Snack Foods," June 2015, http://ers.usda.gov/data-products/fruit-and-vegetable-prices.aspx#33646; U.S. Department of Agriculture, ChooseMyPlate.gov, "Smart Shopping for Veggies and Fruits," September 2015, www.choosemyplate.gov/ten-tips-smart-shopping.

(commonly called *food poisoning*) make the news, the food industry has come under fire. The Food Safety Modernization Act, passed into law in 2011, included new requirements for food processors to take actions to prevent contamination of foods. The act gave the FDA greater authority to inspect food-manufacturing facilities and to recall contaminated foods.[46]

Choosing Organic or Locally Grown Foods

Concerns about the health effects of chemicals that are used to grow and produce food have led many people to turn to foods and beverages that are **organic**—produced without the use of toxic and persistent pesticides or fertilizers, antibiotics, hormones, irradiation, or genetic modification. Any food sold in the United States as organic has to meet criteria set

organic Grown without use of toxic and persistent pesticides, chemicals, or hormones.

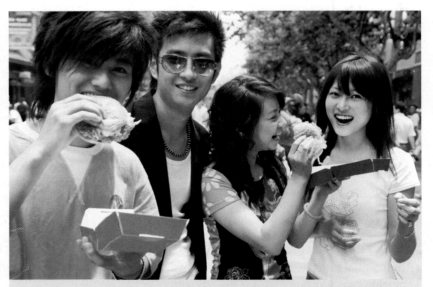

Meals like this one may be convenient, but they are high in saturated fat, sodium, refined carbohydrates, and calories. Even when you are short on time and money, it is possible—and worthwhile—to make healthier choices. If you are ordering fast food, opt for foods prepared by baking, roasting, or steaming; ask for the leanest meat option; and request that sauces, dressings, and gravies be served on the side.

by the USDA under the National Organic Rule and can carry a USDA seal verifying products as "certified organic." Under this rule, a product that is certified may carry one of the following terms:

- "100 percent Organic" (100% compliance with organic criteria)
- "Organic" (must contain at least 95% organic materials)
- "Made with Organic Ingredients" (must contain at least 70% organic ingredients)
- "Some Organic Ingredients" (contains less than 70% organic ingredients, usually listed individually).

In contrast, the term *natural* on food labels is not currently regulated. However, the FDA is investigating concerns related to the use of the term and may shortly develop regulations on its use.[47]

The market for organic foods has been increasing faster than food sales in general for many years. Whereas only a small subset of the population once bought organic, 84 percent of all U.S. families now buy organic foods at least occasionally, and sales of organic foods represent nearly 5 percent of total food sales.[48] In 2015, annual organic food sales were estimated to be over $39 billion.[49]

Is organic food really more nutritious? That depends on what aspect of the food is being studied and how the research is conducted. Two early review studies, both of which examined decades of research into the nutrient quality of organic versus traditionally grown foods, reached opposite conclusions: One found that organic foods were more nutritious; the other did not.[50] These studies confirmed higher pesticide residues on conventionally grown produce. Pesticide exposure is a health risk because various types have been associated with significant adverse effects, from hormonal disorders to an increased risk for cancer.[51] Newer research provides a controversial picture of the benefits of organic meats, dairy and eggs as compared to conventional products. Organic meats provide higher fatty acid levels, but consumer brand preferences, appearance of packaging, and texture appear to influence consumer perceptions more than actual nutritional benefits do.[52] Other research indicates that in terms of food safety, we don't have enough knowledge to say whether or not the higher prices of organic foods are justified for safety reasons alone.[53]

The U.S. Environmental Protection Agency regulates pesticide use, and while this assures Americans that only low levels of pesticide residue remain on conventionally grown foods, consumers are advised to scrub produce under running water and, if possible, peel it.[54]

The word **locavore** has been coined to describe people who mostly eat food that is grown or produced locally, usually within close proximity to their homes. Because these foods are transported only a few miles from farm to market, they are assumed to use fewer resources and cause the emission of a lower level of greenhouse gases as well as to be fresher and to stay fresh longer after they're sold. However, consumers should not assume that these foods are organic or that they are less likely to be contaminated with microorganisms. Pesticide residues and harmful bacteria can be found both in foods shipped to markets from distant countries and in foods purchased from local farms.[55] Additionally, issues about the transport and refrigeration of locally or regionally grown foods have been raised, as regulations and enforcement policies are often not in place.

Foodborne Illnesses

Are you concerned that the chicken you are buying doesn't look pleasingly pink or that your "fresh" fish smells a little *too* fishy? You may have good reason to be worried. The Centers for Disease Control and Prevention (CDC) estimates that foodborne illnesses from 31 pathogens cause 9.4 million illnesses, 55,961 hospitalizations, and 1,351 deaths in the United States annually.[56] Although the incidence of infection with certain microbes has declined, the incidence of infection with other microbes has risen or stayed essentially unchanged; therefore, the CDC reports that foodborne infections are an ongoing public health concern requiring improved prevention.[57]

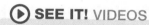
Several common types of bacteria and viruses, including the bacteria *salmonella*, *listeria*, and *campylobacter* and the virus *norovirus*, cause most foodborne infections and illnesses. Foodborne illnesses can also be caused by a toxin in food that was originally produced by a bacterium or other microbe in the food. These toxins can produce illness even if the microbes that produced them have been destroyed. For example, the *Staphylococcus* bacterium produces an intestinal toxin that can cause a self-limiting illness characterized by nausea, vomiting, and diarrhea. In contrast, *Clostridium botulinum*, another bacterium, produces the botulism toxin, which is the most deadly nerve toxin known. Botulism is rare, and most cases occur in home-canned vegetables; however, store-bought foods from cans that are dented, pierced, leaking, or bulging may also harbor the botulism toxin.[58]

Signs of foodborne illnesses vary tremendously and usually include one or several symptoms: diarrhea, nausea, cramping, and vomiting. Depending on the amount and virulence of the pathogen, symptoms may appear as early as 30 minutes after eating contaminated food or as long as several days or weeks later. Most of the time, symptoms occur 5 to 8 hours after eating and last only a day or two. Foodborne diseases can be fatal for certain populations, such as the very young;

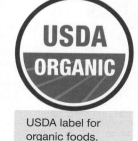

older adults; and people with severe illnesses such as cancer, diabetes, kidney disease, or AIDS.

Several factors contribute to foodborne illnesses, including inadequate oversight of both foreign and domestic suppliers by uncoordinated and underfunded federal agencies. Moreover, federal agencies can be slow to identify and respond to outbreaks.[59] The task is enormous: Food can become contaminated in the field by contaminated irrigation water or runoff from nearby animal feedlots, or during harvesting if farm laborers have not washed their hands properly after using the toilet. Food-processing equipment, facilities, or workers may contaminate food, or it can become contaminated if not kept clean and cool during transport or on store shelves. The bacterium *Escherichia coli*, species of which produce a dangerous toxin, is present in unprocessed cow manure, which is commonly used as a fertilizer on both organic and conventional farms. Although its level drops significantly within 60 days, *E. coli* can survive on fields for up to 120 days and can even be resuscitated after heavy rains.[60] No regulations prohibit farmers from using animal manure to fertilize crops. In addition, *E. coli* quickly reproduces in the summer months as cattle await slaughter in crowded, overheated pens. This increases the chances of meat coming to market already contaminated.

Avoiding Risks in the Home

Although 75 percent of cases of foodborne illness are caused by foods consumed in restaurants, delis, or banquet facilities, about 9 percent result from unsafe handling of food at home.[61] Four basic steps reduce the likelihood of contaminating your food (see **FIGURE 10.9**). Among the most basic precautions are washing your hands and washing all produce before eating it.

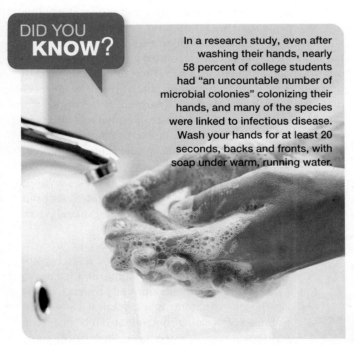

DID YOU KNOW?

In a research study, even after washing their hands, nearly 58 percent of college students had "an uncountable number of microbial colonies" colonizing their hands, and many of the species were linked to infectious disease. Wash your hands for at least 20 seconds, backs and fronts, with soap under warm, running water.

Source: Data are from K.J. Prater et al., "Poor Hand Hygiene by College Students Linked to More Occurrences of Infectious Diseases, Medical Visits, and Absence from Classes," *American Journal of Infection Control* 44, no. 1 (2016): 66–70.

CLEAN   SEPARATE   COOK   CHILL

FIGURE 10.9 **The Four Core Practices** This logo reminds consumers how to prevent foodborne illness.

Source: Partnership for Food Safety Education, 2017, www.fightbac.org/safe-food-handling.

Also, avoid cross-contamination in the kitchen by using separate cutting boards and utensils for meats and produce. Temperature control is also important; refrigerators must be set at 40°F or lower. Cook meats to the recommended temperature to kill contaminants before eating. Keep hot foods hot and cold foods cold to avoid unchecked bacterial growth. Eat leftovers within 3 days, and if you're unsure how long something has been sitting in the fridge, don't take chances. When in doubt, throw it out. See the **Skills for Behavior Change** box for more tips about reducing risk of foodborne illness.

SKILLS FOR
BEHAVIOR CHANGE

Reduce Your Risk For Foodborne Illness

◉ When shopping, put perishable foods in your cart last. Check for cleanliness throughout the store, especially at the salad bar and at the meat and fish counters. Never buy dented cans of food. Check the "sell by" or "use by" date on foods.

◎ Once you get home, put dairy products, eggs, meat, fish, and poultry in the refrigerator immediately. If you don't plan to eat meats within 2 days, freeze them. You can keep an unopened package of hot dogs or luncheon meats for about 2 weeks.

◎ When refrigerating or freezing raw meats, make sure their juices can't spill onto other foods.

◎ Never thaw frozen foods at room temperature. Put them in the refrigerator to thaw, or thaw them in the microwave, following manufacturer's instructions.

◎ Wash your hands with soap and warm water before preparing food. Wash fruits and vegetables before peeling, slicing, cooking, or eating them, but do not wash meat, poultry, or eggs. Wash cutting boards, countertops, and other utensils and surfaces with detergent and hot water after food preparation.

◎ Use a meat thermometer to ensure that meats are completely cooked. To find proper cooking temperatures for different types of meat, visit http://food-safety.gov/keep/charts/mintemp.html.

◎ Refrigeration slows the secretion of bacterial toxins into foods. Never leave leftovers out for more than 2 hours. On hot days, don't leave foods out for longer than 1 hour.

Food Sensitivities, Allergies, and Intolerances

Although many people today *think* they have a food allergy, it is estimated that only 5 percent of children and 4 percent of adults actually do.[62] A **food allergy**, or hypersensitivity, is an abnormal response to a component—usually a protein—in food that is triggered by the immune system. Symptoms of an allergic reaction vary in severity and may include a tingling sensation in the mouth; swelling of the lips, tongue, and throat; difficulty breathing; skin hives; vomiting; abdominal cramps; and diarrhea. A severe reaction called *anaphylaxis* can cause widespread inflammation, difficulty breathing, and cardiovascular problems such as a sudden drop in blood pressure that can be life threatening.[63] Anaphylaxis may occur within seconds to hours after eating a food to which one is allergic.

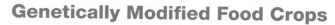

Peanuts are among the eight most common food allergens.

The Food Allergen Labeling and Consumer Protection Act requires food manufacturers to label foods clearly to indicate the presence of (or possible contamination by) any of the eight major food allergens: milk, eggs, peanuts, wheat, soy, tree nuts (walnuts, pecans, cashews, pistachios, etc.), fish, and shellfish. Although over 160 foods have been identified as allergy triggers, these eight foods account for 90 percent of all food allergies in the United States.[64]

Celiac disease is an immune disorder that causes malabsorption of nutrients from the small intestine in genetically susceptible people. It is thought to affect as many as 1 in every 141 Americans, most of whom are undiagnosed.[65] When a person with celiac disease consumes gluten—a protein found in wheat, rye, and barley—the person's immune system responds with inflammation. This degrades the lining of the small intestine and reduces nutrient absorption. Pain, abdominal cramping, diarrhea, constipation, nausea, vomiting, and other symptoms are common. Untreated, celiac disease can lead to long-term health problems, such as nutritional deficiencies, tissue wasting, osteoporosis, seizures, liver disease, and cancer of the small intestine. Blood tests and intestinal biopsies are used to diagnose celiac disease. Individuals who have been diagnosed are encouraged to consult a dietitian for help designing a gluten-free diet. For more information on gluten-free diets, read Health Headlines: Gluten-Free Diets.

Food intolerance can cause symptoms of digestive upset, but the upset is not the result of an immune system response. Probably the best example of a food intolerance is *lactose intolerance*, an inability to adequately digest the disaccharide lactose, which is in dairy products. The problem is common, although the number of Americans with the condition is unknown.[66] Lactase is an enzyme produced by the small intestine that helps to break the bonds in the lactose molecule. If you don't have enough lactase, undigested lactose remains in the small intestine, drawing water by osmosis. This dilates the small intestine and speeds the transit of the food mass, resulting in diarrhea. When the undigested lactose reaches the large intestine, gut bacteria ferment it. Gas is formed, and the person experiences bloating and abdominal pain.

If you suspect that you have a food allergy, celiac disease, or a food intolerance, see your doctor. Because these diseases can have some common symptoms as well as sharing symptoms with other gastrointestinal disorders, clinical diagnosis is essential.

Genetically Modified Food Crops

Genetically modified crop farming is expanding rapidly around the world. Genetic modification involves the insertion or deletion of genes into the DNA of an organism. In the case of **genetically modified (GM) foods**, this genetic cutting and pasting process is typically done to enhance production, for example, by increasing a crop's tolerance to common herbicides (weed killers), making plants disease- or insect-resistant, or improving yield. In fact, GM crops grow faster and have average yields 22 percent higher than those of traditional crops and are credited with contributing to the global decline in hunger prevalence since their widespread adoption in the 1990s.[67] In addition, GM foods are sometimes created to boost the level of specific nutrients. For example, currently under development is a GM variety of rice that is high in vitamin A and iron. Another use under development is the production and delivery of vaccines through GM foods.

The long-term safety of GM foods—for humans, other species, and the environment—is still in question. The American Association for the Advancement of Science reports that foods containing GM ingredients are no more of a risk than are the same foods composed of crops modified over time through conventional plant breeding techniques, and the World Health Organization states that no adverse effects on human health have been shown from consumption of GM foods in countries that have approved their use.[68] The debate surrounding GM foods is not likely to end soon; see the **Points of View** box for more on this debate.

food allergy Overreaction by the immune system to normally harmless proteins in foods, which are perceived as allergens. In response, the body produces antibodies, triggering allergic symptoms.

celiac disease An inherited immune disorder that causes malabsorption of nutrients from the small intestine and is triggered by the consumption of gluten, a protein found in certain grains.

food intolerance Adverse effects that result when people who lack the digestive chemicals needed to break down certain substances eat those substances.

genetically modified (GM) foods Foods derived from organisms whose DNA has been altered through genetic engineering techniques.

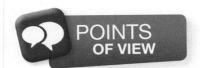
GENETICALLY MODIFIED FOODS
Boon or Bane?

Farmers in the United States have widely accepted genetically modified (GM) crops. GM crops do not occur naturally but have been altered by introducing a gene from a different organism. Soybeans and cotton are the most common GM crops, followed by corn. On supermarket shelves, an estimated 75 percent of processed foods have GM ingredients. Even much of the produce you buy in stores has been genetically modified, including tomatoes, corn, potatoes, squash, and soybeans.

State governments, industry, and scientists tout the benefits of GM foods for health, agriculture, and the ecosystem, including feeding the world's population. In contrast, consumer activists, environmental organizations, religious groups, and health advocates warn of unexpected health risks and environmental and socio-economic consequences. Consumers question whether GM plants are safe to eat. By 2014, two states—Connecticut and Maine—had enacted GMO-labeling laws. However, the legislation doesn't go into effect until nearby states enact similar labeling laws. The FDA continues to evaluate the safety issues of GM foods and future regulations to protect the world's food supply.

Following are some of the main points for and against the development of GM food:

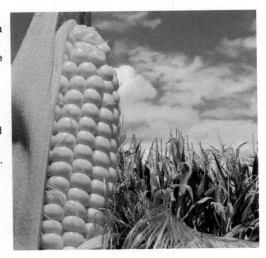

Arguments for the Development of GM Foods

- People have been manipulating food crops—primarily through selective breeding—since the beginning of agriculture. Genetic modification is fundamentally the same thing, just more targeted and precise.
- GM fruits and vegetables produce higher levels of antioxidants, which reduce the risk of heart disease and cancer, and vitamin A, which may prevent blindness.
- GM seeds and products are tested for safety, and there has never been a substantiated claim for a human illness resulting from consumption of a GM food.
- GM crops have the potential to reduce world hunger: They can be created to grow more quickly than conventional crops, increasing productivity and allowing for faster cycling of crops, which means more food yield. In addition, nutrient-enhanced crops can address malnutrition, and crops that have been engineered to resist spoiling or damage can allow for transportation to areas affected by drought or natural disaster.

Arguments against the Development of GM Foods

- Genetic modification may cause an allergic reaction. Allergic reactions occur in humans when their immune system recognizes a protein as a foreign invader. In vitro research studies suggests that some GM foods may cause allergic reactions.
- GM foods have the potential to reduce absorption of essential nutrients. For example, if the gene inserted to make the new GM food increases the phytate content of the food, that will reduce the absorption of certain minerals, such as calcium and iron. Modified soy products may also produce lower amounts of phytoestrogens, which are known to reduce the risk of heart disease and cancer.
- Plants naturally produce low levels of substances that are toxic to humans. While these toxins do not produce problems for humans, there is a concern that adding a new gene to produce a GM plant may cause the new plant to produce toxins at higher levels that could be dangerous if eaten. For instance, GM potatoes produce higher levels of glycoalkaloids.

WHERE DO YOU STAND?

- Do you think GM foods are more helpful or harmful?
- What are your greatest concerns about GM foods? What do you think are their greatest benefits?
- In what ways could the creators of GM foods address the concerns of the people who oppose them?
- What sort of regulation do you think the government should have with

regard to the creation, cultivation, and sale of GM foods?
- Currently, there are no GM livestock; however, many livestock are fed GM feed or feed that includes additives and vaccines produced by GM microorganisms. Do you feel any differently about directly consuming GM crops versus eating the flesh, milk, or eggs of an animal that has been fed on GM crops?

Sources: U.S. Department of Agriculture, Economic Research Service, "Adoption of Genetically Engineered Crops in the U.S.," October 2016, www.ers.usda.gov/data-products/adoption-of-genetically-engineered-crops-in-the-us.aspx; Center for Food Safety, "About Genetically Engineered Foods," Accessed March 2017, www.centerforfoodsafety.org/issues/311/ge-foods/about-ge-foods; A. Bakshi, "Potential Adverse Health Effects of Genetically Modified Crops," Journal of Toxicology and Environmental Health, Part B: Critical Reviews 6, no. 3 (2003): 211–25.

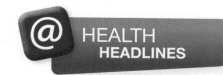

GLUTEN-FREE DIETS

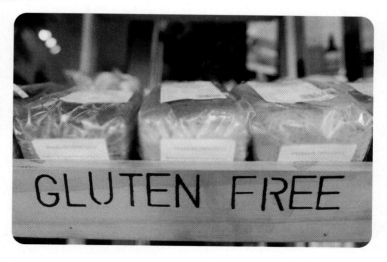

Gluten-free diets have become a fad. The number of individuals following a gluten-free diet is fueling a market of gluten-free products. In a 5-year period ending in 2014, sales of gluten-free products grew by more than 34 percent. According to a 2015 national poll, 1 in 5 Americans purchases gluten-free foods, and 1 in 6 actively avoids foods with gluten. This is far more people than the number who have been clinically diagnosed with celiac disease or nonceliac gluten sensitivity (NCGS). Is this wise?

A gluten-free diet entirely excludes gluten, which is found in breads, cereals, and other grain products made with wheat, barley, and rye, as well as in many processed foods. The diet is highly restrictive, but for people with celiac disease, it is essential to survival.

In contrast, for people who do not have celiac disease or NCGS, a gluten-free diet does not provide any nutritional benefits over a varied diet containing gluten. In fact, many whole-grain foods that contain gluten provide more dietary fiber, vitamins, and minerals than gluten-free versions. These versions are often made with refined, unenriched sorghum and rice flours, which are low in essential nutrients and fiber and high in calories—not to mention expensive. In fact, people who follow a gluten-free diet may have inadequate intakes of several micronutrients, including iron, calcium, and the B vitamins riboflavin, thiamin, folate, and niacin.

If you have been diagnosed with celiac disease or NCGS, consult a dietitian for advice on avoiding gluten while still following a healthy eating pattern.

Many nutritious foods are naturally free of gluten, including beans, peas, lentils, all other vegetables, fruits, nuts, seeds, all animal-based foods, and even several grains such as oats, cornmeal, brown rice, and quinoa. In buying foods for a gluten-free diet, fresh, unprocessed foods are the best choice. When you are buying packaged foods, look for the words "certified gluten-free." The FDA requires that, to have a gluten-free label, the product must contain less than 20 parts per million of gluten. For all other packaged foods, carefully study the ingredients list before buying, as many unfamiliar food ingredients contain gluten.

Sources: Packaged Facts, *Gluten-free Foods and Beverages in the US*, 5th ed. (Rockville, MD: Packaged Foods, 2015), Available from www .packagedfacts.com/Gluten-Free-Foods-8108350; R. Riffkin, "One in Five Americans Include Gluten-Free Foods in Diet," Gallup, Inc., July 23, 2015, www.gallup.com/poll/184307/one-five-americans-include-gluten-free-foods-diet.aspx; S.J. Shepherd and P.R. Gibson, "Nutritional Inadequacies of the Gluten-free Diet in Both Recently-Diagnosed and Long-Term Patients with Celiac Disease," *Journal of Human Nutrition and Dietetics* 26, no. 4 (2013): 349–58.

ASSESS | YOURSELF

How Mindful and Healthy Are Your Eating Habits?

1 Why do I eat? What is driving my eating?

2 When do I feel like eating? When do I think about eating? When do I decide to eat?

3 What do I eat?

Keep a food diary for 5 days, writing down everything you eat and drink. Be sure to include the approximate amount or portion size. Add up the number of servings from each of the major food groups on each day, and enter them into the chart below.

Number of Servings:

	Day 1	Day 2	Day 3	Day 4	Day 5	Average
Fruits						
Vegetables						
Grains						
Protein foods						
Dairy						
Fats and oils						
Sweets						

4 How do I eat? How, specifically, do I get the food I've chosen into my body?

5 Evaluate Your Mindful Eating and Your Food Intake

First, take notes on your mindful eating patterns. Do you get up early enough to eat a nutritious breakfast? Do you eat in the car, in front of the television, or while reading your tablet? Do you eat slowly and savor your foods?

Now compare your consumption patterns to the MyPlate recommendations. Look at Table 10.1 (page 274) and Figure 10.5 (page 285) and visit www.choosemyplate.gov to evaluate your daily caloric needs and the recommended consumption rates for the different food groups. How does your diet match up?

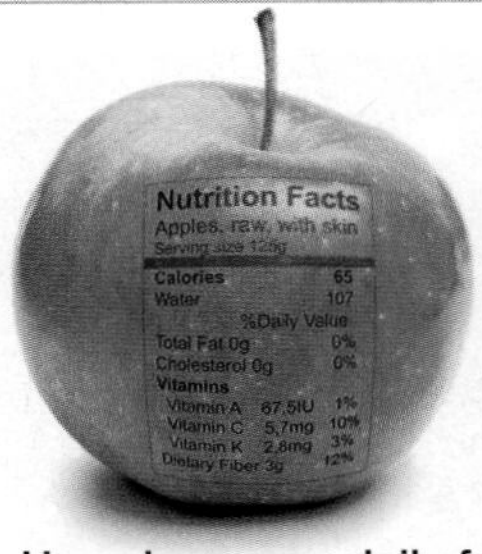

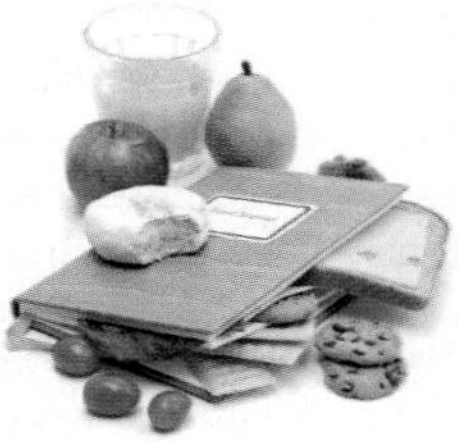

	Less Than the Recommended Amount	About Equal to the Recommended Amount	More Than the Recommended Amount
1. How does your daily fruit consumption compare to the recommendation for you?	○	○	○
2. How does your daily vegetable consumption compare to the recommendation for you?	○	○	○
3. How does your daily grain consumption compare to the recommendation for you?	○	○	○
4. How does your daily protein food consumption compare to the recommendation for you?	○	○	○
5. How does your daily dairy food consumption compare to the recommendation for you?	○	○	○
6. How does your daily calorie consumption compare to the recommendation for your age and activity level?	○	○	○

Scoring

If you found that your food intake is consistent with the MyPlate recommendations, congratulations! If you are falling short in a major food group or are overdoing it in certain categories, consider taking steps to adopt healthier eating habits.

Source: J.S. Blake, K.D. Munoz, and S. Volpe, *Nutrition: From Science to You*, 3rd ed., © 2016. Reprinted and electronically reproduced by permission of Pearson Education, Inc., Upper Saddle River, New Jersey.

YOUR PLAN FOR **CHANGE**

The **ASSESS YOURSELF** activity gave you the chance to evaluate your current mindful eating and nutritional habits. Once you have considered these results, you can decide whether you need to make changes in your daily eating for long-term health.

TODAY, YOU CAN:

☐ Notice when you're hungry and when you're full.

☐ Start keeping a more detailed food log. The easy-to-use SuperTracker at www.supertracker.usda.gov can help you keep track of your food intake and analyze what you eat. Take note of the nutritional content of the various foods you eat, and write down particulars about the number of calories, grams of saturated fat, grams of sugar, milligrams of sodium, and other elements of each food. Try to find specific weak spots: Are you consuming too many calories or too much salt or sugar? Do you eat too little calcium or iron? Use the SuperTracker to plan a healthier food intake to overcome these weak spots.

☐ Take a field trip to the grocery store. Forgo your fast-food dinner, and instead spend time in the produce section of the supermarket. Purchase your favorite fruits and vegetables, and try something new to expand your tastes.

WITHIN THE NEXT TWO WEEKS, YOU CAN:

☐ Practice to be more present when you eat and slow down your eating. Savor the flavor of food, and enjoy every bite to allow the brain time to receive signals that you are becoming full.

☐ Plan at least three meals that you can make at home or in your dorm room, and purchase the ingredients you'll need ahead of time. Something as simple as a chicken sandwich on whole-grain bread will be more nutritious and probably cheaper than heading out for a fast-food meal.

☐ Start reading labels. Be aware of the amount of calories, sodium, sugars, and saturated fats in prepared foods; aim to buy and consume those that are lower in all of these and are higher in micronutrients and fiber.

BY THE END OF THE SEMESTER, YOU CAN:

☐ Eat at the table without distractions from my computer, phone, or television for most meals of the week. Enjoy discussing events with my friends while you eat.

☐ Get in the habit of eating a healthy breakfast every morning. Combine whole grains, proteins, and fruit in your breakfast; for example, eat a bowl of cereal with soy milk and bananas or a cup of low-fat yogurt with granola and berries. Eating a healthy breakfast will jump-start your metabolism, prevent drops in blood glucose levels, and keep your brain and body performing at their best through your morning classes.

☐ Commit to one or two healthful changes to your eating patterns for the rest of the semester. You might resolve to eat five servings of fruits and vegetables every day, to switch to low-fat or nonfat dairy products, to stop drinking soft drinks, or to use only olive oil in your cooking. Use your food diary to help you spot places where you can make healthier choices on a daily basis.

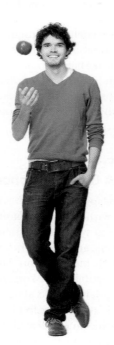

STUDY **PLAN**

Visit the Study Area in Mastering Health to enhance your study plan with MP3 Tutor Sessions, Practice Quizzes, Flashcards, and more!

CHAPTER **REVIEW**

LO 1 | Essential Nutrients for Health

- Nutrition is the science of the relationship between physiological function and the essential elements of the foods we eat. The Dietary Reference Intakes (DRIs) are recommended nutrient intakes for healthy people.
- The essential nutrients are water, proteins, carbohydrates, fats, vitamins, and minerals. Water makes up the majority of our body weight and is necessary for nearly all life processes. Proteins are major components of our cells and tissues and are key elements of antibodies, enzymes, and hormones. Carbohydrates are our primary sources of energy. Fats provide energy while we are at rest and for long-term activity. They also play important roles in maintaining body temperature, cushioning and protecting organs, and promoting healthy cell function. Vitamins are organic compounds, and minerals are inorganic elements. We need these micronutrients in small amounts to maintain healthy body structure and function.

LO 2 | Nutritional Guidelines

- A healthful diet is adequate, moderate, balanced, varied, and nutrient dense. The USDA developed the Dietary Guidelines for Americans and the MyPlate plan provide guidelines for healthy eating. These recommendations place emphasis on balancing calories and understanding which foods to increase and which to decrease.
- The Nutrition Facts label on food labels identifies the serving size, number of calories per serving, and amounts of various nutrients, as well as the %DV, which is the percentage of recommended daily values those amounts represent.

LO 3 | How Can I Eat More Healthfully?

- With a little menu planning, vegetarianism can be a healthful lifestyle choice, providing plenty of nutrients plus fiber and phytochemicals, typically with less saturated fat and fewer calories.
- Although some people may benefit from taking vitamin and mineral supplements, a healthy diet is the best way to give your body the nutrients it needs.
- College students face unique challenges in eating healthfully. Learning to make better choices, to eat healthfully on a budget, and to eat nutritionally in the dorm are all possible when you use the information in this chapter.

LO 4 | Food Safety: A Growing Concern

- Organic foods are grown and produced without the use of toxic and persistent synthetic pesticides, fertilizers, antibiotics, hormones, or genetic modification. The USDA offers certification of organic farms and regulates claims about organic ingredients used on food labels.
- Foodborne illnesses can be traced to contamination of food at any point from the field to the consumer's kitchen. To keep food safe at home, follow four steps: Clean, separate, cook, and chill.
- Food allergies, celiac disease, food intolerances, genetically modified foods, and other food safety and health concerns are becoming increasingly important to health-conscious consumers. Recognizing potential risks and taking steps to prevent problems are part of a sound nutritional plan.

POP **QUIZ**

LO 1 | Essential Nutrients for Health

1. What is the most crucial nutrient for life?
   a. Water
   b. Fiber
   c. Minerals
   d. Starch

2. Which of the following nutrients is critical for the repair and growth of body tissue?
   a. Carbohydrates
   b. Proteins
   c. Vitamins
   d. Fats

3. Which of the following substances helps move food through the digestive tract?
   a. Folate
   b. Fiber
   c. Minerals
   d. Starch

4. What substance provides energy, promotes healthy skin and hair, insulates body organs, helps to maintain body temperature, and contributes to healthy cell function?
   a. Fats
   b. Fibers
   c. Proteins
   d. Carbohydrates

5. Which of the following fats is a healthier fat to include in the diet?
   a. *Trans* fat
   b. Saturated fat
   c. Unsaturated fat
   d. Hydrogenated fat

6. Which vitamin maintains bone health?
   a. B_{12}
   b. D
   c. B_6
   d. Niacin

LO 2 | Nutritional Guidelines

7. Which of the following foods would be considered a healthy, nutrient-dense food?
   a. Butter
   b. Peanut butter
   c. Soft drink
   d. Potato chips

8. The *2015–2020 Dietary Guidelines for Americans* recommend that you
   a. stop smoking and walk daily.
   b. listen to your gut and consume only as many vegetables as you feel like.
   c. keep sodium intake under 2,300 mg/day
   d. increase your intake of animal products.

LO 3 | How Can I Eat More Healthfully?

9. Carrie eats dairy products and eggs, but she does not eat fish, poultry, or meat. Carrie is considered a(n)
   a. vegan.
   b. lacto-ovo-vegetarian.
   c. ovo-vegetarian.
   d. pesco-vegetarian.

LO 4 | Food Safety: A Growing Concern

10. Lucas's doctor diagnoses him with celiac disease. Which of the following foods should Lucas cut out of his diet to eat gluten free?
    a. Shellfish
    b. Eggs
    c. Peanuts
    d. Wheat

Answers to the Pop Quiz can be found on page A-1. If you answered a question incorrectly, review the section tagged by the Learning Outcome. For even more study tools, visit **Mastering Health**.

THINK ABOUT IT!

LO 1 | Essential Nutrients for Health

1. Which factors influence a person's dietary patterns and behaviors? What factors have had the greatest influences on your eating behaviors?

2. What are the major types of nutrients that you need to obtain from the foods you eat? What happens if you fail to get enough of some of them? Are there significant differences between men and women in particular areas of nutrition? If so, what are they?

LO 2 | Nutritional Guidelines

3. What are the main recommendations from the *2015–2020 Dietary Guidelines for Americans*? What can you do to balance your kilocalories to maintain a healthy body weight?

4. What are the major food groups in the MyPlate plan? From which groups do you eat too few servings? What can you do to increase or decrease your intake of selected food groups?

LO 3 | How Can I Eat More Healthfully?

5. Distinguish among varieties of vegetarianism. Which types are most likely to lead to nutrient deficiencies? What can be done to ensure that even the most strict vegetarian diet provides enough of the major nutrients?

6. What are the major problems that many college students face when trying to eat the right foods? List five actions that you and your classmates could take immediately to improve your eating.

LO 4 | Food Safety: A Growing Concern

7. What are the major risks for foodborne illnesses? What can you do to protect yourself?

8. How does a food intolerance differ from a food allergy?

ACCESS YOUR HEALTH ON THE INTERNET

Visit Mastering Health for links to the websites and RSS feeds.

The following websites explore further topics and issues related to nutrition.

Academy of Nutrition and Dietetics. The academy provides information on a full range of dietary topics, including sports nutrition, healthful cooking, and nutritional eating. The site also links to scientific publications and information on scholarships and public meetings. **www.eatright.org**

U.S. Food and Drug Administration (FDA). The FDA provides information for consumers and professionals in the areas of food safety, supplements, and medical devices. There are links to other sources of information about nutrition and food. **www.fda.gov**

Food and Nutrition Information Center. This site offers a wide variety of information related to food and nutrition. **http://fnic.nal.usda.gov**

National Institutes of Health: Office of Dietary Supplements. This is the site of the International Bibliographic Database of Information on Dietary Supplements, updated quarterly. **http://dietary-supplements.info .nih.gov**

U.S. Department of Agriculture, USDA: Choose MyPlate. The USDA offers a personalized nutrition and physical activity plan based on the MyPlate program, sample menus and recipes, and a full discussion of the Dietary Guidelines for Americans. **www .choosemyplate.gov**

U.S. Department of Health and Human Services: Food Safety. This is the official gateway site to food safety information provided by the federal government, including recalls and alerts, news, and tips for reporting problems. **www .foodsafety.gov**

11 Reaching and Maintaining a Healthy Weight

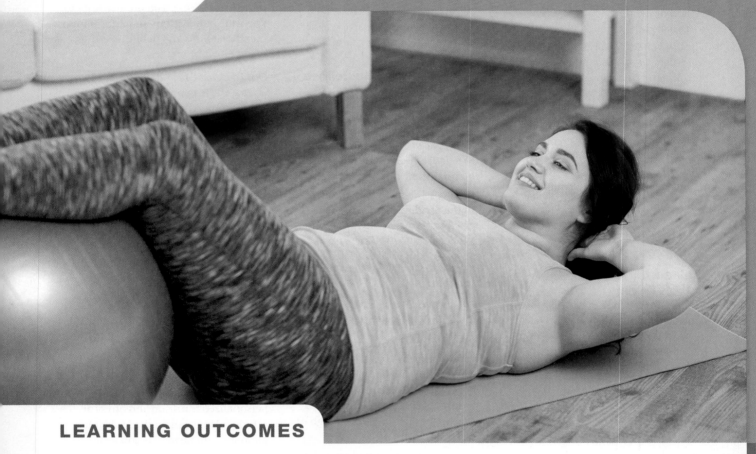

LEARNING OUTCOMES

LO **1** Describe the current epidemic of overweight and obesity in the United States and globally and the health risks associated with excess weight.

LO **2** Describe factors that put people at risk for problems with obesity, distinguishing between controllable and uncontrollable factors.

LO **3** Discuss reliable options for determining a healthy weight and body fat percentage.

LO **4** Explain the effectiveness and potential pros and cons of various weight control strategies, including exercise, diet, lifestyle modification, supplements and diet drugs, surgery, and other options.

It may be easy to grab a handful of chips or pick up a medium vanilla latte between classes, but unless you are physically active and forgo part of your calories at mealtime, those extra calories matter! Eating 500 extra calories a day—less than a latte and bagel with cream cheese—can lead to a pound of weight gain in just a week's time. A 150-pound person would need to walk for about 90 minutes at 4 mph to burn that off. If you walked more slowly, it would take even longer.

Over 30 percent of the world's population is overweight or obese. In spite of major efforts to stem the tide of "fatness," no country's obesity rates have been successfully reduced in the last 33 years. In the United States, between 1980 and 2013, obesity skyrocketed from 29 percent to 37 percent for men and from 30 percent to 38 percent for women. The obese population in the United States also accounts for the highest share of the obese population worldwide at 13 percent, followed by China and India, whose populations together make up 15 percent of the obese population of the world.[1]

Young and old, rich and poor, rural and urban, educated and uneducated, Americans share one thing in common: They are fatter than virtually all previous generations.[2] The word **obesogenic** refers to environmental conditions that promote obesity, such as the availability and marketing of unhealthy foods and social and cultural norms that lead to high calorie consumption and lack of physical activity—an apt descriptor of American society and a growing list of others.

LO 1 | OVERWEIGHT AND OBESITY: A GROWING HEALTH THREAT

Describe the current epidemic of overweight and obesity in the United States and globally and the health risks associated with excess weight.

obesogenic Environmental conditions that promote obesity, such as the availability of unhealthy foods, social and cultural norms that lead to high calorie consumption and lack of physical activity.

obesity Having a body weight more than 20 percent above healthy recommended levels; in an adult, a BMI of 30 or more.

body mass index (BMI) A number calculated from a person's weight and height that is used to assess risk for possible present or future health problems.

overweight Having a body weight more than 10 percent above healthy recommended levels; in an adult, having a BMI of 25 to 29.9.

What do we mean when we use the terms *overweight* and *obesity*? Categorized by class (reflecting both severity and increasing risks based on percent body fat), **obesity** refers to a body weight that is more than 20 percent above recommended levels for health, or a **body mass index (BMI)**—a description of body weight relative to height that we cover in more depth later—over 30. *Class 1 obesity* refers to individuals with a BMI greater than 30 but less than 35. *Class 2 obesity* includes those with a BMI of greater than 35 but less than 40, and *Class 3 obesity* includes those with a BMI greater than 40, who are often referred to as *morbidly obese*.[3] Less extreme but still damaging is **overweight**, which is body weight more than 10 percent above healthy levels or a BMI between 25 and 29.

Overweight and Obesity in the United States

FIGURE 11.1 illustrates the prevalence of obesity in Americans over age 20 years, as a percentage of the population, by age and

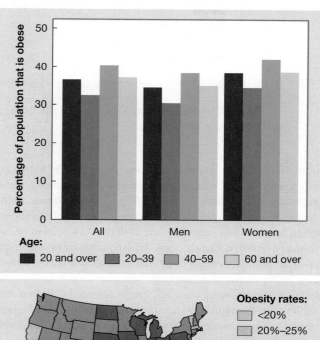

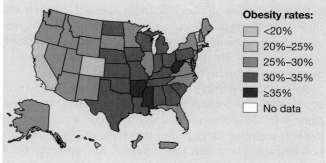

FIGURE 11.1 Obesity in the United States

Sources: Figure 11.1 Prevalence of Obesity in Adults Aged >20 Years by Age, Sex, and Age Group. Source: E. J. Benjamin et al., "Heart Disease and Stroke Statistics—2017 Update: A Report from the American Heart Association," *Circulation* 135, no. 10 (2017): e146–e603.

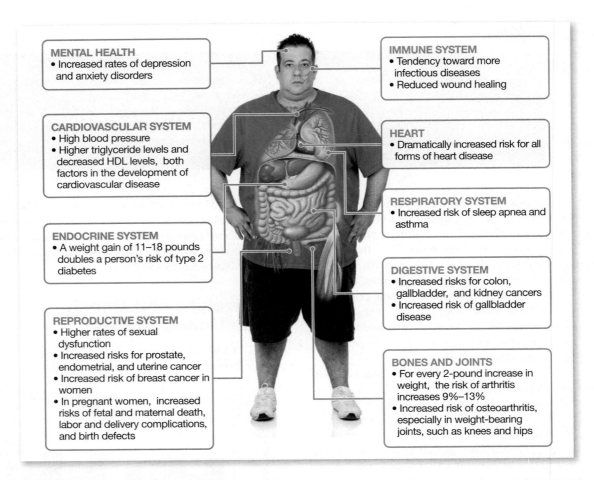

MENTAL HEALTH
• Increased rates of depression and anxiety disorders

IMMUNE SYSTEM
• Tendency toward more infectious diseases
• Reduced wound healing

CARDIOVASCULAR SYSTEM
• High blood pressure
• Higher triglyceride levels and decreased HDL levels, both factors in the development of cardiovascular disease

HEART
• Dramatically increased risk for all forms of heart disease

ENDOCRINE SYSTEM
• A weight gain of 11–18 pounds doubles a person's risk of type 2 diabetes

RESPIRATORY SYSTEM
• Increased risk of sleep apnea and asthma

DIGESTIVE SYSTEM
• Increased risks for colon, gallbladder, and kidney cancers
• Increased risk of gallbladder disease

REPRODUCTIVE SYSTEM
• Higher rates of sexual dysfunction
• Increased risks for prostate, endometrial, and uterine cancer
• Increased risk of breast cancer in women
• In pregnant women, increased risks of fetal and maternal death, labor and delivery complications, and birth defects

BONES AND JOINTS
• For every 2-pound increase in weight, the risk of arthritis increases 9%–13%
• Increased risk of osteoarthritis, especially in weight-bearing joints, such as knees and hips

FIGURE 11.2 Potential Negative Health Effects of Overweight and Obesity

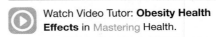 Watch Video Tutor: **Obesity Health Effects** in Mastering Health.

state. Indeed, the prevalence of obesity has steadily increased in recent decades, with disproportionate risks among some populations.[4] Children age 2 to 5 years have shown slight decreases or appear to have stabilized in prevalence in recent years; however, rates remain high, with over 9.4 percent of our youngest children already obese. Obesity rates are up in almost all other groups. Nearly 17.5 percent of children age 6–11 years and 20.6 percent of adolescents aged 12–19 years are obese today, with increasing rates of extreme obesity.[5] Children and adolescents living in low-income, low-education, and higher-unemployment homes are at significantly greater risk of developing obesity, while those from higher-income homes with more educated parents have decreasing risk.[6]

Research also points to higher rates of overweight and obesity among some adult populations in the United States. Hispanic men (79.6 percent) and non-Hispanic white men (73 percent) are more likely to be overweight or obese than are non-Hispanic black men (69 percent).[7] Non-Hispanic black women (82.2 percent) and Hispanic women (77.1 percent) are more likely to be overweight or obese than are non-Hispanic white women (63.7 percent).[8] In sharp contrast, 46.6 percent of Asian men and 34.6 percent of Asian women in the United States are overweight or obese.[9]

globesity Global rates of obesity.

An Obesogenic World

The United States is not alone in the obesity epidemic. In fact, obesity has more than doubled globally since 1980, with over 1.9 billion overweight adults and 600 million obese adults.[10] Obesity was once predominantly a problem in high-income countries, but today increasing numbers of low- and middle-income countries have overweight and obesity problems.[11] The global epidemic of high rates of overweight and obesity in multiple regions of the world has come to be known as **globesity**. Increases in sedentary occupations, mass marketing of high-fat, high-carbohydrate foods, and an increase in the food energy supply to the world's population through international distribution has contributed to the rise in obesity.[12]

Health Risks of Excess Weight

Although smoking is still the leading cause of preventable death in the United States, obesity is rapidly gaining ground. Obesity is linked to cardiovascular disease (CVD), stroke, cancer, hypertension, diabetes, depression, digestive problems, gallstones, sleep apnea, osteoarthritis, decreased mobility, restrictions on activities of daily living, and loss of independence.[13] FIGURE 11.2 summarizes these and other potential health consequences of obesity.

Consider the following facts about specific risks for obese individuals compared to their nonobese counterparts:[14]

- They have a 104 percent increase in risk of heart failure.
- BMI greater than 30 reduces their life expectancy by 2 to 4 years.
- BMI greater than 40 costs 8 to 10 years of life expectancy—similar to what happens to a long-term smoker.
- Nearly 55 percent of obese children are still obese in adolescence, and 80 percent of obese adolescents will be obese adults; 70 percent of those will continue to be obese after age 30.[15]

Diabetes, which is strongly associated with overweight and obesity, is another major concern. Over 29 million Americans have diabetes, and an estimated 25 percent of them don't know it. Another 86 million adults have prediabetes, and one-third of them don't know it.[16] **Focus On: Minimizing Your Risk for Diabetes** discusses the devastating effects of obesity on diabetes-related risks and the benefits of prevention. (See the Money & Health box for information on the costs of obesity.)

CVD, cancers, and other chronic diseases are not the only risks associated with overweight and obesity. Others are pregnancy complications, inflammation, asthma, elevated blood lipids, musculoskeletal issues, increased risks of falls and disability, fatty liver and gall bladder problems, polycystic ovary syndrome, depression, reproductive health problems, and sexual dysfunction.[17] The costs of social isolation, bullying in school, stigmatization, discrimination, and diminished quality of life due to overweight and obesity can also be devastating.

LO 2 | FACTORS CONTRIBUTING TO OVERWEIGHT AND OBESITY

Describe factors that put people at risk for problems with obesity, distinguishing between controllable and uncontrollable factors.

The reasons for our soaring rates of overweight and obesity are not as simple as "calories in and calories burned" formulas, even though these are factors. Other factors, including genetics and physiology, social influences, sleep, and potential pathogens, are also important. Newer thinking about reducing obesity risk involves a more ecological approach that seeks to change obesogenic environmental and contextual factors. Learned behaviors in the home; influences at school and in social environments; media influences; and the environments where we live, work, and play are important to our weight profiles.[18]

satiety The feeling of fullness or satisfaction at the end of a meal.

Physiological, Genetic, and Hormonal Factors

Are some people born to be fat? Obese people may be more likely than thin people to satisfy their appetite and eat for reasons other than nutrition. In fact, obesity appears to involve complex genetic, hormonal, physiological, and environmental interactions.[19]

FTO, Ghrelin, and Leptin: Genes and Hormones at Work? New research suggests that there is a genetic basis for our appetite and that some people inherit a lower sensitivity to **satiety**, or feeling full.[20] These people may be more prone to grazing and food cravings than others. One gene in particular, the *fat mass and obesity-associated (FTO)* gene, may be among the most important.[21] Much research has centered on the role of genes such as FTO on regulating *ghrelin*, a hormone that has been shown to play a key role in metabolism, specifically in determining appetite and food intake control (particularly in controlling satiety), gastrointestinal motility, gastric acid secretion, endocrine and exocrine pancreatic secretions, glucose and lipid metabolism, and cardiovascular and immunological processes.[22]

Another hormone that has gained increased attention and research is *leptin*, an appetite regulator produced by fat cells in mammals. As fat tissue increases, levels of leptin in the blood increase, and when levels of leptin in the blood rise, appetite drops. Scientists believe leptin serves as a form of *adipostat* that signals that you are getting full, slows food intake, and promotes energy. When leptin levels are low, researchers believe

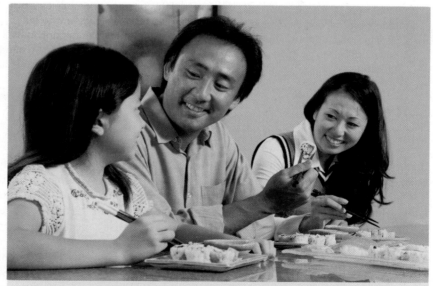

Many factors help to determine weight and body type, including heredity and genetic makeup, environment, and learned eating patterns, which are often connected to family habits.

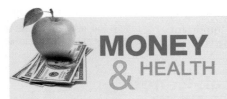

MONEY & HEALTH | THE ECONOMIC COSTS OF OBESITY

Scientific literature points to evidence that as BMI increases, health care consumption and associated costs also increase. Consider the following:

- At current rates, almost half of the world's adult population could be overweight or obese by 2030, imposing tremendous personal, social, and economic costs on society.

- Obesity is responsible for nearly 5 percent of all deaths each year globally. Its economic impact hits international gross domestic product hard, costing nearly $2.0 trillion—right up there with smoking ($2.1 trillion), and alcoholism ($1.4 trillion).

- Obese populations have a 42 percent higher annual health care cost than healthy-weight populations. Severely obese or morbidly obese adults have 81 percent higher health care costs per capita than healthy adults. Lifetime medical costs for major diseases increase by over 50 percent for obese individuals—twice that amount for severely obese. Longer hospital stays, recovery, and increased medications are all part of these costs.

- Obese populations incur 37 percent higher prescription drug costs than healthy-weight populations and are twice as likely to be taking multiple prescriptions.

- Obese individuals miss nearly 2 days of work more than their healthy-weight counterparts, accounting for between 6.5 and 12.6 percent of total absenteeism costs each year.

- Costs of an ER visit for chest paints is 41 percent higher for a severely obese individual than a healthy adult; they're 28 percent higher for an obese individual and 22 percent higher for an overweight individual. The increased numbers of tests run, greater likelihood of admittance to the hospital, and increased monitoring and drugs, often for comorbid conditions (e.g., diabetes, hypertension), increase costs. The greater the level of obesity, the greater the likelihood of multiple visits in a given year.

- Obesity may mean increased transportation costs for more fuel consumption and larger vehicles or seats, bigger ambulances, and other issues.

- A recent study of 150,000 Swedish brothers indicated that being obese is as costly as not having an undergraduate degree; an "obesity penalty" is equivalent to earning over 16 percent less than their normal-weight counterparts.

Many insurance companies are charging more for people who are overweight and refuse to participate in available wellness programs or restricting coverage to those who are likely to

be at greatest risk. Some workplaces offer counseling and free gym memberships for employees who are struggling with their weight. Are these increased charges and benefits fair? Many people argue that such penalties unfairly reflect a form of obesity stigma and size discrimination; others argue that people who are within a normal weight range shouldn't have to subsidize excess costs. Still others argue that this is a slippery slope on the way to paying more for factors such as eating high-fat foods and having high cholesterol, having too many beers in a week, or even unintended pregnancy. What do you think?

Currently, there is much debate about these extra costs, even as many insurers and businesses grapple with ways to motivate employees to increase their activity and improve their diets.

Sources: Robert Wood Johnson Foundation. "The Healthcare Costs of Obesity," 2016, stateofobesity.org/healthcare-costs-obesity; A. Dee et al., "The Direct and Indirect Costs of Both Overweight and Obesity: A Systematic Review," *BMC Research Notes* 7, no. 1 (2014): 242; T. C. Roberts et al., "Patchy Progress on Obesity Prevention: Emerging Examples, Entrenched Barriers and New Thinking," *Lancet* 385, no. 9985 (2015): 2400–09; McKinsey & Company, "How the World Could Better Fight Obesity," November 2014, www.mckinsey.com/insights/economic_studies/how_the_world_could_better_fight_obesity.

that people will be more prone to overeating and weight gain. More research on leptin's role is necessary.

Obese people seem to have excess ghrelin production and faulty leptin receptors, although the exact reasons why these hormones function improperly is not clear. It may be that environmental and psychological cues are stronger than biological signals in some individuals.[23] Specifically, people with certain genetic variations may tend to graze for food more often, eat more meals, consume more calories every day, and display patterns of seeking out high-fat food groups. Also, different genes may influence weight gain at certain periods of

life, particularly during adolescence and young adulthood.[24] Rather than acting individually, the effects of the genes may be in clusters, influencing the regulation of food intake through action in the central nervous system, as well as influencing fat cell synthesis and functioning.

So if your genes play a key role in obesity tendencies, are you doomed to a lifelong battle with your weight? Probably not. A healthy lifestyle may be able to override "obesity" genes. Results of a recent study of 5,079 adult twin pairs indicates that physical activity suppresses genetic variability in BMI, indicating that exercise may override genetic influences on risk of obesity.[25]

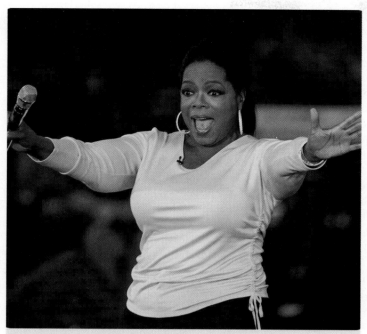

Oprah Winfrey has been candid about her struggles with yo-yo dieting. Such a pattern disrupts the body's metabolism and makes future weight loss more difficult and permanent changes even harder to maintain.

Thrifty and Spendthrift: Impact on Weight Loss

New research appears to support the theory that the ease with which one person loses weight and another hangs onto it may be influenced by individual biology. In a carefully controlled lab study, 12 obese men and women were asked to fast for one day and remain as inpatients for 6 weeks, consuming 50 percent of their normal calories each day. The individuals who lost the least during the time period were those whose metabolism slowed down significantly in response to caloric restriction.[26] New research that focused on the epidemic of obesity in Samoan populations supports this theory.[27]

Individuals in these studies have what researchers refer to as *thrifty metabolism*. In contrast, those with a *spendthrift metabolism* had metabolisms that kept chugging along when caloric intake decreased, losing significantly more weight than the thrifty group. Researchers are unsure whether these responses to dieting have a genetic basis or develop over time in individuals. Regardless, it appears that some obese individuals may have a harder time losing weight than others and that fasting and extreme low-calorie diets may actually slow the metabolism, making weight loss more difficult.

Metabolic Rates

Several aspects of your metabolism also help to determine whether you gain, maintain, or lose weight. Each of us has an innate energy-burning capacity called **basal metabolic rate (BMR)**, which is the minimum rate at which the body uses energy to maintain basic vital functions. A BMR for the average, healthy adult is usually between 1,200 and 1,800 calories per day. Technically, to measure BMR, a person would be awake but all major stimuli (including stressors to the sympathetic nervous system and digestion) would be at rest. Usually, the best time to measure BMR is after 8 hours of sleep and after a 12-hour fast.

A more practical way of assessing your energy expenditure levels is the **resting metabolic rate (RMR)**. Slightly higher than the BMR, the RMR includes the BMR plus any additional energy expended through daily sedentary activities such as food digestion, sitting, studying, or standing. The **exercise metabolic rate (EMR)** accounts for the remaining percentage of all daily calorie expenditures and refers to the energy expenditure that occurs during physical activity. For most of us, these calories come from light daily activities such as walking, climbing stairs, and mowing the lawn.

Your BMR and RMR fluctuate through life, and are highest during infancy, puberty, and pregnancy. Generally, the younger you are, the higher your BMR, partly because cells undergo rapid subdivision during periods of growth, consuming lots of energy. After age 30, a person's BMR slows down 1 to 2 percent a year; older people commonly find an extra helping of ice cream harder to burn off. Slower BMR, coupled with less activity, age-related muscle loss, and shifting priorities from fitness to family and career obligations contribute to the weight gain of many middle-aged people.

Anyone who has ever lost weight only to reach a point at which, try as they might, they can't lose another ounce may be a victim of **adaptive thermogenesis**, whereby the body slows metabolic activity and energy expenditure as a form of defensive protection against possible starvation. With increased weight loss may come increased hunger sensations, slowed energy expenditure, and a tendency to regain weight or make further weight loss more difficult.

In a recent study of *The Biggest Loser* participants, some who engaged in the program of restricted diet and intense exercise showed significant short-term weight loss during the program but had difficulties in maintaining their weight loss months and years after the intervention.[28] In addition, participants experienced significant reduction in their RMR at the conclusion of the intervention. Surprisingly, those with initial lowered RMR maintained their lowered RMR months and even years after the intervention. These individuals experienced challenges keeping their weight off and/or losing more weight. Individuals who undergo rapid and highly restricted regimens for weight loss may find it harder to lose subsequent weight and maintain losses in the future. Without sufficient support, they may actually regain weight.[29]

In **yo-yo dieting**, the person cycles between periods of

basal metabolic rate (BMR) The rate of energy expenditure by a body at complete rest in a neutral environment.

resting metabolic rate (RMR) The energy expenditure of the body under BMR conditions plus other daily sedentary activities.

exercise metabolic rate (EMR) The energy expenditure that occurs during exercise.

adaptive thermogenesis The theoretical mechanism by which the brain regulates metabolic activity according to caloric intake.

yo-yo dieting Cycles in which people diet and regain weight.

weight loss and gain. Typically, after weight loss, BMR is lower because the body has less muscle mass and weight and requires less energy for basic functioning. When dieters resume eating a normal diet after their weight loss, calories burn more slowly as a result of the BMR decrease, and the dieters regain weight. Repeated cycles of dieting and regaining weight may actually increase the likelihood of gaining weight over time. Increased age and overall loss of muscle mass through inactivity also tend to result in lowered BMR.

On the other side of the BMR equation is **set point theory**, which suggests that our bodies fight to maintain weight around a narrow range or set point. If we go on a drastic starvation diet or fast, BMR slows to conserve energy. Set point theory suggests that our own bodies may sabotage our weight-loss efforts by holding onto calories, explaining why people tend to stay near a certain weight threshold and why moving to a different level of weight loss is difficult. The good news is that set points can be changed; however, these changes may take time to be permanent.

Fat Cells and Predisposition to Fatness

Some obese people may have excessive numbers of fat cells. Where an average-weight adult has approximately 25 billion to 35 billion fat cells and a moderately obese adult 60 billion to 100 billion, an extremely obese adult has as many as 200 billion.[30] This condition, **hyperplastic obesity**, usually appears in early childhood and perhaps, as a result of the mother's dietary habits, even before birth. The most critical periods for the development of hyperplasia are the last 2 to 3 months of fetal development, the first year of life, and the period between ages 9 and 13. Central to this theory is the belief that the number of fat cells in a body does not increase appreciably during adulthood. However, the ability of each of these cells to swell (**hypertrophy**) and shrink does carry over into adulthood. People with large numbers of fat cells may be able to lose weight by decreasing the size of each cell in adulthood, but with the next calorie binge, the cells swell and sabotage weight-loss efforts. Weight gain may be tied to both the number of fat cells in the body and the capacity of individual cells to enlarge.

Environmental Factors

Environmental factors have come to play a large role in weight maintenance. Automobiles, remote controls, desk jobs, and sedentary habits contribute to decreased physical activity and energy expenditure. Coupled with our culture of eating more, it's a recipe for weight gain.

Greater Access to High-Calorie Foods

More foods that are high in calories and low in nutrients exist today than in the past. There are many environmental factors that can prompt us to consume them:

- Because of constant advertising, we are bombarded with messages to eat, eat, eat, and flavor often trumps nutrition.
- Super-sized portions are now the norm (see the Student Health Today box), leading to increased calorie and fat intake.
- Widespread availability of high-calorie coffee and sugary drinks lure people in for a form of break or reward between meals, which really add up in calories over time.
- Misleading food labels confuse consumers about serving sizes.

OVER 34%

of children and adolescents in the United States get a significant portion of their nutrition from high-fat, high-carbohydrate, PROCESSED FAST FOOD each day.

Although Americans still consume about 500 calories per day more today than we did in 1970, daily consumption of some healthy foods has increased, with noteworthy declines in others. In 2014, each American had access to an average of 57 more pounds of commercially grown vegetables than they did in 1970 (385 in 2014); a full 17 more pounds of fruit (238 in 2014) 11 more pounds of meat, fish, eggs and nuts (312 in 2014), 12 more pounds of sugar and sweeteners, and 30 more pounds of fats and oils (90 in 2014).[31] If we are consuming healthier foods in some groups, why aren't we seeing major changes in obesity rates? One possibility is that we are exercising less than ever.

Lack of Physical Activity

Although heredity, metabolism, and environment all have an impact on weight management, the way we live our lives is also responsible. In general, Americans are eating more and moving less than ever before, becoming overweight as a result.

According to data from the 2016 *National Health Interview Survey*, just over 52.8 percent of adults age 18 and over in the United States met the guidelines for aerobic activity through involvement in leisure-time activity.[32] Just over 22 percent met the minimum guidelines for both aerobic exercise and muscle strengthening.[33]

set point theory The theory that a form of internal thermostat controls our weight and fights to maintain this weight around a narrowly set range.

hyperplastic obesity A condition characterized by an excessive number of fat cells.

hypertrophy The act of swelling or increasing in size, as with cells.

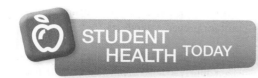
BEWARE OF PORTION INFLATION AT RESTAURANTS

From burgers and fries to meat-and-potato or pasta meals, today's popular restaurant foods dwarf their earlier counterparts. For example, a 25-ounce prime rib dinner served at one local steak chain contains nearly 3,000 calories and 150 grams of fat. That's 1.5 times the calories and two to three times the fat that most adults need in a whole day!

Many researchers believe that the main reason Americans are gaining weight is that people no longer recognize a normal serving size. The National Heart, Lung, and Blood Institute has developed a pair of "Portion Distortion" quizzes that show how today's portions compare with those of 20 years ago. Test your knowledge of portion size online at www.nhlbi.nih .gov/health/educational/wecan/eat-right/ portion-distortion.htm.

To make sure you're not overeating when you dine out, follow these strategies:

- Order the smallest size available. Focus on taste and quality rather than quantity. When you eat huge amounts at the all-you-can-eat buffet, focus on how you feel. Get used to eating less, eating slowly, and enjoying what you eat.

20 years ago	Today
333 kcal	590 kcal
210 kcal	610 kcal

Today's bloated portions.

Source: Data are from National Heart, Lung, and Blood Institute, "Portion Distortion," March 2017, www.nhlbi.nih.gov/health/educational/wecan/eat-right/portion-distortion.htm.

- Take your time, and let your fullness indicator have a chance to kick in while there is still time to stop eating before you go too far. Chew more, talk more, and set your fork down more often between bites.

- Order condiments and dressings on the side, and don't use the entire container. Lightly dip your food in dressings or gravies rather than pouring on extra calories.
- Order a healthy, protein-rich appetizer as your main meal and a small salad or vegetable. Happy hour menus often offer great smaller choices.
- Split an entrée with a friend, and order a side salad for each of you. Alternatively, put half of your meal in a takeout box immediately, and finish the rest at the restaurant.
- Avoid buffets and all-you-can-eat establishments. If you go to them, use small plates and fill them with salads, vegetables, and high-protein, low-calorie, low-fat options. Pay careful attention to newly required menu labeling for fast-food restaurants. These can be helpful in making sure you choose the best alternative for healthy dining.

Source: Data are from National Heart, Lung, and Blood Institute, "Portion Distortion," Accessed April 1, 2015, www.nhlbi.nih.gov/health/educational/wecan/eat-right/portion-distortion.htm.

Psychosocial and Socioeconomic Factors

The relationship between weight problems and emotional insecurities, needs, and wants remains difficult to assess. What we do know is that eating tends to be a focal point of people's lives and is in part a social ritual associated with companionship, celebration, and enjoyment. *Comfort food* is used to help us feel good when other things in life are not going well. Our friends and loved ones are often key influences in our eating behaviors. In fact, according to recent research, young adults who are overweight and obese tend to befriend and date overweight and obese people in much the same way that smokers or exercisers tend to hang out with other smokers or exercisers. Gaining or losing weight may be affected by other people's support for weight loss or social undermining of weight-loss attempts ("Let's order pizza!").[34] According to nutrition and weight control expert Walter Willett, external factors may have an equal or greater impact on our obesity epidemic than individual factors.[35] Family, friends, work, and environment provide the social settings and influences to create an "eating"

culture that even the most motivated find difficult to overcome. According to Willett, it's no accident that your chances of becoming obese increase by 57 percent if a close friend is obese, by 40 percent if a sibling is obese, and by 37 percent if your partner or spouse is obese.[36]

Socioeconomic status can have a significant effect on obesity risk. People in poverty may have less access to fresh, nutrient-dense foods and opt for less expensive, high-calorie processed food. People who work multiple jobs, work odd hours, and have long commutes may not have the time or energy to cook nutritious food. Gyms may be too expensive or inconveniently located. Lack of lighting, sidewalks, trails and other places to walk or bike can make it unsafe and difficult to exercise.[37]

Emerging Theories on Obesity Risks

There is much emerging research on factors that may increase your obesity risk. The results may offer opportunities for prevention and control.

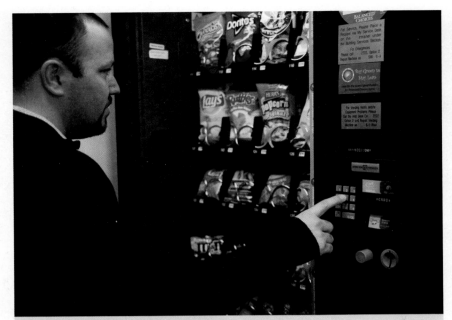

The easy availability of high-calorie foods, such as those found in most vending machines, is one of the environmental factors contributing to the obesity problem in the United States today

mechanisms for each type of drug is important for prevention efforts.[40]

Sleep Deprivation People who are sleep deprived tend to have significant drops in leptin, which plays a role in metabolism, insulin sensitivity, and other weight-related changes as well as disruptions in circadian rhythms which may increase obesity risks.[41] (See Chapter 4 for leptin's role in sleep.)

LO 3 | ASSESSING BODY WEIGHT AND BODY COMPOSITION

Discuss reliable options for determining a healthy weight and body fat percentage.

Everyone has his or her own ideal weight, based on individual variables such as body structure, height, and fat distribution. Traditionally, experts used measurement techniques such as height–weight charts to determine whether an individual was an ideal weight, overweight, or obese. These charts can be misleading because they don't take body composition—a person's ratio of fat to lean muscle—or fat distribution into account. More accurate measures of evaluating healthy weight and disease risk focus on a person's percentage of body fat and how that fat is distributed in his or her body.

It's important to remember that body fat isn't all bad. In fact, some fat is essential for healthy body functioning. Fat regulates body temperature, cushions and insulates organs and tissues, and is the body's main source of stored energy. Body fat is composed of two types: essential fat and storage fat. *Essential fat* is the fat necessary for maintenance of life and reproductive functions. *Storage fat*, the nonessential fat that many of us try to shed, makes up the remainder of our fat reserves.

Being **underweight**, or having extremely low body fat, can cause a host of problems, including hair loss, visual disturbances, skin problems, a tendency to fracture bones easily, digestive system disturbances, heart irregularities, gastrointestinal problems, difficulties in maintaining body temperature, and loss of menstrual period in women.

Pathogens and Environmental Toxins

Several researchers have studied the role of viruses and other pathogens in a form of *infectobesity*. Most of this research focuses on the effect of viruses and bacteria in altering intestinal flora, metabolism, and insulin sensitivity. Obese and nonobese individuals have different intestinal flora, and research is examining possible mechanisms for increased risk.[38]

Researchers are also examining how over three dozen chemicals may alter bacteria in the gastrointestinal tract and predispose people to obesity. Paints, pesticides, floor coverings, and other chemical-containing products are among possible culprits in increased obesity risk.[39]

Drugs

Several studies have examined the role of prescription drugs such as antidepressants, allergy medications, antibiotics, heart and high blood pressure pills, diabetes drugs, and cancer meds in increased weight gain and weight fluctuation. Finding the underlying

underweight Having a body weight more than 10 percent below healthy recommended levels; in an adult, having a BMI below 18.5.

69%
of U.S. adults are **OVERWEIGHT OR OBESE**. Nearly 37% of adults overall—36.3% of those aged 20 and over, 32.3% of those 20–39, 40.4% of those 40–59 and 37% of those 60 plus—are obese.

Body Mass Index (BMI)

As was mentioned earlier, BMI is a description of body weight relative to height—numbers that are highly correlated with your total body fat. Find your BMI in inches and pounds in **FIGURE 11.3**, or calculate your BMI by dividing your weight in kilograms by height in meters squared. The mathematical formula is

$$BMI = weight\ (kg)/height\ squared\ (m^2)$$

A BMI calculator is also available from the National Heart, Lung, and Blood Institute at www.nhlbi.nih.gov/guidelines/obesity/BMI/bmicalc.htm.

Desirable BMI levels may vary with age and by sex; however, most BMI tables for adults do not account for such variables. **Healthy weight** is defined as having a BMI of 18.5 to 24.9, the range of lowest statistical health risk.[42] A BMI of 25 to 29.9 indicates overweight and potentially significant health risks.[43] A BMI of 30 to 39.9 is classified as obese.[44] A BMI of 40 to 49.9 is **morbidly obese**, and a new category of BMI of 50 or higher—one increasing in numbers—has been labeled as **super obese**.[45] Nearly 5 percent of obese men and almost 10 percent of obese women are morbidly obese (see **TABLE 11.1**).[46]

Limitations of BMI Like other assessments of fatness, the BMI has its limitations. Water, muscle, and bone mass are not included in BMI calculations, and BMI levels don't account for the fact that muscle weighs more than fat. BMI levels can be inaccurate for people who are under 5 feet tall, are highly muscled, or are older and have little muscle mass. Although a combination of measures might be most reliable in assessing fat levels, BMI continues to be a quick, inexpensive, and useful tool for developing basic health recommendations.[47]

Height (feet and inches)	100		120		140		160		180		200		220		240		260
4'6"	24	27	29	31	34	36	39	41	43	46	48	51	53	55	58	60	63
4'8"	22	25	27	29	31	34	36	38	40	43	45	47	49	52	54	56	58
4'10"	21	23	25	27	29	31	33	36	38	40	42	44	46	48	50	52	54
5'0"	20	22	23	25	27	29	31	33	35	37	39	41	43	45	47	49	51
5'2"	18	20	22	24	26	27	29	31	33	35	37	38	40	42	44	46	48
5'4"	17	19	21	22	24	26	28	29	31	33	34	36	38	40	41	43	45
5'6"	16	18	19	21	23	24	26	27	29	31	32	34	36	37	39	40	42
5'8"	15	17	18	20	21	23	24	26	27	29	30	32	33	35	37	38	40
5'10"	14	16	17	19	20	22	23	24	26	27	29	30	32	33	34	36	37
6'0"	14	15	16	18	19	20	22	23	24	26	27	29	30	31	33	34	35
6'2"	13	14	15	17	18	19	21	22	23	24	26	27	28	30	31	32	33
6'4"	12	13	15	16	17	18	20	21	22	23	24	26	27	28	29	30	32
6'6"	12	13	14	15	16	17	19	20	21	22	23	24	25	27	28	29	30
6'8"	11	12	13	14	15	17	18	19	20	21	22	23	24	25	26	28	29
6'10"	11	12	13	14	15	16	17	18	19	20	21	22	23	24	25	26	27
7'0"	10	11	12	13	14	15	16	17	18	19	20	21	22	23	24	25	26

Weight (pounds)

Key:
Underweight
Normal weight
Overweight
Obese

FIGURE 11.3 Body Mass Index (BMI)

healthy weight A BMI of 18.5 to 24.9, the range of lowest statistical health risk.

morbidly obese Having a body weight 100 percent or more above healthy recommended levels; in an adult, having a BMI of 40 or more.

super obese Having a body weight higher than morbid obesity; in an adult, having a BMI of 50 or more.

Youth and BMI Today, over 30 percent of youth in America are obese, three times higher than rates in the 1980s.[48] Although the labels *obese* and *morbidly obese* have been used for years for adults, there is growing concern that such labels increase bias and obesity stigma against youth. According to a recent study, when subjected to bias and discrimination, the person who is the recipient of stigma is actually likely to eat more rather than less.[49] BMI ranges above a normal weight for children and teens are often labeled differently—as "at risk of overweight" and "overweight"—to avoid the sense of shame such words may cause. In addition, BMI ranges for children and teens take into account normal differences in body fat between

TABLE 11.1 | Weight Classifications Based on BMI, Waist Circumference, and Associated Risks

			Disease Risk* Relative to Normal Weight and Waist Circumference	
	BMI (kg/m^2)	Obesity Class	Men 102 cm (40 in.) or Less Women 88 cm (35 in.) or Less+	Men > 102 cm cm (40 in.) Women > 88 cm cm (35 in.)
Underweight	< 18.5		–	–
Normal	18.5–24.9		–	–
Overweight	25.0–29.9		Increased	High
Obesity	30.0–34.9	I	High	Very high
	35.0–39.9	II	Very high	Very high
Extreme/Morbid Obesity	40.0+	III	Extremely high	Extremely high

* Disease risk for type 2 diabetes, hypertension, and CVD.
+ Increased waist circumference also can be a marker for increased risk, even in people of normal weight.

Source: National Heart, Lung and Blood Institute, "Classification of Overweight and Obesity by BMI, Waist Circumference, and Associated Disease Risks," Accessed March 2017, https://www.nhlbi.nih.gov/health/educational/lose_wt/BMI/bmi_dis.htm.

boys and girls and the differences in body fat that occur at various ages. Specific guidelines for calculating youth BMI are available at the Centers for Disease Control and Prevention website (www.cdc.gov).

Waist Circumference and Ratio Measurements

Knowing where your fat is carried may be more important than knowing how much you carry. Men and postmenopausal women tend to store fat in the upper regions of the body, particularly in the abdominal area. Premenopausal women usually store fat in the lower regions of their bodies, particularly the hips, buttocks, and thighs. Waist circumference measurements, including *waist circumference* only, the *waist circumference-to-hip ratio*, and the *waist circumference-to-height ratio*, have all been used to measure abdominal fat as an indicator of obesity and health risk. Where you carry the weight may be of particular importance in determining whether you develop diabetes, cardiovascular disease, hypertension, or stroke.[50]

A waistline greater than 40 inches (102 centimeters) in men and greater than 35 inches (88 centimeters) in women may be particularly indicative of greater health risk.[51] If a person is less than 5 feet tall or has a BMI of 35 or above, waist circumference standards used for the general population might not apply.

The waist circumference-to-hip ratio measures regional fat distribution. The higher your waist-to-hip ratio is, the greater your chance of having increased health risks.[52] Newer research has pointed to waist-to-hip ratio being more effective than waist circumference alone or BMI use in measuring body fat in children and adolescents.[53] A waist circumference-to-height ratio is a simple screening tool that says that your waist should be approximately half of your height; if you were 70 inches tall, your waist shouldn't be more than 35 inches.

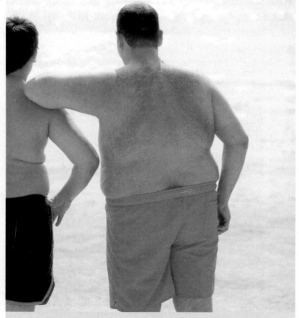

Abdominal obesity puts individuals at increased risk of CVD, stroke, and diabetes, particularly among men.

Measures of Body Fat

There are numerous ways to assess whether your body fat levels are too high. One low-tech way is simply to look in the mirror or consider how your clothes fit now in comparison with how they fit last year. For those who wish to take a more precise measurement of their percentage of body fat, more accurate techniques are available, several of which are described and depicted in **FIGURE 11.4**. These methods usually involve the help of a skilled professional and typically must be done in a

Underwater (hydrostatic) weighing: Measures the amount of water a person displaces when completely submerged. Fat tissue is less dense than muscle or bone, so body fat can be computed within a 2%–3% margin of error by comparing weight underwater and out of water.

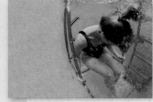

Skinfolds: Involves "pinching" a person's fold of skin (with its underlying layer of fat) at various locations of the body. The fold is measured using a specially designed caliper. When performed by a skilled technician, it can estimate body fat with an error of 3%–4%.

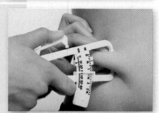

Bioelectrical impedance analysis (BIA): Involves sending a very low level of electrical current through a person's body. As lean body mass is made up of mostly water, the rate at which the electricity is conducted gives an indication of a person's lean body mass and body fat. Under the best circumstances, BIA can estimate body fat with an error of 3%–4%.

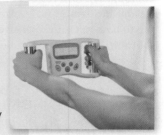

Dual-energy X-ray absorptiometry (DXA): The technology is based on using very-low-level X ray to differentiate between bone tissue, soft (or lean) tissue, and fat (or adipose) tissue. The margin of error for predicting body fat is 2%–4%.

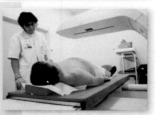

Bod Pod: Uses air displacement to measure body composition. This machine is a large, egg-shaped chamber made from fiberglass. The person being measured sits in the machine wearing a swimsuit. The door is closed and the machine measures how much air is displaced. That value is used to calculate body fat, with a 2%–3% margin of error.

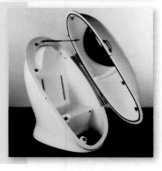

FIGURE 11.4 Overview of Various Body Composition Assessment Methods

Source: Adapted from J. Thompson and M. Manore, *Nutrition: An Applied Approach*, 4th edition, © 2015. Printed and electronically reproduced by permission of Pearson Education, Inc., Upper Saddle River, New Jersey.

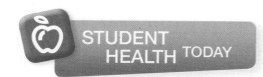
WHO WINS IN LOSING?
Characteristics of Successful Losers

Millions of Americans start their New Year with the most popular resolution: to lose weight and keep it off. Even so, the majority who lose some weight ultimately regain it. But what about those few who manage to keep the weight off?

In general, the literature indicates success rates between 2 and 15 percent, using a variety of weight and BMI parameters, as well as timelines for defining success. According to recent studies, characteristics of those likely to be successful include the following:

- The people who have strong initial weight loss in the first month are most likely to be successful at one year; hence, having supports for change and having incentives to keep going are critical to early and sustained success.
- Those who attend group sessions for support in those first months are more likely to be successful.
- High self-esteem and self-efficacy (success breeds success) are important.
- A strong locus of control—being motivated by internal rather than external factors—increases the chance of success.
- Knowing the health risks of obesity and the health benefits of good nutrition is helpful
- Knowing how to access and utilize community resources is important.
- People who journal and track calories, nutrients, and/or portion sizes, and monitor weight regularly are more likely

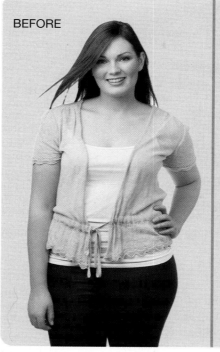

BEFORE   AFTER

to be successful. Using electronic tracking/monitoring devices shows great promise in motivating change.
- Making a commitment to follow a healthy, realistic eating and exercise pattern is crucial.
- Staying positive, practicing self-compassion, and avoiding becoming discouraged by setbacks are ways to improve the likelihood of success.
- Using weight-loss programs that include exercise increases the chances of success.

Sources: CDC, "Keeping It Off," May 15, 2015, www.cdc.gov/healthyweight/losing_weight/keepingitoff.html; C. Pellegrini et al., "Smartphone Applications to Support Weight Loss: A Current Perspective," *Journal of Medical Internet Research* 1 (2015): 13–22; S. Guendelman, M. Rittermann Weintraub, and M. Kaufer-Horwitz, "Weight Loss Success among Overweight and Obese Women of Mexican-Origin Living in Mexico and the United States: A Comparison of Two National Surveys," *Journal of Immigrant and Minority Health* (2016): 1–9; M. Ortner Hadziabdic et al., "Factors Predictive of Drop-out and Weight Loss Success in Weight Management for Obese Patients," *Journal of Human Nutrition and Dietetics* 28, no. 2 (2015): 24–32; J. M. Laitner et al., "The Role of Self-monitoring in the Maintenance of Weight Loss Success," *Eating Behaviors* 21 (2016):193–197.

lab or clinical setting. Before undergoing any procedure, make sure you understand the expense, potential for accuracy, risks, and training of the tester. Also, consider why you are seeking this assessment and what you plan to do with the results.

LO 4 | MANAGING YOUR WEIGHT: INDIVIDUAL ROLES

Explain the effectiveness and potential pros and cons of various weight control strategies, including exercise, diet, lifestyle modification, supplements and diet drugs, surgery, and other options.

At some point, almost all of us will decide to lose weight. Many will have mixed success. Failure is often related to thinking about losing weight in terms of short-term "dieting" rather than

adjusting long-term behaviors. Drugs and intensive counseling can contribute to positive weight loss, but even then, many people regain weight after treatment. Maintaining a healthful body takes constant attention and nurturing. The Student Health Today box looks at characteristics of successful weight losers.

Understanding Calories and Energy Balance

A *calorie* is a unit of measure that indicates the amount of energy gained from food or expended through activity. Each time you consume 3,500 calories more than your body needs to maintain weight, you gain a pound of storage fat. Conversely, each time your body expends an extra 3,500 calories, you lose a pound of fat. If you

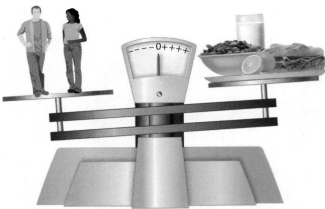

Energy expenditure = Energy intake

FIGURE 11.5 The Concept of Energy Balance If you consume more calories than you burn, you gain weight. If you burn more calories than you consume, you lose weight. If your consumption and burning of calories are equal, your weight will not change.

consume 140 calories (the amount in one can of regular soda) more than you need every single day and make no other changes in diet or activity, you would gain 1 pound in 25 days (3,500 calories ÷ 140 calories per day = 25 days). Conversely, if you walk for 30 minutes each day at a pace of 15 minutes per mile (172 calories burned) in addition to your regular activities, you would lose 1 pound in 20 days (3,500 calories ÷ 172 calories per day = 20.3 days). **FIGURE 11.5** illustrates the concept of energy balance.

Diet and Eating Behaviors

Successful weight loss requires shifting your energy balance. The first part of the equation is to reduce calorie intake through modifying eating behaviors using a variety of strategies.

Being Mindful of Your Eating Triggers

When you sit down to eat, is your mind actually "out to lunch"? If you are like the 66 percent of American adults who eat in front of the TV or computer, it should be no surprise that you are eating faster and eating more, with more awareness of the TV than of your food.[54] *Mindless eating*, or putting food in your mouth that you don't really taste or notice while consuming more than you should, may be a key contributor to excess calorie consumption and weight gain. When we eat mindlessly, we may miss feelings of satiety and ignore tendencies we might have to use restraint in shoving potato chips into our mouths.

▶ **SEE IT! VIDEOS**

Do you snack like crazy when you're watching an exciting movie? Watch **Fast-Paced Movies, Television Shows May Lead to More Snacking** in the Study Area of Mastering Health.

Eating mindfully means eating with awareness—awareness of *why* we are eating (was it a trigger, or are we really hungry?), *what* we are eating (should we really be eating this?), and *how much* we are eating (stop! put it down!).

Before you can change an unhealthy eating habit, you must first determine what triggers you to eat. Keeping a log of eating triggers—*when, what, where,* and *how much* you eat—for 2 to 3 days can help you identify what is pushing those "eat everything in sight" buttons for you.

Typically, dietary triggers center on patterns and problems in everyday living rather than real hunger pangs. Many people eat compulsively when stressed; however, for other people, the same circumstances diminish their appetite, causing them to lose weight. When your mind wanders, you may find yourself grazing in the refrigerator or pulling into a fast-food drive-through. Ask yourself: Are you really hungry, or are you eating

WHAT DO YOU THINK?

If you wanted to lose weight, what strategies would you most likely choose?

■ Which strategies, if any, have worked for you before?

■ What factors might serve to help or hinder your weight-loss efforts?

If your trigger is . . .	then →	try this strategy . . .
A stressful situation		Acknowledge and address feelings of anxiety or stress, and develop stress management techniques to practice daily.
Feeling angry or upset		Analyze your emotions and look for a noneating activity to deal with them, such as taking a quick walk or calling a friend.
A certain time of day		Change your eating schedule to avoid skipping or delaying meals and overeating later; make a plan of what you'll eat ahead of time to avoid impulse or emotional eating.
Pressure from friends and family		Have a response ready to help you refuse food you do not want, or look for healthy alternatives you can eat instead when in social settings.
Being in an environment where food is available		Avoid the environment that causes you to want to eat: Sit far away from the food at meetings, take a different route to class to avoid passing the vending machines, shop from a list and only when you aren't hungry, arrange nonfood outings with your friends.
Feeling bored and tired		Identify the times when you feel low energy and fill them with activities other than eating, such as exercise breaks; cultivate a new interest or hobby that keeps your mind and hands busy.
The sight and smell of food		Stop buying high-calorie foods that tempt you to snack, or store them in an inconvenient place, out of sight; avoid walking past or sitting or standing near the table of tempting treats at a meeting, party, or other gathering.
Eating mindlessly or inattentively		Turn off all distractions, including phones, computers, television, and radio, and eat more slowly, savoring your food and putting your fork down between bites so you can become aware of when your hunger is satisfied.
Spending time alone in the car		Get a book on tape to listen to, or tape your class notes and use the time for studying. Keep your mind off food. Don't bring money into the gas station where snacks are tempting.
Alcohol use		Drink plenty of water and stay hydrated. Seek out healthy snack choices. After a night out, brush your teeth immediately upon getting home and stay out of the kitchen.
Feeling deprived		Allow yourself to eat "indulgences" in moderation, so you won't crave them; focus on balancing your calorie input to calorie output.
Eating out of habit		Establish a new routine to circumvent the old, such as taking a new route to class so you don't feel compelled to stop at your favorite fast-food restaurant on the way.
Watching television		Look for something else to occupy your hands and body while your mind is engaged with the screen: Ride an exercise bike, do stretching exercises, doodle on a pad of paper, or learn to knit.

FIGURE 11.6 Avoid Trigger-Happy Eating

for comfort and distraction? Focus on why you have your hand on the chips. If you eat while working or watching TV, limit what you put on your plate, and put the rest away. Finally, eat slowly. Focus on what you are putting in your mouth. Taste your food and savor the flavor.

See the Skills for Behavior Change box for tips on healthy snacking, and see FIGURE 11.6 for ways to adjust your eating triggers.

Choosing a Diet Plan Once you have determined your triggers, devise a plan for improved eating by doing the following:

- Seek assistance from reputable sources such as *MyPlate* (www.choosemyplate.gov), a registered dietitian, a physician, health educators, or exercise physiologists with nutritional training.
- Be wary of nutritionists or nutritional life coaches, since there is no formal credential for those titles and their training is often limited.
- Avoid weight-loss programs that promise quick or "miracle" results or that are run by people who offer short courses on nutrition and exercise that are designed to sell products or services.

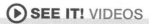

▶ **SEE IT!** VIDEOS
Could a diet high in protein and fats lead to weight loss? Watch **Low-Carb Diet Trumps Low Fat in Weight-Loss Study** in the Study Area of Mastering Health.

TABLE 11.2 | The Top Five Healthy Diets in 2017

Diet Name	Basic Principles	Good for Diabetes and Heart Health?	Weight-Loss Effectiveness	Pros, Cons, and Other Things to Consider
DASH (Dietary Approaches to Stop Hypertension)	A balanced plan developed to fight high blood pressure reduce risks of CVD and diabetes. Eat fruits, vegetables, whole grains, lean protein, and low-fat dairy. Limit sweets, saturated fats, red meat, and sodium.	Yes	Not specifically designed for weight loss but a balanced approach that does lead to loss	A balanced, safe, and healthy diet, rated the number one best diet overall by *U.S. News & World Report* in 2016 and 17. Very effective in improving cholesterol levels and other biomarkers over the long term.
TLC (Therapeutic Lifestyle Change)	Developed by NIH. Focus on CVD risk reduction with fruits and vegetables, lean protein, low fat, etc. Balanced and effective.	Yes	Weight loss likely; cholesterol is key.	Safe, balanced, and healthy diet, tied for number four overall diet with the, Mayo Clinic and Weight Watchers diet by *U.S. News & World Report* in 2017. Particularly good for heart health and cholesterol reduction.
Mediterranean	A plan that emphasizes fruits, vegetables, fish, whole grains, beans, nuts, legumes, olive oil, and herbs and spices. Poultry, eggs, cheese, yogurt, and red wine can be enjoyed in moderation. Sweets and red meat are saved for special occasions.	Yes	Very Effective, safe and easy to follow	Widely considered to be one of the most healthy, safe, and balanced diets. Weight loss may not be as dramatic, but long-term health benefits have been demonstrated. Second best rated by *U.S. News & World Report* in 2017.
Weight Watchers	New "Beyond the Scale" program, which emphasizes three components: eating healthier, fitness that fits your life, and "developing skills and supportive connections to help you stay on track." Involves tracking food, nutritional values, and exercise. In-person group meetings or online membership are options.	Yes (depending on individual choices)	Very Effective, safe	Consistently rated by experts as one of the top three or four most effective weight-loss programs. Flexible programs that don't deny foods but rather teach about healthy choices. Works for both short- and long-term weight loss. Support groups are available, but participants can meet with coaches online in the privacy of their homes. Check your campus or community for meetings, and watch for specials, as some plans involve membership fees. Rated number one weight-loss diet by *U.S. News & World Report* in 2016.
MIND Diet	Combines the best elements of the DASH and Mediterranean diets into a healthy dietary regimen.	Yes	Effective, focus on real food	Number three best overall diet rating by *U.S. News and World Report* in 2017. Noteworthy for potential to boost brain power and reduced risk of cognitive decline.
Flexitarian Diet	High scores for nutritional completeness and easy-to-follow approach for long-term success for all members of the family.	Yes	Very Effective	Ranked among the top five diets in 2017 as safe, effective, and sustainable.

Sources: Opinions on diet pros and cons are based on *U.S. News & World Report*, "Best Diets Overall," 2017, http://health.usnews.com/best-diet/best-overall-diets?int=9c2508. Dietary reviews, particularly of fad diets, are available online from registered dieticians at the Academy of Nutrition and Dietetics, 2016. See also B. Johnson et al., "Comparisons of Weight Loss among Diet Programs in Overweight and Obese Adults: A Meta-Analysis," *Journal of the American Medical Association* 312, no. 9 (2014): 923–33.

■ Assess the nutrient value of any prescribed diet, verify dietary guidelines are consistent with reliable nutrition research, and analyze the suitability of the diet to your tastes, budget, and lifestyle.

Any diet that requires radical behavior changes or sets up artificial dietary programs through prepackaged products or stringent restrictions is likely to fail. The most successful plans allow you to make food choices in real-world settings and do not ask you to sacrifice everything you enjoy. See **TABLE 11.2** for an analysis of some popular diets that are being marketed today. For information on other plans, check out the regularly updated list of reviews on the website of the Academy of Nutrition and Dietetics (formerly the American Dietetic Association) at www .eatright.org.

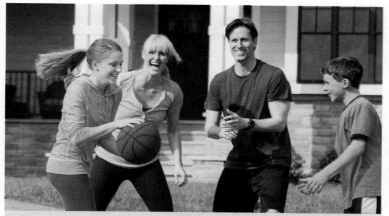

Engaging in regular physical activity at a young age and continuing through all stages of adulthood are critical to weight management and risk reduction

Including Exercise

Although a healthy diet may be the most important factor in weight loss, diet and exercise combine to help people lose weight and increase muscle mass and to maintain any weight loss they have achieved.[55] Because lean (muscle) tissue is more metabolically active than fat tissue, having more muscle mass means that you burn more calories. Exact estimates vary, but experts currently think each pound of muscle burns 2 to 50 more calories per day than each pound of fat tissue. Thus, the base level of calories needed to maintain a healthy weight varies greatly from person to person.

The number of calories spent through physical activity depends on three factors:

- The number and proportion of muscles used
- The amount of weight moved
- The length of time the activity takes.

An activity that involves both the arms and the legs burns more calories than one that involves only the legs. An activity performed by a heavy person burns more calories than the same activity performed by a lighter person. And an activity performed for 40 minutes requires twice as much energy as the same activity performed for only 20 minutes.

Keeping Weight Control in Perspective

Weight loss is seldom easy. To reach and maintain a healthy weight, develop a program of exercise and healthy eating behaviors that you can maintain. Remember that you didn't gain your weight in a week, and it is both unrealistic and potentially dangerous to take drastic weight-loss measures. Instead, try to lose a healthy 1 to 2 pounds during the first week, and keep a slow, easy regimen. Adding exercise and cutting back on calories to expend about 500 calories more than you consume each day will help you lose weight at a rate of 1

very-low-calorie diets (VLCDs) Diets with a daily caloric value of 400 to 700 calories.

pound per week. See the **Tech & Health** box for apps to help you track activity and intake. See the Skills for Behavior Change box for strategies to help your weight management program succeed.

Considering Drastic Weight-Loss Measures?

When nothing seems to work, people become frustrated and pursue high-risk, unproven methods of weight loss or seek medical interventions. Dramatic weight loss may be recommended in cases of extreme health risk. Drastic dietary, pharmacological, or surgical measures should be discussed with several knowledgeable, licensed health professionals working in accredited facilities.

Very-Low-Calorie Diets In severe cases of obesity that are not responsive to traditional dietary strategies, medically supervised, powdered formulas with daily values of 400 to 700 calories plus vitamin and mineral supplements may be given to patients. Many of these diets emphasize high levels of protein and very low amounts of carbohydrates. Such **very-low-calorie diets (VLCDs)**

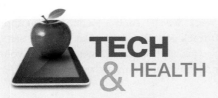

TECH & HEALTH

TRACKING YOUR DIET OR WEIGHT LOSS? *There's an App for That*

Studies consistently report that people who keep detailed food and exercise journals lose more weight and keep it off longer than those who do not. Do you want to track what you ate today in terms of total calories and amount of nutrients? There's an app for that. Do you want to track your walking, running, swimming, lifting, and sleeping activities? There are apps for those, too.

The best programs combine food and physical activity logs so that if you splurge on dessert, you can figure out how many miles you'll need to jog to burn it off. These apps often feature calculators for determining daily calorie intake goals as well as barcode scanners that allow you to quickly add packaged foods to your log. Here are just a few:

- **My Fitness Pal Calorie Counter and Diet Tracker.** An easy-to-use app for tracking details of diet, calories, and exercise. Includes easy data entry, barcode scanning via phone to analyze food purchases, and meal logs to help you assess progress and set goals.
- **Fooducate.** Uses a combination of food lists and barcode scanning via phone to help you determine what is in the food you eat, helping you make healthy food choices while watching calories and daily intake.
- **Instant Heart Rate.** Want to know what your heart rate is as you begin and maintain a diet and exercise regimen? Want to do it without wearing or strapping on all kinds of devices during the day? This app allows you to use your smartphone as a heart rate monitor. Just put your finger on the camera lens to get your pulse. Allows you to track resting heart rate, track progress, and set goals aimed at an optimum heart rate.
- **Fitocracy.** "Fitocrats" play against each other on this app to help motivate them to follow healthy diet and exercise regimens. In the game, users begin at the first level, and, depending on how frequently, how long, and how hard they work out, they earn points, eventually moving to the next level. They also offer support and advice to each other to keep them on track.

should never be undertaken without strict medical supervision. They do not teach healthy eating, and people who manage to lose weight on VLCDs may experience significant weight regain. Problems associated with any form of severe caloric restriction include blood sugar imbalance, cold intolerance, constipation, decreased BMR, dehydration, diarrhea, emotional problems, fatigue, headaches, heart irregularities, kidney infections and failure, loss of lean body tissue, weakness, and the potential for coma and death.

One particularly dangerous potential complication of VLCDs occurs when the person's cells don't have enough of the glucose they need for energy. When this happens, the body begins to burn fat for energy, producing *ketones*—acidic chemicals that can cause major risks to health. Over time on VLCDs or starvation diets, these ketones can increase, the person may not feel hungry or thirsty, and weight loss may occur. As ketones increase and ketosis progresses, *ketoacidosis* or acidic blood levels are likely. This is a potentially dangerous complication of VLCD diets or starvation diets.

Weight-Loss Supplements and Over-the-Counter Drugs
Thousands of over-the-counter supplements and drugs that claim to make weight loss fast and easy are available for purchase. It's important to note that U.S. Food and Drug Administration (FDA) approval is not required for over-the-counter "diet aids" or supplements. The lack of regular and continuous monitoring of supplements in the United States leaves consumers vulnerable to fraud and potentially toxic "remedies." Most dietary supplements contain stimulants, such as caffeine, or diuretics, and their effectiveness in promoting weight loss has been largely untested and unproved by any scientific studies. In many cases, the only thing that

users lose is money. Virtually all people who used supplements and diet pills in review studies regained their weight once they stopped taking them.[56]

Supplements containing *Hoodia gordonii*, an African, cactus-like plant, have become popular in recent years; these supplements may also contain more unproven ingredients such as bitter orange and other stimulants. To date, *Hoodia gordonii* is not FDA approved.

Products containing *ephedra* can cause rapid heart rate, tremors, seizures, insomnia, headaches, and raised blood pressure, all without significant effects on long-term weight control. *St. John's wort* and other alternative medicines reported to enhance serotonin, suppress appetite, and reduce the side effects of depression have also not been shown to be effective in weight loss.

Until relatively recently, FDA-approved diet pills were available only by prescription and were closely monitored. This changed in 2007 when the FDA approved the first over-the-counter weight-loss pill: a half-strength version of the prescription drug orlistat (brand name Xenical), marketed as Alli. This drug inhibits the action of lipase, an enzyme that helps the body to digest fats, causing about 30 percent of fats consumed to pass through the digestive system undigested, leading to reduced overall caloric intake. Known side effects of orlistat include gas with watery fecal discharge; oily stools and spotting; frequent, often unexpected, bowel movements; and possible deficiencies of fat-soluble vitamins.

Prescription Weight-Loss Drugs
Several FDA-approved weight-loss drugs are now available after more than 10 years of inactivity. Belviq and Qsymia, which were among the first available, were met with much controversy and carry

several warnings and restrictions. Qsymia is an appetite suppressant and antiseizure drug that reduces the desire for food. Belviq affects serotonin levels, helping patients feel full. Newer drugs, such as Contrave, combine antidepressants with other approved drugs and carry warnings specific to both. Today, there are nearly 65 prescription, over-the-counter, alternative, and off-label options. When used as part of a long-term, comprehensive weight-loss program, weight-loss drugs can potentially help severely obese individuals to lose weight and keep it off; however, few of these drugs are without side effects. Investigate side effects and check with your doctor before using any of these drugs.[57]

Surgery When all else fails, particularly for people who are severely overweight and have weight-related diseases, a person may be a candidate for weight-loss surgery. Generally, these surgeries fall into one of two major categories: *restrictive surgeries*, such as gastric banding or lap banding, which limit food intake, and *malabsorption surgeries*, such as gastric bypass, which decrease the absorption of food into the body.

To select the best option, a physician will consider that operation's benefits and risks, the patient's age, BMI, eating behaviors, obesity-related health conditions, mental history, dietary history, and previous operations. Like drugs prescribed for weight loss, surgery for obesity carries risks for consumers. Some health advocates have proposed that obesity be classified as a disability (see the **Points of View** box), which could factor into a physician's recommendations about surgery and could affect insurance coverage.

In *gastric banding* and other restrictive surgeries, the surgeon uses an inflatable band to partition off part of the stomach. The band is wrapped around that part of the stomach and is pulled tight, like a belt, leaving only a small opening between

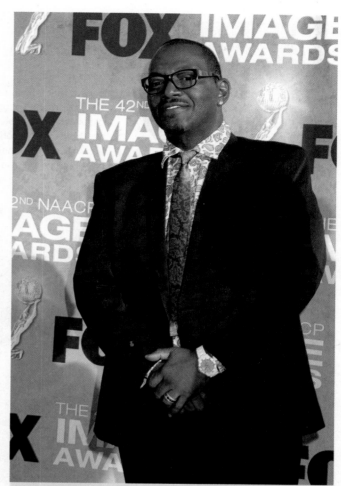

Former *American Idol* judge and record producer Randy Jackson and NBC weatherman Al Roker have undergone gastric bypass surgery to shed well over 100 pounds and reduce the risks of serious chronic diseases such as type 2 diabetes.

the two parts of the stomach. The upper part of the stomach is smaller, so the person feels full more quickly, and food digestion slows so the person also feels full longer. Although the bands are designed to stay in place, they can be removed surgically. They can also be inflated to different levels to adjust the amount of restriction.

Sleeve gastrectomy is a form of restrictive weight-loss surgery that is often done laparoscopically. In this surgery, about 75 percent of the stomach is removed, leaving only a tube (about the size of a banana) or sleeve that is connected directly to the intestines. Usually, this procedure is done on extremely obese or ill patients who need an interim, less invasive procedure before more invasive gastric bypass. However, this procedure isn't reversible, and its potential risks may be higher than those of gastric banding.

Gastric bypass is one of the most common types of weight-loss surgery; it combines restrictive and malabsorption elements. It can be done laparoscopically or via full open surgery. In this surgery, a major section (as much as 70 percent) of the stomach is sutured off, restricting the amount of food the

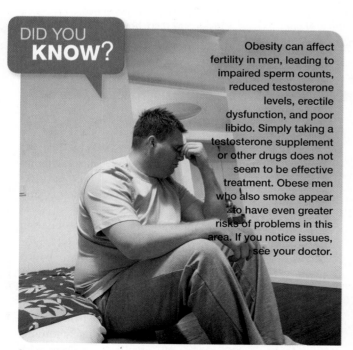

DID YOU KNOW?

Obesity can affect fertility in men, leading to impaired sperm counts, reduced testosterone levels, erectile dysfunction, and poor libido. Simply taking a testosterone supplement or other drugs does not seem to be effective treatment. Obese men who also smoke appear to have even greater risks of problems in this area. If you notice issues, see your doctor.

Source: V. Stokes et al., "How Does Obesity Affect Fertility in Men—and What Are the Treatment Options?," *Clinical Endocrinology* 82, no. 5 (2015): 633–38.

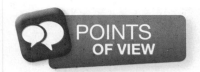
OBESITY *Is It a Disability?*

A person who is 150 to 200 pounds overweight can have difficulty walking, running, standing, and doing other daily tasks. Some people believe that obesity should be considered a disability, legally entitling individuals to certain health benefits and accommodations. Others believe that labeling obesity a disability would add to its stigma and create more problems than it solves.

The federal Americans with Disabilities Act (ADA) defines *disability* as "a physical or mental impairment that substantially limits one or more of the major life activities of [an] individual." Currently, people must have BMIs over 40 or be at least 100 pounds overweight with an underlying disorder before the ADA classifies them as disabled. These strict criteria mean that the ADA currently supports few valid claims relating to obesity.

Arguments Favoring Disability Status for Obese People

- Labeling obesity as a disability would provide obese individuals with increased options for health insurance.
- Labeling obesity as a disability would protect individuals against weight-based discrimination.
- Labeling obesity as a disability would help people with chronic diseases that require use of walkers, wheelchairs, and other special accommodations at work or home to receive them.

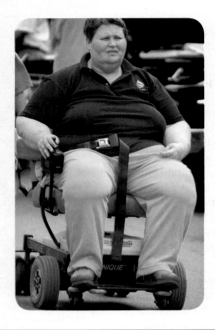

Arguments Opposing Disability Status for Obese People

- Some doctors worry that defining obesity as a disability would make them vulnerable to lawsuits from obese patients who don't want to discuss their weight. Such a threat would prevent doctors from discussing obesity with their overweight patients and recommending specific actions.
- Issues of unfair insurance or job practices could be handled with antidiscrimination laws, not disability status.
- Not all obese people are disabled by their weight, so labeling them all as such would be discriminatory.

WHERE DO YOU STAND?

What consequences might result from classifying overweight or obese individuals as disabled?

- Do you think labeling obesity as a disability would alter the way our society perceives and behaves toward overweight and obese individuals? If so, how?

---

person can eat and absorb. The remaining pouch is hooked up directly to the small intestine. Results are fast and dramatic; health issues related to obesity, such as diabetes, high blood pressure, arthritis, sleep apnea, and other problems, diminish drastically in a short time.

While weight loss tends to be maintained and health problems decline after gastric bypass surgery, it poses many risks, including nutritional deficiencies, blood clots in the legs, a leak in a staple line in the stomach, pneumonia, infection, and, although rare, even death. Another risk is rapid gastric emptying, commonly referred to as "dumping," in which undigested foods rush through the small intestine, causing cramping and problems with uncontrollable diarrhea.[58] Because the stomach pouch that remains after surgery is only the size of a lime, the person can drink only a few tablespoons of liquid and consume only a very small amount of food at a time. For this reason, other possible side effects include nausea, vitamin and mineral deficiencies, and dehydration. Additional risks include the potential for excess bleeding, ulcers, hernia, and the typical risks from anesthesia.

A technique that is gaining in popularity because it is even more effective than gastric bypass for rapid weight loss is the *biliopancreatic diversion* or *duodenal switch procedure*, which combines elements of restrictive and malabsorption surgeries. The patient receives a partial gastrectomy to reduce the size of the stomach (less than the reduction in gastric bypass) while bypassing less of the small intestine. The pyloric valve remains intact, which helps to prevent dumping syndrome, ulcers, blockages, and other problems that can occur with other techniques. This surgery is one of the most difficult and highest-risk surgeries for patients, the risk of death and other complications being higher than with other options.[59]

Considerable research has demonstrated exciting, unexpected results from gastric surgeries: Even before weight loss, patients have shown complete remission of type 2 diabetes in the majority of cases, with drastic reductions in blood glucose levels in others. Add postsurgical exercise to the formula, and both weight loss and relief of type 2 diabetes occur.[60] Although these results are extremely promising, newer research indicates that about one-third of people who have gastric surgery with remission of diabetic symptoms will relapse and begin to show diabetic symptoms within 5 years after surgery. For those at high risk from these diseases, the choice of undergoing a high-risk surgery may ultimately be similar to the risk of maintaining their current weight.

Bariatric arterial embolization is a new nonsurgical alternative to gastric bypass in which a catheter is inserted through the wrist or groin and targets blood vessels in the stomach where the "hunger hormone" ghrelin is produced. Tiny, microscopic beads designed to block ghrelin production are injected in the vessels, causing the patient to be less hungry. With lifestyle and dietary modifications as well as exercise, results of limited early trials appear promising. Options for weight loss via surgical or nonsurgical treatments are not a panacea in and of themselves, and all have risks. Diet and exercise as part of a sound weight control program constitute the best option for most people who want to lose weight.

Unlike surgeries that help to make weight loss easier, *liposuction* is a surgical procedure in which fat cells are actually removed from specific areas of the body. Generally, liposuction is considered cosmetic surgery rather than true weight-loss surgery, even though people who undergo liposuction lose weight. Liposuction is not risk free. If you are considering this procedure, check the credentials of the surgeon, the certification of the facility, and the proximity to emergency care in case problems should arise.

Things to Consider when Considering Surgery
If you are thinking about surgical remedies for obesity, it is important that you think carefully about your options. Ask yourself:

1. Have you exhausted all of the non-surgical strategies for weight loss? Why are you opting for surgery now?
2. What are your goals? (preventing diabetes or other health risks, getting off diabetes or heart medications, wanting to improve your overall health, or wanting to feel better about yourself)
3. What are the costs? According to a recent study assessing costs of gastric bypass or adjustable bands procedures, the costs could easily be over $30,000 with the average cost of $15,000 dollars.[61] Does your insurance pay for it? Under what circumstances, if any?
4. Have you considered where you would have the surgery? What questions should you ask before opting to have a particular procedure? Like most surgeries, the best results are likely to occur in accredited facilities, with board certified surgeons who do large numbers of these procedures each year, have comprehensive pre-surgical counseling and follow-up care, as well as support staff. Hospitals that have emergency and intensive care facilities for those who have surgical complications as well as a documented history of infection control policies and procedures are among those most likely to have positive outcomes.

Trying to Gain Weight

For some people, trying to gain weight is a challenge. If you have this problem, the first priority is to determine why you cannot gain weight. Perhaps you're an athlete and you burn more calories than you eat. Perhaps you're stressed out and skip meals to increase study time. Among older adults, the senses of taste and smell may decline, making food less pleasurable to eat. Visual problems and other disabilities may make meals more difficult to prepare, and dental problems may make eating more difficult. People who engage in extreme energy-burning sports and exercise routines may be at risk for caloric and nutritional deficiencies, which can lead not only to weight loss, but also to immune system problems and organ dysfunction; weakness, which leads to falls and fractures; slower recovery from diseases; and a host of other problems. Underweight individuals need to examine their diet and exercise behaviors and take steps to achieve and maintain a healthy weight.

LIVE IT! ASSESS YOURSELF

An interactive version of this assessment is available online in Mastering Health.

ASSESS | YOURSELF

Are You Ready to Start a Weight-Loss Program?

If you are overweight or obese, complete each of the following questions by circling the responses that best represents your situation or attitudes, then total your points for each section.

1 Family, Weight, and Diet History

1. **How many people in your immediate family (parents or siblings) are overweight or obese?**

   a. None (0 points)

   b. One person (1 point)

   c. Two people (2 points)

   d. Three or more people (3 points)

2. **During which periods of your life were you overweight or obese? (Circle all that apply.)**

   a. Birth through age 5 years (1 point)

   b. Ages 6 to 11 years (1 point)

   c. Ages 12 to 13 years (1 point))

   d. Ages 14 to 18 years (2 points)

   e. Ages 19 years to present (2 points)

3. **How many times in the last year have you made a major effort to lose weight but had little or no success?**

   a. None (0 points)

   b. I've thought about it, but never tried. (1 point)

   c. I have tried 2 to 3 times. (1 point)

   d. I have tried at least once a month. (2 points)

   e. I have tried too many times to count. (3 points)

   Total points: _____

Scoring

A score higher than 4 suggests that you may have several challenges ahead as you begin a weight-loss program. Your weight is often a product of learned patterns of eating and exercise. If you have tried repeatedly to lose weight and have not been successful, you may have to reframe your thinking and try something new.

2 Readiness to Change

1. **What is/are your main reason(s) for wanting to lose weight? (Circle all that apply.)**

   a. I want to please someone I know or attract a new person. (0 points)

   b. I want to look great and/or fit into smaller-size clothes for an upcoming event (wedding, vacation, date, etc.). (1 point)

   c. Someone I know has had major health problems because of being overweight/obese. (1 point)

   d. I want to improve my health and/or have more energy. (2 points)

   e. I was diagnosed with a weight-related health problem. (2 points)

2. **What do you think about your weight and body shape? (Circle all that apply.)**

   a. I'm fine with being overweight, and if others don't like it, tough! (0 points)

   b. My weight hurts my energy levels and my performance. (1 point)

   c. I feel good about myself, but think I will be happier if I lose weight. (1 point)

   d. I'm self-conscious about my weight and uncomfortable in my skin. (1 point)

   e. I'm really worried that I will have a major health problem if I don't change my behaviors now. (2 points)

3. **Which of the following statements describes you? (Circle all that apply.)**

   a. I think about food several times a day, even when I'm not hungry. (0 point)

   b. There are some foods or snacks that I can't stay away from, and I eat them even when I'm not hungry. (0 point)

   c. I tend to eat more meat and fatty foods and seldom get enough fruits and vegetables. (0 points)

   d. I've thought about the weaknesses in my diet and have some ideas about what I need to do. (1 point)

   e. I haven't really tried to eat a balanced diet, but I know that I need to start now. (1 point)

4. **When you binge or eat things you shouldn't, what are you likely to do? (Circle all that apply.)**

   a. Not care and go off of my diet. (0 points)

   b. Feel guilty for a while, but then do it again the next time I am out. (0 points)

   c. Fast for the next day or two to help balance the high consumption day. (0 points)

   d. Plan ahead for next time and have options in mind so that I do not continue to overeat. (1 point)

   e. Acknowledge that I have made a slip and get back on my program the next day. (1 point)

5. **On a typical day, what are your eating patterns? (Circle all that apply.)**

   a. I skip breakfast and save my calories for lunch and dinner. (0 point)

   b. I never really sit down for a meal. I am a "grazer" and eat whatever I find that is readily available. (0 point)

   c. I try to eat at least five servings of fruits and vegetables and restrict saturated fats in my diet. (1 point)

   d. I eat several small meals, trying to be balanced in my portions and getting foods from different food groups. (1 point)

6. **How would you describe your current support system for helping you lose weight? (Circle all that apply.)**

   a. I believe I can do this best by doing it on my own. (0 points)

   b. I am not aware of any sources that can help me. (0 points)

   c. I have two to three friends or family members I can count on to help me. (1 point)

   d. There are counselors on campus with whom I can meet to plan a successful approach to weight loss. (1 point)

   e. I have the resources to join Weight Watchers or other community or online weight-loss programs. (1 point)

7. **How committed are you to exercising? (Circle all that apply.)**

   a. Exercise is uncomfortable and embarrassing, and/or I don't enjoy it. (0 points)

   b. I don't have time to exercise. (0 points)

   c. I would like to exercise, but I'm not sure how to get started. (1 point)

   d. I have visited my campus recreation center or local gym to explore my options. (2 points)

   e. There are specific sports or physical activities I do already, and I can plan to do more of them. (2 points)

8. **What statement best describes your motivation to start a weight loss and lifestyle change program?**

   a. I have no interest in trying to lose weight. (0 points)

   b. I am thinking about doing it sometime in the future, but I have no idea when. (0 points)

   c. I am considering starting in the next few weeks; I just need to make a plan. (1 point)

   d. I would like to start in the next few weeks, and I'm working on a plan. (2 points)

   e. I already have a plan in place, and I'm ready to begin tomorrow or have already started. (3 points)

   Total points: _____

Scoring

A score higher than 8 indicates that you may be ready to change; the higher your score above 8, the more successful you may be. Take a close look at areas that you could work on. Your behaviors, resources, readiness to change, and overall plan for change may give you the extra edge necessary to be successful.

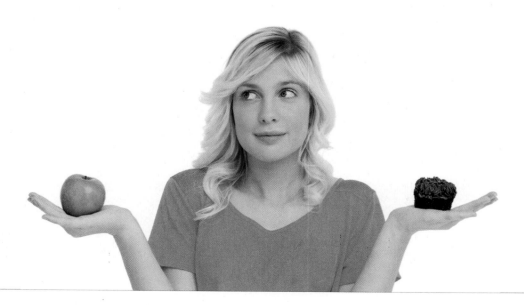

YOUR PLAN FOR CHANGE

The **ASSESS YOURSELF** identifies six areas of importance in determining your readiness for weight loss. If you wish to lose weight to improve your health, understanding your attitudes about food and exercise will help you succeed.

TODAY, YOU CAN:

☐ Set SMART goals for weight loss and give them a reality check: Are they **s**pecific, **m**easurable, **a**chievable, **r**elevant, and **t**ime oriented? For example, rather than aiming to lose 15 pounds this month (which probably wouldn't be healthy or achievable), set a more comfortable goal to lose 1 pound per week by diet and exercise changes.

☐ Keep a food log to identify the triggers that influence your eating habits. Think about what you can do to eliminate or reduce the influence of your two most common food triggers.

WITHIN THE NEXT TWO WEEKS, YOU CAN:

☐ Get in the habit of incorporating more fruits, vegetables, and whole grains in your diet and eating less fat. The next time you make dinner, look at the proportions on your plate. If vegetables and whole grains do not take up most of the space, replace 1 cup of the meat, non-whole grains, or cheese in your meal with 1 cup of legumes, salad greens, or a favorite vegetable.

☐ Ramp up your exercise in small increments. Visit your campus recreation center or a local gym, and familiarize yourself with the equipment and facilities that are available. Try a new machine or sports activity, and experiment until you find something you really like.

BY THE END OF THE SEMESTER, YOU CAN:

☐ Get in the habit of grocery shopping every week and buying healthy, nutritious foods while avoiding high-fat, high-sugar, and overly processed foods. As you make healthy foods more available and unhealthy foods less available, you'll find it easier to eat better.

☐ Chart your progress, and reward yourself as you meet your goals. Instead of rewarding yourself with food, do something fun like seeing a movie or buying that new pair of skinny jeans you've been wanting (which will likely fit better than before!).

STUDY PLAN

CHAPTER REVIEW

LO 1 | Overweight and Obesity: A Growing Health Threat

■ Overweight, obesity, and weight-related health problems have reached epidemic levels. Globesity, or global rates of obesity, threatens the health of many countries. Societal costs from obesity include increased health care costs and lowered worker productivity. Individual health risks from overweight and obesity include increased chance of developing cardiovascular diseases, arthritis, stroke, diabetes, gastrointestinal problems, low back pain, and a number of other diseases. Overweight individuals frequently struggle with depression, low self-esteem, and high levels of stress.

LO 2 | Factors Contributing to Overweight and Obesity

■ It is important to consider environmental, cultural, and socioeconomic factors in working to prevent obesity. In addition to genetics, metabolism, hormonal influences, excess fat cells, and physical risks, key environmental influences, such as poverty, socioeconomic status, education level, and lack of access to nutritious food, and lifestyle factors, including sedentary lifestyle and high calorie consumption, all make weight loss challenging.

LO 3 | Assessing Body Weight and Body Composition

■ Percentage of body fat is a fairly reliable indicator for levels of overweight and obesity. There are many different methods of assessing body fat. Body mass index (BMI) is one of the most commonly accepted measures of weight based on height. *Overweight* is most commonly defined as a BMI of 25 to 29.9 and *obesity* as a BMI of 30 or greater. Waist circumference, or the amount of fat in the belly region, is believed to be related to the risk for several chronic diseases, particularly type 2 diabetes.

LO 4 | Managing Your Weight: Individual Roles

■ Increased physical activity, a balanced, healthy diet that controls caloric intake, and other strategies are recommended for controlling your weight. When these options fail and risks increase, doctor-recommended prescription medications, weight-loss surgery, and other strategies can be used to maintain or lose weight. However, sensible eating behavior, aerobic exercise, and exercise that builds muscle mass offer the best options for weight loss and maintenance.

POP QUIZ

LO 1 | Overweight and Obesity: A Growing Health Threat

1. Which of the following statements is *false*?
   a. Hispanic men and non-Hispanic white men are more likely to be overweight/obese than are non-Hispanic Black or Asian men.
   b. Children and adolescents living in higher-income homes where parents are more educated have a greatly increased risk of obesity in comparison to children and adolescents living in low-income homes where parents are less educated and/or unemployed.
   c. Non-Hispanic black women and Hispanic women are more likely to be overweight or obese than non-Hispanic white women.
   d. The United States has the distinction of being one of the fattest developed nations on earth.

LO 2 | Factors Contributing to Overweight and Obesity

2. The rate at which your body consumes food energy to sustain basic functions is your
   a. basal metabolic rate.
   b. resting metabolic rate.
   c. body mass index.
   d. set point.

3. Which of the following statements is *false*?
   a. A slowing basal metabolic rate may contribute to weight gain after age 30 years.
   b. Hormones are increasingly implicated in hunger impulses and eating behavior.
   c. The more muscles you have, the fewer calories you will burn.
   d. Yo-yo dieting can make weight loss more difficult.

LO 3 | Assessing Body Weight and Body Composition

4. The proportion of your total weight that is made up of fat is called
   a. body composition.
   b. lean mass.
   c. percentage of body fat.
   d. BMI.

5. Which of the following statements about BMI is *false*?
   a. BMI is based on height and weight measurements.
   b. BMI is accurate for everyone, including athletes with high amounts of muscle mass.
   c. Very low and very high BMI scores are associated with greater risk of mortality.
   d. BMI stands for "body mass index."

6. Which of the following body circumferences is most strongly associated with risk of heart disease and diabetes?
   a. Hip circumference
   b. Chest circumference
   c. Waist circumference
   d. Thigh circumference

LO 4 | Managing Your Weight: Individual Roles

7. One pound of additional body fat is created through consuming how many extra calories?
   a. 1,500 calories
   b. 3,500 calories
   c. 5,000 calories
   d. 7,000 calories

8. To lose weight, you must establish a(n)
   a. negative caloric balance.
   b. isocaloric balance.
   c. positive caloric balance.
   d. set point.

9. Successful weight maintainers are most likely to do which of the following?
   a. Eat two large meals a day before 1:00 P.M.
   b. Skip meals
   c. Drink diet sodas
   d. Eat high-volume but low-calorie-density foods

10. Successful, healthy weight loss is characterized by
    a. a lifelong pattern of healthful eating and exercise.
    b. cutting out all fats and carbohydrates and eating a lean, mean, high-protein diet.
    c. never eating foods that are considered bad for you and rigidly adhering to a plan.
    d. a pattern of repeatedly losing and regaining weight.

Answers to the Pop Quiz can be found on page A-1. If you answered a question incorrectly, review the section tagged by the Learning Outcome. For even more study tools, visit **Mastering Health**.

THINK ABOUT IT!

LO 1 | Overweight and Obesity: A Growing Health Threat

1. Why are obesity rates are rising in both developed and less-developed regions of the world? What strategies can we take collectively and individually to reduce risks of obesity nationally? Internationally?

LO 2 | Factors Contributing to Overweight and Obesity

2. List the risk factors for your being overweight or obese right now. Which seem factors most likely to determine whether you will be obese in middle age? If newer theories prove true, how might they influence future weight-loss efforts?

LO 3 | Assessing Body Weight and Body Composition

3. Which measurement would you choose to assess your fat levels? Why?

LO 4 | Managing Your Weight: Individual Roles

4. Are you satisfied with your body weight? If so, what do you do to maintain a healthy weight? What lifestyle changes could you make to improve your weight and overall health?

ACCESS YOUR HEALTH ON THE INTERNET

Visit Mastering Health for links to the websites and RSS feeds.

The following websites explore further topics and issues related to weight.

Academy of Nutrition and Dietetics. This site includes recommended dietary guidelines and other current information about weight control. **www.eatright.org**

Weight Control Information Network. This is an excellent resource for diet and weight control information. **http://win .niddk.nih.gov/index.htm**

The Rudd Center for Food Policy and Obesity. This website provides excellent information on the latest in obesity research, public policy, and ways we can stop the obesity epidemic at the community level. **www.uconnruddcenter.org**

The Obesity Society. This is a key site for information/education about our national obesity epidemic, including statistics, research, consumer issues, and fact sheets. **www.obesity.org**

Enhancing Your Body Image

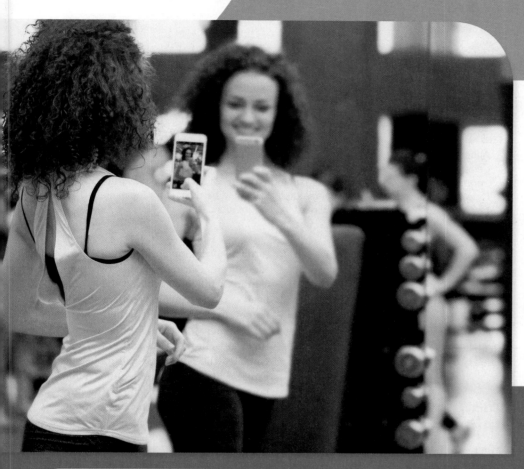

LEARNING OUTCOMES

LO **1** Define body image, list the factors that influence it, and identify the difference between being dissatisfied with one's appearance and having body dysmorphic disorder.

LO **2** Describe the signs and symptoms of disordered eating as well as the physical effects and treatment options for anorexia nervosa, bulimia nervosa, and binge-eating disorder.

LO **3** List the criteria, symptoms, and treatment for exercise disorders and syndromes such as muscle dysmorphia and female athlete triad.

WHY SHOULD I CARE?

Dissatisfaction with one's appearance and shape can foster unhealthy attitudes and thought patterns, as well as disordered eating and compulsive exercise behaviors.

When you look in the mirror, do you like what you see? If you feel dissatisfied, frustrated, or even angry, you're not alone. In a recent national poll, 67 percent of women and 53 percent of men reported worrying about their appearance regularly—women more than every other issue in their lives and men more than every issue but finances.[1] For both women (69 percent) and men (52 percent), the body part of greatest concern is the abdomen.[2] Concerns about weight and shape are central to many people's body dissatisfaction. As body mass increases, dissatisfaction increases, particularly during transitional periods in life. Females, in particular, seem to experience peak levels of body dissatisfaction when transitioning from high school to young adulthood.[3] Sadly, dissatisfaction with your body can result in behaviors that disrupt your relationships, undermine your goals, affect your mental health, and lead to life-threatening illness. By contrast, developing and maintaining a healthy body image can enhance your interactions with other people, reduce stress, give you an increased sense of personal empowerment, and bring confidence and joy to your life.[4]

LO 1 | WHAT IS BODY IMAGE?

Define body image, list the factors that influence it, and identify the difference between being dissatisfied with one's appearance and having body dysmorphic disorder.

Your **body image** is what you believe or emotionally feel about your body's shape, weight, and general appearance. More than what you see in the mirror, it includes the following:

- How you see yourself in your mind
- What you believe about your own appearance (including beliefs about how others view you)
- How you feel about your body, including your height, shape, and weight
- How you sense and control your body as you move
- How you behave in relation to your thoughts and feelings about your body.

A *negative body image* is defined as either a distorted perception of your shape and appearance or feelings of discomfort, shame, or anxiety about your body. It may involve being certain that only people other than you are attractive and that your body is a sign of personal failure. In contrast, a *positive body image* is a true perception of your appearance: You see yourself as you really are. You understand that everyone is different, and you celebrate your uniqueness—including your perceived "flaws," which you know have nothing to do with your value as a person. Keep in mind that having a healthy, realistic goal to change your body and a healthy plan to make the change does not indicate a negative body image.

body image How you see yourself in your mind, what you believe about your appearance, how you feel about your body, and how you behave in response.

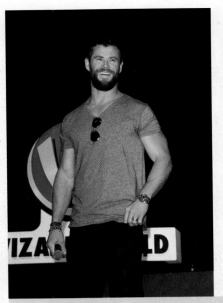 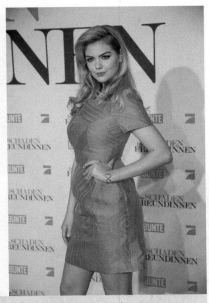

Although the exact nature of the "in" look may change from generation to generation, unrealistic images of both male and female celebrities are nothing new. *People* magazine's 2014's Sexiest Man and Woman Alive, Chris Hemsworth and Kate Upton, both exhibit physical features that would be difficult for the average person to achieve, no matter how hard they might work.

Is your body image negative or positive—or somewhere in between? Researchers have developed a body image continuum that may help you decide (see **FIGURE 1**). Notice that the continuum identifies behaviors associated with particular states, from total dissociation with one's body to body not being an issue.

Many Factors Influence Body Image

You're not born with a body image, but you do begin to develop one at an early age. Let's look at the factors that play a role in body image development. As you read this section, think about the factors that have had the most significant impact on your body image. Also, be mindful of how you handle the negative influences on body image that are prevalent in our culture.

The Media and Popular Culture

Media images tend to set the standard for what we find attractive, leading some people to go to dangerous extremes to have bigger biceps or fit into smaller jeans. Changing our bodies to better achieve what current society identifies as "attractive" has long been part of American culture. During the early twentieth century, while men idolized the strong, hearty outdoorsman President Teddy Roosevelt, women pulled their corsets ever tighter to achieve unrealistically tiny waists. In the 1920s and 1930s, men emulated the burly cops and robbers in gangster films, while women dieted and bound their breasts to achieve the boyish "flapper" look. By the 1960s, tough guys were the male ideal, whereas rail-thin models such as Twiggy embodied the standard of female beauty. Today's societal obsession around appearance—even when many images are airbrushed or Photoshopped—isn't much different.

Social media activity has also increased concerns about negative body images.[5] While many social media sites actively warn against posts that

30%

of college males and **45%** of college females **REPORT DIETING** in the past 30 days to lose weight.

Body hate/ disassociation	Distorted body image	Body preoccupied/ obsessed	Body acceptance	Body is not an issue
I often feel separated and distant from my body—as if it belonged to someone else.	I spend a significant amount of time exercising and dieting to change my body.	I weigh and measure myself a lot.	I pay attention to my body and my appearance because it is important to me, but it only occupies a small part of my day.	I feel fine about my body.
I hate my body, and I often isolate myself from others.	My body shape and size keeps me from dating or finding someone who will treat me the way I want to be treated.	I spend a significant amount of time viewing myself in the mirror.	I would like to change some things about my body, but I spend most of my time highlighting my positive features.	I don't worry about changing my body shape or weight.
I don't see anything positive or even neutral about my body shape and size.	I have considered changing (or have changed) my body shape and size through surgical means.	I compare my body to others.		I never weigh or measure myself.
I don't believe others when they tell me I look okay.	I wish I could change the way I look in the mirror.	I have days when I feel fat.	My self-esteem is based on my personality traits, achievements, and relationships—not just my body image.	My feelings about my body are not influenced by society's concept of an ideal body shape.
I hate the way I look in the mirror.		I accept society's ideal body shape and size as the best body shape and size.		I know that the significant others in my life will always love me for who I am, not for how I look.
		I'd be more attractive if I were thinner, more muscular, etc.		

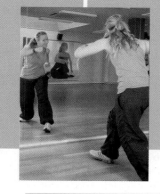

FIGURE 1 **Body Image Continuum** This continuum shows a range of attitudes and behaviors toward body image, from full acceptance to disassociation.

Source: Adapted from Smiley/King/Avery, "Eating Issues and Body Image Continuum," Campus Health Service 1996. Copyright © 1997 Arizona Board of Regents for University of Arizona.

 Watch Video Tutor: **Body Image Continuum** in Mastering Health.

promote or glorify self-harm, messages promoting unhealthy body images are common. Such messages are often disguised as a type of encouragement; for instance, catch phrases telling people to get "thin" or be "fit" might be coupled with images of unrealistically thin bodies.[6] See Student Health Today for more on "thinspiration."

With more than two-thirds of American adults 20 years and older overweight or obese, a significant disconnect exists between the media's idealized images and the typical American body.[7] The images of "beauty" that continually bombard us unrealistic for all but a small fragment of the population. These messages can damage our body image, as no amount of dieting or exercise can shift a person to the size or shape of a Photoshopped body.

Family, Community, and Cultural Groups

People with whom we interact regularly strongly influence the way we see ourselves. Parents are especially influential in body image development. For instance, it's common and natural for fathers of adolescent girls to experience feelings of discomfort related to their daughters' changing bodies. If the men are able to navigate these feelings and validate the acceptability of their daughters' appearance throughout puberty, they will help their daughters maintain a positive body image.[8] Even subtle judgments from her father about her changing body may prompt a girl to question how males see her. Mothers who model body acceptance or body ownership may be more likely to foster a positive

body image in their daughters, whereas mothers who are frustrated with or ashamed of their own bodies may foster negative attitudes in their children.[9]

Interactions with siblings and other relatives, peers, teachers, coworkers, and other community members can also influence body image development. Being overweight is now the most commonly reported reason why children are bullied at school,[10] and peer harassment (teasing and bullying) is widely acknowledged to contribute to a negative body image. Associations within one's cultural group are also an influence on body image. For example, studies have found that white females experience the highest rates of body dissatisfaction and that the body dissatisfaction levels of minority women increase the more they are acculturated within and exposed to mainstream media.[11]

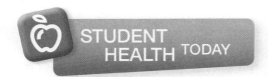
THINSPIRATION AND THE ONLINE WORLD OF ANOREXIA

The pro-anorexia movement has a host of websites, chatrooms, blogs, and discussion boards, most of them created and hosted by girls and women who are struggling with eating disorders. One study found that 13 percent of young females had visited a pro–eating disorder website and that the sites had been Googled 13 million times in the past year. Along with dangerous and incorrect information about restrictive eating, metabolism, bingeing, and laxative abuse, many of these sites feature "thinspiration"—pictures and quotes intended to inspire visitors to thinness—as well as tips and tricks to hide and maintain disordered eating. This is not the type of inspiration girls and women need.

We can be inspired, however, by some changes in the modeling industry. To prevent the use of excessively thin models, the French government passed a law that models must have a BMI of 18 or over. The bill also requires that Photoshopped images—in particular those that make a model's silhouette narrower or wider—be labeled as "retouched."

In the United States, the retailer Modcloth had its employees of all shapes and sizes model the site's new swimsuits; Calvin Klein recently featured a size 10 model in its "Perfect Body" campaign; and in 2016, the cover of the Sports Illustrated swimsuit issue featured a plus-sized model, Ashley Graham. The tag "real-sized" (instead of "plus-sized") is now

commonly used for popular models such as Tocarra Jones and Robyn Lawley. This acceptance of a variety of beauty is the kind of inspiration we need.

Sources: National Eating Disorder Information Centre; MPA website, Accessed May 2015, www.myproana.com/index.php/blogs; M. Persad, "Average-Size Models Could Be Better for Business, Study Says" May 14, 2015, http://www.huffingtonpost.com/2015/05/14/average-size-models-study-advertising_n_7275376.html; Vogue News, "France Passes Model Health Law," December 21, 2015, http://www.vogue.co.uk/news/2015/12/21/french-model-law-bmi-medical-certificate-for-models-in-france; S. Jett et al., "Impact of Exposure to Pro-Eating Disorder Websites on Eating Behavior in College Women," *European Eating Disorders Review* 18 (2010): 410–16.

Physiological and Psychological Factors

Research in neurology suggests that people who have been diagnosed with a body image disorder show differences in the brain's ability to regulate mood-linked chemicals called *neurotransmitters*.[12] Poor regulation of neurotransmitters is also involved in depression, anxiety disorders, and obsessive-compulsive disorder. One study linked distortions in body image to a malfunction in the brain's visual processing region.[13] Another theory suggests that there may be genetic differences in the level of the neurotransmitter serotonin in the brain of individuals with a body image disorder.[14] These findings suggest that some people are more biologically susceptible to developing a body image disorder. They also indicate that a small number of people could benefit from medication, such as SSRIs (which increase the level of available serotonin in the brain), to improve their body image.[15]

Building a Positive Body Image

To develop a more positive body image, start by challenging some commonly

held myths and attitudes in contemporary society.[16]

- **Myth 1:** How you look is more important than who you are.

Fact: Your appearance does not determine who you are or what you are capable of.

- **Myth 2:** You can look like the celebrities if you work at it hard enough.

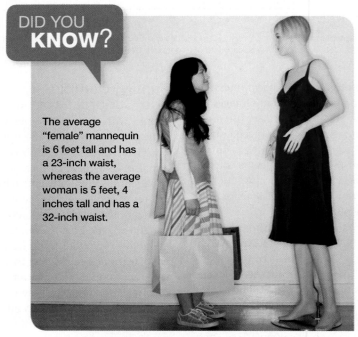

DID YOU **KNOW**?

The average "female" mannequin is 6 feet tall and has a 23-inch waist, whereas the average woman is 5 feet, 4 inches tall and has a 32-inch waist.

Sources: R. Duyff, *American Dietetic Association Complete Food and Nutrition Guide*, 4th ed. (Hoboken, NJ: John Wiley & Sons, Inc., 2012), 50; C. Fryar, Q. Gu, and C. Ogden, "Anthropometric Reference Data for Children and Adults: United States, 2007–2010," National Center for Health Statistics, *Vital and Health Statistics*, Series 11, no. 252 (2012), www.cdc.gov/nchs/data/series/sr_11/sr11_252.pdf.

BEHAVIOR CHANGE

Ten Steps To A Positive Body Image

One way to turn negative thoughts positive is to think about how to look more healthfully and happily at yourself and your body. The more you try, the better you will feel about who you are and the body you naturally have.

Step 1. Appreciate all of the amazing things your body does for you: running, dancing, breathing, laughing, dreaming.

Step 2. Make a list of things you like about yourself—things that aren't related to how much you weigh or how you look. Add to it as you notice things.

Step 3. Remind yourself that true beauty is not skin deep. When you feel good about yourself and who you are, you carry yourself with a sense of confidence, self-acceptance, and openness that is attractive.

Step 4. Look at yourself as a whole person. When you see yourself in a mirror or in your mind, choose not to focus on specific body parts.

Step 5. Surround yourself with positive people. It is easier to feel good about yourself when you are around people who are supportive and who recognize the importance of liking yourself as you naturally are.

Step 6. Shut down those voices in your head that tell you your body is not "right" or that you are a "bad" person.

Step 7. Wear comfortable clothes that make you feel good about your body. Work with your body, not against it.

Step 8. Become a critical viewer of social and media messages. Pay attention to images, slogans, and attitudes that make you feel bad about your appearance.

Step 9. Show appreciation for your body. Take a bubble bath, make time for a nap, or find a peaceful place outside to relax.

Step 10. Use the time and energy you might have spent worrying about food, calories, and your weight to do something to help other people. Reaching out to others can help you feel better about yourself and make a positive change in our world.

Source: "10 Steps to Positive Body Image," from National Eating Disorders Association website, Accessed February 13, 2016; National Eating Disorders Association. Reprinted with permission. For more information, visit www.NationalEatingDisorders.org or call NEDA's helpline at 1-800-931-2237.

Fact: While exercise and healthy eating can improve anyone's health status, not everyone has the genes to be muscular, tall, or curvy. We can exercise and eat our way to good health but not to a particular shape.

- **Myth 3:** Extreme dieting is an effective weight-loss strategy.

Fact: Extreme dieting is dangerous, and quick weight loss is rarely sustainable. (See Chapter 6 for more on weight loss techniques.)

- **Myth 4:** Things will go better for you after you achieve the perfect body.

Fact: Attaining a certain shape or weight is not the key to a happy, wonderful life. Investing in healthy relationships and working toward life goals can bring lasting happiness.

For ways to bust these toxic myths and attitudes and to build a more positive body image, check out the Skills for Behavior Change box.

Body Dysmorphic Disorder

Although most Americans report being dissatisfied with some aspect of their

body dysmorphic disorder (BDD) A psychological disorder characterized by an obsession with one's appearance and a distorted view of one's body or with a minor or imagined flaw in appearance.

appearance, very few have a true body image disorder. The difference lies in the degree of dissatisfaction and the actions taken to chase satisfaction. Approximately 2 percent of people in the United States suffer from **body dysmorphic disorder (BDD)**.[17] People with BDD are obsessively concerned with their appearance and have a distorted view of their own body to the extent that it impairs their social or occupational functioning. Although the cause of the disorder isn't known, an anxiety disorder or obsessive–compulsive disorder is often also present. (See Chapter 2 for more discussion of anxiety disorders.) Contributing factors may include genetic susceptibility, childhood teasing, physical or sexual abuse, low self-esteem, and rigid sociocultural expectations of attractiveness.[18] Males and females show similar prevalence,

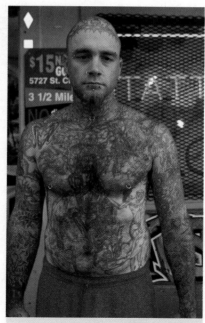

It's not always easy to spot people who are highly dissatisfied with their bodies. People who cover their bodies with tattoos may have a strong sense of self-esteem. Alternatively, extreme tattooing can be an outward sign of a severe body image disturbance known as body dysmorphic disorder.

Eating disordered	Disruptive eating patterns	Food preoccupied/ obsessed	Concerned in a healthy way	Food is not an issue
I worry about what I will eat or when I will exercise all the time.	My food and exercise concerns are starting to interfere with my school and social life.	I think about food a lot.	I pay attention to what I eat in order to maintain a healthy body.	I am not concerned about what or how much I eat.
I follow a very rigid eating plan and know precisely how many calories, fat grams, or carbohydrates I eat every day.	I use food to comfort myself.	I'm obsessed with reading books and magazines about dieting, fitness, and weight control.	Food and exercise are important parts of my life, but they only occupy a small part of my time.	I feel no guilt or shame no matter what I eat or how much I eat.
I feel incredible guilt, shame, and anxiety when I break my diet.	I have tried diet pills, laxatives, vomiting, or extra time exercising in order to lose or maintain my weight.	I sometimes miss school, work, and social events because of my diet or exercise schedule.	I enjoy eating, and I balance my pleasure with my concern for a healthy body.	Exercise is not really important to me. I choose foods based on cost, taste, and convenience, with little regard to health.
I regularly stuff myself and then exercise, vomit, or use laxatives to get rid of the food.	I have fasted or avoided eating for long periods of time in order to lose or maintain my weight.	I divide food into "good" and "bad" categories.	I usually eat three balanced meals daily, plus snacks, to fuel my body with adequate energy.	My eating is very sporadic and irregular.
My friends and family tell me I am too thin, but I feel fat.	If I cannot exercise to burn off calories, I panic.	I feel guilty when I eat "bad" foods or when I eat more than what I feel I should be eating.	I am moderate and flexible in my goals for eating well and being physically active.	I don't worry about meals; I just eat whatever I can, whenever I can.
I am out of control when I eat.	I feel strong when I can restrict how much I eat.	I am afraid of getting fat.	Sometimes I eat more (or less) than I really need, but most of the time I listen to my body.	I enjoy stuffing myself with lots of tasty food at restaurants, holiday meals, and social events.
I am afraid to eat in front of others.	I feel out of control when I eat more than I wanted to.	I wish I could change how much I want to eat and what I am hungry for.		
I prefer to eat alone.				

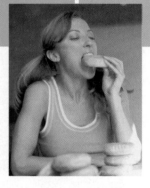
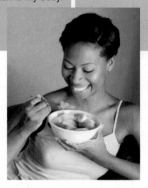

FIGURE 2 **Eating Issues Continuum** This continuum shows the progression from eating disorders to normal eating. Being concerned with eating in a healthy way is the goal rather than functioning at either extreme.

Source: Adapted from Smiley/King/Avery, "Eating Issues and Body Image Continuum," Campus Health Service 1996. Copyright © 1997 Arizona Board of Regents for University of Arizona.

although they usually focus on different perceived defects.[19]

People with BDD may try to fix their perceived flaws through abuse of steroids, excessive bodybuilding, cosmetic surgeries, extreme tattooing, or other appearance-altering behaviors. It is estimated that 10 percent of people who seek dermatology or cosmetic treatments have BDD.[20] Not only do such actions fail to address the underlying problem, but they also are actually considered diagnostic signs of BDD. Psychiatric treatment, including psychotherapy and/or antidepressant medications, can help.

LO 2 | DISORDERED EATING AND EATING DISORDERS

Describe the signs and symptoms of disordered eating as well as the physical effects and treatment options for anorexia nervosa, bulimia nervosa, orthorexia nervosa, and binge-eating disorder.

People with a negative body image may fixate on a wide range of self-perceived "flaws." The so-called flaw that distresses the majority of people with negative body image is feeling overweight.

Some people channel weight-related anxiety into self-defeating thoughts and harmful behaviors. The far left of the eating issues continuum (FIGURE 2) identifies a pattern of thoughts and behaviors associated with **disordered eating**, including chronic dieting, rigid eating patterns, abusing diet pills and laxatives, self-induced vomiting, and many others.

disordered eating A pattern of atypical eating behaviors that is used to achieve or maintain a lower body weight.

A small number of people who exhibit disordered eating patterns progress to a clinical **eating disorder**. The eating disorders defined by the American Psychiatric Association (APA) in the fifth edition of the *Diagnostic and Statistical Manual of Mental Disorders (DSM-5)* are *anorexia nervosa*, *bulimia nervosa*, *binge-eating disorder*, and a cluster of less-distinct conditions that are collectively referred to as *other specified feeding or eating disorder (OSFED)*.[21]

Twenty million women and 10 million men in the United States will suffer from some sort of eating disorder over their lifetimes.[22] Although anorexia nervosa and bulimia nervosa primarily affect people in their teens and 20s, other age groups can be affected from children to the elderly.[23] In 2015, 2.6 percent of college students reported having been diagnosed with anorexia or bulimia.[24] While anyone can have an eating disorder, they are more common among ballet dancers and athletes, particularly athletes in sports with an aesthetic component (e.g., figure skating or gymnastics), lean sports (e.g., cross-country running), or sports tied to a weight class (e.g., tae kwon do or wrestling).[25]

Eating disorders are on the rise among men, who make up nearly 25 percent of all anorexia and bulimia patients.[26] Many men suffering from eating disorders fail to seek treatment because these illnesses are traditionally thought of as a female problem.

What factors put individuals at risk? Many people with eating disorders feel controlled in other aspects of their lives and try to gain a sense of power through food. Many are clinically depressed, suffer from obsessive-compulsive disorder, or have other psychiatric problems. In addition, individuals with low self-esteem, negative body image, and a high tendency for perfectionism are at risk.[27]

Anorexia Nervosa

Anorexia nervosa is a persistent, chronic eating disorder characterized by deliberate food restriction and severe, life-threatening weight loss. It has the highest death rate (20 percent) of any psychological illness.[28] It involves self-starvation motivated by an intense fear of gaining weight and an extremely distorted body image. Initially, most people with anorexia nervosa lose weight by reducing total food intake, particularly of high-calorie foods. Eventually, they progress to restricting their intake of almost all foods. The little they do eat, they may purge through vomiting using laxatives, or even excessive exercise. Although they lose weight, people with anorexia nervosa never feel thin enough. An estimated 0.9 to 2.0 percent of females suffer from anorexia nervosa in their lifetime.[29] FIGURE 3 illustrates physical symptoms and negative health consequences associated with anorexia nervosa.

Causes of anorexia nervosa are complex and variable. Many people with anorexia have coexisting psychiatric problems, including low self-esteem, depression, an anxiety disorder such as obsessive-compulsive disorder, and substance abuse.[30] Some people have a history of being physically or sexually abused, and others have troubled interpersonal relationships. Cultural norms that value appearance and glorify thinness as beauty are factors, as are weight-based shame, peer comparisons, and weight bias.[31] Physical factors are thought to include an imbalance of neurotransmitters and genetic susceptibility.[32]

Bulimia Nervosa

Individuals with **bulimia nervosa** often binge on large amounts of food—often with a feeling of being out of control—and

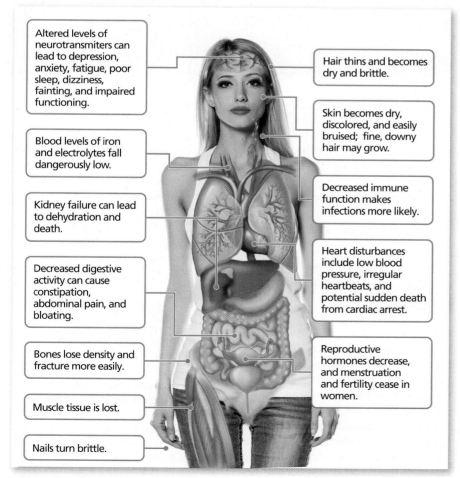

Altered levels of neurotransmitters can lead to depression, anxiety, fatigue, poor sleep, dizziness, fainting, and impaired functioning.

Blood levels of iron and electrolytes fall dangerously low.

Kidney failure can lead to dehydration and death.

Decreased digestive activity can cause constipation, abdominal pain, and bloating.

Bones lose density and fracture more easily.

Muscle tissue is lost.

Nails turn brittle.

Hair thins and becomes dry and brittle.

Skin becomes dry, discolored, and easily bruised; fine, downy hair may grow.

Decreased immune function makes infections more likely.

Heart disturbances include low blood pressure, irregular heartbeats, and potential sudden death from cardiac arrest.

Reproductive hormones decrease, and menstruation and fertility cease in women.

FIGURE 3 What Anorexia Nervosa Can Do to the Body

eating disorder A psychiatric disorder characterized by severe disturbances in body image and eating behaviors.

anorexia nervosa An eating disorder characterized by deliberate food restriction, self-starvation or extreme exercising to achieve weight loss, and an extremely distorted body image.

bulimia nervosa An eating disorder characterized by binge eating followed by inappropriate purging measures or compensatory behavior, such as vomiting or excessive exercise, to prevent weight gain.

then engage in some kind of purging or compensatory behavior, such as vomiting, taking laxatives, or exercising excessively, to lose the calories they have just consumed. People with bulimia are obsessed with their bodies, weight gain, and appearance, but unlike those with anorexia, their problem is often hidden from the public eye because their weight may fall within a normal range or they may be overweight. Bulimia nervosa is most common among adolescents and young adults. Up to 3 percent of adolescents girls and young women have bulimia; rates among young men are about 10 percent of the rates among young women.[33] **FIGURE 4** illustrates the physical symptoms and negative health consequences associated with bulimia nervosa.

A combination of genetic and environmental factors is thought to cause bulimia nervosa.[34] A family history of obesity, an underlying anxiety disorder, and an imbalance in neurotransmitters are all possible contributing factors. In support of the role of neurotransmitters, a study showed that brain circuitry involved in regulating impulsive behavior seems to be less active in women with bulimia than in healthy women.[35] However, it is unknown whether such differences exist before bulimia develops or arise as a consequence of the disorder.

Binge-Eating Disorder

Individuals with **binge-eating disorder** binge on food like those who have bulimia nervosa but do not purge or take excessive measures to lose the weight gained. Therefore, they are often clinically obese. Binge-eating episodes are typically characterized by eating large amounts of food rapidly, even

---

binge-eating disorder A type of eating disorder characterized by binging on food once a week or more, but not typically followed by a purge.

other specified feeding or eating disorder (OSFED) Eating disorders that are a true psychiatric illness but do not fit the strict diagnostic criteria for anorexia nervosa, bulimia nervosa, or binge-eating disorder.

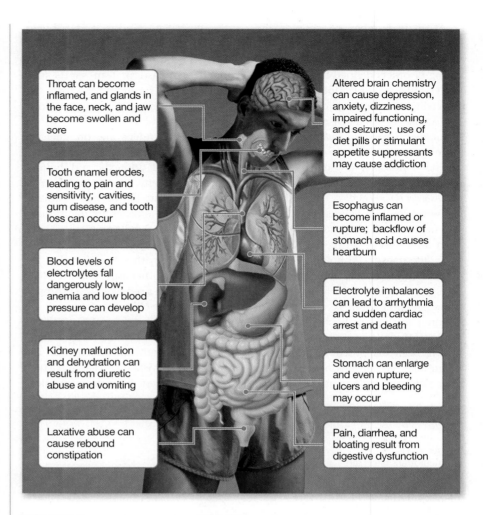

Throat can become inflamed, and glands in the face, neck, and jaw become swollen and sore

Tooth enamel erodes, leading to pain and sensitivity; cavities, gum disease, and tooth loss can occur

Blood levels of electrolytes fall dangerously low; anemia and low blood pressure can develop

Kidney malfunction and dehydration can result from diuretic abuse and vomiting

Laxative abuse can cause rebound constipation

Altered brain chemistry can cause depression, anxiety, dizziness, impaired functioning, and seizures; use of diet pills or stimulant appetite suppressants may cause addiction

Esophagus can become inflamed or rupture; backflow of stomach acid causes heartburn

Electrolyte imbalances can lead to arrhythmia and sudden cardiac arrest and death

Stomach can enlarge and even rupture; ulcers and bleeding may occur

Pain, diarrhea, and bloating result from digestive dysfunction

FIGURE 4 What Bulimia Nervosa Can Do to the Body

when the person does not feel hungry, and feeling guilty or depressed after overeating.[36]

A national survey reported a lifetime prevalence of binge-eating disorder in the study participants of 1.4 percent.[37]

Other Specified Feeding or Eating Disorder

The APA recognizes that some patterns of disordered eating qualify as a legitimate psychiatric illness but don't fit into the strict diagnostic criteria for anorexia, bulimia, or binge-eating disorder. Called **other specified feeding or eating disorders (OSFED)**, this group of disorders includes five specific subtypes: *night eating syndrome, purging disorder, binge-eating disorder of low frequency/limited duration, bulimia nervosa*

of low frequency/duration, and *atypical anorexia nervosa*. Atypical anorexia nervosa is defined in this category as displaying anorexic features without low weight.[38] All of these subtypes can cause remarkable distress or impairment but don't involve the full criteria of another feeding or eating disorder.

WHAT DO **YOU** THINK?

Is attention to the national obesity epidemic likely to worsen problems with eating disorders? Why or why not?

- What do you think can be done to increase awareness of eating disorders in the United States?
- Can you think of ways to prevent eating disorders?

Orthorexia Nervosa

Orthorexia nervosa is an unhealthy obsession with what would otherwise be healthy eating. The term *orthorexia* means "correct appetite," but in this disorder, what typically begins as a simple attempt to eat more healthfully can become a fixation with food quality and purity. People with orthorexia nervosa become hyperfocused on what and how much to eat and how to deal with eating mistakes. Although the DSM-5 does not categorize orthorexia nervosa as an eating disorder, the person's food choices eventually become so restricted that his or her health can suffer. Problems with social relationships and interactions might also result because the individual is obsessed with food.

Treatment for Eating Disorders

Because eating disorders are caused by a combination of factors, there are no simple solutions. Without treatment, approximately 20 percent of people with a serious eating disorder will die as a result; this is the highest fatality risk of any psychiatric disorder. With treatment, long-term full recovery rates range from 44 to 76 percent for anorexia nervosa and from 50 to 70 percent for bulimia nervosa.[39]

Treatment often focuses first on reducing the threat to life. Once the patient has been stabilized, long-term therapy focuses on the psychological, social, environmental, and physiological factors that led to the problem. Through therapy, the patient works on adopting new eating behaviors, building self-confidence, and finding healthy ways to deal with life's problems. Support groups can help the family and the individual learn positive actions and interactions. Treatment of an underlying anxiety disorder or depression may also be a focus.

Helping Someone with Disordered Eating

Although every situation is different, there are several things you can do if you suspect that someone you know is struggling with disordered eating or an eating disorder:[40]

- **Know the facts** about weight, nutrition, exercise, disordered eating, and eating disorders. Accurate information can help you reason against excuses the person may use to maintain a disordered eating pattern.
- **Recognize that eating disorders are more than the eating patterns** and that it is important to address all aspects of the disorder. Encouraging someone to simply change eating habits does not address the underlying problems that contributed to the development and maintenance of the disorder.
- **Be honest** and talk openly about your concerns.
- **Be caring, but be firm** because caring about your friend or loved one does not mean allowing him or her to manipulate you. The person must be responsible for his or her actions and the consequences of those actions. Avoid making threats that you cannot or will not uphold. Don't badger or get angry. Stay calm and be reassuring.
- **Compliment** the person's personality, successes, and accomplishments.
- **Be a good role model** for healthy eating, exercise, and self-acceptance.
- **Tell someone**, and don't wait until your friend or loved one's life is in danger. Addressing disordered eating patterns in their beginning stages offers the person the best chance for working through these issues and becoming healthy again.

There are many resources for people who are considering seeking help or finding out if they are at risk for developing an eating disorder. The National Eating Disorders Association has a general online screening tool that allows individuals to assess their own patterns to determine whether they should seek professional help (www.national eatingdisorders.org/online-eating-disorder-screening). The organization also has additional information and a helpline (1-800-931-2237) for guidance, treatment referrals, and support.[41]

orthorexia nervosa An eating disorder characterized by fixation on food quality and purity.

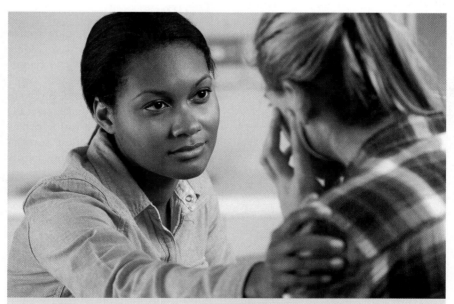

When talking to a friend about an eating disorder or disordered eating patterns, avoid casting blame, preaching, or offering unsolicited advice. Instead, be a good listener, let the person know that you care, and offer your support.

LO 3 | CAN TOO MUCH EXERCISE BE UNHEALTHY?

List the criteria, symptoms, and treatment for exercise disorders and syndromes such as muscle dysmorphia and female athlete triad.

Although exercise is generally beneficial, in excess it can be a problem. In addition to being a common compensatory behavior used by people with anorexia or bulimia, exercise can become a compulsion or contribute to a more complex disorder or syndrome such as muscle dysmorphia or the female athlete triad.

Compulsive Exercise

In a recent study, researchers showed that participants used excessive exercise or **compulsive exercise** as a way to regulate their emotions.[42] *Anorexia athletica* is characterized by obsessive exercise, which is not a *desire* to exercise but a *compulsion*. The person struggles with guilt and anxiety if he or she doesn't work out. Compulsive exercisers, like people with eating disorders, often define their self-worth externally. They overexercise to feel more in control of their lives. Disordered eating or an eating disorder is often part of the picture.

Compulsive exercise can contribute to a variety of injuries. It can also put

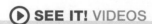

▶ SEE IT! VIDEOS

Can you go too far with extreme exercise? Watch **Young Boys Exercising to Extremes** on Mastering Health.

---

compulsive exercise A disorder characterized by a compulsion to engage in excessive amounts of exercise and feelings of guilt and anxiety if the level of exercise is perceived as inadequate.

muscle dysmorphia A body image disorder in which the person (usually a man) believes that his body is insufficiently lean or muscular.

female athlete triad A syndrome of three interrelated health problems seen in some female athletes: disordered eating, amenorrhea, and poor bone density.

amenorrhea The absence of menstruation.

significant stress on the heart, especially if combined with disordered eating. Psychologically, people who engage in compulsive exercise are often plagued by anxiety and/or depression. Their social lives and academic success can suffer as they fixate more and more on exercise.

Muscle Dysmorphia

Muscle dysmorphia is a form of body image disturbance and exercise disorder in which a person (usually male) believes that his body is insufficiently lean or muscular.[43] Men who have muscle dysmorphia believe, despite looking normal or even unusually brawny, that they look "puny." Because of their adherence to a meticulous diet and time-consuming workout schedule and their shame over their perceived appearance flaws, important social or occupational activities may fall by the wayside. Other behaviors characteristic of muscle dysmorphia include comparing oneself unfavorably to others, checking one's appearance in the mirror, and camouflaging one's appearance. Men with muscle dysmorphia also are likely to abuse anabolic steroids and dietary supplements.[44]

The Female Athlete Triad

In an effort to be the best, some women may put themselves at risk for developing a syndrome called the **female athlete triad**. *Triad* means "three," and the three interrelated problems are low energy (food) intake, typically prompted by disordered eating behaviors; menstrual dysfunction such as **amenorrhea**; and poor bone density (**FIGURE 5**).[45]

This cycle begins when a chronic pattern of low energy intake and intensive exercise alters normal body functions. For example, when a female athlete restricts her eating, she can deplete her body stores of essential nutrients. At the same time, her body begins to burn its stores of fat tissue for energy. Because adequate body fat is essential to maintaining healthy levels of the female reproductive hormone *estrogen*, when

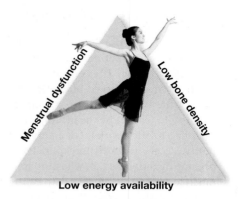

Low energy availability

FIGURE 5 The Female Athlete Triad

an athlete isn't getting enough food, estrogen levels decline. The body, using all calories to keep the athlete alive, then shuts down nonessential body functions, such as menstruation, causing amenorrhea and increasing her risk for future infertility. In addition, fat-soluble vitamins, calcium, and estrogen, all essential for dense, healthy bones, are not stored, so their depletion weakens her bones, leaving her at high risk for fracture and early osteoporosis.

Health at Every Size

Too many college students and their friends and loved ones struggle with disordered eating, eating disorders, and unhealthy exercise patterns. They fail to get proper nourishment and strengthen their bodies for the days and years to come. At the same time, most Americans who are overweight put on their extra pounds through high calorie intake and low energy expenditure. One model that takes all of these issues into account is the Health At Every Size (HAES) philosophy.[46] HAES posits that well-being and healthy eating and exercise habits are more important than any number on a scale, so all of us, no matter our size, should accept our size and not wait to be a different weight to begin self-acceptance. Thus, we can adopt a healthy lifestyle full of movement, nutritious foods, and mindful eating while embracing size diversity.

We need to recognize that humans come in a variety of shapes and sizes, and all of us need to work toward our healthiest selves, which are all deserving of love and respect.

LIVE IT! ASSESS YOURSELF

An interactive version of this assessment is available online in Mastering Health.

ASSESS YOURSELF

Are Your Efforts to Be Thin Sensible—Or Are You Spinning Out of Control?

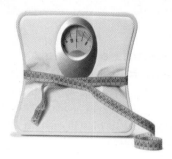

1. I constantly calculate numbers of fat grams and calories.   T   F
2. I weigh myself often and find myself obsessed with the number on the scale.   T   F
3. I exercise to burn calories and not for health or enjoyment.   T   F
4. I sometimes feel out of control while eating.   T   F
5. I often go on extreme diets.   T   F
6. I engage in rituals to get me through mealtimes and/or secretively binge.   T   F
7. Weight loss, dieting, and controlling my food intake have become my major concerns.   T   F
8. I feel ashamed, disgusted, or guilty after eating.   T   F
9. I constantly worry about the weight, shape, and/or size of my body.   T   F
10. I feel that my identity and value are based on how I look or how much I weigh.   T   F

If any of these statements is true for you, you could be dealing with disordered eating. If so, talk about it. Tell a friend, parent, teacher, coach, youth group leader, spiritual mentor, doctor, counselor, or nutritionist what you're going through. Check out the NEDA's Sharing with EEEase handout at www .nationaleatingdisorders.org/sharing-eeease for help planning what to say the first time you talk to someone about your eating and exercise habits.

Source: Adapted from "NEDA Screening for Eating Disorders" by the National Eating Disorders Association (NEDA) and Screening for Mental Health, Inc. (SMH), from NEDA website. Copyright © 2013 NEDA and SMH. Reprinted with permission.

YOUR PLAN FOR CHANGE

The ASSESS YOURSELF activity gives you a chance to evaluate your feelings about your body. Following are some steps you can take to improve your body image.

TODAY, YOU CAN:

☐ Talk back to the media. Write letters to advertisers and magazines that depict unhealthy and unrealistic body types. Boycott their products, or start a blog commenting on harmful body image messages in the media.

☐ Just for today, eat the recommended number of servings from every food group at every meal, and enjoy the recommended amount of physical activity without counting calories.

WITHIN THE NEXT TWO WEEKS, YOU CAN:

☐ Find a photograph of a person you admire for his or her contributions to humanity. Put it up next to your mirror to remind yourself that true beauty comes from within and benefits others.

☐ Start a journal. Each day, record one thing you are grateful for that has nothing to do with your appearance. At the end of each day, record one small thing you did to make someone else's world a little brighter.

BY THE END OF THE SEMESTER, YOU CAN:

☐ Establish a group of friends who support you for who you are, not what you look like, and who get the same support from you. Form a group on a favorite social networking site, and keep in touch, especially when you feel troubled by self-defeating thoughts or have the urge to engage in unhealthy behaviors.

☐ Borrow from the library or purchase one or more of the many books on body image now available, and read them.

STUDY **PLAN**

CHAPTER **REVIEW**

LO **1** | What Is Body Image?

■ Body image refers to what you believe or emotionally feel about your body's shape, weight, and general appearance and how you behave in response to your beliefs and thoughts about your body.

LO **2** | Disordered Eating and Eating Disorders

■ Millions of Americans struggle with an eating disorder at some point in their lives. Media, family, community, cultural groups, and psychological and physiological factors all influence body image.

■ Anorexia nervosa is a persistent, chronic eating disorder characterized by deliberate food restriction and severe, life-threatening weight loss.

■ Individuals with bulimia nervosa rapidly consume large amounts of food and purge either with vomiting or laxative abuse or by using nonpurging techniques such as excessive exercise and/or fasting.

■ Individuals with binge-eating disorder binge on food but do not take excessive measures to lose weight.

■ Orthorexia nervosa is an unhealthy obsession with a rigid diet focused on food quality and purity.

■ Eating disorders are caused by a combination of many factors, and there are no simple solutions. Without treatment, approximately 20 percent of people with a serious eating disorder will die from it. Long-term treatment focuses on the psychological, social, environmental, and physiological factors that have led to the problem.

LO **3** | Can Too Much Exercise Be Unhealthy?

■ Compulsive exercise is used as a way to regulate emotions. *Anorexia athletica* is characterized by a compulsion to exercise, resulting in guilt and anxiety when one doesn't work out.

■ Muscle dysmorphia, typically found in men, is characterized by a distorted belief that the person's body is insufficiently muscular or lean. As a result, the person spends an inordinate amount of time working out or using unhealthy methods to increase muscle mass.

■ The female triad syndrome occurs when female athletes restrict their food intake and train intensively, altering their normal body functions. Three interrelated problems occur: low energy intake; menstrual dysfunction, and poor bone density.

■ Treatment requires a multidisciplinary approach involving the coach, psychologist, and family members.

POP **QUIZ**

LO **1** | What Is Body Image?

1. Which of the statements about body image is false?
   a. The obsession with having big biceps or being able to wear size zero skinny jeans began in the late 1990s.
   b. Concerns about weight seems to be central to many people's dissatisfaction with their body.
   c. People who have been diagnosed with a body image disorder show differences in their brain's ability to regulate neurotransmitters.
   d. Having a positive body image is possessing a true perception of your appearance.

LO **2** | Disordered Eating and Eating Disorders

2. Orthorexia nervosa is
   a. an excessive focus on eating foods that are high in calcium and vitamin D.
   b. characterized by a fixation on the quality and purity of food.
   c. an obsession with bone health.
   d. a condition that results from binging and purging.

LO **3** | Can Too Much Exercise Be Unhealthy?

3. Muscle dysmorphia
   a. is a muscular disease that results from an autoimmune disorder.
   b. occurs only in women.
   c. results in menstrual dysfunction.
   d. occurs most often in men.

*Answers to the Pop Quiz questions can be found on page A-1. If you answered a question incorrectly, review the section identified by the Learning Outcome. For even more study tools, visit **Mastering Health**.*

12

Improving Your Personal Fitness

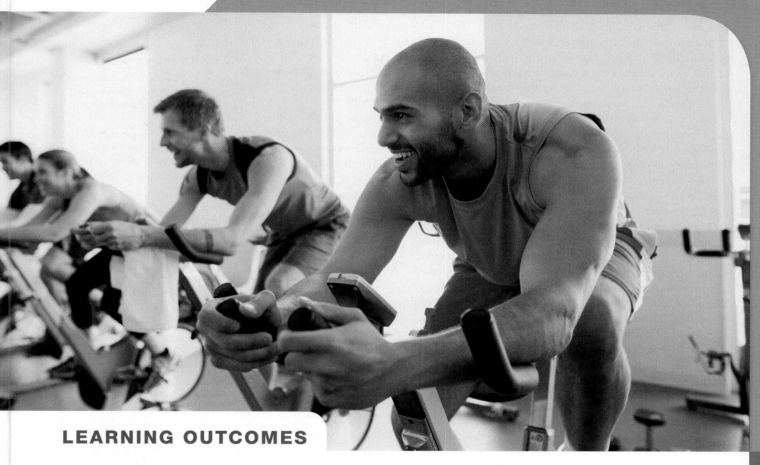

LEARNING OUTCOMES

LO **1** Describe the health benefits of being physically active.

LO **2** Distinguish between the types of physical activity required for health, physical fitness, and performance.

LO **3** Identify lifestyle obstacles to physical activity, describe ways to surmount them, and make a commitment to getting physically fit.

LO **4** Understand and be able to use the FITT (frequency, intensity, time, and type) principles for the health-related components of physical fitness.

LO **5** Devise a plan to implement your safe and effective fitness program.

LO **6** Describe optimal food and fluid consumption recommendations for exercise and recovery.

LO **7** Explain how to prevent and treat common exercise injuries.

Most Americans are aware of the wide range of physical, social, and mental health benefits of physical activity and know that they should be physically active on a regular basis. The physiological changes in the body that result from regular physical activity reduce the likelihood of coronary artery disease, high blood pressure, type 2 diabetes, obesity, and other chronic diseases. Furthermore, regularly engaging in physical activity helps to control stress, increases self-esteem, and contributes to positive mood.

Despite knowing the importance of physical activity for health and wellness, most people are not active enough to get these optimal health benefits. Recent statistics indicate that 50.9 percent of American adults met the 2008 Physical Activity Guidelines for Americans for aerobic exercise, and 30.4 percent met the guidelines for strengthening exercise.[1] However, only 20.5 percent reported meeting the guidelines for both aerobic and strengthening exercise, and 25.9 percent reported no leisure-time physical activities.[2] These statistics are based on activity reported during one's "down" time in the previous month.[3] The growing percentage of Americans who live physically inactive lives has been linked to the current high incidences of obesity, type 2 diabetes, and other chronic physical and mental health diseases.[4]

In general, college students are more physically active than older adults, but a recent survey indicated that 41.6 percent of college women and 49 percent of college men do not perform the recommended 3 to 5 days of moderate to vigorous physical activity per week.[5] Extracurricular activities, screen time, studying, and social activities can be physical activity barriers for college students.

LO 1 | PHYSICAL ACTIVITY FOR HEALTH

Describe the health benefits of being physically active.

Physical activity is all body movements produced by skeletal muscles that result in substantial increases in energy expenditure. Physical activities can be light, moderate, or vigorous in intensity. For example, walking on a flat surface at a casual pace requires little effort (light), whereas walking uphill is more intense and harder to do (moderate). Jogging and running are examples of vigorous physical activities. There are three general categories of physical activity, defined by the purpose for which they are done: leisure-time physical activity, occupational physical activity, and lifestyle physical activity.

Exercise is defined as planned, repetitive, and structured bodily movement undertaken to maintain or improve health or any number of physical fitness components—for

physical activity All body movements produced by skeletal muscles, resulting in substantial increases in energy expenditure.

exercise Planned, structured, and repetitive bodily movement done to improve or maintain one or more components of physical fitness.

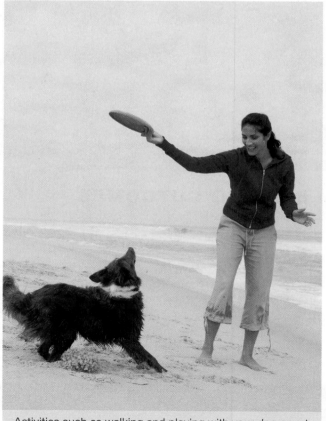

Activities such as walking and playing with your dog count toward your recommended daily physical activity.

example, cardiorespiratory fitness, muscular strength or endurance, or flexibility. Although all exercise is physical activity, not all physical activity would be considered exercise. For example, walking from your car to class is physical activity, whereas going for a brisk 30-minute walk to maintain a healthy body weight is considered exercise, which is also classified as leisure-time physical activity.

Adding more physical activity to your day can benefit your health.[6] We know that physical activity is good for health, and we also know that physical inactivity contributes to increased risk of negative health outcomes. Physical inactivity is defined as not meeting the minimum activity recommendations for health (see **TABLE 12.1**).[7] When considering major chronic diseases, it is estimated that physical inactivity is responsible for 30 percent of the cases of ischemic heart disease, 27 percent of cases of type 2 diabetes, and 21 to 25 percent of cases of breast and colon cancer worldwide.[8]

Sedentary time is generally considered time spent while sitting or reclining in an activity that does not increase energy expenditure more than 1.5 times the resting level (1.5 **METs**, or metabolic equivalents).[9] However, sedentary time should not be confused with inactivity. Common sedentary activities include screen time, reading, and driving. Keep in mind that someone who gets regular activity can also participate in high levels of sedentary behaviors. Individuals who exercise but still report a lot of sedentary time have been referred to as "active couch potatoes."[10]

Although regular exercise and high levels of physical activity can protect against disease and premature death, sedentary time has an independent effect on disease and mortality.[11] Research shows that risk for cardiovascular disease, cancers, and type 2 diabetes increases with high amounts of sitting time.[12]

Regular participation in physical activity improves more than 50 different physiological, metabolic, and psychological

ONLY 20.5% of American adults **MEET GUIDELINES** for both cardiorespiratory and muscular fitness.

sedentary Activity that expends no more than 1.5 times the resting energy level while seated or reclined.

MET A metabolic equivalent or resting level of energy expenditure ($3.5 \text{ ml·kg}^{-1}\text{·min}^{-1}$).

TABLE 12.1 | 2008 Physical Activity Guidelines for Americans*

	Key Guidelines for Health**	For Additional Fitness or Weight Loss Benefits**	Additional Exercises
Adults	150 min/week moderate-intensity physical activity OR 75 min/week of vigorous-intensity physical activity OR Equivalent combination of moderate- and vigorous-intensity physical activity (e.g., 100 min moderate intensity + 25 min min vigorous intensity)	300 min/week moderate-intensity physical activity OR 150 min/week of vigorous-intensity physical activity OR Equivalent combination of moderate- and vigorous-intensity physical activity (e.g., 200 min moderate intensity + 50 min vigorous intensity) OR More than the previously described amounts	Muscle-strengthening activities for all the major muscle groups at least 2 days/week
Older adults	If unable to follow above guidelines, then as much physical activity as their condition allows	If unable to follow above guidelines, then as much physical activity as their condition allows	In addition to muscle-strengthening activities, those with limited mobility should add exercises to improve balance and reduce risk of falling.
Children and youth	60 min or more of moderate- or vigorous-intensity physical activity daily; should include at least 3 days/week or vigorous activity	At least 60 min of moderate- or vigorous-intensity physical activity on every day of the week	Include muscle-strengthening activities at least 3 days/week. Include bone-strengthening activities at least 3 days/week.

*An advisory committee has been established to review research related to the current guidelines and health and to discuss the guidelines with the public. The goal is to have the second edition of the *Physical Activity Guidelines for Health* available for the public in 2018. Check out the website for more information (https://health.gov/paguidelines/second-edition).

**Avoid inactivity (some activity is better than none), accumulate physical activity in sessions of 10 minutes or more at one time, and spread activity throughout the week.

Source: Office of Disease Prevention and Health Promotion, U.S. Department of Health and Human Services, *2008 Physical Activity Guidelines for Americans: Be Active, Healthy, and Happy!* (Washington, DC: U.S. Department of Health and Human Services, 2008), ODPHP Publication no. U0036, www.health.gov.

aspects of human life. **FIGURE 12.1** summarizes some of these major health-related benefits.

Reduced Risk of Cardiovascular Diseases

Aerobic activity is good for your cardiovascular system (the heart, lungs, and blood vessels) and it reduces the risk for heart-related diseases and premature death. High blood pressure (hypertension), unhealthy cholesterol profiles (dyslipidemia), coronary heart disease, and stroke are among the cardiovascular conditions prevented or improved by physical activity. Additionally, regularly getting enough physical activity eases the performance of everyday tasks.

Regular physical activity of moderate intensity can reduce hypertension, or chronic high blood pressure, a cardiovascular disease itself and a significant risk factor for other cardiovascular diseases and stroke.[13] Regular aerobic activity also improves the blood lipid profile. It typically increases high-density lipoproteins (HDLs, or "good" cholesterol), which are associated with

lower risk for coronary artery disease because of their role in removing plaque buildup in the arteries.[14] Triglycerides (a blood fat) typically decrease with aerobic activity. Low-density lipoproteins (LDLs, or "bad" cholesterol) and total cholesterol are also often improved with exercise.[15]

Reduced Risk of Metabolic Syndrome and Type 2 Diabetes

Regular physical activity reduces the risk of *metabolic syndrome*, a combination of risk factors that produces a synergistic increase in risk of heart disease and diabetes.[16] Specifically, metabolic syndrome includes high blood pressure, abdominal obesity, low levels of HDLs, high levels of triglycerides, and impaired glucose tolerance.[17] Regular participation in moderate-intensity physical activities reduces risk for each factor individually and collectively.[18]

Research indicates that a healthy dietary intake combined with sufficient physical activity could prevent many of the current cases of type 2 diabetes.[19] Meeting the recommendation

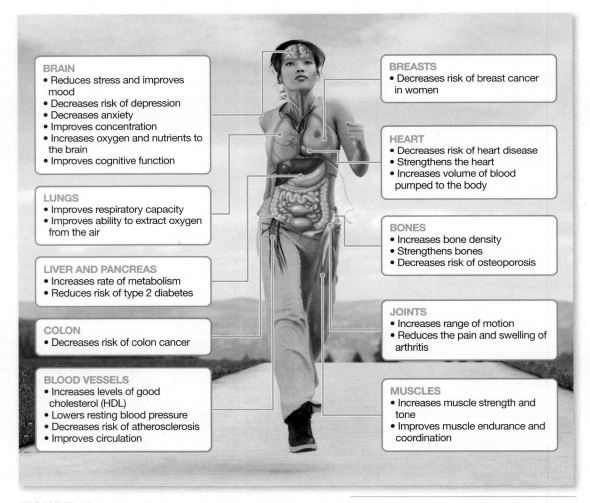

BRAIN
• Reduces stress and improves mood
• Decreases risk of depression
• Decreases anxiety
• Improves concentration
• Increases oxygen and nutrients to the brain
• Improves cognitive function

LUNGS
• Improves respiratory capacity
• Improves ability to extract oxygen from the air

LIVER AND PANCREAS
• Increases rate of metabolism
• Reduces risk of type 2 diabetes

COLON
• Decreases risk of colon cancer

BLOOD VESSELS
• Increases levels of good cholesterol (HDL)
• Lowers resting blood pressure
• Decreases risk of atherosclerosis
• Improves circulation

BREASTS
• Decreases risk of breast cancer in women

HEART
• Decreases risk of heart disease
• Strengthens the heart
• Increases volume of blood pumped to the body

BONES
• Increases bone density
• Strengthens bones
• Decreases risk of osteoporosis

JOINTS
• Increases range of motion
• Reduces the pain and swelling of arthritis

MUSCLES
• Increases muscle strength and tone
• Improves muscle endurance and coordination

FIGURE 12.1 Some Health Benefits of Regular Exercise

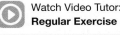 Watch Video Tutor: **Health Benefits of Regular Exercise** in Mastering Health.

of 150 minutes of moderate- to vigorous-intensity aerobic activity per week has been shown to improve glucose tolerance and insulin sensitivity to manage diabetes.[20] (See **Focus On: Minimizing Your Risk for Diabetes** for more.)

Reduced Cancer Risk

After decades of research, most cancer epidemiologists believe that 25 to 37 percent of cancers can be avoided by healthier lifestyle and environmental choices.[21] Recent research assessing the impact of sedentary time on cancer indicates that the risk for several types of cancer is associated with high levels of sedentary time.[22] The American Cancer Society reports that approximately 20 percent of cancers are linked to physical inactivity and dietary choices. Research shows that up to 30 percent of some cancers could be prevented with regular physical activity and healthy diet choices (the number varies according to cancer site).[23] For more see Chapter 13.

Improved Bone Mass and Reduced Risk of Osteoporosis

A common affliction for older people is *osteoporosis*, a disease characterized by low bone mass and deterioration of bone tissue, which increases fracture risk. Regular weight-bearing and strength-building physical activities are recommended to maintain bone health and prevent osteoporotic fractures. However, it appears that the full bone-related benefits of physical activity can be achieved only with sufficient hormone

levels (estrogen in women, testosterone in men) and adequate calcium, vitamin D, and total caloric intakes.[24]

Improved Weight Management

For many people, the desire to lose weight or maintain a healthy weight is the main reason for physical activity. On the most basic level, physical activity requires your body to generate energy through calorie expenditure; if calories expended exceed calories consumed over a span of time, the net result will be weight loss. **FIGURE 12.2** shows the caloric cost of various activities when done for 30 minutes.

Physical activity also has a direct positive effect on metabolic rate, keeping it elevated for several hours after vigorous physical activities.[25] This increase in metabolic rate can lead to body composition changes that favor weight management. After you lose weight, increased physical activity also improves your chances of maintaining the weight loss. If you are currently at a healthy body weight, regular physical activity can prevent significant weight gain.

Improved Immunity

Research shows that regular moderate-intensity physical activity reduces individual susceptibility to disease through improving the body's ability to fight infections.[26] Regular exercise has also been shown to reduce body inflammation that is associated with higher risk of chronic conditions such as cardiovascular disease or cancer.[27] Often, the relationship of physical activity to immunity or, more specifically to disease

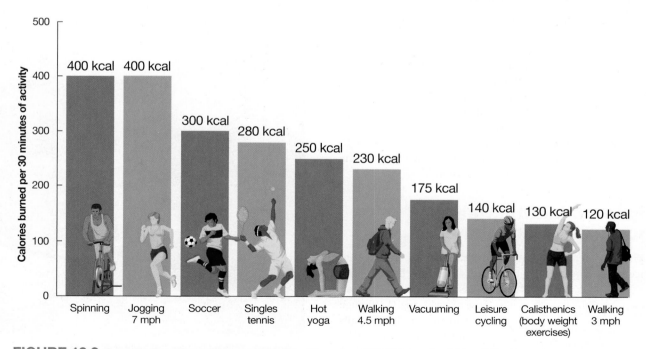

FIGURE 12.2 Calories Burned by Different Activities The more difficult your physical activity, the more energy you expend. The estimated number of calories burned by engaging in various moderate and vigorous activities are listed for 30 minutes of activity. Note that the number of calories burned depends on body weight. Generally, the higher your body weight, the greater the number of calories you'll burn.

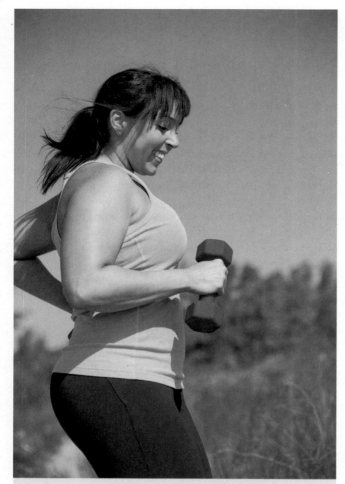

If you want to lose weight, you need to move more and often.

susceptibility is described as a J-shaped curve. Susceptibility to disease decreases with moderate activity but then increases as you move to extreme levels of physical activity or exercise or if you continue to exercise without adequate recovery time and/or dietary intake.[28] Athletes engaging in marathon-type events or very intense physical training programs have been shown to be at greater risk for upper respiratory tract infections in the first 8 hours after an intense exercise session.[29]

Improved Mental Health and Stress Management

People who engage in regular physical activity are likely to notice psychological benefits, such as feeling better about themselves and an overall sense of well-being.[30] Although these mental health benefits are difficult to quantify, they are frequently mentioned as reasons for continuing to be physically active. Learning new skills, developing increased

⏵ **SEE IT!** VIDEOS

Get moving to benefit your brain in a variety of ways! Watch **New Study Shows Exercise May Build Brain Power** in the Study Area of Mastering Health.

ability and capacity in recreational activities, and sticking with a physical activity plan also improve self-esteem.[31] In addition, regular physical activity can improve a person's physical appearance, further increasing self-esteem.[32]

There is increasing evidence that regular physical activity positively affects cognitive function across the lifespan. Research has associated regular activity and fitness (aerobic and muscular) levels with improved academic performance in school, and higher levels of sedentary time have been associated with poorer performance on some measures.[33] Study-related fatigue and performance on laboratory tasks to assess executive cognitive functions improved with regular aerobic exercise, and these effects were seen both immediately after the intervention and during follow-ups 1 and 3 months later.[34] Further, first-year medical students who reported using the recreation center frequently in the 3 weeks before an exam had higher scores on exams than did those using the rec center less frequently.[35] The most frequent use was associated with the highest exam scores.[36] Regular aerobic activity, even when initiated as an adult, has also been associated with reduced risk for and improvement of dementia and Alzheimer's disease in adults.[37]

Longer Lifespan

Experts have long debated the relationship between physical activity and longevity. Several studies indicate significant decreases in long-term health risk and increases in years lived, particularly among people who have several risk factors and who use physical activity as a means of risk reduction.[38] The greatest benefits from physical activity occur in sedentary

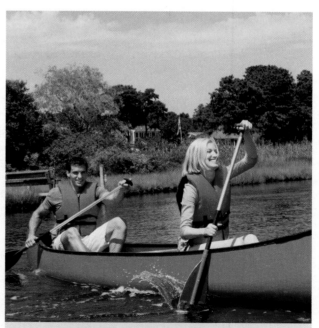

Although physical activity stimulates the stress response, a physically fit body adapts efficiently to the eustress of it, and as a result is better able to tolerate and effectively manage stress.

individuals who add a little physical activity to their lives, with additional benefits as physical activity levels increase.[39] Additionally, data from a national sample show that a sedentary lifestyle is associated with a reduced ability to perform activities of daily living.[40] The more sedentary time adults report, the greater the reduction in their ability to perform activities of daily living. It is not just structured exercise that is important, but moving as much as possible and sitting as little as possible.

PHYSICAL ACTIVITY FOR FITNESS AND PERFORMANCE

Distinguish between the types of physical activity required for health, physical fitness, and performance.

Physical fitness refers to a set of attributes that are either health or skill related.

Health-Related Components of Physical Fitness

The health-related attributes—cardiorespiratory fitness, muscular strength and endurance, flexibility, and body composition—allow you to perform moderate- to vigorous-intensity physical activities on a regular basis without getting too tired and with energy left over to handle physical or mental emergencies. FIGURE 12.3 identifies the major health-related components of physical fitness.

Cardiorespiratory Fitness **Cardiorespiratory fitness** is the ability of the heart, lungs, and blood vessels to supply the body with oxygen efficiently. The primary category of physical activity that is known to improve cardiorespiratory fitness is **aerobic exercise**. The word *aerobic* means "with oxygen" and describes any type of exercise that requires oxygen to make energy for prolonged activity. Aerobic activities, such as swimming, cycling, and jogging, are among the best exercises for improving or maintaining cardiorespiratory fitness.

Cardiorespiratory fitness is measured by determining **aerobic capacity (power)**, the volume of oxygen the muscles consume during exercise. Maximal aerobic power (commonly written as VO_{2max}) is defined as the maximum volume of oxygen that the muscles consume per minute during maximal exercise. The most common measure of maximal aerobic capacity is a walk or run test on a treadmill. For greatest accuracy, this is done in a lab with specialized equipment and technicians to measure the precise amount of oxygen entering and exiting the body during the exercise session. To get a more general sense of cardiorespiratory fitness, submaximal tests performed in the classroom or field can predict maximal aerobic capacity.

Muscular Strength **Muscular strength** is the amount of force a muscle or group of muscles can generate in one contraction. The most common way to assess the strength of a particular

physical fitness A balance of health-related attributes that allows you to perform moderate to vigorous physical activities on a regular basis and complete daily physical tasks without undue fatigue.

cardiorespiratory fitness The ability of the heart, lungs, and blood vessels to supply oxygen to skeletal muscles during sustained physical activity.

aerobic exercise Prolonged exercise that requires oxygen to make energy for activity.

aerobic capacity (power) The functional status of the cardiorespiratory system; refers specifically to the volume of oxygen the muscles consume during exercise.

muscular strength The maximal force that a muscle is capable of exerting in one contraction.

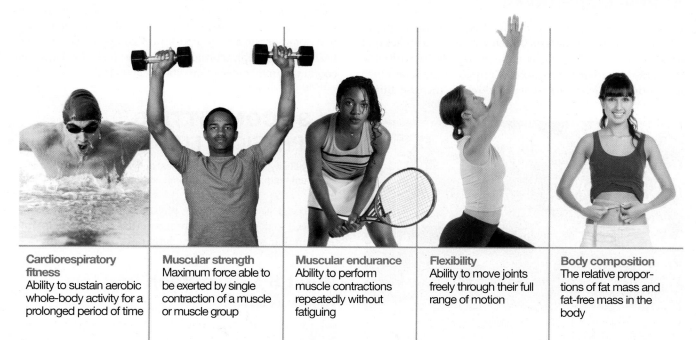

Cardiorespiratory fitness
Ability to sustain aerobic whole-body activity for a prolonged period of time

Muscular strength
Maximum force able to be exerted by single contraction of a muscle or muscle group

Muscular endurance
Ability to perform muscle contractions repeatedly without fatiguing

Flexibility
Ability to move joints freely through their full range of motion

Body composition
The relative proportions of fat mass and fat-free mass in the body

FIGURE 12.3 Health-Related Components of Physical Fitness

**one repetition maximum
(1 RM)** The amount of weight or resistance that can be lifted or moved only once.

muscular endurance A muscle's ability to exert force repeatedly without fatiguing or the ability to sustain a muscular contraction for a length of time.

flexibility The range of motion, or the amount of movement possible, at a particular joint or series of joints.

body composition The relative proportions of fat and fat-free (muscle, bone, water, organs) tissues in the body.

muscle or muscle group is to measure the maximum amount of weight you can move one time (and no more), or your **one repetition maximum (1 RM)**.

Muscular Endurance

Muscular endurance is the ability of a muscle or group of muscles to exert force repeatedly without fatigue or the ability to sustain a muscular contraction. The more repetitions you can perform successfully (e.g., push-ups) or the longer you can hold a certain position (e.g., flexed arm hang), the greater your muscular endurance.

Flexibility

Flexibility refers to the range of motion, or the amount of movement possible, at a particular joint or series of joints. The greater the range of motion, the greater is the flexibility. Various tests measure the flexibility of the body's joints, including range-of-motion tests for specific joints.

Body Composition

Body composition is the fifth and final health-related component of physical fitness. Body composition describes the relative proportions and distribution of fat and fat-free (muscle, bone, water, organs) tissues in the body. (For more details on body composition, including its measurement, see Chapter 11.)

Skill-Related Components of Physical Fitness

In addition to the five health-related components of physical fitness, physical fitness for athletes involves attributes that improve the ability to perform athletic tasks. These attributes, called the *skill-related components* of physical fitness, also help recreational athletes and general exercisers increase fitness

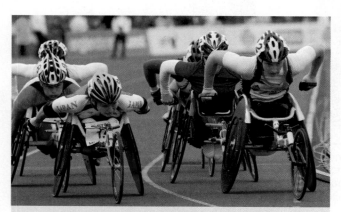

It is important for all people, including those with disabilities, to develop optimal levels of physical fitness and participate in physical activities they enjoy, possibly including competitive sports.

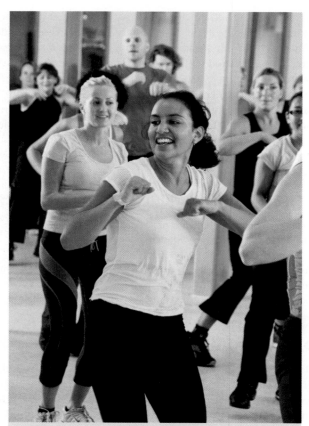

One great way to motivate yourself is to sign up for an exercise class. The structure, schedule, social interaction, and challenge of learning a new skill can be the motivation you need to get moving.

levels and their ability to perform daily tasks. The skill-related components of physical fitness (also called sport skills) are *agility, balance, coordination, power, speed,* and *reaction time.* Note that some of the skill-related fitness components can affect health. For example, consider the importance of balance and coordination for older adults who are at increased risk for falls.

LO 3 | COMMITTING TO PHYSICAL FITNESS

Identify lifestyle obstacles to physical activity, describe ways to surmount them, and make a commitment to getting physically fit.

To succeed at incorporating physical fitness into your life, you need to design a fitness program that takes obstacles into account that is founded on the activities you enjoy most.

What If I Have Been Inactive for a While?

If you have been physically inactive for the past few months or longer, first make sure that your health care provider clears you for exercise. Consider consulting a personal trainer or fitness instructor to help you get started. In this phase of a fitness program, known as the *initial conditioning stage*, you may begin at levels that are lower than those recommended for physical fitness. For example, you might start your cardiorespiratory program by simply moving more each day and reducing your sedentary time. As you make the decision to be more active and reduce your sedentary time, assess your environment to evaluate how it supports and/or impedes physical activity. Be mindful of your physical and social environments to determine how you can become more active. You might notice that you walk past the stairs to get to the elevator in your dorm or that your friends sit more than they move in their free time.

Small changes can get you started on a path to increased activity and improved health. Take the stairs instead of the elevator, walk farther from your car to the store, and plan for organized movement each day, such as a 10- to 15-minute walk. In addition, you can start your muscle fitness program with simple body weight exercises, emphasizing proper technique and body alignment before adding any resistance.

Overcoming Common Obstacles to Physical Activity

People have real and perceived barriers that prevent regular physical activity, ranging from personal ("I do not have time") to environmental ("I do not have a safe place to be active") to social ("I do not have a workout partner"). Some people may be reluctant to exercise if they are overweight, feel embarrassed to work out with their more "fit" friends, or feel that they lack the knowledge and skills required.

Think about your obstacles to physical activity, and write them down. Consider anything that gets in your way of exercising, however minor. Be as specific as possible, and be honest with yourself. Once you have honestly evaluated why you are not as physically active as you want to be, review **TABLE 12.2** for suggestions on overcoming your hurdles.

Incorporating Physical Activity in Your Life, Mindfully

When you design your fitness program, there are several factors to consider. Here are a few ways to incorporate physical activity into your daily life, mindfully:

- **Be Mindful of Your Own Preferences.** Choose activities that are appropriate for you, that are convenient, and that you genuinely enjoy. For example, you might choose jogging because you like to run and there are beautiful trails nearby. Don't swim if you don't like the water and the pool is difficult to get to.

TABLE 12.2 | Overcoming Obstacles to Physical Activity

Obstacle	Possible Solution
Lack of time	■ Look at your schedule. Where can you find 30-minute time slots? Perhaps you need to focus on shorter times (10 minutes or more) throughout the day. ■ Multitask. Read while riding an exercise bike, or listen to lectures or podcasts while walking. ■ Be physically active during your lunch and study breaks as well as between classes. Skip rope, or throw a Frisbee with a friend. ■ Select activities that require less time, such as brisk walking or jogging. ■ Ride your bike to class, or park (or get off the bus) farther from your destination.
Social influence	■ Invite family and friends to be active with you. ■ Join an exercise class to meet new people. ■ Explain the importance of exercise and your commitment to physical activity to people who may not support your efforts. ■ Find a role model to support your efforts. ■ Plan for physically active dates. Go for a walk, dancing, or bowling.
Lack of motivation, willpower, or energy	■ Schedule your workout time just as you would any other important commitment. ■ Enlist the help of an exercise partner to make you accountable for working out. ■ Give yourself an incentive. ■ Schedule your workouts when you feel most energetic. ■ Remind yourself that exercise gives you more energy. ■ Get things ready; for example, if you choose to walk in the morning, set out your clothes and shoes the night before.
Lack of resources	■ Select an activity that requires minimal equipment, such as walking, jogging, jumping rope, or calisthenics. ■ Identify inexpensive resources on campus or in the community. ■ Use active forms of transportation. ■ Take advantage of no-cost opportunities, such as playing catch in the park or green space on campus.

Source: Adapted from National Center for Chronic Disease Prevention and Health Promotion, "How Can I Overcome Barriers to Physical Activity?," Updated May 2011, www.cdc.gov.

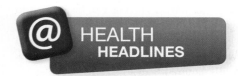
TRANSPORT YOURSELF!

Many people are embracing a movement toward more active transportation. *Active transportation* means using your own power to get from place to place—whether walking, riding a bike, skateboarding, or roller skating. A bicycle is an excellent and cost-effective way to get to and around campus. Check at http://bikeshare.com to see whether your city has a bike share program. Here are a few reasons to make active transportation a bigger part of your life:

- **You will exercise more.** People who use active forms of transportation to complete errands are more likely to meet physical activity guidelines. Research shows that cycling for active transport is associated with lower risk for cardiovascular disease, cancer, and all-cause mortality.
- **It can save you money.** It is much cheaper to own a bike than a car when you consider gas and maintenance. It is estimated that it is costs 30 times more to maintain a car than a bike.
- **It may save you time.** Commutes of 3 to 5 miles are usually as fast or faster by bike than by car.

Hop on that bike and join the green revolution! Active transportation is an excellent want to add physical activity to your day, especially on nonexercise days.

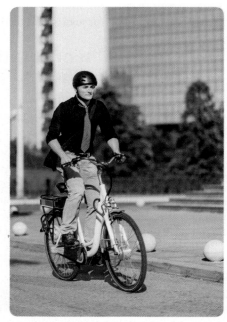

- **You will enjoy being outdoors.** Research is emerging on the physical and mental health benefits of nature

and being outdoors. We spend so much time inside, with recirculated air and artificial lighting, that our bodies are deficient in fresh air and sunlight.

- **It's good for the planet.** More active commuters means fewer cars on the roads and less traffic congestion. Transportation accounts for approximately 30 percent of greenhouse gas emission, so choosing to walk or bike instead of driving can have a significant impact on the environment. Swapping waking or cycling for the car when taking short trips is estimated to save over 10 billion gallons of fuel per year.

Sources: C. Celis-Morales et al., "Association between Active Commuting and Incident Cardiovascular Disease, Cancer, and Mortality: Prospective Cohort Study," *BMJ* 357 (2017): 1456; Momentum Staff, "The Top 10 Reasons Everyone Should Bike to Work," June 2, 2015, https://momentummag.com/top-10-reasons-you-should-bike-to-work; Rails-to-Trails Conservancy, "Investing in Trails: Cost-Effective Improvements—for Everyone," 2013, www.railstotrails.org/resourcehandler.ashx?id=3629; U.S. Environmental Protection Agency, "Climate Change: What You Can Do: On the Road," Updated April 2014, www.epa.gov/climatechange/wycd/road.html; B. McKenzie, "Modes Less Traveled—Bicycling and Walking to Work in the United States: 2008–2012," U.S. Department of Commerce, May 2014, www.census.gov/prod/2014pubs/acs-25.pdf.

- **Be Mindful of Your Current Fitness Level.** Choose activities that make sense for your current fitness level. If you are overweight or have not exercised in months, start slowly, plan fun activities, and progress to more challenging physical activities as your physical fitness improves. You may choose to simply walk more in an attempt to achieve the recommended goal of 10,000 steps per day. Keep track with a pedometer or activity tracker.
- **Be Mindful of Opportunities to Increase Your Activity Levels.** Do you sit all day? Choose the elevator over the stairs? Park as close as you can to the front door or the store entrance? All of these instances could be opportunities for activity. Try to make physical activity a part of your routine by incorporating it into something you already have to do, such as getting to class or work.
- **Green Your Routine.** Outdoor exercise (sometimes called green exercise) is a great way to get mental health benefits on top of the physical ones.[41] Your campus surroundings may offer many opportunities to be active—and present. Take a walk through the campus, purposefully noticing your outdoor spaces. Open green space is a great place for a

yoga mat or meditating. Stadium stairs and benches can be incorporated into an exercise routine, and even trees can become exercise equipment.

See the Health Headlines box for more on using your surroundings and transportation for fitness.

LO 4 | CREATING YOUR OWN FITNESS PROGRAM

Understand and be able to use the FITT (frequency, intensity, time, and type) principles for the health-related components of physical fitness.

The first step in creating a personal physical fitness program is identifying your goals. Are you most concerned with being better at sports or feeling better about your body? Is your goal to manage stress or reduce your risk of chronic diseases? Perhaps your most vital goal will be to establish a realistic schedule of diverse physical activities that you can maintain and enjoy throughout your life. Your physical fitness goals and objectives should be both achievable for you and in line with what you truly want.

Set SMART Goals

To set successful goals, try using the SMART system. SMART goals are **s**pecific, **m**easurable, **a**ction-oriented, **r**ealistic, and **t**ime-oriented.

A vague goal would be "I will improve my fitness by exercising more." A SMART goal would be as follows:

- *Specific.* "I will participate in a resistance-training program that targets all of the major muscle groups 3 to 5 days per week."
- *Measurable.* "I will improve my fitness classification from the average classification to the above average classification."
- *Action-oriented.* "I will meet with a personal trainer to learn how to safely do resistance exercises and to plan a workout for the gym and home."
- *Realistic.* "I will increase the weight I can lift by 20 percent."
- *Time-oriented.* "I will try my new weight program for 8 weeks, then reassess."

Use the FITT Principle

To improve your health-related physical fitness (or performance-related physical fitness), use the **FITT** (frequency, intensity, time, and type)[42] principle to define your exercise program. The FITT prescription (**FIGURE 12.4**) uses the following criteria:

- **Frequency** refers to the number of times per week you need to engage in particular exercises to achieve the desired level of physical fitness in a particular component.

- **Intensity** refers to how hard your workout must be to achieve the desired level of physical fitness.
- **Time**, or *duration*, refers to how many minutes or repetitions of an exercise are required at a specified intensity during any one session to attain the desired level of physical fitness for each component.
- **Type** refers to what kind of exercises should be performed to improve the specific component of physical fitness.

The FITT Principle for Cardiorespiratory Fitness

The most effective aerobic exercises for building cardiorespiratory fitness are whole-body activities involving all the large muscle groups. The FITT prescription for cardiorespiratory fitness includes 3 to 5 days per week of vigorous, rhythmic, continuous activity at 64 to 96 percent of your estimated maximal heart rate for 20 to 60 minutes.[43]

Frequency The frequency of your program is related to your intensity. If you choose to do moderate-intensity exercises, you should aim for a frequency of at least 5 days (frequency drops to at least 3 days per week with vigorous-intensity activities). Newcomers to exercise can still improve by doing less-intense exercise (light to moderate level) but doing it more days each week. In this case, follow the recommendations from the Centers for Disease Control and Prevention for moderate physical activity (refer to **TABLE 12.1**).

Intensity The most commonly used methods to determine the intensity of cardiorespiratory endurance exercises are target heart rate, rating of perceived exertion, and the talk test. The exercise intensity required to improve cardiorespiratory endurance is a heart rate between 64 and 96 percent of your maximum heart rate (moderate to vigorous intensity). Before calculating your

> **FITT** The acronym for frequency, intensity, time, and type; the terms that describe the essential components of a program or plan to improve a health-related component of physical fitness.
>
> **frequency** As part of the FITT prescription, refers to how many days per week a person should exercise.
>
> **intensity** As part of the FITT prescription, refers to how hard or how much effort is needed when a person exercises.
>
> **time** As part of the FITT prescription, refers to the duration of an exercise session.
>
> **type** As part of the FITT prescription, refers to what kind of exercises a person needs to do.

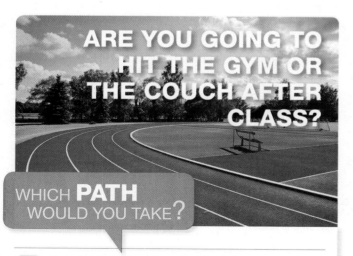

ARE YOU GOING TO HIT THE GYM OR THE COUCH AFTER CLASS?

WHICH **PATH** WOULD YOU TAKE?

▶ Go to Mastering Health to play Which Path Would You Take? and see where decisions like these lead you!

150 MINUTES

of moderate physical activity a week—along with strength exercises 2 days a week—provides substantial **HEALTH BENEFITS**. More is even better!

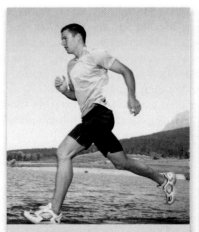
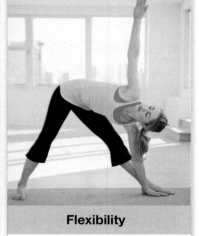
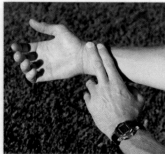

	Cardiorespiratory Endurance	Muscular Fitness	Flexibility
Frequency	3–5 days per week	2–3 days per week	Minimally 2–3 days per week
Intensity	64%–96% of maximum heart rate	60%–80% of 1 RM	To the point of mild tension
Time	20–60 minutes	8–10 exercises, 2–4 sets, 8–12 reps	10–30 seconds per stretch, 2–3 reps
Type	Any moderate to vigorous rhythmic, continuous activity	Resistance training (with body weight and/or external resistance) for all major muscle groups	Stretching, dance, or yoga exercises for all major muscle groups

FIGURE 12.4 The FITT Principle Applied to Cardiorespiratory Fitness, Muscular Strength and Endurance, and Flexibility

target heart rate, you must first estimate your maximal heart rate with the formula [207 − 0.7(age)]. The following example is based on a 20-year-old. Substitute your age to determine your own maximal heart rate, then multiply by 0.64 and 0.94 to determine the lower and upper limits of your target range.

1. $207 − 0.7(20) = $ maximal heart rate for a 20-year old
2. $207 − 14 = 193$ (maximal heart rate)
3. $193(0.64) = 123.52$ (lower target limit)
4. $193.5(0.94) = 185.28$ (upper target limit)
5. Target range $= 124$ to 186 beats per minute

To determine how close you are to your target heart rate, determine your heart rate. As technology has advanced, it has become much easier to monitor heart rate with your cell phone or activity tracker. If you do not have your phone while exercising, see **FIGURE 12.5** for the procedures for taking your carotid or radial pulse. Take your heart rate while exercising, if possible, or immediately after you stop exercising, as your heart rate decreases rapidly when you stop.

target heart rate The heart rate range of aerobic exercise that leads to improved cardiorespiratory fitness (i.e., 64 to 96 percent of maximal heart rate).

perceived exertion The subjective perception of effort during exercise that can be used to monitor exercise intensity.

Another way to determine the intensity of cardiorespiratory exercise intensity is to use Borg's rating of perceived exertion (RPE) scale. **Perceived exertion** refers to how hard you feel you are working, which you might base on your heart rate, breathing rate, sweating, and level of fatigue. This scale uses a rating from 6 (no exertion at all) to 20 (maximal exertion). An

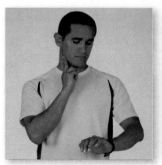

ⓐ Carotid pulse ⓑ Radial pulse

FIGURE 12.5 Taking a Pulse Palpation of the carotid (neck) or radial (wrist) artery is a simple way of determining heart rate. Take a 10-second pulse, and multiply the number by 6 to get beats per minute. Start your count with 1 if using a running watch and with 0 if using a stopwatch.

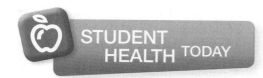
IS HIGH INTENSITY INTERVAL TRAINING RIGHT FOR YOU?

CrossFit and high-intensity interval training (HIIT) are two methods of training that are increasing in popularity. CrossFit is a strength and conditioning program that utilizes a broad range of high-intensity functional movements and activities. CrossFit is typically performed in a CrossFit gym or "Box" in a group or class. It is an intense, specialized training program, so there are special requirements and certifications to become a CrossFit trainer or coach.

HIIT is a type of training that combines alternating high-intensity bouts and active rest bouts in your exercise session. For example, after the warm-up phase, you might do 2 minutes of a near-maximal-paced run, and then jog for 2 minutes to rest. This type of training can provide a very efficient workout. The volume of exercise is generally less than a continuous bout at a constant pace, but similar fitness gains can be seen with

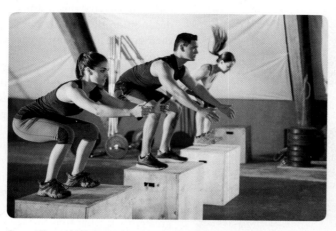

CrossFit and high-intensity interval training are two methods of training that are increasing in popularity. If you're healthy enough—and up for the challenge—they might be right for you.

the lower volume of exercise as with the tradition exercise bout. The intervals can be varied to suit your fitness level and goals.

How do you know whether either type of training is right for you? If you are a beginner, have risk factors for cardiovascular disease or musculoskeletal disorders, are obese, or have been sedentary, make sure you get clearance from your

health care provider. After getting checked out, find a fitness professional who can help you get started. Both types of training can be modified to accommodate varying levels of fitness.

If you like a challenge, a variety of exercises, and the motivation of the gym, CrossFit might be right for you. HIIT might be a good option if time is a barrier or you are trying to improve your performance. Because both are high-intensity activities, it is important to allow your body time to rest and recover to reduce the risk of injury. Using different activities on consecutive days and not doing more than three consecutive days of exercise are recommendations for CrossFit. HIIT should be alternated with other activities throughout the week. If you are up for the challenge, give one of these nontraditional training programs a try.

Sources: CrossFit, "What Is Crossfit?" Accessed April 2016, www.crossfit.com; L. Kravitz, "High-Intensity Interval Training," ACSM, 2014, www.acsm.org/docs/brochures/high-intensity-interval-training.pdf.

RPE of 12 to 16 is generally recommended for training the cardiorespiratory system.

The easiest method of measuring cardiorespiratory exercise intensity is the talk test. A moderate level of exercise (heart rate at 64 to 76 percent of maximum) means that you can hold an intermittent conversation. At this level, you are able to talk with a partner while exercising. If you can talk, but only in short fragments and not sentences, you may be at a vigorous level of exercise (heart rate at 76 to 96 percent of maximum). If you are breathing so hard that speaking at all is difficult, the intensity of your exercise may be too high. Conversely, if you can sing or laugh heartily while exercising, the intensity of your exercise is light and may be insufficient for maintaining or improving cardiorespiratory fitness.

Time For cardiorespiratory fitness benefits, the American College of Sports Medicine (ACSM) recommends that vigorous activities be performed for at least 20 minutes at a time, and moderate activities for at least 30 minutes.[44] Free time for exercise can vary from day to day, so you can set a time goal for the entire week as long as you keep your sessions to at least 10

minutes (150 minutes per week for moderate intensity and 75 minutes per week for vigorous intensity). You can also combine moderate and vigorous activity. For example, you can do 3 days of moderate intensity exercise and 1 or two days of vigorous intensity exercise. See the Student Health Today box for information on a few exercise programs that can really give you a lot of bang for your buck.

Type Any sort of rhythmic, continuous, and physical activity that can be done for 20 or more minutes will improve cardiorespiratory fitness. Examples include walking briskly, cycling, jogging, fitness classes, and swimming.

The FITT Principle for Muscular Strength and Endurance

The FITT prescription for muscular strength and endurance includes 2 to 3 days per week when you perform exercises that train the major muscle groups, using enough sets, repetitions, and resistance to maintain or improve muscular strength and endurance.[45]

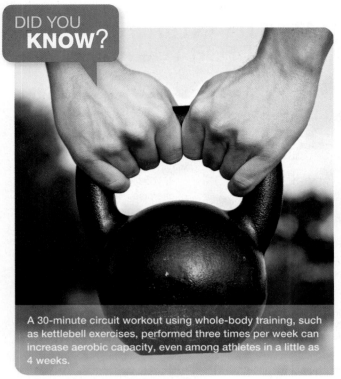

DID YOU KNOW?

A 30-minute circuit workout using whole-body training, such as kettlebell exercises, performed three times per week can increase aerobic capacity, even among athletes in a little as 4 weeks.

Source: J.A. Falatic et al., "Effects of Kettlebell Training on Aerobic Capacity," *Journal of Strength and Conditioning Research* 29, no. 7 (2015): 143–147.

Frequency For frequency, training the major muscle groups 2 to 3 days a week is recommended. It is believed that overloading the muscles, a normal part of resistance training described below, causes microscopic tears in muscle fibers, and the rebuilding process that increases the muscle's size and

capacity takes about 24 to 48 hours. Thus, resistance training exercise programs should include at least 1 day of rest between workouts before the same muscles are overloaded again. But don't wait too long between workouts: One of the important principles of strength training is the idea of *reversibility*. Reversibility means that if you stop exercising, the body responds by deconditioning. Within 2 weeks, muscles begin to revert to their untrained state for novice exercisers.[46] The saying "use it or lose it" applies!

Intensity Resistance exercise is based on a percentage of your one repetition max (1 RM). Because most individuals will not do a 1 RM test, intensity is generally prescribed as the repetition RM (e.g., 10 RM is the weight that be lifted a maximum of 10 times)[47] Muscular strength is improved when resistance loads are greater than 60 percent of your 1 RM, whereas muscular endurance is improved by using loads less than 50 percent of your 1 RM.

To become stronger, you must *overload* your muscles, that is, regularly create a degree of tension in your muscles that is greater than what they are accustomed to. Overloading them forces your muscles to adapt by getting larger, stronger, and capable of producing more tension. If you "underload" your muscles, you will not increase strength. If you create too great an overload, you may experience muscle injury, muscle fatigue, and potentially a loss in strength.

Time The time recommended for muscular strength and endurance exercises is measured not in minutes of exercise but rather in repetitions and sets.

- **Repetitions and sets.** To increase muscular strength, you need higher intensity and fewer repetitions and sets. It is estimated that 60 to 80 percent of your 1 RM is equivalent to an 8 to 12 RM. Performing 8 to 12 repetitions per set

TABLE **12.3** | Methods of Providing Muscular Resistance

Body Weight Resistance (Calisthenics)	Fixed Resistance	Variable Resistance
- Uses your own body weight to develop muscular strength and endurance - Improves overall muscular fitness and, in particular, core body strength and overall muscle tone	- Provides a constant resistance throughout the full range of movement - Requires balance and coordination; promotes development of core body strength	- Resistance altered so that the muscle's effort is consistent throughout the full range of motion - Provides more controlled motion and isolates certain muscle groups
Examples: Push-ups, pull-ups, curl-ups, dips, leg raises, chair sits, etc.	**Examples:** Free weights, such as barbells, dumbbells, medicine balls, and kettlebells	**Examples:** Weight machines in gyms and homes

with two to four sets performed overall is recommended for general health and strength. If improving muscular endurance is your goal, use less resistance and more repetitions: Perform one to two sets of a 15 to 25 RM repetitions for a resistance that is less than 50 percent of your 1 RM.

- **Rest periods.** Resting between exercises is crucial to reduce fatigue and help with performance and safety in subsequent sets. A rest period of 2 to 3 minutes is recommended when you are using the guidelines for general health benefits. However, the rest period when you are working to develop strength or endurance will vary. Note that the rest period refers specifically to the muscle group being exercised. For example, you can alternate a set of push-ups with a set of curl-ups, as the muscle groups worked in one set can rest while you are working the other muscle groups.

Type To improve muscular strength or endurance, resistance training should use either the body's weight or devices that provide a fixed or variable resistance (see **TABLE 12.3**). In selecting strength-training exercises, there are three important principles to bear in mind: specificity, exercise selection, and exercise order. According to the *specificity principle*, the effects of resistance exercise training are specific to the muscles being exercised; therefore, to improve total body strength, include exercises for all the major muscle groups.

The second important concept is *exercise selection*. It is important to select exercises that will meet your goals.

Selecting eight to ten exercises targeting all major muscle groups is generally recommended. This will ensure that exercises are balanced for opposing muscle groups.

Finally, for optimal training effects, pay attention to *exercise order*. When you are training all major muscle groups in a single workout, complete large muscle group exercises (e.g., the bench press or leg press) before small muscle group exercises, multiple-joint exercises before single-joint exercises (e.g., biceps curls, triceps extension), and high-intensity exercises before lower-intensity exercises.

The FITT Principle for Flexibility

Although often overshadowed by cardiorespiratory and muscular fitness training, flexibility is important. Inflexible muscles are susceptible to injury, and flexibility training reduces the incidence and severity of lower back problems and muscle or tendon injuries.[48] Improved flexibility also means less tension and pressure on joints, resulting in less joint pain and joint deterioration.[49] Thus, remaining flexible can help to prevent the decreased physical function that often occurs with aging.[50]

Frequency The FITT principle calls for a minimum of 2 to 3 days per week for flexibility training.

Intensity Intensity recommendations for flexibility are that you perform or hold stretching positions at an individually

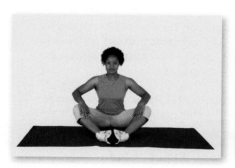
ⓐ Stretching the inside of the thighs

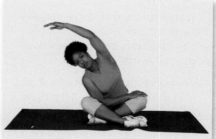
ⓑ Stretching the upper arm and the side of the trunk

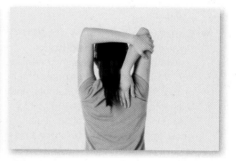
ⓒ Stretching the triceps

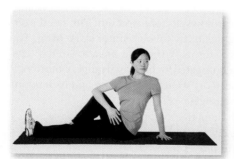
ⓓ Stretching the trunk and the hip

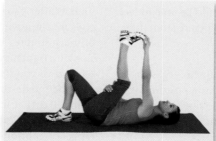
ⓔ Stretching the hip, back of the thigh, and the calf

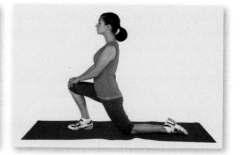
ⓕ Stretching the front of the thigh and the hip flexor

FIGURE 12.6 Stretching Exercises to Improve Flexibility Use these stretches as part of your cool-down. Hold each stretch for 10 to 30 seconds, and repeat two to four times for each limb.

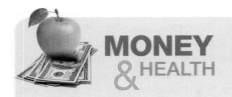

MONEY & HEALTH | ALL CERTIFICATIONS ARE NOT CREATED EQUAL

Using a personal trainer or fitness trainer is a great way to get on track with a new exercise program. So how do you select the best fit for you and your goals?

First, make sure your trainer is certified and carries personal liability insurance, but be careful! There are a lot of certifications available, and not all are reputable. You can use the Internet to review the organizations that award certifications. Consider the following characteristics when you review certifications:

- **Quality of Certification.** Avoid using a trainer with a certification that is very easily obtainable. The reputable certifications have workshops, test review materials, online study materials, and minimum standards to qualify (e.g., a high school diploma). The National Commission for Certifying Agencies, an accrediting agency for health professions (www.credentialingexcellence.org/p/cm/ld/fid=121), lists accredited fitness certifications.

- **Continuing Education Credits.** Review the continuing education requirements to maintain the certification. Workshops, professional conferences, tests in scientific journals, and online courses should be options for maintaining the certification. It's a good sign when other certifying bodies use an organization's conferences and classes for continuing education.

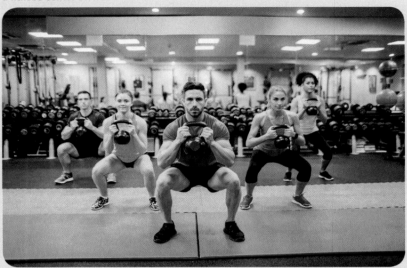

Before you sign on the dotted line, check out the classes, equipment, and personnel a fitness center offers.

- **Readily Available Information.** You should be able to readily find information about the certification or organization that provides the certification.

  In addition to certification, consider characteristics of the trainer, and get recommendations from people whose judgment you trust.

- The trainer's area of specialty should fit with your goals (e.g., weight loss, improved athletic performance).
- The trainer should teach you about fitness and not just give you a workout plan. The trainer should explain things

to you at a level you understand. Consider the trainer's education level.
- You should not feel judged by the trainer.
- The trainer's style should match your needs. For example, if you need a lot of encouragement and reinforcement, select a trainer who will provide those things.

Sources: ACE, "How to Choose the Right Personal Trainer," 2015, www.acefitness.org/acefit/healthy_living_fit_facts_content.aspx?itemid=19; ACSM, "Using a Personal Trainer," www.acsm.org/docs/default-source/brochures/using-a-personal-trainer.pdf?sfvrsn=4.

---

determined "point of mild tension." You should be able to feel tension or mild discomfort in the muscle(s) you are stretching, but the stretch should not hurt.[51]

Time The time recommended to improve flexibility is based on time per stretch. Once you are in a stretching position, you should hold at the point of tension for 10 to 30 seconds for each stretch and repeat two to four times in close succession.[52]

Type The most effective exercises for increasing flexibility involve stretching the major muscle groups of your body when the body is already warm,

such as after your cardiorespiratory workout. The safest exercises for improving flexibility involve **static stretching**. The primary strategy is to decrease the resistance to stretch (tension) in a tight muscle targeted for increased range of motion.[53] To do this, you repeatedly stretch the muscle and its tendons of attachment to elongate them. With each repetition of a static stretch, your range of motion improves temporarily due to the slightly lessened sensitivity of tension receptors in the stretched muscles; when stretching is done regularly,

static stretching Stretching techniques that slowly and gradually lengthen a muscle or group of muscles and their tendons.

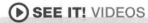 **SEE IT! VIDEOS**

Can you use some tips on stretching before and after exercise? Watch **The Do's and Don'ts of Stretching** in the Study Area of Mastering Health.

range of motion increases. **FIGURE 12.6** illustrates some basic stretching exercises to increase flexibility.

LO 5 | IMPLEMENTING YOUR FITNESS PROGRAM

Devise a plan to implement your safe and effective fitness program.

As your physical fitness improves, you need to adjust the frequency, intensity, time, and type of your exercise to maintain or continue to improve your level of physical fitness. Following are a few suggestions to get started and stay on track. If you're looking for a little more direction, the **Money & Health** box offers suggestions on choosing a personal trainer or fitness coach.

Develop a Progressive Plan

Experts recommend beginning an exercise regimen by picking an exercise you enjoy and gradually increasing the frequency or time of your workouts. For example, in week 1, you might exercise 3 days for 20 minutes per day and then move to 4 days in week 3 or 4. Then, consider increasing your duration to 30 minutes per session over the next couple of weeks. Gradual increases in intensity are typically made once the duration and frequency goals have been met.

Finding a variety of exercises can reduce the risk of overuse injuries. Choosing different exercises for your workouts will also provide for a more complete training program by targeting more muscle groups. Reevaluate your physical fitness goals and action plan monthly to ensure that they are still working for you. A mistake many people make when they decide to become more physically active (or to make any other behavior change) is putting so much effort into getting started that they allow their efforts to dwindle once they are in the action phase. The **Skills for Behavior Change** box offers more tips on starting and sticking with an exercise plan.

Because some goals take several weeks to achieve, be mindful of the benefits you are getting in the meantime to keep yourself motivated. Focus on how you feel after a brisk walk or run. Is your breathing fast and is your face flushed? Do you feel warm and can you feel your heart beating? Focus on the warmth of your skin and how your muscles feel. Inhale deeply. Exhale. Repeat several times. Notice how your body is relaxing yet you feel more alive, more energized, and less stressed. Allow yourself to bask in the moment. Make note of how exercise made you feel. Do you sleep better after exercise? Do you feel more relaxed after a stressful day? Journaling these simple benefits can keep you on track as you work toward bigger goals.

Design Your Exercise Session

A comprehensive workout should include a warm-up, cardiorespiratory and/or resistance training, and then a cool-down to finish the session.

Warm-Up The warm-up prepares the body physically and mentally for cardiorespiratory and/or resistance training. A warm-up should involve large body movements, generally using light cardiorespiratory activities, followed by range-of-motion exercises of the muscle groups that will be used during the exercise session. Usually 5 to 15 minutes long, a warm-up is shorter when you are geared up and ready to go and longer when you are struggling to get moving or your muscles are cold or tight. The warm-up provides a transition from rest to physical activity by slowly increasing the heart rate, blood pressure, breathing rate, and body temperature. These gradual changes improve joint lubrication, increase muscle and tendon

---

SKILLS FOR BEHAVIOR CHANGE

Plan It, Start It, Stick With It!

The most successful physical activity program is one that you enjoy, that is realistic, and that is appropriate for your skill level and needs.

- **Make it enjoyable.** Pick activities you like to do so that you will make the effort and find the time to do it.

- **Start slowly.** If you have been physically inactive for a while, any type and amount of physical activity is a step in the right direction. Start slowly, letting your body adapt so that there is not too much pain the next day.

- **Make only one lifestyle change at a time.** It is not realistic to change everything at once. Furthermore, success with one behavioral change will increase your confidence and encourage you to make other positive changes.

- **Set reasonable expectations for yourself and your physical fitness program.** You will not become fit overnight. Focus on the changes you do see immediately (e.g., improved sleep, feeling relaxed, stress management, feeling good about yourself). These things will help you stay motivated while working to meet long-term goals. Be patient and enjoy!

- **Choose a time to be physically active and stick with it.** Learn to establish priorities and keep to a schedule. Try different times of the day to learn what works best for you. Be flexible so if something comes up that you cannot work around, you will still find time to do some physical activity.

- **Record your progress.** Include the intensity, time, and type of physical activities; your emotions; and your personal achievements.

- **Take lapses in stride.** Sometimes life gets in the way. Start again, and do not despair; your commitment to physical fitness has ebbs and flows like most everything else in life.

- **Reward yourself.** Find meaningful and healthy ways to reward yourself when you reach your goals.

elasticity, and enhance blood flow throughout the body, facilitating performance during the next stage of the workout.

Cardiorespiratory and/or Resistance Training

The next stage of your workout may involve cardiorespiratory training, resistance training, or a little of each. If you are completing aerobic and resistance exercise in the same session, it is often recommended that you perform the aerobic exercise first. This order will provide additional warm-up for the resistance session, and your muscles will not be fatigued for the aerobic workout.

Cool-Down and Stretching

A cool-down is an essential component of a fitness program; it involves another 10 to 15 minutes of activity time. Start your cool-down with 5 to 10 minutes of moderate- to low-intensity activity, and follow it with approximately 5 to 10 minutes of stretching. Because of the body's increased temperature, the cool-down is an excellent time to stretch to improve flexibility. The purpose of the cool-down is to gradually reduce your heart rate, blood pressure, and body temperature to pre-exercise levels. In addition, the cool-down reduces the risk of blood pooling in the extremities and facilitates quicker recovery between exercise sessions.

Explore Activities That Develop Multiple Components of Fitness

Some forms of activity can improve several components of physical fitness and thus improve your everyday functioning ("functional" exercises). For example, core strength training improves posture and can prevent back pain. In addition, yoga, tai chi, and Pilates improve flexibility, muscular strength and endurance, balance, coordination, and agility. They also develop the mind–body connection through concentration on breathing and body position.

Core Strength Training

The body's core muscles are the foundation for all movement.[54] These muscles include the deep back, abdominal, and hip muscles that attach to the spine and pelvis. The contraction of these muscles provides the basis of support for movements of the upper and lower body and powerful movements of the extremities. A weak core generally results in poor posture, low back pain, and muscle injuries. A strong core provides a more stable center of gravity and, as a result, a more stable platform for movements, thus reducing the chance of injury.

You can develop core strength by doing various exercises, including calisthenics, yoga, or Pilates. Holding yourself in a front or reverse plank (an upward-facing version of a push-up position) and doing abdominal curl-ups are examples of exercises that increase core strength. Increased core strength does not happen from one single exercise but rather from a structured regime of postures and exercises.[55] The use of instability devices (e.g., a stability ball, wobble boards) and exercises to train the core have become popular.[56]

Yoga Yoga, based on ancient Indian practices, blends the mental and physical aspects of exercise in a union of mind and body that participants often find relaxing and satisfying. The practice of yoga focuses attention on controlled breathing as well as physical exercise and incorporates a complex array of static stretching and strengthening exercises expressed as postures (*asanas*). Done regularly, yoga improves flexibility, vitality, posture, agility, balance, coordination, and core muscular strength and endurance. Many people also report an improved sense of general well-being.

Tai Chi Tai chi is an ancient Chinese form of exercise that combines stretching, balance, muscular endurance, coordination, and meditation. It increases range of motion and flexibility while reducing muscular tension. It involves continuously performing a series of positions called *forms*. Tai chi is often described as "meditation in motion" because it promotes serenity through gentle movements that connect the mind and body.

Pilates The Pilates style of exercises was developed by Joseph Pilates in 1926 to combine stretching with movement against resistance, frequently aided by devices such as tension springs or heavy rubber bands. It differs from yoga and tai chi in that it includes a component specifically designed to increase strength. Some movements are carried out on specially designed equipment; others can be performed on mats. It teaches body awareness, good posture, and easy, graceful body movements while improving flexibility, coordination, core strength, muscle tone, and economy of motion.

Resistance training to improve muscular strength and endurance can be done with free weights, machines, or even your own body weight.

Assess Your Social Environment

Beyond setting SMART goals and developing a workout plan, it helps to assess your social environment. The important people in your social network should be used as a support system.

It is important that you know who can offer support and that you let them know what type of support you need. Do you need an exercise buddy? An accountability partner? Or just someone to give encouragement? Keep in mind that your needs vary depending on your specific situation. Pay attention to your inner circle to make sure you get the needed support. Know that you can also connect with a support network using social media.

| TAKING IN PROPER NUTRITION FOR EXERCISE

Describe optimal food and fluid consumption recommendations for exercise and recovery.

It's important to evaluate your eating habits considering your exercise habits. Whether you're a seasoned fitness buff or a beginner, the importance of proper nutrition for exercise can't be overstated.

Foods for Exercise and Recovery

To make the most of your workouts, follow the recommendations of the U.S. Department of Agriculture's MyPlate plan, and make sure that you eat sufficient carbohydrates, the body's main source of fuel. Your body stores carbohydrates as glycogen primarily in the muscles and liver and then uses this stored glycogen for energy when you are physically active. Fats are also an important source of energy, packing more than double the amount of energy per gram compared to carbohydrates. Protein plays a role in muscle repair and growth but is not normally a source of energy.

When you eat is almost as important as what you eat. Eating a large meal before exercising can cause upset stomach, cramping, and diarrhea because your muscles have to compete with your digestive system for energy. After a large meal, wait 3 to 4 hours before you begin exercising. Smaller meals (snacks) can be eaten about an hour before activity. Not eating at all before a workout can cause low blood sugar levels, which in turn cause weakness and slower reaction times.

After your workout, help your muscles recover by eating a snack or meal that contains plenty of carbohydrates and a little protein. Today, there is a burgeoning market for dietary supplements that claim to deliver the nutrients needed for muscle recovery as well as additional "performance-enhancing" ingredients. One thing to keep in mind, especially if you consider these products, is that there are few standards for these products, and virtually no U.S. Food and Drug Administration approval is needed for many of them to grace store shelves. (See Chapter 10 on nutrition for more on supplements).

Fluids for Exercise and Recovery

In addition to eating well, staying hydrated is crucial. How much fluid do you need? Keep in mind that the goal of fluid replacement is to prevent excessive dehydration (more than 2

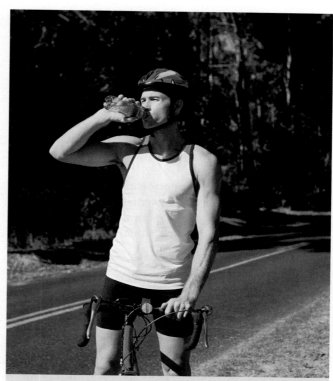

The American College of Sports Medicine and the National Athletic Trainers' Association recommend consuming 14 to 22 ounces of fluid several hours before exercising and about 6 to 12 ounces per 15 to 20 minutes during exercise, assuming that you are sweating.

percent loss of body weight). The ACSM and the National Athletic Trainers Association recommend consuming 5 to 7 milliliters per kilogram of body weight (approximately 0.7 to 1.07 ounces per 10 pounds body weight) 4 hours before exercising.[57] A good way to monitor how much fluid you need to replace is to weigh yourself before and after your workout. The difference in weight is how much you should drink. For example, if you lost 2 pounds during a training session, you should drink 32 ounces of fluid.[58]

hyponatremia Overconsumption of water, which leads to a dilution of sodium concentration in the blood, with potentially fatal results; also known as *water intoxication.*

For exercise sessions lasting less than 1 hour, plain water is sufficient for rehydration. If your exercise session exceeds 1 hour and you sweat profusely, consider a sports drink that contains electrolytes. The electrolytes in these products are minerals and ions such as sodium and potassium that are needed for proper functioning of your nervous and muscular systems. Replacing electrolytes is particularly important for endurance athletes. In endurance events lasting more than 4 hours, an athlete's overconsumption of plain water can lead to electrolyte imbalances diluting the sodium concentration in the blood with potentially fatal results, an effect called **hyponatremia,** or water intoxication.

Although water is the best choice in most cases, there are situations in which you might need to choose something different. Some people are likely to consume more when their drink is flavored, a point that may be significant in ensuring proper hydration. Recently, research has considered low-fat chocolate milk as a recovery drink.[59] Chocolate milk is a liquid that not only hydrates, but also is a source of sodium, potassium, carbohydrates, and protein. Consuming carbohydrates and protein immediately after exercise will help to replenish muscle and liver glycogen stores and stimulate muscle protein synthesis for better recovery from exercise. The protein in milk, whey protein, is ideal because it contains all of the essential amino acids and is rapidly absorbed by the body. Low-fat chocolate milk is a good choice to hydrate and recover after exercise.

LO 7 | PREVENTING AND TREATING FITNESS-RELATED INJURIES

Explain how to prevent and treat common exercise injuries.

Two basic types of injuries stem from fitness-related activities: traumatic injuries and overuse injuries. **Traumatic injuries** occur suddenly and usually by accident. Typical traumatic injuries are broken bones, torn ligaments and muscles, contusions, and lacerations. If a traumatic injury causes a noticeable loss of function and immediate pain or pain that does not go away after 30 minutes, consult a physician.

Overuse injuries result from the cumulative effects of day-after-day stresses. These injuries occur most often in repetitive activities such as swimming, running, bicycling, and step aerobics. The forces that occur normally during physical activity are not enough to cause a ligament sprain or muscle strain as in a traumatic injury, but when these forces are applied daily for weeks or months, they can result in an overuse injury. Factors such as overweight or obesity, running mechanics, and poor choice of shoe can also contribute to overuse injury.

The three most common overuse injuries are *runner's knee*, *shin splints*, and *plantar fasciitis*. Runner's knee is a general term describing a series of problems involving the muscles, tendons, and ligaments around the knee. Shin splints is a general term used for any pain that occurs below the knee and above the ankle in the shin. Plantar fasciitis is an inflammation of the plantar fascia, a broad band of dense, inelastic tissue in the foot. Rest, variation of routine, and stretching are the first lines of treatment for any of these overuse injuries. If pain continues, visit a physician. Orthotics, physical therapy, or steroid shots are possible treatment options.

Preventing Injuries

To reduce your risk of overuse or traumatic injuries, use common sense and the proper gear and equipment. Vary your physical activities throughout the week, setting appropriate and realistic short- and long-term goals. Listen to your body when you are working out. Warning signs include muscle stiffness and soreness, bone and joint pains, and whole-body fatigue that simply does not go away.

Appropriate Footwear Proper footwear, replaced in a timely manner, can decrease the likelihood of foot, knee, hip, or back injuries. Running, jumping, and other high-impact activities put significant stress on your joints. Consider the impact for a runner who has poor mechanics or an overweight individual who participates in weight-bearing activities. The force that is not absorbed by the running shoe is transmitted upward into the foot, leg, thigh, and back. Our bodies can absorb forces such as these but may be injured by the cumulative effect of repetitive impact (such as running 40 miles per week). Thus, the shoes' ability to absorb shock is critical—not just for people who run, but for anyone who engages in weight-bearing activities.

In addition to absorbing shock, an athletic shoe should provide a good fit for maximal comfort and performance—see FIGURE 12.7. To get the best fit, shop at a sports or fitness specialty store where there is a large selection and the salespeople are trained in properly fitting athletic shoes. Try on shoes later in the day, when your feet are largest, and check to make sure there is a little extra room in the toe and that the width is appropriate. Because different activities place different stresses on your feet and joints, you should choose shoes specifically designed for your sport or activity. Shoes of any type should be replaced once they lose their cushioning. A common rule of thumb is that running shoes ought to be replaced after 300 to 500 miles of use, which is typically between 3 and 9 months, depending on your activity level.

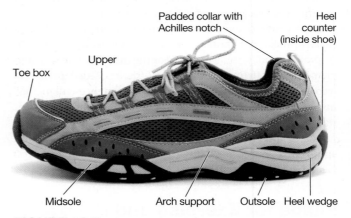

Padded collar with Achilles notch

Heel counter (inside shoe)

Upper

Toe box

Midsole

Arch support

Outsole

Heel wedge

FIGURE 12.7 Anatomy of a Running Shoe A good running shoe should fit comfortably, allow room for your toes to move, have a firm but flexible midsole, and have a firm grip on your heel to prevent slipping.

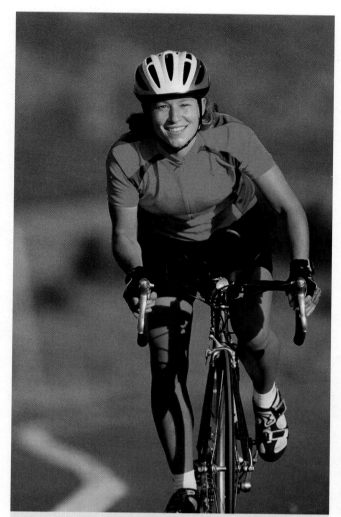

Reducing your risk for exercise injuries requires common sense and preventive measures, including wearing protective gear (helmets, knee pads, elbow pads, eyewear).

Appropriate Protective Equipment It is essential to use well-fitted, appropriate protective equipment for your physical activities. For example, using the correct racquet with the proper tension helps prevent the general inflammatory condition known as tennis elbow. Eye injuries can occur in virtually all physical activities, although some activities (such as baseball, basketball, and racquet sports) are riskier than others.[60] As many as 90 percent of eye injuries could be prevented by wearing appropriate eye protection, such as goggles with polycarbonate lenses.[61]

Wearing a helmet while bicycle riding is an important safety precaution. An estimated 66 to 88 percent of head injuries among cyclists can be prevented by wearing a helmet.[62] In a recent study of college students, 39.1 percent of students who rode a bicycle in the past 12 months reported never wearing a helmet, and 24.3 percent said they wore one only sometimes or rarely.[63] The direct medical costs from cyclists' failure to wear helmets is an estimated $81 million a year.[64] Cyclists aren't the only ones who should be wearing helmets. People who skateboard, ski, in-line skate, snowboard, play contact sports, or use kick-scooters should also wear helmets. Look for helmets that meet the standards established by the American National Standards Institute or the Snell Memorial Foundation.

Exercising in the Heat

Exercising in hot or humid weather increases your risk of a heat-related illness. In these conditions, your body's rate of heat production can exceed its ability to cool itself. The three heat stress illnesses, progressive in their level of severity, are heat cramps, heat exhaustion, and heatstroke.

Heat cramps (heat-related involuntary and forcible muscle contractions that cannot be relaxed), the least serious heat-related illness, can usually be prevented by adequate fluid replacement and a dietary intake that includes the electrolytes that are lost during sweating.

Heat exhaustion is actually a mild form of shock in which the blood pools in the arms and legs away from the brain and major organs of the body. It is caused by excessive water loss because of intense or prolonged exercise or work in a hot and/or humid environment. Symptoms of heat exhaustion include nausea, headache, fatigue, dizziness and faintness, and, paradoxically, goose bumps and chills. When you are suffering from heat exhaustion, your skin will be cool and moist.

Heatstroke, often called *sunstroke*, is a life-threatening emergency condition with a high morbidity and mortality rate.[65] Heatstroke occurs during vigorous exercise when the body's heat production significantly exceeds its cooling capacities. The core body temperature can rise from normal (around 98.6°F) to 105°F to 110°F within minutes after the body's cooling mechanism shuts down. A rapid increase in core body temperature can cause brain damage, permanent disability, and death. Common signs of heatstroke are dry, hot, and usually red skin; very high body temperature; and rapid heart rate. If you experience any of these symptoms, stop exercising immediately. Move to the shade or a cool spot to rest, and drink plenty of cool fluids for heat cramps and exhaustion. If heatstroke is suspected, seek medical attention immediately.

You can prevent heat stress by following certain precautions. First, acclimatize yourself to hot or humid climates. The process of heat acclimatization, which increases your body's cooling efficiency, requires about 10 to 14 days of gradually increased physical activity in the hot environment. Second, reduce your risk of dehydration by replacing fluids before, during, and after exercise. Third, wear clothing appropriate for the activity and the environment. Most athletic clothing companies make clothing for different environmental conditions. Check the descriptions and labels for the appropriate clothing to dissipate heat and help maintain body temperature when exercising in hot environments. Finally, use common sense. On days when the temperature is 85°F and the humidity is

heat cramps Involuntary and forcible muscle contractions that occur during or following exercise in hot and/or humid weather.

heat exhaustion A heat stress illness caused by significant dehydration resulting from exercise in hot and/or humid conditions.

heatstroke A deadly heat stress illness resulting from dehydration and overexertion in hot and/or humid conditions.

around 80 percent, postpone physical activity until the evening when it is cooler, or exercise in an indoor space where the temperature and humidity level are controlled.

Exercising in the Cold

When you exercise in cool weather, especially in windy and damp conditions, your body's rate of heat loss is frequently greater than its rate of heat production. These conditions may lead to **hypothermia**—a condition in which the body's core temperature drops below 95°F.[66] Temperatures need not be frigid for hypothermia to occur; it can also result from prolonged, vigorous exercise in 40°F to 50°F temperatures, particularly if there is rain, snow, or a strong wind.

As the body's core temperature drops from the normal 98.6°F to about 93.2°F, shivering begins. Shivering—the involuntary contraction of nearly every muscle in the body—increases body temperature by using the heat given off by muscle activity. You may also experience cold hands and feet, poor judgment, apathy, and amnesia. Shivering ceases in most hypothermia victims as core temperatures drop to between 87°F and 90°F, a sign that the body has lost its ability to generate heat. Death usually occurs at core temperatures between 75°F and 80°F.[67]

To prevent hypothermia, analyze weather conditions before you engage in outdoor physical activity. Remember that wind and humidity are as significant as temperature. Have a friend join you for safety when exercising outdoors in cold weather, and wear layers of appropriate clothing to prevent excessive heat loss and frostbite (polypropylene or woolen undergarments, a windproof outer garment, and a wool hat and gloves). Keep your head, hands, and feet warm. Finally, do not allow yourself to become dehydrated.[68]

Treating Injuries

First-aid treatment for virtually all fitness training–related injuries involves **RICE**: **r**est, **i**ce, **c**ompression, and **e**levation.

- **Rest** is required to avoid further irritation of the injured body part.
- **Ice** is applied to relieve pain and constrict the blood vessels to reduce internal or external bleeding. To prevent frostbite, wrap the ice or cold pack in a layer of wet toweling or elastic bandage before applying it to your skin. A new injury should be iced for approximately 20 minutes of every hour for the first 24 to 72 hours.
- **Compression** of the injured body part can be accomplished with a 4- or 6-inch-wide elastic bandage; this applies indirect pressure to damaged blood vessels to help stop bleeding. Be careful, though, that the compression wrap does not interfere with normal blood flow. Throbbing or pain indicates that the compression wrap should be loosened.
- **Elevation** of an injured extremity above the level of your heart also helps to control internal or external bleeding by making the blood flow upward to reach the injured area.

Applying ice to an injury such as a sprain can help to relieve pain and reduce swelling. Never apply the ice directly to the skin, as that could lead to frostbite.

LIVE IT! ASSESS YOURSELF

An interactive version of this assessment is available online in Mastering Health.

ASSESS YOURSELF

How Physically Fit Are You?

1 Evaluating Your Cardiorespiratory Endurance (1.5-Mile Run Test)

This test assesses your cardiorespiratory endurance level.

Procedure

Find a local track, typically a quarter of a mile per lap, to perform your test. Run 1.5 miles, and time yourself. If you become

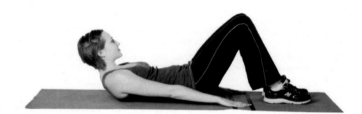

extremely fatigued during the test, slow your pace or walk—do not overstress yourself! If you feel faint or nauseated or experience any unusual pains in your upper body, stop and notify your instructor. Use the chart below to estimate your cardiorespiratory fitness level based on your age and sex. Note that women have lower standards for each fitness category because they have higher levels of essential fat than men do.

Fitness Categories for 1.5-Mile Run Test

Men, Ages	Excellent	Good	Fair	Poor	Very Poor	Women, Ages	Excellent	Good	Fair	Poor	Very Poor
20–29	< 10:17	10:17–11:41	11:42–12:51	12:52–14:13	>14:13	20–29	<12:51	12:51–14:24	14:25–15:26	15:27–16:43	>16:33
30–39	<10:48	10:48–12:20	12:21–13:36	13:37–14:52	>14:52	30–39	<13:43	13:43–15:08	15:09–15:57	15:58–17:14	>17:14
40–49	<11:45	11:45–13:14	13:15–14:29	14:30–15:41	>15:41	40–49	<14:31	14:31–15:57	15:58–16:58	16:59–18:00	>18:00
50–59	<12:52	12:52–14:24	14:25–15:26	15:27–16:43	>16:43	50–59	<15:57	15:57–16:58	16:59–17:54	17:55–18:49	>18:49

Source: Page 5-2, Federal Air Marshal Service Pre-Training Guide, Produced by the Office of Training and Workforce Programs, Department of Homeland Security, Transportation Security Administration, Federal Air Marshal Service.

2 Evaluating Your Muscular Strength and Endurance (Partial Curl-Up Test)

Your abdominal muscles are important for core stability and back support. This test assesses their muscular endurance.

Procedure

Lie on a mat with your arms by your sides, palms flat on the mat, elbows straight, and fingers extended. Bend your knees at a 90-degree angle. Your instructor or partner will mark your starting finger position with a piece of masking tape aligned with the tip of each middle finger. He or she will also mark with tape your ending position, 10 centimeters (4 inches) away from the first piece of tape—one ending position tape for each hand.

Set a metronome to 50 beats per minute, and curl up at this slow, controlled pace: one curl-up every two beats (25 curl-ups per minute). Curl your head and upper back upward, lifting your shoulder blades off the mat (your trunk should make a 30-degree angle with the mat) and reaching your arms forward along the mat to touch the ending tape. Then curl back down so that your upper back and shoulders touch the floor. During the entire curl-up, your fingers, feet, and buttocks should stay on the mat. Your partner will count the number of correct repetitions you complete. Perform as many curl-ups as you can in 1 minute without pausing, to a maximum of 25.

Healthy Musculoskeletal Fitness: Norms and Health Benefit Zones: Curl-Ups

Men, years	Excellent	Good	Fair	Needs Improvement	Women, years	Excellent	Good	Fair	Needs Improvement
20–29	25	21–24	11–20	≤10	20–29	25	18–24	5–17	≤4
30–39	25	18–24	11–17	≤10	30–39	25	19–24	6–18	≤5
40–49	25	18–24	6–17	≤5	40–49	25	19–24	4–18	≤3
50–59	25	17–24	8–16	≤7	50–59	25	19–24	6–18	≤5
60–69	25	16–24	6–15	≤5	60–69	25	17–24	3–16	≤2

Source: From Canadian Physical Activity, Fitness & Lifestyle Approach: CSEP-Health & Fitness Program's Appraisal and Counselling Strategy, 3rd edition, © 2003. Reprinted with permission from the Canadian Society for Exercise Physiology.

3 Evaluating Your Flexibility (Sit-and-Reach Test)

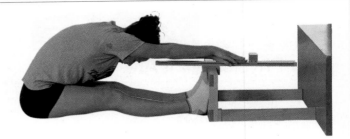

This test measures the general flexibility of your lower back, hips, and hamstring muscles.

Procedure

Warm up with some light activity that involves the total body, range-of-motion exercises, and stretches for the lower back and hamstrings. For the test, start by sitting upright, straight-legged on a mat with your shoes removed and soles of the feet flat against a flexometer (sit-and-reach box) at the 10.25-inch mark. The inner edges of the soles are placed within 0.75 inch of the measuring scale.

Have a partner on hand to record your measurements. Stretch your arms out in front of you and, keeping the hands parallel to each other, slowly reach forward with both hands as far as possible, holding the position for approximately 2 seconds. Your fingertips should be in contact with the measuring portion of the sit-and-reach box. To facilitate a longer reach, exhale and drop your head between your arms while reaching forward. Keep your knees extended the whole time, and breathe normally.

Your score is the most distant point (in inches) reached with the fingertips; have your partner make note of this number for you. Perform the test twice, record your best score, and compare it with the norms presented in the following table.

Healthy Musculoskeletal Fitness: Norms and Health Benefit Zones: Sit-and-Reach Test*

Men, years	Excellent (inches)	Very Good (inches)	Good (inches)	Fair (inches)	Needs Improvement (inches)	Women, years	Excellent (inches)	Very Good (inches)	Good (inches)	Fair (inches)	Needs Improvement (inches)
20–29	≥15.5	13.5–15.5	12–13	10–11.5	≤10	20–29	≥16	14.5–15.5	13–14	11–12.5	≤10.5
30–39	≥15	13–14.5	11–12.5	9–10.5	≤9	30–39	≥16	14–15.5	12.5–13.5	10.5–12	≤10
40–49	≥13.5	11.5–13.5	9.5–11	7–9	≤6.5	40–49	≥15	13.5–14.5	12–13	10–11.5	≤9.5
50–59	≥13.5	11–13.5	9.5–10.5	6–9	≤6	50–59	≥15.5	13–15	12–12.5	10–11.5	≤9.5
60–69	≥13	10–12.5	8–9.5	6–7.5	≤5.5	60–69	≥13.5	12–13.5	10.5–12	9–10	≤8.5

*Note: These norms are based on a sit-and-reach box in which the zero point is set at 10.25 inches. When using a box in which the zero point is set at 9 inch, subtract 1.2 inch from each value in this table.

Source: From *Canadian Physical Activity, Fitness & Lifestyle Approach: CSEP-Health & Fitness Program's Appraisal and Counselling Strategy*, 3rd edition, © 2003. Reprinted with permission from the Canadian Society for Exercise Physiology.

YOUR PLAN FOR **CHANGE**

The **ASSESS YOURSELF** activity helped you determine your current level of physical fitness. On the basis of your results, you may decide that you should take steps to improve one or more components of your physical fitness.

TODAY, YOU CAN:

☐ Visit your campus fitness facility (or its website), and familiarize yourself with the equipment and resources. Find out what classes it offers, and take home (or print out) a copy of the schedule.

☐ Walk between your classes, making an extra effort to take the long way to get from building to building. Use the stairs instead of the elevator or escalator.

☐ Take an activity break. Spend 5 to 10 minutes between homework projects or just before bed doing some type of activity, such as abdominal crunches, push-ups, or yoga poses.

WITHIN THE NEXT TWO WEEKS, YOU CAN:

☐ Shop for comfortable workout clothes and appropriate athletic footwear.

☐ Look into group activities on your campus or in your community that you might enjoy.

☐ Ask a friend to join you in your workout once a week. Agree on a date and time in advance so that you both will be committed to following through.

☐ Plan for a physically active outing with a friend or date, such as dancing, bowling, or shooting hoops. Use active transportation (e.g., walk or cycle) to get to a movie or go out for dinner.

BY THE END OF THE SEMESTER, YOU CAN:

☐ Establish a regular routine of engaging in physical activity or exercise at least three times a week. Mark your exercise times on your calendar and keep a log to track your progress.

☐ Take your workouts to the next level. If you have been working out at home, try going to a gym or participating in an exercise class. If you are walking, try walking up hills, intermittent jogging, or sign up for a fitness event such as a charity 5K.

STUDY PLAN

Visit the Study Area in Mastering Health to enhance your study plan with MP3 Tutor Sessions, Practice Quizzes, Flashcards, and more!

CHAPTER REVIEW

LO 1 | Physical Activity for Health

■ Benefits of regular physical activity include reduced risk of cardiovascular diseases, metabolic syndrome, type 2 diabetes, and cancer, as well as improved blood lipoprotein levels, bone mass, weight control, immunity to disease, mental health, and stress management and a longer lifespan.

LO 2 | Physical Activity for Fitness and Performance

■ Physical fitness involves achieving minimal levels necessary for good health and improved daily functioning in the health-related components of fitness: Skill-related components of fitness, are essential for elite and recreational athletes to increase performance in and enjoyment of sport.

LO 3 | Committing to Physical Fitness

■ Incorporate fitness activities into your life. If you are new to exercise, start slowly, keep your fitness program simple, and consider consulting your health care provider and/or a fitness instructor for recommendations. Overcome your barriers or obstacles to exercise by identifying them and then planning specific strategies to address them. Choose fun and convenient activities to increase your likelihood of sticking with them.

LO 4 | Creating Your Own Fitness Program

■ The FITT principle can be used to develop a progressive program of physical fitness. Every adult should participate in moderate-intensity activities for 30 minutes at least 5 days a week. To improve cardiorespiratory fitness, engage in vigorous, continuous, and rhythmic activities 3 to 5 days per week at an intensity of 64 to 96 percent of your maximum heart rate for 20 to 30 minutes.

■ Muscular strength is improved by engaging in resistance-training exercises two to three times per week, using an intensity of greater than 60 percent of 1 RM, and completing two to four sets of 8 to 12 repetitions. Muscular endurance is improved by engaging in resistance-training exercises two to three times per week, using an intensity of less than 50 percent of 1 RM, and completing one to two sets of 15 to 25 repetitions.

■ Flexibility is improved by engaging in two to four repetitions of static stretching exercises at least 2 to 3 days a week, where each stretch is held for 10 to 30 seconds.

LO 5 | Implementing Your Fitness Program

■ To improve physical fitness, set goals and design a program to achieve these goals. A comprehensive workout should include a warm-up with some light stretching, strength-development exercises, aerobic activities, and a cool-down period. Core strength training is important for mobility, stability, and preventing back injury.

LO 6 | Taking in Proper Nutrition for Exercise

■ Fueling properly for exercise involves eating a balance of healthy foods 3 to 4 hours before exercise. In exercise sessions lasting an hour or more, performance can benefit from some additional calories ingested during the session. Hydrating properly for exercise is important for performance and injury prevention.

LO 7 | Preventing and Treating Fitness-Related Injuries

■ The most common overuse injuries are plantar fasciitis, shin splints, and runner's knee. Proper footwear and protective equipment help to prevent injuries. Exercising in the heat or cold requires taking special precautions. Minor exercise injuries should be treated with RICE (rest, ice, compression, and elevation).

POP QUIZ

LO 1 | Physical Activity for Health

1. What is physical fitness?
   a. The ability to respond to routine physical demands
   b. Having enough physical reserves to cope with a sudden challenge
   c. A balance of cardiorespiratory, muscle, and flexibility fitness
   d. All of the above

2. Which of the following is *not* a health benefit of regular exercise?
   a. Reduced risk for some cancers
   b. Reduced risk for cardiovascular diseases
   c. Elimination of chronic diseases
   d. Improved mental health

LO 2 | Physical Activity for Fitness and Performance

3. The maximum volume of oxygen consumed by the muscles during exercise defines
   a. the target heart rate.
   b. muscular strength.
   c. aerobic capacity.
   d. muscular endurance.

4. Flexibility is the range of motion around
   a. specific bones.
   b. a joint or series of joints.
   c. the tendons.
   d. the muscles.

LO 3 | Committing to Physical Fitness

5. Miguel is thinking about becoming more active. What is *not* a good piece of advice to offer him?
   a. Incorporate physical activity into your daily life.
   b. Make multiple changes to diet and exercise routines simultaneously.
   c. Identify obstacles to being active.
   d. Set SMART goals.

LO 4 | Creating Your Own Fitness Program

6. Janice has been lifting 95 pounds while doing three sets of six leg curls. To become stronger, she began lifting 105 pounds while doing leg curls. What principle of strength development does this represent?
   a. Reversibility
   b. Overload
   c. Flexibility
   d. Specificity of training

7. The talk test measures
   a. exercise intensity.
   b. exercise time.
   c. exercise frequency.
   d. exercise type.

LO 5 | Implementing Your Fitness Program

8. At the start of an exercise session, you should always
   a. stretch before doing any activity.
   b. do 50 crunches to activate your core muscles.
   c. warm up with light cardiorespiratory activities.
   d. eat a meal to ensure that you are fueled for the activity.

LO 6 | Taking in Proper Nutrition for Exercise

9. Chocolate milk is good for
   a. a preworkout energy boost.
   b. postworkout recovery.
   c. slimming down.
   d. staying hydrated during exercise.

LO 7 | Preventing and Treating Fitness-Related Injuries

10. Overuse injuries can be prevented by
    a. monitoring the quantity and quality of your workouts.
    b. engaging in only one type of aerobic training.
    c. working out daily.
    d. working out with a friend.

Answers to the Pop Quiz can be found on page A-1. If you answered a question incorrectly, review the section identified by the Learning Outcome. For even more study tools, visit **Mastering Health**.

THINK ABOUT IT!

LO 1 | Physical Activity for Health

1. How do you define physical fitness? Identify at least four physiological and psychological benefits of physical activity. How would you promote these benefits to nonexercisers?

LO 2 | Physical Activity for Fitness and Performance

2. How are muscle strength and muscle endurance different? How might you work to increase muscle strength and muscle endurance?

LO 3 | Committing to Physical Fitness

3. What do you do to motivate yourself to engage in physical activity on a regular basis? What and who helps you to be physically active?

LO 4 | Creating Your Own Fitness Program

4. Describe the FITT prescription for cardiorespiratory fitness, muscular strength and endurance, and flexibility training.

LO 5 | Implementing Your Fitness Program

5. Why is core strength important? What are some ways to increase your core strength every day?

LO 6 | Taking in Proper Nutrition for Exercise

6. Why is *when* you eat as important as *what* you eat?

LO 7 | Preventing and Treating Fitness-Related Injuries

7. What precautions do you need to take when exercising outdoors in the heat and in the cold?

ACCESS YOUR HEALTH ON THE INTERNET

For links to the websites below, visit the Study Area in Mastering Health.

The following websites explore further topics and issues related to personal fitness.

American College of Sports Medicine. This site is the link to the American College of Sports Medicine and all its resources. **www.acsm.org**

American Council on Exercise. Information is found here on exercise and disease prevention. **www.acefitness.org**

Centers for Disease Control and Prevention, National Center for Chronic Disease Prevention and Health Promotion, Division of Nutrition, Physical Activity, and Obesity. This site is a great resource for current information on exercise and health. **www.cdc.gov/nccdphp/dnpao**

National Strength and Conditioning Association. This site is a resource for personal trainers and other people who are interested in conditioning and fitness. **www.nsca-lift.org**

13 Reducing Your Risk of Cardiovascular Disease and Cancer

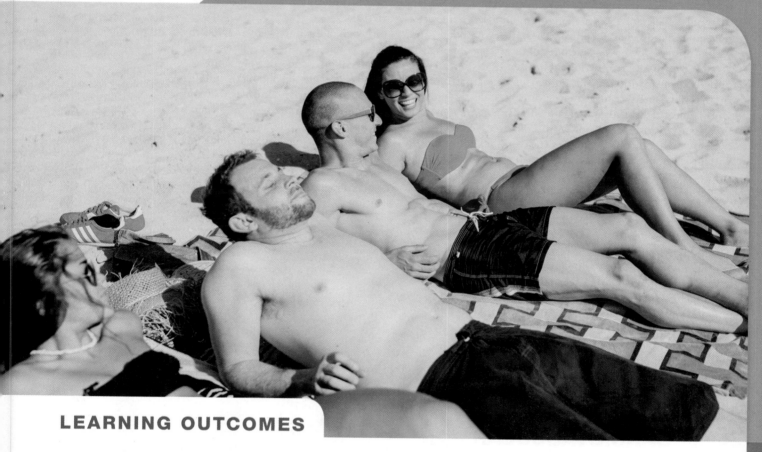

LEARNING OUTCOMES

LO **1** Discuss the social, physical, and economic burden of cardiovascular disease in the United States and globally, as well as the importance of ideal cardiovascular health.

LO **2** Describe the anatomy and physiology of the heart and circulatory system and the importance of healthy heart function.

LO **3** Review major types of cardiovascular disease, their symptoms, and their prevalence.

LO **4** Describe the modifiable and nonmodifiable risk factors for cardiovascular disease and methods of prevention.

LO **5** Examine current strategies for diagnosis and treatment of cardiovascular disease.

LO **6** Describe cancer and how it develops, as well as its impact compared to other major health problems in terms of morbidity/mortality, costs, and overall effectiveness of prevention and control.

LO **7** Explain key risk factors for cancer, and identify which risks are preventable, given current knowledge in the field.

LO **8** Describe symptoms, populations at risk, and key methods of prevention for the most common types of cancer.

LO **9** Discuss the most current and effective methods of cancer detection and treatment, including areas of significant progress and future challenges.

When we think of the major fatal diseases, we tend to picture a very old person dying after a long battle with cancer or succumbing to a fast, painful death from cardiovascular disease (CVD) such as a heart attack or stroke. In reality, more often than not, cancer and CVD are long-term illnesses that exact a huge toll on individuals young and old, their loved ones, and society. In fact, these two categories of disease are among the greatest contributors to the **global burden of disease (GBD)**, a method of quantifying the burden of premature morbidity, disability, and death for a given disease or disease group.[1] GBD is measured in **disability-adjusted life years (DALYs)**, or years lived in ill health or with disability.[2] Today, people in many higher-income regions of the world often live longer with diseases such as cancer and CVD as a result of earlier diagnosis, better treatments, and improved medicines.

Both CVD and cancer are **chronic diseases**, meaning that they are prolonged, do not resolve spontaneously, and are rarely cured completely. As such, they are responsible for significant rates of disability, lost productivity, and physical and emotional suffering, not to mention soaring health care costs. CVDs in particular are closely related to lifestyle factors such as obesity, sedentary behavior, poor nutrition, stress, lack of sleep, tobacco use, and excessive alcohol use. The good news is that in many cases, these lifestyle factors can be changed or modified to decrease disease risks for both CVD and cancer and result in more healthy years.

LO 1 | CARDIOVASCULAR DISEASE IN THE UNITED STATES

Discuss the physical, social, emotional, and economic burden of cardiovascular disease in the United States and globally, as well as the importance of ideal cardiovascular health.

In 2015–2016, the American Heart Association (AHA) reported that death rates from **cardiovascular disease (CVD)**—diseases associated with the heart and blood vessels, such as high blood pressure, coronary heart disease (CHD), heart failure, stroke, and congenital cardiovascular defects—had declined in the United States by nearly 33 percent in the last decade.[3] In spite of the promising decline, over 92 million American adults, more than 1 in every 3 adults, suffer from one or more types of CVD.[4]

Much of the improvement in death rates is due to better diagnosis, early intervention, and steadily improving treatments, including a multibillion-dollar market in drugs that are designed to keep the heart and circulatory system ticking along. We have also improved our understanding of how diet, activity, and other behaviors affect the risk of CVD and have created policies and programs designed to reduce risks. Yet CVD continues to be a threat (**FIGURE 13.1**).[5]

global burden of disease (GBD) A method of quantifying the burden of premature morbidity, disability, and death for a given disease or disease group.

disability-adjusted life years (DALYs) A measure of overall disease burden expressed as the number of years lost due to ill health.

chronic disease An illness that is prolonged, does not resolve spontaneously, and is rarely cured.

cardiovascular disease (CVD) Disease of the heart and/or blood vessels.

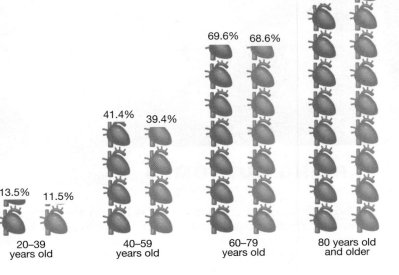

Men with CVD; each heart = 10% of the population

Women with CVD; each heart = 10% of the population

FIGURE 13.1 Prevalence of Cardiovascular Diseases (CVDs) in Adults Aged 20 and Older by Age and Sex

Source: Data from E. Benjamin et al., "Heart Disease and Stroke Statistics—2017 Update: A Report from the American Heart Association," *Circulation* 135, no. 10 (2017): e146–e603.

$1.1 TRILLION

is the projected **STAGGERING COST OF CVD** in the United States by 2035 based on the fact that 45% of the population will have at least one cardiovascular problem.

Even though rates of death from many diseases have declined and people may live longer, CVD continues to be the leading cause of death in the world, killing more than 17 million people each year and exacting a heavy toll on the physical and emotional health of survivors and their families. The reality is that CVD has been the leading killer of both men and women in the United States every year since 1918 (in that year, a pandemic flu killed more people).[6] If current trends continue, a staggering 45 percent of the U.S. population will have one or more forms of CVD by 2035 at a cost of over 1.1 trillion dollars. Millions of people may find themselves shut out of the early diagnosis and expensive treatment regimens that may save their lives.[7] Some populations are disproportionately affected; almost 50 percent of African American adults have some form of cardiovascular disease.[8]

Recognizing that selected risk factors are key to changing the future course of CVD, the AHA has established goals designed to improve Americans' cardiovascular health by 20 percent and to reduce deaths from CVDs and stroke by 20 percent—all by the year 2020.[9] As part of this strategy, the AHA is focusing on goals of **ideal cardiovascular health (ICH)** rather than mortality rates and the disease process. ICH is defined as the absence of clinical indicators of CVD and the simultaneous presence of the following seven behavioral and health factor metrics[10]:

Behaviors:
1. Not smoking
2. Sufficient physical activity
3. A healthy diet
4. An appropriate energy balance and normal body weight.

Health Factors:
5. Optimal total cholesterol without medication
6. Optimal blood pressure without medication
7. Optimal fasting blood glucose without medication.

Essentially, ICH is a recipe for reducing CVD risk. While it might sound easy enough, we're not doing so well with respect to these measures. Only 13 percent of U.S. adults meet five or more metrics with ideal levels; fewer than 1 percent meet all seven.[11]

While we clearly have a long way to go, understanding how the cardiovascular system works and how your actions can affect its functioning is an important first step.

LO 2 | UNDERSTANDING THE CARDIOVASCULAR SYSTEM

Describe the anatomy and physiology of the heart and circulatory system and the importance of healthy heart function.

The **cardiovascular system** is the network of organs and vessels through which blood flows as it carries oxygen and nutrients to all parts of the body. It includes the *heart, arteries, arterioles* (small arteries), *veins, venules* (small veins), and *capillaries* (minute blood vessels).

The Heart: A Mighty Machine

The heart is a muscular pump, roughly the size of your fist. It is a highly efficient, extremely flexible organ that contracts over 100,000 times daily and pumps the equivalent of 2,000 gallons of blood through the body. In a 70-year lifetime, an average human heart beats 2.5 billion times.

Under normal circumstances, the human body contains approximately 6 quarts of blood, which transports nutrients, oxygen, waste products, hormones, and enzymes throughout the body. Blood also helps to regulate body temperature, cellular water levels, and acidity levels of body components, and it helps to defend the body against toxins and harmful microorganisms. An adequate blood supply is essential to good health and well-being.

The heart has four chambers that work together to circulate blood constantly throughout the body. The two upper chambers of the heart, called **atria**, are large collecting chambers that receive blood from the rest of the body. The two lower chambers, known as **ventricles**, pump the blood out again. Small valves both regulate the steady, rhythmic flow of blood and prevent leakage or backflow between chambers.

> **ideal cardiovascular health (ICH)** The absence of clinical indicators of CVD and the presence of certain behavioral and health factor metrics.
>
> **cardiovascular system** The organ system, consisting of the heart and blood vessels, that transports nutrients, oxygen, hormones, metabolic wastes, and enzymes throughout the body.
>
> **atria** The heart's two upper chambers, which receive blood; singular: atrium.
>
> **ventricles** The heart's two lower chambers, which pump blood through the blood vessels.

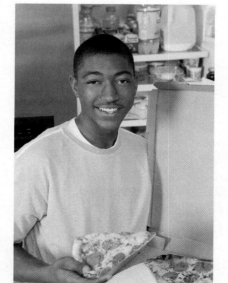

About 25 percent of your blood cholesterol level comes from foods you eat, and this is where you can make real improvements.

arteries Vessels that carry blood away from the heart to other regions of the body.

arterioles Branches of the arteries.

capillaries Minute blood vessels that branch out from the arterioles and venules; their thin walls permit exchange of oxygen, carbon dioxide, nutrients, and waste products among body cells.

veins Vessels that carry blood back to the heart from other regions of the body.

venules Branches of the veins.

sinoatrial node (SA node) A cluster of electrical pulse–generating cells that serves as a natural pacemaker for the heart.

Heart Function

Heart activity depends on a complex interaction of biochemical, physical, and neurological signals. There are four basic steps involved in heart function (see FIGURE 13.2):

1. Deoxygenated blood enters the right atrium after circulating through the body.
2. Blood moves to the right ventricle and is pumped through the pulmonary artery to the lungs, where it receives oxygen.
3. Oxygenated blood returns to the left atrium of the heart.
4. Blood from the left atrium moves into the left ventricle. The left ventricle pumps blood through the aorta to all body parts.

Various blood vessels perform different parts of this process. **Arteries** carry blood away from the heart; all arteries carry oxygenated blood *except* pulmonary arteries, which carry deoxygenated blood to the lungs, where the blood picks up oxygen and gives off carbon dioxide. As the arteries branch off from the heart, they branch into smaller blood vessels called **arterioles** and then into even smaller blood vessels known as **capillaries**. Capillaries have thin walls that permit the exchange of oxygen, carbon dioxide, nutrients, and waste products with body cells. Carbon dioxide and other waste products are transported to the lungs and kidneys through **veins** and **venules** (small veins).

For the heart to function properly, the four chambers must beat in an organized manner. Your heartbeat is governed by an electrical impulse that directs the heart muscle to move when the impulse travels across it, resulting in a sequential contraction of the four chambers. This signal starts in a small bundle of highly specialized cells, the **sinoatrial node (SA node)**, located in the right atrium. The SA node serves as a natural pacemaker for the heart. People with a damaged SA node must often have a mechanical pacemaker implanted to ensure the smooth passage of blood through the heartbeat's sequential phases.

At rest, the average adult heart beats 70 to 80 times per minute; a well-conditioned heart may beat only 50 to 60 times per minute to achieve the same results. If your resting heart rate is routinely in the high 80s or 90s, it may indicate that you are out of shape or suffering from some underlying illness. When overly stressed, a heart may beat more than 200 times per minute. A healthy heart functions more efficiently and is less likely to suffer damage from overwork.

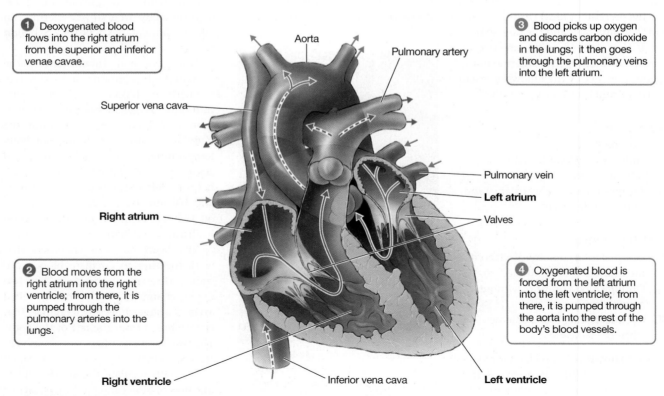

❶ Deoxygenated blood flows into the right atrium from the superior and inferior venae cavae.

❸ Blood picks up oxygen and discards carbon dioxide in the lungs; it then goes through the pulmonary veins into the left atrium.

❷ Blood moves from the right atrium into the right ventricle; from there, it is pumped through the pulmonary arteries into the lungs.

❹ Oxygenated blood is forced from the left atrium into the left ventricle; from there, it is pumped through the aorta into the rest of the body's blood vessels.

Aorta

Pulmonary artery

Superior vena cava

Pulmonary vein

Left atrium

Right atrium

Valves

Right ventricle

Inferior vena cava

Left ventricle

FIGURE 13.2 Blood Flow within the Heart

LO 3 | THE MAJOR CARDIOVASCULAR DISEASES

Review major types of cardiovascular disease, their symptoms, and their prevalence.

Although there are several types of CVD and its derivatives, the key ones we will consider are *hypertension, atherosclerosis, peripheral arterial disease (PAD), coronary heart disease (CHD), angina pectoris, arrhythmia, congestive heart failure,* and *stroke.* FIGURE 13.3 shows the prevalence of CVD-related deaths among adults in the United States.

Hypertension

Blood pressure is a measure of how hard blood pushes against the walls of vessels as your heart pumps. Sustained high blood pressure is called **hypertension**. Known as the "silent killer," it has few overt symptoms. Untreated hypertension damages blood vessels and increases your chance of angina, heart failure, peripheral artery disease, stroke, and heart attack. Hypertension can also cause kidney damage and contribute to vision loss, erectile dysfunction, and memory problems.[12]

In late 2017, several professional groups approved new National Hypertension guidelines in the United States. A key provision of these guidelines was to lower the numbers for labeling a person hypertensive. Effectively, this change will mean that nearly 50 percent of adults in the U.S. are likely to be labeled as hypertensive. See Table 13.1 and this URL for more details.[13] There are large disparities in self-reported hypertension by race/ethnicity, age, sex, level of education, and state. Currently approximately 45 percent, African Americans have the highest rates of high blood pressure in the United States and globally.[14] Rates are also much higher among older adults, men, and people who have less than a high school education.[15] Although awareness of hypertension has increased and most diagnosed individuals are using hypertension medications, only 53 percent of those taking medications have their hypertension under control.[16]

Blood pressure is measured by two numbers; for example, a blood pressure of 110/80 mmHg means "110 over 80 millimeters of mercury." The top number, **systolic blood pressure**, refers to the pressure of blood in the arteries when the heart muscle contracts, sending blood to the rest of the body. The bottom number, **diastolic blood pressure**, refers to the pressure of blood on the arteries when the heart muscle relaxes, as blood is reentering the heart chambers. Normal blood pressure varies depending on the person's age, weight, and physical condition. High blood pressure will now be diagnosed when systolic pressure is 130 or above (see **TABLE 13.1**). When only systolic pressure is high, the condition is known as *isolated systolic hypertension (ISH),* the most common form of high blood pressure in older Americans.

Systolic blood pressure tends to increase with age, whereas diastolic blood pressure typically increases until age 55 and then declines. Currently, men under the age of 45 have nearly twice the risk of becoming hypertensive as their female counterparts.[17] Men and women have nearly the same rates of high blood pressure between the ages of 45 and 64.[18] Women have

> **hypertension** Sustained elevated blood pressure.
>
> **systolic blood pressure** The upper number in the fraction that measures blood pressure, indicating pressure on the walls of the arteries when the heart contracts.
>
> **diastolic blood pressure** The lower number in the fraction that measures blood pressure, indicating pressure on the walls of the arteries during the relaxation phase of heart activity.

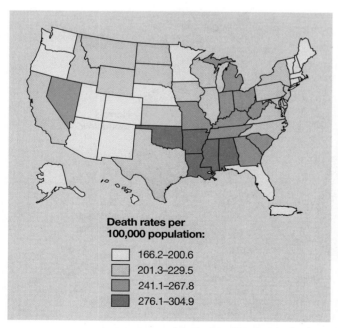

Death rates per 100,000 population:

- 166.2–200.6
- 201.3–229.5
- 241.1–267.8
- 276.1–304.9

FIGURE 13.3 Major Cardiovascular Disease Age-Adjusted Death Rates by State

Source: E. Benjamin et al., "Heart Disease and Stroke Statistics—2017 Update: A Report from the American Heart Association," *Circulation* 135, no. 10 (2017): e146–e603.

TABLE **13.1** | Blood Pressure Classifications

Blood Pressure Category	Systolic (mmHg)		Diastolic (mmHg)
Normal	less than 120	and	less than 80
Elevated	120–129	or	<80
High blood pressure (hypertension) stage 1	30–139	or	80–89
High blood pressure (hypertension) stage 2	140 or higher	or	90 or higher
Hypertensive crisis (emergency care needed)	Higher than 180	or	Higher than 120

Source: P. Welton et al. 2017 ACC/AHA/AAPA/ABC/ACPM/AGS/APhA/ASH/NMA/PCNA Guidelines for the Prevention, Detection, Evaluation and Management of High Blood Pressure in Adults. Journal of the American College of Cardiology. 2017. doi:10.1016/j.jacc.2017.11.006.

arteriosclerosis A general term for thickening and hardening of the arteries.

atherosclerosis A condition characterized by deposits of fatty substances (plaque) on the inner lining of an artery.

plaque The buildup of deposits in the arteries.

ischemia Reduced oxygen supply to a body part or organ.

higher rates after age 65.[19] New guidelines will increase the rates of both sexes.

New guidelines have eliminated the term "prehypertensive" and replaced it with the word "*elevated*", meaning that their blood pressure is above normal but not yet in the hypertensive range. These individuals have a significantly greater risk of becoming hypertensive.[20]

Over 17 percent of people with high blood pressure don't know it.[21] The majority of those who take medication to control their hypertension do not have it under control.[22] Young adults aged 18 to 39 are the worst of all age groups when it comes to following recommendations to control hypertension. Variable blood pressure readings, costs of treatment, denial of the seriousness of the problem, and resistance to drug side effects appear to be among reasons for poor control.[23]

Atherosclerosis

Arteriosclerosis, which is thickening and hardening of arteries, is a condition that underlies many cardiovascular health problems. **Atherosclerosis** is a type of arteriosclerosis in which fatty substances, cholesterol, cellular waste products, calcium, and fibrin (a clotting material in the blood) accumulate in the inner lining of an artery. *Hyperlipidemia* (abnormally high blood levels of *lipids*, which are non-water-soluble molecules such as fats and cholesterol) is a key factor in this process, and the resulting buildup is referred to as **plaque**.

As plaque accumulates, it adheres to the inner lining of the blood vessels. Vessel walls become narrow and may eventually block blood flow or rupture. This is similar to putting your thumb over the end of a hose while water is running through the hose. Pressure builds within arteries just as pressure builds in the hose. If vessels are weakened and pressure persists, the artery may become weak and eventually burst. Fluctuation in the blood pressure levels within arteries may actually damage their internal walls, making it even more likely that plaque will accumulate.

Atherosclerosis is the most common form of *coronary artery disease (CAD)*. It occurs as plaques are deposited in vessel walls and restrict blood flow and oxygen to the body's main coronary arteries on the outer surface of the heart, often eventually resulting in a heart attack (see **FIGURE 13.4**). When circulation is impaired and blood flow to the heart is limited, the heart may become starved for oxygen—a condition commonly referred to as **ischemia**. Sometimes coronary artery disease is referred to as *ischemic heart disease*.

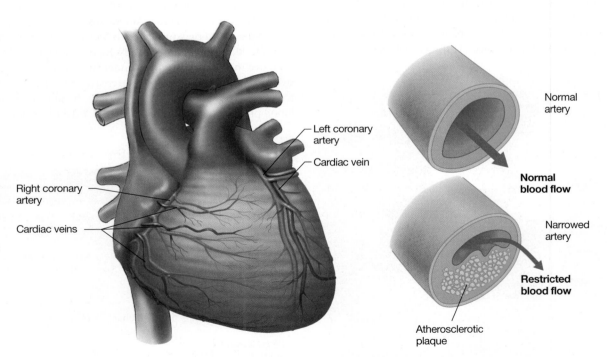

FIGURE 13.4 Atherosclerosis and Coronary Heart Disease The coronary arteries, which are located on the exterior of the heart, supply blood and oxygen to the heart muscle itself. In atherosclerosis, arteries become clogged by a buildup of plaque. When atherosclerosis occurs in coronary arteries, blood flow to the heart muscle is restricted, and a heart attack may occur.

Sources: Adapted from Joan Salge Blake, *Nutrition & You*, and Michael D. Johnson, *Human: Biology: Concepts and Current Issues*, 7th ed. Both copyright © 2014 Pearson Education, Inc. Reprinted by permission.

 Watch Video Tutor: **Atherosclerosis and Coronary Artery Disease** in Mastering Health.

Peripheral Artery Disease

When atherosclerosis or injury occurs in the upper or lower extremities, such as in the arms, feet, calves, or legs, and causes narrowing or complete blockage of arteries, it is often called **peripheral artery disease (PAD)**. In the United States, over 8.5 million people have PAD, particularly those who smoke, have diabetes, have high cholesterol, have high blood pressure, are over 65, are non-Hispanic black, and/or are male. Sometimes PAD can be caused by trauma, certain diseases, radiation therapy or surgery, inflammation, or combined risks from atherosclerosis. Many people with PAD receive no treatment because they are asymptomatic or don't recognize symptoms until they have a heart attack or stroke.[24] Others have pain and aching in the legs, calves, or feet upon walking or exercising that is relieved by rest (known as *intermittent claudication*). PAD is a leading cause of disability in people over age 50, and men develop it more frequently than women do.[25]

Coronary Heart Disease

Over 16.5 million Americans age 20 or older have **coronary heart disease (CHD)**. Of all the major cardiovascular diseases, CHD is the greatest killer, accounting for nearly 1 in 7 deaths (over 360,000 people) in the United States each year.[26] In addition, there are over 580,000 new coronary events and 210,000 reoccurrences each year.[27] Increasing numbers of people survive their heart attacks, thanks to medical intervention; however, treatment of CHD and heart attack are among the ten most expensive medical treatments, running in excess of $200 million dollars and projected to double by 2030.[28] A **myocardial infarction (MI)**, or *heart attack*, involves an area of the heart that suffers permanent damage because its normal blood supply has been blocked, often by a **coronary thrombosis** (formation of a clot) or an atherosclerotic narrowing that blocks a coronary artery. When a clot, or **thrombus**, becomes dislodged and moves through the circulatory system, it is called an **embolus**. Whenever blood does not flow readily, there is a corresponding decrease in oxygen flow to tissue below the blockage. If the blockage is extremely minor, an otherwise healthy heart will adapt over time by enlarging existing blood vessels and growing new ones to reroute needed blood through other areas. This system, called *collateral circulation*, is a form of self-preservation that allows an affected heart muscle to cope with damage.

When heart blockage is more severe, however, the body is unable to adapt on its own, and outside lifesaving support is

750,000

Americans have a **HEART ATTACK** each year in the United States; 116,000 of whom die and 200,000 of whom will have another heart attack within 5 years.

critical. See the Skills for Behavior Change box to learn what to do in case of a heart attack.

Arrhythmias

Over the course of a lifetime, most people experience some type of **arrhythmia**, an irregularity in heart rhythm that occurs when the electrical impulses in the heart that coordinate heartbeat don't work properly. Often described as a heart "fluttering" or racing, these irregularities send many people to the emergency room, only to find that they are fine. A racing heart in the absence of exercise or anxiety may be experiencing *tachycardia*, the medical term for abnormally fast heartbeat. On the other end of the continuum is *bradycardia*,

peripheral artery disease (PAD) Atherosclerosis occurring in the lower extremities, such as in the feet, calves, or legs, or in the arms.

coronary heart disease (CHD) A narrowing of the small blood vessels that supply blood to the heart.

myocardial infarction (MI) A blockage of normal blood supply to an area in the heart; also referred to as a *heart attack*.

coronary thrombosis Blood clot formation.

thrombus A blood clot.

embolus A clot that has been dislodged and can move through the circulatory system.

arrhythmia An irregularity in heartbeat.

or abnormally slow heartbeat. When a heart goes into **fibrillation**, it beats in a sporadic, quivering pattern, resulting in extreme inefficiency in moving blood through the cardiovascular system. If untreated, fibrillation may be fatal. The most common type of arrhythmias, **preventricular contractions (PVCs)**—premature heart beats in the ventricles—are on the rise among all age groups. Teens, young adults, and athletes seem particularly susceptible to PVCs.[29]

Not all arrhythmias are life threatening. In many instances, stress, lack of sleep, or excessive caffeine or nicotine consumption can trigger an episode. However, severe cases may require drug therapy and/or an *ablation procedure*, in which a catheter is inserted into the heart at the place where faulty electrical signals originate, and electricity zaps those areas to prevent the arrhythmia and subsequent heart damage. If you notice heart palpitations or have dizziness and other symptoms, check with your health care provider.

Angina Pectoris

Angina pectoris is a symptom of CHD that occurs when not enough oxygen supplies the heart muscle and is an indicator of underlying heart disease. Over 10 million people in the United States suffer from angina symptoms, ranging from heartburn-like symptoms to palpitations and crushing chest pain.[30] Mild cases may be treated with rest. Drugs such as *nitroglycerin* can dilate veins and provide pain relief. Other medications such as *calcium channel blockers* can relieve cardiac spasms and arrhythmias, lower blood pressure, and slow heart rate. *Beta-blockers* can control potential overactivity of the heart muscle.

Cardiomyopathy and Heart Failure

Cardiomyopathy occurs when the heart muscle is damaged or overworked, becomes enlarged, and lacks the strength to keep blood circulating normally through the body. Blood and fluids begin to back up into the lungs and other body tissues, such as the feet, ankles, and legs, resulting in swelling. Additionally, shortness of breath and tiredness may occur as the disease progresses. *Heart failure*, or **congestive heart failure**, is often the diagnosis in these cases. Cardiomyopathy is increasingly common, particularly among people with a history of arrhythmia, uncontrolled hypertension or

heart attack, sleep apnea, or respiratory problems. Certain prescription drugs such as NSAIDs and diabetes medications also increase risks, as do chronic drug abuse and alcohol abuse. In some cases, radiation or chemotherapy treatments for cancer can cause damage to the heart or the protective covering around the heart. Nearly 5.1 million adults have heart failure in the United States, and the number of cases is expected to approach 10 million by 2030.[31]

Untreated, heart failure can be fatal. However, most cases respond well to treatment that includes *diuretics* ("water pills") to relieve fluid accumulation; drugs such as *digitalis* that increase the pumping action of the heart; and drugs called *vasodilators*, which expand blood vessels and decrease resistance, allowing blood to flow more freely and making the heart's work easier.

Stroke

Like heart muscle, brain cells require a continuous supply of oxygen. A **stroke** (also called a *cerebrovascular accident*) occurs when the blood supply to the brain is interrupted. Strokes may be either *ischemic* (caused by plaque formation that narrows a blood vessel or a clot that obstructs a blood vessel) or *hemorrhagic* (due to a weakening of a blood vessel that causes it to bulge or rupture). An **aneurysm** (a widening or bulge in a blood vessel that may become hemorrhagic) is the best-known type of hemorrhagic stroke. When any of these events occurs, oxygen deprivation kills brain cells.

Some strokes are mild and cause only temporary dizziness or slight weakness or numbness. More serious interruptions in blood flow may impair speech, swallowing, memory, or motor control in the long term. Other strokes affect parts of the brain that regulate heart and lung function, killing within minutes. Fortunately, the incidence of strokes has declined by nearly 29 percent since 2004, largely as a result of factors

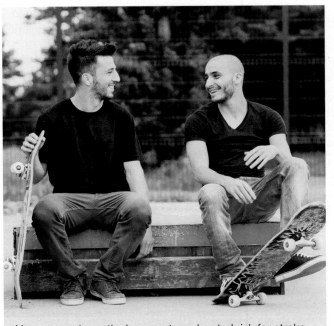

Young men, in particular, are at an elevated risk for stroke.

fibrillation A sporadic, quivering pattern of heartbeat that results in extreme inefficiency in moving blood through the cardiovascular system.

preventricular contractions (PVCs) Premature heart beats in the ventricles.

angina pectoris Chest pain occurring as a result of reduced oxygen flow to the heart.

cardiomyopathy The condition in which the heart muscle is damaged or overworked, becomes enlarged, and lacks the strength to keep blood circulating normally through the body.

congestive heart failure (CHF) An abnormal cardiovascular condition that reflects impaired cardiac pumping and blood flow; pooling blood leads to congestion in body tissues.

stroke A condition that occurs when the brain is damaged by disrupted blood supply; also called *cerebrovascular accident*.

aneurysm A weakened blood vessel that may bulge under pressure and, in severe cases, burst.

attention, improvements in emergency medicine protocols and medicines, and a greater emphasis on fast rehabilitation and therapy have helped many people to survive. Newer treatments include *tissue plasminogen activator (tPA)*, the only FDA-approved treatment for ischemic stroke; this medication dissolves clots and improves blood flow to affected areas, resulting in less damage and better chances of recovery. *Intra-arterial treatment (IAT)* is a technique in which a catheter delivers clot-dissolving drugs such as tPA right to the site of injury, allowing for quick blood restoration and less long-term damage. One promising new treatment, *stent retriever therapy*, involves inserting a catheter in the groin and snaking it through the body to the blocked artery. Once there, a wire mesh device opens and grabs the clot, often immediately restoring blood flow. Techniques like these result in minimal or no disability in 91 percent of patients if used quickly after a stroke diagnosis.[34] New ambulances equipped with the ability to scan for, diagnose, and treat strokes immediately offer the promise of better outcomes for patients. Preventing strokes and other cardiovascular diseases before they occur, by controlling blood pressure and reducing salt consumption, are among the best and least expensive options. The earlier you start, the better!

transient ischemic attacks (TIAs) A brief interruption of the blood supply to the brain that causes only temporary impairment; often an indicator of impending major stroke.

cardiometabolic risks Risk factors that affect both the cardiovascular system and the body's biochemical metabolic processes.

metabolic syndrome (MetS) A group of metabolic conditions occurring together that increase a person's risk of heart disease, stroke, and diabetes.

LO 4 | REDUCING YOUR RISKS

Describe the modifiable and nonmodifiable risk factors for cardiovascular disease and methods of prevention.

According to the U.S. Burden of Disease Collaborators, the greatest contributor to CVD is suboptimal diet, followed by tobacco smoking, high body mass index (BMI), high blood pressure, high fasting plasma glucose, and physical inactivity.[35] Newer research indicates that for people age 12 to 39, hypertension, smoking, high body fat, and high blood glucose increase the chances of dying from CVD-related complications before age 60.[36]

Cardiometabolic risks are the combined risks that indicate physical and biochemical changes that can lead to both CVD and type 2 diabetes. Some of these risks result from choices and behaviors and therefore are modifiable. Others are inherited or intrinsic (such as age and gender) and cannot be modified.

Metabolic Syndrome: Quick Risk Profile

A cluster of combined cardiometabolic risks, variably labeled as *syndrome X, insulin resistance syndrome*, and, most recently, **metabolic syndrome (MetS)** are believed to increase the risk for atherosclerotic heart disease by as much as three times the normal rates.[37] Women are more likely than men to have metabolic syndrome.[38] The highest prevalence occurs among

such as reductions in smoking, decreases in high-fat diets, and improvements in diagnosis and treatment. Despite overall decreases in occurrence, stroke still affects nearly 7 million Americans every year and kills 133,000 people, making it the fifth leading cause of death in the United States.[32] Ten percent of all strokes occur in people age 18 to 50. Strokes are on the increase among young adults, meaning significant increases in costs associated with long-term treatment and medication.[33]

Many strokes are preceded days, weeks, or months by **transient ischemic attacks (TIAs)**, brief interruptions of the blood supply to the brain that cause only temporary impairment. Symptoms of TIAs include dizziness, particularly on first rising in the morning; weakness; temporary paralysis or numbness in the face or other regions; temporary memory loss; blurred vision; nausea, headache; slurred speech; or other unusual physiological reactions. While some people may experience unexpected falls or have blackouts, others may have no obvious symptoms. TIAs often indicate an impending major stroke. The earlier a stroke is recognized, the more effective treatment will be (best results are seen if treatment begins within the first 1 to 2 hours). See the Skills for Behavior Change box for tips on recognizing signs and symptoms of a possible stroke.

Stroke survival rates have improved significantly in recent years, in part because of a greater recognition that *time is critical*. Greater awareness of stroke symptoms and faster medical

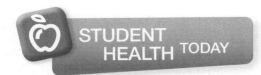
EMERGING CONCERN *Is Gut Bacteria a Culprit in CVD Risk?*

While the high levels of saturated fat in red meat and high-fat dairy can lead to clogged arteries, new research suggests that it's the way the bacteria in your gut process these substances that might put you at risk for CVD, not the fat level itself.

According to researchers, a chemical by-product created by digesting animal products may harm the linings of blood

vessels, contributing to atherosclerosis. The by-product, known as trimethylamine (TMA), changes into trimethylamine-N-oxide (TMAO) in the liver, apparently doubling the risk of heart attack, stroke, and death. While we need good bacteria in the gut, bacterial interactions with substances found in animal cells end up contributing to TMAO development and cholesterol accumulation on vessel walls.

If a blood test shows that levels of TMAO are elevated, reductions in high-fat animal products may be warranted. It's just one more reason to cut the levels of saturated fat in your diet to less than 10 percent of total calories.

Source: J. Brown and S. Hazen, "The Gut Microbial Endocrine Organ: Bacterially Derived Signals Driving Cardiometabolic Diseases," *Annual Review of Medicine* 66 (2015): 343.

Hispanics, followed by non-Hispanic whites and blacks.[39] As age increases, so does the incidence of MetS, which affects over 18 percent of 20- to 39-year-olds and nearly 47 percent of those age 60.[40] A person with three or more of the following risks is diagnosed with metabolic syndrome[41]:

- Abdominal obesity (waist measurement of more than 40 inches in men or 35 inches in women)
- Elevated blood fat (triglycerides greater than 150) or on drug treatment for elevated triglyceride
- Low levels of HDL ("good") cholesterol (less than 40 in men and less than 50 in women) or on drug treatment for HDL reduction
- Elevated blood pressure greater than 130/85 mmHg or on drug treatment for blood pressure reduction
- Elevated fasting glucose greater than 100 mg/dL (a sign of insulin resistance or glucose intolerance) or on drug treatment for elevated glucose.

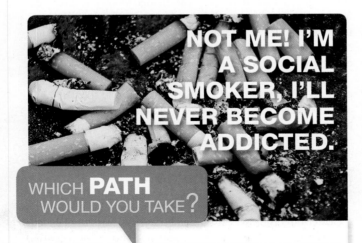

NOT ME! I'M A SOCIAL SMOKER, I'LL NEVER BECOME ADDICTED.

WHICH **PATH** WOULD YOU TAKE?

 Go to Mastering Health to see how your actions today affect your future health.

Modifiable Risks for CVD

It may surprise you that CVD is not something you get as you hit middle age. In fact, you are a CVD work in progress right now. From the first moments of your life, you were genetically preprogrammed with some risks. How that genetic predisposition plays out is influenced significantly by your lifestyle. Your behaviors set the stage for risks in your thirties, forties, and beyond. Making certain lifestyle modifications can have a significant effect on your future health profile.[42]

Avoid Tobacco
Since the 1960s, smoking prevalence in the United States has dropped dramatically, down from 51 percent of all males smoking to 16.7 percent today and down from 34 percent of women to 13.6 today.[43] Only 13.3 percent of male college students and 8.3 percent of female college students report smoking in the last 30 days.[44] Just how great a risk is smoking when it comes to CVD? Consider these facts[45]:

- Smokers are two to four times more likely to develop CHD than nonsmokers.
- Cigarette smoking doubles a person's stroke risk.
- Smokers are over ten times more likely than nonsmokers to develop peripheral vascular diseases.

Smoking is thought to damage the heart in several ways. Nicotine increases heart rate, blood pressure, and oxygen use by heart muscles; over time, this forces the organ to work harder. Additionally, chemicals in smoke may damage and inflame coronary arteries, increasing blood pressure and allowing plaque to accumulate more easily. The benefits of quitting smoking are significant. (See Chapter 9 on the health risks of smoking.)

Changing Fat and Cholesterol Recommendations
Cholesterol is a fatty, waxy substance found in the bloodstream and in body cells that is believed to be a factor in over 2.6 million deaths in the United States each year.[46] Cholesterol plays an important role in the production of cell membranes and hormones, among other beneficial functions.

How do we determine whether a behavior or substance is a risk factor for a disease? Should programs be enacted to reduce the risk or stop the behavior?

■ Do you think that there should be legislation banning tanning booths in all 50 states? Why or why not? Would you favor such a bill if it banned tanning for minors only?

For years, cholesterol has been seen as a key culprit in CVD risk rather than an essential part of our diets. However, in early 2016, surprising reversals in the "cholesterol is bad" mantra emerged with the new *Dietary Guidelines*.[47]

As a result of years of study, the new *2015–2020 Dietary Guidelines for Americans*, Eighth Edition, published in early 2016, eased up on recommendations focused on cutting cholesterol. It turns out that, with 75 percent of blood cholesterol produced by your liver and other cells—mostly out of your control as part of your genetic risk—much of your CVD risk may not have as much to do with dietary cholesterol intake as other factors, such as physical activity, body weight, intake of saturated and *trans* fat, heredity, age, and sex.[48] Eggs and other cholesterol-rich foods are now on the "eat in moderation" list as experts put the emphasis on reducing saturated fat from high-fat meats and dairy to 10 percent of the daily diet.[49] See the Student Health Today box for one more reason to cut saturated fat levels in your diet.

Still, just because eggs are off the "bad" list doesn't mean you can gorge on bacon or high-fat steak or burgers on a regular basis. Many factors influence the other 25 percent of cholesterol in your bloodstream—most important, the amount of saturated fat and *trans* fat in the diet. High-fat dairy, red meat, and other sources of saturated fat continue to be of concern for increased CVD risk. Moderation is the key, and new recommendations focus more on a healthy diet with leaner meats, poultry, nuts, fish, and shellfish and drastic reductions in refined carbohydrates, sugar, and salt.[50]

To help guide public behavior, the AHA and the American College of Cardiology came up with new cardiovascular prevention guidelines recommending that people work with their health care provider and assess their risk. A new risk equation assesses factors such as gender, race, age, current blood pressure control and medications, total cholesterol, HDL cholesterol, diabetes, smoking status, overall lifestyle, and genetic/family CVD risks. For certain risk factors, your doctor may prescribe *statins*—medications designed to lower cholesterol and significantly reduce stroke and CVD risk.

Currently, about 45 percent of adults age 20 and over have cholesterol levels at or above 200 mg/dL, and another 16 percent have levels in excess of 240 mg/dL.[51] More than 28 percent of Americans over the age of 40 in the United States are taking a cholesterol-lowering prescription; 93 percent of those are on statins.[52] A new survey indicates that many people with high cholesterol know their risks but either don't know how to keep their cholesterol level under control or aren't confident enough to do so. Compliance with medication is often sporadic, and nearly 47 percent of respondents hadn't had a cholesterol check in the last year.[53]

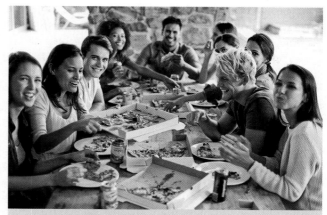

Excess sodium consumption is a key factor in hypertension risks in the United States. Major dietary sodium sources include yeast breads, chicken dishes, cold cuts, condiments, sausage, hot dogs, bacon, and cheeses.

Historically, total cholesterol hasn't been the only level of concern; the focus has also been on the two major types of blood cholesterol: *low-density lipoprotein (LDL)* and *high-density lipoprotein (HDL)*. Low-density lipoprotein, often referred to as "bad" cholesterol, is believed to build up on artery walls. In contrast, high-density lipoprotein, or "good" cholesterol, appears to remove cholesterol from artery walls, thus serving as a protector. In theory, if LDL levels got too high or HDL levels too low, cholesterol would accumulate inside arteries and lead to cardiovascular problems. There is still controversy over whether this long-held theory is valid or not.

TABLE 13.2 | Recommended Cholesterol Levels for Lower/Moderate-Risk Adults

Total Cholesterol Level (lower numbers are better)	
Less than 200 mg/dL	Desirable
200–239 mg/dL	Borderline high
240 mg/dL and above	High
HDL Cholesterol Level (higher numbers are better)	
Less than 40 mg/dL (for men)	Low
60 mg/dL and above	Desirable
LDL Cholesterol Level (lower numbers are better)	
Less than 100 mg/dL	Optimal
100–129 mg/dL	Near or above optimal
130–159 mg/dL	Borderline high
160–189 mg/dL	High
190 mg/dL and above	Very high
Triglyceride Level (lower numbers are better)	
Less than 150 mg/dL	Normal/desirable

Source: National Heart Lung and Blood Institute, "What Is Cholesterol?" April 2016, http://www.nhlbi.nih.gov/health/health-topics/topics/hbc/diagnosis.

In general, LDL (or "bad" cholesterol) is more closely associated with cardiovascular risk than is total cholesterol. Until recently, most authorities agreed that looking only at LDL ignored the positive effects of "good" cholesterol (HDL) and that raising HDL was an important goal. There has been general agreement that the best method of evaluating risk is to examine the ratio of HDL to total cholesterol. If the level of HDL is lower than 35 mg/dL, cardiovascular risk increases dramatically. To reduce risk, the goal has been to manage the ratio of HDL to total cholesterol by lowering LDL levels, raising HDL, or both. New research indicates that trying to raise HDL as a means of preventing negative CVD outcomes may not be as beneficial as was once thought.[54] However, many professional groups continue to believe that reducing LDL levels through aggressive drug therapy such as using statins is the right goal for many at-risk populations, along with increased exercise levels, weight control, healthy diet, and avoidance of tobacco.[55]

Triglycerides continue to be a focus of attention as a key factor in CVD risk. When you consume extra calories, the body converts them to triglycerides, which are stored in fat cells. Hormones release triglycerides throughout the day to provide energy. High levels of blood triglycerides are often found in people who have high cholesterol levels, heart problems, or diabetes or who are overweight. As people get older, heavier, or both, their triglyceride and cholesterol levels tend to rise. It has been recommended that a baseline cholesterol test (known as a lipid panel or lipid profile) be taken at age 20, with follow-ups every 5 years. This test, which measures triglyceride levels as well as HDL, LDL, and total cholesterol levels, requires that you fast for 12 hours before the test, are well hydrated, and avoid coffee and tea before testing. Men over the age of 35 and women over the age of 45 have been advised to have their lipid profile checked annually, with more frequent tests for those at high risk. Whether any or all of these recommendations will still be in force after the *Dietary Guidelines* are considered for their clinical implications remains unclear. See **TABLE 13.2** for current recommended levels of cholesterol and triglycerides.

Strive for a Heart-Healthy Diet Research continues into dietary modifications that may affect heart health. The DASH (Dietary Approaches to Stop Hypertension) eating plan from the National Heart, Lung, and Blood Institute (**FIGURE 13.5**) has strong evidence to back up its recommendations. DASH guidelines include the following:

- Reduce salt intake. Sodium chloride (salt) is hidden in many popular foods. Levels of sodium in breads, pasta sauces, processed meats such as hot dogs and some ethnic foods can be extremely high.
- Consume 5 to 10 milligrams per day of soluble fiber from sources such as oat bran, fruits, vegetables, and seeds. This may result in a 5 percent drop in LDL levels.
- Consume about 2 grams per day of plant sterols, which are naturally present in many plant-based foods. Intake of plant sterols can reduce LDL by another 5 percent. The Health Headlines box presents benefits of some other heart-healthy superfoods.

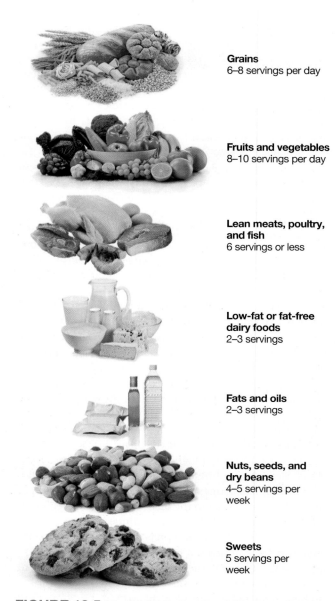

Grains
6–8 servings per day

Fruits and vegetables
8–10 servings per day

Lean meats, poultry, and fish
6 servings or less

Low-fat or fat-free dairy foods
2–3 servings

Fats and oils
2–3 servings

Nuts, seeds, and dry beans
4–5 servings per week

Sweets
5 servings per week

FIGURE 13.5 The DASH Eating Plan This plan is based on a 2,000-calorie/day diet. All serving suggestions are per day unless otherwise noted.

Source: National Heart, Lung, and Blood Institute, "Following the DASH Eating Plan," September 2015, www.nhlbi.nih.gov/health/health-topics/topics/dash/followdash.html.

Maintain a Healthy Weight Overweight people are more likely to develop heart disease and stroke even if they have no other risk factors. This is especially true if for people who are "apples" (thicker around the upper body and waist) rather than "pears" (thicker around the hips and thighs).

Exercise Regularly Even modest levels of low-intensity physical activity—walking, gardening, housework, dancing—are beneficial if done regularly and over the long term. Exercise can increase HDL, lower triglycerides, and reduce coronary risks in several ways.

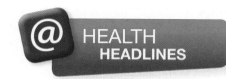

HEART-HEALTHY SUPER FOODS

The foods you eat play a major role in your risk for CVD. While many foods can increase your risk, several have been shown to reduce the chances that cholesterol will be absorbed in the cells, reduce levels of LDL cholesterol, or enhance the protective effects of HDL cholesterol. To protect your heart, include the following in your diet:

- **Dark chocolate.** Dark chocolate contains 70 percent or more of flavonoid-rich cocoa and much less sugar than milk chocolate. If you must indulge, buy chocolate with the highest percentage of cocoa you can find, and savor 1 to 2 ounces a bit at a time. Moderation is the key.
- **Fish high in omega-3 fatty acids.** Consumption of fish such as salmon, sardines, and herring may help to reduce blood pressure and the inflammation that leads to plaque formation. However, new research is showing

conflicting results about the benefits of omega-3 fatty acid supplements.
- **Olive oil.** Using monounsaturated fats in cooking, particularly extra virgin olive oil, helps to lower total cholesterol and raise your HDL levels.
- **Whole grains and fiber.** Getting enough fiber in the form of 100 percent whole wheat, oats, oat bran, flaxseed, fruits, and vegetables helps to lower LDL or bad cholesterol. Soluble fiber, in particular, seems to keep cholesterol from being absorbed in the intestines.
- **Nuts.** Walnuts are naturally high in omega-3 fatty acids, which are important in lowering triglyceride levels and good for the blood vessels themselves.
- **Red wine.** Many observational studies have indicated that one glass of red wine may be protective and reduce the risk of CVD. The American Heart Association recommends dietary modification, exercise, and stress reduction while supporting additional research.

Although one drink of red wine might be protective, adding additional doses of wine doesn't appear to help.

Sources: A. Tresserra-Rimbau et al., "Moderate Red Wine Consumption Is Associated with Lower Prevalence of the Metabolic Syndrome in the PREDIMED Population," *British Journal of Nutrition* 113, no. S2 (2015): S121–S130; American Heart Association, "Alcoholic Beverages and Cardiovascular Disease," 2015, www.heart.org/HEARTORG/ GettingHealthy/NutritionCenter/HealthyEating/ Alcohol-and-Heart-Health_UCM_305173_Article. jsp; S. Kalesi, J. Sun, and N. Buys, "Green Tea Catechins and Blood Pressure: A Systematic Review and Meta Analysis of Randomized Controlled Trials," *European Journal of Nutrition* (2014), doi:10.1007/s00394-014-0720-1; M. Murray, C. Walcuk, M. Suh, and P. J. Jones, "Green Tea Catechins and Cardiovascular Risk Factors: Should a Health Claim Be Made by U.S. FDA?," *Trends in Food Science and Technology* 41, no. 2 (2015): 188–97; American Heart Association, "Fish and Omega 3 Fatty Acids," June 15, 2015, www.heart. org/HEARTORG/General/Fish-and-Omega-3-Fatty-Acids_UCM_303248_Article.jsp.

Control Diabetes Heart disease death rates among adults with diabetes are two to four times higher than the rates for adults without diabetes. At least 65 percent of people with diabetes die of some form of heart disease or stroke.[56] Through a prescribed regimen of diet, exercise, and medication, they can control much of their increased risk for CVD. See **Focus On: Minimizing Your Risk for Diabetes** for more on preventing and controlling diabetes.

Control Your Blood Pressure In general, the higher your blood pressure, the greater your risk for CVD. Key factors in increasing blood pressure include obesity, lack of exercise, atherosclerosis, kidney damage from diabetes complications, certain arrhythmias, and other factors.[57] Treatment of hypertension should involve dietary changes, particularly lowering the amount of sodium, which plays a key role in increasing blood pressure.

Manage Stress and Get More Sleep In recent years, scientists have shown compelling evidence that both acute and chronic stress may trigger acute cardiac events or even sudden cardiac death, as well as increasing risks of hypertension, stroke, and elevated cholesterol levels.[58] Multiple life stressors can have tsunami-like effects on people young and old, and sleep deprivation may increase risks.[59]

(See Chapter 3 for more on the effects of stress and coping with stress.)

Nonmodifiable Risks

Unfortunately, not all risk factors for CVD can be prevented or controlled. The most important nonmodifiable risk factors are the following:

- **Race and ethnicity.** African Americans tend to have the highest overall rates of CVD and hypertension and the lowest rates of physical activity. Mexican Americans have the highest percentage of adults with cholesterol levels exceeding 200 mg/dL and the highest rates of obesity and overweight.[60]
- **Heredity.** A family history of heart disease increases the risk of CVD significantly. The amount of cholesterol you produce, tendencies to form plaque, and other factors seem to have genetic links. The difficulty comes in distinguishing genetic influences from the modifiable factors shared by family members, such as environment, stress, and dietary habits. Newer research has focused on studying the interactions between nutrition and genes (*nutrigenetics*) and the role that diet may play in increasing or decreasing risks among certain genetic profiles.[61]

- **Age.** Advanced age and multiple risk factors increase the risk of CVD for everyone.[62]
- **Gender.** Men are at greater risk for CVD until about age 60, when women begin to catch up, taking the lead at age 80. Otherwise healthy women under age 35 have a fairly low risk, although oral contraceptive use and smoking increase risks. After menopause or after estrogen levels are otherwise reduced (for example, because of hysterectomy), women's LDL levels tend to go up, which increases the chance for CVD. Women also have poorer health outcomes and higher death rates than men after a heart attack.[63]

Other Risk Factors Being Studied

Although risk factors for CVD are widely known, most people who die suddenly of a heart attack haven't had obvious symptoms before the heart attack happens. New tests and emerging risk factors are being studied. Two fairly new CVD risks include high levels of inflammation in the vessels and homocysteine levels.

Inflammation and C-Reactive Protein Occurring when tissues are injured by bacteria, trauma, toxins, or heat, among other things, inflammation is increasingly being considered a culprit in atherosclerotic plaque formation. Injured vessel walls are more prone to plaque formation. To date, several factors, including cigarette smoke, high blood pressure, high LDL cholesterol levels, diabetes mellitus, certain forms of arthritis, gastrointestinal problems, and exposure to toxic substances have been linked to increased risk of inflammation. However, the greatest risk appears to be from certain infectious disease pathogens, most notably *Chlamydia pneumoniae*, a common cause of respiratory infections; *Helicobacter pylori*, a bacterium that causes ulcers; herpes simplex virus, a virus that most of us have been exposed to; and *Cytomegalovirus*, another herpes virus infecting most Americans before the age of 40. During an inflammatory reaction, **C-reactive proteins** tend to be present at high levels. A recent meta-analysis of over 38 studies with nearly 170,000 subjects has shown a strong association between C-reactive proteins in the blood and increased risks for atherosclerosis and CVD.[64] Blood tests can test these proteins by using a highly sensitive assay called *hs-CRP* (high-sensitivity C-reactive protein); if levels are high, action can be taken to reduce inflammation.

The FDA recently approved a new, nonfasting blood test that predicts heart attack in people with no history of heart disease. Known as *PLAC*, the test measures activity of inflammatory enzymes in the blood, which cause plaque to form. More inflammatory enzymes mean more plaque in blood vessels—and greater risk. The PLAC test could increase our ability to spot and treat potential heart attacks early in the process.[65]

The AHA and other groups have recommended fish oil,

C-reactive protein (CRP) A protein whose blood levels rise in response to inflammation.

homocysteine An amino acid normally present in the blood that, when found at high levels, may be related to higher risk of cardiovascular disease.

flax, and other foods high in omega-3 fatty acids for their anti-inflammatory properties, but newer research raises questions about the role of omega-3 fatty acids in reducing risk of CHD and other cardiovascular problems.[66]

In spite of conflicting reports, major professional organizations continue to recommend dietary omega-3 fatty acid supplementation for risk reduction.[67] More research is necessary to determine the actual role that inflammation plays in increased risk of CVD and whether there is something unique about inflammation that omega-3 fatty acids may work to counter.[68]

Homocysteine In the last decade, an increasing amount of attention has been given to the role of **homocysteine**—an amino acid normally present in the blood—in increasing the risk for CVD. When present at high levels, homocysteine may be related to higher risk of coronary heart disease, stroke, and peripheral artery disease. Although more research is needed, scientists hypothesize that homocysteine works like C-reactive proteins, inflaming the inner lining of the arterial walls, promoting fat deposits on the damaged walls, and encouraging blood clot development.[69] When early studies indicated that folic acid and other B vitamins may help break down homocysteine in the body, food manufacturers responded by adding folic acids to a number of foods and touting the CVD benefits. With conflicting research, the jury is still out on the role of folic acid in CVD risk reduction. In fact, professional groups such as the AHA indicate that although folic acid supplements appear to have a modest positive effect on stroke risk, there appears to be neither benefit nor harm in taking folic acid supplements to lower risk of CHD.[70] For now, a healthy diet is the best preventive action.

LO 5 | DIAGNOSING AND TREATING CARDIOVASCULAR DISEASE

Examine current strategies for diagnosis and treatment of cardiovascular disease.

Today, patients with CVD have many diagnostic, treatment, prevention, and rehabilitation options that were not available a generation ago. Medications can strengthen the heartbeat, control arrhythmias, remove fluids, reduce blood pressure, improve heart function, and reduce pain. Among the most common groups of drugs are statins, which are used to lower blood cholesterol levels; ACE inhibitors, which cause the muscles surrounding blood vessels to contract, thereby lowering blood pressure; and beta-blockers, which reduce blood pressure by blocking the effects of the hormone epinephrine. New treatment procedures and techniques are saving countless lives. Even long-standing methods of cardiopulmonary resuscitation (CPR) have been changed to focus primarily on chest compressions rather than mouth-to-mouth breathing. The thinking behind this is that people will be more likely to do CPR if the risk for exchange of body fluids is reduced, and any effort to save a person in trouble is better than inaction.

Techniques for Diagnosing Cardiovascular Disease

Several techniques are used to diagnose CVD, including electrocardiogram, angiography, and positron emission tomography scans. An **electrocardiogram (ECG)** is a record of the electrical activity of the heart. Patients may undergo a *stress test*—standard exercise on a stationary bike or treadmill with an electrocardiogram and no injections—or a *nuclear stress test*, which involves injecting a radioactive dye and taking images of the heart to reveal problems with blood flow. In **angiography** (often referred to as *cardiac catheterization*), a needle-thin tube called a *catheter* is threaded through heart arteries, a dye is injected, and an X-ray image is taken to discover which areas are blocked. *Positron emission tomography (PET)* produces three-dimensional images of the heart as blood flows through it. Other tests include the following:

- **Magnetic resonance imaging (MRI).** This test uses powerful magnets to look inside the body. Computer-generated pictures can help physicians identify damage from a heart attack and evaluate disease of larger blood vessels such as the aorta.
- **Ultrafast computed tomography (CT).** This is an especially fast form of X-ray imaging of the heart designed to evaluate bypass grafts, diagnose ventricular function, and measure calcium deposits.
- **Cardiac calcium score.** This test measures the amount of calcium-containing plaque in the coronary arteries, a marker for overall atherosclerotic buildup. The greater the amount of calcium, the higher your calcium score and the greater your risk of heart attack. Concerns have been raised over higher than average exposure to radiation from these tests.

Surgical Options: Bypass Surgery, Angioplasty, and Stents

Coronary bypass surgery has helped many patients who suffered coronary blockages or heart attacks. In a *coronary artery bypass graft (CABG)*, referred to as a "cabbage," a blood vessel is taken from another site in the patient's body (usually the saphenous vein in the leg or the internal thoracic artery in the chest) and implanted to bypass blocked coronary arteries and transport blood to heart tissue.

Another procedure, **angioplasty** (sometimes called *balloon angioplasty*), carries fewer risks. As in angiography, a thin catheter is threaded through blocked heart arteries. The catheter has a balloon at the tip, which is inflated to flatten fatty deposits against the artery walls, allowing blood to flow more freely. A *stent* (a meshlike stainless steel tube) may be inserted to prop open the artery. Although highly effective, stents can lead to inflammation and tissue growth in the area that can actually lead to more blockage and problems. In about 30 percent of patients, the treated arteries become clogged again within 6 months. Newer stents are usually medicated to reduce this risk. Nonetheless, some surgeons argue that given this high rate of recurrence, bypass may be a more effective treatment. Newer forms of laser angioplasty and *atherectomy*, a procedure that removes plaque, are being done in several clinics.

Changing Aspirin Recommendations and Other Treatments

Although aspirin has been touted for its blood-thinning qualities and for possibly reducing risks for future heart attacks among people who already have had MI events, the benefits of an aspirin regimen for otherwise healthy adults has been controversial. New recommendations focus on those over the age of 50, as the evidence for aspirin use in younger, low-risk adults is inconclusive. Older individuals with a history of heart attack or who are at risk for a heart attack or stroke should consult with a doctor to discuss aspirin use. Those with risks of gastrointestinal bleeding or a history of stroke due to bleeding in the brain should discuss risks versus benefits with their health care provider before use. Ultimately, the FDA indicates that aspirin may be helpful for those who have had a heart attack or stroke in preventing a recurrence; however, it shouldn't be taken forever.[71] Furthermore, once a patient has taken aspirin regularly for possible protection against CHD, stopping this regimen may in fact increase the person's risk.[72]

Beyond aspirin, if a patient reaches an emergency room and is diagnosed fast enough, a form of clot-busting therapy called **thrombolysis** can be performed. Thrombolysis involves injecting an agent such as tPA to dissolve the clot and restore some blood flow to the heart (or brain), thereby reducing the amount of tissue that dies from ischemia.[73] These drugs must be administered within 1 to 3 hours after a cardiovascular event.

LO 6 | AN OVERVIEW OF CANCER

Describe cancer and how it develops, as well as its impact compared to other major health problems in terms of morbidity/mortality, costs, and overall effectiveness of prevention and control.

Cancer is the general term for a large group of diseases characterized by the uncontrolled growth and spread of abnormal cells. If these cells aren't stopped, they can impair vital functions of the body and lead to death. After heart disease, cancer is the greatest killer in the United States.[74] In 2017, there were nearly 1.7 million *new* cancer diagnoses, and nearly 601,000 deaths.[75] Cancers of the lungs, colon, pancreas, female breasts, liver, and prostate account for the largest percentage of cancer

---

electrocardiogram (ECG) A record of the electrical activity of the heart; may be measured during a stress test.

angiography A technique for examining blockages in heart arteries.

coronary bypass surgery A surgical technique whereby a blood vessel taken from another part of the body is implanted to bypass a clogged coronary artery.

angioplasty A technique in which a catheter with a balloon at the tip is inserted into a clogged artery; the balloon is inflated to flatten fatty deposits against artery walls, and a stent is typically inserted to keep the artery open.

thrombolysis Injection of an agent to dissolve clots and restore some blood flow, thereby reducing the amount of tissue that dies from ischemia.

cancer A large group of diseases characterized by the uncontrolled growth and spread of abnormal cells.

death.[76] While those numbers may sound bleak, we've made remarkable progress in cancer death rates in recent years, and more people are surviving cancer today than ever before.

The **5-year relative survival rate** (the percentage of people alive 5 years after diagnosis divided by the percentage expected to be alive and cancer-free according to normal life expectancy) has increased greatly from the 50 percent of past generations. Today, about 68 percent of whites and 61 percent of blacks diagnosed with cancer each year will be alive 5 years after diagnosis.[77] But 5-year survival rate should be viewed with caution. Relative survival rate doesn't distinguish between people who are truly cancer-free, those in **remission** (responding to treatment with cancer under control), those who have relapsed, those still in treatment whose cancer is not controlled, and those beginning new treatment regimens.[78]

Although treatments and survival statistics have improved dramatically, there continue to be huge disparities based on age, socioeconomic status, insurance status, race, geographical location, and other variables.[79] In the following sections, we look at factors that increase risk of cancer and discuss ways to reduce those risks.

How Does Cancer Develop?

When something interrupts normal cell function, uncontrolled growth and abnormal cellular development result in a **neoplasm**, a new growth of tissue that serves no physiological function. This neoplasmic mass often forms a clumping of cells known as a **tumor**.

Not all tumors are **malignant** (cancerous); in fact, most are **benign** (noncancerous). Benign tumors are generally harmless unless they grow to obstruct or crowd out normal tissues. A benign tumor of the brain, for instance, is life threatening when it grows enough to restrict blood flow and cause a stroke. The only way to determine whether a tumor is malignant is through **biopsy**, or microscopic examination of cell development.

Benign tumors generally consist of ordinary-looking cells enclosed in a fibrous shell or capsule that prevents their spreading. Malignant tumors are usually not enclosed in a protective capsule and can therefore spread to other organs (**FIGURE 13.6**). This process, known as **metastasis**, makes some forms of cancer particularly aggressive. By the time they are diagnosed, malignant tumors have frequently metastasized throughout

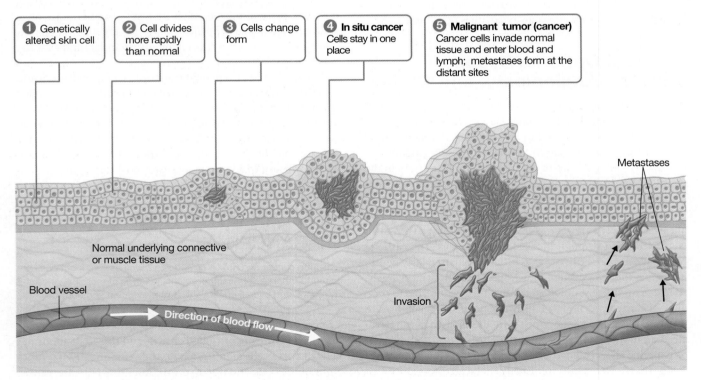

① **Genetically altered skin cell**

② **Cell divides more rapidly than normal**

③ **Cells change form**

④ **In situ cancer** Cells stay in one place

⑤ **Malignant tumor (cancer)** Cancer cells invade normal tissue and enter blood and lymph; metastases form at the distant sites

Metastases

Normal underlying connective or muscle tissue

Blood vessel

Direction of blood flow

Invasion

FIGURE 13.6 Metastasis A mutation to the genetic material of a skin cell triggers abnormal cell division and changes cell formation, resulting in a cancerous tumor. If the tumor remains localized, it is considered in situ cancer. If the tumor spreads, it is considered a malignant cancer.

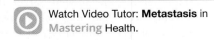

Watch Video Tutor: **Metastasis** in Mastering Health.

the body, making treatment extremely difficult. Malignant cells invade surrounding tissue, emitting clawlike protrusions that disturb the RNA and DNA within normal cells. Disrupting these substances, which control cellular metabolism and reproduction, produces **mutant cells** that differ in form, quality, and function from normal cells.

How Is Cancer Classified?

Cancer staging is a classification system that describes how much a cancer has spread at the time it is diagnosed; it helps doctors and patients decide on appropriate treatments and estimate a person's life expectancy. Cancers are typically staged based on the size of a tumor, how deeply it has penetrated , the number of affected lymph nodes, and the degree of metastasis or spread, known as the TNM (for *tumor*, *node*, and *metastasis*) staging system. The most commonly known staging system assigns a number from 0 to IV to the disease, IV being most advanced and often having the worst prognosis. Other staging systems are often used (see **TABLE 13.3**). In addition to staging, many tumors are assigned a grade based on the degree of cell abnormality. Typically, the lower the stage and grade, the better the prognosis.[80]

LO 7 | WHAT CAUSES CANCER?

Explain the suspected causes of cancer, and identify which risks are preventable, given current knowledge in the field.

Causes are generally divided into two categories of risk factors: *hereditary* and *acquired* (environmental). Although we cannot change our hereditary predisposition to certain cancers, we do have control over some factors in our lives, such as our exposure to certain infectious agents, dietary factors that increase risk, whether to have diagnostic procedures that find cancers at their earliest stages, drug and alcohol consumption, smoking status, amount of sun exposure, and exposure to **carcinogens** (cancer-causing agents) in food and in our immediate environment. Where we live, the water we drink, the air we breathe, and exposures in the workplace are often part of broader life choices. Some populations have fewer choices and greater risks than others.

TABLE 13.3 | Cancer Stages

Stage	Definition
0	Early cancer, when abnormal cells remain only in the place they originated.
I	Higher numbers indicate more extensive disease:
II	Larger tumor size and/or spread of the cancer
III	beyond the organ in which it first developed to nearby lymph nodes and/or organs adjacent to the location of the primary tumor.
IV	Cancer has spread to other organs.

Source: National Cancer Institute, National Institutes of Health, "Fact Sheet, Cancer Staging, 2015," January 6, 2015, www.cancer.gov/cancertopics/diagnosis-staging/staging/staging-fact-sheet.

mutant cells Cells that differ in form, quality, or function from normal cells.

cancer staging A classification system that describes how far a person's disease has advanced.

carcinogens Cancer-causing agents.

lifetime risk The probability that a person will develop or die from a given disease.

Lifestyle Risks

Cancer occurs in all age groups, but the older you are, the greater is your risk. In fact, 78 percent of all cancers are diagnosed in adults over age 55.[81] Cancer researchers refer to one's cancer risk when they assess risk factors. **Lifetime risk** refers to the probability that an individual, over the course of a lifetime, will develop cancer. In the United States, men have a lifetime risk of about 42 percent; women have a lifetime risk of 33 percent.[82] Risks also vary by race, socioeconomic status, education, occupation, geographic location, and several other factors.

Relative risk is a measure of the strength of the relationship between risk factors and a particular cancer. Basically, it compares your risk of

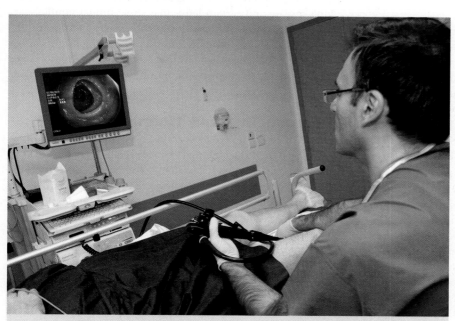

Physicians usually order biopsies of tumors, in which sample cells are taken from the tumor and studied under a microscope to determine whether they are cancerous. Newer techniques, such as the minimally invasive optical biopsy shown here, allow for the microscopic examination of tissue without doing a physical biopsy.

cancer if you engage in certain known risk behaviors with the risk of someone who does not. For example, men and women who smoke have 25 times the risk of lung cancer of a nonsmoker—a relative risk of 25.[83]

Over the years, researchers have found that certain types of diet, a sedentary lifestyle, overconsumption of alcohol, tobacco use, stress, and other factors play a key role in the incidence (number of new cases) of cancer. Keep in mind that a high relative risk does not guarantee cause and effect. It merely indicates the likelihood of a particular risk factor being related to a particular outcome.

Tobacco Use

Smoking is associated with increased risk of at least 15 different cancers. According to the 2014 *Surgeon General's Report on the Health Consequences of Smoking*, several compelling associations between smoking and cancer were reported, including causal relationships between smoking and liver cancer, colorectal polyps, oral cancer, and colorectal cancer.[84]

Over the years, cigarette smoking has declined in many regions of the world, largely as a result of efforts aimed at prevention and control through education, policy development programs that mandate plain packaging and less glamorous appeal, media campaigns, advertising bans, and taxation. Still, developing countries continue to be disproportionately affected by increasing numbers of cancer cases and high smoking rates. In fact, over 60 percent of the world's total cancer cases and 70 percent of cancer deaths occur in Africa, Asia, and Central and South America, particularly in low- and middle-income countries.[85] Lung cancer continues to be the leading cause of cancer deaths globally in spite of massive efforts to prevent or control smoking.[86]

Alcohol and Cancer Risk

Countless studies have implicated alcohol as a risk factor for cancer, particularly cancers of the oral cavity and pharynx, esophagus, colon and rectum, liver, larynx, and female breast. There is increasing evidence that moderate to high levels of drinking are associated with some other cancers, such as pancreas and prostate cancer and melanoma.[87] Both men and women who binge-drink (more than 8 drinks per week for women and more than 15 drinks per week for men) significantly increase their risks of cancer.[88]

Poor Nutrition, Physical Inactivity, and Obesity

Nearly one-third of annual cancer deaths in the United States may be due to lifestyle factors such as overweight or obesity, physical inactivity, and poor nutrition. In fact, obesity may be a key contributor in 1 out of 5 cancer deaths.[89] Dietary choices and physical activity are some of the most important modifiable determinants of cancer risk. Several studies indicate a relationship between a high BMI and death rates from cancers of the esophagus, colon, rectum, liver, stomach, kidney, pancreas, and others, as well as a high risk of endometrial cancer among younger women age 18 to 25 with higher BMIs and rapid weight gain.[90] Numerous other studies support the link between various forms of cancer and obesity.[91] The higher the BMI, the greater the cancer risk.[92]

Stress and Psychosocial Risks

Although a recent large meta-analytic study found no relationship between job strain and risk for colorectal, lung, breast, or prostate cancer, people who are under chronic, severe stress or who suffer from depression or other persistent emotional problems do show higher rates of cancer than their healthy counterparts.[93] Sleep disturbances, an unhealthy diet, and emotional or physical trauma may weaken the body's immune system, increasing susceptibility to cancer. Other possible contributors to cancer are poverty and the health disparities associated with low socio-economic status.

Genetic and Physiological Risks

Scientists believe that between 5 and 10 percent of all cancers are strongly hereditary.[94] It seems that some people may be more predisposed to the malfunctioning of genes that ultimately cause cancer.[95]

Our DNA includes multiple genes that contribute to normal cell growth. Mutated forms of these genes, called **oncogenes**, may cause the uncontrolled growth of cancer cells. Similarly, our DNA includes tumor suppressor genes that help limit cell growth. Mutated forms of these genes are unable to suppress the formation of tumors. These gene mutations may be inherited or may be triggered by exposure to carcinogens such as pollution, viruses, and radiation.

Certain cancers, particularly those of the breast, stomach, colon, prostate, uterus, ovaries, and lungs, appear to run in families. For example, a woman runs a much higher risk of breast cancer and/or ovarian cancer if her mother or sisters (primary relatives) have had the disease or if she inherits the breast cancer susceptibility genes (*BRCA1* or *BRCA2*). Hodgkin's disease and certain leukemias show similar familial patterns. The complex interaction of hereditary predisposition, lifestyle, and environment on the development of cancer makes it a challenge to determine a single cause. Even among people predisposed to genetic mutations, avoiding risks may decrease chances of cancer development.

Reproductive and Hormonal Factors

The effects of reproductive factors on breast and cervical cancers have been well documented. Increased numbers of fertile or menstrual cycle years (early menarche, late menopause), not having children or having them later in life, recent use of birth control pills or hormone replacement therapy, and opting not to breast-feed all appear to increase risks of breast cancer.[96] While these factors appear to play a significant role in increased risk for non-Hispanic white women, they do not appear to have as strong an influence on Hispanic women, who may have more protective reproductive patterns (an overall lower age at first birth and a greater number of births). Hispanic women also tend to use less hormone replacement therapy and have a lower utilization rate for mammograms, making comparisons difficult.[97]

Inflammation and Cancer Risks

According to some researchers, the vast majority of cancers (90 percent) are caused by cellular mutations and environmental factors that occur as a result of inflammation.[98] These same researchers believe that up to 20 percent of cancers are the result of chronic infections, 30 percent are the result of tobacco smoking and inhaled particulates such as asbestos, and 35 percent are due to dietary factors and obesity.[99]

The common denominator in these threats is inflammation that primes the system for cancer to gain a foothold and spread. Inflammation appears to be a key factor in colorectal cancer; inflammatory bowel disease, Crohn disease, colitis, and other gastrointestinal tract inflammatory problems are implicated in a higher risk of cancer development.[100] If inflammation is indeed a key factor, reducing inflammation via stress reduction, sleep, dietary supplements, low-dose aspirin, and other behaviors may prove beneficial in reducing cancer risks.

Occupational and Environmental Risks

Several workplace hazards are known to cause cancer when exposure levels are high or prolonged. Asbestos (a fibrous material once widely used in the construction, insulation, and automobile industries), nickel, chromate, and chemicals such as benzene, arsenic, and vinyl chloride have been shown to be carcinogens. People who routinely work with certain dyes and radioactive substances may have increased risks for cancer. Working with coal tars, as in the mining profession, or with inhalants, as in the auto-painting business, or with herbicides and pesticides increases cancer risks. Several federal and state agencies are responsible for monitoring such exposures and ensuring compliance with standards designed to protect workers.

Radiation Ionizing radiation (IR)—radiation from X-rays, radon, cosmic rays, and ultraviolet radiation (primarily ultraviolet B, or UVB, radiation)—is the only form of radiation that has been proven to cause human cancer. Evidence that high-dose IR causes cancer comes from studies of atomic bomb survivors, patients receiving radiotherapy, and certain occupational groups (e.g., uranium miners). Virtually any part of the body can be affected by IR, but bone marrow and the thyroid are particularly susceptible. Radon exposure in homes can increase lung cancer risk, especially in cigarette smokers. To make sure you get the lowest dose possible, ask for the newest machines, which tend to have lower radiation levels than older models. Limit unnecessary medical and dental exams and ask questions when these are recommended.

Nonionizing radiation produced by radio waves, cell phones, microwaves, computer screens, televisions, electric blankets, and other products has been a topic of great concern in recent years, but research to date has not proven excess risk. A wide range of studies have been conducted. None had shown a consistent link between cell phone use and cancers of the brain until publication of a new study in rats exposed to similar radio frequencies and modulations (RF-EMFs) in 2017. This study showed a relationship between RF-EMFs exposure and malignant brain and heart tumor development.[101] Stay tuned, as more studies are

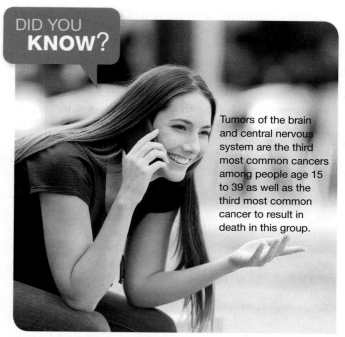

under way.[102] (See Chapter 16 for more on the potential environmental and health hazards of radiation.)

Chemicals in Foods Much of the concern about chemicals in food centers on the possible harm caused by pesticide and herbicide residues. Whereas some of these chemicals cause cancer at high doses in experimental animals, the government considers the very low concentrations found in some foods to be safe. Continued research on pesticide and herbicide use is essential, and scientists and consumer groups stress the importance of a balance between chemical use and the production of high-quality food products.

Infectious Diseases and Cancer

Over 10 percent of all cancers in the United States are caused by infectious agents such as viruses, bacteria, or parasites.[103] Worldwide, approximately 15 to 20 percent of human cancers have been traced to infectious agents.[104] Infections are thought to influence cancer development in several ways, most commonly through chronic inflammation, suppression of the immune system, or chronic stimulation.

Hepatitis B, Hepatitis C, and Liver Cancer

Viruses such as hepatitis B (HBV) and hepatitis C (HCV) are believed to stimulate the growth of cancer cells in the liver because they are chronic diseases that inflame liver tissue, potentially priming the liver for cancer or making the liver more hospitable for cancer development. In addition, HCV has been implicated in increased risks for non-Hodgkin lymphoma and prostate and renal cancers. Global increases in HBV and HBC rates and concurrent rises in liver cancer rates seem to provide evidence of such an association.

Human Papillomavirus and Cervical Cancer

Every year in the United States, nearly 28,500 men and women get cancer linked to *human papillomavirus (HPV)* infection. HPV causes most cervical, vulvar, vaginal, anal, and oropharyngeal cancers in females and most oropharyngeal, anal, and penile cancers in males. HPV vaccinations would prevent many of these infections as well as HPV-caused cancers of the back of the throat, tongue, and tonsils.[105] Although vaccines don't completely prevent all of these cancers, they seem to be effective in reducing risks of cervical and penile cancer.[106] (For more on the HPV vaccine, see the discussion in Chapter 14.)

Helicobacter Pylori and Stomach Cancer

Helicobacter pylori is a potent bacterium found in the stomach lining of approximately 30 percent of Americans.[107] It causes inflammation, scarring, and ulcers, damaging the lining of the stomach and leading to cellular changes that may lead to cancer. More than half of all cases of stomach cancer are thought to be linked to *H. pylori* infection, even though most infected people don't develop cancer.[108] Treatment with antibiotics often cures the ulcers, and this appears to reduce risk of new stomach cancer.[109]

LO 8 | TYPES OF CANCERS

Describe symptoms, populations at risk, and key methods of prevention for the most common types of cancer.

Cancers are grouped into four broad categories based on the type of tissue from which each cancer arises:

- **Carcinomas.** Epithelial tissues (tissues covering body surfaces and lining most body cavities) are the most common sites for cancers called *carcinomas*. These cancers affect the outer layer of the skin and mouth as well as the mucous membranes. They metastasize through the circulatory or lymphatic system initially and form solid tumors.

- **Sarcomas.** Sarcomas occur in the mesodermal, or middle, layers of tissue—for example, in bones, muscles, and general connective tissue. They metastasize primarily via the blood in the early stages of disease. These cancers are less common but generally more virulent than carcinomas. They also form solid tumors.

- **Lymphomas.** Lymphomas develop in the lymphatic system—the infection-fighting regions of the body—and metastasize through the lymphatic system. Hodgkin's disease is an example. Lymphomas also form solid tumors.

- **Leukemias.** Cancer of the blood-forming parts of the body, particularly the bone marrow and spleen, is called leukemia. A nonsolid tumor, leukemia is characterized by an abnormal increase in white blood cells.

FIGURE 13.7 shows the most common sites of cancer and the estimated number of new cases and deaths from each type in 2017. A comprehensive discussion of the many different forms of cancer is beyond the scope of this book, but we discuss the most common types in the next sections.

Estimated New Cases of Cancer*		Estimated Deaths from Cancer*	
Female	Male	Female	Male
Breast 246,660 (29%)	Prostate 180,890 (21%)	Lung & bronchus 72,160 (26%)	Lung & bronchus 85,920 (27%)
Lung & bronchus 106,470 (13%)	Lung & bronchus 117,920 (14%)	Breast 40,450 (14%)	Prostate 26,120 (8%)
Colon & rectum 63,670 (8%)	Colon & rectum 70,820 (8%)	Colon & rectum 23,170 (8%)	Colon & rectum 26,020 (8%)
Uterine corpus 60,050 (7%)	Urinary bladder 58,950 (7%)	Pancreas 20,330 (7%)	Pancreas 21,450 (7%)
Thyroid 49,350 (6%)	Melanoma of the skin 46,870 (6%)	Ovary 14,240 (5%)	Liver & intrahepatic bile duct 18,280 (6%)
Non-Hodgkin lymphoma 32,410 (4%)	Non-Hodgkin lymphoma 40,170 (5%)	Uterine corpus 10,470 (4%)	Leukemia 14,130 (4%)
Melanoma of the skin 29,510 (3%)	Kidney & renal pelvis 39,650 (5%)	Leukemia 10,270 (4%)	Esophagus 12,720 (4%)
Leukemia 26,050 (3%)	Oral cavity & pharynx 34,780 (4%)	Liver & intrahepatic bile duct 8,890 (3%)	Urinary bladder 11,820 (4%)
Kidney & renal pelvis 23,050 (3%)	Leukemia 34,780 (4%)	Non-Hodgkin lymphoma 8,630 (3%)	Non-Hodgkin lymphoma 11,520 (4%)
All Sites 843,820 (100%)	Liver & intrahepatic bile duct 28,410 (3%)	Brain & other nervous system 6,610 (2%)	Brain & other nervous system 9,440 (3%)
	All Sites 841,390 (100%)	All Sites 281,400 (100%)	All Sites 314,290 (100%)

*Excludes basal and squamous cell skin cancers and in situ carcinoma except urinary bladder. Percentages may not total 100% due to rounding.

FIGURE 13.7 Leading Sites of New Cancer Cases and Deaths, 2017 Estimates

Source: Data from American Cancer Society, *Cancer Facts and Figures 2017* (Atlanta, GA: American Cancer Society, 2017), 10. Note that percentages do not add up to 100, owing to omissions of certain rare cancers as well as rounding of statistics.

Lung Cancer

Lung cancer is the leading cause of cancer deaths for both men and women in the United States. It killed an estimated 155,870 Americans in 2017, accounting for nearly 1 in 4 cancer deaths.[110] Since 1987, more women have died each year from lung cancer than breast cancer, which had been the leading cause of cancer deaths in women for the previous 40 years.[111] Declining smoking rates and policies limiting environmental pollutants have been key factors in reducing lung cancer rates.[112]

Detection, Symptoms, and Treatment

Symptoms of lung cancer include a persistent cough, blood-streaked sputum, chest pain or back pain, and recurrent attacks of pneumonia or bronchitis. Treatment depends on the type and stage of the cancer. Surgery, radiation therapy, and chemotherapy are all options. If the cancer is localized, surgery is usually the treatment of choice. If the cancer has spread, surgery is combined with radiation and chemotherapy and other targeted drug treatments. Fewer than 15 percent of lung cancer cases are diagnosed at the early, localized stages.[113] Despite advances in medical technology, survival rates 1 year after diagnosis are only 44 percent overall.[114] The 5-year survival rate for all stages combined is only 17 percent.[115]

Risk Factors and Prevention

Risks for cancer increase dramatically based on the quantity of cigarettes smoked and the number of years smoked, often referred to as *pack-years*. The greater the number of pack-years smoked, the greater is the risk of developing cancer. Quitting smoking does substantially reduce the risk of developing lung cancer.[116] Exposure to industrial substances or radiation also greatly increases the risk for lung cancer. In fact, as many as 20% of all lung cancer deaths occur in people who have never smoked.

Breast Cancer

Women have a 1 in 8 lifetime risk of being diagnosed with breast cancer.[117] For women from birth to age 49, the chance is about 1 in 53; the rates are significantly higher after menopause.[118] In 2016, approximately 252,710 women and 2,500 men in the United States were diagnosed with invasive breast cancer for the first time.[119] In addition, 63,500 new cases of in situ breast cancer, a more localized cancer, were diagnosed.[120] Over 41,000 women and 460 men died of breast cancer, making it the second leading cause of cancer death for women.[121]

Detection, Symptoms, and Treatment

The earliest signs of breast cancer are usually observable on mammograms, often before lumps can be felt. However, mammograms are not foolproof, and there is debate about the age at which women should start getting them regularly. A newer form of 3D mammogram and an MRI appear to be more accurate than mammograms, particularly in women with genetic risks for tumors.[122]

For decades, monthly breast self-exams were also recommended for cancer screening. In 2016, the U.S. Preventive Services Task Force approved new recommendations for breast self-exams and mammography screenings.[123] Although breast self-exams are not formally recommended, many professional groups recommend that women do them regularly. Learn how to do them, and if you desire, do them to know your body and be able to recognize changes. FIGURE 13.8 describes how to do a breast self-exam.

If breast cancer grows large enough, it can produce the following symptoms: a lump in the breast or surrounding lymph nodes, thickening, dimpling, skin irritation, distortion, retraction or scaliness of the nipple, nipple discharge, or tenderness.

Treatments range from a lumpectomy to radical mastectomy to various combinations of radiation or chemotherapy. Among nonsurgical options, promising results have been noted among women using *selective estrogen-receptor*

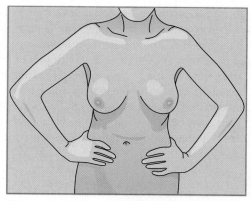

❶ Face a mirror and check for changes in symmetry.

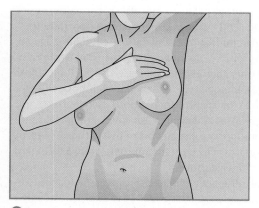

❷ Either standing or lying down, use the pads of the three middle fingers to check for lumps. Follow an up and down pattern on the breast to ensure all tissue gets inspected.

FIGURE 13.8 Breast Awareness and Self-Exam

Source: Adapted from Breast Self-Exam Illustration Series, National Cancer Institute Visuals Online Collection, U.S. National Institutes of Health, 1984.

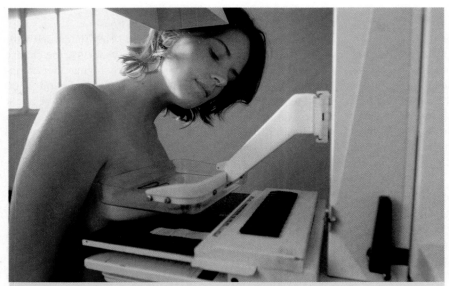

Regular checkups and early detection using the latest equipment with the lowest radiation exposure greatly increase a woman's chance of surviving breast cancer.

Colon and Rectal Cancers

Colorectal cancers (cancers of the colon and rectum) are the second most commonly diagnosed cancer in both men and women as well as the second leading cause of cancer deaths.[129] In 2017, there were 95,520 cases of colon cancer and 39,910 cases of rectal cancer diagnosed in the United States, as well as 50,260 deaths attributed to colon or rectal cancer.[130] While rates of colon cancer appear to be declining in people over age 50, they are increasing among people under age 50, largely driven by increased rates of rectal cancer.[131] Younger men and women have approximately a 1 in 300 risk of developing colon and rectal cancer from birth to age 49, increasing to about 1 in 21 to 22 later in life.[132]

modulators (SERMs) such as tamoxifen and raloxifene, particularly women whose cancers appear to grow in response to estrogen. These drugs, as well as new *aromatase inhibitors*, work by blocking estrogen. The 5-year survival rate for people with localized breast cancer has risen from 80 percent in the 1950s to over 90 percent today, although statistics vary dramatically depending on the stage of cancer when it is first detected. Black women's survival rate is 11 percent lower overall than that of white women, largely owing to stage at diagnosis.[124]

Risk Factors and Prevention The incidence of breast cancer increases with age. Risk factors that are well supported by research include family history of breast cancer, menstrual periods that started early and ended late in life, weight gain after the age of 18, obesity after menopause, recent use of oral contraceptives or postmenopausal hormone therapy, never having children or having a first child after age 30, consuming two or more alcoholic drinks per day, and physical inactivity. Other factors that increase risk include smoking, having dense breasts, type 2 diabetes, high bone mineral density, shift work and sleep deprivation, dietary risks, and exposure to high-dose radiation.[125] Although the *BRCA1* and *BRCA2* gene mutations are rare and occur in less than 1 percent of the population, they account for approximately 5 to 10 percent of all cases of breast cancer.[126]

International differences in breast cancer incidence correlate with variations in diet, especially fat intake, although a causal role for these dietary factors has not been firmly established. Sudden weight gain has also been implicated. Research also shows that regular exercise, particularly at higher than recommended rates, can reduce risks of breast cancer, colon cancer, diabetes, and CVD.[127] Additionally, exercise has proven to help breast cancer survivors cope with their treatment and related psychological aspects of the disease.[128]

Detection, Symptoms, and Treatment Because colorectal cancer tends to spread slowly, the prognosis is quite good if it is caught in the early stages. Later stages may have symptoms such as stool changes, bleeding, cramping or pain in the lower abdomen, and unusual fatigue, but colorectal cancers usually have no symptoms in the early stages. Colonoscopies and other screening tests should begin at age 50 for most people. Virtual colonoscopies and fecal DNA testing are newer diagnostic techniques that have shown promise. Treatment often consists of radiation or surgery. Chemotherapy, although not used extensively in the past, is increasingly used.

Risk Factors and Prevention Anyone can get colorectal cancer, but people who are over age 50, who are obese, who smoke, who have a family history of colon and rectal cancer, who have a personal or family history of polyps (benign growths) in the colon or rectum, or who have type 2 diabetes or inflammatory bowel problems such as colitis are at increased risk. Among the most promising prevention strategies are regular exercise; a diet with lots of fruits, vegetables, and grains; limiting consumption of red and processed meats; maintaining a healthy weight; avoiding tobacco products, and moderation in alcohol consumption. However, other factors, such as use of nonsteroidal anti-inflammatory drugs (NSAIDs), diet, vitamins, and calcium have shown conflicting results in studies.[133]

Skin Cancer

Skin cancer is the most common form of cancer in the United States today, although the exact numbers of cases remain in question because skin cancer is not reported to cancer registries.[134] The good news is that most cases of basal cell and squamous cell carcinoma are highly treatable, and not life threatening. Most skin cancer deaths—nearly 10,000

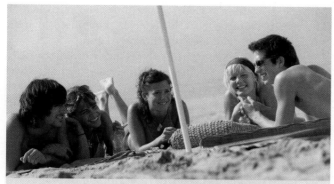

There is no such thing as a "safe" tan, because a tan is visible evidence of UV-induced skin damage. According to the American Cancer Society, tanned skin provides only about the equivalent of sun protection factor (SPF) 4 sunscreen—much too weak to be considered protective.

in 2017—are from a much more serious form of skin cancer known as *melanoma*, which affects over 87,000 people in the United States each year.[135]

Detection, Symptoms, and Treatment

Basal and squamous cell carcinomas typically develop on the face, ears, neck, arms, hands, and legs as warty bumps, colored spots, or scaly patches. Bleeding, itching, pain, or oozing are other symptoms that warrant attention. Surgery may be necessary to remove them, but they are seldom life threatening.

Although malignant melanoma may initially appear to be a harmless form of cancer, it often undergoes distinctive changes in size, shape, and color over time. Unless one takes note of these changes, it can invade body organs and tissues with devastating consequences. Early diagnosis and treatment are key to survival. If melanoma has not yet penetrated the underlying layers of skin, chances of survival are over 98 percent. However, if it is diagnosed after deeper layers of skin have been penetrated and it has spread to other organs, the survival rate falls to 17 percent.[136] FIGURE 13.9 compares melanoma with basal cell and squamous cell carcinomas. The *ABCDE* rule can help you remember the warning signs of melanoma:[137]

- **Asymmetry.** One half of the mole or lesion does not match the other half.

- **Border irregularity.** The edges are uneven, notched, or scalloped.
- **Color.** Pigmentation is not uniform. Melanomas may vary in color from tan to deeper brown, reddish black, black, or deep bluish black.
- **Diameter.** Diameter is greater than 6 millimeters (about the size of a pea).
- **Evolving.** The symmetry, size, shape, color, border, or other characteristics have changed over time.

malignant melanoma A virulent cancer of the melanocytes (pigment-producing cells) of the skin.

Treatment of skin cancer depends on the type of cancer, its stage, and its location. Surgery, laser treatments, topical chemical agents, *electrodesiccation* (tissue destruction by heat), and *cryosurgery* (tissue destruction by freezing) are all common forms of treatment. Melanoma treatments have advanced significantly in recent years, with targeted therapies showing much promise in addition to newer surgical, radiation, and chemotherapy regimens.

Risk Factors and Prevention

Anyone who has been overexposed to ultraviolet radiation without adequate protection is at risk for skin cancer. The risk is greatest for people who fit the following categories:

- Have fair skin; blonde, red, or light brown hair; blue, green, or gray eyes; lots of moles
- Always burn before tanning or burn easily and peel readily
- Don't tan easily but spend lots of time outdoors
- Use outdated or low sun protection factor (SPF) sunscreens or suntan lotions and don't put on enough of either.
- Have previously been treated for skin cancer or have a family history of skin cancer
- Have experienced severe sunburns during childhood.

Preventing skin cancer is a matter of limiting exposure to harmful UV rays found in sunlight. What happens when you expose yourself to sunlight? Biologically, the skin responds to photodamage by increasing its thickness and the number of pigment cells (melanocytes), which produce the "tan" look. The skin's cells that ward off infection are also prone to photodamage, lowering the normal immune protection of our skin and priming it for cancer. Photodamage also causes wrinkling by impairing

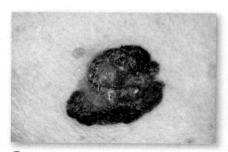

ⓐ Malignant melanoma

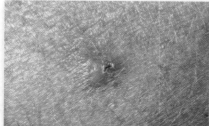

ⓑ Basal cell carcinoma

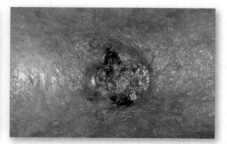

ⓒ Squamous cell carcinoma

FIGURE 13.9 Types of Skin Cancers Preventing skin cancer includes keeping a careful watch for any new pigmented growths and for changes to any moles. The ABCD warning signs of melanoma (a) include asymmetrical shapes, irregular borders, color variation, and an increase in diameter. Basal cell carcinoma (b) and squamous cell carcinoma (c) should be brought to your health care provider's attention but are not as deadly as melanoma.

the elastic substances (collagens) that keep skin soft and pliable. Stay safe in the sun by limiting sun exposure when its rays are strongest, between 10:00 A.M. and 4:00 P.M., and by liberally applying an SPF 15 or higher sunscreen before going outside.

Despite the risk of skin cancer, many Americans are still working to get tan. Many believe that tanning booths are safer than sitting in the sun. The truth is that there is no such thing as a safe tan from *any* source. Every time you tan, you are exposing your skin to harmful UV light rays. All tanning lamps emit UVA rays, and most emit UVB rays as well; both types can cause long-term skin damage and contribute to cancer. Even worse, some salons do not calibrate the UV output of their tanning bulbs properly, which can cause more or less exposure than you paid for.

▶ **SEE IT!** VIDEOS

Is there such a thing as a safe tan? Watch **Extreme Tanning**, available on Mastering Health.

Prostate Cancer

After skin cancer, prostate cancer is the most frequently diagnosed cancer in American males, with an estimated 151,360 new cases in 2017.[138] It is the third leading cause of cancer deaths in men, killing an estimated 26,730 men in 2017.[139] However, with improved screening and early diagnosis, 5-year survival rates are nearly 100 percent for all but the most advanced cases, which have a much more bleak outcome, with only 29 percent surviving.[140]

Detection, Symptoms, and Treatment The prostate is a muscular, walnut-sized gland that surrounds part of a man's urethra, the tube that transports urine and sperm out of the body. As part of the male reproductive system, its primary function is to produce seminal fluid. Symptoms of prostate cancer include weak or interrupted urine flow; difficulty starting or stopping urination; feeling the urge to urinate frequently; pain on urination; blood in the urine; or pain in the low back, pelvis, or thighs. Many men have no symptoms in the early stages.

Men over the age of 40 should have an annual digital rectal prostate examination. Another screening method for prostate cancer is the **prostate-specific antigen (PSA)** test, which is a blood test that screens for an indicator of prostate cancer. However, the U.S. Preventive Services Task Force recommends that otherwise asymptomatic men no longer receive the routine PSA test because, overall, it does not save lives and may lead to painful, unnecessary cancer treatments. If you have a family history or symptoms of prostate cancer, consult with your health care provider.

Risk Factors and Prevention Increasing age is one of the biggest risks for prostate cancer, most cases occurring in men over the age of 50. Other risk factors are African ancestry and a family history of prostate cancer.[141]

Black men in the United States and Caribbean men of African descent have the highest documented prostate cancer incidence rates in the world. Genetics may account for

between 5 and 10 percent of prostate cancers overall.[142] These men are also more likely to be diagnosed at more advanced stages than men of other racial groups.[143]

Having a father or brother with prostate cancer more than doubles a man's risk of getting prostate cancer. Men who have had several relatives with prostate cancer, especially those with relatives who developed prostate cancer at younger ages, are also at higher risk.[144]

Eating more fruits and vegetables, particularly those containing *lycopene*, a pigment found in tomatoes and other red fruits, may lower the risk of death from prostate cancer; however, more research is necessary to determine the validity of these claims.[145] The best advice is to follow the dietary recommendations of the U.S. Department of Agriculture, maintain a healthy weight, and refrain from smoking.

Ovarian Cancer

Ovarian cancer is the fifth leading cause of cancer deaths for women, with an estimated 23,000 diagnoses in 2017 and just over 14,000 deaths.[146] Ovarian cancer causes more deaths than any other cancer of the reproductive system because women tend not to discover it until the cancer is at an advanced stage, for which the 5-year survival is only 29 percent.[147] Younger women (under the age of 45) are much more likely to survive 5 years compared to those age 65 or older. For all stages, the 5-year survival is 46 percent.[148]

Ovarian cancer typically has no early symptoms; however, some women may complain of feeling bloated, having pain in the pelvic area, feeling full quickly, or feeling the need to urinate more frequently. Some women with ovarian cancer may experience persistent digestive disturbances. Other symptoms include fatigue, pain during intercourse, unexplained weight loss, unexplained changes in bowel or bladder habits, and incontinence.

Primary relatives (mother, daughter, sister) of a woman who has had ovarian cancer are at increased risk, as are those with a family or personal history of breast or colon cancer. Women who have never been pregnant are more likely to develop ovarian cancer than are those who have had a child. The use of fertility drugs may increase a woman's risk.

General prevention strategies such as focusing on a healthy diet, exercise, sleep, stress management, and weight control are good ideas to lower your risk. Getting annual pelvic examinations is important, and women over the age of 40 should have a cancer-related checkup every year.

Cervical and Endometrial (Uterine Corpus) Cancer

Most uterine cancers develop in the body of the uterus, usually in the endometrium. The rest develop in the cervix, located at the base of the uterus. In 2017, an estimated 13,000 new cases of cervical cancer and over 60,000 cases of endometrial cancer were diagnosed in the United States, with nearly 15,000 deaths from the two types of cancer.[149] As more women have regular

Pap test screenings—a procedure in which cells taken from the cervical region are examined for abnormal activity—rates should decline even further. As of 2017, it is recommended women get a Pap test every 2 years beginning at age 21. Between ages 30 and 65, women should have an HPV and Pap test every 5 years and a Pap test alone every 3 years. Women with parents and/or siblings with breast cancer or those with *Lynch syndrome*, a hereditary predisposition to colon or endometrial cancer, should talk with their health care provider about having tests more frequently.

Pap tests are very effective for detecting early-stage cervical cancer but less effective for detecting cancers of the uterine lining. Women have a lifetime risk of 1 in 157 for being diagnosed with cervical cancer and a 1 in 36 risk of being diagnosed with uterine corpus cancer.[150] Early warning signs of uterine cancer include bleeding outside the normal menstrual period or after menopause or persistent unusual vaginal discharge.

Risk factors for cervical cancer include early age at first intercourse, multiple sex partners, cigarette smoking, and a history of infection with HPV (the cause of genital warts). Today, both young men and young women have the option of getting vaccinated with either Gardasil or Cervarix, which are designed to protect against the two types of HPV that cause most cervical cancers. For endometrial cancer, age is a risk factor; however, estrogen and obesity (particularly abdominal obesity) are also strong risk factors. In addition, risks are increased by treatment with tamoxifen for breast cancer, metabolic syndrome, late menopause, never bearing children, a history of polyps in the uterus or ovaries, a history of other cancers, and race (white women are at higher risk).[151]

Testicular Cancer

Testicular cancer is one of the most common types of solid tumors found in young adult men, affecting an estimated 8,720 young men in 2017.[152] Over half of all cases occur between the ages of 20 and 34, with steady increases in this group over the last few years.[153] However, with a 95.4 percent 5-year survival rate, testicular cancer is one of the most curable forms of cancer, particularly if it is caught in localized stages.[154] Although the cause of testicular cancer is unknown, several risk factors have been identified. Men with undescended testicles appear to be at greatest risk. HIV and a family history of testicular cancer are also possible risk factors.[155]

In general, testicular tumors first appear as an enlargement of one or both of the testes caused by a lump or thickening in testicular tissue. Some men report a heavy feeling, a dull ache, or pain that extends to the lower abdomen or groin area. Testicular self-exams have long been recommended as a means of detecting testicular cancer (**FIGURE 13.10**). However, recent studies have shown that findings from monthly self-exams result in testing for noncancerous conditions and therefore are not cost-effective. For this reason, the U.S. Preventive Services Task Force stopped recommending self-exams. Regardless, most cases of testicular cancer are discovered through self-exam; there is currently no other screening test for the disease.

The testicular self-exam is best done after a hot shower, which relaxes the scrotum. Standing in front of a mirror, hold

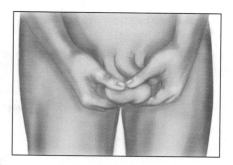

FIGURE 13.10 Testicular Self-Exam

Source: From Michael Johnson, *Human Biology: Concepts and Current Issues*, 3rd ed. Copyright © 2006. Reprinted with permission of Pearson Education, Inc.

the testicle with one hand while gently rolling its surface between the thumb and fingers of your other hand. Feel underneath the scrotum for the tubes of the epididymis and blood vessels that sit close to the body. Repeat with the other testicle. Feel for any lump, thickening, or pealike nodules, paying attention to any areas that may be painful over the entire surface of the scrotum. When done, wash your hands with soap and water. Consult your health care provider if you note anything that is unusual.

> **Pap test** A procedure in which cells taken from the cervical region are examined for abnormal activity.

Pancreatic Cancer: Deadly and on the Rise

Pancreatic cancer is one of the deadliest forms of cancer; only 8 percent of people with this cancer survive 5 years after diagnosis. Even among those who are diagnosed at the earliest stages, the 5-year survival rate is only 29 percent.[156] Although most cases occur after age 50, there are increasing numbers of cases at earlier ages. Rates are higher in men, in African Americans, and in populations with lower socioeconomic status and lower education levels.

Tobacco use appears to be a key risk factor, as are obesity, consumption of high levels of red meat, and a high-fat diet. Family history, possible genetic links, and a history of chronic inflammation of the pancreas (*pancreatitis*) over the years seem to increase the risk of pancreatic cancer. There also appears to be a greater risk among diabetics and people who have had infections with hepatitis B and C and the *Helicobacter* bacteria. Because pancreatic cancer has few early symptoms, there is no reliable test to detect it in its early stages. Often, by the time it is diagnosed, it is too advanced to treat effectively.

LO 9 | FACING CANCER

Discuss the most current and effective methods of cancer detection and treatment, including areas of significant progress and future challenges.

The earlier cancer is diagnosed, the better the prospect for survival. Policies that ensure health care for everyone would make

TABLE **13.4** | Screening Guidelines for Early Cancer Detection in Average Risk and Asymptomatic People

Cancer Site	Screening Procedure	Age and Frequency of Test
Breast	Mammograms	The NCI recommends that women in their forties and older have mammograms every 1 to 2 years. Women who are at higher than average risk of breast cancer should talk with their health care provider about whether to have mammograms before age 40 and how often to have them.
Cervix	Pap test (Pap smear)	Testing is generally recommended to begin at age 21 and to end at age 65 if recent results have been normal. Most women should have a Pap test at least once every 3 years.
Colon and rectum	Fecal occult blood test: Sometimes cancer or polyps bleed. This test can detect tiny amounts of blood in the stool. Sigmoidoscopy: Checks the rectum and lower part of the colon for polyps. Colonoscopy: Checks the rectum and entire colon for polyps and cancer.	People age 50 and older should be screened. People who have a higher than average risk of cancer of the colon or rectum should talk with their health care provider about whether to have screening tests before age 50 and how often to have them.
Prostate	Prostate-specific antigen (PSA) test	Some groups encourage yearly screening for men over age 50, and some advise men who are at a higher risk for prostate cancer to begin screening at age 40 or 45. Many expert groups no longer recommend routine PSA testing, as studies have shown little or no effect on prostate cancer death rates, and it leads to overdiagnosis and overtreatment. Currently, Medicare provides coverage for an annual PSA test for all men age 50 and older.

Source: National Cancer Institute, National Institutes of Health, "Screening Tests," March 24, 2015, http://www.cancer.gov/about-cancer/screening/screening-tests.

it possible for uninsured and underinsured people to get recommended screening tests earlier in the disease course. Do you have insurance that pays for preventive care and diagnostic care? If not, check out available options and costs. Make a realistic assessment of your own risk factors, focus on current lifestyle behaviors that increase risk, and make changes now. Even if you have significant risks, there are factors you can control. Do you have a family history of cancer? If so, what types? Make sure you know which symptoms to watch for, avoid known carcinogens—such as tobacco—and other environmental hazards, and follow the recommendations for self-exams and medical checkups outlined in **TABLE 13.4.**

If you are at high risk for developing cancer or you notice possible cancer symptoms, your health care provider might use one or more tests to diagnose or rule out cancer. **Magnetic resonance imaging (MRI)** uses a huge electromagnet to detect hidden tumors by mapping the vibrations of the various atoms in the body on a computer screen. Another key weapon is the **computed tomography (CT) scan,** which uses X-rays to examine parts of the body. In both of these painless, noninvasive procedures, cross-sectioned pictures can reveal a tumor's shape and location more accurately than can conventional X-ray images. *Prostatic ultrasound* (a rectal probe using ultrasonic waves to produce an image of the prostate) is being investigated as a means to increase the early detection of prostate cancer. New three-dimensional mammogram machines offer significant improvements in imaging and breast cancer detection but deliver nearly double the radiation risk of conventional mammograms at increased costs.

magnetic resonance imaging (MRI) A device that uses magnetic fields, radio waves, and computers to generate an image of internal tissues of the body for diagnostic purposes without the use of radiation.

computed tomography (CT) scan A scan by a machine that uses radiation to view internal organs that are not normally visible on X-ray images.

stereotactic radiosurgery A type of radiation therapy that can be used to zap tumors. Also known as *gamma knife surgery.*

radiotherapy Use of radiation to kill cancerous cells.

chemotherapy Use of drugs to kill cancerous cells.

⊙ SEE IT! VIDEOS

Researchers and physicians are rethinking procedures for early detection of cancer. Watch **How Effective Is Breast Cancer Early Detection?** in the Study Area of Mastering Health.

Cancer Treatments

Cancer treatments vary according to the type of cancer and the stage at which it is detected. Surgery, in which the tumor and surrounding tissue are removed, is one common treatment. New **stereotactic radiosurgery,** also known as *gamma knife surgery,* uses a targeted dose of gamma radiation to destroy the DNA of tumors with pinpoint accuracy without blood loss or need for a scalpel. It is most commonly used to treat brain tumors. **Radiotherapy** (the use of radiation) and **chemotherapy** (the use of drugs) to kill cancerous cells are common types of treatment for cancer. When cancer has spread throughout the body, chemotherapy is necessary.

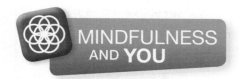

COPING WITH CANCER

MINDFULNESS AND YOU

Imagine that you have just noticed a lump somewhere on your body. After probing, scans, and a biopsy, your worst fear has become reality: you have cancer. You can't shake the feeling of dread. You are scared and feel alone. Facing such a diagnosis, many people go through similar stages of emotional turmoil. They feel pain and anxiety during treatment, and even if they're cleared of cancer, fear may remain. Is the cancer really gone, or is it still lurking?

Increasingly, cancer experts realize that people need help battling that alien entity in their bodies—the one that is beating them up physically and emotionally, sapping their strength when they need it most. Some efforts have focused on *mindfulness-based interventions (MBIs)* for cancer survivor care. MBIs have consistently proven effective in helping

people deal with diagnosis, treatment, and life as survivors. MBIs help individuals cope with loss of control, uncertainty about the future, fear of recurrence, and the psychological and physiological realities of treatment, including pain, anxiety, anger, sleeplessness, fatigue, and depression.

MBI participants learn skills to help them refocus on things that are important to them in the present moment. Through meditation, mindfulness-based stress reduction (MBSR), yoga and other spirituality-based techniques, survivors can move through the stages of grieving for themselves and focus outward. MBSR programs are typically 8 weeks long with sessions that last for 2 to 3 hours each week, usually in small groups. Mindfulness-based cancer recovery programs that focus specifically on the unique challenges

in coping with cancer survivorship are also available, and results are promising. Most cancer treatment programs have mindfulness-based stress reduction, relaxation, and meditation programs for survivors and family members.

Sources: L. Carlson, "Mindfulness-Based Cancer Recovery: The Development of an Evidence-based Psychosocial Oncology Intervention," *Oncology Exchange* 12, no. 2 (2013): 21–5; M. Zhang et al., "Effectiveness of Mindfulness-based Therapy for Reducing Anxiety and Depression in Patients with Cancer: A Meta-analysis," *Medicine* 94, no. 45 (2015): e0897; L. Carlson, *Mindfulness-Based Cancer Recovery: A Step-by-Step MBSR Approach to Help You Cope with Treatment and Reclaim Your Life* (Oakland, CA: New Harbinger, 2011); J. Kabat-Zinn and Thich Nhat Hanh, *Full Catastrophe Living: Using the Wisdom of Your Body and Mind to Face Stress, Pain, and Illness* (New York: Bantam, 2013).

Whether used alone or in combination, virtually all cancer treatments have side effects, including nausea, nutritional deficiencies, hair loss, and general fatigue. The more aggressive the cancer, the more likely it is that there will be side effects from powerful drugs and invasive procedures. In the process of killing malignant cells, some healthy cells are also destroyed, and long-term damage to the cardiovascular system, kidneys, liver, and other body systems can be significant. Cancer has emotional side effects too. See the **Mindfulness and You** box for some ways to cope.

New ways of killing tumors and new chemotherapeutic drug cocktails are being developed regularly. Promising areas of research include *immunotherapy*, which enhances the body's

own disease-fighting mechanisms; *cancer-fighting vaccines* to combat abnormal cells; *gene therapy* to increase the patient's immune response; and treatment with various substances that block cancer-causing events along the cancer pathway. Another promising avenue of potential treatment is *stem cell research*, although controversy around the use of stem cells continues to slow research. Because our knowledge of cancer treatment is constantly evolving, people who have been diagnosed with cancer and their loved ones should look for information on the best cancer centers for specific types of cancer, new treatments being developed, and whether or not they are eligible for new clinical trials and experimental treatments that might be available for particularly aggressive cancers.

LIVE IT! ASSESS YOURSELF

An interactive version of this assessment is available online in Mastering Health.

ASSESS | YOURSELF

CVD and Cancer: What's Your Personal Risk?

1 Evaluating Your CVD Risk

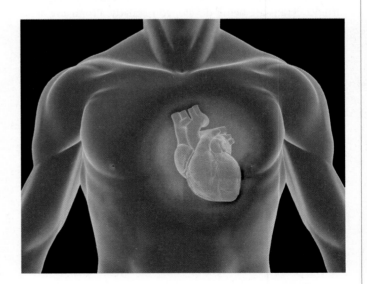

Complete each of the following questions and total your points in each section.

A: Your Family Risk for CVD

	Yes (1 point)	No (0 point)	Don't Know
1. Do any of your primary relatives (parents, grandparents, siblings) have a history of heart disease or stroke?	○	○	○
2. Do any of your primary relatives have diabetes?	○	○	○
3. Do any of your primary relatives have high blood pressure?	○	○	○
4. Do any of your primary relatives have a history of high cholesterol?	○	○	○
5. Would you say that your family consumed a high-fat diet (lots of red meat, whole dairy, butter/margarine) during your time spent at home?	○	○	○

Total points: _____

B: Your Lifestyle Risk for CVD

1. Is your total cholesterol level higher than it should be?	○	○	○
2. Do you have high blood pressure?	○	○	○
3. Have you been diagnosed as prediabetic or diabetic?	○	○	○
4. Would you describe your life as being highly stressful?	○	○	○
5. Do you smoke?	○	○	○

Total points: _____

C: Your Additional Risks for CVD

1. **How would you describe your current weight?**
   a. Lower than it should be for my height and weight (0 points)
   b. About what it should be for my height and weight (0 points)
   c. Higher than it should be for my height and weight (1 point)

2. **How would you describe the level of exercise that you get each day?**
   a. Less than I should get each day (1 point)
   b. About what I should get each day (0 points)
   c. More than I should get each day (0 points)

3. **How would you describe your dietary behaviors?**
   a. Eating only the recommended number of calories each day (0 points)
   b. Eating less than the recommended number of calories each day (0 points)
   c. Eating more than the recommended number of calories each day (1 point)

4. **Which of the following best describes your typical dietary behavior?**
   a. I eat from the major food groups, especially trying to get the recommended fruits and vegetables. (0 points)
   b. I eat too much red meat and consume too much saturated and *trans* fats from meat, dairy products, and processed foods each day. (1 point)
   c. Whenever possible, I try to substitute olive oil or canola oil for other forms of dietary fat. (0 points)

5. Which of the following (if any) describes you?
   a. I watch my sodium intake and try to reduce stress in my life. (0 points)
   b. I have a history of chlamydia infection. (1 point)
   c. I try to eat 5 to 10 mg of soluble fiber each day and try to substitute a nonanimal source of protein (beans, nuts, soy) in my diet at least once each week. (0 points)

Total points: _____

Scoring Part 1

If you scored between 1 and 5 in any section, consider your risk. The higher the number, the greater your risk will be. If you answered Don't Know for any question, talk to your parents or other family members as soon as possible to find out whether you have any unknown risks.

2 Evaluating Your Cancer Risk

Read each question, and circle the number corresponding to Yes or No for each. Individual scores for specific questions should not be interpreted as a precise measure of relative risk, but the totals in each section will give a general indication of risk.

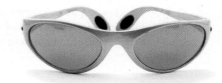

A: Cancers in General

	Yes	No
1. Do you smoke cigarettes on most days of the week?	2	1
2. Do you consume a diet that is rich in fruits and vegetables?	1	2
3. Are you obese or do you lead a primarily sedentary lifestyle?	2	1
4. Do you live in an area with high air pollution levels or work in a job in which you are exposed to several chemicals on a regular basis?	2	1
5. Are you careful about the amount of animal fat in your diet, substituting olive oil or canola oil for animal fat whenever possible?	1	2
6. Do you limit your overall consumption of alcohol?	1	2
7. Do you eat foods rich in lycopenes (such as tomatoes) and antioxidants?	1	2
8. Are you "body aware" and alert for changes in your body?	1	2
9. Do you have a family history of ulcers or of colorectal, stomach, or other digestive system cancers?	2	1
10. Do you avoid unnecessary exposure to radiation and microwave emissions?	1	2

Total points: _____

B: Skin Cancer

	Yes	No
1. Do you spend a lot of time outdoors, either at work or at play?	2	1
2. Do you use sunscreens with an SPF rating of 15 or more when you are in the sun?	1	2
3. Do you use tanning beds or sun booths regularly to maintain a tan?	2	1
4. Do you examine your skin once a month, checking any moles or other irregularities, particularly in hard-to-see areas such as your back, genitals, neck, and under your hair?	1	2
5. Do you purchase and wear sunglasses that adequately filter out harmful sun rays?	1	2

Total points: _____

C: Breast Cancer

	Yes	No
1. Do you check your breasts at least monthly using breast self-exam procedures?	1	2
2. Do you look at your breasts in the mirror regularly, checking for any irregular indentations/lumps, discharge from the nipples, or other noticeable changes?	1	2
3. Has your mother, sister, or daughter been diagnosed with breast cancer?	2	1
4. Have you ever been pregnant?	1	2
5. Have you had a history of lumps or cysts in your breasts or underarm?	2	1

Total points: _____

D: Cancers of the Reproductive System

Men	Yes	No
1. Do you examine your penis regularly for unusual bumps or growths?	1	2
2. Do you perform regular testicular self-examinations?	1	2
3. Do you have a family history of prostate or testicular cancer?	2	1
4. Do you practice safe sex and wear condoms during every sexual encounter?	1	2
5. Do you avoid exposure to harmful environmental hazards such as mercury, coal tars, benzene, chromate, and vinyl chloride?	1	2

Total points: _____

Women	Yes	No
1. Do you have regularly scheduled Pap tests?	1	2
2. Have you been infected with HPV, Epstein-Barr virus, or other viruses believed to increase cancer risk?	2	1
3. Has your mother, sister, or daughter been diagnosed with breast, cervical, endometrial, or ovarian cancer (particularly at a young age)?	2	1
4. Do you practice safer sex and use condoms with every sexual encounter?	1	2
5. Are you obese, taking estrogen, or consuming a diet that is very high in saturated fats?	2	1

Total points: _____

Scoring Part 2

Look carefully at each question for which you received a 2. Are there any areas in which you received mostly 2s? Did you receive total points of 11 or higher in A? Did you receive total points of 6 or higher in B through D? If so, you have at least one identifiable risk. The higher the score, the more risks you may have.

YOUR PLAN FOR **CHANGE**

The **ASSESS YOURSELF** activities evaluated your risk of heart disease and cancer. Depending on your results, you may need to take steps to reduce your risk for these diseases and improve your future health.

TODAY, YOU CAN:

☐ Get up and move! Take a walk in the evening, use the stairs instead of the elevator, or ride your bike to class. Think of ways to incorporate more physical activity into your daily routine.

☐ Improve your dietary habits by reading labels and choosing low-sodium foods, low-fat foods, and nutrient-dense fruits and vegetables. Replace meat and processed foods with a serving of fresh fruit or soy-based protein and leafy green vegetables several times per week. Eat more monounsaturated fat and foods with lower cholesterol counts. Watch your total calorie consumption.

☐ Assess your personal risks for specific cancers, looking at lifestyle as well as your genetic risks. For which cancers might you be most at risk?

WITHIN THE NEXT TWO WEEKS, YOU CAN:

☐ Buy a bottle of broad-spectrum sunscreen (with SPF 15 or higher). Apply it liberally as part of your daily routine. (Be sure to check the expiration date, particularly on sale items.) Also, stay in the shade when the sun is strongest, from 10 A.M. to 4 P.M.

☐ Find out your family health history. Talk to your parents, grandparents, and any aunts or uncles to find out whether family members have developed cancer or CVD. Ask whether they know their latest LDL and HDL cholesterol levels. Do you have a family history of diabetes?

☐ Begin a regular exercise program. Set small goals and try to meet them. (See Chapter 9 for ideas.)

☐ Practice a new stress management technique. (See Chapter 3 for ideas for managing stress.)

☐ Make sure you get at least 8 hours of sleep per night.

BY THE END OF THE SEMESTER, YOU CAN:

☐ Get a full lipid panel for yourself, and have your blood pressure checked. Once you know your levels, you'll have a better sense of what risk factors to address. If your levels are high, talk to your health care provider about how to reduce them.

☐ Stop smoking, avoid secondhand smoke, and limit your alcohol intake.

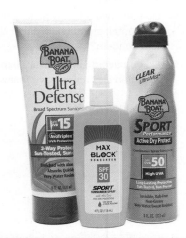

STUDY PLAN

Visit the Study Area in Mastering Health to enhance your study plan with MP3 Tutor Sessions, Practice Quizzes, Flashcards, and more!

CHAPTER REVIEW

LO 1 | Cardiovascular Disease in the United States

- Cardiovascular disease is the leading cause of death in the United States, and it puts a huge economic burden on our society. CVD is also a leading cause of death globally and is an increasing threat in the developing world.

LO 2 | Understanding the Cardiovascular System

- The cardiovascular system consists of the heart and circulatory system and is a carefully regulated, integrated network of vessels that supplies the body with nutrients and oxygen.

LO 3 | The Major Cardiovascular Diseases

- Cardiovascular diseases include atherosclerosis, coronary artery disease, peripheral artery disease, coronary heart disease, stroke, hypertension, angina pectoris, arrhythmias, congestive heart failure, and congenital and rheumatic heart disease.

LO 4 | Reducing Your Risks

- Cardiometabolic risks are combined factors that increase a person's chances of CVD and diabetes.
- Many risk factors can be modified, such as cigarette smoking, lack of exercise, poor diet, and emotional stress. Some risk factors, such as age, gender, and heredity, cannot be modified.

LO 5 | Diagnosing and Treating Cardiovascular Disease

- Coronary bypass surgery is an established treatment for heart blockage; increasing numbers of angioplasty procedures and stents are being used with great success. Increasing numbers of pharmacological interventions such as statins are being used to reduce risk and prevent problems.

LO 6 | An Overview of Cancer

- Cancer is a group of diseases characterized by uncontrolled growth and spread of abnormal cells.
- Cancer is the second most common cause of death in the United States. The current 5-year survival rates for cancer have greatly improved from those of previous generations.

LO 7 | What Causes Cancer?

- Lifestyle factors for cancer include smoking and obesity as well as poor diet, lack of exercise, and other factors. Biological factors include inherited genes, age, and gender. Potential environmental carcinogens include asbestos, radiation, preservatives, and pesticides. Infectious agents may also increase your risks for cancer.

LO 8 | Types of Cancers

- Common cancers include that of the lung, breast, colon and rectum, skin, prostate, testis, ovary, and uterus; leukemia; and lymphomas. Each has different risks and strategies for prevention.

LO 9 | Facing Cancer

- The most common treatments for cancer are surgery, chemotherapy, and radiation. Newer therapies, including biologicals, smart drugs, and immunotherapy, show promising results.
- Early diagnosis improves survival rate. Self-exams for breast, testicular, and skin cancer aid in early diagnosis.

POP QUIZ

LO 1 | Cardiovascular Disease in the United States

1. Which of the following is true about CVD?
   a. It is a problem only in developed nations.
   b. Risks are highest in Asian American populations.
   c. Risk factors are an issue only starting at age 50.
   d. It is the leading cause of death in the United States.

LO 2 | Understanding the Cardiovascular System

2. Which type of blood vessels carry oxygenated blood away from the heart?
   a. Ventricles
   b. Arteries
   c. Pulmonary arteries
   d. Venules

LO 3 | The Major Cardiovascular Diseases

3. Which of these statements is *not* true about strokes?
   a. High blood pressure is a leading cause.
   b. Strokes are increasing among young adults, with young women having higher stroke risk than young men.
   c. Strokes occur when blood flow to the brain has been compromised.
   d. Stress is a major factor in hypertension and possible stroke development.

LO 4 | Reducing Your Risks

4. Which of the following statements is *not* correct?
   a. High-density lipoprotein is believed to be protective in cardiovascular risk.
   b. Inflammation is believed to be protective in cardiovascular risk.
   c. LDL cholesterol is believed to increase CVD risks.
   d. Genetics and diet are key factors in cholesterol levels.

LO 5 | Diagnosing and Treating Cardiovascular Disease

5. The surgery in which a blood vessel is taken from another site in the patient's body and implanted to bypass a blocked artery is called

a. atherosclerosis surgery.
b. thrombolysis.
c. coronary bypass surgery.
d. angioplasty.

LO 6 | An Overview of Cancer

6. Overall, which cancer has the worst 5-year survival rate today?
   a. Prostate
   b. Pancreas
   c. Melanoma
   d. Breast

7. When cancer cells have metastasized,
   a. they have grown into a malignant tumor.
   b. they have spread.
   c. they are dying off.
   d. the tumor is localized and considered in situ.

LO 7 | What Causes Cancer?

8. One of the biggest factors in increased risk for cancer is
   a. increasing age.
   b. not having children.
   c. having long-lived parents.
   d. increased consumption of fruits and vegetables.

LO 8 | Types of Cancers

9. The cancer that causes the most deaths for men and women in the United States is
   a. colorectal cancer.
   b. pancreatic cancer.
   c. lung cancer.
   d. stomach cancer.

LO 9 | Facing Cancer

10. Which of the following treatment methods uses drugs to kill cancerous cells?
    a. Radiotherapy
    b. Chemotherapy
    c. Stem cell therapy
    d. Stereotactic radiosurgery

Answers to the Pop Quiz can be found on page A-1. If you answered a question incorrectly, review the section identified by the learning outcome. For even more study tools, visit Mastering Health.

THINK ABOUT IT!

LO 1 | Cardiovascular Disease in the United States

1. Why might hypertension rates be rising among college students?

LO 2 | Understanding the Cardiovascular System

2. What can your resting heart rate tell you about your overall health? Why might a person's resting heart rate might be higher or lower than the median?

LO 3 | The Major Cardiovascular Diseases

3. Why do some populations have higher rates of CVD than others? What are your risk factors, if any?

LO 4 | Reducing Your Risks

4. Discuss the role that exercise, stress management, dietary changes, medical checkups, sodium reduction, and other factors can play in reducing the risk for CVD.

LO 5 | Diagnosing and Treating Cardiovascular Disease

5. Describe some of the diagnostic, preventive, and treatment alternatives for CVD. If you had a heart attack today, which treatment would you prefer? Explain why.

LO 6 | An Overview of Cancer

6. What accounts for the improvement in 5-year survival rates for people with cancer in recent years?

LO 7 | What Causes Cancer?

7. What can you do to reduce your cancer risks? What risk factors do you share with family members?

LO 8 | Types of Cancers

8. What are the differences between carcinomas, sarcomas, lymphomas, and leukemia? Why is it important that you know the stage of your cancer?

LO 9 | Facing Cancer

9. Why are breast and testicular self-exams especially important for college students? What could you do to make sure you do regular self-exams?

ACCESS YOUR HEALTH ON THE INTERNET

For links to the websites below, visit Mastering Health.

The following websites explore further topics and issues related to CVD and cancer.

American Heart Association. This site provides information, statistics, and resources on cardiovascular care, including an opportunity to test your risk for CVD. www.heart.org

National Heart, Lung, and Blood Institute. This valuable resource provides information on all aspects of cardiovascular health and wellness. www.nhlbi.nih.gov

Watch, Learn and Live. This joint effort by the American Heart Association and the American Stroke Association provides a wealth of video demonstrations of a wide variety of cardiovascular conditions and procedures. watchlearnlive.heart.org

American Cancer Society. Here, you'll find information, statistics, and resources about cancer and cancer prevention. www.cancer.org

National Cancer Institute. On this site, you will find cancer facts, research, and the Physician Data Query (PDQ), a comprehensive database of cancer treatment information. www.cancer.gov

Oncolink. This site offers cancer patients and their families information on support services, cancer causes, screening, prevention, and common questions. www.oncolink.com

Susan G. Komen for the Cure. Up-to-date information about breast cancer, issues in treatment, and support groups are presented here, along with a wealth of videos and information. www.komen.org

National Coalition for Cancer Survivorship. Cancer survivors share their experiences during and after cancer treatment. www.canceradvocacy.org

Minimizing Your Risk for Diabetes

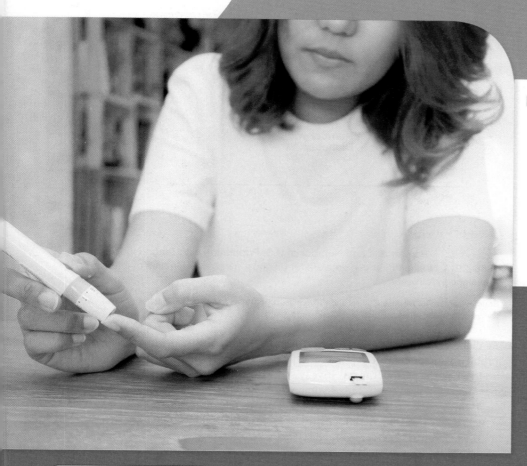

LEARNING OUTCOMES

1 Explain trends in diabetes, describe the effect of diabetes on the body, and differentiate among types of diabetes and their risk factors.

2 Describe the symptoms of, complications associated with, and main tests for diabetes.

3 Explain how diabetes can be prevented and treated.

WHY SHOULD I CARE?

The health care costs of treating and managing diabetes and its complications are over $825 billion per year globally. Over $105 billion of these costs are incurred in the United States for people with diagnosed diabetes. As diabetes rates increase, the impact on our health care system, insurance rates, and consumers will be staggering.

Source: C. Bommer et al., "The Global Economic Burden of Diabetes in Adults Aged 20–79 Years: A Cost of Illness Study," *Lancet Diabetes & Endocrinology* 5, no. 6 (2017): 423–30.

Last week, Nora's mother called to say that she'd just been diagnosed with type 2 diabetes. Her voice sounded shaky as she mentioned her own mother's death from kidney failure—a complication of diabetes—at age 52. Later, Nora searched online for information about her own risks. Her Hispanic ethnicity, family history of diabetes, high stress level and lack of sleep, excessive weight, and sedentary lifestyle made her a prime candidate.

Nora made an appointment for a diabetes screening and was told to fast the night before. At her visit, the nurse practitioner took a blood sample. A few days later, the nurse practitioner called to tell Nora that her blood glucose was elevated, and although she wasn't diabetic yet, she needed to make lifestyle changes to reduce her risks.

Over the past two decades, diabetes rates in the United States have increased dramatically[1] (see **FIGURE 1**). The Centers for Disease Control and Prevention estimate that nearly 30 million people—almost 10 percent of the U.S. population—have diabetes and that 25 percent of them don't know it. Another 86 million have *prediabetes*.[2] At current rates, more than 1 in 3 Americans will have diabetes by 2050. Diabetes kills more Americans each year than breast cancer and AIDS combined, and millions of people suffer the consequences of dealing with this difficult disease.[3]

Rates of diabetes increase with age and weight; approximately 2.4 percent of persons age 18 to 44 years, 12.3 percent of those age 45 to 64, 22.1 percent of those 65 to 74, and 19.8 percent of those age 75 and over have diabetes.[4] Globally, diabetes rates are skyrocketing, with over 422 million adults diagnosed—half of whom are located in five countries: China, India, the United States, Brazil, and Indonesia. In contrast, the lowest diabetes rates are in Switzerland, the Netherlands, Denmark, Austria, and Belgium.[5]

The combined economic burden of all types of diabetes was over $322 billion in 2012.[6] For more on the personal financial toll of diabetes, see the Money & Health box.

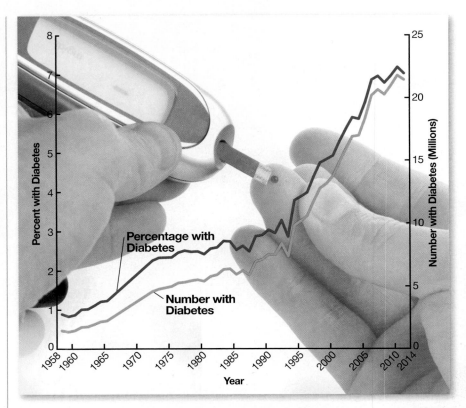

FIGURE 1 **Percentage and Number of U.S. Population with Diagnosed Diabetes, 1958–2014** Notice that these data are for diagnosed cases. Estimates of actual prevalence are higher.

Source: Centers for Disease Control and Prevention, "Long-term Trends in Diabetes," April 2016, www.cdc.gov/diabetes/statistics/slides/long_term_trends.pdf.

LO 1 | WHAT IS DIABETES?

Explain trends in diabetes, describe the effect of diabetes on the body, and differentiate among types of diabetes and their risk factors.

Diabetes mellitus is a group of diseases, each with its own mechanism, all characterized by a persistently high level of glucose, a type of sugar, in the blood. One sign of diabetes is the production of an abnormal level of glucose in the urine, a fact reflected in the name: *Diabetes* derives from a Greek word meaning "to flow through," and *mellitus* is Latin for "sweet." The high blood glucose levels—or **hyperglycemia**—seen in diabetes can lead to serious health problems and premature death.

In a healthy person, the digestive system breaks down eaten carbohydrates into glucose—a main energy source—which it releases into the bloodstream for use by body cells. The red blood cells can use only glucose to fuel functioning, and brain and other nerve cells prefer glucose over other fuels. When glucose levels drop below normal, certain mental functions, such as concentration, may be impaired. When more glucose is available than required to meet immediate needs, the excess is stored as glycogen in the liver and muscles for later use.

Glucose can't cross cell membranes on its own. Instead, cells have structures that transport glucose across in response to a signal generated by the **pancreas**, an organ located just beneath the stomach. Whenever a surge of glucose enters the bloodstream, the pancreas secretes a hormone called **insulin**. Insulin stimulates cells to take up glucose from the bloodstream and carry it into the cell, where it is used for immediate energy. Insulin also assists the conversion of glucose to glycogen for storage in the liver and muscles. When levels of glucose fall, the pancreas stops secreting insulin until more glucose arrives.

Type 1 Diabetes

The more serious and less prevalent form of diabetes, called **type 1 diabetes (T1D)** (or insulin-dependent diabetes), is an autoimmune disease in which the

diabetes mellitus A group of diseases characterized by elevated blood glucose levels.

hyperglycemia Elevated blood glucose level.

pancreas The organ that secretes digestive enzymes into the small intestine and hormones, including insulin, into the bloodstream.

insulin A hormone secreted by the pancreas and required by body cells for the uptake and storage of glucose.

type 1 diabetes (T1D) A form of diabetes mellitus in which the pancreas is not able to make insulin, and therefore blood glucose cannot enter the cells to be used for energy.

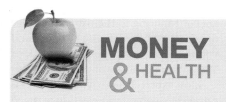

MONEY & HEALTH

DIABETES
At What Cost?

One in every five health care dollars is spent on diabetes care today. Costs of doctor visits, testing supplies, laboratory results, medicine, and other necessities are often only partially covered. If you are underinsured or uninsured, the *diabetes drain* on your bank account could be major, particularly if your diabetes is difficult to control and/or you don't improve your lifestyle.

Costs of treatment vary tremendously. Your deductibles and copays, your proximity to pharmacies that can supply generic drugs, and the number and dosage of drugs necessary to control your blood glucose are all factors. Prices for drugs have increased dramatically in the last few years. Newer drugs may not be more effective yet may cost significantly more. To give you an idea of what it might cost someone without insurance who is diagnosed with type 2 diabetes, consider these very conservative monthly estimates.

Diabetic Health Care Need	Estimated Monthly Cost
Doctor visit for monitoring and testing	$200 to $1,000, depending on number of visits and specialists seen
Lab tests: fasting glucose blood test, glucose tolerance, A1C tests	$50 to $250 for fasting blood glucose; $100 to $200 for A1C
Home glucose meter, test strips	Meter: $35 to $50 Test strips: roughly $2 each. Average: $100/month
Lancets and lancing devices, alcohol wipes	$5 to $$10/month
Oral medications such as metformin (depends on dosage and type), Actos (depends on dosage), or Januvia (depends on dosage)	Metformin: $13 to $15 (at low end) per month. Less at big box stores, more for different dosage; Actos: $220 to $370/month; Januvia: $265/month
Insulin pumps and supplies	$7,000 or more without insurance; copays may run $2,000 or more

The American Diabetes Association estimates costs of between $350 and $1,000 per month for the typical person with type 2 diabetes. However, those whose diabetes is difficult to control and those who must use insulin or use multiple drug therapy may have costs that are two to three times higher.

Source: American Diabetes Association. "The Costs of Diabetes," May 2017, http://www.diabetes.org/advocacy/news-events/cost-of-diabetes.htm.

---

individual's immune system attacks and destroys the pancreas's insulin-making cells. This causes a dramatic reduction or total cessation of insulin production. Without insulin, cells cannot take up glucose, leaving blood glucose levels permanently elevated.

Only about 5 percent of diabetic cases are type 1.[7] People inherit a predisposition to type 1 diabetes, and something in the environment triggers it.[8] Type 1 diabetes is more common in predominantly white European populations, people with a genetic predisposition, those living in cold climates, children who are not breastfed, and people with a history of certain viral infections.[9] People with type 1 diabetes require daily insulin injections or infusions and must carefully monitor their diet and exercise levels. They often face particular challenges as the lesser known diabetic type, with fewer research funds available and fewer treatment options.

Type 2 Diabetes

Type 2 diabetes (T2D) (non-insulin-dependent diabetes) accounts for 90 to 95 percent of all cases. In type 2, either the pancreas does not make sufficient insulin or body cells are resistant to its effects—a condition called **insulin resistance**—and don't use it efficiently (**FIGURE 2**). Genetics and lifestyle play significant roles in its development.[10]

Development of Type 2 Diabetes

Type 2 diabetes usually develops slowly. In its early stages, cells throughout the body begin to resist the effects of insulin; over time, the body may not produce enough insulin. An overabundance of free fatty acids concentrated in a person's fat cells (as may be the case

type 2 diabetes(T2D) A form of diabetes mellitus in which the pancreas does not make enough insulin or the body is unable to use insulin correctly.

insulin resistance The situation in which body cells fail to respond to the effects of insulin; obesity increases the risk that cells will become insulin resistant.

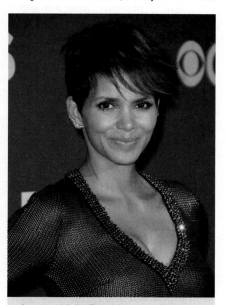

Actress Halle Berry is one of many Americans diagnosed with type 2 diabetes.

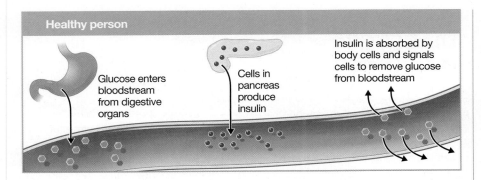

Healthy person

Glucose enters bloodstream from digestive organs

Cells in pancreas produce insulin

Insulin is absorbed by body cells and signals cells to remove glucose from bloodstream

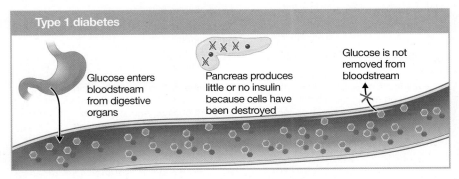

Type 1 diabetes

Glucose enters bloodstream from digestive organs

Pancreas produces little or no insulin because cells have been destroyed

Glucose is not removed from bloodstream

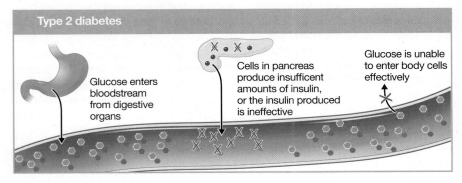

Type 2 diabetes

Glucose enters bloodstream from digestive organs

Cells in pancreas produce insufficient amounts of insulin, or the insulin produced is ineffective

Glucose is unable to enter body cells effectively

FIGURE 2 Diabetes: What It Is and How It Develops In a healthy person, a sufficient amount of insulin is produced and released by the pancreas and used efficiently by the cells. In type 1 diabetes, the pancreas makes little or no insulin. In type 2 diabetes, either the pancreas does not make enough insulin or cells are resistant to insulin and are not able to use it efficiently.

 Watch Video Tutor: How Diabetes Develops in Mastering Health.

in an obese individual) inhibit glucose uptake by body cells and suppress the liver's sensitivity to insulin. As a result, the liver's ability to self-regulate its conversion of glucose into glycogen begins to fail, and blood levels of glucose gradually rise.

The pancreas attempts to compensate by producing more insulin, but it cannot maintain hyper-production indefinitely. More and more pancreatic insulin-producing cells become nonfunctional, insulin output declines, and blood glucose levels rise high enough to warrant a diagnosis of type 2 diabetes.

Nonmodifiable Risk Factors

Type 2 diabetes is associated with a cluster of nonmodifiable risk factors including age, ethnicity, family history, and genetic and biological factors. Nearly 26 percent of adults over the age of 65 have a form of diabetes.[11] Although T2D used to be referred to as *adult-onset diabetes*, today it is increasingly diagnosed among children and teens.[12] Currently, diabetes is one of the leading chronic diseases in youth, affecting over 208,000 people under the age of 20, or 1 in every 400 youth.[13] Rising rates of obesity among adolescents and youth

are contributing to the rising incidence of type 2 diabetes among children and young adults, quadrupling the risk of T2D in those who are obese.[14]

Most experts believe type 2 diabetes is caused by a complex interaction between environmental factors, lifestyle, and genetic susceptibility. According to the most recent study, rates of T2D are up significantly among youth age 10 to 19, particularly among members of minorities. Rates for Hispanics, Native American, Asian/Pacific Islanders, non-Hispanic Blacks and non-Hispanic whites, in that order, have increased dramatically.[15] Having a close relative with type 2 diabetes is a significant risk factor. Although numerous genes have been identified as likely culprits in increased risk, the mechanisms by which inherited diabetes develops remain poorly understood.[16] A recent global report on diabetes prevention indicates that governments and society need to work together and consider the impact of policies in trade, agriculture, finance, transportation, education, and urban planning in the belief that health improves or worsens as a result of both individual and macroenvironmental behaviors.[17]

Modifiable Risk Factors

Body weight, dietary choices, level of physical activity, sleep patterns, and stress level are all diabetes-related factors that people have some control over. In adults, a body mass index (BMI) of 25 or greater increases risks, with significantly higher risks for each 5 kg/m^2 increase.[18] Excess weight around the waistline—a condition called *central adiposity*—is a significant risk factor for older women and younger adults.[19] People with T2D who lose weight and increase their physical activity can significantly improve their blood glucose levels.

Inadequate sleep may contribute to the development of both obesity and type 2 diabetes, possibly because sleep-deprived people tend to engage in less physical activity.[20] People who are routinely sleep deprived are also at higher risk for *metabolic syndrome* (see Chapter 13: Reducing Your Risk of Cardiovascular Disease and Cancer), a cluster of risk factors that include poor glucose

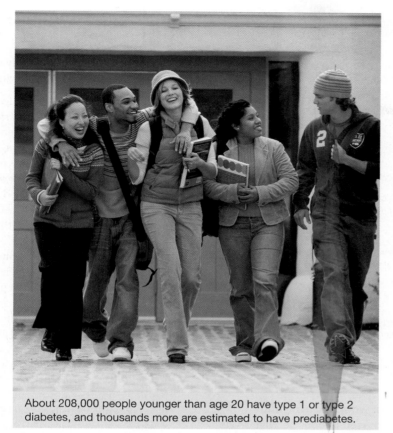

About 208,000 people younger than age 20 have type 1 or type 2 diabetes, and thousands more are estimated to have prediabetes.

Source: E. Mayor-Davis et al. "Increasing Trends of Type 1 and Type 2 Diabetes among Youth, 2002–2012." *New England Journal of Medicine* 376(2017):1419-29.

WHAT DO YOU THINK?

Why is type 2 diabetes is increasing in the United States?

- Why is the rate of T2D increasing among young people?
- Do you think young people are generally aware of what diabetes is and their own susceptibility for it?

complications.[30] See tips for halting or slowing the progression of diabetes in the Skills for Behavior Change box.

Gestational Diabetes

Gestational diabetes is a state of high blood glucose levels during pregnancy, which poses risks for both mother and child. Gestational diabetes is thought to be associated with metabolic stresses that occur in response to changing hormonal levels, and as many as 18 percent of pregnancies are affected by this type of diabetes.[31] Between 40 and 50 percent of women who develop gestational diabetes may develop type 2 diabetes within a decade of initial diagnosis if they don't make lifestyle changes. If the women never loses excess weight, her higher "normal" weight increases the risk of progression to type 2 diabetes with subsequent pregnancies.[32]

Women with gestational diabetes also have increased risk of high blood pressure, high blood acidity, increased infections, and death.[33] As a result of excess fat accumulation, women can give birth to large babies, increasing the risk of birth injuries and the need for cesarean sections. High blood glucose and excess weight in a pregnant woman can trigger high insulin levels and blood glucose fluctuations in the newborn. Babies born to women with gestational diabetes are also at risk for malformations of the heart, nervous system, and bones; respiratory distress; and fetal death.[34]

prediabetes The situation in which blood glucose levels are higher than normal, but not high enough to be classified as diabetes.

gestational diabetes A form of diabetes mellitus in which women who have never had diabetes have high blood glucose levels during pregnancy.

metabolism.[21] A recent review of the accumulated research indicates that T2D risk increases among people who are experiencing trauma or stressful working conditions, those with chronically high inflammation levels, those with a history of depression, and those with confrontational personalities.[22]

In addition, diabetes is more common among people with low socioeconomic status (SES) and members of racial and ethnic minorities, independent of current SES.[23]

Prediabetes

An estimated 86 million Americans age 20 or older—37 percent of the population over 20, and 51 percent of those over 65—have **prediabetes**, a condition involving higher than normal blood glucose levels, but not high enough to be classified as diabetes. Current rates of prediabetes in college students are unknown, but rising obesity rates indicate increasing risks. Many college students underestimate their risks.[24]

Prediabetes is clearly linked to lifestyle, including overweight and obesity profiles constituting *metabolic syndrome*, a cluster of risk factors that contribute to several health problems. A person with metabolic syndrome is five times more likely to develop type 2 diabetes than is a person without it.[25] In the United States, Mexican Americans have the highest rates of metabolic syndrome, with white Americans and African Americans not far behind.[26] Women with uterine fibroids or ovarian cysts also are at increased risk.[27]

Without weight loss and increases in moderate physical activity, 15 to 30 percent of people with prediabetes will develop type 2 diabetes within 5 years.[28] Lack of knowledge—over 90 percent of people with prediabetes don't know it and less than 14 percent of the healthy population knows what prediabetes is—poses a major challenge.[29] A prediabetes diagnosis represents an opportunity to adjust your lifestyle. Increasing physical activity can reduce risks of type 2 diabetes, hypertension, and other diabetic

LO 2 | WHAT ARE THE SYMPTOMS OF DIABETES?

Describe the symptoms of, complications associated with, and main tests for diabetes.

The symptoms of diabetes are similar for both T1D and T2D. They include the following:

- **Thirst.** The kidneys filter excessive glucose by diluting it with water. This can pull too much water from the body and result in dehydration.
- **Excessive urination.** For the same reason, the person with diabetes feels an increased need to urinate.
- **Increased hunger.** Because so many calories are lost in the glucose that passes into the urine, a person with diabetes often feels hungry.
- **Weight loss.** Despite eating more, weight loss is typical.
- **Fatigue.** When glucose cannot enter cells, fatigue and weakness occur.
- **Nerve damage.** A high glucose concentration damages blood vessels, including those that supply the nerves in the hands and feet. This can cause numbness and tingling in the extremities.
- **Poor wound healing and increased infections.** High levels of glucose can affect the body's ability to ward off infections and overall immune system functioning.

Complications of Diabetes

The main complications of poorly controlled diabetes include the following:[35]

- **Diabetic coma.** A coma from high blood acidity known as *diabetic ketoacidosis* can occur when, in the absence of glucose, body cells break down stored fat for energy. The process produces acidic molecules called *ketones*. Too many ketones can raise blood acid level dangerously high. The diabetic person slips into a coma and, without medical intervention, will die.
- **Cardiovascular disease.** Because many diabetics are also overweight or obese, hypertension is often present. Blood vessels become damaged, and essential nutrients and other substances are not transported as effectively.
- **Kidney disease.** Diabetes is the leading cause of kidney failure. The kidneys become scarred by overwork and high blood pressure. More than 247,000 Americans currently live with diabetes-caused kidney failure—35 percent of diabetics 20 years or older.[36] Many are on dialysis or waiting for a kidney transplant that may never come.

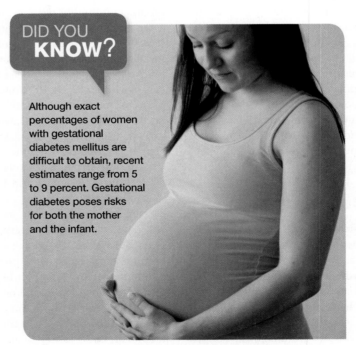

DID YOU KNOW?

Although exact percentages of women with gestational diabetes mellitus are difficult to obtain, recent estimates range from 5 to 9 percent. Gestational diabetes poses risks for both the mother and the infant.

Source: C. Desisto et al., "Prevalence Estimates of Gestational Diabetes in the United States: Pregnancy Risk Assessment Monitoring System (PRAMS) 2007–2010," *Preventing Chronic Disease* 11 (2014): 130415, doi:10.5888/pcd 11.130415.

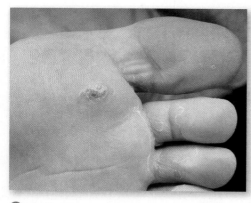

(a) Diabetics are prone to wounds that don't heal on the feet as nerves may be damaged, healing impaired, and sensation diminished. Blisters, infections, and other irritants can easily progress to more serious problems.

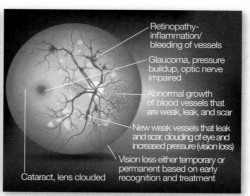

Retinopathy-inflammation/bleeding of vessels

Glaucoma, pressure buildup, optic nerve impaired

Abnormal growth of blood vessels that are weak, leak, and scar

New weak vessels that leak and scar; clouding of eye and increased pressure (vision loss)

Vision loss either temporary or permanent based on early recognition and treatment

Cataract, lens clouded

(b) Uncontrolled diabetes can damage the eye, causing swelling and rupture of blood vessels.

FIGURE 3 Complications of Uncontrolled Diabetes: Amputation and Eye Disease

- **Amputations.** An impaired immune response, damaged blood vessels, and neuropathy in hands and feet makes it easier for people with diabetes not to notice injury until damage is extensive. Lack of circulation increases risk of infection and difficulty of treatment, leading to tissue death and amputation. More than 60 percent of nontraumatic amputations of legs, feet, and toes are due to diabetes[37] (see **FIGURE 3**). Each year, nearly 73,000 nontraumatic lower-limb amputations are performed on people with diabetes (180 per day).[38]

- **Eye disease and blindness.** High blood glucose levels damage microvessels in the eye, leading to vision loss. Nearly 7.7 million people over the age of 40 have early-stage retinopathy, swelling of capillaries in the eye, which can lead to blindness (**FIGURE 3b**).[39] Dry eyes and infections are also common.

30%

percent of people with type 1 diabetes and **10–40%** of those with type 2 diabetes will eventually develop **KIDNEY FAILURE**.

- **Infectious diseases.** People with diabetes have increased susceptibility to infectious diseases, particularly influenza and pneumonia. Once infection occurs, it may be more difficult to treat.

- **Tooth and gum diseases.** People with diabetes are more susceptible to bacterial infections of the mouth that can lead to *gingivitis* (an early stage of gum disease) and *periodontitis*—a more serious inflammation of the gums that can lead to decay, tooth loss, and a variety of other health risks.[40] Emerging research suggests that the relationship between diabetes and gum disease may be a two-way street, with those who have gum disease being more susceptible to problems with blood glucose control, increasing the risk of progression to diabetes.[41]

- **Other complications.** Many people with diabetes suffer from nerve damage known as *diabetic neuropathy*, which can be extremely painful and cause difficulty driving, walking, and other activities. About half of all people with diabetes have some degree of nerve damage.[42] People with diabetes are more likely to suffer from depression, making intervention and treatment more difficult, and depressed individuals are more likely to develop type 2 diabetes.

Diagnosing Diabetes

Diabetes and prediabetes are diagnosed when a blood test reveals elevated blood glucose levels. Generally, a physician orders one of the following blood tests:

- The *fasting plasma glucose (FPG) test* requires fasting for 8 to 10 hours. Then a small blood sample is tested for glucose concentration. An FPG level of 100 mg/dL or more indicates prediabetes, and a level of 126 mg/dL or more indicates diabetes (**FIGURE 4**).

- The *oral glucose tolerance test (OGTT)* requires the patient to drink concentrated glucose 2 hours before having blood drawn. A reading of 140 mg/dL or more indicates prediabetes; a reading of 200 mg/dL or more indicates diabetes.

- A third test, *A1C* or *glycosylated hemoglobin test (HbA1C)*, gives the average value of a patient's blood glucose over the past 2 to 3 months instead of just at one moment in time. In general, an A1C of 5.7 to 6.4 means a high risk for diabetes or prediabetes. If A1C is 6.5 or higher, then diabetes may be diagnosed.[43] **Estimated average glucose (eAG)** shows how A1C numbers correspond to blood glucose numbers. For example, someone with an A1C value of 6.1 would be able to look at a chart and see that his or her average blood glucose was around 128—a high level that should prompt healthy lifestyle modifications.

People with diabetes need to check their blood glucose levels several times each day to help them stay within their target range. To check blood glucose, they prick one of their fingers to obtain a drop of blood. A handheld glucose meter can then evaluate the blood sample.

estimated average glucose (eAG) A1C test results that gives the average blood glucose levels for the testing period using the same units (milligrams per deciliter [mg/dL]) that patients are used to seeing in self-administered glucose tests.

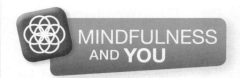

MINDFULNESS AND YOU

PUTTING A LITTLE "ZEN" INTO PREVENTING AND CONTROLLING TD2

The emotions that come with discovering that you are prediabetic or have type 2 diabetes can be overwhelming. And making lifestyle changes, taking medications, and avoiding stressors is tough for even the healthiest among us. *Mindfulness-based interventions (MBIs)* are increasingly seen as effective complementary strategies that enhance the effectiveness of day-to-day dietary, exercise, and pharmacological recommendations—from passing up the extra ice cream and eating more vegetables to exercising regularly and making time for meditation. Mindfulness helps people work through feelings of guilt, anxiety, self-blame, or depression and take positive, compassionate steps to reduce their risks of diabetes.

Because stress, sleep deprivation, and depression symptoms are implicated in increased risk for TD2, research assessing the effectiveness of mindfulness-based stress reduction (MBSR) programs in reducing these risks in overweight and obese women is promising. After a 16-week, randomized, controlled MBSR program, participants had significant reduction in fasting glucose, improvement in quality of life, and reductions in sleep impairments, depression, anxiety, and overall psychological distress compared to controls. In the New England Family study, participants who measured high on mindfulness attention reported increased control of their diabetes course through exercise, dietary changes, and medication adherence.

Although these results are promising, longer-term trials are necessary to fully understand the potential benefits of MBIs.

Sources: W.L. Medina et al., "Effects of Mindfulness on Diabetes Mellitus: Rationale and Overview," *Current Diabetes Reviews* 13, no. 2 (2017):141–47; N. Raja-Khan et al., "Mindfulness-based Stress Reduction Decreases Fasting Glucose in Overweight and Obese Women," *Endocrine Society, Obesity-Clinical Trials II* (2015): FRI-550; E.B. Loucks et al., "Associations of Mindfulness with Glucose Regulation and Diabetes," *American Journal of Health Behavior* 40, no. 2 (2016): 258–67.

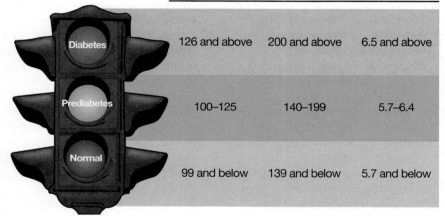

	FPG Levels	OGTT Levels	A1C Levels
Diabetes	126 and above	200 and above	6.5 and above
Prediabetes	100–125	140–199	5.7–6.4
Normal	99 and below	139 and below	5.7 and below

FIGURE 4 Blood Glucose Levels in Prediabetes and Untreated Diabetes
The fasting plasma glucose (FPG) test measures levels of blood glucose after a person fasts overnight. The oral glucose tolerance test (OGTT) measures levels of blood glucose after a person consumes a concentrated amount of glucose.

Source: American Diabetes Association, "Diagnosing Diabetes and Learning about Prediabetes," Accessed May 2017, www.diabetes.org/diabetes-basics/diagnosis.

LO 3 | PREVENTING AND TREATING DIABETES

Explain how diabetes can be prevented and treated.

Treatment options for people with prediabetes and diabetes vary according to disease type and progression.

Lifestyle Changes

Studies show that lifestyle changes can prevent or delay the development of type 2 diabetes by up to 58 percent.[44] Even for people with type 2 diabetes, lifestyle changes can sometimes prevent or delay the need for medication or insulin injections. See the **Mindfulness and You** box for information on mindfulness-based interventions.

Losing Weight

In a landmark clinical trial, the Diabetes Prevention Program (DPP) study, regular exercise and losing as little as 5 to 7 percent of body weight significantly reduced the risk of people with prediabetes progressing to type 2 diabetes.[45] Weight loss and exercise can improve your blood glucose and other health indicators.

Adopting a Healthy Diet

To prevent surges in blood sugar, people with diabetes must pay attention to the glycemic index and glycemic load of the foods they eat. The *glycemic index* compares the potential of foods containing the same amount of carbohydrate to

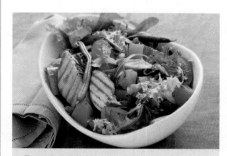

People with diabetes don't have to give up all the foods they love. Careful monitoring of portions and balancing carbohydrate, fat, and protein intake are key.

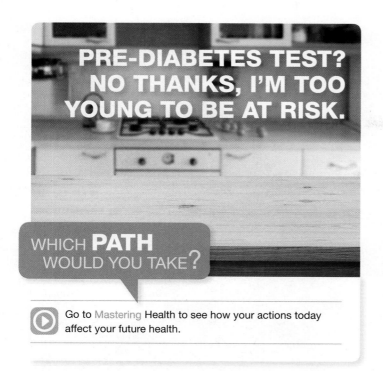

PRE-DIABETES TEST? NO THANKS, I'M TOO YOUNG TO BE AT RISK.

WHICH **PATH** WOULD YOU TAKE?

Go to Mastering Health to see how your actions today affect your future health.

raise blood glucose. Scientists developed the concept of *glycemic load* to simultaneously describe the quality (glycemic index) and quantity of carbohydrate in a meal.[46] By learning to combine high— and low—glycemic index foods, people with diabetes can help to control their average blood glucose levels.

Researchers have studied a variety of foods for their effect on blood glucose levels. Here is a brief summary of foods that may reduce T2D risks[47]:

- **Low-fat dairy.**
- **Nuts.** Almonds and walnuts are particularly good for this.
- **Whole grains.**[48]
- **High-fiber foods.** Berries, beans, and vegetables are among the best options.[49]
- **Fatty fish.** Research has linked fish that is high in omega-3 fatty acids with decreased progression of insulin resistance. However, further research has called into question this connection between high fish intake

▶ SEE IT! VIDEOS

Could fewer, larger meals be better for people with diabetes? Watch **Two Meals a Day Could Help Diabetics Control Blood Sugar** in the Study Area of Mastering Health.

and risk reduction.[50] More research is necessary.[51]

Increasing Physical Fitness

In late 2016, the American Diabetes Association changed its exercise recommendations for diabetes prevention, calling for at least 3 minutes of light activity every 30 minutes during long sitting stretches. Rather than prescribing 90 minutes of exercise over several days, getting people up and moving at more regular intervals is key to glucose control.[52] Exercise increases sensitivity to insulin. The more muscle mass you have and the more you use your muscles throughout the day, the more efficiently cells use glucose, meaning that less glucose is circulating in the bloodstream.

Medical Interventions

Many people use medication to control diabetes. When medications are less effective, bariatric surgery may be an option for slowing or halting the progression of prediabetes and type 2 diabetes.

Oral Medications

When lifestyle changes fail to control type 2 diabetes or the person cannot maintain the necessary lifestyle changes, oral medications may be

prescribed. Some medications reduce the liver's glucose production; others slow the absorption of carbohydrates from the small intestine. Other medications increase insulin production, and still others work to increase the insulin sensitivity of cells. SGLT2 inhibitors cause the kidneys to excrete more glucose, lowering levels of glucose circulating in the body.

Some people use diabetes medications without altering their lifestyle, thinking that the drugs are taking care of the problem. However, with time, medications become less effective, and treatment options become increasingly scarce. It is best to follow the American Diabetes Association recommendations on diet, exercise, and lifestyle.

Currently, there is much discussion about whether people with prediabetes should use the drug metformin, along with lifestyle intervention and counseling, as an early intervention. Although sources indicate potential benefits, metformin is not without risks, particularly for those with a history of gastrointestinal, cardiovascular, or kidney problems. Always consult your doctor about the best drug regimen, weight loss program, and exercise program for you.[53]

Weight Loss Surgery

People who undergo gastric or bariatric surgery have shown remarkable reductions in blood glucose and diabetes symptoms more than 2 years after surgery.[54] Those who combined gastric bypass or sleeve gastrectomy with intensive medical therapy had similar outcomes.[55] In many cases, former diabetics can stop taking some medications and their diabetes symptoms subside altogether. Consensus is growing about potential short- and long-term benefits of these more drastic methods.[56] (See Chapter 11 for more on gastric bypass surgeries.)

Insulin Injections

For people with type 1 diabetes, insulin injections or infusions are absolutely essential for daily functioning because their pancreas can no longer produce enough insulin. People with type 2 diabetes whose blood glucose levels cannot be adequately controlled with other treatment options also require insulin injections. Because insulin is a protein and would be digested in the gastrointestinal tract, it cannot be taken orally and must be injected into the fat layer under the skin; from there, it is absorbed into the bloodstream.

People with T1D used to need two or more daily insulin injections. Now, many use an *insulin infusion pump* to deliver tiny amounts of insulin throughout the day. The external portion of the pump is only about the size of an MP3 player and can easily be hidden by clothes; and a thin tube and catheter are inserted under the patient's skin. Infusion over time is less painful and more effective than a few larger doses of insulin.

To overcome current limitations of insulin therapy, researchers are working to link glucose monitoring and insulin delivery by developing an artificial pancreas. An artificial pancreas would mimic the way a healthy pancreas detects changes in blood glucose levels, responding automatically to secrete appropriate amounts of insulin. Although the first prototype devices have received approval from the U.S. Food and Drug Administration, they may not be available until late 2017 or beyond.[57] Stay tuned!

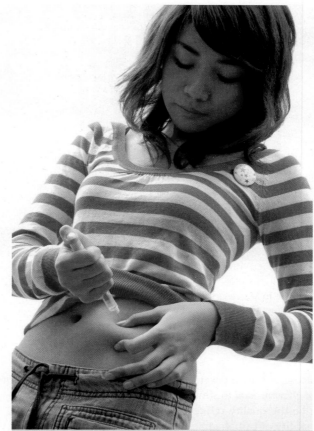

Some people with type 2 diabetes can control their condition with changes in diet and lifestyle habits or with oral medications. However, some people with type 2 diabetes and all people with type 1 diabetes require insulin injections or infusions.

New Research in the Battle to Cure TD2

Although prevention is always the best option, those who develop TD2 have a growing arsenal of treatment options. Although treatment is good; finding a possible cure would be even better. A new drug is showing promising results in the when given to mice with insulin resistance (when the body doesn't produce enough or can't use insulin and blood glucose levels rise).[58] Exploring the idea that a specific enzyme found in the liver (known as low molecular weight protein tyrosine phosphate or LMPTP) interacts with cells and makes them resistant to insulin, scientists developed a new drug that would keep LMPTP from negatively affecting insulin receptors. In other words, less LMPT, more effective insulin, and more normal blood glucose. Insulin resistance was canceled out and blood glucose levels remained within normal ranges.

Mice used in the study had been fed high fat diets and developed obesity and TD2. The good news was that the orally administered drug resulted in no apparent side effects in the mice! Of course, this study is just the first step. Clinical trials in humans will test whether this "cure" for mice may actually be the next step in finding a cure for TD2 in humans. Stay tuned!

ASSESS | YOURSELF

Are You at Risk for Diabetes?

LIVE IT! ASSESS YOURSELF

An interactive version of this assessment is available online in Mastering Health.

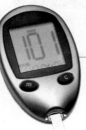

Certain characteristics place people at greater risk for diabetes. Take the following quiz to help determine your risk for diabetes. If you answer yes to three or more of the questions, consider seeking medical advice.

	Yes	No
1. Do any of your primary relatives (parents, siblings, grandparents) have diabetes?	○	○
2. Are you overweight or obese?	○	○
3. Do you smoke?	○	○
4. Have you been diagnosed with high blood pressure?	○	○
5. Are you typically sedentary (seldom, if ever, engaging in vigorous aerobic exercise)?	○	○
6. Have you noticed an increase in your craving for water or other beverages?	○	○
7. Have you noticed that you have to urinate more frequently than you used to during a typical day?	○	○
8. Have you noticed any tingling or numbness in your hands and feet that might indicate circulatory problems?	○	○
9. Do you often feel a gnawing hunger during the day even though you usually eat regular meals?	○	○
10. Are you often so tired that you find it difficult to stay awake?	○	○
11. Have you noticed that you are losing weight but don't seem to be doing anything in particular to make this happen?	○	○
12. Have you noticed that you have skin irritations more frequently and that minor infections don't heal as quickly as they used to?	○	○
13. Have you noticed any unusual changes in your vision (e.g., blurring, difficulty in focusing)?	○	○
14. Have you noticed unusual pain or swelling in your joints?	○	○
15. Do you often feel weak or nauseated when you awaken in the morning or if you wait too long to eat a meal?	○	○
16. If you are a woman, have you had several vaginal yeast infections during the past year?	○	○

YOUR PLAN FOR CHANGE

If the results of the ASSESS YOURSELF activity "Are You at Risk for Diabetes?" indicate that you need to take further steps to decrease your risks, then follow this plan.

TODAY, YOU CAN:

☐ Talk to your parents and find out whether there is a history of prediabetes or diabetes mellitus in your family.

☐ Take stock of other risk factors you may have for diabetes. Do you exercise regularly and watch your weight? Do you eat healthfully? Have you ever had your blood glucose measured?

WITHIN THE NEXT TWO WEEKS, YOU CAN:

☐ Make an appointment with your health care provider to have your blood glucose levels tested.

☐ If you smoke, begin devising a plan to quit. (Chapter 8 can give you some ideas.)

BY THE END OF THE SEMESTER, YOU CAN:

☐ Pay attention to what you eat. Increase your intake of whole grains, fruits, and vegetables, and decrease your consumption of saturated fats, *trans* fats, and sugar.

☐ Make physical activity and exercise part of your daily routine, aiming for at least 30 minutes 5 days a week.

STUDY **PLAN**

Visit the Study Area in Mastering Health to enhance your study plan with MP3 Tutor Sessions, Practice Quizzes, Flashcards, and more!

CHAPTER **REVIEW**

LO **1** | What Is Diabetes?

- Diabetes mellitus is a group of diseases, each with its own mechanism. All the diseases are characterized by a persistently high level of glucose, a type of sugar, in the blood.
- Complications can range from cardiovascular disease to eye and gum problems, neuropathy, poor wound healing, and a host of other health problems.

LO **2** | What Are the Symptoms of Diabetes?

- Symptoms of diabetes may include increased thirst, excessive urination, increased hunger, weight loss, fatigue, nerve damage, poor wound healing, and increased infections, among others.
- Key tests for diabetes include a fasting plasma glucose test taken after an 8- to 10-hour fast, an oral glucose tolerance test, taken 2 hours after consuming a concentrated glucose drink, and an estimated average glucose test.

LO **3** | Preventing and Treating Diabetes

- Prevention of diabetes include lifestyle changes such as a healthy and balanced diet, a healthy weight, regular exercise, sufficient sleep, and stress reduction.
- Treatment of diabetes may include oral or injectable medications such as insulin, use of infusion pumps and other technologies, appropriate visits to the doctor, monitoring of glucose levels, and possibly weight loss surgery.

POP **QUIZ**

LO **1** | What Is Diabetes?

1. Which of the following is *not* correct?
   a. Type 1 diabetes is an autoimmune disease in which the body does not produce insulin.
   b. Type 2 diabetes is a disease in which the body may not produce sufficient amounts of insulin or the insulin may not be utilized properly.
   c. Gestational diabetes is a problem for the mother only while she is pregnant.
   d. Increased weight gain, high stress, lack of sleep, and sedentary lifestyle are key contributors to risks for type 2 diabetes.

LO **2** | What Are the Symptoms of Diabetes?

2. Which of the following is *not* an accurate match between blood glucose level and diabetes-related problems in adults?
   a. A fasting blood glucose level of 100 to 126 mg/dL indicates prediabetes.
   b. A fasting blood glucose level of 50 to 70 mg/dL is an ideal blood glucose level.
   c. A fasting blood glucose level of less than 90 to 99 mg/dL is normal.
   d. An A1C test of 5.7 is normal.

LO **3** | Preventing and Treating Diabetes

3. Which of the following statements is *correct*?
   a. People with type 2 diabetes must eliminate sweets or high-sugar foods from their diets.
   b. Skipping meals and eating two high-protein meals or no-carbohydrate meals per day is the best way to control blood sugar.
   c. Regular exercise, weight control, a balanced diet, adequate sleep, and stress management are key factors in blood glucose control.
   d. Most people with prediabetes know that they have it.

*Answers to the Pop Quiz questions can be found on page A-1. If you answered a question incorrectly, review the section identified by the Learning Outcome. For even more study tools, visit **Mastering Health**.*

14

Protecting Against Infectious Diseases and Sexually Transmitted Infections

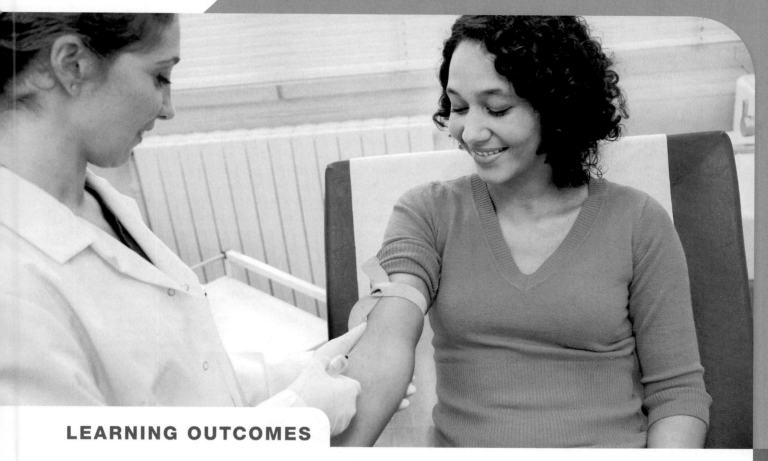

LEARNING OUTCOMES

LO **1** Describe the process of infection and the factors that increase your risk for infectious diseases.

LO **2** Explain how your immune system protects you, factors that diminish its effectiveness, and what you can do to boost its effectiveness.

LO **3** Describe the most common pathogens infecting humans today, key diseases caused by each, and the threat of growing antimicrobial resistance as well as individual- and community-based strategies for prevention and control of infectious diseases.

LO **4** Explain the risk factors for sexually transmitted infections and actions that can prevent their spread.

LO **5** Describe common types of sexually transmitted infections, including their symptoms and treatment methods.

LO **6** Discuss human immunodeficiency virus (HIV) and acquired immune deficiency syndrome (AIDS), trends in infection and treatment, and the impact of these diseases on special populations.

An increasing number of chronic diseases are being linked to the inflammation that occurs when certain pathogens invade. Avoiding infections and their inflammatory side effects now has the added benefit that it may help you avoid certain chronic diseases later. Getting an STI can be painful, and you can infect your current partner with it. In the long term, it could affect the health of your children or your ability to have children.

Pathogens—disease-causing agents—are everywhere. We inhale them, swallow them, rub them in our eyes, and are constantly in a hidden, high-stakes battle with them. Although many pathogens have existed as long as there has been life on the planet, new varieties emerge all the time. Some infectious diseases, such as the common cold, are **endemic**, meaning that they are present at expected prevalence rates in virtually all populations on Earth, with rates that rise and fall predictably each season. Historically, many infectious diseases become **epidemic**, meaning that they occur at rates that are much greater than expected, causing illness and possibly death in large percentages of populations. For example, the *bubonic plague*, popularly known as the "Black Death", began as an epidemic in China and spread along major trade routes to many regions of the world, eventually reaching **pandemic** (global epidemic) status, killing over 60 percent of the population of Europe in the 1300s. HIV/AIDS is a major pandemic of the 20th and 21st centuries.

Despite constant bombardment by pathogens, our immune systems are usually adept at protecting us. Millions of microorganisms live in and on our bodies, usually in a peaceful, sometimes even symbiotic coexistence. Exposure to invading microorganisms helps us build pathogen resistance. Generally harmless to healthy people, these organisms can cause serious health problems in those with weakened immune systems.

When pathogens gain entry into the body, they are apt to produce an infection or illness. The more **virulent** the pathogen, the more likely it will be to breach the body's defenses and sustain itself, increasing the chances of disease. By keeping your immune system strong, you improve your ability to resist and fight off even the most virulent pathogen.

pathogen A disease-causing agent.

endemic A disease that is always present to some degree.

epidemic A disease outbreak that affects many people in a community or region at the same time.

pandemic A global epidemic of a disease.

virulent Strong enough to overcome host resistance and cause disease.

infection The state of pathogens being established in or on a host and causing disease.

epidemiological triad of disease The process by which a disease is likely to occur, including characteristics of the host (health of immune system, etc.), the agent (pathogen and its virulence), and the environment (whether conditions are conducive to spread).

opportunistic infections Infections that occur more often and with greater severity in people with compromised immune systems.

immunocompromised Having an immune system that is impaired.

LO 1 | THE PROCESS OF INFECTION

Describe the process of infection and the factors that increase your risk for infectious diseases.

Most infectious disease are *multifactorial*, that is, caused by the interaction of several factors inside and outside the person. For an **infection** to occur, three key conditions known as the **epidemiological triad of disease** (FIGURE 14.1) must be met. First, *the host (the person) must come into contact with a pathogen (infectious agent)* that is virulent enough to overcome the body's elaborate defenses and capable of sustaining itself long enough to cause an infection.

Second, *the host must be susceptible*, or in some way vulnerable to infection. In other words, the pathogen must be so virulent that it overcomes a typical healthy immune system, or, in an **opportunistic infection**, a normal pathogen overcomes an **immunocompromised** immune system—one that has been weakened or is nonfunctional. As an example, a person on

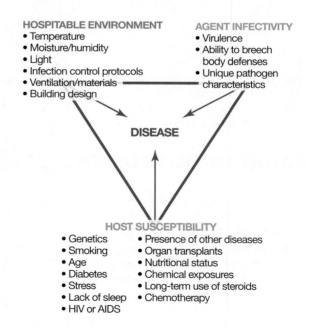

FIGURE 14.1 Epidemiological Triad of Disease For a disease to occur, the agent, host, and environment must be conducive to overcoming the body's elaborate defense systems.

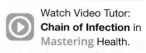

Watch Video Tutor: **Chain of Infection** in Mastering Health.

TABLE 14.1 | Routes of Disease Transmission

Transmission Mode	Description
Contact	Either direct (e.g., skin or sexual contact) or indirect (e.g., infected blood or body fluid)
Food-borne or waterborne	Eating, drinking, washing, and unsanitary food preparation
Airborne	Infection spreads by inhaling droplets from an infected person's sneezes or coughs
Vector-borne	Blood-sucking insects such as mosquitoes, fleas, flies, or ticks pass along pathogens when they bite human victims.
Perinatal	Similar to contact infection; happens in the uterus, as the baby passes through the birth canal, or through breastfeeding

antirejection drugs after an organ transplant may be severely immunocompromised and would be vulnerable to any number of pathogens, be they lurking in a hospital room or carried in on well-wishing visitors.

Finally, *the environment must be hospitable* to the pathogen in terms of temperature, light, moisture, and other requirements. Although pathogens pose a threat if they gain entry and begin to grow in your body, the chances that they will do serious, long-term harm are normally quite small.

Routes of Transmission: How Do Pathogens Gain Entry?

Pathogens may enter the body by *direct contact* between infected persons or by *indirect contact*, such as touching an object an infected person has touched. **TABLE 14.1** lists common routes of transmission. You may also **autoinoculate** yourself, or transmit a pathogen from one part of your body to another—for example, by touching a herpes sore on your lip with a finger and then touching your eye with that finger.

Dogs, cats, livestock, and wild animals can directly or indirectly spread infections to each other and to humans, known as *animal-borne (zoonotic) infections*. Companion animals such as cats and dogs can carry fleas and ticks into homes; when these insects bite humans, diseases such as Lyme disease can occur. Untreated puppies and dogs can be infested with worms that can be transmitted to humans via saliva or through fecal residue on bedding, household carpets, or furniture. Every year, pet outbreaks send thousands of people to their veterinarian, worried about their pet and about whether they themselves might get a disease from their animals. Although you can get some illnesses from your pet, such as certain forms of influenza, salmonellosis, leptospirosis, and rabies, *interspecies transmission*—transmission between humans and animals—is fairly rare, owing to vaccination of pets, basic hygiene, and using care in contacting animal fluids. Washing your hands after contact with pets, keeping your pets off your pillow, and not letting your dog share your ice cream cone are important examples of prevention.[1]

Risk Factors You Can Control

Surrounded by pathogens, how can you be sure you don't get sick? Too much stress, poor diet, a low fitness level, lack of sleep, misuse or abuse of drugs, poor personal hygiene, and unprotected sex significantly increase the risk for many diseases. College students are at higher risk because of their close living conditions, All these factors create higher risk for exposure to pathogens. The Skills for Behavior Change box lists some actions you can take to minimize your risk of infection.

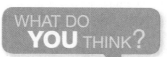

WHAT DO YOU THINK?

Do you have any risks for infectious disease that you may have been born with? Do you have any that are the result of your lifestyle?

- What actions can you take to reduce your risks?
- What behaviors do you or your friends engage in that might make you more susceptible to various infections?
- Are your risks greater today than before you entered college? Why or why not?

autoinoculate Transmit a pathogen from one part of your body to another part.

Hard to Control Risk Factors

Unfortunately, some risk factors are difficult or impossible to control. Following are the most common of these:

- **Heredity.** It is often unclear whether hereditary diseases are due to inherited genetic traits or to inherited insufficiencies in the immune system. If we inherit the quality of our immune system, some people are naturally more resistant or more susceptible to infection and disease.
- **Age.** Thinning of the skin, reduced sweating, and other physical changes can make people more susceptible to disease as they age. Older adults and very young children are particularly vulnerable.
- **Environmental conditions.** A growing body of research points to climate change as a major contributor to infectious diseases. As temperatures rise, insect populations may rise, potentially increasing cases of mosquito-borne diseases such as West Nile virus, malaria, dengue fever, chikungunya virus, and others. Dwindling water supplies where there is little water turnover or flow contribute to an environment that fosters pathogen growth. When animals move to new environments in search of water and congregate near water sources, they are exposed to new species of animals with a new set of pathogens. In these environments, disease spreads quickly. Scientists argue that changing environmental conditions such as drought, flooding, fires, and other natural and human-caused events may increase disease spread and hasten the chances of interspecies transmission in humans.[2] Chronic exposure to toxic chemicals in pesticides, herbicides, mercury, and lead and other threats such as radiation exposure can damage the immune system and increase disease susceptibility.
- **Organism virulence and resistance.** Even tiny numbers of a particularly virulent organism can make the hardiest of us ill. Other organisms have mutated and become resistant to medical treatments. This kind of **drug resistance** occurs when pathogens grow and proliferate in the presence of chemicals that would normally slow their growth or kill them. See the Health Headlines box for more on antibiotic and antimicrobial resistance and superbugs.

drug resistance Occurs when microbes such as bacteria, viruses, or other pathogens grow and proliferate in the presence of chemicals that would normally kill them or slow their growth.

LO 2 | YOUR BODY'S DEFENSES AGAINST INFECTION

Explain how your immune system protects you, factors that diminish its effectiveness, and what you can do to boost its effectiveness.

To gain entry into your body, pathogens must overcome barriers that prevent their entrance, mechanisms that weaken organisms, and substances that counteract the threat that these organisms pose. FIGURE 14.2 summarizes some of the body's defenses against invasion and disease.

Physical and Chemical Defenses

Layered to provide an intricate web of barriers, the skin—our most critical early defense system—allows few pathogens to enter. Enzymes in body secretions such as sweat provide additional protection, destroying microorganisms on skin surfaces by producing inhospitable pH levels. Only through cracks or breaks in the skin can pathogens gain easy access to the body.

The internal linings, structures, and secretions of the body provide further protection. Mucous membranes in the respiratory tract, for example, trap and engulf invading organisms. Cilia, hairlike projections in the lungs and respiratory tract, sweep invaders toward body openings, where they are expelled. Nose hairs trap airborne invaders with a sticky film. Tears, earwax, and other secretions contain enzymes that destroy or neutralize pathogens.

The Immune System: Your 24/7 Protector

Immunity is a condition of being able to resist a particular disease by counteracting the substance that produces the disease. Any substance that is capable of triggering an immune response—a virus, a bacterium, a fungus, a parasite,

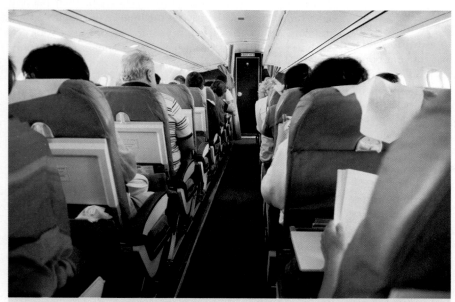
Crowded public transportation, trains, and airplanes are key areas where infectious diseases can be transmitted. Washing your hands and keeping your hands away from your face will help to reduce risks.

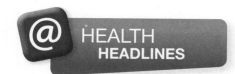

@ HEALTH HEADLINES

ANTIMICROBIAL RESISTANCE
Bugs Versus Drugs

According to the WHO, **antimicrobial resistance (AMR)** is defined as "the ability of a microorganism (e.g., bacteria, viruses, and some parasites) to stop an antimicrobial (antibiotics, antivirals, etc.) from working against it." Pathogens, particularly bacteria, evolve and develop ways to survive drugs that previously killed them. Some microorganisms that were easily dealt with a few decades ago are becoming "superbugs" that cannot be stopped with existing medications.

Why Is Antibiotic Resistance on the Rise?

- **Overuse of antibiotics in food production.** About 70 percent of antibiotics produced today are fed to animals or fish living in crowded feedlots or fish farms to encourage their growth and fight off disease. Water runoff and sewage from feedlots can contaminate the water in rivers and streams with antibiotics. Antibiotic-resistant bacteria may also spread beyond farms via dried particles of animal manure that disperse in the wind.

- **Improper use of antibiotics by humans and unnecessary prescriptions.** Humans also contaminate waterways and soil through dumping their unused prescription drugs down the toilet or tossing them into the garbage. The CDC estimates that one third to one half of the 150 million antibiotic prescriptions written each year are unnecessary, resulting in bacterial strains that are tougher than the drugs used to fight them. Growing awareness of the

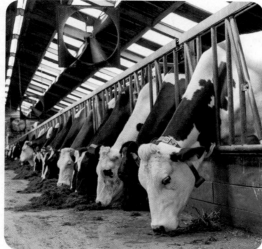

Widespread use of antibiotics in industrial food production has been a key factor in antibiotic resistance.

problem has led patients and doctors to be more careful in their requests for and dispersal of antibiotics.

- **Misuse and overuse of antibacterial soaps and other cleaning products.** Preying on the public's fear of germs and disease, the cleaning industry adds antibacterial ingredients to many soaps and household products. Just how much these products contribute to overall resistance is difficult to assess; as with antibiotics, the germs these products do not kill may become stronger than before.

What Can You Do?

- **Be responsible with medications.** Use antibiotics only when prescribed for you and for the disease for which they are intended. Ask your doctor if there is an older-generation antibiotic

that still works to treat the illness and save the newer drugs for the most difficult problems.

- **Finish the entire bottle of a drug as prescribed.** Antibiotic regimens are designed to kill entire colonies of bacteria if taken exactly as prescribed. If you stop early, the hardiest bacteria may survive and reproduce, leading to increased chances of drug-resistant pathogens.

- **Use regular soap when washing your hands.** Research suggests that antibacterial agents contained in soaps may actually kill normal bacteria found on the skin that does not cause disease, thus creating an environment for resistant, mutated bacteria that are impervious to antibacterial cleaners and antibiotics to colonize the skin.

- **Avoid food treated with antibiotics.** Buy organic meat and poultry, particularly those with labels that say that they have not been fed antibiotics or hormones. If you buy farmed fish, choose fish grown in U.S. coastal waters, where there is less likelihood of questionable fish-feeding practice and less chance of contaminated water and antibiotics or growth hormones.

Sources: Centers for Disease Control and Prevention, "Fast Facts: Get Smart about Antibiotics," April 2017, www.cdc.gov/getsmart /community/about/index.html; World Health Organization, "Antimicrobial Resistance," May 2017, http://www.who.int/antimicrobial-resistance /en; Centers for Disease Control and Prevention, "Antibiotic/Antimicrobial Resistance," April, 14, 2017, https://www.cdc.gov/drugresistance.

---

a toxin, a tissue or cell from another organism, or even chemicals from the environment—is called an **antigen**. When a pathogen breaches the initial external defenses, the body first analyzes the antigen, verifying that it isn't part of the body itself. It then responds by forming **antibodies** specific to that antigen, much as a key is matched to a lock. These antibodies are designed to destroy or weaken the antigen. This process is part of a system called *humoral immune responses*. **Humoral immunity** is the body's major defense against many bacteria and the poisonous substances—**toxins**—they produce.

In **cell-mediated immunity**, specialized white blood cells called **lymphocytes** attack and destroy the foreign invader. Lymphocytes constitute the body's main defense against viruses, fungi, parasites, and some bacteria; they are found in the blood, lymph nodes, bone marrow, and certain glands. Another key

antibiotic/antimicrobial resistance (AMR) The ability of microbes to resist the effects of drugs, to grow and proliferate, even in the face of our best weapons.

antigen A substance that is capable of triggering an immune response.

antibodies Immune-system proteins that are individually matched to specific antigens.

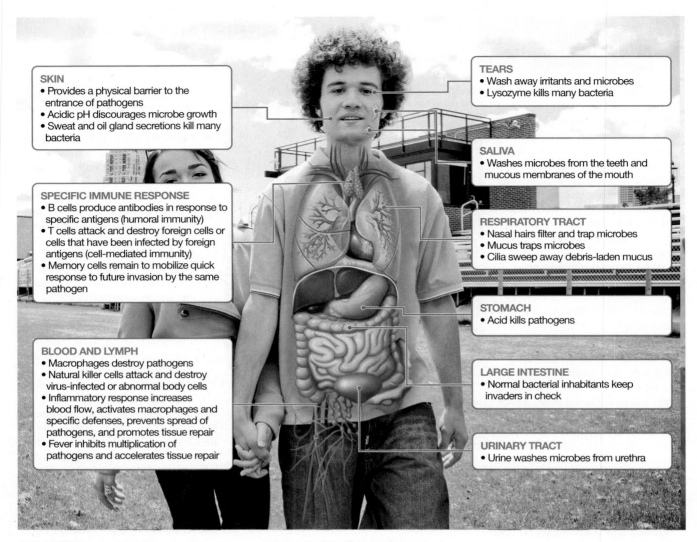

FIGURE 14.2 The Body's Defenses against Disease-Causing Pathogens To protect against a steady onslaught by pathogens, the body has developed an elaborate defense system to keep invaders out.

The labels in the figure read:

SKIN
- Provides a physical barrier to the entrance of pathogens
- Acidic pH discourages microbe growth
- Sweat and oil gland secretions kill many bacteria

SPECIFIC IMMUNE RESPONSE
- B cells produce antibodies in response to specific antigens (humoral immunity)
- T cells attack and destroy foreign cells or cells that have been infected by foreign antigens (cell-mediated immunity)
- Memory cells remain to mobilize quick response to future invasion by the same pathogen

BLOOD AND LYMPH
- Macrophages destroy pathogens
- Natural killer cells attack and destroy virus-infected or abnormal body cells
- Inflammatory response increases blood flow, activates macrophages and specific defenses, prevents spread of pathogens, and promotes tissue repair
- Fever inhibits multiplication of pathogens and accelerates tissue repair

TEARS
- Wash away irritants and microbes
- Lysozyme kills many bacteria

SALIVA
- Washes microbes from the teeth and mucous membranes of the mouth

RESPIRATORY TRACT
- Nasal hairs filter and trap microbes
- Mucus traps microbes
- Cilia sweep away debris-laden mucus

STOMACH
- Acid kills pathogens

LARGE INTESTINE
- Normal bacterial inhabitants keep invaders in check

URINARY TRACT
- Urine washes microbes from urethra

---

humoral immunity The aspect of immunity that is mediated by antibodies secreted by white blood cells.

toxins Poisonous substances produced by certain microorganisms that cause various diseases.

cell-mediated immunity The aspect of immunity that is mediated by specialized white blood cells that attack pathogens and antigens directly.

lymphocyte A type of white blood cell involved in the immune response.

macrophage A type of white blood cell that ingests foreign material.

autoimmune disease A disease caused by an overactive immune response against the body's own cells.

player in this immune response are **macrophages** (a type of phagocytic, or cell-eating, white blood cell).

Two forms of lymphocytes in particular, the *B lymphocytes* (B cells) and *T lymphocytes* (T cells), are involved in the immune response. *Helper T cells* are essential for activating B cells to produce antibodies. They also activate other T cells and macrophages. *Killer T cells* directly attack infected or malignant cells. *Suppressor T cells* turn off or suppress the activity of B cells, killer T cells, and macrophages. After a successful attack on a pathogen, some attacker T and B cells are preserved as *memory T and B cells*, enabling the body

to recognize and respond quickly to subsequent attacks by the same kind of organism. Once having survived certain infectious diseases, a person will likely not develop these diseases again. **FIGURE 14.3** provides a summary of the cell-mediated immune response.

When the Immune System Misfires: Autoimmune Diseases

Sometimes the process for recognizing and ignoring the body's own cells goes awry, and the immune system targets its own tissues. This is known as **autoimmune disease** (*auto* means "self"). There are over 80 different types of autoimmune diseases that affect humans, and millions of new cases occur each year. In these cases, people's *autoantibodies* fail to recognize "self" and attack the body's own tissues. The presence of autoantibodies can indicate autoimmunity, in many cases well before the symptoms of autoimmune diseases actually begin.[3] Rheumatoid arthritis, lupus erythematosus, type 1 diabetes, and multiple sclerosis are some common autoimmune disorders.

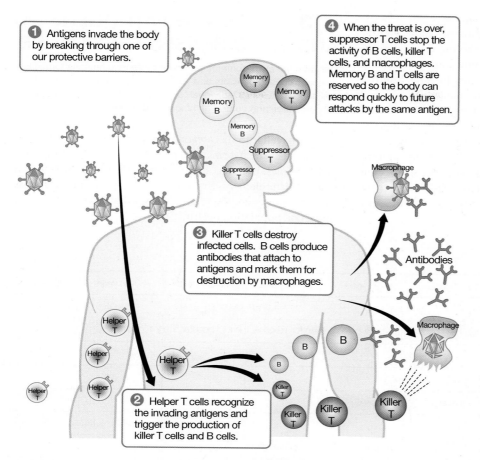

① Antigens invade the body by breaking through one of our protective barriers.

② Helper T cells recognize the invading antigens and trigger the production of killer T cells and B cells.

③ Killer T cells destroy infected cells. B cells produce antibodies that attach to antigens and mark them for destruction by macrophages.

④ When the threat is over, suppressor T cells stop the activity of B cells, killer T cells, and macrophages. Memory B and T cells are reserved so the body can respond quickly to future attacks by the same antigen.

FIGURE 14.3 The Cell-Mediated Immune Response

Inflammatory Response, Pain, and Fever

If an infection is localized, pus formation, redness, swelling, and irritation often occur. These symptoms are components of the body's inflammatory response and indicate that the invading organisms are being fought. The four cardinal signs of inflammation are *redness*, *swelling*, *pain*, and *heat*.

Pain is often one of the earliest signs that an injury or infection has occurred. Pathogens kill or injure tissue at the site of infection, causing swelling that puts pressure on nerve endings in the area, resulting in pain. Although pain is unpleasant, it plays a valuable role in the body's response to injury or invasion by causing a person to avoid activity that may aggravate the injury and cause additional damage.

In addition to *inflammation*, another frequent indicator of infection is *fever*, or a body temperature above the average norm of 98.6°F. Caused by toxins secreted by pathogens that interfere with the control of body temperature, a fever also stimulates the body to produce more white blood cells. A mild fever is protective; raising the body temperature by one or two degrees provides an environment that destroys some disease-causing organisms. As fever increases, more pathogens are destroyed. However, for babies and small children, when a fever goes higher than 101°F, medical attention should be sought. When fevers rise above 103°F for adults, medical attention is warranted.

Vaccines Bolster Immunity

Vaccination is based on the principle that once people have been exposed to a specific pathogen and have had a successful immune response, subsequent attacks will activate their "immune memory" and allow them to fight the pathogen off.

A *vaccine* consists of killed or weakened versions of a disease-causing microorganism or an antigen that is similar to, but less dangerous than the disease antigen. The dose given produces antibodies against future attacks—without actually causing the disease (or by causing a very minor case of it). Vaccines typically are given orally or by injection, and this form of immunity is termed *artificially acquired active immunity* in contrast to *naturally acquired active immunity* (which is obtained by exposure to antigens in the normal course of daily life) or *naturally acquired passive immunity* (as occurs when a mother passes immunity to her fetus via their shared blood supply or to an infant via breast milk). Concern about the safety of vaccines among certain Americans has led to a drop in vaccination and an increase in serious diseases such as the measles and pertussis—diseases that have rarely been seen in the United States since vaccines first became available in the 1950s and 1960s.

Specific vaccination schedules have been established for various population groups. See **TABLE 14.2** for recommended

vaccination Inoculation with killed or weakened pathogens or similar, less dangerous antigens to prevent or lessen the effects of a particular disease.

TABLE **14.2** | Recommended Vaccinations for Teens and College Students

Tetanus, diphtheria, pertussis vaccine (Td/Tdap)
Meningococcal vaccine (booster at age 16)
HPV vaccine series
Hepatitis B vaccine series
Polio vaccine series
Measles-mumps-rubella (MMR) vaccine series
Varicella (chickenpox) vaccine series
Influenza vaccine
Pneumococcal polysaccharide (PPV) vaccine
Hepatitis A vaccine series (for high-risk groups)

Source: Centers for Disease Control and Prevention, "Preteen and Teen Vaccines," July 2014, www.cdc.gov/vaccines/who/teens/vaccines/index.html; Centers for Disease Control and Prevention, "Vaccine Information for Adults," September 2014, www.cdc.gov/vaccines/adults/rec-vac/index.html.

vaccines for teens and college students ages 19 to 26. **FIGURE 14.4** shows the recommended vaccination schedule for the general adult population. Childhood vaccine schedules are available at the Centers for Disease Control and Prevention (CDC) website, as are requirements that vary by state. International travel recommendations are also available.

Because of their close living quarters, high stress levels, and poor sleep habits, college students face a higher-than-average risk of infection from largely preventable diseases. Vaccines that should be a high priority among 20-somethings include tetanus-diphtheria-pertussis vaccine (Tdap), meningococcal conjugate vaccine (MCV4), vaccine against the human papillomavirus, and the yearly influenza vaccine.[4]

LO 3 | TYPES OF PATHOGENS AND THE DISEASES THEY CAUSE

Describe the most common pathogens infecting humans today, key diseases caused by each, and the threat of growing antimicrobial resistance as well as individual- and community-based strategies for prevention and control of infectious diseases.

Pathogens fall into six categories: bacteria, viruses, fungi, protozoans, parasitic worms, and prions. **FIGURE 14.5** shows several examples. Each has a particular route of transmission and characteristic elements that make it unique. Herein, we discuss these categories and highlight diseases that have a significant impact on population health.

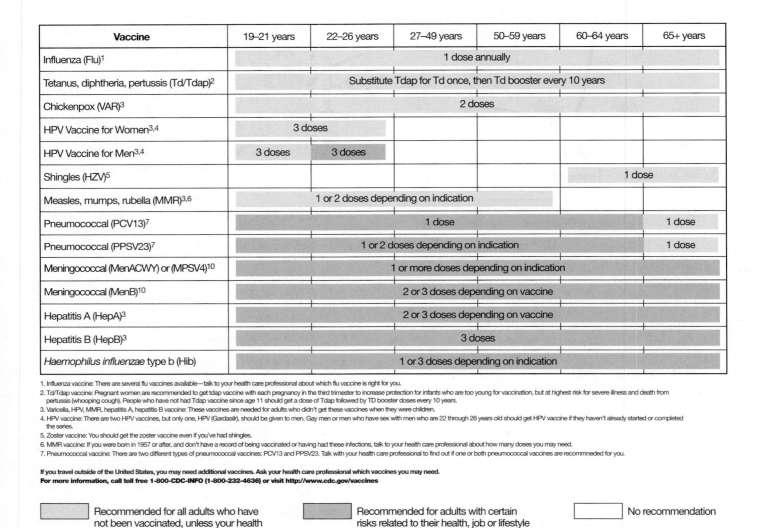

Vaccine	19–21 years	22–26 years	27–49 years	50–59 years	60–64 years	65+ years
Influenza (Flu)[1]	1 dose annually					
Tetanus, diphtheria, pertussis (Td/Tdap)[2]	Substitute Tdap for Td once, then Td booster every 10 years					
Chickenpox (VAR)[3]	2 doses					
HPV Vaccine for Women[3,4]	3 doses					
HPV Vaccine for Men[3,4]	3 doses	3 doses				
Shingles (HZV)[5]					1 dose	
Measles, mumps, rubella (MMR)[3,6]	1 or 2 doses depending on indication					
Pneumococcal (PCV13)[7]	1 dose					1 dose
Pneumococcal (PPSV23)[7]	1 or 2 doses depending on indication					1 dose
Meningococcal (MenACWY) or (MPSV4)[10]	1 or more doses depending on indication					
Meningococcal (MenB)[10]	2 or 3 doses depending on vaccine					
Hepatitis A (HepA)[3]	2 or 3 doses depending on vaccine					
Hepatitis B (HepB)[3]	3 doses					
Haemophilus influenzae type b (Hib)	1 or 3 doses depending on indication					

1. Influenza vaccine: There are several flu vaccines available—talk to your health care professional about which flu vaccine is right for you.
2. Td/Tdap vaccine: Pregnant women are recommended to get tdap vaccine with each pregnancy in the third trimester to increase protection for infants who are too young for vaccination, but at highest risk for severe illness and death from pertussis (whooping cough). People who have not had Tdap vaccine since age 11 should get a dose of Tdap followed by TD booster doses every 10 years.
3. Varicella, HPV, MMR, hepatitis A, hepatitis B vaccine: These vaccines are needed for adults who didn't get these vaccines when they were children.
4. HPV vaccine: There are two HPV vaccines, but only one, HPV (Gardasil), should be given to men. Gay men or men who have sex with men who are 22 through 26 years old should get HPV vaccine if they haven't already started or completed the series.
5. Zoster vaccine: You should get the zoster vaccine even if you've had shingles.
6. MMR vaccine: If you were born in 1957 or after, and don't have a record of being vaccinated or having had these infections, talk to your health care professional about how many doses you may need.
7. Pneumococcal vaccine: There are two different types of pneumococcal vaccines: PCV13 and PPSV23. Talk with your health care professional to find out if one or both pneumococcal vaccines are recommneded for you.

If you travel outside of the United States, you may need additional vaccines. Ask your health care professional which vaccines you may need.
For more information, call toll free 1-800-CDC-INFO (1-800-232-4636) or visit http://www.cdc.gov/vaccines

Recommended for all adults who have not been vaccinated, unless your health care professional tells you that you cannot safely receive the vaccine or that you do not need it.

Recommended for adults with certain risks related to their health, job or lifestyle that put them at higher risk for serious diseases. Talk to your halth care professional to see if you are at higher risk.

No recommendation

FIGURE 14.4 Recommended Adult Immunization Schedule, by Vaccine and Age Group, 2015

Source: Centers for Disease Control and Prevention, "Recommended Adult Immunization Schedule—United States, 2017," Updated February 2017, http://www.cdc.gov/vaccines/schedules/downloads/adult/adult-schedule.pdf.
Note: Important explanations and additions to these recommendations should be checked by consulting the latest schedule at www.cdc.gov.

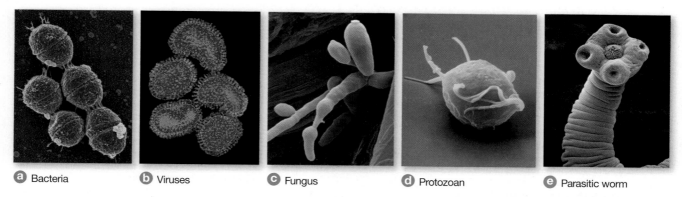

ⓐ Bacteria   ⓑ Viruses   ⓒ Fungus   ⓓ Protozoan   ⓔ Parasitic worm

FIGURE 14.5 **Examples of Five Major Types of Pathogens** (a) Color-enhanced scanning electron micrograph (SEM) of *Streptococcus* bacteria, magnified 40,000×. (b) Colored transmission electron micrograph (TEM) of influenza (flu) viruses, magnified 32,000×. (c) Color SEM of *Candida albicans*, a yeast fungus, magnified 50,000×. (d) Color TEM of *Trichomonas vaginalis*, a protozoan, magnified 9,000×. (e) Color-enhanced SEM of a tapeworm, magnified 50×.

Bacteria

Bacteria (singular: *bacterium*) are simple, single-celled organisms. There are three major types of bacteria, classified by shape: *cocci*, *bacilli*, and *spirilla*. Although there are several thousand known species of bacteria, they (and the toxins they produce) cause just over 100 human diseases.

After Alexander Fleming discovered penicillin in 1928, bacteria were in a losing battle with their enemy: **antibiotics**. With each decade thereafter, newer, more potent, and more specialized antibiotics decimated generation after generation of bacterial diseases. However, the battle is not over. Because many doctors prescribe antibiotics for conditions they were not designed to treat and because many patients do not take even necessary antibiotics as instructed, generations of bacteria survived, mutated, changed, and developed into "superbugs" that can overcome many of the drugs that were originally used to fight them.

Today, **antibiotic/antimicrobial resistance**—the ability of microbes to resist the effects of drugs, to grow and proliferate, even in the face of our best weapons—is one of the world's most pressing problems, with over 2 million people infected and 23,000 deaths per year in the United States alone.[5] **FIGURE 14.6** outlines the ways in which antibiotic resistance spreads.

Staphylococcal Infections

Staphylococci are present on the skin or in the nostrils of 20 to 30 percent of us at any given time. They usually cause no problems for otherwise healthy people. The presence of bacteria on or in a person without infection is called **colonization**. A colonized person may spread the bacteria to other people, some of whom may develop infections, yet the colonized person may never develop the disease. For example, colonized individuals can inadvertently touch their noses and spread bacteria from the nose onto a door handle, causing people who touch the handle to get sick. When the pathogen is present on the skin surface, a cut or break in the skin can allow it to gain entry to the body, where **infection** develops. If you have ever suffered from acne,

boils, styes (infections of the eyelids), or infected wounds, you have probably had a "staph" infection. If you pick at pimples and don't wash your hands, you can transmit those same bacteria to your eyes or to other people. If you don't wash your hands after flossing or after using the toilet, your hands may be teeming with bacteria and other organisms that could infect other people. Simple changes in personal hygiene reduce risks for all.

One form of staph, **methicillin-resistant *Staphylococcus aureus* (MRSA)**, has come under intense international scrutiny as numerous cases have arisen globally, especially in the United States. As the name implies, this bacteria has grown resistant to the class of drugs normally used to treat staph infections. Symptoms of MRSA infection often start with a rash or a pimple-like skin irritation. Within hours, early symptoms may progress to redness, inflammation, pain, and deeper wounds. If untreated, MRSA may invade the blood, bones, joints, surgical wounds, heart valves, and lungs, and it can be fatal.

Health care–associated MRSA, also known as *health care–acquired MRSA* has become one of the leading **health care–associated infections (HAIs)** in the United States. It is found in significant numbers in hospitals, nursing homes, and clinics where invasive treatments, infectious pathogens, and weakened immune systems converge. Today, 5 to 10 percent of hospitalized patients—over

> **bacteria** Simple, single-celled microscopic organisms (singular: bacterium). About 100 known species of bacteria cause disease in humans.
>
> **antibiotics** Medicines used to kill microorganisms such as bacteria.
>
> **antibiotic/antimicrobial resistance** The ability of microbes to resist the effects of drugs, allowing the germs to grow and proliferate.
>
> **staphylococci** A group of round bacteria, usually found in clusters, that cause a variety of diseases in humans and other animals.
>
> **colonization** The process in which bacteria or some other infectious organisms establish themselves in a host without causing infection.
>
> **methicillin-resistant *Staphylococcus aureus* (MRSA)** Highly resistant form of staph infection that is growing in international prevalence.
>
> **health care–associated infections (HAIs)** Infections that patients acquire in a health care setting while receiving treatment for a different condition.

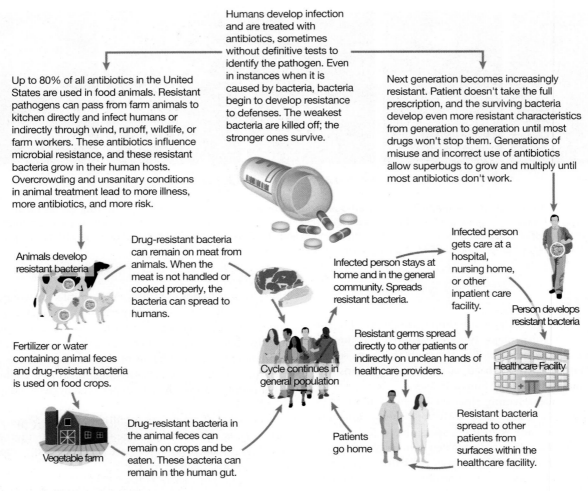

Humans develop infection and are treated with antibiotics, sometimes without definitive tests to identify the pathogen. Even in instances when it is caused by bacteria, bacteria begin to develop resistance to defenses. The weakest bacteria are killed off; the stronger ones survive.

Up to 80% of all antibiotics in the United States are used in food animals. Resistant pathogens can pass from farm animals to kitchen directly and infect humans or indirectly through wind, runoff, wildlife, or farm workers. These antibiotics influence microbial resistance, and these resistant bacteria grow in their human hosts. Overcrowding and unsanitary conditions in animal treatment lead to more illness, more antibiotics, and more risk.

Next generation becomes increasingly resistant. Patient doesn't take the full prescription, and the surviving bacteria develop even more resistant characteristics from generation to generation until most drugs won't stop them. Generations of misuse and incorrect use of antibiotics allow superbugs to grow and multiply until most antibiotics don't work.

Animals develop resistant bacteria

Drug-resistant bacteria can remain on meat from animals. When the meat is not handled or cooked properly, the bacteria can spread to humans.

Infected person gets care at a hospital, nursing home, or other inpatient care facility.

Infected person stays at home and in the general community. Spreads resistant bacteria.

Person develops resistant bacteria

Fertilizer or water containing animal feces and drug-resistant bacteria is used on food crops.

Resistant germs spread directly to other patients or indirectly on unclean hands of healthcare providers.

Cycle continues in general population

Healthcare Facility

Vegetable farm

Drug-resistant bacteria in the animal feces can remain on crops and be eaten. These bacteria can remain in the human gut.

Patients go home

Resistant bacteria spread to other patients from surfaces within the healthcare facility.

FIGURE 14.6 How Antibiotic Resistance Spreads

Source: Adapted from Centers for Disease Control and Prevention, "About Antimicrobial Resistance: Examples of How Antibiotic Resistance Spreads," September 8, 2015, http://www.cdc.gov/drugresistance/about.html.

1.7 million people yearly—get HAIs while in treatment, suffering costly, prolonged stays due to these illnesses. Over 99,000 people die from HAIs each year.[6] Many of these people died of HA-MRSA.[7]

Even though HA-MRSA is on the decline, *community-acquired MRSA (CA-MRSA)* is on the rise in homes, workplaces, and other places in the communities where we live. Although the exact number of people with CA-MRSA is not known, studies show that 1 in 3 people harbor staph bacteria in their nose, most of the time without any signs of illness.[8] Two percent of people carry MRSA.[9]

Often, CA-MRSA appears as a skin infection that becomes red, inflamed, and painful and may be filled with pus or fluids. The initial irritated spot may be mistaken for a spider bite or boil or an infection due to a cut or other injury. Although it can occur anywhere, irritation often appears in the groin area, beard, buttocks, underarm, or scalp. Because the initial site of infection may mimic other things, many people with CA-MRSA delay treatment and unknowingly infect other people. Prevention of CA-MRSA involves keeping the hands away from the nose (since the nose often harbors the staph organism);

good personal hygiene; and not sharing razors, towels, pillows, or other personal products. Careful attention to unusual sores on the body is key to risk reduction.

A type of MRSA that appears to spread among people who work closely with livestock in other countries is known as *livestock-associated MRSA*, or LA-MRSA.

Clostridium difficile One of the most common and difficult to treat health care–associated bacterial infections in the United States is *Clostridium difficile*, sometimes called *C-diff*. Symptoms include major inflammation of the colon, complete with watery diarrhea, fever, pain, bloating, and nausea. Ironically, the antibiotics used to treat bacterial infection are the major cause of *C. difficile* development; with long-term antibiotic use, some of the good bacteria that help keep the system running smoothly may be killed. Older adults, particularly those whose immune systems are compromised and/or are living in long term care or nursing facilities are at particular risk. Although rates of *C. difficile* infection are declining as a result of improved infection control protocols and more conservative antibiotic regimens, it is still regarded as an urgent threat.[10]

Today, there are nearly 500,000 new cases and 30,000 deaths from this disease each year. New drugs designed to reduce reoccurrences are being tested.[11]

Streptococcal Infections

At least five types of the *Streptococcus* microorganism are known to cause bacterial infections. *Group A streptococci (GAS)* cause the most common diseases, such as streptococcal pharyngitis ("strep throat") and scarlet fever. One particularly virulent group of GAS can lead to a rare but serious disease called *necrotizing fasciitis* ("flesh-eating strep"). Group B streptococci can cause illness in newborn babies, pregnant women, older adults, and adults with illnesses such as diabetes or liver disease. Because about 1 in 4 pregnant women have *group B strep* in their rectum or vagina, the CDC recommends testing for it in the last weeks of pregnancy.[12] Expectant mothers who are group B positive can be treated with antibiotics to prevent problems in their newborn.

The species *Streptococcus pneumoniae* is responsible for thousands of cases of bacterial meningitis and pneumonia each year and is the primary culprit in most ear infections. Although antibiotic treatments are still effective, an increasing number of cases are becoming resistant.

Meningitis

Meningitis is an inflammation of the *meninges*, the protective membranes that surround the brain and spinal cord. There are a variety of causes, including bacterial, viral, parasitic, and fungal infections, as well as noninfectious causes such as trauma to the brain, cancer, lupus, drugs, or brain surgery.

One virulent form of bacterial meningitis that is prevalent on college campuses, *meningococcal meningitis* is among the most serious. Spread through contact with saliva, nasal discharge, feces, or respiratory and throat secretions, it is highly contagious. Sharing eating utensils, drinking glasses, cigarettes, and vaping devices, kissing, and not covering your mouth and nose when you cough or sneeze are common ways of infecting others. Globally, meningococcal meningitis

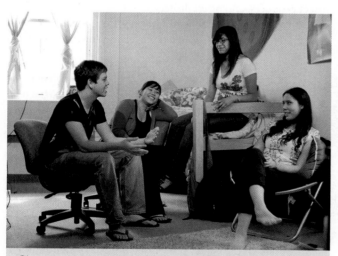

Close quarters, such as college dorms, are prime breeding grounds for some contagious diseases such as meningococcal meningitis.

results in death within 24 to 48 hours for between 5 and 10 percent of those infected, despite treatment. Up to 20 percent of infected individuals are left with neurological issues.[13] There were nearly 500 cases of meningococcal disease in the United States in 2016.[14] Children, adolescents, and young adults between 16 and 23 years old are among the most likely to be infected and to have serious complications.[15]

Bacterial meningitis progresses rapidly; can cause brain damage, hearing loss, and death; and needs immediate medical attention. *Viral meningitis* is much less dangerous, and symptoms usually diminish in 3 to 5 days in otherwise healthy people. There is no vaccine or treatment for viral meningitis. Fortunately, vaccines exist for *pneumococcal meningitis*, the most common form of bacterial meningitis, and *meningococcal meningitis*. The other vaccine-preventable form of bacterial meningitis is *Haemophilus influenzae* type b (Hib). Most campuses require vaccinations against four forms of the disease; however, requirements vary by state. The strain of organism present on your campus might not be one you are vaccinated against. Check with your health center for more information, and see your immunization table for more information about vaccines.

Typical signs of meningitis are sudden fever, severe headache, and a stiff neck, particularly stiffness that causes difficulty touching your chin to your chest. People who are suspected of having meningitis should receive immediate, aggressive medical treatment. Talk to the professionals at your student health center to learn what vaccine may protect people in your area.

Prevention of meningitis involves universal infection control behaviors, such as frequent hand washing; sneezing into your arm; using disposable tissues rather than reusable handkerchiefs; keeping your hands away from your nose; and keeping "high touch" surfaces, such as phones, doorknobs, and remote controls clean and free of bacteria.

Pneumonia

Pneumonia is a general term for a wide range of conditions that result in inflammation of the lungs and difficulty breathing. It is characterized by chronic cough, chest pain, chills, high fever, fluid accumulation, and eventual respiratory failure. Although bacterial and viral pathogens are the most common culprits, pneumonia can also be caused by fungi, occupational exposure to chemicals, or trauma.

Bacterial pneumonia responds readily to antibiotic treatment in early stages but can be deadly in more advanced stages. Forms of pneumonia caused by other organisms are more difficult to treat. Although medical advances have reduced the overall incidence of pneumonia, it continues to be a major threat in the United States and throughout the world.

Tuberculosis

Only HIV/AIDS is a greater infectious killer than **tuberculosis (TB)** in the global population.[16] With

Streptococcus A round bacterium, usually found in chain formation.

meningitis An infection of the meninges, the membranes that surround the brain and spinal cord.

pneumonia An inflammatory disease of the lungs characterized by chronic cough, chest pain, chills, high fever, and fluid accumulation; may be caused by bacteria, viruses, fungi, chemicals, or other substances.

tuberculosis (TB) A disease caused by bacterial infiltration of the respiratory system.

multidrug-resistant TB A form of TB that is resistant to at least two of the best antibiotics available.

extensively drug-resistant TB A form of TB that is resistant to nearly all existing antibiotics.

Lyme disease A bacterial disease transmitted by the black-legged tick with symptoms of inflammation, rash, muscle aches, headache in early stages and arthritis, neurological disabilities, and other problems in later stages.

rickettsia A bacterium that produces toxins that multiply in small blood vessels and causes Rocky Mountain spotted fever when carried by a tick and typhus when carried by a louse, flea, or tick

Powassan A tick-borne disease that can result in encephalitis or other brain issues.

Babesiosis a tick-borne disease with potentially severe flu-like symptoms.

over 10.4 million new cases and 1.8 million deaths in 2015, an astounding one third of the world's population is infected with TB.[17] Although infection rates have decreased dramatically in the United States since the 1950s, there were still nearly 9,300 new cases in 2016.[18] Tuberculosis is one of the top five killers of women of reproductive age worldwide and the leading cause of death among HIV-positive patients.[19] Poverty and lack of access to treatment are key risk factors.

Historically, people used the term *consumption* to refer to a bacterial respiratory disease with symptoms that include wasting or weight loss, fever, chronic cough and blood streaked sputum, fluid- and blood-filled lungs, and eventual spread throughout the body. That term is still used in some parts of the world today; however, TB is now widely recognized for these same symptoms. Airborne transmission via the respiratory tract is the primary mode of infection. Infected people may either have the *latent form*—meaning that they carry TB but it is not active and not contagious—or TB that may or may not show symptoms and is contagious.

The current recommended treatment for TB involves taking four drugs for 6 to 9 months; a 12-dose regimen is available for high-risk populations.[20] Medications may cause side effects ranging from minor stomach irritation to liver failure. The side effects, lengthy treatment, and barriers (including cost) to obtaining drugs and care in many developing areas leads to missed doses and treatments that are stopped before the infection is cured. This, in turn, breeds drug-resistant tuberculosis. Although a newer vaccine, *the BCG vaccine*, is given in many countries where TB rates are high, it is not recommended in the United States except for high-risk individuals.[21]

Multidrug-resistant TB is resistant to at least two of the best anti-TB drugs in use today, and **extensively drug-resistant TB** is resistant to nearly all current TB drugs. These newer strains of TB are reaching epidemic proportions in at least 58 countries.[22]

The Rise of The Ticks: Multiple Disease Threats

When we think of tick borne diseases, we historically have focused on bacterially causes diseases, such as **Lyme disease**, a major threat to pets and humans in many regions of the United States. Symptoms of Lyme disease may be very subtle or may include flulike symptoms, a rash that may look like a bull's eye, arthritis, blindness, and long-term physical and mental disability.

Rickettsia is a bacterium that produces toxins that multiply in small blood vessels and causes Rocky Mountain spotted fever when carried by a tick and *typhus* when carried by a louse, flea, or tick. These diseases produce similar symptoms, including high fever, weakness, rash, and coma, and both can be life threatening.

Ehrlichiosis, another bacterially caused disease spread by ticks, has symptoms that progress rapidly with respiratory difficulties, flulike symptoms, and even death. Fortunately, for many of these bacterially caused diseases, early recognition and prompt antibiotic treatment can reduce risks.

Powassan, a virally caused tick-borne disease, is discussed later in this chapter.

Babesiosis, a tick-borne disease caused by a protozoan, has garnered increased attention in the upper Midwest and northeastern United States. When symptoms occur, they often mimic flulike aches, headache, fatigue, and nausea. Because the babesiosis parasite attacks and destroys red blood cells, anemia may result. Older adults and people with weakened immune systems are at greatest risk of complications.

The bottom line is this: If you have flulike symptoms in what are typically the non-flu months of the year, particularly if you have been in areas where ticks live, get checked out.

The best protection against insect-borne diseases is to stay indoors at dusk and early morning to avoid hours of high insect activity. To prevent tick-borne diseases, remember to stay out of grass, brushy areas from late spring to fall, when ticks are most active. Use insect repellents that contain 20 to 30 percent DEET, picaridin, oil of lemon eucalyptus, PMD (p-menthane-3,8-diol), IR3535, natural oils, or pyrethrins that you put on your clothing. Wear long sleeves and long pants, and tuck your pants into your socks. Do tick checks by examining your genitals, buttocks, scalp, and other places ticks like to hide. Bathe or shower to wash off ticks within 1 hour of coming indoors. Check your clothing and your pets.

If you travel in areas of the world where other insect-borne diseases such as malaria are prevalent, consider taking bed nets, U.S. Environmental Protection Agency (EPA) –registered insect products, and other protective measures. Stay informed. Consult a travel doctor, who might prescribe preventive medications, depending on the area of travel and the risks involved.

Escherichia coli **O157:H7** *Escherichia coli* O157:H7 is one of over 170 types of *E. coli* bacteria that can infect humans. Most *E. coli* organisms are harmless and live in the intestines of healthy animals and humans. *E. coli* O157:H7, however, produces a lethal toxin and can cause severe illness or death. You can get it from eating undercooked ground beef, drinking unpasteurized milk or juice, or swimming in sewage-contaminated water. Outbreaks in the United States have been caused by contaminated

Tick-borne diseases such as Lyme disease, Rocky Mountain spotted fever, Powassan, ehrlichiosis, and babesiosis are on the rise in many parts of the United States. Protect yourself with insecticides and protective clothing.

frozen pizza and quesadillas, organic spinach and spring mix lettuce, cheese, poultry, and other foods.

A symptom of *E. coli* infection is nonbloody diarrhea, usually 2 to 8 days after exposure; however, asymptomatic (symptom-free) cases have been noted. Children, older adults, and people with weakened immune systems are particularly vulnerable to serious side effects such as kidney failure, intestinal damage, or death.

Strengthened regulations on chlorine levels in pools and cooked meat temperatures have helped to reduce *E. coli* infections. Difficulties in isolating the source of infections have prompted a close examination of labeling and distribution of food products. The U.S. Department of Agriculture as well as the EPA, Food and the U.S. Drug Administration, and others are all involved in developing food and transportation policies designed to keep food safe.

Viruses

Viruses are the smallest known pathogens, approximately 1/500th the size of bacteria; hundreds of viruses cause diseases in humans. Essentially, a virus consists of a protein structure that contains either *ribonucleic acid (RNA)* or *deoxyribonucleic acid (DNA)*. Viruses are incapable of carrying out any life processes on their own. To reproduce, they must invade a host cell, inject their own DNA or RNA into it, and force the cell to make copies of itself containing the virus. The new viruses then erupt out of the host cell and seek other cells to invade.

Viral diseases can be difficult to treat because many viruses can withstand heat, formaldehyde, and large doses of radiation. Some viruses have **incubation periods** (the length of time required to develop fully and cause symptoms in their hosts) that last for years, which delays diagnosis. Drug treatment for viral infections is also limited. Drugs that are powerful enough to kill viruses generally kill the host cells too, although some medications block stages in viral reproduction without damaging the host cells.

The Common Cold Some experts claim there may be over 200 different viruses responsible for the common cold. Colds are the main reason for missed work and missed school in the United States, with millions of cases each year.[23] Although most colds occur in the winter and spring, you can actually get a cold any time. Adults have an average of two to three colds per year, and children have even more.[24] If you get a cold, the most likely cause is the *rhinovirus*, which causes 10 to 40 percent of all colds, followed by the *coronavirus*, which is responsible for 20 percent of all colds. The cause of colds is not known in up to 20 percent of all cases.[25] Colds are always present to some degree, with increasing prevalence in colder weather as people spend more time indoors. Otherwise healthy people carry cold viruses in their noses and throats most of the time, held in check until immune defenses are weakened. It is possible to "catch" a cold—through airborne transmission, skin-to-skin touching, or mucous membrane contact—and the hands are the single greatest way of transmitting colds and other viruses. Obviously, then, covering your nose and mouth with a tissue, a handkerchief, or even the crook of your elbow when you sneeze is better than using your hand. Washing your hands with soap and water is key to prevention. Contrary to popular belief, you cannot catch a cold from getting a chill or being out in the cold, but the chill may lower your immune system's resistance to a virus if one is present.

Influenza **Influenza**, or flu, is a contagious respiratory illness that includes fever and chills along with other cold symptoms. While death rates from the flu are only estimates, since influenza is not a reportable disease, common estimates range from 3,000 to 49,000 per year.[26] Although a rapid diagnosis flu test is available, doctors typically diagnose influenza on the basis of symptoms.

Although many people don't realize it, there are actually many different types of influenza, including the most common *seasonal variety* and some other less common types. Fortunately, most types of flu are not readily transmitted to humans.

For seasonal flu, although symptoms are always more serious than those of a cold, most adolescents and adults recover after a week or two. However, seasonal flu can be deadly to the very young, people over age 65, and those with weakened immune systems. Occasionally, a particularly deadly strain of influenza evolves and spreads rapidly, killing many.

Five to 20 percent of Americans get the flu each year; of these, 200,000 will need hospitalization.[27] Once a person gets the flu, treatment is *palliative*, that is, focused on relief of symptoms rather than cure.

The best way to avoid the flu is to get an annual vaccination. There are numerous and constantly mutating flu strains,

> **viruses** Minute microbes consisting of DNA or RNA that invade a host cell and use the cell's resources to reproduce themselves.
>
> **incubation period** The time between exposure to a disease and the appearance of symptoms.
>
> **influenza** A common viral disease of the respiratory tract.

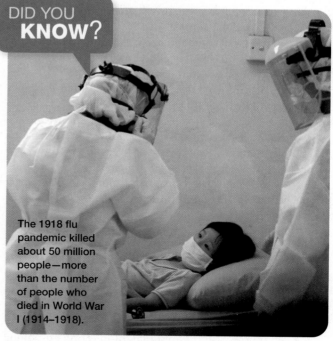

DID YOU KNOW?

The 1918 flu pandemic killed about 50 million people—more than the number of people who died in World War I (1914–1918).

Source: Centers for Disease Control and Prevention, "Past Pandemics," November 2, 2017, https://www.cdc.gov/flu/pandemic-resources/basics/past-pandemics.html.

so vaccines are formulated for the few strains that are most likely to be prevalent in an upcoming season. If researchers correctly predict strains, vaccines are thought to be 70 to 90 percent effective in healthy adults for about a year. If the prediction is off, a shot is less beneficial.[28]

In spite of minor risks, the CDC now recommends that everyone over the age of 6 months get the seasonal flu vaccine annually. Unfortunately, many people don't follow the recommendation; only about 170 million people are projected to have had vaccinations for the 2015 to 2016 season.[29] Flu shots take 2 to 3 weeks to become effective, so it's best to get the shot in the fall, before the flu season begins. Today, you have options for vaccination, including a standard shot, a high-dose shot if you are over age 65 or at risk, or the Flublok shot if you are allergic to the eggs that are used to produce vaccines. Another popular option, FluMist, is a nasal spray used by those who opt out of the shot vaccination. However, in June 2016, the CDC recommended that FluMist not be given for the next flu season, as its effectiveness has been called into question until more research has been conducted.[30]

Hepatitis
One of the most highly publicized viral diseases is **hepatitis**, an inflammation of the liver. Symptoms include fever, headache, nausea, loss of appetite, skin rashes, pain in the upper right abdomen, dark yellow urine with a brownish tinge, and jaundice. Internationally, viral hepatitis is a major contributor to liver disease and accounts for high rates of morbidity and mortality. There are several known forms (A, B, C, D, and E); hepatitis A, B, and C have the highest rates of incidence.

Hepatitis A (HAV) is contracted by eating food or drinking water contaminated with human feces. Many people who contract HAV are asymptomatic. Since vaccinations became available, HAV rates had been steadily declining until 2013, when they again began to increase. In 2015, there were nearly 2,800 reported new cases of HAV.[31] Hepatitis A can also be spread through sexual contact with HAV-positive individuals or through the use of contaminated needles. Fortunately, individuals infected with HAV do not become chronic carriers, and vaccines for the disease are available.

Hepatitis B (HBV) is spread through body fluid exchange during unprotected sex, from sharing needles when injecting drugs, through needlesticks on the job, or, in the case of a newborn baby, from an infected mother during birth. Hepatitis B can lead to chronic liver disease or liver cancer. HBV is currently the 15th leading cause of death globally, with 240 million chronically infected.[32] Increasing numbers of younger people getting vaccinated; this has reduced new cases. Needle exchange programs are believed to be an important part of risk reduction for HBV, HCV, and HIV infection in the last decade.[33]

Rates of HBV are on the decline in the United States; however, an estimated 20,000 cases are reported each year, and nearly 1.4 million people are chronic carriers.[34] The highest rates of infection are among males ages 30 to 39 and black non-Hispanics; the lowest rates

are among Asian Pacific Islanders and Hispanics.[35] Because the hepatitis B virus is considered 50 to 100 times more virulent than HIV, efforts to increase global vaccination rates have become a major priority.

Hepatitis C (HCV) infections are on an epidemic rise in many regions of the world as resistant forms emerge. Some cases can be traced to blood transfusions or organ transplants. An estimated 33,900 new cases of HCV occurred in 2015, and the estimated number of chronic cases of HCV may be as high as 3.5 million.[36] Of those infected, 75 to 85 percent will develop chronic hepatitis C, and 60 to 70 percent will develop chronic liver disease.[37] Of those who develop chronic liver disease, 5 to 20 percent will develop cirrhosis of the liver.[38] One in 5 people will die from cirrhosis or liver cancer.[39] Because there are several different genotypes of HCV, careful testing and appropriate treatment regimens are essential. Seeing a physician who is an HCV specialist is recommended for best results. For a complete listing of current treatment guidelines, go to http://www.hcvguidelines.org.[40]

To prevent the spread of HBV and HCV, use latex condoms correctly every time you have sex; don't share personal care items that could have blood on them, such as razors or toothbrushes; get a blood test for HBV so you know your status; never share needles; and if you get tattoos or piercings, go to reputable shops that follow established sterilization and infection control protocols.

Zika
In late 2015 and early 2016, reports of the explosive spread of a little-known virus in Central and South America surfaced. Known as the **Zika virus**, this mosquito-borne virus was reported to be transmitted by infected women during pregnancy, resulting in a higher than expected rate of babies born with *microcephaly*, a condition in which a baby's head is unusually small at birth because of a lack of development of brain tissue. The World Health Organization estimates that 61 countries have reported infections, 1 million people are already infected

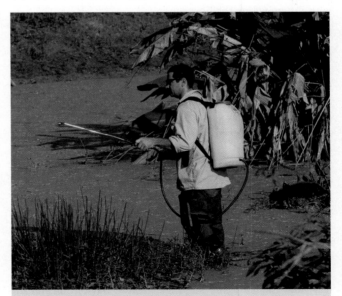

Careful monitoring and control of mosquito and other insect populations is important to combat emerging diseases such as Zika and West Nile virus.

hepatitis A viral disease in which the liver becomes inflamed, producing symptoms such as fever, headache, and possibly jaundice.

Zika virus An emerging threat from bite of the Aedes mosquito in the United States and globally, particularly for pregnant women.

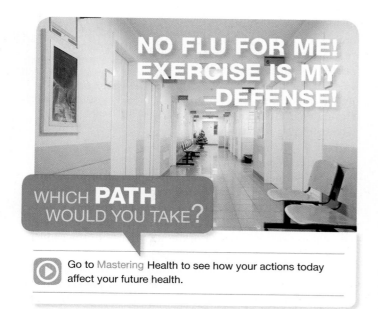

NO FLU FOR ME! EXERCISE IS MY DEFENSE!

WHICH **PATH** WOULD YOU TAKE?

Go to Mastering Health to see how your actions today affect your future health.

in South America, and as many as 5 million additional people might be infected in 2017 as temperatures rise, flooding and rainfall levels increase, and mosquito populations increase.[41] Although the global community is mobilizing to kill mosquitoes, reduce breeding grounds, and protect populations, cases of Zika are likely to increase as politicians in the United States stall on the funding of prevention measures.

Other Pathogens

While bacteria and viruses account for many common diseases, other organisms can also infect people. Among these are fungi, protozoans, parasitic worms, and prions.

Fungi Hundreds of species of **fungi** exist. While many of these unicellular or multicellular organisms are beneficial—such as edible mushrooms, penicillin, and yeast used in bread—others are the causes of disease such as candidiasis, athlete's foot, ringworm, jock itch, and toenail fungus. Another fungal disease that is increasing in the United States is *valley fever* (coccidioidomycosis), a potentially life-threatening respiratory disease that is common in the desert Southwest, where the fungus lives in the soil. Fungal spores in homes may be inhaled and cause respiratory problems, including issues with allergies and asthma. Other fungal diseases may be spread to humans and pets via breathing in fungal spores. With most fungal diseases, keeping the affected area clean and dry and treating it promptly with the appropriate medication will generally bring relief. Fungal diseases are typically transmitted via physical contact, so avoid going barefoot in public showers, hotel rooms, and other areas where fungus may be present, and use care in choosing where you go for pedicures.

Protozoans **Protozoans** are single-celled organisms that cause diseases such as malaria and African sleeping sickness. These diseases are largely controlled in the United States,

though a common waterborne protozoan disease in many regions of the country is *giardiasis*. People who drink contaminated water may be exposed to the *giardia* pathogen and will suffer intestinal pain and discomfort weeks after initial infection. Protection of water supplies is the key to prevention.

Parasitic Worms **Parasitic worms** are the largest pathogens. Ranging in size from small pinworms, typically found in children, to large tapeworms that can stretch much of the length of the human intestines, most parasitic worms are more nuisance than threat. Of special note are the worm infestations associated with eating raw fish (as in some forms of sushi). You can prevent worm infestations by cooking fish and other foods to temperatures high enough to kill the worms and their eggs. Other preventive measures include getting your pets checked for worms, being careful while swimming in international areas known for these infections, and wearing shoes in parks or places where animal feces are present.

Prions A **prion** is a self-replicating, protein-based agent that can infect humans and other animals. One such prion is believed to be the underlying cause of spongiform diseases such as *bovine spongiform encephalopathy (BSE)*, popularly known as "mad cow disease." Humans who eat contaminated meat from cattle with BSE may develop a mad cow–like disease known as *variant Creutzfeld-Jakob disease (vCJD)*. Symptoms of vCJD include loss of memory, tremors, and muscle spasms or "tics." Over time, depression, difficulty walking, seizures, and severe dementia can lead to death in both cows and humans. An increasing number of infected cattle have been found in the United States and globally. However, to date, there have been no confirmed human infections from U.S. beef.

Emerging and Resurgent Diseases

Although our immune systems are adept at responding to challenges, microbes and other pathogens constantly evolve and develop new tactics in their natural drive to survive. Within the past decade, rates for many infectious diseases have increased. This trend can be attributed to a combination of widely recognized factors. *Economic development and land use* (humans encroaching on delicate ecosystems and upsetting microbial balances established over the centuries); *human behaviors* that overuse, pollute, overfish, and overconsume natural resources, upsetting species balances, the earth's ability to regenerate and heal, and contributing to climate change; and the *proliferation of international travel* contributing to the transport and intermingling of microbes that have been separated by natural barriers over the centuries all are factors in

fungi A group of multicellular and unicellular organisms that obtain their food by infiltrating the bodies of other organisms, both living and dead; several microscopic varieties are pathogenic.

protozoans Microscopic single-celled organisms that can be pathogenic.

parasitic worms The largest of the pathogens, most of which are more a nuisance than they are a threat.

prion A self-replicating, protein-based pathogen.

emergent and resurgent diseases. In addition, overpopulation, inadequate health care, increasing poverty, loss of habitat, microbial mutation and change, and antibiotic resistance all lead to assaults on our immune systems.

Significant increases in cases of vaccine-preventable diseases such as pertussis, meningococcal meningitis, measles, chicken-pox, and hepatitis A as well as increases in the number of people opting out of vaccinations in recent years are causing concern throughout the country. Increased hospitalizations and deaths of children from vaccine-preventable diseases and more families using the "personal belief exemption" from vaccination prompted California to reinstate mandatory vaccinations of school-age children in May 2015.[42] Stay tuned as other states move to protect the population through similar vaccine mandates in schools.

Measles and Mumps

The best-known symptom of **mumps** is swelling of the salivary glands. In severe cases, mumps can cause hearing loss or male sterility. **Measles**, known for a high fever and itchy red rash, is increasingly common, particularly on college campuses. Increased incidences of these and other vaccine-preventable diseases between 2015 and 2016 are reason for significant concern in many regions of the country. A growing number of children and young adults have not been vaccinated against the viruses that cause measles or mumps because their parents believed that the diseases are gone and the risk of a vaccine is greater than the risk of contracting the disease. See the Health Headlines box for more on the growing vaccine controversy.

West Nile Virus

Several thousand cases of West Nile virus occur in the United States each year. In 2016, there were 2,038 cases in the United States. Over 56 percent of people infected with the *neuroinvasive* type have more serious symptoms of meningitis or encephalitis, which can lead to disability and death, and 44 percent have the non-neuroinvasive form of the disease with headache and other flulike symptoms that are less severe.[43] Today, only Alaska and Hawaii remain free of the disease in the United States. Because West Nile virus is spread by infected mosquitoes, the best way to avoid infection is through mosquito eradication programs, wearing mosquito repellant, and avoiding mosquito-infested areas altogether, especially at peak mosquito feeding times. There is no vaccine or specific treatment.

Avian (Bird) Flu and Swine (Pig) Flu

Avian influenza is an infectious disease of birds. Birds infect other birds during migrations, spreading the disease internationally as they fly among different locations. Strains of the virus that are capable of crossing the species barrier can cause severe illness in humans who come into contact with bird droppings or fluids. Bird flu appears to have originated in Asia and spread via migrating bird populations.[44] Although the virus has yet to mutate into a form that is highly infectious to humans, outbreaks have occurred in rural areas of the world, where people live in close proximity to poultry and other animals. By the end of 2016, the World Health Organization had recorded 859 cumulative cases of bird flu in humans, with 453 deaths, an indication of the severity of this disease.[45]

H1N1 (formerly referred to as "swine flu") or one of its variants is a respiratory infection that was believed initially to be found primarily in pigs but that eventually combined with a human flu virus. Between 2009 and 2010, there were over 60 million cases of a variant of the H1N1 virus in the United States, killing nearly 12.5 thousand people.[46]

Today, various strains of influenza hit different regions of the world each year. Scientists must accurately predict which strains will occur in the United States at least a year ahead of their arrival and come up with a vaccine that will protect people. Although success rates are high, there are years when vaccines do not meet expected levels of protection.[47]

Powassan Virus

Today, we know that ticks don't just carry bacteria. They can latch on, pierce the skin, and inject bacteria, viruses, protozoan, nematodes, rickettsiae, spirochetes, and toxins into the body in varying combinations—all with a single bite. One new tick-borne disease that has been striking fear in the Northeast and upper Midwest is a viral disease known as Powassan, which is related to West Nile virus. Powassan attacks the brain of those bitten, causing encephalitis. Unlike other tick borne diseases, infection with the Powassan virus can occur when a tick is attached to the person for less than an hour.

Mindfulness: A New Ally in Bolstering Defenses?

Although several lifestyle variables have been shown to positively affect immune system function—including a healthy diet, exercise, stress reduction, and sleep—an emerging body of research indicates that mindfulness may be another weapon in your arsenal against infectious and chronic diseases.

A recent systematic review of the accumulated research indicates that mindfulness appears to have a positive effect on cell-mediated immunity, immune cell aging, and overall immune system functioning; however, more research is necessary to examine these effects.[48] Another recent study indicates that *early life adversity* is associated with higher risks of diseases overall in adulthood. Long-term adversity may result in cumulative pathologies, including inflammation, autoimmune diseases, allergies, and asthma, as well as alterations in immune function related to higher stress and sleep disturbances.[49]

Yet another new study analyzes the accumulated research showing the link between emotions and the immune system, indicating that infectious diseases can affect emotions and

► **SEE IT!** VIDEOS

A brief history of measles presents fascinating facts from 1657 to the present day. Watch **A Brief History: Measles in America** in the Study Area of Mastering Health.

mumps A once common viral disease that is controllable by vaccination.

measles A viral disease that produces symptoms such as an itchy rash and a high fever.

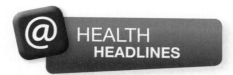

VACCINE CONTROVERSY
Should Parents Be Allowed to Opt Out?

In 2000, the United States claimed that measles was no longer of concern on U.S. soil. In 2015, nearly 4 percent of children were allowed to skip measles vaccines. When a particularly nasty bout of measles swept through Disneyland, 169 people from over 20 states became ill—most of them unvaccinated. This outbreak and an unrelated 2014 outbreak of measles in Ohio among unvaccinated Amish children raised major concerns in many states.

In response, in 2015, California passed one of the strictest laws in the country, mandating vaccinations of all school-age children. Several other states are examining their own policies about exemptions as rates of unvaccinated have grown with corresponding increases in vaccine-preventable diseases. As rates of measles, pertussis, and other vaccine-preventable diseases rise and large numbers of unvaccinated individuals travel to the United States, more states are considering the rights of parents versus the safety of the general population. In fact, vaccination percentages in 2016 were actually up in the United States overall, coming closer to the *Healthy People 2020* national goal of a 95 percent vaccination rate.

Immunizations against killer diseases are one of the greatest public health success stories of all time. Most people have never seen or heard of anyone having diseases such as smallpox that once wiped out entire populations, and they question why they should get a vaccination for a disease that isn't around anymore. Others opt out for religious, personal, or medical reasons, while still others consider vaccinations to be a government intrusion into their individual rights. Many people mistakenly believe that they are doing the right thing by avoiding vaccination. Others fail to complete the entire series of shots for a vaccine and thus may not be immune.

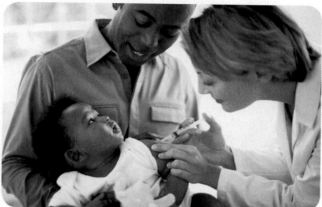

Some parents have concerns over vaccination safety, but research shows that vaccines are safe and effective for most individuals as well as crucial for maintaining good community health.

Undervaccination rates are highest among people with health insurance and incomes above $75,000,and who are college educated and white. Although all 50 states require some vaccinations, 48 states have religious or medical exemptions, and several have personal belief options. Much initial vaccine anxiety was fueled by an article in *Lancet* in 1998 that linked the MMR vaccine to increased risk of autism and bowel disease. The article prompted many people to refuse the vaccine in the United States and elsewhere, and the resulting dropoff in immunizations led to epidemic increases of measles in many parts of the world. Over 10 years later, after a thorough investigation of ethical and factual issues with the research, *Lancet* retracted the article as false. The lead author was fired from his research position and had his license to practice revoked.

Today, anyone who is against vaccination can post on a blog or website that looks reputable even though it has little scientific validity. Conspiracy theories abound. When in doubt, check out peer-reviewed journals or national databases for information. To date, the CDC has found *no* evidence to substantiate claims that vaccines lead to conditions such as autism, multiple sclerosis, or sudden infant death syndrome. Virtually all medical and public health organizations support vaccinations, pointing to stringent safety controls in the manufacturing and testing of vaccines, as well as ongoing safety monitoring and the long history of vaccines in wiping out killer diseases. If large numbers of people were to avoid vaccinations, old killers would probably reemerge, and people who were sick or weak from other conditions would be extremely vulnerable.

The CDC's Immunization Safety Office monitors complaints and investigates potential problems with vaccines as they occur.

Still, the danger of major complications from getting vaccinations is extremely low and generally pales in comparison to the effects of contracting the diseases that the vaccinations protect against. For an interactive and updated comparison of how your state compares to others on vaccine exemptions, see http://www.nvic.org/vaccine-laws/state-vaccine-requirements.aspx. To find out how your state is doing when it comes to vaccination rates, check out the ChildVaxView (https://www.cdc.gov/vaccines/imz-managers/coverage/childvaxview/data-reports/index.html) for complete information by disease.

Sources: Centers for Disease Control and Prevention, "Vaccine Coverage in the United States," February 2016, http://www.cdc.gov/vaccines/imz-managers/coverage/imz-coverage.html; R Seither et al., "Vaccination Coverage among Children in Kindergarten—United States, 2015–16 School Year," *Morbidity and Mortality Weekly Report* 65 (2016); Centers for Disease Control and Prevention, National Center for Health Statistics "Early Release of Selected Estimates Based on Data From the 2016 National Health Interview Survey," May 22, 2017, https://www.cdc.gov/nchs/nhis/releases/released201705.htm; National Vaccine Information Center, "State Law and Vaccine Requirements, Accessed June, 2017, http://www.nvic.org/vaccine-laws/state-vaccine-requirements.aspx; Editors of the *Lancet*, "Retraction—Ileal-Lymphoid-Nodular Hyperplasia, Non-specific Colitis, and Pervasive Development Disorder in Children," *Lancet* 375, no. 9713 (2010): 445.

that emotions can alter immune function. Thus, mindfulness and other anxiety- and stress-relieving strategies appear to have great potential for reducing the risks of disease initiation and progress.[50]

LO 4 | SEXUALLY TRANSMITTED INFECTIONS

Explain the risk factors for sexually transmitted infections and actions that can prevent their spread.

Although more than 20 million cases of **sexually transmitted infections (STIs)** are reported each year, many others are never diagnosed or reported, often because the people who are infected are asymptomatic.[51] Some STIs, particularly chlamydia, gonorrhea, and syphilis, are increasing at alarming rates, particularly among young adults.[52] Huge disparities in rates exist by age, race, income, and gender.[53]

Sexually transmitted infections affect people of all backgrounds and socioeconomic levels, but they disproportionately affect women, minorities, and infants.[54] Young people age 15 to 24 acquire half of all new STIs, making this age group the most at risk group for STIs overall.[55] Reasons for the higher rates of STIs in this population include a range of behavioral, biological, socioeconomic, and cultural reasons. Barriers to prevention and treatment, such as lack of access to affordable health care, confidentiality, and transportation, as well as peer norms and media influences, risk-taking behaviors, and social and cultural norms that promote and influence sexual interest and activity, are some of the factors that put adolescents and young adults at risk.[56]

Early symptoms of an STI are often mild and unrecognizable.

sexually transmitted infections (STIs) Infections transmitted through some form of intimate, usually sexual, contact.

Decisions to be intimate should take into consideration risks from highly infectious sexually transmitted diseases such as chlamydia, gonorrhea, and syphilis, which are skyrocketing among young adults.

Although both men and women feel the effects of STIs, long-term health consequences are most serious for young women, with 24,000 infertility cases each year.[57] Men can face sterility too. Left untreated, some STIs can also cause blindness, central nervous system destruction, disfigurement, and even death. Infants born to mothers carrying these infections are at risk for a variety of health problems.

What's Your Risk?

Generally, the more sex partners a person has, the greater is the person's risk for contracting an STI. Four out of ten sexually active teen girls have been infected with an STI, and while rates of HIV are low among adolescents, males age 13 to 19 make up 80 percent of HIV diagnosis in this group.[58] Shame and embarrassment often keep infected people from seeking treatment. Unfortunately, they usually continue to be sexually active, thereby infecting unsuspecting partners. People who are uncomfortable discussing sexual issues may also be less likely to use or ask their partners to use condoms to protect against STIs and pregnancy. Another reason proposed for the STI epidemic is our casual attitude about sex.

Ignorance—about the infections, their symptoms, and the fact that someone can be asymptomatic but still infected—is also a factor. By the time someone realizes that something is wrong and seeks medical help, he or she may have infected several other people. In addition, many people mistakenly believe that certain sexual practices—oral sex, for example—carry no risk for STIs. In fact, oral sex practices among young adults may be responsible for increases in herpes and other infections. FIGURE 14.7 shows the continuum of disease risk for various sexual behaviors. The Skills for Behavior Change box offers tips for ways to practice safer sex.

High-risk behaviors	Moderate-risk behaviors	Low-risk behaviors	No-risk behaviors
Unprotected vaginal, anal, and oral sex—any activity that involves direct contact with bodily fluids, such as ejaculate, vaginal secretions, or blood—are high-risk behaviors.	Vaginal, anal, or oral sex with a latex or polyurethane condom and a water-based lubricant used properly and consistently can greatly reduce the risk of STI transmission. Dental dams used during oral sex can also greatly reduce the risk of STI transmission.	Mutual masturbation, if there are no cuts on the hand, penis, or vagina, is very low risk. Rubbing, kissing, and massaging carry low risk, but herpes can be spread by skin-to-skin contact from an infected partner.	Abstinence, phone sex, talking, and fantasy are all no-risk behaviors.

FIGURE 14.7 Continuum of Disease Risk for Various Sexual Behaviors There are different levels of risk for various behaviors and various sexually transmitted infections. However, no matter what, any sexual activity involving direct contact with blood, semen, or vaginal secretions is high risk.

 Watch Video Tutor: **Signs and Symptoms of STIs** in Mastering Health.

BEHAVIOR CHANGE

Safe is Sexy

The following behaviors will help you reduce your risk of contracting a sexually transmitted infection (STI) when considering a sexual encounter:

- Avoid multiple sexual encounters.

- Remember that oral sex is *not* safe sex! While the risks of contracting an STI are lower with oral sex than with vaginal or anal intercourse, the risk is not zero. It is entirely possible to contract HIV from oral sex as well as herpes, gonorrhea, syphilis, genital warts, and other diseases. Beyond common STIs, it is also possible to spread or contract intestinal parasites and other diseases, depending on hygiene and the presence of other organisms.

- Just say NO to casual sex. Know what you will say ahead of time. An example might be "No. Sorry. I'm attracted to you, but I don't have sex with anyone I don't know well."

- Insist on using a latex condom or a dental dam (a sensitive latex sheet, about the size of a tissue, that can be placed over the female genitals to form a protective layer) during vaginal, oral, or anal sex.

- Get tested. Know your status and your partner's.

- Avoid injury to body tissue, including abrasions and microscopic tears during sexual activity. Anal sex is particularly risky, as the anus tears easily. However, any rough sex increases risks. Don't be afraid to say, "That hurts. Stop."

- Make handwashing a habit, insisting that both you and your partner wash hands before sex, petting, or masturbation and afterward. Herpes and genital warts can easily be spread by someone touching the sore on their mouth or their genitals and then touching yours. As a rule, use soap and water, and count to 20 when washing your hands before and after sexual encounters. Urinate after sexual relations and, if possible, wash your genitals.

- Abstinence is the only way to be 100 percent sure you don't transmit or contract an STI. If you have any doubt about the potential risks of having sex, consider other means of intimacy (at least until you can ensure your safety). Some possibilities are massage, dry kissing, hugging, holding and touching, and masturbation (alone or with a partner).

- Get vaccinated for HPV, hepatitis B, and hepatitis C.

- If you contract an STI, ask your health care provider for advice on notifying past or potential partners.

Sources: American College of Obstetricians and Gynecologists, *How to Prevent Sexually Transmitted Diseases: Frequently Asked Questions*, FQ009 (Washington, DC: American College of Obstetricians and Gynecologists, 2015), Available at http://www.acog.org/~/media/For%20Patients/faq009.pdf?dmc=; American Sexual Health Association, "Reduce Your Risk," Accessed March 2016, http://www.ashasexualhealth.org/stdsstis/reduce-your-risk.

Routes of Transmission

Sexually transmitted infections are generally spread through intimate sexual contact. Less common modes of transmission are mouth-to-mouth contact and contact with fluids from body sores. Although each STI is a different infection caused by a different pathogen, all STI pathogens prefer dark, moist places, especially the mucous membranes lining reproductive organs. Most of these pathogens are susceptible to light, extreme temperature, and dryness, and many die quickly on exposure to air. Like other communicable infections, STIs have both pathogen-specific incubation periods and periods of communicability—times during which transmission is most likely.

LO 5 | COMMON TYPES OF SEXUALLY TRANSMITTED INFECTIONS

Describe common types of sexually transmitted infections, including their symptoms and treatment methods.

There are more than 20 known types of STIs—once referred to as *venereal diseases* and then *sexually transmitted diseases*. Today, you will see the terms STI and STD used interchangeably; however, the term STI is more reflective of the number and types of infections and of the fact that they are caused by pathogens. STI rates for several diseases are currently at the highest rates in our history.[59] Here, we turn to some of the most common STIs.

Chlamydia

Chlamydia, an infection caused by the bacterium *Chlamydia trachomatis*, is the most commonly reported STI in the United States. In 2015, over 1.5 million chlamydia infections were reported—the largest number of yearly cases of anything the CDC has ever recorded. Experts believe the actual number may be closer to 3 million cases, with soaring unreported numbers among young adults.[60]

Signs and Symptoms In men with symptoms, there may be painful urination, an urge to urinate frequently, or difficult urination, as well as a watery, pus-like discharge from the penis. Women with

> **chlamydia** A bacterially caused STI of the urogenital tract.

2 MILLION+

is the number of new cases of **SYPHILIS, CHLAMYDIA, GONORRHEA, AND CHANCROID** in the United States in 2015—the highest numbers ever!

symptoms may have a yellowish discharge, spotting between periods, and occasional spotting after intercourse.

Complications Men can suffer injury to the prostate gland, seminal vesicles, and bulbourethral glands, as well as arthritis-like symptoms and inflammatory damage to the blood vessels and heart. Men can also experience *epididymitis*—inflammation of the area near the testicles. In women, chlamydia-related inflammation can injure the cervix or fallopian tubes, causing sterility, and can damage the inner pelvic structure, leading to **pelvic inflammatory disease (PID).** If an infected woman becomes pregnant, she has a high risk for miscarriage and stillbirth. Women with chlamydia are at greater risks for urinary tract infections. Chlamydia may also be responsible for one type of *conjunctivitis*, an eye infection that affects not only adults but also infants, who can contract the disease from an infected mother during delivery. Untreated conjunctivitis can cause blindness.

Diagnosis and Treatment A sample of urine or fluid from the vagina or penis is collected and tested to identify the presence of the bacteria. Unfortunately, chlamydia tests are not a routine part of many health clinics' testing procedures. If detected early, chlamydia is easily treatable with antibiotics.

Gonorrhea

Gonorrhea is also on the rise in the United States, with nearly 400,000 new infections each year.[61] Like chlamydia, gonorrhea is likely largely underreported; estimates of the actual number of cases approach double the number of reported cases. Over two thirds of reported cases occur in 15- to 24-year-olds.[62] Caused by the bacterial pathogen *Neisseria gonorrhoeae*, gonorrhea primarily infects the linings of the urethra, genital tract, pharynx, and rectum. It may spread to the eyes or other body regions by the hands or through body fluids, typically during vaginal, oral, or anal sex. It most frequently occurs in people in their early 20s.

Signs and Symptoms While some men who have gonorrhea are asymptomatic, a typical symptom is a white, milky discharge from the penis accompanied by painful, burning urination 2 to 9 days after contact (**FIGURE 14.8**). Epididymitis can also occur as a symptom of infection.

Most women with gonorrhea do not experience any symptoms; some may have vaginal discharge or a burning sensation on urinating. The organism can remain in the woman's vagina, cervix, uterus, or fallopian tubes for long periods with no apparent symptoms other than an occasional slight fever. Thus, a woman can be unaware that she has been infected and is infecting her sex partners.

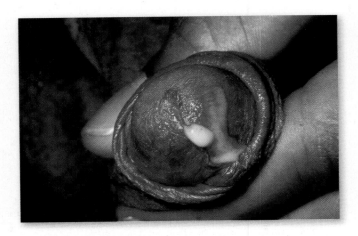

FIGURE 14.8 Gonorrhea One common symptom of gonorrhea in men is a milky discharge from the penis, accompanied by burning sensations during urination. These symptoms will cause most men to seek diagnosis and treatment. By contrast, women with gonorrhea are often asymptomatic, so they might not be aware they are infected.

Complications Gonorrhea may spread to the prostate, testicles, urinary tract, kidneys, and bladder in men, and scar tissue may cause sterility. In some cases, the penis develops a painful curvature during erection. If the infection goes undetected in a woman, it can spread to the fallopian tubes and ovaries, causing sterility or severe inflammation and PID. If untreated, the gonorrhea can spread through the blood and cause *disseminated gonococcal infection*, which can result in arthritis and problems with bones and joints, as well as cardiovascular and brain issues—problems that can be life threatening.[63] If an infected woman becomes pregnant, the infection can be transmitted to her baby during delivery, potentially causing blindness, joint infection, or a life-threatening blood infection in the child.

Diagnosis and Treatment Diagnosis of gonorrhea requires a sample of either urine or fluid from the vagina or penis to detect the presence of the bacteria. In its early stages, gonorrhea is treatable with antibiotics, but antimicrobial resistance is posing an even greater threat. Chlamydia and gonorrhea often occur at the same time, but different antibiotics are needed to treat each infection separately.

Syphilis

Syphilis is caused by a bacterium called *Treponema pallidum*. The incidence of syphilis is highest in adults age 20 to 39, and is particularly high among African Americans and men who have sex with men. There were nearly 75,000 reported new cases of syphilis in 2014, up significantly from the 17,375 cases in 2013.[64] Because it is extremely delicate and dies readily on exposure to air, dryness, or cold, the organism is generally transferred only through direct sexual contact or from mother to fetus. The incidence of syphilis in newborns has continued to increase in the United States.[65]

pelvic inflammatory disease (PID) One of various infections of the female reproductive tract.

gonorrhea The second most common bacterial STI in the United States; if untreated, it may cause sterility.

syphilis One of the most widespread bacterial STIs; characterized by distinct phases and potentially serious, even life-threatening results.

Signs and Symptoms

Syphilis is known as "the great imitator," because its symptoms resemble those of several other infections. It should be noted, however, that some people experience no symptoms at all. Syphilis can occur in four distinct stages[66]:

- **Primary syphilis.** The first stage of syphilis is often characterized by the development of a **chancre** (pronounced "shank-er"), a bacteria-oozing sore located at the infection site that usually appears about a month after initial infection (see **FIGURE 14.9**). In men, the site of the chancre tends to be the penis or scrotum; in women, the site of infection is often internal, on the vaginal wall or high on the cervix, where the chancre is not readily apparent, making the likelihood of detection small. In both men and women, the chancre will disappear in 3 to 6 weeks.
- **Secondary syphilis.** If the infection is left untreated, secondary symptoms may appear a month to a year after the chancre disappears, including a rash or white patches on the skin or on the mucous membranes of the mouth, throat, or genitals. Hair loss may occur, lymph nodes may enlarge, and the victim may develop a slight fever or headache. In rare cases, bacteria-containing sores develop around the mouth or genitals.
- **Latent syphilis.** After the secondary stage, if the infection is left untreated, the syphilis spirochetes begin to invade body organs, causing lesions called *gummas*. At this stage, the infection is rarely transmitted to others, except during pregnancy, when it can be passed to the fetus.
- **Tertiary/late syphilis.** Years after syphilis has entered the body, its effects become all too evident if it is still untreated. Indications of late-stage syphilis include heart and central nervous system damage, blindness, deafness, paralysis, dementia, and possible death.

Complications

Pregnant women with syphilis can experience premature births, miscarriages, or stillbirths or may transmit the infection to the unborn child. An infected pregnant woman may transmit to her unborn child *congenital syphilis*, which can cause death; severe birth defects such as blindness, deafness, or disfigurement; developmental delays; seizures; and other health problems. Because in most cases the fetus does not become infected until after the first trimester, treatment of the mother during this time will usually prevent infection of the fetus.

Diagnosis and Treatment

Syphilis can be diagnosed with a blood test or by collecting a sample from the chancre. It is easily treated with antibiotics, usually penicillin, for all stages except the late stage.

Herpes

Herpes is a general term for a family of infections characterized by sores or eruptions on the skin caused by the *herpes simplex virus*. While herpes can be transmitted by sexual contact,

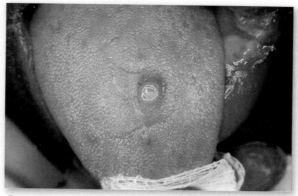

(a) Primary syphilis

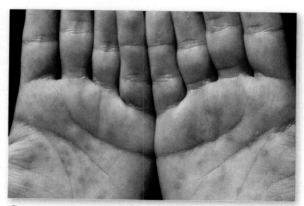

(b) Secondary syphilis

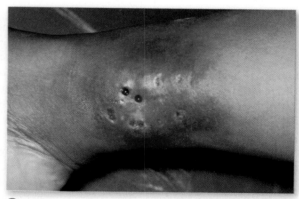

(c) Latent syphilis

FIGURE 14.9 Syphilis (a) A chancre on the site of the initial infection is a symptom of primary syphilis. (b) A rash is characteristic of secondary syphilis. (c) Lesions called gummas are often present in latent syphilis.

kissing or sharing eating utensils can also transmit the infection. Herpes infections range from mildly uncomfortable to extremely serious. **Genital herpes** affects approximately 16 percent of the population age 14 to 49 in the United States, with over 776,000 new cases overall each year in the United States.[67]

> **chancre** A sore often found at the site of syphilis infection.
>
> **genital herpes** A sexually transmitted infection caused by the herpes simplex virus.

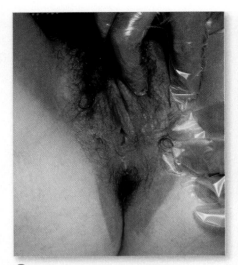

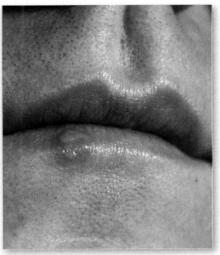

(a) Genital herpes is a highly contagious and incurable STI. It is characterized by recurring cycles of painful blisters on the genitalia.

(b) Oral herpes, caused by the same virus as genital herpes, is extremely contagious and can cause painful sores and blisters around the mouth.

FIGURE 14.10 Herpes Both genital and oral herpes can be caused by either herpes simplex virus type 1 or 2.

There are two types of herpes simplex virus.[68] Only about 1 in 6 Americans are believed to have HSV-2; however, exact numbers are difficult to assess.[69] HSV-1 is believed to be much more common, potentially infecting between 50 and 80 percent of all adults.[70] Both types can infect any area of the body (**FIGURE 14.10**).[71]

Signs and Symptoms

The precursor phase of a herpes infection is characterized by a burning sensation and redness at the site of infection. By the second phase, a blister filled with a clear fluid containing the virus forms. If you pick at this blister or otherwise touch the site, you can autoinoculate other body parts. Particularly dangerous is the possibility of spreading the infection to your eyes, as blindness can occur.

Over a period of days, the unsightly blister will crust over, dry up, and disappear, and the virus will travel to the base of an affected nerve supplying the area and become dormant. Only when the victim becomes overly stressed, when diet and sleep are inadequate, when the immune system is overworked, or when excessive exposure to sunlight or other stressors occur will the virus become reactivated (at the same site every time) and begin the blistering cycle all over again. Each time a sore develops, it casts off (sheds) viruses that can be highly infectious, but a herpes site can shed the virus even when no overt sore is present.

human papillomavirus (HPV)
A group of viruses, many of which are transmitted sexually; some types of HPV can cause genital warts or cervical cancer.

genital warts Warts that appear in the genital area or the anus; caused by the human papillomavirus.

Complications

Many physicians recommend cesarean deliveries for pregnant women who are infected with herpes, as it can be passed to the baby during birth. Additionally, women with a history of genital herpes appear to have a greater risk of developing cervical cancer and may have regular flare-ups during the menstrual cycle or in times of high stress.

Diagnosis and Treatment

Diagnosis of herpes can be determined by collecting a sample from the suspected sore or by performing a blood test. Although there is no cure for herpes at present, antiviral medications can prevent or shorten outbreaks. Certain prescription drugs such as acyclovir and over-the-counter medications such as Abreva can be used to treat symptoms. The effectiveness of other treatments, such as L-lysine, is largely unsubstantiated. Other drugs, such as famciclovir, may reduce viral shedding between outbreaks, potentially reducing risks to the infected person's sex partners. Although vaccines are being tested, there is currently no commercially available vaccine that is protective against genital herpes.[72]

Human Papillomavirus (HPV) and Genital Warts

Human papillomavirus (HPV) is one of a group of over 150 related viruses—each of which has a number indicating its type. HPV is the type that causes **genital warts** (also known as *venereal warts* or *condylomas*). HPV infections are so common that most sexually active men and women will have at least one form of HPV during their lives.[73] More than 40 types of HPV can infect the genital or anal areas of humans via skin-to-skin contact, making vaginal, anal, and oral sex all risky behaviors.[74] While genital warts are the most common result of the infection, HPV can cause cervical cancer; cancer of the vulva, penis, anus, vagina, back of the throat, and tongue can also occur. Because HPV is often asymptomatic in the early stages, the risk of infection is great, particularly among people who are immunocompromised, such as those with HIV or AIDS.

Signs and Symptoms

The typical incubation period for HPV is 6 to 8 weeks after contact. People infected with low-risk types of HPV may develop genital warts, a series of bumps or growths on the genitals ranging in size from small pinheads to large cauliflower-like growths (**FIGURE 14.11**). Warts on the penis may be flat and difficult to see. Cancer may develop years after sexual contact and may be symptomless for years.

Complications Cervical cancers often result from HPV infection, particularly infection with HPV-16 and HPV-18.[75] As such, with prevention, and early detection through a Pap test, cervical cancer may be detected at its earliest stages. These tests can also identify women who are at risk for rare cervical cancers (adenocarcinomas) that Pap tests may miss.[76] Ask your doctor if your Pap test includes an HPV test; if not, discuss whether one might be right for you.

In addition, HPV may also pose a threat to a fetus that is exposed to the virus during birth. Cesarean deliveries may be considered in serious cases. Human papillomavirus can cause cancers—called *oropharyngeal cancers*—around the tonsils or the base of the tongue with oral sex as the suspected culprit. Over 9000 people are diagnosed each year, men being about four times more likely to develop this form of cancer than women.[77]

Diagnosis and Treatment Diagnosis of genital warts from low-risk types of HPV is determined through a visual examination. High-risk types can be diagnosed in women through microscopic analysis of cells from a Pap smear or by collecting a sample from the cervix to test for HPV DNA. There is currently no HPV DNA test for men.

Treatment is available only for the low-risk forms of HPV that cause genital warts. Most warts can be treated with topical medication or can be frozen with liquid nitrogen and then removed; large warts may require surgical removal. See the Student Health Today box for more information about HPV vaccines.

> ▶ **SEE IT!** VIDEOS
> Learn more about the surprising prevalence of oral HPV. Watch **Oral HPV** in the Study Area of Mastering Health.

Candidiasis (Moniliasis)

Most STIs are caused by pathogens that come from outside the body; however, the yeast-like fungus *Candida albicans* is a normal inhabitant of the vaginal tract in most women. (See Figure 14.5c for a micrograph of this fungus.) Only when the normal chemical balance of the vagina is disturbed will these organisms multiply and cause the fungal disease **candidiasis**, also sometimes called *moniliasis* or a *yeast infection*.

Signs and Symptoms Symptoms of candidiasis include severe itching and burning of the vagina and vulva and a white, cheesy vaginal discharge. When this microbe infects the mouth, whitish patches form, and the condition is referred to as *thrush*. Thrush infection can also occur in men and is easily transmitted between sex partners. Symptoms of candidiasis can be aggravated by contact with soaps, douches, perfumed toilet paper, chlorinated water, and spermicides.

Diagnosis and Treatment Diagnosis of candidiasis is usually made by collecting a vaginal sample and analyzing it to identify the pathogen. Antifungal drugs applied on the surface or by suppository usually cure candidiasis in just a few days.

Trichomoniasis

Unlike many STIs, **trichomoniasis** is caused by a protozoan, *Trichomonas vaginalis*. (See Figure 14.5d for a micrograph of this organism.) The "trich" organism can be spread by sexual contact and by contact with items that have discharged fluids on them. An estimated 3.7 million new cases occur in the United States each year, although only about one third of people who contract trichomoniasis experience symptoms. The good news is that it is one of the most curable STIs if diagnosed and treated.[78]

Signs and Symptoms Symptoms of trichomoniasis among women include a foamy, yellowish, unpleasant-smelling discharge accompanied by a burning sensation, itching, and painful urination. Most men with trichomoniasis do not have any symptoms, though some men experience irritation inside the penis, mild discharge, and a slight burning after urinating.[79]

Diagnosis and Treatment Diagnosis of trichomoniasis is determined by collecting fluid samples from the penis or vagina to

> **candidiasis** A yeast-like fungal infection that is often transmitted sexually; also called *moniliasis* or *yeast infection*.
>
> **trichomoniasis** A protozoan STI characterized by foamy, yellowish discharge and an unpleasant odor.

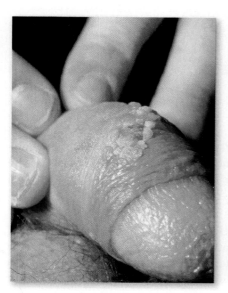
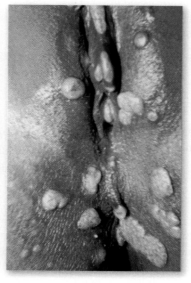

FIGURE 14.11 Genital Warts Genital warts are caused by certain types of the human papillomavirus. Not all warts are this obvious. Flat warts may be nearly invisible yet are contagious.

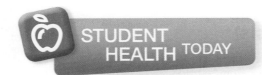
Q&A ON HPV VACCINES

Every year in the United States, about 12,000 women are diagnosed with cervical cancer, and almost 4,000 die from this disease. There are currently two HPV vaccines that can help prevent women from becoming infected with HPV and subsequently developing cervical cancer.

■ **Who should get the HPV vaccine?** There are two vaccines currently available: Cervarix and Gardasil. Human papillomavirus vaccines are recommended for 11- and 12-year-old girls but can be given to girls as young as 9 years old. The vaccines are also recommended for girls and women age 13 to 26 who have not yet been vaccinated. Ideally, females should get a vaccine before they become sexually active. Females who are sexually active may get less benefit from it because they may have already contracted an HPV type targeted by the vaccines. One of the HPV vaccines, Gardasil, is also licensed, safe, and effective for males age 9 to 26. The CDC recommends Gardasil for all boys 11 or 12 years old and for males age 13 to 21 who did not get any or all of the three recommended doses when they were younger. All men may receive the vaccine through the age of 26, but it is recommended that they speak with their doctor to find out whether getting vaccinated is right for them.

■ **How are the HPV vaccines similar and how are they different?** Both Cervarix and Gardasil are very effective against high-risk HPV types 16 and 18, which cause 70 percent of cervical cancer cases. Both vaccines are given as shots and require three doses. But only Gardasil protects against low-risk HPV types 6 and 11. These HPV types cause 90 percent of cases of genital warts in females and males, so Gardasil is approved for use by males as well as females.

■ **What do the two vaccines *not* protect against?** The vaccines do not protect against all types of HPV, so about 30 percent of cervical cancers will not be prevented by the vaccines. It will be important for women to continue getting screened for cervical cancer through regular Pap tests. Also, the vaccines do not prevent other STIs.

■ **How safe are the HPV vaccines?** The vaccines are licensed by the FDA and approved by the CDC as safe and effective. They have been studied in thousands of females (age 9 to 26) around the world, and the CDC and the FDA continue to monitor their safety.

■ **Are there side effects?** Side effects are rare. When they occur, they may include pain, redness and swelling in the arm where the shot was given, fever, headache, fatigue, nausea, or muscle pain. These usually go away

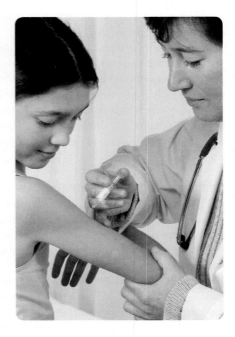

within a short time. People with a history of allergies should talk to their doctor before getting the HPV vaccines.

Sources: Centers for Disease Control and Prevention, "HPV Vaccine Information for Young Women," January 17, 2017, http://www.cdc.gov /std/hpv/STDFact-HPV-vaccine-young-women .htm; Centers for Disease Control and Prevention "HPV Vaccine—Questions & Answers," November 2016, https://www.cdc.gov/hpv/parents/questions -answers.html.

---

test. Treatment includes oral metronidazole, usually given to both sex partners to avoid the possible "ping-pong" effect of repeated cross-infection.

Pubic Lice

Pubic lice, often called "crabs," are small parasitic insects that are usually transmitted during sexual contact (**FIGURE 14.12**). More annoying than dangerous, they have an affinity for pubic hair and attach themselves to the base of these hairs, where they deposit their eggs (nits). One to 2 weeks later, these nits develop into adults that lay eggs and migrate to other body parts.

pubic lice Parasitic insects that can inhabit various body areas, especially the genitals.

Signs and Symptoms Symptoms of pubic lice infestation include itchiness in the area covered by pubic hair, bluish-gray skin color in the pubic region, and sores in the genital area.

Diagnosis and Treatment Diagnosis of pubic lice involves an examination by a health care provider to identify the eggs in the genital area. Treatment begins with application of a topical lice-killing product. All clothing and linens that may harbor the eggs must be machine-washed in hot water and dried on high heat. Items that cannot be washed should be dry cleaned or stored in a sealed plastic bag for 2 weeks to kill all larval forms.

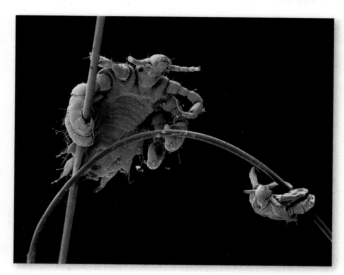

FIGURE 14.12 Pubic Lice Pubic lice, also known as "crabs," are small parasitic insects that attach themselves to pubic hair. They may also move and end up infesting other body hair, even as far away as eyebrows or the hair on the head.

LO 6 | HIV/AIDS

Discuss human immunodeficiency virus (HIV) and acquired immune deficiency syndrome (AIDS), trends in infection and treatment, and the impact of these diseases on special populations.

Acquired immune deficiency syndrome (AIDS) was first recognized over 37 years ago. Since its discovery, approximately 78 million people worldwide have become infected with **human immunodeficiency virus (HIV)**, the virus that causes AIDS, and 35 million have died.[80] Today, 37 million people worldwide are living with HIV, with 2.1 million new infections and 1.1 million deaths in 2015.[81] Of these, approximately 18.2 million people have access to HIV treatment.[82] The vast majority of HIV-infected individuals (25.8 million) are in sub-Saharan Africa, making up nearly 70 percent of all new cases in the world.[83] Globally, the numbers of people living with HIV have decreased, the numbers of new infections and deaths have declined, and the numbers of people receiving treatments have increased.[84]

In the United States, over 1.2 million people are infected with HIV, and over 1 in 8 of them don't know they are infected.[85] There are approximately 40,000 new HIV infections each year, down significantly from the nearly 130,000 new cases per year in the 1980s.[86] Since HIV was first discovered, nearly 700,000 people in the United States have died of AIDS, with just over 12,000 deaths each year.[87] Because of improved treatments, more people are living with HIV than ever before. However, we have not yet developed a vaccine to completely prevent HIV, nor have we found a cure for this disease.

How HIV Is Transmitted

HIV typically enters the body when another person's infected body fluids (e.g., semen, vaginal secretions, blood) gain entry through a breach in body defenses. If there is a break in

mucous membranes of the genitals or anus (as can occur during sexual intercourse, particularly anal intercourse), the virus enters and begins to multiply, invading the bloodstream and cerebrospinal fluid. It progressively destroys helper T cells, weakening the body's resistance to disease.

HIV is not highly contagious. It cannot reproduce outside a living host, except in a laboratory, and does not survive well in open air. As a result, it cannot be transmitted through casual contact such as sharing food utensils, musical instruments, toilet seats, towels, or the like. Research also provides overwhelming evidence that insect bites do not transmit HIV.

Engaging in High-Risk Behaviors

During the early days of the AIDS pandemic, it appeared that HIV infected only homosexuals. However, it quickly became apparent that the disease was related to certain high-risk behaviors rather than to groups of people. **FIGURE 14.13** shows the breakdown of new HIV diagnoses for the most-affected populations.

Men who have sex with men (MSM), particularly young black MSM, are most seriously affected by HIV.[88] Overall, African Americans, Hispanics, and white

acquired immunodeficiency syndrome (AIDS) A disease caused by a retrovirus, the human immunodeficiency virus (HIV), that attacks the immune system, reducing the number of helper T cells and leaving the victim vulnerable to infections, malignancies, and neurological disorders.

human immunodeficiency virus (HIV) The virus that causes AIDS by infecting helper T cells.

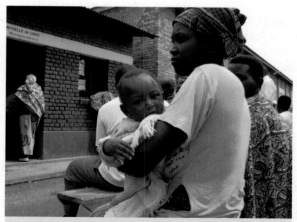

HIV/AIDS remains a devastating problem throughout the world. Over 70 percent of the new cases of HIV globally occur in sub-Saharan Africa. The woman and child shown here await treatment outside a clinic in Rwanda.

Source: UNAIDS, "Fact Sheet, 2015," accessed June 2017, Available at http://www.unaids.org/en/resources/campaigns /HowAIDSchangedeverything/factsheet.

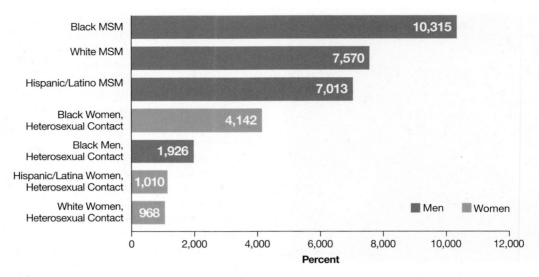

Black MSM		10,315
White MSM		7,570
Hispanic/Latino MSM		7,013
Black Women, Heterosexual Contact	4,142	
Black Men, Heterosexual Contact	1,926	
Hispanic/Latina Women, Heterosexual Contact	1,010	
White Women, Heterosexual Contact	968	

■ Men   ■ Women

0   2,000   4,000   6,000   8,000   10,000   12,000

Percent

FIGURE 14.13 Estimates of New HIV Diagnoses in the United States for Most Affected Subpopulations, 2015

Source: Centers for Disease Control and Prevention, "HIV Diagnoses in the United States: At a Glance," June 9, 2017, https://www.cdc.gov/hiv/statistics/overview/ataglance.html.

Americans bear the greatest burden of HIV infection in the United States. People of color have poorer HIV/AIDS outcomes than whites, owing to a number of social and economic barriers and challenges, such as lack of access to early diagnosis and treatment, discrimination, stigma, homophobia, and poverty.

The majority of HIV infections arise from the following:

■ **Exchange of body fluids.** Substantial research indicates that blood, semen, and vaginal secretions are the major fluids of concern. The vaginal area is more susceptible to microtears, and a woman is exposed to more semen than a man is to vaginal fluids. In fact, 80 percent of HIV in women is through heterosexual contact.[89] In rare instances, the virus has been found in saliva, but most health officials state that saliva is a less significant risk than other shared body fluids.

■ **Contaminated needles.** Although users of illicit drugs are the most obvious members of this category, people with diabetes who inject insulin or athletes who inject steroids may also share needles. Sharing needles and engaging in high-risk sexual activities increase the risks dramatically. Tattooing and body piercing can also be risky (see the Student Health Today box).

Before 1985, blood donations were not checked for HIV, and some people contracted the virus from transfusions. Because of massive screening efforts, the risk of receiving HIV-infected blood is now almost nonexistent in developed countries.

Mother-to-Child (Perinatal) Transmision

Mother-to-child transmission of HIV can occur during pregnancy, during labor and delivery, or through breastfeeding. Without antiretroviral treatment, approximately 15 to 45 percent of HIV-positive pregnant women will transmit the virus to their infant.[90] With appropriate interventions during

pregnancy, labor, birth, and breastfeeding, the transmission rate can be lowered to 5 percent.[91]

Signs and Symptoms of HIV/AIDS

A person may go for months or years after infection before any significant symptoms appear, and incubation time varies greatly from person to person. Without treatment, it typically takes an average of 8 to 10 years for the virus to cause the slow, degenerative changes in the immune system that are characteristic of AIDS. During this time, the person may experience *opportunistic infections* (infections that gain a foothold when the immune system is not functioning effectively). Colds, sore throats, fever, tiredness, nausea, night sweats, and other generally non–life-threatening pre-AIDS symptoms may occur. As HIV progresses, wasting syndrome, swollen lymph nodes, and neurological problems may occur. A diagnosis of AIDS, the final stage of HIV infection, is made when the infected person either has a dangerously low CD4 (helper T) cell count (below 200 cells per cubic milliliter of blood) or has contracted one or more opportunistic infections that are characteristic of the disease, such as Kaposi's sarcoma, tuberculosis, recurrent pneumonia, or invasive cervical cancer.

Testing for HIV: Newer Options

Today, three categories of tests exist for people who are concerned they may be infected with HIV: antibody

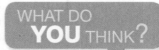

WHAT DO YOU THINK?

Why is HIV testing important?

■ Do you want your potential sex partners to be tested for HIV or other STIs? How would you ask someone to get tested?

■ How can you protect yourself from HIV?

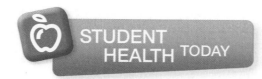
TATTOOS AND BODY PIERCING
Potential Risks

Today, 3 in 10 people have at least one tattoo. During body piercing or tattooing, the use of unsterile needles—which can transmit staph, HIV, hepatitis B and C, tetanus, and other diseases—poses a very real risk.

Laws and policies regulating body piercing and tattooing vary greatly by state. A beautiful tattoo and painless piercing don't always mean a "safe" procedure. There is a good reason why anyone who receives a tattoo or body piercing cannot donate blood for 1 year! If you opt for tattooing or body piercing, take the following safety precautions:

- Look for clean, well-lighted work areas. Ask about sterilization procedures and equipment and how they ensure safety.
- Watch to ensure that the needles and tubing used on you are new, in their original packaging with the sterile logo confirmation. Needles should be used once, then discarded. A piercing gun should not be used because it cannot be sterilized properly.
- Immediately before piercing or tattooing, the body area should be carefully sterilized. Handwashing before and after the procedure and new latex gloves for each client should be the norm. Gloves should be changed if anything else is touched during the procedure.

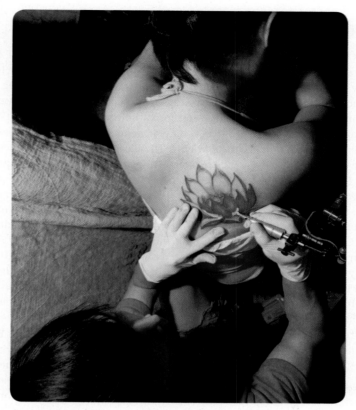

Use caution when selecting a tattoo artist and facility to ensure that proper infection control procedures are in place.

- Leftover tattoo ink should be discarded after each procedure. Do not allow the artist to double dip ink used for other customers. Used needles should be disposed of in a "sharps" container, with the biohazard symbol clearly visible.

Source: FDA, "Think Before You Ink: Are Tattoos Safe?" May 2017, https://www.fda.gov /ForConsumers/ConsumerUpdates/ucm048919.htm.

---

tests, combination fourth-generation tests, and nucleic acid tests. The tests may involve blood, body fluid, or urine testing, depending on the test.[92]

Antibody Tests If infected, the body produces antibodies 18 to 84 days after infection. Known as *the window period*, this is the general timeframe it may take for sufficient antibodies to be detectable. Get tested on day 34 or even day 65, and you may have a negative test, even though you may test positive after day 84. A new rapid antibody test provides results from blood in 30 minutes, and the OraQuick test kit can provide results within 20 minutes, provided that the window period has been long enough. The Home Access HIV-1 Test System requires a finger prick of blood to be sent to a lab. Results are generally available anonymously after 24 hours. Again, the window of time when you can be reasonably sure that your negative is negative and positive is positive is about 3 months.

Combo or Fourth-Generation Tests These tests look for HIV antibodies and antigens produced when the body reacts to foreign invaders. The window for detection is shorter (usually 2 to 4 weeks or 13 to 42 days) for antigens and antibodies to be detected. There is a rapid combo fourth generation test available online; however, it is considerably more expensive than antibody tests.

Nucleic Acid Tests (NAT) and HIV p24 Antigen Test These newer, quicker, more costly tests look for the virus (NAT) and antigens for the virus (HIV p24) and are available to the public. However, these are not usually recommended for initial screening. A benefit of these tests is that picking up the infection sooner prevents the infected person from unknowingly infecting others.

New Hope and Treatments

New drugs have slowed the progression from HIV to AIDS and have prolonged life expectancies for most AIDS patients. In fact, the U.S. death rate from AIDS has dropped nearly 83 percent since the 1990s.[93] However, these drugs are expensive. With recent price increases, the average cost for antiretroviral therapy may range from $4000 to $48,000 per year, depending on drug newness and pharmaceutical pricing. These costs are just for the drugs and do not include regular testing and doctor's visits. Soaring drug prices affect treatment availability for many patients.[94]

Current treatments combine selected drugs, especially protease inhibitors and reverse transcriptase inhibitors. *Protease inhibitors* (e.g., amprenavir, ritonavir, saquinavir) prevent the production of the virus in chronically infected cells that HIV has already invaded and seem to work best in combination with other therapies. Other drugs, such as AZT, ddI, ddC, d4T, and 3TC, inhibit the HIV enzyme *reverse transcriptase* before the virus has invaded the cell, thereby preventing the virus from infecting new cells. Drug options change frequently, and no combination has proven effective for all people.[95]

Preventing HIV Infection

The only way to prevent HIV infection is through the choices you make in sexual behaviors and drug use and by taking responsibility for your own health and the health of your loved ones. You can't determine the presence of HIV by looking at a person. You also can't tell by questioning the person unless he or she has been tested recently and is giving an honest answer. So what should you do? The simplest answer is abstinence. If you do decide to have sex, the next best option is to use a condom.

Newer Prevention Strategies for Persons at High Risk for HIV Infection There is currently no vaccine to prevent HIV and no cure, though numerous labs are working on these issues. When abstinence, protection, and other prevention strategies are inconsistent—or when your risks of HIV are increased because of multiple sex partners, high-risk sex partners, and other risks—new options are available. Studies have shown promising results from the use of **preexposure prophylaxis (PrEP) for HIV**. Individuals who aren't HIV positive and are engaging in high-risk sex with multiple partners or with someone who is HIV positive can reduce their risk of sexually transmitted HIV by nearly 90 percent and of HIV from drug injection by 70 percent.[96] PrEP use involves taking a daily HIV combination pill known as Truvada to prevent infection. It is important to remember that Truvada is not 100 percent effective. The key to its effectiveness is taking it consistently, using condoms and other prevention strategies, and getting regular medical checkups..[97]

Where to Go for Help If you are concerned about your risk or that of a friend, arrange a confidential meeting with the health educator or other health professional at your college health service. He or she will provide you with the information that you need to decide whether you should be tested for HIV antibodies and the pros and cons of PrEP use. Local public health departments or community STI clinics can also provide this information.

LIVE IT! ASSESS YOURSELF

An interactive version of this assessment is available online in Mastering Health.

ASSESS | YOURSELF

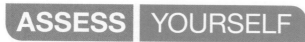

STIs: Do You Really Know What You Think You Know?

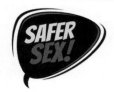

The following quiz will help you evaluate whether your beliefs and attitudes about sexually transmitted infections lead you to behaviors that increase your risk of infection. Indicate whether you believe that each of the following items is true or false. Then consult the answer key that follows.

		True	False
1.	You can always tell when you've got an STI because the symptoms are so obvious.	○	○
2.	Some STIs can be passed on by skin-to-skin contact in the genital area.	○	○
3.	Herpes can be transmitted only when a person has visible sores on his or her genitals.	○	○
4.	Oral sex is safe sex.	○	○
5.	Condoms reduce your risk of both pregnancy and STIs.	○	○
6.	As long as you don't have anal intercourse, you can't get HIV.	○	○
7.	All sexually active females should have a regular Pap smear.	○	○
8.	Once genital warts have been removed, there is no risk of passing on the virus.	○	○
9.	You can get several STIs at one time.	○	○
10.	If the signs of an STI go away, you are cured.	○	○
11.	People who get an STI are those who have a lot of sex partners.	○	○
12.	All STIs can be cured.	○	○
13.	You can get an STI more than once.	○	○

Answer Key

1. False. The unfortunate fact is that many STIs show no symptoms. This has serious implications For one thing, you can be passing on the infection without knowing it. For another, the pathogen may be damaging your reproductive organs without your knowing it.

2. True. Some viruses are present on the skin around the genital area. Herpes and genital warts are the main culprits.

3. False. Herpes is most easily passed on when the sores and blisters are present, because the fluid in the lesions carries the virus. But it can also be spread when no sores are present but the virus is still active. The virus can also be present on the genitals, and people may contract it through oral sex or touching these areas and not washing their hands.

4. False. Oral sex is not safe sex. Herpes, genital warts, and chlamydia can all be passed on through oral sex. Condoms should be used on the penis. Dental dams should be placed over the female genitals during oral sex.

5. True. Condoms significantly reduce the risk of pregnancy when used correctly. They also reduce the risk of STIs. It is important to point out that abstinence is the only behavior that provides complete protection against pregnancy and STIs.

6. False. HIV is present in blood, semen, and vaginal fluid. Any activity that allows for the transfer of these fluids is risky. Anal intercourse is a high-risk activity, especially for the receptive (passive) partner, but other sexual activity is also a risk. To be safe, condoms are your best option.

7. True. A Pap smear is a simple procedure involving the scraping of a small amount of tissue from the surface of the cervix (at the upper end of the vagina). The sample is tested for abnormal cells that may indicate cancer. All sexually active women should have regular Pap smears.

8. False. Genital warts, which may be present on the penis, the anus, and inside and outside the vagina, can be removed.

However, people with no apparent warts may still carry the virus. The virus that caused the warts will always be present in the body and can be passed on to a sex partner.

9. True. It is possible to have many STIs at one time. In fact, having one STI may make it more likely that a person will acquire more STIs. For example, the open sore from herpes creates a place for HIV to be transmitted.

10. False. The symptoms may go away, but your body is still infected. For example, syphilis is characterized by various stages. In the first stage, a painless sore called a chancre appears for about a week and then goes away.

11. False. If you have sex once with an infected partner, you are at risk for an STI.

12. False. Some STIs are viruses and therefore cannot be cured. There is no cure at present for herpes, HIV/AIDS, or genital warts. These STIs are treatable (to lessen the pain and irritation of symptoms) but not curable.

13. True. Experiencing one infection with an STI does not mean that you can never be infected again. A person can be reinfected many times with the same STI. This is especially true if a person does not get treated for the STI and thus keeps reinfecting his or her partner with the same STI, so they swap the infection back and forth.

Sources: Adapted from Jefferson County Public Health, "STD Quiz," modified March 2009, www.co.jefferson.co.us/health /health_T111_R69.htm; Adapted from Family Planning Victoria, "Play Safe," updated July 2005, www.fpv.org.au/1_2_2.html.

YOUR PLAN FOR **CHANGE**

After completing the **ASSESS YOURSELF** activity, you can begin to change behaviors that may be putting you at risk for STIs and for infection in general.

TODAY, YOU CAN:

☐ Put together an "emergency" supply of condoms. Outside of abstinence, condoms are your best protection against an STI. If you don't have a supply on hand, visit your local drugstore or health clinic. Remember that both men and women are responsible for preventing the transmission of STIs.

☐ To prevent infections in general, get in the habit of washing your hands regularly. After you cough, sneeze, blow your nose, use the toilet, or prepare food, find a sink, wet your hands with warm water, and lather up with soap. Scrub your hands for about 20 seconds (count to 20 or recite the alphabet), rinse well, and dry your hands.

WITHIN THE NEXT TWO WEEKS, YOU CAN:

☐ Talk with your significant other honestly about your sexual history. Make appointments to get tested if either of you think you may have been exposed to an STI.

☐ Adjust your sleep schedule so that you're getting enough rest every night. Being well rested is one key aspect of maintaining a healthy immune system.

BY THE END OF THE SEMESTER, YOU CAN:

☐ Check your immunization schedule, and make sure you're current with all recommended vaccinations. Make an appointment with your health care provider if you need a booster or vaccine.

☐ If you are due for an annual pelvic exam, make an appointment. Ask your partner whether he or she has had an annual exam, and encourage him or her to make an appointment if not.

STUDY **PLAN**

Visit the Study Area in Mastering Health to enhance your study plan with MP3 Tutor Sessions, Practice Quizzes, Flashcards, and more!

CHAPTER **REVIEW**

LO 1 | The Process of Infection

- To become infected with a disease, a person must come into contact with a pathogen, and the pathogen must get past the body's immune system defenses to establish infection.

LO 2 | Your Body's Defenses against Infection

- The skin is the body's major barrier against infection, helped by enzymes and body secretions.
- If pathogens get inside the body, the immune system finds the foreign cells or particles and creates antibodies to destroy them. Inflammation and fever also play a role in defending the body against infections.
- Vaccines bolster the body's immune system against specific diseases.

LO 3 | Types of Pathogens and the Diseases They Cause

- The major classes of pathogens are bacteria, viruses, fungi, protozoans, parasitic worms, and prions. Bacterial infections include staphylococcal infections, streptococcal infections, meningitis, pneumonia, tuberculosis, and tick-borne diseases. Major viral infections include the common cold, influenza, mononucleosis, and hepatitis.
- Emerging and resurgent diseases such as West Nile virus, and avian flu potentially pose significant threats for future generations. Many factors contribute to these risks.

LO 4 | Sexually Transmitted Infections

- Sexually transmitted infections (STIs) are spread through vaginal intercourse, oral–genital contact, anal intercourse, hand–genital contact, and sometimes mouth-to-mouth contact.
- Every year, there are at least 20 million new cases of STIs in the United States. STIs affect people of all backgrounds and socioeconomic levels, but rates are disproportionately higher among young adults, women, minorities, and infants.
- Generally, the more sex partners one has, the greater is one's risk of contracting an STI. Reduce risk of contraction by using condoms and dental dams and avoiding sexual activities that allow blood, semen, or other body fluid to enter breaks in the skin or breach mucous membranes.

LO 5 | Common Types of Sexually Transmitted Infections

- Major STIs include chlamydia, gonorrhea, syphilis, herpes, human papillomavirus (HPV) and genital warts, candidiasis, trichomoniasis, and pubic lice.

LO 6 | HIV/AIDS

- Acquired immunodeficiency syndrome (AIDS) is caused by the human immunodeficiency virus (HIV). HIV/AIDS is a global pandemic.
- Anyone can get HIV by engaging in unprotected sexual activities or by injecting drugs (or by having sex with someone who does).

POP **QUIZ**

LO 1 | The Process of Infection

1. Jennifer touched her viral herpes sore on her lip and then touched her eye. She ended up with the herpes virus in her eye as well. This is an example of
   a. acquired immunity.
   b. passive spread.
   c. autoinoculation.
   d. self-vaccination.

2. One of the best ways to prevent contagious viruses from spreading is to
   a. wash your hands frequently.
   b. cover your mouth when sneezing and dispose of your tissues.
   c. keep your hands away from your mouth and eyes.
   d. All of the above

LO 2 | Your Body's Defenses against Infection

3. Which of the following do *not* assist the body in fighting disease?
   a. Antigens
   b. Antibodies
   c. Lymphocytes
   d. Macrophages

LO 3 | Types of Pathogens and the Diseases They Cause

4. Which of the following is a viral disease?
   a. Lyme disease
   b. Powassan
   c. Malaria
   d. Streptococcal infection

5. Which of the following diseases is caused by a prion?
   a. Shingles
   b. Listeria
   c. Mad cow disease
   d. Trichomoniasis

LO 4 **Sexually Transmitted Infections**

6. What type of environment do STI pathogens prefer?
   a. Any environment
   b. Dark, moist environments
   c. Light, dry environments
   d. Cold, dry environments

LO 5 **Common Types of Sexually Transmitted Infections**

7. Which of the following is *correct* about HPV?
   a. It is a virus.
   b. Most sexually active men and women will develop it at some time in their lives.
   c. It is the leading cause of cervical cancer.
   d. All of the above

8. Which of the following STIs cannot be treated with antibiotics?
   a. Chlamydia
   b. Gonorrhea
   c. Syphilis
   d. Herpes

LO 6 **HIV/AIDS**

9. Which of the following is *not* a true statement?
   a. PrEP is a newly developed treatment for HIV/AIDS.
   b. Almost 40 years after its discovery, we still don't have a vaccine to prevent or a treatment to cure HIV/AIDS.
   c. Women are much more likely to be in infected with HIV during heterosexual sex than men.
   d. Several new home screening tests for HIV are currently available.

10. After HIV/AIDS, which infectious disease kills more people than any other disease in the global population?
    a. Malaria
    b. Avian influenza
    c. Tuberculosis
    d. Hepatitis C

*Answers to the Pop Quiz can be found on page A-1. If you answered a question incorrectly, review the section identified by the Learning Outcome. For even more study tools, visit **Mastering Health**.*

THINK ABOUT IT!

LO 1 **The Process of Infection**

1. What are three lifestyle changes you could make right now that would reduce your risk of developing an infectious disease? How can you help to reduce antibiotic resistance in the world today?

LO 2 **Your Body's Defenses against Infection**

2. What are pathogens, antigens, and antibodies? Discuss noncontrollable and controllable risk factors that can make you more or less susceptible to infectious pathogens in your immediate surroundings.

LO 3 **Types of Pathogens and the Diseases They Cause**

3. What are some differences between bacteria and viruses?

LO 4 **Sexually Transmitted Infections**

4. What are the key risk factors for STI infections? What kind of behaviors should you avoid to cut down on the risk of contracting a sexually transmitted infection?

LO 5 **Common Types of Sexually Transmitted Infections**

5. Identify five STIs and their symptoms. How are they transmitted? What are their potential long-term effects?

LO 6 **HIV/AIDS**

6. Why are women more susceptible to HIV infection than men? What implications does this have for prevention, treatment, and research?

ACCESS YOUR HEALTH ON THE INTERNET

Visit Mastering Health for links to the websites and RSS feeds.

The following websites explore further topics and issues related to infectious diseases and STIs.

Centers for Disease Control and Prevention (CDC). This government agency is dedicated to disease intervention and prevention. The site links to all the latest data and publications put out by the CDC. **www.cdc.gov**

Association for Professionals in Infection Control and Epidemiology (APIC). This is an excellent resource for health professionals and consumers. It covers a wide range of infectious disease issues in health care, workplaces, schools, and the personal environment. **www.apic .org**

World Health Organization (WHO). You'll gain access to the latest information on world health issues and direct access to publications and fact sheets at WHO's site. **www.who.int**

American Sexual Health Association. This site provides facts, support, and referrals about sexually transmitted infections and diseases. **www.ashastd.org**

AVERT. This is an international site with information on HIV/AIDS, global STI statistics, interactive quizzes, and graphics displaying current statistics for vulnerable populations. **www.avert .org**

Reducing Risks for Chronic Diseases and Conditions

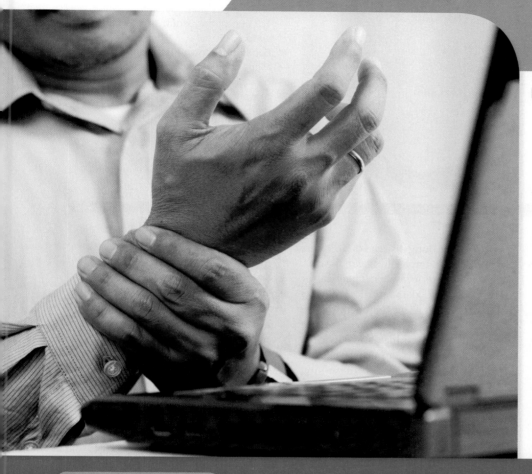

LEARNING OUTCOMES

1 Describe the prevalence and symptoms of key respiratory diseases such as bronchitis, emphysema, and asthma, including their risk factors and impact on society.

2 Describe the allergic response, as well as key types of allergy, potential complications, and susceptibility.

3 Explain common neurological disorders, including headaches and seizure disorders, risk factors, possible causes, and methods of prevention and control.

4 Summarize key digestive disorders, their risks, symptoms, and strategies for prevention.

5 Explain the risk factors and symptoms of major musculoskeletal diseases, including arthritis and low back pain, and suggest strategies for prevention.

WHY SHOULD I CARE?

Chronic conditions represent the single greatest threat to health in the United States, responsible for 7 out of 10 deaths and over 86 percent of our nation's health care costs.[1] The good news is that many chronic conditions are preventable or manageable.

Chronic diseases and conditions take time to develop, cause progressive damage to the body, and are not easily cured. Typically, they are not transmitted by pathogens; you don't "catch" them from other people. Genetics, the environment, lifestyle, and aging are often implicated as underlying causes. However, the causes of many chronic diseases and conditions remain a mystery. Healthy changes in lifestyle; public health efforts aimed at research, prevention, and control; and an ever-growing pharmaceutical arsenal can minimize the effects of these diseases. Policies that protect the environment and keep

chronic diseases Diseases or conditions that take time to develop, cause progressive damage to the body, and are not easily cured.

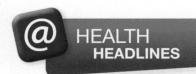
BE ECO-CLEAN AND ALLERGEN FREE

Exposure to household chemicals may exacerbate asthma, allergies, and other respiratory problems. You can reduce exposure and create a clean, comfortable home by using less toxic cleaning supplies. Read labels carefully, and look for independent certifications such as the Green Seal and the Environmental Protection Agency's Design for the Environment program.

- For a handy glass and surface cleaner, mix 1/2 cup of white vinegar with 4 cups of water. Pour the solution into a spray bottle, and keep the remainder for a quick and cheap refill.

Making your own cleansers from natural products such as vinegar and water, ensures that they are not harmful to your health.

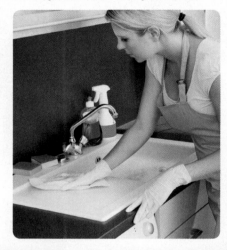

- Use baking soda to remove odors from carpets and to scour sinks, toilets, and bathtubs.
- Instead of bleach, use 1/2 cup of hydrogen peroxide in your laundry, or try oxygen-based bleaches.
- Make an all-purpose cleaner with 1/2 cup of borax and 1 gallon of hot water.
- For air fresheners, use essential oils. Place a few drops of essential oils on a piece of tissue paper, in a bowl of warm water, or in a store-bought diffuser.

---

us safe from chemicals can also make a difference. In this chapter, we highlight several chronic diseases and actions you can take to reduce your risks.

LO 1 | COPING WITH CHRONIC LOWER RESPIRATORY (LUNG) DISEASES

Describe the prevalence and symptoms of key respiratory diseases such as bronchitis, emphysema, and asthma, including their risk factors and impact on society.

Chronic lower respiratory disease is the third leading cause of death in the United States (right after heart disease and cancer), killing over 147,000 people in 2017.[2]

dyspnea Shortness of breath, usually associated with disease of the heart or lungs.

chronic obstructive pulmonary diseases (COPD) A collection of chronic lung diseases, including emphysema and chronic bronchitis, in which some form of obstruction interferes with the person's ability to breathe.

Essentially, lung diseases or disorders are those that impair lung function. A single exposure to a toxic chemical or severe heat can damage the lungs, as can years of inhaling the chemicals in tobacco smoke. Exposure to asbestos, silica dust, paint fumes and lacquers, pesticides, and a host of other environmental substances can also cause lung damage. When the lungs are impaired, a condition known as **dyspnea**, a choking type of breathlessness, can occur, even with mild exertion. As the lungs are oxygen deprived, the heart must work harder. Over time, cardiovascular problems, suffocation, and death can occur.

Chronic Obstructive Pulmonary Disease

Chronic obstructive pulmonary disease (COPD) is a progressive lung disease that gradually makes it more difficult for the person to breathe. In the United States, the term *COPD* refers to two specific diseases, *chronic bronchitis* and *emphysema*, which often occur together and can lead to problems with inhalation and exhalation. Currently, nearly 13 million people age 18 and over have been diagnosed with

COPD; however, this is believed to be a gross underestimate of the actual number of people with the disease.[3]

There is no cure for COPD, but much can be done to prevent it. Exercising, quitting smoking, and avoiding obesity can all help your lungs function more effectively, as can avoiding secondhand smoke, toxic aerosols, radon, and other chemicals. The Health Headlines box describes actions you can take to reduce risks from common exposures in your home.

Major improvements in air cleaning and ventilation systems have reduced occupational exposure to chemicals in recent years. Reading labels,

147 MILLION

people die each year from **CHRONIC LOWER RESPIRATORY DISEASES**.

wearing protective devices, and making sure areas where toxins accumulate are ventilated during spraying of chemicals and cleaning products are important.

Bronchitis

Bronchitis involves inflammation and eventual scarring of the lining of the bronchial tubes (*bronchi*) that connect the windpipe to the lungs. When the bronchi become inflamed or infected, less air flows from the lungs, and heavy mucus begins to form. *Acute bronchitis* is the most common bronchial disease. Symptoms often improve in a week or two after sources have been removed and inflammation or infection has been treated.

When symptoms of bronchitis last for at least 3 months of the year for 2 consecutive years, the condition is considered *chronic bronchitis*. In some cases, symptoms go undiagnosed for years, particularly in smokers who consider "smoker's cough" to be a normal part of their lives. Over 9.3 million Americans—the majority of them women—suffer from chronic bronchitis; over 30 percent are under age 45.[4] African Americans and whites experience more chronic bronchitis than other groups. Poverty, lack of education, and higher smoking rates are likely contributors in to the prevalence of chronic bronchitis.[5]

Emphysema

Emphysema involves the gradual, irreversible destruction of the lungs' alveoli (tiny air sacs through which gas exchange occurs). Over 3.5 million Americans suffer from emphysema, more of them women than men.[6] As the alveoli are destroyed, the affected person finds it increasingly difficult to exhale. People with emphysema liken this experience to engaging in heavy exercise while breathing through a straw. What most of us take for granted—the easy, rhythmic flow of air into and out of the lungs—becomes a continuous, anxious, and life-threatening struggle. (For more on emphysema and smoking, see Chapter 9.)

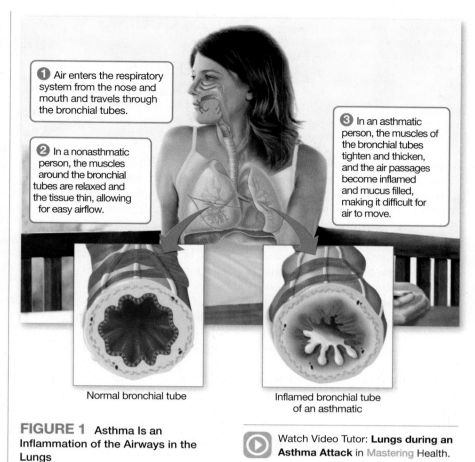

1 Air enters the respiratory system from the nose and mouth and travels through the bronchial tubes.

2 In a nonasthmatic person, the muscles around the bronchial tubes are relaxed and the tissue thin, allowing for easy airflow.

3 In an asthmatic person, the muscles of the bronchial tubes tighten and thicken, and the air passages become inflamed and mucus filled, making it difficult for air to move.

Normal bronchial tube

Inflamed bronchial tube of an asthmatic

FIGURE 1 **Asthma Is an Inflammation of the Airways in the Lungs**

Watch Video Tutor: **Lungs during an Asthma Attack** in Mastering Health.

Asthma

Asthma is a long-term, chronic disorder that inflames and blocks lung airflow (see **FIGURE 1**). Tiny airways in the lungs overreact with spasms, resulting in wheezing, difficulty breathing, shortness of breath, and coughing spasms. Approximately 18.5 million adults and over 6 million children in the United States have asthma.[7] The most common chronic disease of childhood, asthma affects nearly 9 percent of all children in the United States and nearly 7.5 percent of adults.[8] Rates are significantly higher among women, particularly those who are obese.[9] In childhood, asthma strikes more boys than girls; in adulthood, it strikes more women than men. Even with advances in treatment, asthma deaths among young people have more than doubled, with over 3,700 deaths last year in the United States.[10]

There are two distinctly different types of asthma. The more common form, known as *extrinsic or allergic asthma*, is typically associated with allergic triggers; it tends to run in families

bronchitis An inflammation and eventual scarring of the lining of the bronchial tubes.

emphysema A respiratory disease in which the alveoli become distended or ruptured and are no longer functional.

asthma A long-term, chronic inflammatory disorder characterized by attacks of wheezing, shortness of breath, and coughing spasms.

and develop in childhood. Often, by adulthood, a person has few episodes, or the disorder completely goes away. *Intrinsic or nonallergic asthma* may be triggered by anything except an allergy.

Several factors—including medical conditions, animal dander and saliva, mold, cockroach allergens, dust mites, perfumes, exercise, smoke, food allergies, weather changes, pollen, and air pollution—can trigger asthma flare-ups. In fact, even anger, fear, or stress can trigger an asthma attack.[11] Genetics may play a role in asthma development. If a close relative has asthma or a history of allergies, you are more likely to have asthma yourself. If you had respiratory infections when you were younger, such

allergy A hypersensitivity reaction to a specific antigen in which the body produces antibodies to a normally harmless substance in the environment.

allergen An antigen that induces a hypersensitive immune response.

histamine A chemical substance that dilates blood vessels, increases mucous secretions, and produces other symptoms of allergies.

as colds, the flu, or sinus infections, or if you are exposed to environmental allergens and irritants, you are more likely to develop asthma.[12] Certain medications, particularly fever reducers or anti-inflammatory drugs such as nonsteroidal anti-inflammatory drugs (NSAIDs), beta-blockers, and angiotensin-converting enzyme inhibitors, which are used to treat cardiovascular problems may also be triggers.[13]

Poverty, low education, and risky home and work environments as well as limited access to health care lead to clear disparities in asthma treatment and control. African Americans have the highest rates of asthma in the United States at 10.3 percent, followed by whites at 7.8 percent, and Hispanics at 6.6 percent.[14] See the Skills for Behavior Change box for ways to avoid or reduce asthma attacks.

LO 2 | COPING WITH ALLERGIES

Describe the allergic response, as well as key types of allergy, potential complications, and susceptibility.

Allergies are characterized by an overreaction of the immune system to a foreign protein substance (**allergen** or *antigen*) that is swallowed, breathed into the lungs, injected, or touched.[15] When foreign pathogens such as bacteria or viruses enter the body, the body responds by producing *antibodies* to destroy them. Normally, antibody production is a good thing. However, for unknown reasons, sometimes the body develops an overly elaborate protective mechanism against relatively harmless substances.

Most commonly, these *hypersensitivity*, or allergic, reactions occur as a

response to environmental antigens such as molds, animal dander (hair and dead skin), pollen, ragweed, particulate matter, air pollution, dust, insect bites, and certain foods and medications. Although food allergies such as lactose intolerance and gluten intolerance have captured national attention and marketers have launched massive campaigns to sell food allergy–related products and services, recent research indicates that food allergies may affect fewer than 4 percent of Americans.[16]

Although symptoms vary by individual, in a true allergic response, antibodies trigger the release of **histamine**, a chemical that dilates blood vessels; increases mucus secretions; causes tissues to swell; and produces rashes, difficulty breathing, and other allergy

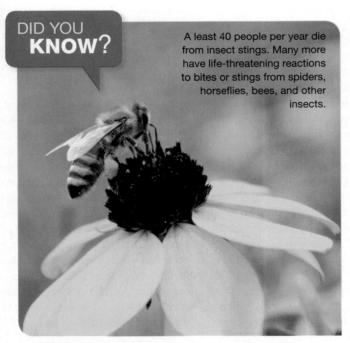

DID YOU KNOW?

A least 40 people per year die from insect stings. Many more have life-threatening reactions to bites or stings from spiders, horseflies, bees, and other insects.

Source: Asthma and Allergy Foundation of America, "Allergy Facts and Figures," Accessed June 2017, http://www.aafa.org/display .cfm?id=9&sub=30#mort

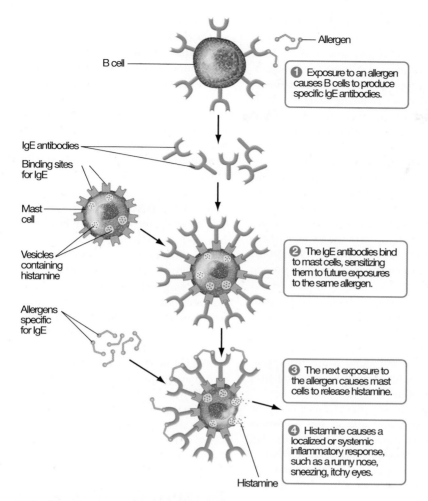

① Exposure to an allergen causes B cells to produce specific IgE antibodies.

B cell

IgE antibodies

Binding sites for IgE

Mast cell

Vesicles containing histamine

② The IgE antibodies bind to mast cells, sensitizing them to future exposures to the same allergen.

Allergens specific for IgE

③ The next exposure to the allergen causes mast cells to release histamine.

④ Histamine causes a localized or systemic inflammatory response, such as a runny nose, sneezing, itchy eyes.

Histamine

FIGURE 2 Steps in an Allergic Response

Source: Adapted from Johnson, Michael D., *Human Biology: Concepts and Current Issues*, 7th Ed., © 2014, p. 211. Printed and electronically reproduced by permission of Pearson Education, Inc., Upper Saddle River, New Jersey.

symptoms (**FIGURE 2**). Sometimes *anaphylaxis*—a potentially life-threatening set of serious allergy symptoms—can result.

Globally, between 40 and 50 percent of school-aged children are sensitized to one or more common allergens.[17] Prevention of allergies usually focuses on preventing exposure to allergens. If you are exposed, treatments may be as simple as quickly washing off the substance you came into contact with, taking antihistamines or getting shots to avoid serious reactions, and working with your doctor to come up with a treatment regimen.

Hay Fever

Hay fever, or *allergic rhinitis*, is one of the most common chronic diseases in the United States, affecting over 20 million adults and 6.1 million children each year.[18] Usually considered a seasonal disease, hay fever is most prevalent when ragweed and flowers bloom. Hay fever attacks are characterized by sneezing and itchy, watery eyes and nose; these symptoms result from overzealous immune system reactions to certain substances. You are more likely to have hay fever if you have a family history of allergies or asthma, are male, were born during pollen season, are a first-born child, were exposed to cigarette smoke during your first year of life, or are exposed to dust mites.

Typical over-the-counter treatments for hay fever include antihistamines, which work well for mild cases but may become less effective over time. Air-conditioning, whole-house air filters, and air purifiers, as well as limiting outdoor air exposure during peak pollen seasons can relieve symptoms. To determine whether you have pollen allergy, your best bet is to get tested by an *allergist*—a doctor who specializes in allergies. Typical treatments include prescription medications and/or allergy shots. While allergy shots are effective, side effects are possible, and doctors recommend them for limited time periods.

LO 3 | COPING WITH NEUROLOGICAL DISORDERS

Explain common neurological disorders, including headaches and seizure disorders, risk factors, possible causes, and methods of prevention and control.

More than 600 disorders can affect the nervous systems—from movement, speech, swallowing, and pain to autonomic functions such as heart rate and breathing, ability to learn, memory, sensations, and emotions.[19] At their worst, neurological disorders can cause major disability or even loss of life Some of them—*faulty gene* disorders such as muscular dystrophy and Huntington's

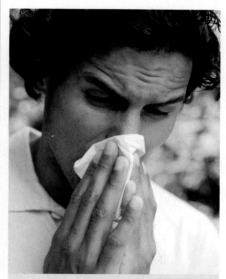

To minimize your risk of hay fever, keep windows closed, stay indoors when pollen counts are highest (typically 10 A.M. to 4 P.M.), and change clothes after spending time outdoors.

disease or *degenerative* disorders such as Alzheimer's disease and Parkinson's disease—are well known, but there are many lesser-known neurological disorders and some that elude diagnosis.

Headaches

Headaches are one of the most common reasons for emergency room visits. Adults age 18 to 44 are more likely to visit emergency rooms for headaches than are other age groups.[20] Most of the time, headaches are not serious and go away fairly quickly. There are over 150 different types of headaches.[21] We'll look at the most common.

Tension-Type Headaches

Up to 80 percent of the population occasionally have *tension-type headaches*. The most common headache symptoms are dull, aching pain on either or both sides of the head; a sensation of tightness or pressure; tenderness of the scalp, neck, and shoulder muscles; and, occasionally, loss of appetite.[22] While causes remain unknown, possible triggers include stress, depression and anxiety,

jaw clenching, and poor posture. Red wine, lack of sleep, extreme fasting, hormonal changes, and certain food additives have also been implicated.[23] Tension-type headaches are most often prevented by reducing triggers. Aspirin, ibuprofen, acetaminophen, and naproxen sodium often relieve pain.

Migraine Headaches

Over 1 billion people globally and 36 million Americans suffer from **migraines**, an inherited neurological disorder characterized by overexcitability of specific areas of the brain, particularly the vascular network.[24] Symptoms include moderate to severe pain on one or both sides of the head, pain with a pulsating or throbbing quality, pain that worsens with physical activity or interferes with regular activity, nausea with or without vomiting, and sensitivity to light and sound. Migraines appear to run in families and occur in 1 in 4 households.[25]

Migraine symptoms vary greatly by individual, and attacks last anywhere from 4 to 72 hours. Roughly one third of people who get migraines can predict an attack on the basis of a sensory warning sign called an *aura*, which may involve flashes of light, flickering vision, blind spots, tingling in the arms or legs, or a sensation of odor or taste.[26] The World Health Organization lists migraines as

one of the ten most disabling illnesses on the planet.[27]

Because migraine triggers vary by individual, treatment varies. Noting when migraine occurs is important in identifying triggers and making appropriate changes. Diet and exercise are important. When true migraines occur, relaxation is only minimally effective as a treatment. Often, prescription pain relievers are necessary.

Cluster Headaches

The severe pain of a cluster headache has been described as "killer" or "suicidal." Usually, these headaches cause excruciating, stabbing pain on one side of the head, behind the eye, or in one defined spot. Fortunately, cluster headaches are relatively rare, though adults between the ages of 20 and 40 tend to be particularly susceptible.[28]

Cluster headaches can last for weeks and may disappear quickly. More commonly, they last for 40 to 90 minutes and occur in the middle of the night, usually during rapid eye movement (REM) sleep. Oxygen therapy, drugs, and even surgery have been used to treat severe cases.[29]

Seizure Disorders

Approximately 5.1 million people in the United States, including about 750,000 children, suffer from epilepsy or some other seizure-related disorder.[30] **Seizure disorders** are generally caused by abnormal electrical activity in the brain and are characterized by loss of control of muscular activity and unconsciousness. Risk factors include taking certain drugs; drug withdrawal; having a high fever and abnormal blood levels of sodium or glucose; or experiencing physical, chemical, or temperature trauma.

Public ignorance and stigma associated with seizure disorders can have a significant impact on sufferers coping

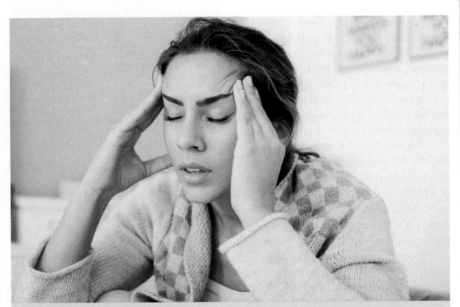

Patients report that migraines can be triggered by a variety of causes. What triggers a migraine in one person may relieve it in another.

migraines Throbbing headaches, often felt in one part of the head, with often debilitating symptoms such as nausea and light or sound sensitivity.

seizure disorders Neurological disorders caused by abnormal electrical activity in the brain and characterized by loss of control of muscular activity and unconsciousness.

with the challenges of daily living. In most cases, people with these disorders can lead normal, seizure-free lives as a result of advancements in diagnosis and treatment.

LO 4 | COPING WITH DIGESTION-RELATED DISORDERS AND DISEASES

Summarize key digestive disorders, their risks, symptoms, and strategies for prevention.

Diseases of the gastrointestinal tract appear to be on the rise among young and old adults. In this chapter, we focus on the more common "gut aches": irritable bowel syndrome and inflammatory bowel disease. See Chapter 10 for information on celiac disease and other gastrointestinal afflictions.)

Irritable Bowel Syndrome

Irritable bowel syndrome (IBS) is a *functional bowel disorder* (affecting how the bowel, including the colon and rectum, works) that affects an estimated 10 to 15 percent of adults in the United States, particularly women. Individuals under the age of 35 are most susceptible.[31] IBS is the second leading cause of work absenteeism after the common cold.[32]

In individuals with IBS, the normal muscular contractions in the intestines don't work properly, and food isn't processed or eliminated as it should be.[33] Characterized by nausea, pain, gas, diarrhea, bloating, or cramps, IBS can be uncomfortable but usually does not permanently harm the intestines unless the symptoms are severe. Symptoms may vary and can fade for long periods of time. Researchers suspect that people with IBS have digestive systems that are overly sensitive to what they eat and drink, to stress, and to certain hormonal changes. Often, because symptoms are so similar to those of other gastrointestinal tract diseases, IBS is diagnosed only after all the other gastrointestinal diseases have been ruled out.

Although there is no cure for IBS, treatments attempt to relieve symptoms.

Stress management, relaxation techniques, regular activity, and diet changes (including gradual increases in fiber and fluids and reductions in fat to help control cramps, diarrhea, and constipation) can help.

Inflammatory Bowel Disease

Inflammatory bowel disease (IBD) is an umbrella term for a group of disorders in which the intestines become inflamed. The most common are *ulcerative colitis* and *Crohn's disease*. Affecting over 1.6 million Americans, these two diseases both result from abnormal immune responses.[34]

Ulcerative Colitis

Ulcerative colitis is a condition that occurs when the lining of the large intestine (*colon*) becomes inflamed. This happens when the immune system misfires and signals "invader" when food or pathogens are introduced, leading to inflammation and ulcers. Signs and symptoms include abdominal pain, diarrhea, which is often bloody, weight loss, and fatigue. Affecting nearly 907,000 Americans and on the increase, ulcerative colitis often first flares up in the teens, and most people who have the disease are diagnosed in their thirties.[35]

Environmental exposure, pathogens, stress, smoking, and genetics are all possible causes of ulcerative colitis. Research indicates that up to 20 percent of people affected have close relatives who have the disorder; it is most common in white populations of European descent and Jewish populations.[36] Determining the cause of colitis is difficult because the disease can go into remission and then recur without apparent reason. This pattern often continues over periods of years and may be related to increased risks for colorectal cancer.[37]

Keeping a food diary and recording potential flare-ups are important parts of prevention. Treatment focuses on relieving symptoms by decreasing foods that are hard to digest (raw vegetables, seeds, nuts, and high-fiber foods), taking probiotics, and taking anti-inflammatory drugs.

Crohn's Disease

Often confused with colitis, **Crohn's disease** can affect any area of the gastrointestinal tract from the mouth to the anus, particularly the small intestine. It causes major pain, inflammation, and bleeding and can lead to tears in the gastrointestinal tract.[38] Genes, environmental exposures, and an autoimmune reaction are among the most likely culprits.[39] Crohn's disease tends to affect individuals age 15 to 35, with increased risk among those who smoke and those with a family history.[40] It is characterized by intense stomach pain, fever, weight loss, joint pain, mouth ulcers, and watery diarrhea. Intestinal bleeding can be serious enough to cause anemia, fatigue, and immune system dysfunction. The most common complication is bowel obstruction due to swelling, scar tissue, and ulcers that erode and form little infection-prone outpouches known as fistulas. People with Crohn's disease must carefully monitor their diet to ensure adequate nutrition, be tuned in to their body, see their doctor if symptoms develop, and take medications to reduce inflammation and prevent infection.[41] Surgery to remove damaged or obstructed portions of the bowel may be necessary.

LO 5 | COPING WITH MUSCULOSKELETAL DISEASES

Explain the risk factors and symptoms of major musculoskeletal diseases, including arthritis and low back pain, and suggest strategies for prevention.

Fifty percent of Americans age 18 and older and 75 percent over age 65 suffer

irritable bowel syndrome (IBS) A functional bowel disorder caused by certain foods or stress that is characterized by nausea, pain, gas, or diarrhea.

inflammatory bowel disease (IBD) A group of disorders in which the intestines become inflamed.

ulcerative colitis An inflammatory bowel disease that affects the mucous membranes of the large intestine and can lead to ulcers, erosion of the outer lining of the colon, and serious bleeding.

Crohn's disease A type of inflammatory bowel disease that can affect several parts of the gastrointestinal tract as well has have significant affects on other body organs and systems.

WHAT DO **YOU** THINK?

What factors are contributing to epidemic rises in musculoskeletal diseases today?

■ What actions should individuals and communities take to stem the tide of these ailments?

■ How do you alleviate pain?

■ What actions can you take to reduce your risks?

from a musculoskeletal disease—significantly higher than the number who suffer from cancer or cardiovascular disease. Although musculoskeletal diseases are less likely to result in death, they can exact a heavy toll on quality of life as well as ability to work and perform activities of daily living. Back pain, trauma or injury, and arthritis are the most common and costly musculoskeletal conditions. With the aging of the U.S. population, epidemic rates of disabling obesity, and increasingly sedentary lifestyles, future increases in musculoskeletal disease may have a staggering effect on our economy and individual lives.

Arthritis

Nearly 23 percent of Americans, or 54.4 million people, have a diagnosed form of **arthritis**.[42] Arthritis consists of more than 100 conditions that wreak havoc on joints, bones, muscles, organs, cartilage, and connective tissues, leading to disability and pain. Unfortunately, arthritis is not just a disease of old age; in fact, nearly two-thirds of people with

arthritis A painful inflammatory disease of the joints.

osteoarthritis Progressive deterioration of bones and joints that has been associated with the wear-and-tear theory of aging; also called *degenerative joint disease*.

rheumatoid arthritis A painful form of arthritis that occurs when the body's immune system attacks its own body cells.

low back pain (LBP) Pain in the lower back that may be mild, involving short-lived muscle spasms, or more severe, involving damage to discs, dislocation, a fracture, or another form of spinal trauma.

arthritis are under the age of 65, with nearly 300,000 children affected.[43] If current rates of obesity and sedentary lifestyle continue, over 78.4 million people will have a doctor-diagnosed form of arthritis by 2040, and over 43 percent of these individuals will have arthritis-attributable activity limitation.[44]

Also called *degenerative joint disease*, **osteoarthritis** is the most common form of arthritis, affecting over 30 million adults in the United States.[45] Before age 45, more men than women have osteoarthritis; after age 45, more women have it.[46] Although age, wear and tear, and injury are all factors, heredity, abnormal joint use, diet and excess weight, abnormalities in joint structure, and impaired blood supply to the joint may also contribute. Weight loss and exercise are key to prevention. For most people, anti-inflammatory drugs and pain relievers such as aspirin and cortisone-related agents ease discomfort. In some sufferers, applications of heat, mild exercise, and massage also help. When joints become

so distorted that they impair activity, surgical intervention is often necessary.

Another major form of arthritis is **rheumatoid arthritis**, in which a person's immune system attacks body tissues, including joints and other organs, causing inflammation, damage to affected areas, and pain/disability. Over 1.5 million people have RA, including nearly three times as many women as men.[47]

Low Back Pain

If you're like 85 to 90 percent of the population, you will at some point experience **low back pain (LBP)**, the number one cause of activity limitation and work absence worldwide.[48] The pain may be mild, involving short-lived muscle spasms, or it may be more severe, involving damage to discs, dislocation, a fracture, or another form of spinal trauma. In about 23 percent of LBP cases, the pain is chronic and comes and goes with activities as varied as sneezing, bending over, and lifting heavy objects.[49] About

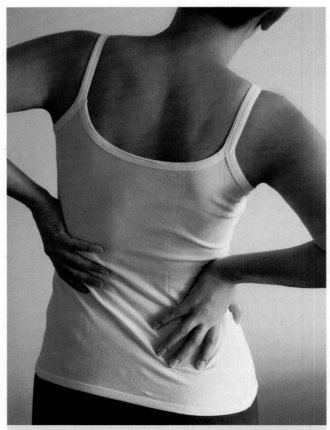

In the United States, low back pain is the second most frequent cause of disability and lost work time, after the common cold.

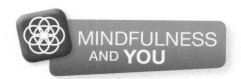
RELIEVING PAIN WITH MINDFULNESS?

Anyone with chronic pain knows how disabling it can be. New research indicates that mindfulness may be the newest pain reliever.

For instance, a Wake Forest Medical Center study using pain ratings and MRI brain imagery of pain centers found that the subjects who practiced mindfulness meditation fared better on pain relief after getting zapped on their skin with a thermal probe at 120 degrees (a level that most people would find very painful) than those who got a placebo or those in a control group.

Additionally, in one large meta-analysis (study of studies) researchers assessed the role of mindfulness strategies, including mindfulness meditation and elements of breath awareness, body awareness, and gentle movement on both pain and depression. After analyzing data from 38 randomized, controlled trials, the authors concluded that mindfulness was significantly effective in reducing both pain and depression. They recommended that larger, more rigorous studies be conducted to examine how mindfulness moderates pain.

Sources: F. Zeiden, "Mindfulness Meditation-based Pain Relief Employs Different Neural Mechanisms Than Placebo and Sham Mindfulness Meditation-induced Analgesia," *Journal of Neuroscience* 35, no. 46 (2015): 15307–25; L. Hilton et al., "Mindfulness Meditation for Chronic Pain: Systematic Review and Meta-analysis," *Annals of Behavioral Medicine* 51, no. 2 (2017): 199–213.

---

12 percent of people with LBP become permanently disabled.[50] Treatment may involve medication, rehabilitation, injections, and surgery, with varying results. A comprehensive analysis of recent research indicates that strength and resistance exercise and exercises focusing on coordination and stabilization, particularly under the guidance of a physical therapist, are among the most effective strategies for long-term LBP relief.[51]

New guidelines, based on the fact that most acute LBP cases resolve without treatment, adopt the "less is more" philosophy. In part because of growing concern over the use of addictive prescription opioid pain pills, patients are advised to forgo these and opt instead for over-the-counter medications such as aspirin, ibuprofen, acetaminophen, and muscle relaxants; to get a massage; to keep moving rather than staying in bed; to apply heat; and to use other lower-risk therapies.

For chronic LBP, recommendations include adding gentle exercise and rehabilitation, acupuncture, progressive relaxation, tai chi, electromyography biofeedback, yoga, low-level laser therapy, operant therapy, cognitive behavioral therapy, spinal manipulation, or mindfulness-based stress reduction. For more, see the **Mindfulness and You** box.[52]

If your LBP isn't relieved by the above measures, talk with your doctor about non-opioid drugs, NSAIDs, and other options.[53]

The following factors contribute to LBP and suggest areas for prevention:

- **Age.** People between the ages of 20 and 45 run the greatest risk of LBP. At age 50, the condition becomes less common. After age 65, the incidence again rises, apparently because of bone and joint deterioration.
- **Body Type.** Many studies indicate that people who are very tall, have a high BMI, or have a lanky body type run an increased risk of LBP.
- **Posture.** Poor posture may be one of the greatest contributors to LBP.
- **Strength and Fitness.** People with LBP tend to have less overall core strength than other people. Staying fit reduces your risks.
- **Psychological Factors.** Depression, apathy, inattentiveness, boredom, emotional upsets, drug abuse, and family and financial problems all heighten risk.
- **Occupational Risk.** Work and working conditions greatly affect risk. For example, truck drivers and desk workers frequently suffer from back pain.

Repetitive Strain/ Motion Injuries

It's the end of the term, and you have finished the last of several papers. After hours of nonstop typing, your hands are numb, and you feel an intense, burning pain in your wrists. If this happens, you may be suffering from a *repetitive strain/motion disorder*. Repetitive strain/motion disorders include carpal tunnel syndrome, bursitis, tendonitis, ganglion cysts, and others.[54] Twisting of the arm or wrist, overexertion, and incorrect posture or position are usually contributors, particularly among people who spend hours texting, gaming, or using other devices. One of the most common repetitive strain/motion disorders is **carpal tunnel syndrome**, which features numbness, tingling, and pain in the fingers, wrists, and hands.

carpal tunnel syndrome An occupational injury in which the median nerve in the wrist becomes irritated, causing numbness, tingling, and pain in the fingers, wrists, and hands.

ASSESS | YOURSELF

Are You at Risk for Chronic Illness?

LIVE IT! ASSESS YOURSELF

An interactive version of this assessment is available online in Mastering Health.

Certain characteristics place people at greater risk for chronic illness. Examine areas below where you have checked *Yes*. If you have several risks for a given problem, think about how to reduce risks, and talk with your doctor about possible concerns.

1 Chronic Lung Disease

Yes No

1. As part of your daily routine, are you exposed to environmental toxins such as tobacco smoke, air pollution, asbestos, or silica dust? ○ ○
2. Do you smoke? ○ ○
3. Does your family have a history of lung disease? ○ ○

2 Allergies

Yes No

1. Were you exposed to cigarette smoke at home? ○ ○
2. Does your family have a history of allergies? ○ ○
3. Do you live in an area where pollen counts are high and/or air-quality levels are less than desirable? ○ ○

3 Headaches

Yes No

1. Do you suffer from higher than normal levels of anxiety or stress? ○ ○
2. Is your desk or chair positioned such that you often have a stiff neck or unusual tension in your head/neck area? ○ ○
3. Does your family have a history of headaches? ○ ○

4 Digestion-Related Disorders

Yes No

1. Do you suffer from symptoms of bowel irregularity such as abdominal pain and/or bloating on a regular basis? ○ ○
2. Do you often experience heartburn, gas, or nausea? ○ ○
3. Does your family have a history of digestion-related disorders? ○ ○

5 Musculoskeletal Diseases

Yes No

1. Are you overweight and/or not getting enough physical activity? ○ ○
2. Do you often carry a backpack or laptop over one shoulder? ○ ○
3. Does your work require that you use one body part such as your wrist or elbow over and over in the same motion? ○ ○
4. Do you have a family history of musculoskeletal disease? ○ ○

YOUR PLAN FOR **CHANGE**

Now that you have completed the **ASSESS YOURSELF** activity and considered your results, you may need to take further steps to understand and address your risks.

TODAY, YOU CAN:

☐ Make an appointment with your doctor to discuss symptoms or potential risk factors.

☐ Find out whether your parents have had similar problems or know of anyone in your family who has.

WITHIN THE NEXT TWO WEEKS, YOU CAN:

☐ If you suffer from migraines, keep a diary of triggers. Create a routine that keeps you out of harm's way.

☐ If you suffer from irritable bowel syndrome, identify the foods or situations that bring it on.

BY THE END OF THE SEMESTER, YOU CAN:

☐ Adjust your routine to avoid environmental toxins. Avoid going to parties where people smoke, for example.

☐ Keep track of allergy-related symptoms to help you identify any likely triggers.

☐ Replace all cleaning products for your house, apartment, or dorm room with ones made from natural ingredients.

STUDY **PLAN**

Visit the Study Area in Mastering Health to enhance your study plan with MP3 Tutor Sessions, Practice Quizzes, Flashcards, and more!

CHAPTER **REVIEW**

LO 1 | **Chronic Lower Respiratory (Lung) Diseases**

- Chronic lower respiratory disease (including bronchitis, emphysema, and asthma) is the third leading cause of death in the United States (right after heart disease and cancer).

LO 2 | **Coping with Allergies**

- Allergies occur as the immune system responds to allergens. They can be triggered by pollens, foods, or other substances. Allergic rhinitis is more common among people with a family history of hay fever or other allergies.

LO 3 | **Coping with Neurological Disorders**

- The most common types of headache are tension, migraine, and cluster. Prevention includes reducing triggers. Treatment includes medication, environmental changes, and behavioral strategies.

LO 4 | **Coping with Digestion-Related Disorders and Diseases**

- Irritable bowel syndrome and other digestive problems affect increasing numbers of adults. Inflammatory bowel disease includes Crohn's disease and ulcerative colitis.

LO 5 | **Coping with Musculoskeletal Diseases**

- Musculoskeletal problems such as arthritis, low back pain, and repetitive motion disorders cause significant pain and disability in millions of people. Many of these problems are preventable.

POP **QUIZ**

LO 1 | **Chronic Lower Respiratory (Lung) Diseases**

1. Margaret experiences occasional wheezing, shortness of breath, and coughing spasms. What chronic respiratory disorder is she likely suffering from?
   a. Emphysema
   b. Bronchitis
   c. Asthma
   d. COPD

LO 2 | **Coping with Allergies**

2. Which of the following is *not* correct?
   a. Allergies are on the increase among most populations in the United States.
   b. Allergies are a result of problems with the immune system.
   c. Food allergies affect approximately 25 percent of the people in the United States.
   d. Eczema is an example of a skin allergy.

LO 3 | **Coping with Neurological Disorders**

3. Which of the following is correct?
   a. Cluster headaches are the most common type of headache.
   b. Tension-type headaches are often described as "suicidal."
   c. Migraine headaches can be preceded by an aura.
   d. Symptoms of epilepsy include wheezing and coughing attacks.

LO 4 | **Coping with Digestion-Related Disorders and Diseases**

4. Which of the following is correct?
   a. Inflammatory bowel syndrome is often mistaken for other intestinal disorders.
   b. Crohn's disease and ulcerative colitis are examples of irritable bowel syndrome.
   c. Digestive diseases are on the decline in the United States because of improved dietary practices.
   d. Smokers have a lower risk of ulcerative colitis.

LO 5 | **Coping with Musculoskeletal Diseases**

5. Which of the following conditions is currently the leading cause of disability throughout the world?
   a. Low back pain
   b. Upper respiratory infections
   c. Asthma
   d. Rheumatoid arthritis

*Answers to the Pop Quiz can be found on page A-1. If you answered a question incorrectly, review the section identified by the Learning Outcome. For even more study tools, visit **Mastering Health**.*

15

Making Smart Health Care Choices

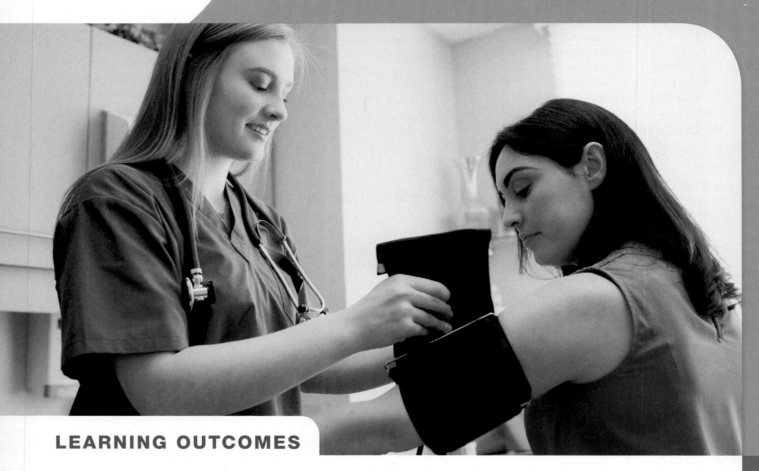

LEARNING OUTCOMES

LO **1** Explain why it is important to be a responsible health care consumer, and identify several factors to consider in making health care decisions.

LO **2** Discuss conventional health care, including types of practitioners and the health care products and treatments available.

LO **3** Describe the U.S. health care system in terms of types of insurance; the changing structure of the systems; and issues of cost, quality, and access to services.

LO **4** Explain key issues facing our health care system today and possible actions that could improve the system.

WHY SHOULD I CARE?

The ultimate choice about health care remains with you. To make sound decisions about what is best for your health, you need to understand as much as you can about your options.

Have you ever wondered whether you were sick enough to go to your campus health clinic? Have you left visits with your health care provider feeling that he or she didn't give you a thorough examination or that you had more questions than you did when you arrived? Do you understand health insurance provisions and what your options are in terms of health care systems and services? What are the current issues with health care in the United States, and what policies, programs, and individual behavior changes might help us reduce cost, improve quality, and ensure access for all? Are you worried that you, your family members, and your close friends do not or will not have health insurance? Would you seek care from complementary and integrative health providers? Are you among the nearly 15 percent of young adults age 18 to 24 in the United States who do not have health insurance?[1]

If the answer to any of these questions is yes, then you will find this chapter valuable for becoming a better consumer of health care. Learning how to navigate the health care system is an important part of taking charge of your health.

LO 1 | TAKING RESPONSIBILITY FOR YOUR HEALTH CARE

Explain why it is important to be a responsible health care consumer, and identify several factors to consider when making health care decisions.

Acting responsibly in times of illness can be difficult. If you are not feeling well, you must first decide whether you need to seek medical advice. For ailments such as colds or minor injuries, self-care may be the best course of action. In more serious cases, not seeking treatment—whether because of high costs or limited coverage or because the person tries to self-medicate when a professional diagnosis and treatment are needed—is potentially dangerous. It's important to know both the benefits and the limits of self-care.

Self-Care

Individuals can practice behaviors that promote health and reduce the risk of disease and can treat minor afflictions without seeking professional help. Self-care consists of knowing your body, paying attention to its signals, and taking appropriate action to stop the progression of illness or injury. Common forms of self-care include the following:

- Diagnosing symptoms or conditions that occur frequently but do not require physician visits (e.g., the common cold, minor abrasions)
- Using over-the-counter remedies to treat mild, infrequent, and unambiguous pain and other symptoms
- Performing first aid for common, uncomplicated injuries and conditions
- Having periodic checks for blood pressure, blood glucose, blood lipids, or other levels as prescribed by a physician
- Learning from reliable self-help books, websites, and videos
- Performing meditation or other relaxation techniques
- Maintaining a healthful diet, getting adequate rest, and exercising an appropriate amount.

A vast array of at-home diagnostic kits are now available to test for pregnancy, allergies, HIV, prediabetes, genetic disorders, and many other conditions. Caution is in order here: Diagnoses from these devices are not always accurate, or you may need professional interpretation to explain the ramifications of test results. Moreover, home health tests are not

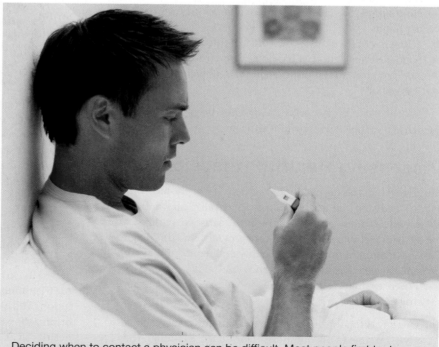

Deciding when to contact a physician can be difficult. Most people first try to diagnose and treat a minor condition themselves.

substitutes for regular, complete examinations by a trained practitioner.

Taking prescription drugs used for a previous illness to treat your current illness, using unproven self-treatment or using other people's medications are examples of inappropriate self-care. Using self-care methods appropriately takes effort, education, and the ability to make informed decisions based on scientific evidence.

When to Seek Help

Effective self-care also means understanding when to seek medical attention and how to access the most cost-effective and appropriate level of care. Generally, you should consult a physician if you experience *any* of the following:

- Serious accident or injury
- Sudden or severe chest pains, especially if they cause breathing difficulties
- Trauma to the head or spine accompanied by persistent headache, blurred vision, loss of consciousness, vomiting, convulsions, or paralysis
- Sudden high fever or recurring high temperature (over 102°F for children and 103°F for adults) and/or sweats
- Tingling sensation in the arm accompanied by slurred speech or impaired thought processes
- Adverse reactions to a drug or insect bite (shortness of breath, severe swelling, or dizziness)
- Unexplained sudden weight loss
- Persistent or recurrent diarrhea or vomiting
- Blue-tinted lips, eyelids, or nail beds
- Any lump, swelling, thickness, or sore that does not subside or that grows for over a month
- Any blood in the stool or urine, significant pain during elimination, or marked, persistent change in bowel or bladder habits
- Yellowing of the skin or the whites of the eyes
- Sudden severe pain that has no apparent cause
- Any symptom that is unusual, persists, or recurs over time
- Pregnancy.

See the Skills for Behavior Change box for pointers on taking an active role in your own health care.

Assessing Health Professionals

Suppose that you do need medical help. How should you go about assessing the qualifications of a health care provider? Numerous studies show that the most satisfied patients are those who feel that their health care provider explains diagnosis and treatment options thoroughly and demonstrates competence as well as genuine concern.[2]

When evaluating health care providers, consider the following questions:

- Do they listen to you, respect you as an individual, and give you time to ask questions? Do you feel as though they are in a rush to finish and move on to the next patient, or are they "tuned in" to you? Do they return your calls,

SKILLS FOR
BEHAVIOR CHANGE

Be Proactive in Your Health Care

The following points help you communicate well with health care providers:

- ◉ Research your personal and family medical history. Visit https://familyhistory.hhs.gov/FHH/html/index.html to create a family health portrait that you can share with your health care providers.
- ◎ Research your condition: causes, physiological effects, possible treatments, and prognosis. Don't rely solely on the health care provider.
- ◎ Write out your questions in advance. Asking questions is your right as a patient.
- ◎ Bring someone with you to appointments to listen, take notes, and ask for clarification if necessary. If you go alone, take notes.
- ◎ Ask the practitioner to explain the problem and possible tests, treatments, and medications. If you don't understand something, ask for clarification.
- ◎ If the health care provider prescribes any medications, ask whether you can take generic equivalents that cost less.
- ◎ Ask for a written summary of the results of your visit and any lab tests.
- ◎ Seek a second opinion about important tests or treatment recommendations.
- ◎ After an appointment, write down an account of what happened and what was said. Include the names of the provider and all other people involved in your care, the date, and the place.
- ◎ When getting prescriptions filled, read the pharmacist-provided drug information sheet that lists medical considerations and details about potential drug and food interactions.

and are they available to answer questions between visits? How quickly could you get in to see them in an emergency? Does your insurance cover their care?

- What professional education and training have they had, and what are their credentials? What license or board certification(s) do they hold? Note an important difference: *Board certified* indicates that the physician has passed the national board examination for his or her specialty (e.g., pediatrics) and has been certified as competent in that specialty. In contrast, *board eligible* merely means that the physician is eligible to take the exam but not that he or she has passed it. Do they have a record of any malpractice claims?
- Are they affiliated with an accredited medical facility or institution? The Joint Commission is an independent nonprofit organization that evaluates and accredits more than 20,500 health care organizations and programs in the United States. Accreditation requires institutions to verify all education, licensing, and training claims of their affiliated practitioners.[3]

▶ **SEE IT!** VIDEOS

Knowing your medical history can keep you informed of health risks. Watch **Your Medical History**, available on Mastering Health.

- Are they open to complementary or integrative strategies? Would they refer you for different treatment modalities if appropriate?
- Do they communicate possible treatment options clearly, the pros and cons of each, and the effectiveness of a given treatment in the short and long terms? Do they explain the possible side effects of a treatment and what symptoms might you expect?
- Who will be responsible for your care when they are away or not on call? Are they part of a practice group with colleagues who can help you when they aren't available?
- Are there professional reviews and information on any lawsuits against them available online?

Being prepared for appointments and asking the right questions will allow you to work in partnership with your health care provider. Many patients find that writing questions down before an appointment helps them get the answers they need. Don't accept a defensive or hostile response; if you are not satisfied with how a practitioner communicates, go elsewhere. It is also important that you provide honest answers to the practitioner's questions about your symptoms, condition, lifestyle, and medical history.

Active participation in your treatment is the only sensible course in a health care environment that encourages

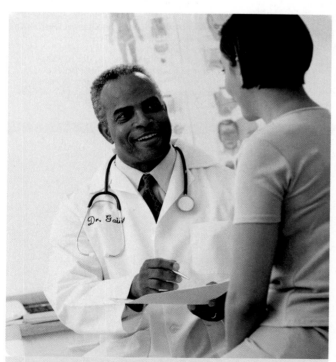

It's important to understand recommendations that your health care provider makes. Questions to ask include how often the practitioner has performed a procedure, the proportion of successful outcomes for the treatment or procedure, and why a test has been ordered.

35.1 MILLION

Americans are **ADMITTED** to a hospital each year.

defensive medicine, in which providers take certain actions primarily to avoid a **malpractice** claim. Today, the third leading cause of death in America is preventable medical error: hospital errors, errors in diagnosis, injuries from medications, and other health care errors.[4] In a complex, often overtaxed health care system, mistakes can happen. Being a savvy health care consumer is the best way to reduce your risks.[5]

Your Rights as a Patient

More than asking questions, being proactive in your health care also means being aware of your rights as a patient:[6]

- The right of **informed consent** means that before receiving care, you should be fully informed of what is planned; risks and potential benefits; and possible alternative forms of treatment, including the option of no treatment. Your consent must be voluntary and given without coercion. It is critical to read consent forms carefully and amend them as necessary before signing.
- You are entitled to know whether the treatment you are receiving is standard or experimental. In experimental conditions, you have the legal and ethical right to know whether any drug is being used as part of a research project for a purpose not approved by the U.S. Food and Drug Administration (FDA) and whether the study is one in which some people receive treatment while others receive a **placebo**. (See the Student Health Today box on this page for more on placebos and the placebo effect.)

malpractice Improper or negligent treatment by a health practitioner that results in loss, injury, or harm to the patient.

informed consent The acknowledgment that you have been told of the potential risks and benefits of a recommended test or treatment, understand what you have been told, and agree to the care.

placebo An inactive substance used as a control in a clinical test to determine the effectiveness of a particular drug; the *placebo effect* occurs when patients who are given a placebo drug or treatment experience an improved state of health owing to the belief that they are receiving something that will be of benefit.

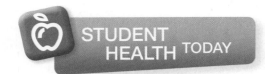
THE PLACEBO EFFECT
Mind Over Matter?

The *placebo effect* is an apparent cure or improved state of health brought about by a substance, product, or procedure that has no generally recognized therapeutic value. Patients often report improvements in a condition based on what they expect, desire, or were told would happen after receiving a treatment, even though the treatment was, for example, simple sugar pills instead of powerful drugs. Placebo-controlled studies are often used to determine the effectiveness of medications. Patients with a particular condition are given either the drug that is being tested or a placebo. If significantly more patients receiving the drug have a significantly better outcome than the patients receiving the placebo, the treatment can be considered effective. Most such studies are double-blind; that is, neither the patients nor the doctors involved are told until the study ends who had the real treatment.

There is also a *nocebo effect*, in which a practitioner's negative assessment of a patient's symptoms leads to a worsening of the condition, such as increased anxiety and pain. Similarly, a negative assessment of a treatment's potential efficacy induces a failure to respond to that treatment.

Researchers are investigating how and why expectation appears to change physiology. Evidence from pain studies suggests that use of a placebo for pain control causes the brain to release the same endogenous (natural) opioids that it releases when the study participant uses a pain medication with an active ingredient. But pain is not the only factor that responds to expectation.

- A study of resting tremor (such as involuntary finger tapping) in patients with Parkinson's disease found that positive or negative expectations of a treatment's effectiveness reduced or increased patient tremor when patients were given the same valid medication or the same placebo.
- A recent review study of thousands of clinical trials of antidepressants concluded that their therapeutic benefits reflect a combination of effects, including those induced pharmacologically and placebo effects.
- Several studies have found a significant placebo effect in trials of medications to treat alcohol dependency. Alcohol-dependent patients consume fewer alcoholic drinks and report less alcohol dependence and cravings, regardless of whether they are receiving the drug or a placebo.

If you're curious about the scientific evidence behind a drug prescribed for you, get online. A quick search using the exact name of the medication and the words "drug studies" should provide links to the information you're looking for.

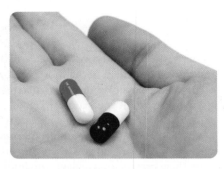

Is it a real medicine or a placebo? In some cases, it may not make a difference.

Sources: T. Bschor and L.L. Kilarski, "Are Antidepressants Effective? A Debate on Their Efficacy for the Treatment of Major Depression in Adults," *Expert Review of Neurotherapeutics* 16, no. 4 (2016): 367–74; L. Colloca and C. Grillon, "Understanding Placebo and Nocebo Responses for Pain Management," *Current Pain and Headache Reports* 18, no. 6 (2014): 419, doi:10.1007/s11916-014-0419-2; A. Keitel et al., "Expectation Modulates the Effect of Deep Brain Stimulation on Motor and Cognitive Function in Tremor-Dominant Parkinson's Disease," *PLoS One* 8, no. 12 (2013): e81878, doi:10.1371/journal.pone.0081878; G.L. Petersen et al., "The Magnitude of Nocebo Effects in Pain: A Meta-Analysis," *Pain* 155, no. 8 (2014), 1426–34, doi:10.1016/j.pain.2014.04.016.

- You have the right to make decisions about the health care that is recommended by the physician.
- You have the right to confidentiality, which includes the source of payment for treatment and care. It also means that you have the right to make personal decisions about all reproductive matters.
- You have the right to receive adequate health care, as well as to refuse treatment and to cease treatment at any time.
- You are entitled to have access to all of your medical records and to have those records remain confidential.
- You have the right to continuity of health care.
- You have the right to seek the opinions of other health care professionals about your condition.
- You have the right to courtesy, respect, dignity, responsiveness, and timely attention to health needs.

AN ESTIMATED
250,000
people **DIE EACH YEAR** from medical errors, making this the third leading cause of death in the US.

LO 2 | CONVENTIONAL HEALTH CARE

Discuss conventional health care, including types of practitioners and the health care products and treatments available.

Conventional health care, also called **allopathic medicine**, mainstream medicine, or traditional Western medical practice, is the dominant type of health care delivered in the United States, Canada, Europe, and much of the developed world. It is based on the premise that illness is a result of exposure to harmful environmental agents or organic changes in the body. The prevention of disease and the restoration of health involve vaccines, drugs, surgery, and other treatments.

Be aware, however, that not all allopathic treatments have had the benefit of the extensive clinical trials and long-term studies of outcomes that would conclusively prove effectiveness in various populations. Even when studies appear to support the benefits of a particular treatment or product, other studies with equal or better scientific validity often refute earlier claims. A comprehensive review of drug studies and medical devices found, for example, that those funded by the pharmaceutical industry are more likely to report positive response to the drug in comparison to studies of the same drug funded by outside sources.[7] This is one reason that later studies without sponsorship bias often refute earlier claims. Also, recommended treatments may change dramatically as new technologies and medical advances replace older practices. Like other professionals, medical doctors must keep up with new research and changing practices in their field(s) of specialty.

One of the ways health care providers ensure the quality of care they provide is by practicing **evidence-based medicine**. Decisions about patient care are based on clinical expertise, patient values, and current best scientific evidence. Clinical expertise refers to the clinician's cumulative experience, education, and clinical skills. The patient brings his or her own personal and unique concerns, expectations, and values. The best evidence is usually found in clinically relevant research conducted using sound methodology.

Conventional Health Care Practitioners

Selecting a **primary care practitioner (PCP)**—a medical practitioner whom you can visit for routine ailments, preventive care, general medical advice, and appropriate referrals—is not an easy task. The PCP for most people is a family practitioner or an internist. For a woman, the PCP might be an obstetrician-gynecologist (ob-gyn). Many people routinely see nurse practitioners or physician assistants who work for an individual doctor or a medical group. Others use nontraditional providers as their primary source of care. As a college student, you may opt to visit a PCP at your campus health center.

Doctors undergo rigorous training before they can begin practicing. After four years of undergraduate work, students typically spend four additional years studying for their doctor of medicine (MD) degree. After this general training, some students choose a specialty, such as pediatrics, cardiology, oncology, radiology, or surgery, and spend another year in an internship and several years doing a residency. Some specialties also require a fellowship, so additional training after receiving a medical degree can take up to eight years. Remember that not all MDs are trained in nutrition, exercise science, health behaviors, and other areas. Seek out care providers who have additional training in prevention, or ask for a referral for nutrition or dietary counseling.

Osteopaths are general practitioners who receive training similar to that of a medical doctor but who place special emphasis on the skeletal and muscular systems. Their treatments may involve manipulation of the muscles and joints. Osteopaths receive the degree of doctor of osteopathy (DO) rather than an MD.

Eye care specialists can be either ophthalmologists or optometrists. An **ophthalmologist** holds a medical degree and can perform surgery and prescribe medications. An **optometrist** typically evaluates visual problems and fits glasses but is not a trained physician. If you

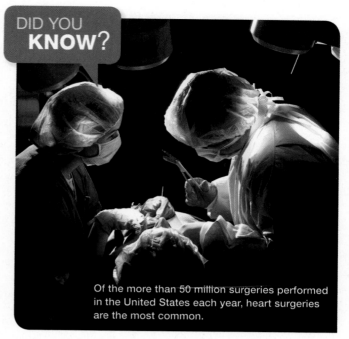

Of the more than 50 million surgeries performed in the United States each year, heart surgeries are the most common.

Source: U.S. Centers for Disease Control and Prevention, "Inpatient Surgery," April, 2016, http://www.cdc.gov/nchs/fastats/inpatient-surgery.htm.

---

allopathic medicine Conventional, Western medical practice; in theory, based on scientifically validated methods and procedures.

evidence-based medicine Decisions about patient care based on clinical expertise, patient values, and current best scientific evidence.

primary care practitioner (PCP) A medical practitioner who provides preventive care and treats routine ailments, gives general medical advice, and makes appropriate referrals when necessary.

osteopath A general practitioner who receives training similar to a medical doctor's but with an emphasis on the skeletal and muscular systems; may use spinal manipulation as part of treatment.

ophthalmologist A physician who specializes in the medical and surgical care of the eyes, including prescriptions for lenses.

optometrist An eye specialist whose practice is limited to prescribing and fitting lenses to correct vision problems.

have an eye condition requiring diagnosis and treatment, see an ophthalmologist.

Dentists diagnose and treat diseases of the teeth, gums, and oral cavity. They attend dental school for four years and receive the title of doctor of dental surgery (DDS) or doctor of medical dentistry (DMD). They must also pass both state and national board examinations before receiving their license to practice. The field of dentistry includes specialties; for example, *orthodontists* specialize in the alignment of teeth, *periodontists* treat diseases of the gums and other tissues surrounding the teeth, and *oral surgeons* perform surgical procedures to correct problems of the mouth, face, and jaw.

Nurses are trained health care professionals who provide a wide range of services for patients and their families, including patient education, counseling, providing community health and disease prevention information, and administration of medications. Registered nurses (RNs) in the United States complete either a four-year program leading to a bachelor of science in nursing (BSN) degree or a two-year associate degree program, and must also pass a national certification exam. Lower-level licensed practical or vocational nurses (LPN or LVN) complete a one- to two-year training program, which may be based in either a community college or hospital, and take a licensing exam.

Nurse practitioners (NPs) are nurses with advanced training obtained through either a master's degree program or a specialized nurse practitioner program. Nurse practitioners have the training and authority to conduct diagnostic tests and prescribe medications (in some states). They work in a variety of settings, including clinics and student health centers, and can specialize in areas such as pediatrics or acute care. Nurses and nurse practitioners may also earn the clinical doctor of nursing degree (ND), doctor of nursing science (DNS and DNSc degrees), or a research-based PhD in nursing.

Physician assistants (PAs) are licensed to examine and diagnose patients, offer treatment, and write prescriptions under a physician's supervision. An important difference between a PA and an NP is that the PA must practice under a physician's supervision. Like other health care providers, PAs are licensed by state boards of medicine.

Conventional Medication

Prescription drugs can be obtained only with a written prescription from a physician or other authorized professional (e.g. an NP or a PA), while over-the-counter drugs can be purchased without a prescription. Making wise decisions about medication is an important aspect of responsible health care.

Prescription Drugs In almost three-fourths of doctor visits, the physician administers or prescribes at least one medication.[8] In fact, prescription drug use has increased steadily over the past decade; over 49 percent of Americans report having used one or more prescription drugs in the previous 30 days, and more than 11 percent of Americans have used five or more.[9] Even though these drugs are administered under medical supervision, the wise consumer still takes precautions. Adverse effects and complications arising from the use of prescription drugs are common, as is failure to respond as expected to a medication.

A variety of resources are available to help consumers make educated decisions about whether to take a certain drug. One of the best resources is the FDA's Center for Drug Evaluation and Research website (www.fda.gov/drugs), which provides current information for consumers on risks and benefits of prescription drugs. Being knowledgeable can help to ensure your safety.

Generic drugs are prescription medications sold under the drug's chemical name rather than a brand name; they contain the same active ingredients as brand-name drugs but are usually much less expensive. Not all drugs are available as generics. If your doctor prescribes medication, ask whether a generic equivalent exists and whether it would be safe and effective for you to try.

Generic drugs need to have approximately the same effects on the body as whatever brand-name drug they are said to be modeled after. Concerns about cheaper drugs necessarily meaning lower quality is misguided. Generic drugs cost less because their manufacturers don't have to pay for clinical trials and costly advertising and promotion of the drug.[10] Always tell your doctor about any reactions you have to medications.

Over-the-Counter Drugs Medications available without a prescription are referred to as *over-the-counter (OTC)* drugs. American consumers spend billions of dollars yearly on OTC preparations for relief of everything from runny noses to ingrown toenails. The most commonly used OTC drugs are pain relievers; cold, cough, and allergy medications; stimulants; sleeping aids and relaxants; and dieting aids.

Despite a common belief that OTC products are safe and effective, they are medications that affect the body, and indiscriminate use and abuse can occur with these drugs as with all others. For example, people who frequently use eye drops to "get the red out" or pop antacids after every meal are likely to become dependent. Many people also experience adverse side effects because they ignore warnings on drug interactions and other cautions printed on labels. The FDA has developed a standard label that appears on most OTC products (see **FIGURE 15.1**). It includes directions for use, active and inactive ingredients, warnings, and other useful information.

dentist A physician who diagnoses and treats diseases of the teeth, gums, and oral cavity.

nurse A health professional who provides patient care in a variety of settings.

nurse practitioner (NP) A nurse with advanced training obtained through either a master's degree program or a specialized nurse practitioner program.

physician assistant (PA) A health care practitioner who is trained to handle most routine care under the supervision of a physician.

generic drugs Medications marketed by their chemical names rather than brand names.

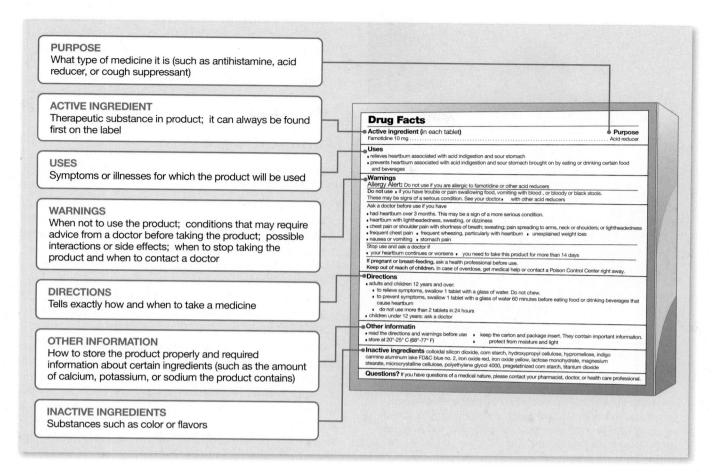

PURPOSE
What type of medicine it is (such as antihistamine, acid reducer, or cough suppressant)

ACTIVE INGREDIENT
Therapeutic substance in product; it can always be found first on the label

USES
Symptoms or illnesses for which the product will be used

WARNINGS
When not to use the product; conditions that may require advice from a doctor before taking the product; possible interactions or side effects; when to stop taking the product and when to contact a doctor

DIRECTIONS
Tells exactly how and when to take a medicine

OTHER INFORMATION
How to store the product properly and required information about certain ingredients (such as the amount of calcium, potassium, or sodium the product contains)

INACTIVE INGREDIENTS
Substances such as color or flavors

Drug Facts
Active ingredient (in each tablet) — Purpose
Famotidine 10 mg .... Acid reducer

Uses
- relieves heartburn associated with acid indigestion and sour stomach
- prevents heartburn associated with acid indigestion and sour stomach brought on by eating or drinking certain food and beverages

Warnings
Allergy Alert: Do not use if you are allergic to famotidine or other acid reducers
Do not use - if you have trouble or pain swallowing food, vomiting with blood, or bloody or black stools. These may be signs of a serious condition. See your doctor. - with other acid reducers
Ask a doctor before use if you have
- had heartburn over 3 months. This may be a sign of a more serious condition.
- heartburn with lightheadedness, sweating, or dizziness
- chest pain or shoulder pain with shortness of breath; sweating; pain spreading to arms, neck or shoulders; or lightheadedness
- frequent chest pain - frequent wheezing, particularly with heartburn - unexplained weight loss
- nausea or vomiting - stomach pain
Stop use and ask a doctor if
- your heartburn continues or worsens - you need to take this product for more than 14 days
If pregnant or breast-feeding, ask a health professional before use.
Keep out of reach of children. In case of overdose, get medical help or contact a Poison Control Center right away.

Directions
- adults and children 12 years and over:
  - to relieve symptoms, swallow 1 tablet with a glass of water. Do not chew.
  - to prevent symptoms, swallow 1 tablet with a glass of water 60 minutes before eating food or drinking beverages that cause heartburn
  - do not use more than 2 tablets in 24 hours
- children under 12 years: ask a doctor

Other informatin
- read the directions and warnings before use - keep the carton and package insert. They contain important informaiton.
- store at 20°-25° C (68°-77° F) - protect from moisture and light

Inactive ingredients colloidal silicon dioxide, corn starch, hydroxypropyl cellulose, hypromellose, indigo carmine aluminum lake FD&C blue no. 2, iron oxide red, iron oxide yellow, lactose monohydrate, magnesium stearate, microcrystalline cellulose, polyethylene glycol 4000, pregelatinized corn starch, titanium dioxide

Questions? If you have questions of a medical nature, please contact your pharmacist, doctor, or health care professional.

FIGURE 15.1 **Over-the-Counter Medicine Label**

Source: Consumer Healthcare Products Association, OTC Label. Courtesy of CHPA Educational Foundation, www.otcsafety.org.

LO 3 | **HEALTH** INSURANCE

Describe the U.S. health care system in terms of types of insurance; the changing structure of the systems; and issues of cost, quality, and access to services.

No matter what medical treatment you get, chances are that you'll use some form of health insurance to pay for your care. Insurance typically allows you, the consumer, to pay into a pool of funds and then bill the insurance carrier for covered charges you incur. The fundamental principle of insurance underwriting is that the cost of health care can be predicted for large populations. This is how health care **premiums** are determined. Policyholders pay premiums into a pool from which insurance companies pay claims. When you are sick or injured, the insurance company pays your care provider out of the pool, regardless of your total contribution to the pool. If you require a great deal of medical care, you may never pay anything close to the actual cost of that care. If you are basically healthy, you may pay more in insurance premiums than the total cost of your medical bills. Health insurance is based on the idea that policyholders pay affordable premiums so that they never have to face catastrophic bills. In profit-oriented systems, insurers prefer to have healthy people in their plans who pour money into risk pools without taking money out.

Private Health Insurance

Originally, health insurance consisted solely of coverage for hospital costs (it was called *major medical*), but it was gradually extended to cover routine physicians' treatment and other services, such as dental, vision care, and pharmaceuticals. These payment mechanisms laid the groundwork for today's steadily rising health care costs as hospitals were reimbursed for the costs of providing care plus an amount for profit. This system provided no incentive to contain costs, limit the number of procedures, or curtail capital investment in redundant equipment and facilities. Physicians were reimbursed on a fee-for-service (indemnity) basis determined by "usual, customary, and reasonable" fees. This system encouraged physicians to charge high fees, raise them often, and perform as many procedures as possible. Until the mid- to late twentieth century, most health insurance did not cover routine or preventive services, and consumers generally

premium A payment made to an insurance carrier, usually in monthly installments, that covers the cost of an insurance policy.

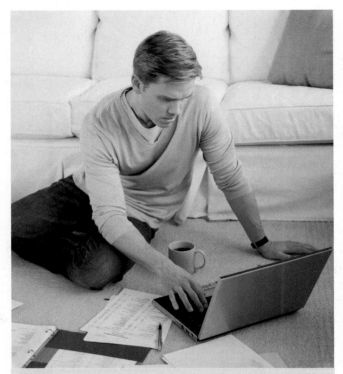

Choosing a health insurance plan can be confusing. Some things to think about include how comprehensive your coverage needs to be, how much you are willing to spend on premiums and co-payments, and whether the services of the plan meet your needs.

waited until illness developed to see a doctor instead of seeking preventive care. Consumers were free to choose any provider or service they wished, including even inappropriate—and often expensive—levels of care.

To limit potential losses, private insurance companies began increasingly using the following cost-sharing mechanisms and coverage limits:

- **Deductibles** are payments (which can range from about $500 to $5,000 annually) you make for health care before insurance coverage kicks in to pay for eligible services.
- **Co-payments** are set amounts that you pay per service or product received, regardless of the total cost (e.g., $20 per doctor visit or per prescription filled).
- **Coinsurance** is the percentage of costs that you must pay based on the terms of the policy (e.g., 20 percent of the total bill).
- Some group plans specify a *waiting period* that cannot exceed 90 days before they will provide coverage. Waiting periods do not apply to plans purchased by individuals.
- All insurers set some limits on the types of *covered services* (e.g., most exclude cosmetic surgery, private rooms, and experimental procedures).
- **Preexisting condition clauses** once limited the insurance company's liability for medical conditions

that a consumer had before obtaining coverage. Under the 2010 Patient Protection and Affordable Care Act (ACA), no one can be discriminated against because of a preexisting condition.
- Some plans imposed an *annual upper limit* or *lifetime limit,* after which coverage would end. The ACA makes this practice illegal.

Managed Care

Managed care describes a health care delivery system consisting of the following:

- A network of physicians, hospitals, and other providers and facilities linked contractually to deliver comprehensive health benefits within a predetermined budget and sharing economic risk for any budget deficit or surplus
- A budget based on an estimate of the annual cost of delivering health care for a given population
- An established set of administrative rules regarding how services are to be obtained from participating health care providers under the terms of the health plan.

Many managed care plans pay their contracted health care providers through **capitation**, a fixed monthly amount paid for each enrolled patient regardless of services provided. Some plans pay health care providers a salary, and some are still fee-for-service plans. Doctors participating in managed care networks are motivated (and sometimes incentivized) to keep their patient pool healthy and avoid preventable catastrophic ailments. Prevention and early intervention are often capstone components of such plans.

The three most common types of managed care available in the United States are *health maintenance organizations (HMOs), preferred provider organizations (PPOs),* and *point of service (POS).*[11]

Health Maintenance Organizations Health maintenance organizations provide a wide range of covered health benefits (e.g., physician visits, lab tests, surgery) for a fixed amount prepaid by the patient, the employer, Medicaid, or Medicare. Usually, HMO premiums are the least expensive form of managed care, but they are also the most restrictive (offering more limited choices of staff and health care facilities). There are low or no deductibles or coinsurance payments, and co-payments are small.

The downside of HMOs is that patients are required to use the plan's doctors and hospitals. Within an HMO, the PCP serves as a *gatekeeper,* coordinating the patient's care and providing referrals to specialists and other services. As more and more people enroll in HMOs, concerns have arisen about care allocation and access to services, profit-motivated medical decision making, and the degree of focus on prevention and intervention.

Preferred Provider Organization Preferred provider organizations are networks of independent doctors and hospitals that contract to provide care at discounted rates. Although they often offer more choices of providers than HMOs do, they are less likely to coordinate a patient's care. Members may choose to see doctors who are not on the preferred list at a higher percentage of out-of-pocket costs.

managed care A type of health insurance plan based on coordination of care and cost-reduction strategies; emphasizes health education and preventive care.

capitation Prepayment of a fixed monthly amount for each patient without regard to the type or number of services provided.

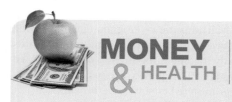

MONEY & HEALTH | HEALTH CARE SPENDING ACCOUNTS

A Flexible Spending Account (FSA) for health care and a Health Savings Account (HSA) are savings plans that give you the opportunity to save money tax free to be used toward qualified health care expenses. If you're not claimed as a dependent on someone else's tax return, you can open either an FSA through your employer or an HSA through your bank.

If you're an employee, when you enroll in an FSA, you identify the amount you want diverted from your paycheck into your FSA before taxes are withheld. The maximum you can contribute varies with different employers and health plans. One drawback to the FSA is that any funds still in the account at the end of the plan year are forfeited. This is known as the "use it or lose it" rule. Therefore, you need to estimate carefully what your out-of-pocket health expenses will be during the plan year.

With an HSA, there is no time limit on when the funds must be used. Contributions to the account can be made from your paycheck by your employer as pre-tax deductions, or you can make them yourself, in which case you can claim them as an above-the-line deduction (a deduction from your gross income) when you file your tax return.

What expenses can you pay for with the money in your account? Deductibles, co-payments, eyeglasses, contact lenses, and prescription drugs are all allowed. Visits to approved health care providers, including dentists and optometrists, are also payable from your account if you have no health insurance coverage for them. You can even use the funds to pay for OTC drugs such as pain relievers or allergy medications if you have a written statement from your care provider.

If you currently pay out of pocket for more than one or two health care visits a year, for a few prescriptions, contact lenses, and so on, and the money you use for these expenses comes from taxable income, then a health care savings plan might be worth a closer look. Contact your employee benefits specialist, your tax preparer, or a customer service provider at your bank.

Point of Service

Point of service (POS)—a hybrid of HMO and PPO plans—provides a more familiar form of managed care for people who are used to traditional indemnity insurance in which services are directly reimbursed. That may explain why it is among the fastest growing of managed care plans. Under POS plans, members select an in-network PCP, but they can go to nonnetwork providers for care without a referral and must pay the extra cost.

Other Types of Managed Care

Independent practice associations (IPAs) comprise independent physicians who maintain their own offices but who also agree to enroll members of an organization for a negotiated fee for each assigned patient or on a negotiated fee-for-service basis. IPAs can help eliminate isolation, risks, and expenses associated with independent private practice. *Exclusive provider organizations (EPOs)* are a type of managed care in which no coverage is typically provided for services received outside the EPO. Treatment or care received outside of the approved network must be paid by the patient.

No matter what type of plan you have, a special savings account for health-related expenses could save you money. See the Money & Health box to find out how they work and whether they're right for you.

Government-Funded Programs

The federal government, through programs such as Medicare and Medicaid, currently funds about 45 percent of total U.S. health care spending.[12]

Medicare

Medicare is a federal insurance program that employees and employers pay into over the course of a person's working life, a form of long-term savings plan for health insurance and care rather than an "entitlement" program. The funds are used to cover a broad range of services, except long-term care. Medicare covers citizens or permanent residents of the United States who are 65 or older, have any of certain disabilities, or have permanent end-stage kidney damage. Currently, 55.3 million people receive Medicare (46.3 million aged 65 or older, and 9 million disabled persons).[13] As the costs of medical care have continued to increase (over $600 billion in 2014), Medicare has placed limits on the amount of reimbursement to providers.[14] As a result, some providers no longer accept Medicare patients or do not accept such patients who are new to their practice, and patients must pay increasing levels of out-of-pocket expenses.

Currently, Medicare is divided into two major parts. Part A is the hospital insurance portion and helps pay for care while in hospitals, skilled nursing facilities, hospice care, and limited home health care. Part B requires monthly payments (typically deducted from the individual's Social Security check). People with a higher income pay more than lower-income individuals. Typically, Part B covers most of your care as long as your provider or facility "accepts assignment"—meaning that they agree to charge only what Medicare reimburses.

To control hospital costs, the federal government set up a prospective payment system based on *diagnosis-related groups (DRGs)* for Medicare as well as other insurance plans. Nearly 500 groupings establish how much a hospital will be reimbursed for caring for a patient diagnosed with particular conditions. DRGs are based on the assumption that patients with similar health status and conditions require a similar amount of hospital resources. If the costs

> **Medicare** A federal health insurance program that covers people over the age of 65, permanently disabled people, and people with end-stage kidney failure.

Medicaid A federal–state matching funds program that provides health insurance to low-income people.

of treating a patient are less than the predetermined amount, the hospital can keep the difference. However, if a patient's care costs more than the set amount, the hospital must absorb the difference. This system motivates hospitals to discharge patients quickly, to provide more ambulatory care, and to admit patients classified into the most favorable (profitable) DRGs. Many private health insurance companies have also adopted reimbursement rates based on DRGs.

Medicare Supplemental Plans
If providers charge more than Medicare allows, either the individual or a so-called *Medigap* plan must make up the difference. Medigap plans cover such "gaps" in charges, as well as certain services that Medicare doesn't cover—such as emergency international travel or additional stays in the hospital.

Medicare Advantage plans (often called Medicare Part C) are private plans that contract with Medicare, which funds their coverage of Medicare Part A and B; however, the plans also typically cover other services and operate like an HMO or PPO, forming a sort of hybrid Medicare plan. Some Advantage plans offer dental, vision, or prescription drug coverage. It is important to note that states differ in types of Advantage plans and coverage and that some health care organizations do not accept Medicare Advantage plans.

In an era of rapidly increasing drug costs, prescription drug coverage is an essential part of any Medicare plan. Part A and Part B Medicare typically cover only minimal drugs, making the purchase of an additional drug plan, known as Medicare Part D, sensible for many individuals. People who opt for Advantage plans must check to find out whether or not their prescriptions are covered.

Medicaid
A federal–state matching funds program, **Medicaid** provides health insurance for approximately 74 million low-income Americans, including children, pregnant women, adults, older adults, and people with disabilities.[15] Because each state determines income eligibility, covered services, and payments to providers, there are vast differences in the way Medicaid operates from state to state. The ACA provides generous federal subsidies to states that expand Medicaid coverage to all Americans with incomes up to 133 percent (and, in some states, 138 percent) of the federal poverty threshold (in 2016 the poverty threshold was $24,300 for a four-person household).[16] Although states are not responsible for the costs to expand Medicaid until 2020, at which time states will be required to fund just 10 percent of the costs, some have refused. However, state compliance with the Medicaid expansion brought insurance coverage to 12.3 million previously uninsured low-income Americans between 2013 and 2015.[17]

The Children's Health Insurance Program (CHIP) provides health insurance coverage to more than 8 million uninsured children whose family income is too high to qualify for Medicaid.[18] Like Medicaid, CHIP is jointly funded by federal and state funds and is administered by state governments.

Insurance Coverage by the Numbers

For 2016, the average family's annual health insurance premium was estimated to exceed $18,142.[19] For workers employed in organizations that offer health care insurance, most of this cost is hidden. The worker pays 15 to 25 percent of the full premium, usually as a deduction from his or her paycheck, and earns lower wages in return for the remaining cost of the coverage. However, people who are self-employed or work in companies that do not provide group health insurance must pay their premiums independently, often at extremely high rates. Despite the implementation of the ACA, 28.2 million uninsured Americans (over 9 percent of Americans) do not find health insurance affordable.[20] These numbers could increase significantly if ACA is changed during this presidential term. The vast majority of uninsured Americans are employed or are dependents of people who are employed.

Lack of health insurance has been associated with delayed health care and increased mortality. *Underinsurance* (the inability to pay out-of-pocket expenses despite having insurance) also may result in adverse health consequences. Among young adults age 18 to 24, nearly 15 percent lack health insurance coverage; among those age 25 to 34, nearly 16 percent lack coverage.[21] College students as a group fare better than non-college adults when it comes to insurance. In a 2016 national survey of college students, 3.4 percent of respondents said they did not have health insurance.[22] People without adequate health care coverage are

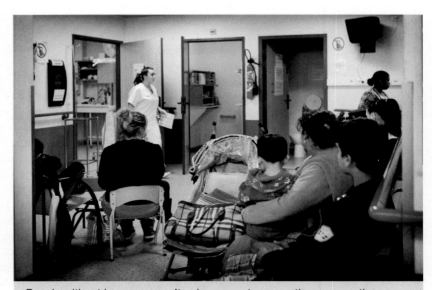

People without insurance can't gain access to preventive care, so they seek care only in an emergency or crisis. Because emergency care is extraordinarily expensive, they often are unable to pay, and the cost is absorbed by those who can pay—the insured or taxpayers.

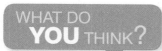

WHAT DO YOU THINK?

Why is it important that private insurance cover preventive or lower-level care as well as hospitalization and high-tech interventions?

- What kinds of incentives would cause you to seek care early rather than delaying care?

less likely than other Americans to have their children immunized, seek early prenatal care, obtain annual blood pressure checks and other screenings, and seek attention for symptoms of health problems. Forgoing preventative care because of cost, they tend to rely on emergency care at later stages of illness. Because emergency care is far more expensive than other types of care, uninsured and underinsured patients are often unable to pay, and the cost is absorbed by "the system" in the form of higher hospital costs, insurance premiums, and taxes for all.

LO 4 | ISSUES FACING TODAY'S HEALTH CARE SYSTEM

Explain key issues facing our health care system today and possible actions that could improve the system.

In 2010, Congress passed the *Patient Protection and Affordable Care Act (ACA)* to provide a means for all Americans to obtain affordable health care. In addition to increasing access to care, the ACA is addressing the high cost of care and improving the overall quality of care.

Access

The most significant factors in determining access to health care are the supply and proximity of providers and facilities and the availability of insurance coverage.

Access to Providers, Facilities, and Treatments

In 2016, there were more than 926,000 physicians in the United States.[23] However, there is an oversupply of higher-paid specialists and a shortage of lower-paid primary care physicians (e.g., family practitioners, internists, pediatricians). Moreover, the majority of nongovernment hospitals in the United States are located in urban areas, leaving many rural communities underserved.[24]

Managed care health plans determine access on the basis of participating providers, health plan benefits, and administrative rules. As a result, consumers have little say in who treats them or what facility they can use.

The ACA and other government investments have helped in training many new health care providers and have encouraged primary care providers to set up their practices in high-need areas. Some of these efforts have included the following:

- Investing in new primary care training programs such as the National Health Service Corps and the Graduate Medical Education program
- Training new primary care providers through increased funding of medical training programs
- Supporting mental and behavioral health training to boost numbers of practitioners in mental and behavioral health.

Access to High-Quality Health Insurance Key provisions in the ACA aim to increase access to quality health insurance among Americans. These include the following:

- Insurers are now required to cover 15 preventive services (22 for women), such as health screenings for breast, cervical, and colorectal cancer; blood glucose and cholesterol screenings for patients of certain ages or with certain health risks; immunizations; contraception; and counseling on topics such as losing weight, quitting smoking, treating depression, and reducing alcohol use.
- Insurers are required to cover young adults on a parent's plan through age 26.
- Coverage is in place for prescription medications, including psychotropic medications.
- Americans with preexisting conditions cannot be denied coverage.
- No annual and lifetime limits on benefits are allowed.
- An online insurance marketplace helps consumers shop for and enroll in plans as well as apply for federal subsidies that lower the cost of premiums for many Americans.
- Small businesses, which typically paid as much as 18 percent more than large businesses, now qualify for special tax credits to help fund insurance plans.

Even before passage of the ACA, Congress provided assistance with insurance coverage for employees who change jobs. Under the Consolidated Omnibus Budget Reconciliation Act (COBRA), former employees, retirees, spouses, and dependents have the option to continue their insurance for up to 18 months at group rates. People who enroll in COBRA do pay a higher amount than they did when they were employed because they are covering both the personal premium and the amount previously covered by the employer.

Cost

Both per capita and as a percentage of gross domestic product (GDP), the United States spends more on health care than any other nation (**FIGURE 15.2**). In 2015, our national health expenditures were estimated to exceed $3.2 trillion, about $9,990 for every man, woman, and child.[25] Health care expenditures are projected to grow by 5.6 percent each year to and climb to over 20 percent of our projected GDP by 2025.[26]

Why are U.S. health care costs so high? Many factors are involved: duplication of services; an aging population; growing rates of obesity, inactivity, and related health problems; demand for new diagnostic and treatment technologies; an emphasis on crisis-oriented care instead of prevention; physician overtreatment; and inappropriate use of services.

Our insurance system is also to blame. Currently, more than 2,000 companies provide health insurance in the United States, each with different coverage structures and administrative requirements. This lack of uniformity prevents our system from achieving the *economies of scale* (bulk purchasing at a reduced cost) and administrative efficiency that are realized in countries with a single-payer delivery system. On average, America's commercial insurance companies spend about 16 percent of

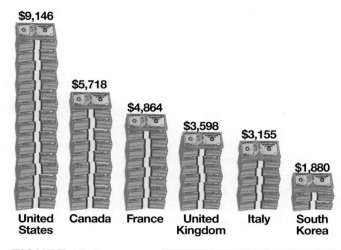

$9,146

$5,718

$4,864

$3,598

$3,155

$1,880

United States Canada France United Kingdom Italy South Korea

FIGURE 15.2 Health Care Spending per Person, 2014

 Watch Video Tutor: Being a Good Health Care Consumer in Mastering Health.

Source: The World Bank, "Health Care Expenditure per Capita," 2016, http://data.worldbank.org/indicator/SH.XPD.PCAP.

their total premiums on administrative costs.[27] These expenses contribute to the high cost of health care. See **FIGURE 15.3** for a breakdown of how our health care dollars are spent.

The ACA's 80/20 rule mandates that insurance companies that spend less than 80 percent of premium dollars on medical care in a given year now must send enrollees a rebate. Also, insurance companies now have to publicly justify their actions if they plan to raise rates by 10 percent or more.

Another way our insurance system contributes to America's high health care costs is through increasing consolidation. Excluding HMOs and other forms of managed care, just four companies dominate 83 percent of the private health insurance market, a market share that expanded from 74 percent a decade ago.[28] Since affordable insurance depends on rivalry within the market, reduced competition promotes higher premiums. Moreover, despite the fact that these large companies serve more patients within a geographic area and thus have been able to negotiate lower charges from hospitals and physicians, they have not passed this savings along to their policyholders in the form of lower premiums.[29]

Quality

The United States has several mechanisms for ensuring the quality of health care services: Providers are assessed according to education, licensure, certification or registration, accreditation, peer review, and the legal system of malpractice litigation.

OTC and prescription medications, as well as medical devices, must be approved by the FDA. Insurance companies and the U.S. Centers for Medicare and Medicaid Services may also require a higher level of quality by linking payment to whether a practitioner is board certified, whether a facility is accredited, or whether a treatment is an approved therapy. In addition, most insurance plans now require prior authorization and/or second opinions, not only to reduce costs, but also to improve quality of care.

Although our health care spending far exceeds that of any other nation, the United States rank far below many other nations in key indicators of health care quality. For example, in 2017, the Central Intelligence Agency ranked the United States 42nd in life expectancy among 224 nations ranked.[30] At a projected 79.8 years, U.S. life expectancy was a decade below that of the top-ranked country, Monaco.[31] And our *infant mortality rate*, at 5.8 deaths per every 1,000 live births, is higher than that of 56 other nations.[32] The ACA is intended to improve the quality of health care in the United States. As a first step, in 2011, the Department of Health and Human Services released to Congress a National Strategy for Quality Improvement in Health Care. Updated annually, the National Quality Strategy emphasizes promoting the safest, most preventive, and most effective care; making care affordable for individuals, families, employers, and governments; increasing communication and coordination among providers; and ensuring that patients and families are engaged as partners in their care.[33]

Still, many health experts believe that our system has failed and should be replaced (see the **Points of View** box for a discussion). For you as a consumer, the best strategy is to read the accumulated evidence on what is and is not working in the health care system and base your decisions on a rational, unbiased approach as we work to improve health care delivery in the United States.

2013 total expenditures = $2.6 trillion

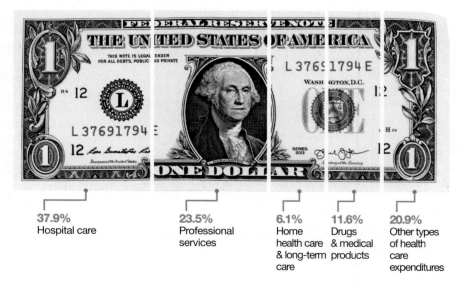

37.9% Hospital care

23.5% Professional services

6.1% Home health care & long-term care

11.6% Drugs & medical products

20.9% Other types of health care expenditures

FIGURE 15.3 Where Do We Spend Our Health Care Dollars?

Source: U.S. Department of Health and Human Services, "Health, United States, 2015," National Center for Health Statistics, May 2016, www.cdc.gov/nchs/data/hus/hus14.pdf.

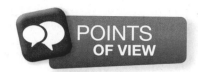
NATIONAL HEALTH CARE
Is It a Government Responsibility?

Whether universal health care coverage will—or should—be achieved in the United States and, if so, through what mechanism remain hotly debated topics. Proponents of reform argue that health care is a basic human right and should be available and affordable for everyone. They point to countries such as Canada, the United Kingdom, France, Israel, Taiwan, and Japan that currently provide health care to all citizens through a national service funded primarily through taxes. Opponents of universal health care feel that health care is not a right, but a commodity. They contend that the high cost of changing the system is more than the United States can afford and that the government should not interfere in what has been largely a free-market industry. In addition, lobbying efforts by the insurance industry, pharmaceutical manufacturers, the medical community, and special interest groups have all played a role in thwarting comprehensive reform.

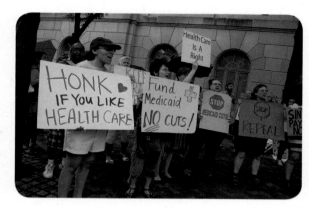

In 2010, Congress passed the Patient Protection and Affordable Care Act (ACA)—a set of initial steps toward increasing the number of insured Americans. Both before and after its passage, the ACA has been the subject of intense and often rancorous debate. The reforms mandated by the ACA are currently being implemented, but their actual effects are still uncertain. Meanwhile, opponents of the ACA have made attempts to repeal or replace it.

Arguments for National Health Insurance

- Health care is a human right. Article 25 of the United Nations Universal Declaration of Human Rights states that "everyone has the right to a standard of living adequate for the health and well-being of oneself and one's family, including . . . medical care."
- Americans would be more likely to engage in health-promoting behaviors. People who are underinsured and uninsured forego preventive care checkups, wait to be seen about troubling symptoms, and fail to take prescribed medications because of cost concerns.
- Medical professionals could concentrate on the care of patients rather than on insurance procedures, malpractice liability, and other administrative distractions.
- Providing all citizens the right to health care is good for economic productivity because it allows them to live longer and healthier lives, thus contributing to society for a longer time.

Arguments against National Health Insurance

- Health care is not a right. It is not covered by the Bill of Rights in the U.S. Constitution, which lists rights that the government cannot infringe upon, not services or goods that the government must ensure for the people. Amending the U.S. Constitution to acknowledge a right to health care would be bad for economic productivity.
- It is the individual's responsibility, not the government's, to ensure personal health. Diseases and health problems can often be prevented by individuals choosing to live healthier lifestyles.
- Expenses for health care would have to be paid for with higher taxes or spending cuts in other areas, such as defense and education.

WHERE DO YOU STAND?

- Do you think that the United States should move toward a system of national health care? Why or why not?
- Is health insurance a private or a public issue?
- Do you currently have health insurance? If you don't, why not? Do you think that people should have the choice to spend their money on other things rather than health insurance, or should it be mandated that everyone pay for insurance?
- If you do have health insurance, are you currently paying for it? If you are not paying for it, who is?
- Do you have a family member or close friend who lives in a country with a national health care system? If so, does this person support national health care or not, and why?

Sources: United Nations, "The Universal Declaration of Human Rights," 1948, www.un.org/en/documents/udhr/index.shtml; P. Krugman, "The Medicaid Cure," New York Times, January 10, 2014; Right to Health Care ProCon.org, "Should All Americans Have the Right (Be Entitled) to Health Care?," Updated February 2017, http://healthcare.procon.org.

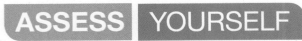
Are You a Smart Health Care Consumer?

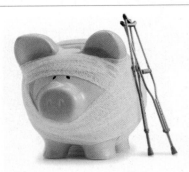

		Yes	No	Not Applicable
1.	Do you have health insurance? (If no, skip to 3.)	◯	◯	◯
2.	Do you understand the coverage available to you?	◯	◯	◯
3.	Do you know which health care services are available for free or at a reduced cost at your student health center or local clinic?	◯	◯	◯
4.	In the last year have you received a prescription for medication? (If no, skip to 9.)	◯	◯	◯
5.	When you received your prescription, did you ask the doctor or pharmacist whether a generic brand could be substituted?	◯	◯	◯
6.	When you received your prescription, did you ask the doctor or pharmacist about potential side effects, including possible food and drug interactions?	◯	◯	◯
7.	If you experienced any unusual drug side effects, did you report them to your health care provider?	◯	◯	◯
8.	Did you take medication as directed?	◯	◯	◯
9.	When you receive a diagnosis, do you seek more information about the diagnosis and treatment?	◯	◯	◯
10.	If your health care provider recommends surgery or an invasive type of treatment, do you seek a second opinion?	◯	◯	◯
11.	Do you seek health information only from reliable and credible sources?	◯	◯	◯
12.	Do you read labels carefully before buying OTC medications?	◯	◯	◯
13.	Do you have a primary health care provider?	◯	◯	◯
14.	Do you think advertising plays a significant role in your decision to purchase health care products and services?	◯	◯	◯

YOUR PLAN FOR **CHANGE**

Once you have considered your responses to the ASSESS YOURSELF questions, you may want to change or improve certain behaviors to get the best treatment from your health care provider and the health care system.

TODAY, YOU CAN:

☐ Research your insurance plan. Find out which health care providers and hospitals you can visit in your area, options for medical care outside your area, co-payment and premium costs, and plan drug coverage.

☐ Update your medicine cabinet. Dispose properly of any expired prescriptions or OTC medications. Keep on hand a supply of basic items, such as pain relievers, antiseptic cream, bandages, cough suppressants, and throat lozenges.

WITHIN THE NEXT TWO WEEKS, YOU CAN:

☐ Find a regular health care provider if you do not have one, and make an appointment for a general checkup.

☐ Do some research on health conditions you have experienced or that run in your family. Write down any unanswered questions for discussion with your health care provider.

BY THE END OF THE SEMESTER, YOU CAN:

☐ Ask whether a generic version is appropriate and available when you fill your next prescription.

☐ Become informed about health care issues in both your state and the country. Write to your state and congressional legislators to express your opinions about needed reforms.

STUDY PLAN

Visit the Study Area in Mastering Health to enhance your study plan with MP3 Tutor Sessions, Practice Quizzes, Flashcards, and more!

CHAPTER REVIEW

LO 1 | Taking Responsibility for Your Health Care

■ Knowing when to take care of yourself and when to seek professional help will save you money and improve your health status. Advance planning can help you navigate health care treatment in unfamiliar situations or emergencies. Assess health professionals by considering their qualifications, their record of treating similar problems, and their ability to work with you.

LO 2 | Conventional Health Care

■ In theory, conventional Western (allopathic) medicine is based on scientifically validated methods and procedures. Medical doctors, specialists of various kinds, nurses, physician assistants, and other health care professionals practice allopathic medicine.

■ Prescription drugs are obtained through a written prescription from a physician. Over-the-counter-drugs can be purchased without a prescription.

LO 3 | Health Insurance

■ Health insurance is based on the concept of spreading risk. Insurance is provided by private insurance companies (which charge premiums) and the government's Medicare and Medicaid programs (which are funded by taxes). Managed care (in the form of HMOs, PPOs, and POS plans) attempts to control costs by streamlining administrative procedures and promoting preventive care, among other initiatives.

LO 4 | Issues Facing Today's Health Care System

■ Concerns about the U.S. health care system involve access, cost, and quality. The Patient Protection and Affordable Care Act was passed by Congress in 2010 to address these issues. Many public health experts believe that it does not go far enough.

POP QUIZ

LO 1 | Taking Responsibility for Your Health Care

1. Of the following conditions, which would be appropriately managed by self-care?
   a. A persistent temperature of 104°F or higher
   b. Sudden weight loss of more than a few pounds without changes in diet or exercise patterns
   c. A sore throat, runny nose, and cough that persist for several days
   d. Yellowing of the skin or the whites of the eyes

2. A component of your rights as a patient includes informed consent. Informed consent means that before you receive any care, you
   a. should be fully informed of what is being planned.
   b. should know the risks and potential benefits.
   c. have the option to refuse treatment.
   d. all of the above.

LO 2 | Conventional Health Care

3. Which medical practice is based on treating the patient's symptoms using scientifically validated methods?
   a. Allopathic medicine
   b. Nonallopathic medicine
   c. Osteopathic medicine
   d. Chiropractic medicine

4. A specialist who diagnoses and treats diseases of the teeth, gums, and oral cavity is a(n)
   a. dentist.
   b. orthodontist.
   c. oral surgeon.
   d. periodontist.

5. Which is a common type of over-the-counter drug?
   a. Antibiotics
   b. Hormonal contraceptives
   c. Antidepressants
   d. Antacids

LO 3 | Health Insurance

6. What is the term for an amount paid directly to a provider by a patient before the patient's insurance carrier will begin paying for services?
   a. Coinsurance
   b. Cost sharing
   c. Co-payment
   d. Deductible

7. The most restrictive type of managed care is
   a. fee-for-service.
   b. health maintenance organizations.
   c. point of service.
   d. preferred provider organizations.

8. The federal health insurance program that covers people over the age of 65, permanently disabled people, and people with end-stage kidney failure is
   a. Medicare.
   b. Medicaid.
   c. COBRA.
   d. HMO.

9. Which of the following is a federal–state funds matching program

providing care for low-income individuals?
a. CHIP
b. Social Security
c. Medicaid
d. Medicare

LO 4 | Issues Facing Today's Health Care System

10. Which of the following is a key provision of the ACA?
    a. Insurers are required to cover only major medical emergencies.
    b. Lifetime limits on benefits are allowed if costs exceed a set amount.
    c. Insurers are required to cover young adults on a parent's plan through age 21.
    d. Americans with preexisting conditions can't be denied coverage.

Answers to the Pop Quiz can be found on page A-1. If you answered a question incorrectly, review the section identifies by the Learning Outcome. For even more study tools, visit **Mastering Health**.

THINK ABOUT IT!

LO 1 | Taking Responsibility for Your Health Care

1. List several conditions for which you wouldn't need to seek medical help. When would you consider each condition to be bad enough to require medical attention? How would you decide where to go for treatment?

2. Describe your rights as a patient. Have you ever received treatment that violated these rights? If so, what action, if any, did you take?

LO 2 | Conventional Health Care

3. What is the most common form of medicine practiced in Northern America? What is the scientific foundation for this form of medicine? What measures do practitioners take to help ensure a high quality of care?

LO 3 | Health Insurance

4. What are the inherent benefits and risks of managed care health insurance plans?

5. Explain the differences between traditional indemnity insurance and managed health care. Should insurance companies dictate reimbursement rates for various medical tests and procedures in an attempt to keep prices down? Why or why not?

LO 4 | Issues Facing Today's Health Care System

6. Discuss how the Affordable Care Act (ACA) has provided access to health care for Americans. What are the key provisions of the ACA?

ACCESS YOUR HEALTH ON THE INTERNET

Visit Mastering Health for links to the websites and RSS feeds.

The following websites explore further topics and issues related to health care.

Agency for Healthcare Research and Quality (AHRQ). This provides links to sites that can address health care concerns and information on what questions to ask, what to look for, and what you should know when making critical decisions about personal care. **www.ahrq.gov**

Food and Drug Administration (FDA). This website provides news on the latest government-approved home health tests and other health-related products. **www.fda.gov**

HealthGrades. This company provides quality reports on physicians as well as hospitals, nursing homes, and other health care facilities. **www.healthgrades.com**

National Committee for Quality Assurance (NCQA). The NCQA assesses and reports on the quality of managed care plans, including HMOs. **www.ncqa.org**

Healthcare.gov. This website provides up-to-date information regarding health care reform in the United States. **www.healthcare.gov**

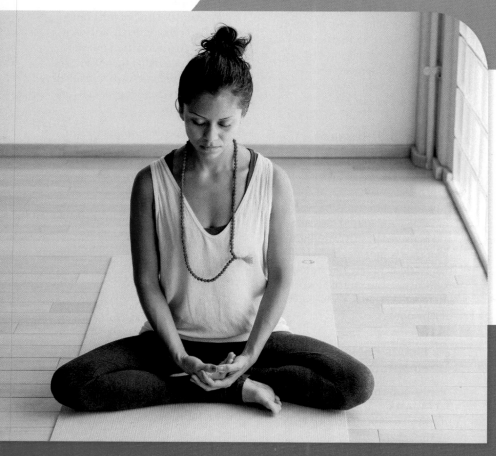

Understanding Complementary and Integrative Health

LEARNING OUTCOMES

1 Distinguish between complementary health approaches, alternative health approaches, and integrative medicine.

2 Describe four complementary medical systems in use in the United States.

3 Discuss several mind and body practices, including manipulative therapies and energy therapies.

4 Explain why caution is important in using natural products.

WHY SHOULD I CARE?

Conventional health care providers undergo rigorous training and licensure, and the medications and other therapies they prescribe are regulated by the FDA. In contrast, training of complementary and integrative health care providers varies, and their products and services do not undergo testing for effectiveness and safety before being marketed and sold. For this reason, you should discuss your use of complementary and integrative health approaches with your primary health care provider.

ncreasingly popular for both self-care and health promotion are a group of diverse medical systems, practices, and products that were developed outside of conventional mainstream Western medicine.[1] Although these offer consumers a broader range of choices and research suggests that some may be effective, the evidence of therapeutic benefits of others is not convincing, and a few have been associated with adverse effects.

LO 1 | WHAT ARE COMPLEMENTARY, ALTERNATIVE, AND INTEGRATIVE HEALTH APPROACHES?

Distinguish between complementary health approaches, alternative health approaches, and integrative medicine.

Complementary health approaches are non-mainstream practices and products that are commonly used along with conventional medicine.[2] A patient with chronic back pain, for example, may combine massage therapy with prescription medication. In contrast, **alternative health approaches** are used in place of conventional medicine, such as treating cancer by taking a herbal remedy or following a special diet instead of using surgery, radiation, or other conventional treatments. The National Center for Complementary and Integrative Health (NCCIH) reports that use of true alternative medicine is rare in the United States; most people who use non-mainstream approaches use them alongside conventional treatments.[3]

Doctors of medicine (MDs), doctors of osteopathy (DOs), nurses, and other allied health professionals practice conventional medicine. These practitioners may recommend massage therapy, nutrient supplements, or other complementary therapies for individual patients. However, some practitioners incorporate complementary therapies into their conventional health care in a coordinated, purposeful way. Increasing in popularity in many health care systems today, this coordinated approach is known as **integrative medicine**.[4]

A survey conducted by the NCCIH revealed that 33 percent of U.S. adults use one or more complementary therapies.[5] FIGURE 1 identifies those most commonly used. Why do so many people find complementary approaches appealing? Many people turn to these therapies to promote their general health and well-being or to relieve unrelenting symptoms associated with a chronic disease or the side effects of conventional medicine.[6] They may also be seeking a **holistic** approach, that is, care that focuses on the mind and the whole body rather than just an isolated symptom or body part. They may also desire an approach to healing that allows them a measure of control. Mindfulness meditation, for example, has been shown to increase patients' sense of control over their symptoms and treatment, reducing individual healthcare utilization as a result.[7] In one study of patients who had been trained in mindfulness, annual health care utilization dropped 43 percent, specifically, the average number of annual visits to the emergency department declined from 3.6 visits to 1.7 on average. By increasing patients' own self-care abilities, mindfulness training is thought to have the potential to substantially reduce overall health care costs.[8]

Although practitioners of most complementary health approaches spend many years in training, each approach has a different set of training standards, guidelines for practice, and licensure procedures. Moreover, there are no national standards, and states differ in their requirements. It is important to remember that a license or certificate does not guarantee effective or safe treatment from any provider, whether complementary or traditional. Consumers must be informed, ask questions, and make sound decisions when selecting any provider for any services. If you are considering any complementary therapy, visit the website of the NCCIH, a division of the National Institutes of Health. Its mission is to study complementary health approaches using rigorous scientific methods and to build an evidence base regarding their safety and effectiveness.

---

complementary health approaches Practices and products that originated outside of, but are used in conjunction with, conventional medicine.

alternative health approaches Practices and products that originated outside of, and are used in place of, conventional medicine.

integrative medicine Medical practice that brings conventional and complementary approaches together in a coordinated way.

holistic Relating to or concerned with the whole body and the interactions of systems rather than treatment of individual parts.

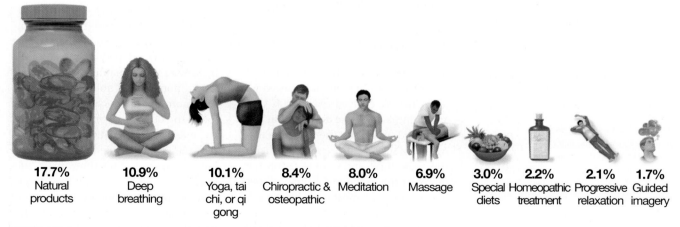

| 17.7% Natural products | 10.9% Deep breathing | 10.1% Yoga, tai chi, or qi gong | 8.4% Chiropractic & osteopathic | 8.0% Meditation | 6.9% Massage | 3.0% Special diets | 2.2% Homeopathic treatment | 2.1% Progressive relaxation | 1.7% Guided imagery |

FIGURE 1 The Ten Most Common Complementary Therapies among U.S. Adults

Source: Data from T.C. Clarke, et al., "Trends in the Use of Complementary Health Approaches among Adults: United States, 2002–2012," *National Health Statistics Reports*, no. 79 (2015). February 2015. Available at www.cdc.gov/nchs/data/nhsr/nhsr079.pdf.

32%

of 18- to 44-year-olds report having used a **COMPLEMENTARY HEALTH** approach.

The NCCIH groups the complementary health approaches into three general categories of practice: *natural products*, *mind and body practices*, and *other complementary health approaches*—what we'll call complementary medical systems.

LO 2

COMPLEMENTARY MEDICAL SYSTEMS

Describe four complementary medical systems in use in the United States.

Complementary medical systems reflect specific theories of physiology, health, and disease that have developed outside the influence of conventional medicine. Many of these systems have been used throughout the world for centuries. For example, Native American, Australian Aboriginal, African, Middle Eastern, South American, and Asian cultures have their own unique healing systems. Here, we discuss those most commonly available in the United States.

complementary medical systems Approaches to health care that reflect specific theories of physiology, health, and disease that have developed outside of conventional medicine.

traditional Chinese medicine (TCM) An ancient comprehensive system of healing that uses herbs, acupuncture, massage, and qigong to bring vital energy, *qi*, into balance and to remove blockages of *qi* that lead to disease.

Ayurveda (Ayurvedic medicine) A comprehensive system of medicine, originating in ancient India, that places equal emphasis on the body, mind, and spirit and strives to restore the body's innate harmony through diet, exercise, meditation, herbs, massage, sun exposure, and controlled breathing.

homeopathy (homeopathic medicine) An unconventional Western system of medicine based on the principle that "like cures like" and the "law of minimum dose."

Traditional Chinese Medicine

The concept of *qi* (pronounced "chee"), or vital energy, is the foundation of **traditional Chinese medicine (TCM)**. When *qi* is in balance, the person is in a state of health; imbalance of *qi* results in disease. Diagnosis is based on personal history, observation of the body (especially the tongue), palpation, and pulse diagnosis, a detailed procedure requiring considerable skill. Techniques such as acupuncture, herbal medicine, massage, and qigong (a form of energy therapy) are among the TCM approaches to health and healing. TCM is complex, and research into its effectiveness is limited.[9] Analyses of Chinese herbal medicines have found some of the medicines to be contaminated by toxic heavy metals, drugs not listed on the label, and other potentially harmful ingredients. Note that herbal supplements are regulated by the U.S. Food and Drug Administration (FDA) but not as foods or drugs. If you are taking a dietary supplement for a specific health problem, it is always best to talk with your health care provider to determine whether the supplement is safe for your health issue.[10]

TCM practitioners in the United States are required to have completed a graduate program in a college or university approved by the Accreditation Commission for Acupuncture and Oriental Medicine. Graduate programs usually involve a 3- or 4-year clinical internship. In addition, the student must pass a national certification and licensing examination.

Ayurveda

Ayurveda (Ayurvedic medicine), is one of the world's oldest medical systems, having evolved over 3,000 years ago in India. Its name derives from Sanskrit words meaning "the science of life." Ayurveda seeks to integrate and balance the body, mind, and spirit to restore harmony in the individual.[11] Practitioners use various diagnostic techniques to determine which of three vital energies, or *doshas*, is dominant in the patient. Treatment plans aim to bring the doshas into balance, thereby reducing symptoms. Dietary modification and herbal remedies drawn from the botanical wealth of the Indian subcontinent are common. Research into Ayurveda is limited, but studies have shown some of its herbal remedies to be effective for certain joint and digestive disorders.[12] However, some have been found tainted with lead, mercury, or arsenic.[13] Other Ayurvedic treatments include yoga, meditation, massage, steam baths, changes in sleep patterns, and controlled breathing.

Training of Ayurvedic practitioners varies. There is no national standard for certification, although professional groups are working toward creating licensing guidelines.

Homeopathy

Homeopathy (homeopathic medicine) is an unconventional Western system of medicine based on the principle that "like cures like." In other words, the same substance that in a large dose produces the symptoms of an illness—and may even be fatal—will in a small dose prompt the body's own defenses to cure the illness. Developed in the late 1700s by Samuel Hahnemann, a German physician, homeopathy follows the "law of minimum dose," which asserts that the lower the dose of a remedy, the greater its effectiveness. Thus, homeopathic remedies, which are derived from a wide range of natural, sometimes toxic, substances such as arsenic and belladonna, may be so diluted that no molecules of the original substance remain.[14] The NCCIH reports that certain foundational concepts in homeopathy are at odds with foundational concepts of physics and chemistry and that little

WHAT DO YOU THINK?

Why do you think so many people are choosing complementary health approaches?

▪ Do you or your friends use any complementary therapies? If so, which ones?

▪ What are the potential benefits of these therapies?

▪ What are the potential risks?

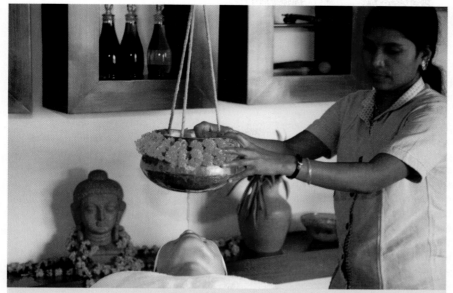

Shirodhara, a traditional Ayurvedic treatment in which warm herbalized oil is poured over the forehead in guided rhythmic patterns, is said to relieve stress and anxiety, treat insomnia and chronic headaches, and improve memory.

evidence supports homeopathy for treatment of any specific condition.[15]

Homeopathic training varies considerably, from diploma programs to correspondence courses. Only Arizona, Connecticut, and Nevada have homeopathic licensing boards. Requirements to practice vary from state to state.

Naturopathy

Naturopathy (naturopathic medicine) is a system of medicine that emphasizes the power of nature to restore health. Naturopathic physicians view their role as supporting the body's innate ability to maintain and restore health, typically by identifying and removing obstacles to these innate processes. They favor prevention and, when treatment is necessary, holistic, natural, and minimally invasive approaches.[16]

Specific approaches to care include diet; dietary supplements; homeopathy; spinal and soft-tissue manipulation; detoxification using fasting, juice diets, colon cleansing, or other means; and therapeutic counseling. Only some of these therapies have been researched, and results have varied; moreover, the complexity of naturopathic care has made this system challenging to study. Limited research suggests that naturopathy may be more effective than

conventional medicine for certain types of chronic pain. However, the efficacy and safety of some practices may not be supported by scientific evidence.[17]

Several major naturopathic schools in the United States and Canada provide training. *Naturopathic physicians* have completed a 4-year graduate program and, in most states, have passed a licensing examination. Naturopaths who are not physicians may have received less training and typically are unlicensed.

LO 3 | MIND AND BODY PRACTICES

Discuss several mind and body practices, including manipulative therapies and energy therapies.

Mind and body practices are a large and diverse group of complementary health approaches that a trained practitioner or teacher often teaches or administers.[18] They include movement reeducation therapies as well as modalities in which the practitioner directly manipulates body tissues, attempts to shift the flow of body energy, or teaches the client techniques to promote relaxation or manage stress. Several mind and body practices—including deep breathing,

yoga, chiropractic, meditation, massage, progressive relaxation, and guided imagery—are among the ten most commonly used complementary therapies in the United States (see Figure 1). One in particular—*mindfulness meditation*—is linked not only to increased psychological and physical health, but also to increased intellectual health, including health in the college classroom. See the **Mindfulness and You** box for more on the unexpected academic benefits of mindfulness.

Manipulative Therapies

Manipulative therapies are approaches based on manipulation or movement of body tissues and structures.

Chiropractic Medicine

Chiropractic medicine has been practiced for more than 100 years and focuses on disorders of the muscular and skeletal system and the use of various modalities to reduce health effects from these disorders.[19] Many health care providers work closely with chiropractors, and many insurance companies pay for chiropractic treatment recommended by a medical doctor.

Chiropractic medicine is based on the principle that energy flows through the nervous system. If the spine is misaligned, energy flow through the spinal cord is disrupted. Chiropractors manipulate the spine into proper alignment so that energy can flow unimpeded. Typically, chiropractors treat low back pain; neck pain; pain in the arms, legs, and feet; and headaches. Studies suggest that chiropractic spinal

naturopathy (naturopathic medicine) A system of medicine in which practitioners work to support the body's innate healing mechanisms and use treatment approaches such as diet, exercise, and massage that are minimally invasive.

mind and body practices A large and diverse group of complementary health approaches administered or taught by a trained practitioner or teacher.

manipulative therapies Treatments involving manipulation or movement of one or more body structures or the whole body.

chiropractic medicine A system of treatment that involves manipulation of the spine and neuromuscular structures to promote proper energy flow.

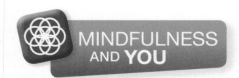

THE SURPRISING ACADEMIC BENEFITS OF MINDFULNESS MEDITATION

It's relatively well known that the regular practice of mindfulness can reduce symptoms of stress, anxiety, and depression and improve physical conditions such as obesity, hypertension, and asthma. But the benefits of mindfulness go beyond your psychological and physical health to intellectual health and even academic success.

A growing body of research links the long-term practice of mindfulness meditation to improvements in both the structure and function of the brain. Over time, mindfulness meditation appears to preserve and even enhance the integrity and connectivity of nerve cells in the white matter of the brain, thereby helping to reduce the amount of age-related brain tissue degeneration that takes place. In particular, the prefrontal cortex—the part of the brain associated with decision making and concentration—enlarges, and its connectivity to other parts of the brain increases. At the same time, the brain's fight-or-flight center, the amygdala, which is associated with fear and the stress response, appears to decrease in size, and its connectivity with other parts of the

brain decreases. The same is true for brain regions involving the perception of pain.

Even among novices, mindfulness meditation has been shown to boost cognitive skills, leading to better classroom performance. In one study, university students who participated in a one-semester mindfulness meditation course experienced significant improvements in both attention and memory, as well as the overall effectiveness of their learning. But a full semester of mindfulness training isn't required; another group that participated in a 2-week mindfulness training program saw improvements in reading comprehension and working memory, as well as less mind wandering. In another study, students who practiced just 6 minutes of meditation before a lecture scored higher on a quiz after the lecture than students who did not meditate. The researchers speculated that meditation before class could be especially helpful to students who have trouble maintaining focus. A similar study found that students who engaged in a 5-minute instructor-led mindfulness meditation at the start of class reported feeling more grounded and more focused on the class content.

So instead of rushing into class at the last possible moment, get there 5 minutes early, close your eyes, breathe deeply, and tune in. You might find that you feel more focused and engaged in class, retain more afterward, and perform better on the next exam.

Sources: M. Goretski and A. Zysk, "Using Mindfulness techniques to Improve Student Well-Being and Academic Performance for University Students: A Pilot Study," *Journal of Australian and New Zealand Student Services Association* 49 (April 2017), http://isana.proceedings.com.au /docs/2014/paper_goretzki.pdf; D. Laneri et al., "Effects of Long-Term Mindfulness Meditation on Brain's White Matter Microstructure and Its Aging," *Frontiers in Aging Neuroscience* 7 (2015); T. Ireland, "What Does Mindfulness Meditation Do to Your Brain?" *Scientific American*, June 12, 2014, https://blogs.scientificamerican.com /guest-blog/what-does-mindfulness-meditation -do-to-your-brain; H.H. Ching et al., "Effects of a Mindfulness Meditation Course on Learning and Cognitive Performance among University Students in Taiwan," *Evidence-Based Complementary and Alternative Medicine* 2015 (2015); M.D. Mrazek et al., "Mindfulness Training Improves Working Memory Capacity and GRE Performance While Reducing Mind Wandering," *Psychological Science* 24, no. 5 (2013): 776–81; J.T. Ramsburg and R.J. Youmans, "Meditation in the Higher-Education Classroom: Meditation Training Improves Student Knowledge Retention during Lectures," *Mindfulness* 5, no. 4 (2014): 431–41.

---

manipulation is as beneficial in easing low back pain as pain relief medications and other common remedies, particularly during the first 6 weeks of transient or acute episodes. However, the evidence for other benefits is less clear, and minor adverse effects of headache, muscle stiffness and pain may increase with manipulation.[20]

Chiropractic training typically begins with a premedical undergraduate degree followed by a 4-year chiropractic program involving intensive coursework similar to that of medical school programs, combined with hands-on clinical training. Graduates must also pass a licensing examination given by the National Board of Chiropractic Examiners. Chiropractic care is licensed and regulated in all 50 states.[21]

massage therapy Soft-tissue manipulation by trained therapists for relaxation and healing.

Massage Therapy

References to massage can be found in numerous ancient texts, including those of Greece, Rome, Japan, China, Egypt, and India.[22] **Massage therapy** is soft tissue manipulation by trained therapists for relaxation and healing. Therapists manipulate the patient's muscles and connective tissues to loosen the fibers and break up adhesions, improve the body's circulation, and remove waste products. The NCCIH reports that research evidence supports the effectiveness of massage therapy to temporarily relieve musculoskeletal pain such as low back and neck pain, and it may help to promote relaxation and relieve depression.[23]

The course of study in massage schools varies greatly by state but typically covers sciences such as anatomy and physiology as well as massage techniques and business, ethical, and

legal considerations.[24] For licensing, many states require a minimum of 500 hours of training and a passing grade on a national certification exam. Massage therapists work in private studios, health spas, medical and chiropractic offices, nursing homes, hotels, and fitness centers. The job outlook for massage therapists is very strong.[25]

Movement Therapies

A broad range of Eastern and Western complementary health approaches use movement, including postural realignment, to increase physical, mental, and emotional well-being and reduce limitations in body functioning. Two commonly available approaches are as follows:

■ The *Alexander technique* is a movement education method designed to release harmful tension in the body

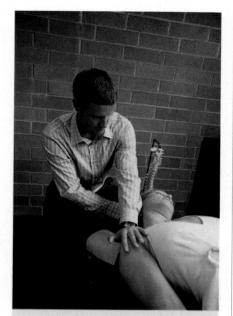

Chiropractic medicine is often used to treat pain. Chiropractors manipulate the alignment of the spine, allowing energy to flow freely throughout the body.

to improve ease of movement, balance, and coordination.

- The *Feldenkrais method* is a system of gentle movements and exercises designed to improve movement, flexibility, coordination, and overall functioning through techniques that enhance the client's awareness and retrain the nervous system.

Energy Therapies

Energy therapies focus either on energy fields thought to originate within the body (biofields) or from other sources (electromagnetic fields). The existence of these fields has not been experimentally proven. Popular examples of energy therapy include acupuncture, acupressure, qigong, Reiki, and therapeutic touch.

Acupuncture

One of the oldest and most popular TCM therapies, **acupuncture** is used to relieve a wide variety of health conditions, from musculoskeletal dysfunction to depression. The therapist stimulates various points on the body with a series of precisely placed and extremely fine needles. The stimulation of these acupuncture points is thought to increase the flow of *qi* through the *meridians*, or energy pathways, in the body.

After receiving acupuncture, most participants in clinical studies report satisfaction with the treatment and improvement in their condition; however, there is significant controversy over whether or not such results are simply a placebo response.[26] A recent review study found acupuncture effective in achieving at least a 50 percent reduction in headache frequency; however, sham acupuncture achieved a 43 percent reduction.[27] Moreover, a 2017 clinical trial found sham acupuncture as effective as true acupuncture for the treatment of irritable bowel syndrome.[28] In contrast, a 2016 review study found acupuncture beneficial for back pain and knee pain.[29]

Acupuncture licensing requirements vary by state; however, most states require a diploma from the National Certification Commission for Acupuncture and Oriental Medicine. In addition, many conventional physicians and dentists practice acupuncture.[30]

Acupressure

Like acupuncture, **acupressure** is based on the principles of the flow of *qi*. Instead of inserting needles, however, the therapist applies pressure. The goal of the therapy is for *qi* to be evenly distributed and flow freely throughout the body. Practitioners of acupressure typically have the

energy therapies Therapies using energy fields such as electromagnetic fields or biofields.

acupuncture A technique of traditional Chinese medicine that involves the placement of long, thin needles to affect the flow of energy (*qi*) along energy pathways (meridians) within the body.

acupressure A technique of traditional Chinese medicine that uses application of pressure to selected points along meridians to balance energy.

same basic training and understanding of meridians and acupuncture points as do acupuncturists.

Other Forms of Energy Therapy

Qigong, a technique of TCM, brings together movement, meditation, and regulation of breathing to increase the flow of *qi*, enhance blood circulation, and improve immune function. A 2015 systematic review of meta-analyses found that the practice of qigong and other meditative movement therapies was associated with statistically significant improvements in pain management and other aspects of health-related quality of life for people recovering from breast cancer as well as people with low back pain, heart failure, and other conditions.[31]

Reiki is a non-touch form of energy therapy that originated in Japan. The name is derived from the Japanese words representing "universal" and "vital

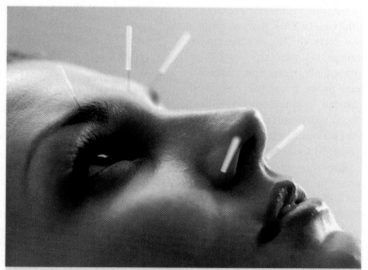

In acupuncture, long, thin needles are inserted into specific points along the body. This is thought to increase the flow of life-force energy, providing many physical and mental benefits.

energy," or *ki*. Reiki is based on the belief that by channeling *ki* to the patient, the practitioner facilitates healing. In two related non-touch energy therapies, *therapeutic touch* and *healing touch*, the therapist attempts to perceive, through his or her hands held just above the patient's body, imbalances in the patient's energy. The therapist promotes healing by increasing the flow of the body's energies and bringing them into balance. Although studies have found at least a partial therapeutic response from non-touch energy therapies, the contribution of patients' expectations and desires to the outcome (a form of placebo effect) is not known.[32]

LO 4 | NATURAL PRODUCTS

Explain why caution is important in using natural products.

Natural products include functional foods and dietary supplements. (For definitions and basic descriptions, see Chapter 10.) They are the most commonly used and perhaps the most controversial of complementary health approaches because of the sheer number of options available, the many claims that are made about their effects, and the fact that they do not undergo FDA approval.

First, although it's tempting to assume that natural products are safe because they are labeled "natural," the FDA has not developed a definition for the term *natural* and cautions consumers to avoid assuming that any food or dietary supplement claiming to be "natural" is safe.[33] For example, in recent years, dietary supplements have caused a variety of health problems, such as liver damage, heart problems, and miscarriage, and some supplements have been found to be contaminated with bacteria, toxic metals, and hidden drug ingredients as well as grass, gluten, or other potential allergens. When you consider taking supplements, choose those labeled with the U.S.

Pharmacopoeia Verified Mark (**FIGURE 2**), a label that means that what it says on the bottle is in the bottle, that the supplement doesn't contain unsafe levels of contaminants, and that the product was created through well-controlled, sanitary manufacturing processes.[34]

The NCCIH "Alerts and Advisories" web page continually releases notifications of natural products that are contaminated or contain hidden drug ingredients. In early 2017, for example, the FDA recalled three weight-loss supplements containing sibutramine, a controlled substance linked to life-threatening surges in blood pressure and pulse, and a fourth containing ephedra, an herb banned for its association with heart attack, stroke, and sudden death.[35] Moreover, the NCCIH warns that some natural products can be dangerous when combined with prescription or over-the-counter drugs, can disrupt the normal action of those drugs, or can cause unusual side effects.[36] It is essential to consult your primary health care provider before using dietary supplements.

In recent years, there have been increasing media claims about the health benefits of various hormones, enzymes, and other biological and synthetic compounds. Although a few products, such as melatonin (a hormone) or zinc lozenges (a mineral), have been widely studied, there

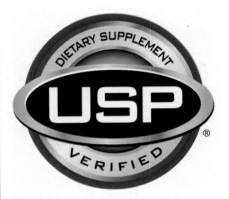

FIGURE 2 **The USP Verified Mark**
The USP Verified Mark is given only to products that meet a set of testing criteria, including accurately labeling content, no unsafe levels of contaminants, and sanitary processes. Registered Trademark of U.S. Pharmacopeial Convention (USP).

Source: Used with permission of The United States Pharmacopeial Convention, 12601 Twinbrook Parkway, Rockville, MD 20851.

is little high-quality research to support the claims of many others. **TABLE 1** gives an overview of some of the most common dietary supplements on the market.

Individuals must take an active role in their health care, which means staying educated. See the Skills for Behavior Change box for tips on how to make smart decisions about integrating complementary therapies into your health care.

TABLE **1** | Common Dietary Supplements: Benefits, Research, and Risks

Herb	Claims of Benefits	Research Findings	Potential Risks
Echinacea (purple coneflower, *Echinacea purpurea*, *E. angustifolia*, *E. pallida*)	Stimulates the immune system and helps fight infection. Used to both prevent and treat colds.	Some studies have provided evidence that taking Echinacea slightly reduces the risk for catching a cold but does not shorten the duration or severity of colds.	Allergic reactions, including rashes and anaphylaxis (a life-threatening allergic reaction), increased asthma, nausea, stomach pain.
Flaxseed (*Linum usitatissimum*) and flaxseed oil	Used to treat constipation, diabetes, and hot flashes and to reduce cholesterol levels and risk of heart disease and cancer.	Flaxseed contains soluble fiber and may have a laxative effect. It has not been shown to be effective in decreasing hot flashes. Insufficient data are available on the effect of flaxseed on diabetes, cholesterol levels, heart disease, or cancer risks.	Flaxseed may have hormonal effects and should not be used during pregnancy or nursing. Can cause diarrhea. Few other side effects. Flaxseed should be taken with plenty of water.
Ginkgo (*Ginkgo biloba*)	Popularly used to prevent cognitive decline, dementia, vision and hearing problems, and vascular disease.	There is no conclusive evidence that ginkgo has any health benefits.	Headache, nausea, upset stomach, and allergic skin reactions. Ginkgo seeds are highly toxic; only products made from leaf extracts should be used.
Ginseng (*Panax ginseng*)	Claimed to increase resistance to stress, boost the immune system, slow aging, and relieve various physical and psychological disorders.	There is no conclusive evidence that ginseng has any health benefits.	Headaches, insomnia, and gastrointestinal problems are the most commonly reported adverse effects.
Green tea (*Camellia sinensis*)	Useful for reducing the risk for heart disease and some cancers, increasing mental alertness, and promoting weight loss.	Green tea contains caffeine and is thought to increase mental alertness. Both green and black tea may reduce heart disease risk factors. Studies of green tea and its effects on cancer are limited, and results are inconsistent. Data suggest that green tea is not effective for weight loss.	Insomnia, anxiety, irritability, headaches, liver problems, abdominal pain.
Zinc (mineral)	Supports immune system; lozenges, syrup, and nasal sprays used to lessen duration and severity of cold symptoms; slow progression of age-related macular degeneration (AMD).	Some research suggests that zinc lozenges or syrup can reduce the severity and duration of a cold if taken within 24 hours of onset of symptoms. Zinc may help slow the progression of AMD.	Use of zinc lozenges or syrup can cause nausea. Use of nasal sprays can results in loss of sense of smell, which can be permanent. Prolonged excessive use can reduce immune function and levels of copper and HDL cholesterol.

Sources: National Center for Complementary and Integrative Health, "Herbs at a Glance," November 2016, https://nccih.nih.gov/health/herbsataglance.htm; Office of Dietary Supplements, National Institutes of Health, "Zinc: Fact Sheet for Consumers," February 2016, https://ods.od.nih.gov/factsheets/Zinc-Consumer.

ASSESS | YOURSELF

Do You Use Complementary Therapies Safely?

LIVE IT! ASSESS YOURSELF
An interactive version of this assessment is available online in Mastering Health.

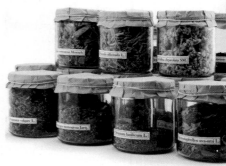

If you are like millions of Americans, you have already tried one or more complementary therapies (including supplements) or may be considering using one. If so, assess yourself: For each item, indicate whether you do or do not practice the recommended safety strategy.

	Yes	No
1. When considering a complementary therapy, do you research the scientific findings on safety and effectiveness?	○	○
2. Before scheduling an appointment with a complementary health practitioner or purchasing a natural product, do you check the NCCIH website for licensing and certification requirements, potential adverse effects, alerts and advisories, and other information?	○	○
3. If you buy dietary supplements, do you choose those with the USP Verified Mark on their label?	○	○
4. Do you tell all your health care providers about the complementary health approaches, including dietary supplements, you use, as well as all over-the-counter and prescription drugs?	○	○
5. Do you follow your practitioner's instructions and the instructions on the label of dietary supplements carefully?	○	○
6. Would you be able to articulate to a friend why a service or product labeled "natural" is not necessarily safe?	○	○

Interpreting Your Score

If you are using, or considering using, any type of complementary health approach, you should be able to answer "Yes" to each question with confidence. "No" responses indicate actions that you can begin to take to use complementary approaches with greater safety. Ultimately, these six strategies can help you take responsibility for your health.

YOUR PLAN FOR **CHANGE**

The **ASSESS YOURSELF** activity gave you the chance to evaluate your responsible use of complementary health approaches. Depending on the results of the assessment, and your own interest, you may consider investigating certain therapies further.

TODAY, YOU CAN:

☐ Close your eyes, and think of a calm place or activity you enjoy for a few minutes. Perhaps you are lying on a beach or are curled up in front of a fireplace. Clear your mind of everything else, and use relaxation to improve your health.

☐ Go to a credible website and look up information on a therapy you might be using or considering. What are the scientific findings? What are the benefits?

WITHIN THE NEXT TWO WEEKS, YOU CAN:

☐ Review your insurance documents or check with your carrier to learn what complementary therapies are covered. Ask which expenses you'll be responsible for and whether you are limited to a certain network of practitioners.

☐ Check with your college's health clinic or wellness center to find out what types of complementary therapies it offers.

BY THE END OF THE SEMESTER, YOU CAN:

☐ Schedule an appointment with your health care provider to discuss any complementary therapies you are considering.

☐ Make relaxation and stress-management techniques part of your everyday life. This can mean practicing meditation, deep breathing, or even taking long walks in nature.

STUDY **PLAN**

CHAPTER **REVIEW**

LO **1** | What Are Complementary, Alternative, and Integrative Health Approaches?

■ Complementary health approaches are used together with conventional medicine, whereas alternative approaches are used in place of conventional medicine. Integrative medicine is a practice that incorporates complementary therapies into conventional care in a coordinated, purposeful way.

LO **2** | Complementary Medical Systems

■ Complementary medical systems are comprehensive approaches to health care that reflect specific theories of physiology, health, and disease that have developed outside of conventional medicine. They include traditional Chinese medicine, Ayurveda, and other culturally based systems, as well as homeopathy and naturopathy.

LO **3** | Mind and Body Practices

■ Mind and body practices are a large and diverse group of complementary health approaches administered or taught by a trainer, practitioner, or teacher. They include manipulative therapies such as chiropractic medicine, movement therapies such as the Alexander technique, energy therapies such as acupuncture, and relaxation and stress-management modalities such as yoga and mindfulness meditation.

LO **4** | Natural Products

■ Natural products include functional foods such as those containing antioxidant phytochemicals or probiotics, as well as dietary supplements, products containing vitamins, minerals, herbs, or other ingredients and taken by mouth. The FDA does not study or approve dietary supplements before they are brought to market; therefore, there is no guarantee of their safety or effectiveness. Moreover, a label claim that a product is "natural" does not mean that the product is safe to use. However, the USP Verified Mark on the label does indicate that a supplement has met certain criteria for ingredient accuracy, product purity, and manufacturing standards.

POP **QUIZ**

LO **1** | What Are Complementary, Alternative, and Integrative Health Approaches?

1. Complementary health approaches typically focus on treating the mind and the whole body, so they are part of a
   a. natural approach.
   b. psychological approach.
   c. holistic approach.
   d. gentle approach.

LO **2** | Complementary Medical Systems

2. What type of medicine addresses imbalances of *qi*?
   a. Chiropractic medicine
   b. Ayurvedic medicine
   c. Traditional Chinese medicine
   d. Homeopathic medicine

LO **3** | Mind and Body Practices

3. Which of the following is a non-touch energy therapy?
   a. Acupressure
   b. Alexander technique
   c. Massage therapy
   d. Reiki

LO **4** | Natural Products

4. Which of the following supplements is claimed to stimulate the immune system to help fight infection?
   a. Echinacea
   b. Ginkgo
   c. Ginseng
   d. Green tea

Answers to the Pop Quiz can be found on page A-1. If you answered a question incorrectly, review the section identified by the Learning Outcome. For even more study tools, visit **Mastering Health.**

Aging, Death, and Dying

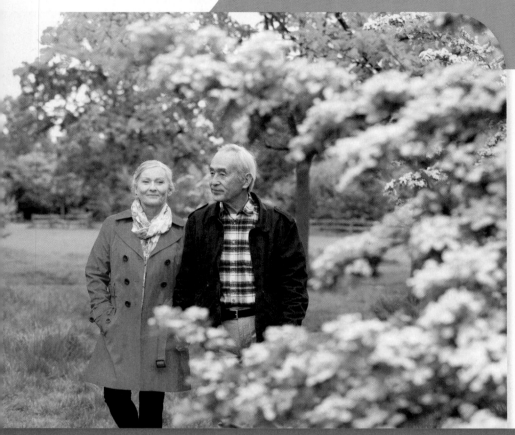

LEARNING OUTCOMES

1 Define aging, describe the physical and mental changes associated with aging, and explain how the growing population of older adults will affect society, including considerations of economics, health care, and living arrangements.

2 List strategies for successful and healthy aging.

3 Define death, and discuss strategies for coping with loss.

4 Explain the ethical concerns that arise from the concepts of the right to die and rational suicide.

5 Review the decisions that need to be made when someone is dying or has died, including hospice care, funeral arrangements, wills, and organ donation.

WHY SHOULD I CARE?

Aging isn't a distant process that will happen sometime in the future—it's happening now, to every one of us, every day of our lives. The way you live your life now has a direct impact on how you will live it in the future. Learning to cope with challenges and changes early in life develops attitudes and skills that contribute to a full and satisfying old age.

In a society that seems to worship youth, researchers have begun to offer good—even revolutionary—news about the aging process. Numerous studies show that people who make even modest beneficial lifestyle changes can reap significant health benefits. In fact, getting older can mean getting better in many ways—particularly socially, psychologically, spiritually, and intellectually.

LO **1** | AGING

Define aging, describe the physical and mental changes associated with aging, and explain how the growing population of older adults will affect society, including considerations of economics, health care, and living arrangements.

- -

Aging has traditionally been described as the patterns of life changes that occur in members of all species as they become older. The study of individual and collective aging processes, known as **gerontology**, explores the reasons

aging The patterns of life changes that occur in members of all species as they grow older.

gerontology The study of individual and collective aging processes.

Older Adults: A Growing Population

The United States and much of the developed world are on the brink of a *longevity revolution*, one that will affect society in many ways. Medical care breakthroughs and improved understanding of fitness and nutrition have steadily increased the human lifespan in the developed world. According to the latest statistics, life expectancy for a child in the United States born in 2016 is 79.8 years—more than 30 years longer than that for a child born in 1900.[1] In 2016, there were 47.8 million people age 65 or older in the United States, making up nearly 15 percent of the total population.[2] In comparison, the number of people age 65 and older has more than tripled since 1900 and is up 30 percent just since 2005! (see **FIGURE 1**).[3] Similar trends are seen throughout the world, and the percentage of people over age 60 worldwide is expected to hit 22 percent by 2050—a doubling or tripling since 2010.[4]

Health Issues for an Aging Society

Meeting the financial and medical needs of an older population, providing health care and adequate housing for older adults, and addressing end-of-life ethical considerations are all of concern in an aging society. Many people fear that the combination of fewer younger workers paying into the Social Security system and more older people drawing benefits for longer than ever before will result in tremendous government budget shortfalls and the potential bankruptcy of the system.

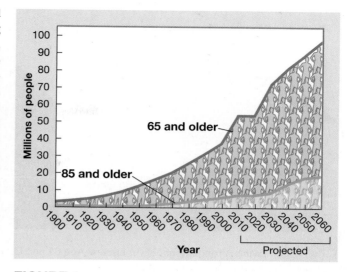

FIGURE 1 **Number of Americans 65 and Older (in millions), 1900–2008 and Projected 2010–2050** Data for 2010–2050 are projections of the population.

Source: Administration on Aging, U.S. Department of Health and Human Services, "Projected Future Growth of the Older Population," Administration on Aging, 2014, https://www.aoa.acl.gov/Aging_Statistics/future_growth/future_growth.aspx.

Health Care Costs

Older Americans averaged $5,756 in out-of-pocket medical expenses in 2016, an increase of 37 percent since 2005.[5] About 68 percent of those costs, on average, went to pay for health insurance itself; drugs and medical services not covered by insurance premiums accounted for roughly one-third of the costs.[6] As people live longer, their chances of developing a costly chronic disease increase, and as technology improves, chronic illnesses that once were quickly fatal may now be treated successfully for years. Most older adults have at least one chronic condition; about 75 percent have hypertension or are taking antihypertensive medication, 53 percent have been diagnosed with arthritis, 35 percent have heart disease, 324 percent have cancer, and 22 percent have diabetes.[7]

Housing and Living Arrangements

Most older adults never live in a nursing home (**FIGURE 2**). However, with increasing age comes an increased likelihood of some form of institutional setting. Just over 1 percent of those age 65 to 74 years, 3 percent of those age 75 to 85 years, and 10 percent of those over age 85 years live in nursing homes.[8] The average cost for institutional care varies tremendously by state and level of care, with a median price of over $92,000 per year for a private room in a nursing home and a median price of nearly $44,000 for an assisted living facility room.[9] But many older adults in the United States live on small fixed incomes, and in 2016, the government estimated that between 10 and 14 percent of older adults lived in poverty, and older women were significantly more

Grow old along with me!
The best is yet to be,
The last of life, for which the first was made . . .
—Robert Browning, *Rabbi Ben Ezra*

3.2%
of older adults live in **SKILLED NURSING CARE** facilities.

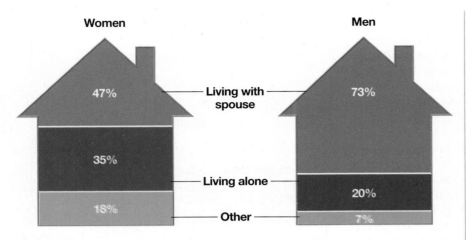

Women

47% — Living with spouse

35%

18%

Men

73% — Living with spouse

Living alone

20%

Other — 7%

FIGURE 2 Living Arrangements of Americans Age 65 and Older Percentages may not total 100 percent because of rounding.

Source: Administration on Aging, U.S. Department of Health and Human Services, "A Profile of Older Americans: Living Arrangements, 2016," 2017, https://www.giaging.org/documents/A_Profile_of_Older_Americans__2016.pdf.

---

osteoporosis A degenerative bone disorder characterized by increasingly porous bones.

likely to live in poverty.[10] Those without means are more likely to be shut out of all but the most meager care situations.

Physical and Mental Changes of Aging

Although the physiological consequences of aging can differ in severity and timing, certain physical, mental, and psychosocial changes occur as a result of the aging process (see **FIGURE 3**).

The Skin

As a normal part of aging, the skin becomes thinner and loses elasticity, particularly in the outer surfaces. Fat deposits, which add to the soft lines and shape of the skin, diminish. Starting at about age 30, lines develop on the forehead as a result of smiling, squinting, and other facial expressions. During one's forties, these lines become more pronounced, with added "crow's feet" around the eyes. In a one's fifties and sixties, the skin begins to thin, sag and lose color, which leads to pallor in one's seventies. Body fat in the underlying layers of skin continues to be redistributed away from the limbs and extremities into the body's trunk region. Age spots become more

numerous because of excessive pigment accumulation under the thinning skin, particularly in areas of the skin that have been exposed to a lot of sunlight.

Bones and Joints

Throughout the lifespan, bones are continually changing as minerals are accumulated and lost. By the third or fourth decade of life, mineral loss from bones becomes more prevalent than mineral accumulation, which results in a weakening and porosity (diminishing density) of bony tissue. **Osteoporosis** is a disease characterized by low bone density and structural deterioration of bone tissue, leaving bones susceptible to fracture and crippling malformation of the spine characteristic of the

"dowager's hump" that is seen in stooped individuals.

More than 54 million Americans have low bone density or osteoporosis. In fact, about 40 percent of women and 15 to 30 percent of men over 50 years of age will break a bone because of osteoporosis.[11] Some of the factors that predispose a person to developing osteoporosis are intrinsic and cannot be controlled, including gender, age, body size, ethnicity, and family history. But there *are* things you can do to prevent the disease. Adequate calcium intake is important, as is vitamin D, which helps the body absorb and use calcium more efficiently. Bone is a living tissue that grows stronger with exercise and weight-bearing activity; therefore, bone loss can be slowed or prevented with regular weight-bearing exercise, such as walking, jogging, and dancing, as well as through strength training. Unhealthy behaviors that contribute to bone loss include smoking, excessive alcohol consumption, and anorexia nervosa.

Another bone condition that afflicts almost 27 million Americans is *osteoarthritis*, a progressive breakdown of joint cartilage that becomes more common

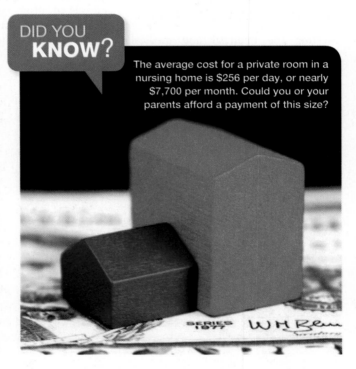

DID YOU KNOW?

The average cost for a private room in a nursing home is $256 per day, or nearly $7,700 per month. Could you or your parents afford a payment of this size?

Source: Genworth, "Compare Long-Term Care Costs across the United States," May 2016, http://newsroom.genworth.com/2016-05-10-Genworth-2016-Annual-Cost-of-Care-Study-Costs-Continue-to-Rise-Particularly-for-Services-in-Home.

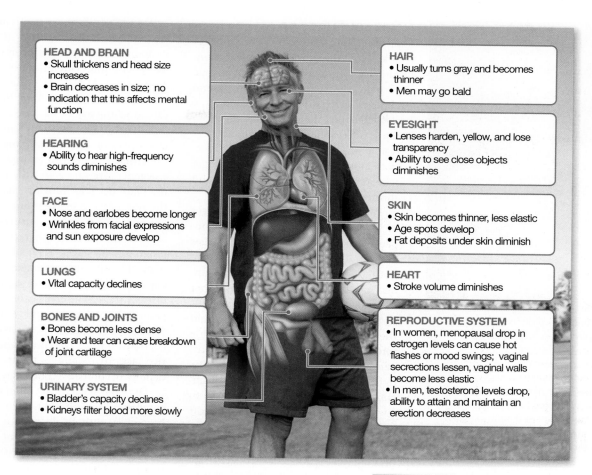

HEAD AND BRAIN
- Skull thickens and head size increases
- Brain decreases in size; no indication that this affects mental function

HEARING
- Ability to hear high-frequency sounds diminishes

FACE
- Nose and earlobes become longer
- Wrinkles from facial expressions and sun exposure develop

LUNGS
- Vital capacity declines

BONES AND JOINTS
- Bones become less dense
- Wear and tear can cause breakdown of joint cartilage

URINARY SYSTEM
- Bladder's capacity declines
- Kidneys filter blood more slowly

HAIR
- Usually turns gray and becomes thinner
- Men may go bald

EYESIGHT
- Lenses harden, yellow, and lose transparency
- Ability to see close objects diminishes

SKIN
- Skin becomes thinner, less elastic
- Age spots develop
- Fat deposits under skin diminish

HEART
- Stroke volume diminishes

REPRODUCTIVE SYSTEM
- In women, menopausal drop in estrogen levels can cause hot flashes or mood swings; vaginal secretions lessen, vaginal walls become less elastic
- In men, testosterone levels drop, ability to attain and maintain an erection decreases

FIGURE 3 Normal Effects of Aging on the Body

 Watch Video Tutor: **Effects of Aging on the Body** in Mastering Health.

with age and is a major cause of disability in the United States.[12]

The Urinary Tract

For about two-thirds of us, the thirties and forties bring a gradual decrease in the size and weight of the kidneys, effectively reducing blood filtering and other functions. In addition, shrinkage and thinning of the bladder and urinary tract affect urination.[13] Besides age, other key factors in these changes include high blood pressure, lead exposure, smoking, inflammation, obesity, and plaque formation. Some changes, such as hormonal decreases in women, may increase bladder and urinary tract changes, leading to **urinary incontinence**, which ranges from passing a few drops of urine while laughing or sneezing to having no control over urination.

However, incontinence is not an inevitable part of aging. Most cases are caused by persistent infections,

medications, treatable neurological problems that affect the central nervous system, weakness in the pelvic floor, and other factors. With treatment for infections and other conditions and exercises to strengthen the pelvic floor, the incontinence is usually resolved.

The Senses

With aging, the senses (vision, hearing, touch, taste, and smell) become less acute. By the time a person reaches age 30, the lens of the eye begins to harden, which can cause problems by the early forties. The lens also begins to yellow and lose transparency, and the pupil shrinks, allowing less light to penetrate. By age 60, depth perception declines, and farsightedness often develops. **Cataracts** (clouding of the lens) and **glaucoma** (elevated pressure within the eyeball) become more likely. Eventually, a tendency toward color blindness may develop, especially for shades of blue and green.

Macular degeneration is the breakdown of the light-sensitive area of the retina responsible for the sharp, direct vision needed to read or drive. Its effects can be devastating to independent older adults. Its causes are still being investigated.

Presbycusis, or age-related hearing loss, is one of the most common chronic conditions of older adults, affecting 25 to 30 percent of people between the ages of 65 and 74 and between 40 and 50 percent of people over 75 years of age.[14]

urinary incontinence The inability to control urination.

cataracts Clouding of the lens that interrupts the focusing of light on the retina, resulting in blurred vision and possibly eventual blindness.

glaucoma Elevation of pressure within the eyeball, leading to hardening of the eyeball, impaired vision, and possible blindness.

macular degeneration Breakdown of the macula, the light-sensitive part of the retina that is responsible for sharp, direct vision.

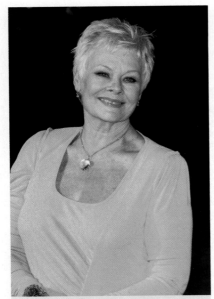

The people we often think of as aging gracefully, such as actress Dame Judi Dench, are those who continue to be active and productive; who are not frightened or ashamed of growing older; who adapt to the changing circumstances of their lives; and who strive to be healthy, vibrant, and alive at any age.

It is estimated that by 2020, 55 percent of people over the age of 70 or older will have presbycusis.[15]

With age, the ear structure also experiences changes and often deteriorates. The eardrum thickens, and the inner ear bones are affected. The inner ear is the portion that controls balance (equilibrium). As a result, it often becomes difficult for a person to maintain balance. Studies have shown that exercises including resistance/strength training, yoga, and tai chi can improve balance in older adults.[16] The ability to hear high-frequency consonants (e.g., *s*, *t*, and *z*) also diminishes with age. Much of the actual hearing loss lies in the inability to distinguish extreme ranges of sound rather than in the inability to distinguish normal conversational tones.

dementias Progressive brain impairments that interfere with memory and normal intellectual functioning.

Alzheimer's disease (AD) A chronic condition involving changes in nerve fibers of the brain that results in mental deterioration.

Sexual Function

As men age, they experience noticeable alterations in sexual function. Although the degree and rate of change vary greatly from man to man, several changes generally occur, including a slowed ability to obtain an erection, diminished ability to maintain an erection, and a decline in angle of the erection. Men may also experience a longer refractory period between orgasms and shortened duration of orgasm.

Women also experience changes in sexual function as they age. Menopause usually occurs between the ages of 45 and 55. Women may experience hot flashes, mood swings, weight gain, development of facial hair, or other hormone-related symptoms. The walls of the vagina become less elastic, and the epithelium thins, possibly making intercourse painful. Vaginal secretions, particularly during sexual activity, diminish. The breasts become less firm, and loss of fat in various areas leads to fewer curves, with a decrease in the soft lines of body contours.

Although these physiological changes may sound discouraging, sex is still an essential component in the lives of people in their mid-fifties and older, and many people remain sexually active throughout their entire adult lives. According to a recent study, the majority of people 50 to 80 years old are still very engaged about sex and intimacy.[17] With the advent of drugs such as Viagra and medical interventions designed to treat sexual dysfunction, many older adults can be sexually active. However, older adults report low percentages of condom use, signifying a need for education about the spread of STIs in the older population.

Mental Function and Memory

Certain physiological conditions or diseases may cause older people to experience memory loss, but in general, the knowledge and memories gained through a lifetime remain intact. Although short-term memory may fluctuate on a daily basis, the ability to remember events from past decades seems to remain largely unchanged in the absence of disease.

Dementing diseases, or **dementias**, are used to describe either reversible symptoms or progressive forms of brain malfunctioning. One of the most common forms is **Alzheimer's disease (AD)**. Affecting an estimated 1 in 10 Americans over the age of 65, or 5.5 million individuals, this disease is one of the most painful and devastating conditions that families can endure.[18] AD is a degenerative illness in which areas of the brain develop "tangles" that impair the way nerve cells communicate with one another, eventually causing the cells to die. This disease characteristically progresses in stages, each of which is marked by increasingly impaired memory and judgment. In later stages of the disease, these symptoms can be accompanied by agitation and restlessness (especially at night), loss of sensory perceptions, muscle twitching, and repetitive actions. Many patients become depressed, combative, and aggressive.

The final stage of AD often includes complete disorientation, with patients becoming entirely dependent on the help of others to dress, eat, and perform other daily activities. Identity loss and speech problems are common. Eventually, control of bodily functions may be lost. Patients with AD live for an average of 4 to 6 years after diagnosis, although the disease can last for up to 20 years.[19]

Researchers are investigating several possible causes of AD, including genetic predisposition, immune system malfunction, a slow-acting virus, chromosomal or genetic defects, chronic inflammation, uncontrolled hypertension, and neurotransmitter imbalance. No current treatment can stop the progression of the disease, but there are medications that can prevent progression of some symptoms for a short period of time or relieve symptoms such as sleeplessness, anxiety, and depression. Some researchers are looking at anti-inflammatory drugs, theorizing that AD may develop in response to an inflammatory ailment. Others are focusing on studying deposits of protein called plaques and their role in damaging and killing nerve cells.

Studies have found that meditation can lead to improvements in attention and memory in older adults.

Mindfulness-based interventions may also help older adults who are struggling with depression and anxiety.[20]

LO 2 | STRATEGIES FOR HEALTHY AGING

List strategies for successful and healthy aging.

You can do many things to prolong and improve the quality of your life. To provide for healthy older years, make each of the following part of your younger years.

Improve Fitness

Just about any moderate-intensity exercise that gets your heart beating faster and increases strength and/or flexibility will maximize your physical health and functional years. One of the physical changes that the body undergoes is *sarcopenia*, age-associated loss of muscle mass. The less muscle you have, the less energy you will burn even while resting. The lower your metabolic rate, the more likely it is that you will gain weight. With regular strength training, you can increase your muscle mass, boost your metabolism, strengthen your bones, prevent osteoporosis, and, in general, feel better and function more efficiently.

Both aerobic and muscle-strengthening activities are crucial for healthy aging. **TABLE 1** lists the basic recommendations for aerobic and strength-training exercises in older adults. In addition to these, the Centers for Disease Control and Prevention recommends that

people who are at risk of falling perform regular balance exercises.[21] Older adults and adults with chronic conditions should also develop an activity plan with a health professional to manage risks and take therapeutic needs into account. This will maximize the benefits of physical activity and ensure safety.

Eat for Longevity

Although other chapters in this text provide detailed information about nutrition and weight control, certain nutrients are especially essential to healthy aging:

- **Calcium.** Bone loss tends to increase in women shortly before menopause. During perimenopause and menopause, this bone loss accelerates rapidly, increasing risks for fracture and disability. Adequate consumption of calcium throughout one's life can help to prevent bone loss.
- **Vitamin D.** Vitamin D is necessary for adequate calcium absorption, yet as people age, they do not absorb vitamin D from foods as readily as they did in their younger years. If vitamin D is unavailable, calcium levels are also likely to be lower.
- **Protein.** Increasingly, research is showing that protein intake can improve people's health. The more protein you eat in a balanced diet, the better your body is at building muscle. So eating a diet high in protein helps to reduce the gradual loss of muscle mass that occurs most markedly after the age of 65.[22] Total calorie intake must be considered.

Many forms of activity can improve physical fitness.

Other nutrients, including vitamin E, folic acid (folate), iron, potassium, and vitamin B_{12} (cobalamin), are important in the aging process. Most of these are readily available in any diet that follows the U.S. Department of Agriculture's (USDA) MyPlate recommendations (www.choosemyplate.gov).

Develop and Maintain Healthy Relationships

Social bonds lend vigor and energy to life. Be willing to give to others, and seek variety in your relationships rather than befriending only people who agree with you. By experiencing diverse people and points of view, we gain broader perspective. Positive relationships are important for well-being at any age, but as people age, support systems decrease, making it particularly important to remain socially active.

Enrich the Spiritual Side of Life

Although some people take the spiritual side of life for granted, cultivating a relationship with nature, the environment, a higher being, and yourself is a key factor in personal growth and

TABLE 1 | Exercise Recommendations for Adults over Age 65

Option 1	Option 2	Option 3
Moderate-intensity aerobic activity (e.g., brisk walking) at least 2 hours and 30 minutes every week	Vigorous-intensity aerobic activity (e.g., jogging or running) at least 1 hour and 15 minutes every week	An equal mix of moderate- and vigorous-intensity aerobic activity
and	*and*	*and*
muscle-strengthening activity, working all major muscle groups, 2 or more days a week	muscle-strengthening activity, working all major muscle groups, 2 or more days a week	muscle-strengthening activity 2 or more days a week

Source: Centers for Disease Control and Prevention, "How Much Physical Activity Do Older Adults Need?," 2015, https://www.cdc.gov/physicalactivity/basics/older_adults/index.htm.

development. Adopt a mindfulness lifestyle. Take time to enjoy sunsets, the sounds of nature, and the energy of life. Taking "me time" will leave you invigorated and refreshed, better able to cope with the ups and downs of life.

LO **3**

UNDERSTANDING THE FINAL TRANSITIONS: DYING AND DEATH

Define death, and discuss strategies for coping with loss.

Throughout history, humans have attempted to determine the nature and meaning of death. Individuals' feelings about death vary widely, depending on many factors, including age, religious beliefs, family orientation, health, personal experience with death, and the circumstances of the death itself.

Defining Death

According to *Merriam-Webster's Collegiate Dictionary*, **death** can be defined as the "a permanent cessation of all vital functions: the end of life."[23] This definition has become more significant as medical advances make it increasingly possible to postpone death. Legal and ethical issues led to the Uniform Determination of Death Act in 1981. This act, which several states have adopted, reads as follows: "An individual who has sustained either (1) irreversible cessation of circulatory and respiratory functions, or (2) irreversible cessation of all functions of the entire brain, including the brain stem, is dead. A determination of death must be made in accordance with accepted medical standards."[24]

The concept of **brain death**, defined as the irreversible cessation of all functions of the entire brainstem, has gained

death The permanent ending of all vital functions.

brain death The irreversible cessation of all functions of the entire brainstem.

dying The process of decline in body functions that results in the death of an organism.

thanatology The study of death and dying.

FIGURE 4 Kübler-Ross's Stages of Dying Elisabeth Kübler-Ross developed this model while working with terminally ill patients. She later expanded the model to apply to people experiencing grief or significant loss of any kind.

increasing credence. As defined by the Ad Hoc Committee of the Harvard Medical School, brain death occurs when the following criteria are met[25]:

- Unreceptivity and unresponsiveness—that is, no response even to painful stimuli
- No movement for a continuous hour after observation by a physician and no breathing after 3 minutes off a respirator
- No reflexes, including brain stem reflexes; fixed and dilated pupils
- A "flat" electroencephalogram (which monitors electrical activity of the brain) for at least 10 minutes
- All of these tests repeated at least 24 hours later with no change
- Certainty that hypothermia (extreme loss of body heat) or depression of the central nervous system caused by use of drugs such as barbiturates are not responsible for these conditions.

The Harvard report provides useful guidelines. However, the definition of death and all its ramifications continue to concern us.

The Process of Dying

Dying is the process of decline in body functions that results in the death of an

WHAT DO YOU THINK?

Why is there so much concern over the definition of death?

- How does modern technology complicate the understanding of when death occurs?

organism. It is a complex process that includes physical, intellectual, social, spiritual, and emotional dimensions.

Kübler-Ross and the Stages of Dying

Much of our knowledge about reactions to dying stems from the work of Elisabeth Kübler-Ross, a pioneer in **thanatology**, the study of death and dying. In 1969, Kübler-Ross published *On Death and Dying*, a sensitive analysis of the reactions of terminally ill patients that encouraged the development of death education as a discipline and prompted efforts to improve the care of dying patients. Kübler-Ross identified five psychological stages (**FIGURE 4**) that people coping with death often experience[26]:

1. **Denial.** ("Not me, there must be a mistake.") A person intellectually accepts that death will soon occur but rejects it emotionally and feels a sense of shock and disbelief. The person is too confused

and stunned to comprehend "not being" and therefore rejects the idea.

2. **Anger.** ("Why me?") The person becomes angry at having to face death when other people, including loved ones, are healthy and not threatened. The dying person perceives the situation as unfair or senseless and may be hostile to friends, family, physicians, or the world in general.

3. **Bargaining.** ("If I'm allowed to live, I promise . . . .") The dying person may resolve to be a better person in return for an extension of life or may secretly pray for a short postponement of death in order to experience a special event, such as a family wedding or birth.

4. **Depression.** ("It's really going to happen to me, and I can't do anything about it.") Depression eventually sets in as the person's deteriorating condition becomes impossible for him or her to deny. Common feelings include doom, loss, a sense of worthlessness, and guilt over the emotional suffering of loved ones and the arduous but seemingly futile efforts of caregivers.

5. **Acceptance.** ("I'm ready.") This is often the final stage. The patient stops battling with emotions and becomes tired and weak. With acceptance, the person does not "give up" and become sullen or resentfully resigned to death but rather becomes calm and open to death.

Some of Kübler-Ross's contemporaries consider her stage theory too neat and orderly. Subsequent research has indicated that the experiences of dying people do not fit easily into specific stages and that patterns vary from person to person. Even if it is not accurate in all its particulars, however, Kübler-Ross's theory offers valuable insights for anyone seeking to understand or deal with the process of dying.

Social Death

The need for recognition and appreciation within a social group is nearly universal. Loss of being valued or appreciated by others can lead to **social death**, a situation in which a person is not treated like an active member of society. Numerous studies indicate that people are treated differently when they are dying, causing them to feel more isolated and unable to talk about their feelings. A decrease in meaningful social interaction often strips dying and bereaved people of their identity as valued members of society at a time when being able to talk, share, and make important decisions or say important things is critical.

Coping with Loss

Coping with the loss of a loved one is extremely difficult. The dying person, as well as close family members and friends, frequently suffers emotionally and physically from the loss of critical relationships and roles.

Bereavement is generally defined as the loss or deprivation that a survivor experiences when a loved one dies. In the lives of the bereaved or of close survivors, the loss of loved ones leaves "holes" and inevitable changes. Understanding normal reactions, time, patience, and support from loved ones can do much to help the bereaved heal and move on.

Grief occurs in reaction to significant loss, including one's own impending death, the death of a loved one, or a *quasi-death* experience (a significant loss such as the end of a relationship or job, which often involves separation, rejection, or a change in personal identity). Grief may be experienced as a mental, physical, social, or emotional reaction and often includes changes in patterns of eating, sleeping, working, and even thinking.

When a person experiences a loss that cannot be openly acknowledged, publicly mourned, or socially supported, coping may be much more difficult. This type of grief is referred to as *disenfranchised*

social death A seemingly irreversible situation in which a person is not treated like an active member of society.

bereavement The loss or deprivation experienced by a survivor when a loved one dies.

grief An individual's reaction to significant loss, including one's own impending death, the death of a loved one, or a quasi-death experience; can involve mental, physical, social, or emotional responses.

mourning The culturally prescribed behavior patterns for the expression of grief.

grief. It may occur among people who experience a miscarriage, who are developmentally disabled, or who are close friends rather than blood relatives of the deceased. It may also include relationships such as extramarital affairs or same-sex relationships.

Symptoms of grief vary in severity and duration, depending on the situation and the individual. However, the bereaved person can benefit from emotional and social support from family, friends, clergy, employers, and traditional support organizations. The larger and stronger the support system, the easier readjustment is likely to be. See the Skills for Behavior Change box to learn about how you can best help a grieving friend or loved one.

The term *mourning* is often incorrectly equated with the term *grief*. As we have noted, grief may involve a wide variety of feelings and actions that occur in response to bereavement. **Mourning**, in contrast, refers to culturally prescribed and accepted time periods and behavior

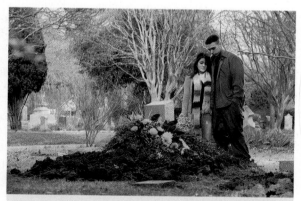

The most important thing you can do for a grieving friend is offer emotional support and a caring presence. Knowing what to say is less important than knowing how to listen.

BEHAVIOR CHANGE

Talking To Loved Ones When Someone Dies

Seeing a loved one grieving is never easy, and talking to someone about their loss can be a challenge. Here are a few ways to show some compassion to friends and loved ones in their time of need:

◉ Don't let your own sense of helplessness keep you from reaching out. Let your genuine concern and caring show. Say that you are sorry about their loss and pain.

◎ Be available to listen, run errands, or help with whatever they need.

◎ Don't change the subject when they mention the person who has died. Allow them to express as much grief as they are feeling and willing to share.

◎ Give reassurance, using whatever you know to be true and positive about the care given.

◎ Don't say you know how they feel. Unless you have suffered a similar loss, you probably don't. Encourage them to be patient with themselves and not worry about things they should be doing.

◎ Avoid comments such as "This is behind you; now it is time to get on with your life," or "Your loved one is in a better place now."

patterns for the expression of grief. In Judaism, for example, *sitting shiva* is a designated mourning period of 7 days that involves prescribed rituals and prayers. Depending on a person's relationship with the deceased, various other rituals may continue for up to a year.

What Is "Typical" Grief?

Grief responses vary widely from person to person but frequently include periodic waves of prolonged physical distress, a feeling of tightness in the throat, choking and shortness of breath, a frequent need to sigh, feelings of emptiness and muscular weakness, or intense anxiety that is described as actually painful. Other common symptoms of grief include insomnia, memory lapses, loss of appetite, difficulty concentrating, a tendency to engage in repetitive or purposeless behavior, a feeling of being removed from reality, difficulty making decisions, lack of organization, excessive

grief work The process of accepting the reality of a person's death and coping with memories of the deceased.

talking, social withdrawal or hostility, guilt feelings, and preoccupation with the image of the deceased. Susceptibility to disease increases with grief and may even be life threatening in severe and enduring cases.

The rate of the healing process depends on the amount and quality of grief work that a person does. **Grief work** is the process of integrating the reality of the loss into everyday life and learning to feel better. Often, the bereaved person must deliberately and systematically work at reducing denial and coping with the pain that comes from remembering the deceased.

Worden's Model of Grieving Tasks

William Worden, a researcher into the death process, developed an active grieving model that suggests four developmental tasks that a grieving person must complete in the grief work process[27]:

1. **Accept the reality of the loss.** This task requires acknowledging and realizing that the person

is dead. Traditional rituals, such as the funeral, help many bereaved people move toward acceptance.

2. **Work through the pain of grief.** It is necessary to acknowledge and work through the pain associated with loss, or it will manifest itself through other symptoms or behaviors.

3. **Adjust to an environment in which the deceased is missing.** The bereaved may feel lonely and uncertain about a new identity without the person who has died. This loss confronts them with the challenge of adjusting their own sense of self.

4. **Emotionally relocate the deceased and move on with life.** Individuals may need help in letting go of the emotional energy that used to be invested in the person who has died, and they may need help in finding an appropriate place for the deceased in their emotional lives.

LO 4 | LIFE-AND-DEATH DECISION MAKING

Explain the ethical concerns that arise from the concepts of the right to die and rational suicide.

When a loved one is dying, many complex and emotional—and often expensive—life-and-death decisions must be made during a highly distressing period in people's lives.

The Right to Die

Many people today believe that they should be allowed to die if their physical condition is terminal and their existence depends on mechanical life-support devices. Artificial life-support techniques that may be legally refused by competent patients include electrical or mechanical heart resuscitation, mechanical respiration by machine, nasogastric tube feedings, intravenous nutrition, gastrostomy (tube feeding directly into the stomach), and medications to treat life-threatening infections.

As long as a person is conscious and competent, he or she has the legal right to refuse treatment even if this decision will hasten death. However, when a person is in a coma or otherwise incapable of speaking on his or her own behalf, medical personnel, family members, and administrative policy will dictate treatment. This issue has evolved into a battle involving personal freedom, legal rulings, health care administration policy, and physician responsibility. The **living will** and other **advance directives** were developed to assist in solving these conflicts.

Even young, apparently healthy people need a living will. Consider Terri Schiavo, who collapsed at age 26 from heart failure that led to irreversible brain damage. Schiavo, unable to survive without life support, had never left any written guidelines about her wishes should she become incapacitated. After a 15-year legal battle between her parents, who wanted her to be kept alive, and her husband, who felt that she should be allowed to die, the courts sided with her husband, and she was removed from life support.

Many legal experts suggest that you take the following steps to ensure that your wishes will be carried out[28]:

- **Be specific.** Complete an advance directive that permits you to make very specific choices about a variety of procedures, including cardiopulmonary resuscitation (CPR); being placed on a ventilator; being given food, water, or medication through tubes; being given pain medication; and organ donation.
- **Name a health care proxy.** Appointing a family member or friend to act as your agent, or *proxy*, by completing a form known as either a *durable power of attorney for health care* or a *health care proxy*, allows the person to make medical decisions for you in the event that you are incapacitated.
- **Discuss your wishes.** Discuss your preferences in detail with your proxy and your doctor.
- **Deliver the directive.** Distribute several copies, not only to your doctor and your proxy, but also to your lawyer and to immediate family members or a close friend. Make sure *someone* knows to bring a copy to the hospital in the event you are hospitalized.

One alternative to the traditional advance directive or living will is a document called "Five Wishes," which meets the legal requirements for advance directive statutes in most states. This document differs from most other living wills because it addresses personal, emotional, and spiritual needs as well as medical needs.[29] It is available at low cost online at www.agingwithdignity.org.

Rational Suicide and Euthanasia

Thousands of terminally ill people every year decide to kill themselves rather than enduring constant pain and slow decay. This alternative to the extended dying process is known as **rational suicide**. To these people, the prospect of an undignified death is unacceptable. This issue has been complicated by advances in death prevention techniques that allow terminally ill patients to exist in an irreversible disease state for extended periods of time.

▶ **SEE IT!** VIDEOS

What are the options to consider at the end of life? Watch **Opting Out of Old Age?** in the Study Area of Mastering Health.

Euthanasia is often referred to as "mercy killing." The term **active euthanasia** refers to ending the life of a person or animal who is suffering greatly and has no chance of recovery. An example might be a physician-prescribed lethal injection, as in physician-assisted suicide. **Passive euthanasia** refers to the intentional withholding of treatment that would prolong life. Deciding not to place a person with massive brain trauma on life support is an example

living will A type of advance directive.

advance directive A document that stipulates an individual's wishes about medical care; used to make treatment decisions when and if the individual becomes physically unable to voice his or her preferences.

rational suicide The decision to kill oneself rather than enduring constant pain and slow decay.

active euthanasia "Mercy killing" in which a person or organization knowingly acts to end the life of a terminally ill person.

passive euthanasia The intentional withholding of treatment that would prolong life.

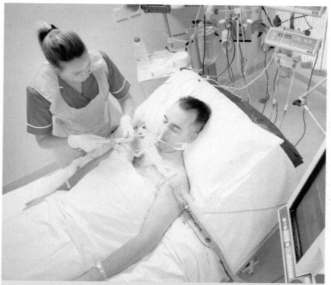

Today's sophisticated life-support technology can prolong a patient's life even in cases of terminal illness or mortal injury, yet not everyone would choose to have their life extended by such means. Living wills, advance directives, and health care proxies can protect your wishes and aid your loved ones should you become incapacitated.

SEE IT! VIDEOS

Should families have group conversations about end-of-life decisions? Watch **The Conversation: A Family's Private Decision**, on Mastering Health.

of passive euthanasia. Advance directives, such as "do not resuscitate" (DNR) orders, can provide legal justification for various forms of passive euthanasia.

LO 5 | MAKING FINAL ARRANGEMENTS

Review the decisions that need to be made when someone is dying or has died, including hospice care, funeral arrangements, wills, and organ donation.

Caring for a dying person and his or her bereaved loved ones involves a wide variety of psychological, legal, social, spiritual, economic, and interpersonal issues.

Hospice Care: Positive Alternatives

Since the mid-1970s, **hospice** programs in the United States have grown from a mere handful to more than 6,100 and are available in nearly every community.[30] These programs are a form of **palliative care** that focuses on reducing pain and suffering while attending to the emotional and spiritual needs of dying individuals and their caregivers. Hospice may help survivors cope better with the death experience.

The primary goals of hospice programs are to relieve the dying person's pain; offer emotional support to the dying person and loved ones; and restore a sense of control to the dying person, family members, and friends. Hospice programs also usually include the following characteristics:

hospice A concept of end-of-life care designed to maximize quality of life and help the dying person have peace, comfort, and dignity.

palliative care Any form of medical care that is focused on relieving the pain, symptoms, and stress of serious illness to improve the quality of life for patients and their families.

intestate Dying without a will.

- There is overall medical direction of the program, with all health care provided under the direction of a qualified physician. Emphasis is on symptom control, primarily the alleviation of pain.
- Services are provided by an interdisciplinary team.
- Coverage is provided 24 hours a day, 7 days a week, with emphasis on the availability of medical and nursing skills.
- Carefully selected and extensively trained volunteers who augment but do not replace staff service are an integral part of the health care team.
- Care of the family extends through the bereavement period.
- Patients are accepted on the basis of their health needs, not their ability to pay.

Making Funeral Arrangements

Anthropological evidence indicates that all cultures throughout human history have developed some sort of funeral ritual. For this reason, social scientists agree that funerals assist survivors of the deceased in coping with their loss. In some faiths, the deceased may be displayed in a *wake* or *viewing* to formalize last respects and increase social support of the bereaved. The funeral service may be held in a church or chapel, at a funeral home, or at the burial site. Some people choose to replace the funeral service with a simple memorial service held within a few days of the burial. Social interaction associated with funeral and memorial services is valuable in helping survivors cope with their losses.

Loved ones must also consider the cost of funeral and memorial options. They usually have to contact friends and relatives, plan for the arrival of guests, choose markers, submit obituary information to newspapers, and deal with many other details. Even though funeral directors are available to facilitate decision making, the bereaved may experience considerable stress, especially if the death is unexpected. People who make their own funeral arrangements ahead of time can save loved ones the difficulty of having to make these decisions during a very stressful time.

Wills

The issue of inheritance should be resolved before the person dies to reduce both conflict and needless expense. Unfortunately, many people die **intestate** (without a will). This is a mistake, especially because the procedure for establishing a legal will is relatively simple and inexpensive. If you don't make a will before you die, the courts (as directed by state laws) will make a will for you. Legal issues, rather than your wishes, will prevail. Furthermore, settling an estate takes longer when a person dies without a will.

Organ Donation

Organ donation takes healthy organs and tissues from one person for transplantation into another. Experts say that the organs from one donor can save or help as many as 50 people.[31] You can donate internal organs, skin, bone and bone marrow, and corneas.

The number of patients waiting for organ donations greatly outnumbers the number of available organs. Although some people are opposed to organ transplants and tissue donation, others experience personal fulfillment from knowing that their organs may extend and improve someone else's life after their own death. The most important step on the road to being an organ donor is to enroll in your state's donor registry. Go to www.organdonor.gov to sign up in your state. It is also a good idea to indicate your decision on your driver's license, tell your family and physician, and include the donation in your will and living will. Uniform donor cards are available through the U.S. Department of Health and Human Services and through many health care foundations and nonprofit organizations.

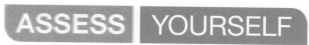
ASSESS YOURSELF

LIVE IT! ASSESS YOURSELF

An interactive version of this assessment is available online in Mastering Health.

Are You Afraid of Death?

How anxious or accepting are you about the prospect of your death? Indicate how well each statement describes your attitude.

Not true at all = **0**   Mainly not true = **1**   Not sure = **2**

Somewhat true = **3**   Very true = **4**

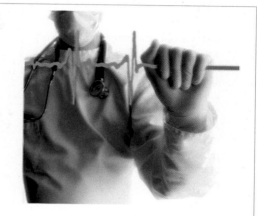

1. I tend not to be very brave in times of crisis situations. 0 1 2 3 4
2. I am something of a hypochondriac. 0 1 2 3 4
3. I tend to be unusually frightened in airplanes at takeoff and landing. 0 1 2 3 4
4. I would give a lot to be immortal in this body. 0 1 2 3 4
5. I am superstitious that preparing for dying might hasten my death. 0 1 2 3 4
6. My experience of friends and family dying has been wholly negative. 0 1 2 3 4
7. I would feel easier being with a dying relative if he or she had not been told he or she was dying. 0 1 2 3 4
8. I have fears of dying alone without friends around me. 0 1 2 3 4
9. I have fears of dying slowly and suffering. 0 1 2 3 4
10. I have fears of dying suddenly. 0 1 2 3 4
11. I have fears of dying young or while my children are still young. 0 1 2 3 4
12. I have fears of what could happen to my family after my death. 0 1 2 3 4
13. I have fears of dying in a hospital or an institution. 0 1 2 3 4
14. I have fears of not getting help with euthanasia. 0 1 2 3 4
15. I have fears of dying without having adequately expressed my love to those I am close to. 0 1 2 3 4
16. I have fears of being given unofficial and unwanted euthanasia. 0 1 2 3 4
17. I have fears of getting insufficient pain control while dying. 0 1 2 3 4
18. I have fears of being overmedicated and unconscious while dying. 0 1 2 3 4
19. I have fears of being declared dead when not really dead or being buried alive. 0 1 2 3 4
20. I have fears of what may happen to my body after death. 0 1 2 3 4

Total points: _____

Interpreting Your Score

If you are extremely anxious (scoring 38 or more), you might consider counseling or therapy. If you are unusually anxious (scoring between 24 and 37), you might want to find a method of meditation, philosophy, or spiritual practice to help experience, explore, and accept your feelings about death. Average anxiety is a score under 24.

YOUR PLAN FOR **CHANGE**

The **ASSESS YOURSELF** activity encouraged you to explore your death-related anxiety. Now that you have considered your results, you may want to take steps to lessen your fears about death and dying.

TODAY, YOU CAN:

- ☐ Learn about advance directives. Visit a low-cost legal clinic for information and a sample. You can also locate samples online, including the "Five Wishes" document, which is available at www.agingwithdignity.org.

- ☐ Fill out an organ donation card. Knowing that you may be able to prolong another person's life after your death can help you feel more at peace with your mortality.

WITHIN THE NEXT TWO WEEKS, YOU CAN:

- ☐ Consider how you would like to be remembered. Are you living in a way that you want to be remembered? What actions can you take now to help ensure that your eulogy reflects your ideal life course?

- ☐ Talk to family members about their life goals. What have they achieved? What do they wish they had done differently? What can you learn from their experiences?

BY THE END OF THE SEMESTER, YOU CAN:

- ☐ Consider how you feel about various medical techniques that might be used in the event you become incapacitated. Do you feel comfortable being kept alive by a machine? Make your wishes on these matters known to family members and friends, and put your wishes in writing.

- ☐ Talk to your parents or grandparents about the arrangements they prefer in the event of their death. Do they want a burial or cremation? A full funeral or a small service? Making these decisions now will save you and your loved ones stress later.

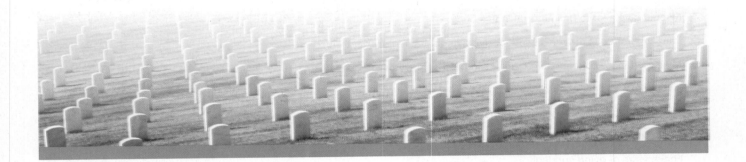

STUDY PLAN

Visit the Study Area in Mastering Health to enhance your study plan with MP3 Tutor Sessions, Practice Quizzes, Flashcards, and more!

CHAPTER REVIEW

LO 1 | Aging

- Aging is the pattern of life changes that occur in members of all species as they grow older. The growing number of older adults (people age 65 and older) has an increasing impact on society in terms of the economy, health care, housing, and ethical considerations.
- Major physical concerns of aging are osteoporosis, urinary incontinence, and changes in eyesight and hearing. Most older people maintain a high level of intelligence and memory. Potential mental problems include Alzheimer's disease.

LO 2 | Strategies for Healthy Living

- Lifestyle choices we make today will affect health status later in life. Choosing to exercise, eat a healthy diet, foster lasting relationships, and enrich your spiritual side will contribute to healthy aging.

LO 3 | Understanding the Final Transitions: Dying and Death

- Death can be defined biologically in terms of brain death or the cessation of vital functions. Dying is a multifaceted emotional process, and individuals may experience emotional stages of dying such as denial, anger, bargaining, depression, and acceptance. Social death results when a person is no longer treated as an active member of society.
- Grief is the state of distress felt after loss. People differ in their responses to grief.

LO 4 | Life-and-Death Decision Making

- Advanced directives assist people who believe they should be allowed to die if their physical condition is terminal and their existence depends on mechanical life-support devices or artificial feeding or hydration systems.
- The right to die by rational suicide involves ethical, moral, and legal issues.

LO 5 | Making Final Arrangements

- Hospice services are available to provide care for the terminally ill and their caregivers. After death, funeral arrangements must be made quickly. Customs vary by family, region, religious affiliation, and cultural background. Decisions made in advance of illness and death, including wills and organ donation decisions, make the process easier for survivors.

POP QUIZ

LO 1 | Aging

1. The progressive breakdown of joint cartilage is known as
   a. osteoporosis.
   b. osteoarthritis.
   c. calcium loss.
   d. vitamin D deficiency.

LO 2 | Strategies for Healthy Living

2. The keys to successful aging include
   a. drinking red wine regularly.
   b. reducing protein intake.
   c. avoiding weight-bearing activities.
   d. eating foods that contain enough calcium and vitamin D.

LO 3 | Understanding the Final Transitions: Dying and Death

3. The Kübler-Ross stage of dying in which the individual rejects death emotionally and feels a sense of shock and disbelief is known as
   a. acceptance.
   b. bargaining.
   c. denial.
   d. anger.

LO 4 | Life-and-Death Decision Making

4. Kerri's elderly grandmother is terminally ill and wants to die without medical intervention. Her family has agreed to withhold treatment that may prolong her life. This is called
   a. rational suicide.
   b. health care proxy.
   c. passive euthanasia.
   d. active euthanasia.

LO 5 | Making Final Arrangements

5. Destiny's grandfather dies intestate. This means that he
   a. had a health care proxy.
   b. did not have a will.
   c. received hospice care.
   d. did not have a trust.

Answers to the Pop Quiz can be found on page A-1. If you answered a question incorrectly, review the section identified by the Learning Outcome. For even more study tools, visit **Mastering Health**.

16 Promoting Environmental Health

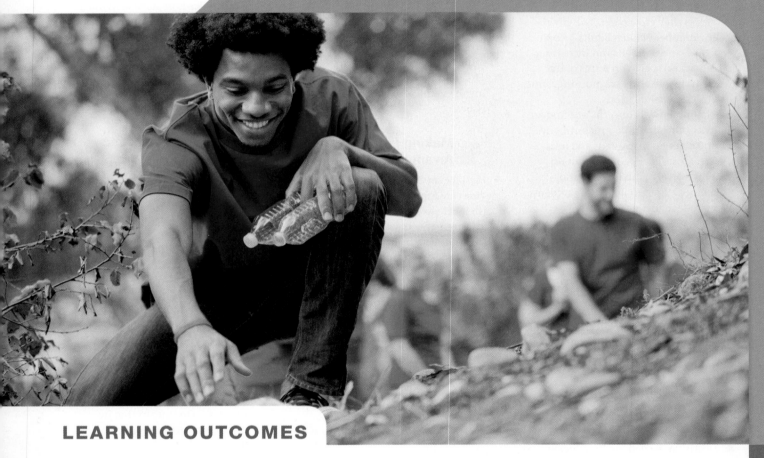

LEARNING OUTCOMES

1 Explain the environmental impact associated with global population growth.

2 Describe major causes of air pollution and the consequences of greenhouse gas accumulation and ozone depletion.

3 Explain climate change and global warming, the underlying causes of each, impacts on health, and how alternative energy and individual actions can reduce risks.

4 Identify sources of pollution and chemical contaminants often found in water.

5 Distinguish between municipal solid waste and hazardous waste, and list strategies for reducing land pollution.

6 List and explain key health concerns associated with ionizing and nonionizing radiation.

Currently, we consume Earth's resources at a rate that is 1.5 times the sustainable rate. What happens when the global population zooms to 9 to 12 million and much of the growth is in high-fertility countries that use increasing amounts of resources? Major challenges lie ahead unless individuals and nations cut consumption, reduce waste, and create policies to curb population growth.

"2014 was the planet's warmest year on record. Now, one year doesn't make a trend, but this does—14 of the 15 warmest years on record have all fallen in the first 15 years of this century."

—Barack Obama, excerpt from January 2015 State of the Union Address.

The global population has grown more in the past 50 years than at any other time in human history. All these people pose a potentially devastating threat to our water, air, food supply, and capacity to survive. Polar ice caps and glaciers are melting at rates that surpass even the most dire predictions of a decade ago, and threats of rising sea levels loom large. According to one report, we have lost 58 percent of the world's mammals, fish, birds, amphibians, and reptiles in the last 40 years.[1] Unsustainable agriculture, overfishing, habitat loss and degradation, and other human-driven activities all contribute.[2] Drought, fires, floods, and a host of other natural disasters create additional stress on dwindling resources. Clean, safe drinking water is becoming scarce in many parts of the world, fossil fuels are being depleted, and the amount of solid and hazardous waste is growing at exponential rates. Is this "fake news"? Virtually the entire scientific community says "no."

This chapter provides an overview of the factors contributing to the global environmental crisis and a blueprint for action. Staying informed, making important behavioral changes, and becoming an advocate for a healthy environment are key things you can do to help.

LO 1 | OVERPOPULATION: THE PLANET'S GREATEST THREAT

Explain the environmental impact associated with global population growth and our global ecological footprint.

The United Nations projects that the world population will grow from its current level of 7 billion people to 9.8 billion by 2050, given recent jumps in **fertility rates**—the average number of births per woman in a specific country or region.[3] Add increases in overall survival, life expectancy at birth, and other variables, and the population may swell to over 12 billion by 2100.[4] Tomorrow's population will be significantly larger, younger on average, and more industrialized. It will consume more resources and produce even more waste than previous generations unless population growth is controlled

and major changes in environmental policy and behavior occur.[5]

Global Population Growth

Key factors leading to population growth are changes in fertility and mortality rates. While many developed countries have shown consistent declines in fertility rates in recent years, other countries, particularly those in the most impoverished areas, continue to have high rates. Although lower fertility rates might slow the rate of population growth, sheer population sizes of countries such as India and China can cause major increases even if fertility rates remain constant or decline (**TABLE 16.1**).[6]

WHAT DO YOU THINK?

Should individuals get tax breaks for having fewer children?

- How would such policies compare to our current policies?
- Can you think of other policies that might be effective in encouraging population control and resource conservation in the United States?

97%

of **GLOBAL POPULATION GROWTH** in the next four decades will happen in Asia, Africa, Latin America, and the Caribbean

Historically, in countries where women have little education and little control over reproductive choices and where birth control is either not available or frowned upon, pregnancy rates continue to rise. As women become more educated, obtain higher socioeconomic status, work more outside the home, and have more control over reproduction—as birth control becomes more accessible—fertility rates decline. Many countries have enacted strict population control measures or have encouraged their citizens to limit the size of their families. Proponents of *zero population growth* believe that each couple should produce only two offspring, allowing the population to stabilize.

fertility rate Average number of births a female in a certain population has during her reproductive years.

TABLE 16.1 | Selected Total Fertility Rates Worldwide, 2015

Country	Number of Children Born per Woman*
Niger	7.6
Somalia	6.4 ↓
India	1.8 ↓
Mexico	2.3 ↓
United States	1.8 ↓
Australia	1.8 ↓
Canada	1.6
China	1.6 ↓
Russia	1.8
European Union	1.6 ↑

*Indicates the average number of children that would be born per woman if all women lived to the end of their childbearing years and bore children according to a given fertility rate at each age.
↓ ↑ Denotes change from 2015 fertility rates. If no arrow, no change.

Source: Data from Population Reference Bureau, "World Population Data Sheet," 2016, http://www.prb.org/pdf16/prb-wpds2016-web-2016.pdf.

Currently, China, with 1.4 billion people, and India, with 1.3 billion people, are the two most populous countries, making up 37 percent of the world's population.[7] Of the world's ten largest nations, Nigeria is growing the fastest.[8]

With a current population of over 326 million and a net gain of one person every 8 seconds, the United States is among the largest and fastest-growing industrialized nations.[9] It also has one of the largest **ecological footprints**—a measure of the biologically productive land and water area an individual or a population occupies and uses—exerting a greater impact on many of the planet's resources than do most other nations.[10]

Measuring the Impact of People

Experts are analyzing the **carrying capacity of the earth**—the largest population that can be supported indefinitely, given the resources available in the environment. At what point will we be unable to restore the balance between humans and nature? Or are we beyond that point?

Since 1996, the global demand for natural resources has doubled. Currently, an estimated 1.6 planets worth of resources are necessary to meet resource demands. By 2030, it will take the equivalent of two planets to meet the demand for

ecological footprint A measure of the biologically productive land and water area an individual, a population, or activity occupies and utilizes.

carrying capacity of the earth The largest population that can be supported indefinitely given the resources available in the environment.

ecosystem The physical (nonliving) and biological (living) components of an environment and the relationships between them.

resources, and by 2100, we may need more than four planets to support human needs. Simply put, we are running out of the natural resources necessary to sustain us, and the problem is growing at an unprecedented rate.[11] Vast differences exist between countries that have the *biocapacity* to sustain their growth and those that are draining the global capacity to sustain life. When essential resources become unavailable, the likelihood of human conflict to ensure survival will increase, along with increased pressure on all living things.

Evidence of the effects of unchecked human population growth is everywhere:

- **Impact on other species.** Changes in the **ecosystem** are resulting in the mass destruction of many species and their habitats.[12] Over 477 vertebrate species have gone extinct since 1900. Vertebrates are declining at rates over 100 times faster than normal rates of extinction, prompting some scientists to predict the *sixth mass extinction of living creatures*, similar to the fifth extinction, which occurred with the demise of the dinosaurs.[13] According to a recent report by the International Union for the Conservation of Nature, nearly 25 percent of Earth's existing known mammal species are threatened with extinction.[14] Over 41% of all currently known amphibians and large numbers of other species are also threatened with extinction.[15] Rapid declines in plant species and habitat are also reasons for concern.[16]

- **Impact on ecosystems.** Aquatic ecosystems are heavily contaminated by chemical and human waste. Our oceans are 30 percent more acidic than they were just 200 years ago, largely owing to human-caused pollutants.[17] Coral reefs that support aquatic life have declined by over 50 percent in the last 27 years, with dead zones stretching for miles.[18]

- **Impact on the food supply.** Globally, oceans are being fished at rates 250 percent faster than they can regenerate. Scientists project a global collapse of all fish species by 2050 and major food shortages.[19] While increasing amounts of the earth's surface are used for agriculture, drought, erosion, and natural disasters make growing food increasingly difficult, and food shortages and famine occur in many regions of the world with increasing frequency.[20]

- **Land degradation and contamination of drinking water.** The per capita availability of freshwater is declining rapidly, and contaminated water remains the greatest single environmental cause of human illness. Unsustainable land use and climate change are increasing land degradation, including erosion, toxic chemical infiltration, nutrient depletion, deforestation, and other problems. Fracking and other processes place additional pressure on increasingly scarce ground and surface water reserves.[21]

- **Energy consumption.** "Use it *and* lose it" is an apt saying for our greedy use of nonrenewable

▶ SEE IT! VIDEOS

What are the environmental and human costs of fashion and what's one solution? Watch **Actress Rosario Dawson's Mission for Sustainable Fashion** in the Study Area of Mastering Health.

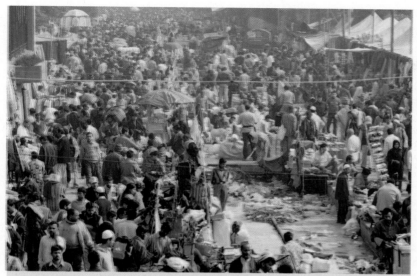

Every year, the global population grows by 115 million, but Earth's resources are not expanding. Population increases are believed to be responsible for most of the current environmental stress.

(cars, trucks, and buses) or *off-road* (sources such as construction equipment). Planes, trains, and watercraft are considered *nonroad* sources.[24] Today, 82 percent of all greenhouse gases are from carbon dioxide (CO_2).[25] In the United States, fossil fuels used to generate electricity contribute 37 percent of greenhouse gases, followed by transportation at 31 percent and industry at 15 percent.[26]

Components of Air Pollution

Congress passed the *Clean Air Act* in 1970 and has amended it several times since then. The act established standards for six of the most widespread air pollutants that seriously affect health: *carbon monoxide, sulfur dioxide, nitrogen dioxide, ground-level ozone, lead* and *particulates* (**TABLE 16.2**).

SEE IT! VIDEOS

How far does China's extreme smog extend from its capital Beijing? Watch **China Smog Creates What Some Call a Kind of Respiratory Nuclear Winter** on Mastering Health.

fossil fuels (oil, coal, and natural gas). On the basis of total population use, the United States is the largest consumer of liquid fossil fuels and natural gas and is among the top four consumers of nuclear power, coal, and hydroelectric power.[22] When ranked on a per person basis, Qatar ranks first in carbon emissions at 14.58 metric tons per person, and the United States ranks twelfth at 4.9 metric tons per person.[23] In many developing regions of the world, movement toward greater industrialization and increasing citizen affluence have resulted in skyrocketing demands for limited fossil fuels.

See the **Mindfulness and You** box for a reflection on *your* impact on the environment.

LO 2 | AIR POLLUTION

Describe major causes of air pollution and the consequences of greenhouse gas accumulation and ozone depletion.

The term *air pollution* refers to the presence of substances (suspended particles, gases, and vapors) not found in perfectly clean air. Air pollution is not new, but the vast array of **pollutants** that now exist and their potential interactive effects are.

Air pollutants are either *naturally occurring* or *anthropogenic* (caused by humans). Naturally occurring air pollutants include *particulate matter*, such as ash from volcanic eruptions, soil, and dust. Anthropogenic sources include those caused by *stationary sources* (e.g., power plants, factories, and refineries) and *mobile sources* such as vehicles. Mobile sources are *on-road*

Photochemical Smog

Smog is a brownish haze produced by the photochemical reaction of sunlight with **hydrocarbons**, nitrogen compounds, and other gases in vehicle exhaust. It is sometimes called *ozone pollution* because ground-level ozone is a main component of smog. Smog tends to form in areas that experience a **temperature inversion**, in which a cool layer of air is trapped under a layer of warmer air, preventing the air from circulating. Smog is most likely to occur in valley areas such as those in Los Angeles or Phoenix. The most noticeable adverse health effects of smog are difficulty breathing, burning eyes, headaches, and nausea. Long-term exposure to smog poses serious health risks, particularly for children, older adults, pregnant women, and people with chronic respiratory disorders.

Air Quality Index

The *Air Quality Index (AQI)*, a measure of how clean or polluted the air is on a given day, focuses on health effects that can happen within a few hours or days after breathing polluted air.

The AQI runs from 0 to 500, and the higher the AQI value, the greater the level of air pollution and associated health risks. When AQI values rise above 100—the level the Environmental Protection Agency (EPA) has set to protect public health—air quality is considered unhealthy. At certain levels,

fossil fuel Carbon-based material used for energy; includes oil, coal, and natural gas.

pollutant A substance that contaminates some aspect of the environment and causes potential harm to living organisms.

smog Brownish haze that is a form of pollution produced by the photochemical reaction of sunlight with hydrocarbons, nitrogen compounds, and other gases in vehicle exhaust.

hydrocarbons Chemical compounds containing carbon and hydrogen.

temperature inversion A weather condition that occurs when a layer of cool air is trapped under a layer of warmer air.

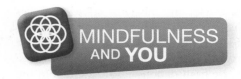

ENVIRONMENTAL MINDFULNESS
It Starts With You

Today's environmental challenges are mainly related to human actions and policies. Environmental Mindfulness means realizing that Earth isn't a "thing" or "place we use while here" but rather a giver of life with which we are intricately connected. We are so caught up in our own daily challenges that we don't pay attention to how our actions affect the planet. Zen master Thich Nhat Hanh has described humans living in a rapidly deteriorating planet as "a group of chickens fighting desperately over a few seeds of grain, unaware that in a few hours, they will all be killed."

We all need to do more to live unselfishly and connect with what is happening around us. We need to focus less on what others are doing and more on what *each of us* is doing as an individual, moment to moment, every day of our lives. We need to walk the proverbial talk about environmental concerns, to slow down, to care more by doing more to preserve and protect the planet for now and for future generations. Of course, it's not enough to just live in the moment; we need to *act* in the moment, by minimizing wasteful behaviors and doing more to tread more lightly on the earth.

There are thousands of ways that you can do your part to reduce your footprint and love the Earth. However you choose to do your part, take the time to notice what you are doing and how it might affect our scarce resources. Choose wisely and set clear goals. What steps will you take today? This week? How can you reduce, reuse, waste less, conserve more, and protect the world you live in—that we all live in? It all starts with you.

Source of quote: Thich Nhat Hanh, "The World We Have," *Lion's Roar: Buddhist Wisdom for Our Time*, April 6, 2017, https://www.lionsroar.com/the-world-we-have.

TABLE **16.2** | Sources, Health Effects, and Environmental Impacts of Six Major Air Pollutants

Pollutant	Description	Sources	Health Effects	Welfare Effects
Carbon monoxide (CO)	Colorless, odorless gas	Motor vehicle exhaust; kerosene- and wood-burning stoves	Headaches, impairment, cardiovascular diseases, death	Contributes to the formation of smog
Sulfur dioxide (SO_2)	Colorless gas that dissolves to form acid; interacts with other gases and particles	Coal-fired power plants, petroleum refineries, manufacture of sulfuric acid, and smelting of ores containing sulfur	Eye irritation, wheezing, chest tightness, shortness of breath, lung damage	Contributes to the formation of acid rain, visibility impairment, plant and water damage,
Nitrogen dioxide (NO_2)	Reddish brown, highly reactive gas	Motor vehicles, electric utilities, and other industrial, commercial, and residential fuel burning sources	Susceptibility to respiratory infections, respiratory symptoms (e.g., cough, chest pain, difficulty breathing)	Contributes to the formation of smog, acid rain, water quality deterioration, global warming, and visibility
Ground-level ozone (O_3)	Component of smog	Vehicle exhaust and other air pollutants in the presence of sunlight	Eye and throat irritation, coughing, respiratory tract problems, asthma, lung damage	Plant and ecosystem damage, global warming
Lead (Pb)	Metallic element	Metal refineries, lead smelters, battery manufacturers, iron and steel producers	Anemia, high blood pressure, cancer, brain, kidney, brain and IQ issues	Affects animals, plants, and the aquatic ecosystem
Particulate matter (PM)	Very small particles of soot, dust, or other matter, including tiny liquid droplets	Diesel engines, power plants, industries, dust, wood stoves	Eye irritation, respiratory problems cancer, heavy metal poisoning, cardiovascular effects	Visibility impairment, atmospheric deposition, aesthetic damage

Source: U.S. Environmental Protection Agency, "Air and Radiation: Air Pollutants," May 18, 2017, www.epa.gov.

it is unhealthy for specific groups of people, and at higher levels, it is unhealthy for everyone.

As **FIGURE 16.1** shows, the EPA has divided the AQI scale into six categories with corresponding color codes. National and local weather reports generally include information on the day's AQI.

Acid Deposition

Acid deposition, formerly called *acid rain*, refers to *wet* (rain, snow, sleet, fog, cloud water, and dew) and *dry* (acidifying particles and gases) acidic components that fall to the earth.[27]

Acid deposition gradually acidifies ponds, lakes, and other bodies of water. Once the acid content of the water reaches a certain level, plant and animal life cannot survive. Ironically, acidified lakes and ponds turn a crystal-clear deep blue, giving the illusion of beauty and health.

Every year, acid deposition destroys millions of trees in Europe and North America. For example, sugar maples and other trees in the northeastern United States are having difficulty replacing seedlings destroyed by these deposits. Much of the world's forestland has now experienced damaging levels of acid deposition.[28]

Acid deposition aggravates and may even cause bronchitis, asthma, and other respiratory problems, and people with emphysema or heart disease may suffer from exposure to acid deposition.[29] It may also be hazardous to fetuses. Acid deposition can cause metals such as aluminum, cadmium, lead, and mercury to **leach** out of the soil. If they make their way into water or food supplies, these metals can cause cancer in humans.

Indoor Air Pollution

Mounting evidence indicates that air pollution levels inside homes and other buildings, where we spend 90 percent of our time, may be two to five times higher than outdoor pollution levels.[30] Potentially dangerous chemical compounds can increase risks of cancer, contribute to respiratory problems, reduce the immune system's ability to fight disease, and increase allergy problems.

When the AQI is in this range:	... air quality conditions are	... as symbolized by this color:
0 to 50	Good	Green
51 to 100	Moderate	Yellow
101 to 150	Unhealthy for sensitive groups	Orange
151 to 200	Unhealthy	Red
201 to 300	Very unhealthy	Purple
301 to 500	Hazardous	Maroon

FIGURE 16.1 Air Quality Index (AQI) The EPA provides individual AQIs for ground-level ozone, particle pollution, carbon monoxide, sulfur dioxide, and nitrogen dioxide. All of the AQIs are presented using the general values, categories, and colors seen in this figure.

Source: U.S. Environmental Protection Agency, "Air Quality Index: AQI Basics," August 2016, https://airnow.gov/index.cfm?action=aqibasics.aqi.

SKILLS FOR BEHAVIOR CHANGE

Avoiding Mold

- Keep indoor humidity levels between 40 and 60 percent.
- Ventilate your living space. Use exhaust fans in the kitchen and bathrooms. Watch for leaks.
- Add mold inhibitors to paints or buy paints with mold-resistant properties. If you notice a musty smell or see mold, call your landlord.
- Do not carpet bathrooms and basements.
- Use a dehumidifier in damp rooms.
- Dry clothing thoroughly before putting away.
- Have a mold inspection performed before buying or renting a house, and check for mold regularly.

Indoor air pollution comes primarily from environmental tobacco smoke, cooking stoves and heat sources, household cleaners, mold, pesticides, asbestos, formaldehyde, radon, and lead. Today, more and more manufacturers offer green building products and furnishings, such as natural fiber fabrics, untreated wood for furniture and floors, and *low-VOC (volatile organic compound)* paints.

Multiple factors, including age, individual sensitivity, preexisting medical conditions, liver function, and immune and respiratory health, contribute to a person's risk for being affected by indoor air pollution.[31] People with allergies may be particularly vulnerable. Health effects may develop over years of exposure or may occur in response to toxic levels of pollutants, particularly in homes where air doesn't circulate freely. Room temperature and humidity also play a role. **TABLE 16.3** lists major sources of indoor air pollution and possible health effects.

Preventing indoor air pollution involves *source control* (eliminating or reducing contaminants), *ventilation improvements* (increasing the amount of outdoor air coming indoors), and *air cleaners* (removing particulates from the air).[32] For ways to reduce your exposure to biological contaminants such as mold, see the **Skills for Behavior Change** box.

Ozone Layer Depletion

The ozone layer is a stratum in the stratosphere—the highest level of Earth's atmosphere, located 12 to 30 miles above the surface—that protects our planet and its inhabitants from ultraviolet B radiation, a primary cause of skin cancer. Such radiation damages DNA and weakens immune systems.

acid deposition The acidification process that occurs when pollutants are deposited by precipitation, clouds, or directly on the land.

leach To dissolve and filter through soil.

TABLE 16.3 | Selected Indoor Air Pollutants, Their Sources, and Their Health Effects

Pollutant	Sources	Health Effects
Asbestos	Deteriorating or damaged insulation; fireproofing, acoustical materials, and floor tiles	Long-term risk of chest and abdominal cancers and lung diseases and lung cancer in smokers.
Lead	Lead-based paint, contaminated soil, dust, and drinking water	≥ 80 µg/dL of blood (high levels) can cause convulsions, coma, and death. Lower levels can cause nervous system, kidney, blood disorders, and impair mental and physical development.
Radon	Uranium in the soil or rock on which homes are built can lead to air exposure inside. Well water also can be a source.	A major nontobacco cause of lung cancer from air and drinking water exposure; also has a synergistic effect with smoking exposure.
Biological contaminants (molds, mildew, pet dander, saliva, dust mites, and cockroaches)	Improper ventilation and moisture buildup, lack of cleanliness/sanitation, contaminated heating systems, faulty construction, pets	Allergic reactions, including hypersensitivity, rhinitis, asthma, coughing, shortness of breath, dizziness, lethargy, fever, digestive problems
Combustion products	Unvented kerosene heaters, woodstoves, fireplaces, gas stoves	Carbon monoxide causes headaches, dizziness, weakness, nausea, confusion and disorientation, chest pain, and death.
Benzene	Paint, new carpet, new drapes, upholstery, fast-drying glues, caulks	Headaches, eye and skin irritation, fatigue, cancer
Formaldehyde	Tobacco smoke, plywood, cabinets, furniture, particleboard, new carpet and drapes, wallpaper, ceiling tile, paneling	Headaches, eye and skin irritation, drowsiness, fatigue, respiratory problems, memory loss, depression, gynecological problems, cancer

Source: U.S. Environmental Protection Agency, "Indoor Air Quality," Updated July 11, 2017.

In the 1970s, scientists began to warn of a breakdown in the ozone layer. Instruments developed to test atmospheric contents indicated that certain chemicals, especially **chlorofluorocarbons (CFCs)**, were contributing to rapid depletion of the ozone layer. In response, the U.S. government banned the use of aerosol sprays containing CFCs. The discovery of an ozone "hole" over Antarctica led to treaties whereby the United States and other nations agreed to further reduce the use of CFCs and other ozone-depleting chemicals. Today, more than 197 United Nations member countries have agreed to basic protocols designed to preserve and protect the ozone layer.[33] Although the ban on CFCs is believed to be responsible for slowing the depletion of the ozone layer, some CFC replacements may also be damaging.

chlorofluorocarbons (CFCs) Chemicals that contribute to the depletion of the atmospheric ozone layer.

climate change A shift in typical weather patterns that includes fluctuations in seasonal temperatures, rain or snowfall amounts, and the occurrence of catastrophic storms.

global warming A type of climate change in which average temperatures increase.

greenhouse gases Gases that accumulate in the atmosphere where they contribute to global warming by trapping heat near the Earth's surface.

enhanced greenhouse effect Warming of Earth's surface as a direct result of human activities that release greenhouse gases into the atmosphere, trapping more of the sun's radiation than is normal.

LO 3 | CLIMATE CHANGE

Explain climate change and global warming, the underlying causes of each, impacts on health, and how alternative energy and individual actions can reduce risks.

Climate change refers to a shift in global weather patterns, including fluctuations in seasonal temperatures and in rain or snowfall amounts and the occurrence of catastrophic storms. **Global warming** is a type of climate change in which average temperatures increase. Over 97 percent of scientists now agree that the planet is warming, driven largely by the burning of fossil fuels.[34] Over the last 100 years, the average temperature of the earth has increased by 1.5°F, with projections of another 2°F to 11.5°F rise expected in the next 100 years.[35]

According to the National Aeronautics and Space Administration (NASA), the National Oceanic and Atmospheric Administration (NOAA), and the National Research Council, climate change poses major risks to lives, and excess **greenhouse gases** are key culprits.[36] Excess carbon dioxide accounts for 82 percent of human-caused greenhouse gases in the United States.[37] In 2015, after years of increases, global CO_2 emissions from fossil fuel use and from steel and cement production was brought to a standstill, largely due to a 2 percent decline in coal burning and reductions in cement production.[38]

The *greenhouse effect* is a natural phenomenon in which certain gases form a layer in the atmosphere and act like the glass in a greenhouse, allowing solar heat to pass through and then trapping some of that heat close to the surface, where it warms the planet. The natural greenhouse effect is important for keeping the planet warm enough to sustain life, but human activities have increased the amounts of greenhouse gases in the atmosphere, resulting in the **enhanced greenhouse effect**, raising the planet's temperature higher than normal by trapping excess heat.

▶ SEE IT! VIDEOS

How is climate change affecting the weather during winter? Watch **Snowstorms in the Forecast**, available on Mastering Health.

Scientific Evidence of Climate Change and Human-Caused Global Warming

According to data from U.S. and international sources, climate responds to changes in naturally occurring greenhouse gases as well as solar output and the earth's orbit. However, recent evidence points to unusual changes in climate that go beyond predictable natural causes. Consider the following[39]:

- Global sea levels rose 6.7 inches in the last 100 years, mostly in the last decade.
- 2016 was the warmest year globally since records have been kept beginning in 1880.
- Sixteen of the 17 warmest years on record occurred since 2001. Since 1981, 20 of the warmest years ever have occurred.
- Greenland is losing 36 to 60 cubic miles of ice per year, and Antarctica is losing 36 cubic miles of ice per year.

Multiple reconstructions of the earth's climate history show that the amounts of greenhouse gases in the atmosphere rose dramatically around the time of the industrial revolution—when humans began burning fossil fuels on a large scale—and correlate very closely with temperature increases.[40] Studies also indicate that large changes in climate can occur within decades rather than taking centuries or thousands of years.[41]

Reducing the Threat of Global Warming

Our current climate change problems are largely rooted in modern energy, transportation, and industrial practices.[42] Beyond increased CO_2 production, rapid deforestation contributes to the rise in greenhouse gases. Trees take in carbon dioxide, transform it, store the carbon for food, and release oxygen into the air. As we lose forests, we lose the capacity to store and dissipate carbon dioxide.[43]

Most experts agree that to slow climate change, reducing consumption of fossil fuels and using mass transportation are crucial, but clean energy, green factories, hybrid and electric vehicles, improved energy efficiency, and governmental regulation are also key. Several global initiatives have been developed not only to reduce climate change, but also to improve lives.

In 2012, nations gathered in Rio de Janeiro at a meeting called *The World We Want* to outline a plan for **sustainable development**—development that meets present needs without compromising future generations. However, leaders of many nations, including the United States, France, Germany, and the United Kingdom, opted not to attend. The resulting plan included a list of general goals without the "teeth" necessary to motivate nations to comply.

Late in 2015, nearly 190 nations, representing over 95 percent of the world's greenhouse gas emissions met in Paris to work toward slowing emissions and spurring the development of alternative energy sources. The *Paris Agreement* allowed countries to come up with their own **intended nationally determined contributions (INDCs)**. The U.S. goal for INDC was to reduce net greenhouse gas emissions to 26 to 28 percent below 2005 levels by 2025.[44] Much of this would come from obtaining compliance with existing policies, along with additional technological advances and improvements.[45]

Early in 2017, President Trump said that the United States was exiting the Paris Agreement. After Nicaragua and Syria signed on to the agreement later in the year, the U.S. became the only country in the world to opt out. Since then, several states, cities, companies, and individuals acting in defiance of the Trump administration's exit indicated that they intended to comply with the agreement to reduce emissions and/or provide funding for special environmental initiatives.

In spite of the Trump administration's actions, many U.S. cities and states are considering a **carbon tax**. A carbon tax is the price a government charges for the carbon content in fuels. Diesel, gas, natural gas, jet fuel, and coal-fired electricity all emit percentages of carbon per unit of fuel. If you use more, you will pay more carbon tax. This should have the effect of motivating individuals to invest in noncarbon power generation such as solar, wind, or hydropower and to drive less, turn down the heat, and air-condition less. The city of Boulder, Colorado, was the first to implement a carbon tax, and others are considering doing so.

Cap and trade policies are designed to set limits, or caps, on how much carbon large industrial polluters can emit. Large emitters would be issued permits for allowable levels of pollutants and then would be taxed on overages unless they were able to acquire, trade, or pay for more allowances from companies that produced lower carbon emissions. Carbon taxes and cap and trade policies are mechanisms for incentivizing green behaviors and motivating those with large carbon footprints to reduce emissions.[46]

More wind, solar, and bioenergy use, movements toward hybrid and electric vehicles, and more alternative energy sources may improve carbon emissions. Still, major fuel-hungry industry development in poorer regions of the world may offset some of the potential decreases in future years.[47]

Many communities and campuses have established plans to reduce their **carbon footprint**, or the amount of CO_2 emissions contributed to the atmosphere through daily life. Creating bicycle lanes, building monitored bike garages to prevent theft and vandalism, and holding "bike to work" days motivate students to

sustainable development
Development that meets the needs of the present without compromising the ability of future generations to meet their own needs.

intended nationally determined contributions (INDCs) Goals that individual countries said they would achieve in order to do their part in the Paris Agreement and reduce global emissions.

carbon tax The price a government charges for the carbon content in fuels used by an individual, industry, or organization.

cap and trade Policies designed to set limits (caps) on how much carbon large industrial polluters can emit. Large emitters are issued permits for allowable levels of pollutants and then taxed on overages unless they are able to acquire allowances from other emitters.

carbon footprint The amount of greenhouse gases contributed to the atmosphere through daily life, usually expressed in equivalent tons of carbon dioxide emissions.

leave cars at home. Some campuses have raised fees for parking permits in the hopes of discouraging cars on campus. Many campuses have taken steps to make their campuses "green" through programs focused on recycling and reusing furniture and other items that are discarded when students leave school in the spring, as well as on buying food locally, which will cut down fossil fuels used in transportation.

LO 4 | WATER POLLUTION AND SHORTAGES

Identify sources of pollution and chemical contaminants often found in water.

Seventy-five percent of the Earth is covered with water, but only 1 to 2 percent of the world's water is freshwater and available for human consumption.[48] Approximately 1.2 percent of freshwater is surface water that comes from lakes, ground ice, swamps, marshes, rivers, and soil moisture.[49] Another 30.1 percent is groundwater from underwater wells and aquifers, and the rest (68.7 percent) is locked in glaciers and ice caps.[50] We draw our drinking water from groundwater and surface water; however, much of this water is too polluted or too difficult to reach.[51] Recent severe drought in many regions and unseasonably hot weather have forced rationing, voluntary water reduction, and community efforts to conserve water by individuals, industry, agriculture, and power generation in recent decades.

Although we have seen improvements in *gallons per capita per day (GPCD)* water usage from agriculture, thermoelectric power, municipal, and industrial sources in the United States—having declined from 1,900 GPCD in 1900 to 1,100 GPCD in 2010—we still exceed most nations in per capita water consumption.[52] Residential use has also declined from nearly 120 GPCD in the 1980s to between 80 and 100 GPCD in 2015.[53] Water-saving toilets, faucets, showerheads, washers, dishwashers, and drip irrigation options are responsible for much of this decline.[54] While these changes are laudable, note that the GPCD residential consumption in parts of Africa is closer to 5 gallons![55] FIGURE 16.2 shows a breakdown of water uses.

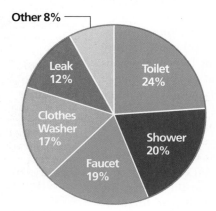

FIGURE 16.2 Individual Water Usage

Source: Environmental Protection Agency, "How We Use Water," Accessed June 2017, https://www.epa.gov/watersense/how-we-use-water.

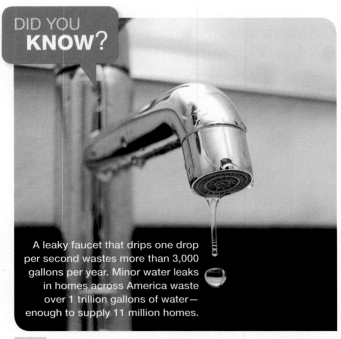

A leaky faucet that drips one drop per second wastes more than 3,000 gallons per year. Minor water leaks in homes across America waste over 1 trillion gallons of water—enough to supply 11 million homes.

Source: Environmental Protection Agency, "Fix a Leak Week," Accessed June 2017, https://www.epa.gov/watersense/fix-a-leak-week.

SKILLS FOR BEHAVIOR CHANGE

Waste Less Water!

In the Kitchen

◉ Turn off the tap while washing dishes. Shut water off after a quick rinse.

◎ Equip faucets with aerators to reduce water use by 4 percent.

◎ Run dishwashers only when they are full, and use the energy-saving mode.

In the Laundry Room

◎ Wash only full loads, or use a washing machine that adjusts to allow a reduced water level for smaller loads.

◎ Upgrade to a high-efficiency washer to use 30 percent less water per load.

In the Bathroom

◎ Replace old toilets with high-efficiency models that use 60 to 80 percent less water per flush.

◎ Take showers instead of baths, and limit showers to the time it takes to lather up and rinse off. Ideally, get wet, shut off the water, lather up, and turn on the water to rinse.

◎ Replace old showerheads with efficient models that use 60 percent less water per minute.

◎ Turn off the tap while brushing your teeth to save up to 8 gallons of water per day.

Over half the global population faces a shortage of clean water. The U.N. estimates that by 2025, two-thirds of the world's population will live in water-stressed areas, increasing competition for scarce reserves and posing a major risk to global food supplies, energy supplies, and survival of all living things.[56]

The Skills for Behavior Change box presents simple conservation measures you can adopt to save water.

Water Contamination

In most parts of the United States, tap water is among the safest in the world. Under the *Safe Drinking Water Act*, the EPA sets standards for drinking water quality and oversees the states, localities, and water suppliers that implement those standards. Cities and municipalities have policies and procedures governing water treatment, filtration, and disinfection to screen out pathogens and microorganisms. However, their ability to filter out increasing amounts of chemical by-products and other substances is in question. According to a 2014 study of over 50 large wastewater sites in the United States, more than half of the samples tested positive for at least 25 of the 56 prescription and over-the-counter drugs monitored.[57] A more recent study estimates that the drinking water of over 41 million Americans in 24 major cities is contaminated with pharmaceuticals.[58] Beyond pharmaceuticals, our aging infrastructure and pipes can also lead to contamination.

Congress uses two terms to describe general sources of water pollution. **Point source pollutants** enter a waterway at a specific location such as a pipe, ditch, culvert, or other conduit. The major sources of point source pollution are sewage treatment plants and industrial facilities. **Nonpoint source pollutants**—commonly known as *runoff* and *sedimentation*—drain or seep into waterways from broad areas of land. Nonpoint source pollution results from a variety of land use practices and includes soil erosion and sedimentation, construction and engineering project waste, pesticide and fertilizer runoff, urban street runoff, acid mine drainage, septic tank leakage, and sewage sludge. TABLE 16.4 presents some of the pollutants causing the greatest potential harm.

point source pollutant A pollutant that enters waterways at a specific point.

nonpoint source pollutant A pollutant that runs off or seeps into waterways from broad areas of land.

LO 5 | LAND POLLUTION

Distinguish between municipal solid waste and hazardous waste, and list strategies for reducing land pollution.

Much of the waste that pollutes water starts out by polluting land. As populations grow, there is more waste, much of which doesn't degrade.

TABLE 16.4 | Selected Water Pollutants and Their Health and Ecosystem Effects

Pollutant	Description	Health Effects
Gasoline and petroleum products	Leaks from underground storage tanks at filling stations; occupational exposures in processing plants and filling stations. Fumes can spark fires and cause respiratory issues.	Can affect nervous system, leading to headaches, dizziness, nausea, skin irritations, and damage to kidneys and blood; benzene in gas has been linked to several cancers in humans as well as being toxic to birds, animals, and aquatic life.
Organic solvents	Chemicals designed to dissolve grease and oil; dry-cleaning fluids, paints, antifreeze, etc. Consumers dump leftovers into the toilet or street drains; industries bury barrels that can leak.	Difficult to clean up; can cause cancer and damage to immune, nervous, and reproductive systems. Harmful to aquatic life and animals that come into contact with them or ingest them.
Fracking by-products	Chemicals used in hydraulic fracking, a method of extracting natural gas from the ground by forcing pressurized liquids into underground rock	Linked to groundwater and surface water contamination; and risks to humans and other species, air pollution, and potential earthquake risk.
Polychlorinated biphenyls (PCBs)	Insulating materials in high-voltage electrical equipment such as transformers and fluorescent lights; no longer manufactured in the United States	Stored in the liver; associated with birth defects, cancer, and skin problems
Dioxins	Formed as contaminant during certain industrial processes, such as the production of some herbicides, the incineration of waste, and the burning of fuels such as wood, coal, or oil.	Accumulate in the body; long-term effects include possible immune system damage and increased risk of infections and cancer. High level short term exposure can cause nausea, vomiting, diarrhea, rashes and sores.
Pesticides	Chemicals designed to prevent, mitigate, or kill any pest, including insects (insecticides) rodents, weeds (herbicides), and microorganisms (algaecides, fungicides, or bactericides) can be dispersed by winds, water runoff, and food contamination.	Can accumulate in the body. Risks include birth defects, cancer, liver and kidney damage, reproductive problems, nervous system and diseases in aquatic, animal, and bird populations; contamination of groundwater and food.

Sources: Environmental Protection Agency. "Drinking Water Contaminants: Standards and Regulations," May 2017, https://www.epa.gov/dwstandardsregulations; U.S. Geological Survey, "Contaminants Found in Ground Water," December 2016, https://water.usgs.gov/edu/earthgwquality.html; Environmental Protection Agency, "Assessment of the Potential Impacts of Hydraulic Fracturing for Oil and Gas on Drinking Water Resources," External Review Draft, EPA/600/R-15/047.

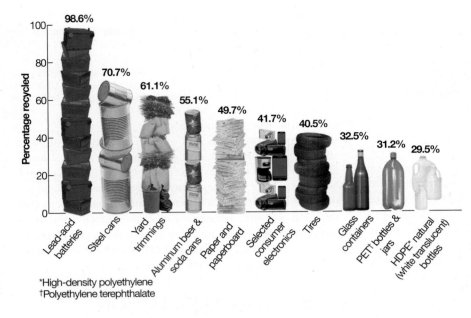

Percentage recycled

- Lead-acid batteries: 98.6%
- Steel cans: 70.7%
- Yard trimmings: 61.1%
- Aluminum beer & soda cans: 55.1%
- Paper and paperboard: 49.7%
- Selected consumer electronics: 41.7%
- Tires: 40.5%
- Glass containers: 32.5%
- PET† bottles & jars: 31.2%
- HDPE* natural (white translucent) bottles: 29.5%

*High-density polyethylene
†Polyethylene terephthalate

FIGURE 16.3 How Much Do We Recycle?

Source: Environmental Protection Agency, "Advancing Sustainable Materials Management: 2014 Fact Sheet," June 2016, www.epa.gov/epawaste/nonhaz/municipal/pubs/2014_advncng_smm_fs.pdf.

Solid Waste

Each day, on average, every person in the United States generates nearly 4.5 pounds of **municipal solid waste (MSW)**, more commonly known as trash or garbage, totaling about 258 million tons of trash each year, with organic materials making up the largest share.[59] Although we recycle only slightly over one-third of the waste we generate, experts believe that we could recycle up to 90 percent (**FIGURE 16.3**).[60] Currently, 34.6 percent of all MSW in the United States is recycled or composted, 12.8 percent is burned at combustion facilities, and the remaining 52.6 percent is disposed of in landfills.[61]

The number of U.S. landfills has decreased in the past decade, but their sheer mass has increased. As communities run out of landfill space, garbage is hauled to other states; dumped illegally in woods, waterways, or oceans, where it contaminates ecosystems; or shipped to landfills in developing countries, where it becomes someone else's problem. To decrease the strain on landfills, communities, businesses, and individuals can adopt strategies to reduce solid waste:

- *Source reduction (waste prevention)* involves altering the design, manufacture, or use of products and materials to reduce the amount and toxicity of waste.
- *Recycling* involves sorting, collecting, and processing materials for reuse in new products and diverts items such as paper, cardboard, glass, plastic, and metals from the waste stream.
- *Composting* involves collecting organic waste, such as food scraps and yard trimmings, and allowing it to decompose with the help of microorganisms (mainly bacteria and fungi), producing a nutrient-rich substance used for soil enhancement. Not all organic waste is composted. See the Student Health Today box for more on food waste.
- *Combustion with energy recovery* typically involves the use of boilers and industrial furnaces to incinerate waste and use the burning process to generate energy.

municipal solid waste (MSW) Solid waste such as containers and packaging; food waste; yard waste; and miscellaneous waste from residential, commercial, institutional, and industrial sources.

hazardous waste Toxic waste that poses a hazard to humans or to the environment.

Superfund A fund established under the Comprehensive Environmental Response Compensation and Liability Act for toxic waste cleanup.

Hazardous Waste

Hazardous waste has properties that make it capable of harming human health or the environment. American manufacturers and individuals generate around 40 million of tons of hazardous waste each year, including commercial chemical refuse, solvents and oils, petroleum-refining by-products, and household wastes such as batteries, cleaning products, and paints.[62] Many wastes are now banned from land disposal sites or are being treated to reduce their toxicity before they become part of land disposal sites. The EPA has developed protective requirements for land disposal facilities, such as double liners, detection systems for substances that may leach into groundwater, and groundwater monitoring systems.

In 1980, the *Comprehensive Environmental Response, Compensation and Liability Act*, known as the **Superfund**, was enacted to provide funds for cleaning up what are typically "abandoned" hazardous waste dump sites. Since then, the Superfund has located and assessed tens of thousands of hazardous waste sites, worked to protect people and the environment from contamination at the worst sites, and involved affected communities, states, and other groups in cleanup. The vast majority of sites have been cleared or "recovered," with over 1729 final or deleted sites and 53 proposed sites needing cleanup as of July 2017.[63] To see Superfund sites in your state, go to https://www.epa.gov/superfund/superfund-national-priorities-list-npl.

WHAT DO YOU THINK?

Do you know anyone who throws recyclable items away instead of recycling them?

- What do you think motivates their behavior?
- What might encourage them to recycle?

▶ **SEE IT!** VIDEOS

Is bottled water better for you? Watch **Americans' Obsession with Bottled Water** available on Mastering Health.

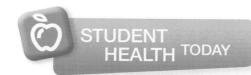
ARE YOU A FOOD WASTER?

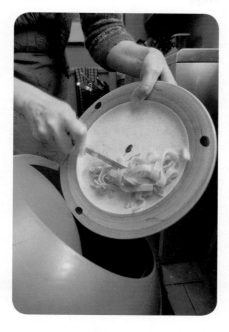

U.S. municipal solid waste. And when we waste food, we also waste all of the time, effort, and resources that went into production and put unnecessary stress on the environment. By wasting less, we put less pressure on our vulnerable habitat.

At a time when food insecurity plagues people throughout the world, a new study by Britain's Institute of Mechanical Engineers indicates that *up to half of the food produced worldwide never makes it into consumer's mouths*.

Over one-third of the world's edible food is lost or wasted annually, and consumer behavior is responsible for much of this waste.

Americans are among the worst of the food wasters, wasting over 40 percent of all edible food. The average person in the United States dumps over 20 pounds of food each month, which when added to others waste, is enough to fill the Rose Bowl stadium every day of the year. If we cut our food waste by just 15 percent, an estimated 26 million food-insecure people in the United States could be fed. And although recent research indicates that Americans know they waste food and even feel guilty about it, many say that they don't have time to be more efficient in their consumption behaviors.

Food waste is the largest source (35.2 million tons) and the most harmful part (in terms of greenhouse gas emission) of

What can you do?

- Be a better food planner. Make a list when shopping and only buy what you will use by expiration dates.
- Buy locally. And use reusable bags!
- Buy ugly produce. It tastes the same, and you can save money! Some cities even have services that deliver boxes of "ugly" fruits and vegetables—those that might not be pretty or that grocery stores have a surplus of.
- Eat leftovers. Make a rule that you can't eat out when there is good food in your fridge or pantry.
- Eat lower on the food chain. By eating more of a plant-based diet, you have a smaller footprint stomping on the planet.

Sources: D. Qi and B. Roe, "Household Food Waste: Multivariate Regression and Principal Components Analyses of Awareness and Attitudes among U.S. Consumers," *PLoS ONE* 11, no. 7 (2016): e0159250; Feeding America, "Food Waste in America," Accessed July 2016, http://www.feedingamerica.org/about-us/how-we-work/securing-meals/reducing-food-waste.html.

LO 6 | RADIATION

List and explain key health concerns associated with ionizing and nonionizing radiation.

Radiation is energy that travels in waves or particles. There are many different types of radiation, ranging from radio waves to gamma rays. They all make up the electromagnetic spectrum, but only some of them pose threats to human health.

Nonionizing Radiation

Nonionizing radiation is radiation at the lower end of the electromagnetic spectrum, which moves in relatively long wavelengths. Examples of nonionizing radiation sources are radio waves, TV signals, cell phones, computer monitors, microwaves, and infrared waves. Concerns have also been raised about the safety of radio-frequency waves generated by cell phones (See the Health Headlines box).[64]

Ionizing Radiation

Ionizing radiation is caused by the release of particles and electromagnetic rays from the nuclei of atoms during the normal process of disintegration. This type of radiation has enough energy to remove electrons from the atoms it passes through. Some naturally occurring elements, such as uranium, emit ionizing radiation. The sun is another source of ionizing radiation, in the form of high-frequency ultraviolet rays.

Radiation exposure is measured in **radiation absorbed doses**, or **rads** (also called *roentgens*). Radiation can cause damage at doses as low as 100 to

> **nonionizing radiation** Electromagnetic waves that have long wavelengths and enough energy to move atoms or cause them to vibrate.
>
> **ionizing radiation** Electromagnetic waves and particles that have short wavelengths and energy high enough to ionize atoms.
>
> **radiation absorbed dose (rad)** The unit of measure of radiation exposure.

258 MILLION

tons of **TRASH** are generated each year in the united states.

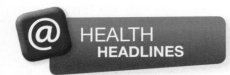

E-CONCERNS

Given that mobile phone use has skyrocketed, only the most apathetic people wouldn't be concerned about *radio-frequency (RF) waves*. But what is the real risk? In theory, RF energy has the potential to penetrate the skull, neck, and upper torso. The risk might be even greater for the very young, whose skulls have not yet fully hardened. However, after over a decade of research trying to prove a solid link to cell phone use and some type of disease, very little conclusive evidence exists. Nevertheless, experts call for additional research. In the interim, it makes good sense to use caution. Go hands free. Check out specific absorption rate (SAR) charts online or from your phone company before buying.

While you are in class, out to dinner, or in bed sound asleep, your cable box and other plugged-in-all-the-time devices are draining electricity unnecessarily, and it can add up. Newer, Energy Star products can save you money. Ask for them. And pay attention to your charging habits. Turn off your chargeable devices when they are fully charged. Unplug electrically powered devices when not using them. Stream more using lower-energy devices.

The global burden of e-waste (discarded computers, televisions, and other electronic devices) has also skyrocketed in recent years. Although there are many avenues for disposing of them, many end up in landfills. What can you do to reduce this waste? Very

simply, hang onto your devices for as long as possible. When you are thinking about *e-recycling*, check out www .ecyclingcentral.com for a state-by-state listing of e-recyclers in your area.

Sources: EPA, "Basic Information about Electronics Stewardship." April 26, 2016, https://www.epa.gov /smm-electronics/basic-information-about -electronics-stewardship#01; National Cancer Institute, "Factsheet: Cell Phones and Cancer Risk," May 27, 2016, www.cancer.gov/cancertopics /factsheet/Risk/cellphones; American Cancer Society, "Cell Phones," Accessed June 2017, https://www.cancer.org/cancer/cancer-causes /radiation-exposure/cellular-phones.html.

---

nuclear meltdown An accident that results when the temperature in the core of a nuclear reactor increases enough to melt the nuclear fuel and breach the containment vessel.

200 rads. At this level, signs of radiation sickness include nausea, diarrhea, fatigue, anemia, sore throat, and hair loss. At 350 to 500 rads, symptoms become more severe, and death may result as white blood cell production is hindered. Doses above 600 to 700 rads are fatal.

Recommended maximum "safe" exposure ranges from 0.5 to 5 rads per year.[65] Approximately 50 percent of the radiation to which we are exposed comes from natural sources, which include radon gas in the air and cosmic radiation. Another 45 percent comes from human-made sources such as diagnostic x-rays, nuclear medicine, and radiation therapy. The remaining 5 percent of exposure comes from nonionizing radiation.[66] Most of us are exposed to far less radiation than the safe maximum dosage per year. The effects of long-term exposure to relatively low levels of radiation are unknown.

Nuclear Power Plants

Proponents of nuclear energy believe that it is a safe and efficient way to generate electricity. The initial costs of building nuclear power plants are high, but actual power generation is

relatively inexpensive in comparison to other forms. Nuclear power also causes reductions in fossil fuel use in heating and discharges less carbon into the air than do fossil fuel–powered generators.

Although there are advantages to nuclear power, there are also clear disadvantages. Disposal of nuclear waste poses significant risks to our environment. In addition, a reactor core meltdown could pose serious threats to all living things.

A **nuclear meltdown** occurs when the temperature in the core of a nuclear reactor increases enough to melt both the nuclear fuel and its containment vessel. Most modern facilities seal the reactors and containment vessels in concrete buildings with pools of cold water at the bottom. If a meltdown occurs, the building and the pool are supposed to prevent radiation from escaping. However, a catastrophic 1986 fire and explosion at Chernobyl's nuclear site in Ukraine killed thousands and left the area uninhabitable for decades.[67] The damage to the Fukushima Daiichi Nuclear Power Station in northern Japan caused by the March 2011 earthquake and tsunami reawakened worldwide fears about nuclear energy. Nonetheless, the use of nuclear power worldwide is expected to double in the next 35 years, particularly in China. Balancing the risks and benefits of nuclear power will continue to be challenging.[68]

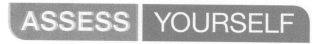

LIVE IT! ASSESS YOURSELF

An interactive version of this assessment is available online in Mastering Health.

Are You Doing All You Can to Protect the Environment?

Environmental problems often seem too big for the actions of one person to make a difference. Each day, however, there are things you can do. For each statement below, indicate how often you follow the described behavior.

	Always	Usually	Sometimes	Never
1. I walk or ride my bicycle rather than driving a car.	1	2	3	4
2. I carpool to school or work.	1	2	3	4
3. I read labels and buy products that have fewer chemicals in their ingredients whenever I buy food, personal care products, and household cleaners.	1	2	3	4
4. I use air-conditioning only as needed on very hot days, and I put on more clothes rather than cranking up the furnace whenever possible.	1	2	3	4
5. I turn off the lights when a room is not being used.	1	2	3	4
6. To reduce e-waste and conserve natural resources, I do not replace my cell phone and other electronics until they are at least 2-3 years old.	1	2	3	4
7. I have water-saving devices installed on my shower, toilet, and sinks.	1	2	3	4
8. I unplug my TV DVR/cable/satellite dish when I'm going to be gone for extended periods.	1	2	3	4
9. I use bath towels more than once before putting them in the laundry.	1	2	3	4
10. I wear my clothes more than once between washings, when appropriate.	1	2	3	4
11. I limit my use of the clothes dryer and line-dry my clothes as often as possible.	1	2	3	4
12. I purchase biodegradable soaps and detergents.	1	2	3	4
13. At home, I use dishes and utensils rather than Styrofoam or plastic.	1	2	3	4
14. When I buy prepackaged foods, I choose the ones with the least packaging.	1	2	3	4
15. I go paperless in my transactions whenever I can.	1	2	3	4
16. I use energy-efficient appliances.	1	2	3	4
17. I bring my own reusable bags to the grocery store.	1	2	3	4
18. I don't run water continuously while washing the dishes, shaving, or brushing my teeth.	1	2	3	4
19. I reuse the blank side of printed papers.	1	2	3	4
20. I try to reuse, recycle, donate, or sell household items when I move.	1	2	3	4
21. I bring my container and get refills instead of buying bottled water or coffee in paper cups.	1	2	3	4
22. I volunteer for cleanup days in my community.	1	2	3	4
23. I consider candidates' positions on environmental issues before casting my vote.	1	2	3	4

For Further Thought

Review your scores. Are your responses mostly 1s and 2s? If not, what actions can you take to become more environmentally responsible? Are there ways to help the environment on this list that you had not thought of? Are there behaviors not on the list that you are already doing?

YOUR PLAN FOR CHANGE

The activity gave you the chance to look at your behavior and consider ways to conserve energy, save water, reduce waste, and otherwise help protect the planet. Now that you have considered these results, you can take steps to become more environmentally responsible.

TODAY, YOU CAN:

☐ Find out how much energy you are using. Visit http://footprint.wwf .org.uk to find out what your carbon footprint is and how your behaviors would affect the planet if other people lived like you. Learn about things you can do to change your carbon footprint.

☐ Reduce paper waste in your mailbox. The Direct Marketing Association's Mail Preference Service site (www .dmachoice.org), 1-888-5-OPT-OUT, and www.catalogchoice.org are all free services that help cut down on unsolicited catalogs, credit card offers, and advertisements.

WITHIN THE NEXT TWO WEEKS, YOU CAN:

☐ Look into joining a local environmental group, attending a campus environmental event, or taking an environmental science course.

☐ Take part in a local cleanup day or recycling drive to meet like-minded people while benefiting the planet.

BY THE END OF THE SEMESTER, YOU CAN:

☐ Check whether your campus dining hall composts or recycles. If it doesn't, ask the managers to start. Follow up on your request.

☐ Make a habit of recycling everything you can, from bottles to batteries.

☐ Let your legislators know how you feel about environmental issues, and vote for candidates with pro-environment records.

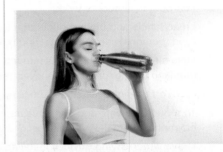

STUDY PLAN

Visit the Study Area in Mastering Health to enhance your study plan with MP3 Tutor Sessions, Practice Quizzes, Flashcards, and more!

CHAPTER REVIEW

LO 1 | Overpopulation: The Planet's Greatest Threat

- Population growth is the single largest factor affecting the environment. Demand for more food, water, and energy—as well as places to dispose of waste—strains the earth's resources.

LO 2 | Air Pollution

- The primary constituents of air pollution are carbon monoxide, sulfur dioxide, nitrogen dioxide, ground-level ozone, lead, and particulate matter. Smog, is caused by the reaction of sunlight with hydrocarbons, nitrogen compounds, and other gases in vehicle exhaust. Indoor air pollution is caused primarily by tobacco smoke, woodstove, and furnace emissions, asbestos, formaldehyde, radon, lead, and mold.

LO 3 | Climate Change

- Climate change is a major environmental threat and is caused by a wide range of factors. Air, water, and solid waste pollution are key contributors, as is our growing dependence on fossil fuels. Sustainable development should be an international goal.

LO 4 | Water Pollution and Shortages

- Water pollution can be caused by point sources (direct entry) or non-point sources (runoff or seepage). Major pollutants include petroleum products, organic solvents, polychlorinated biphenyl (PCBs), dioxins, pesticides, and lead.

LO 5 | Land Pollution

- Municipal solid waste (MSW) includes household trash, plastics, glass, metals, paper and other items. Many can be recycled. Limited landfill space creates problems in dealing with growing volumes of MSW. Hazardous waste is toxic; improper disposal creates health hazards for people in surrounding communities and those downstream.

LO 6 | Radiation

- Nonionizing radiation comes from electromagnetic fields such as those around power lines and is less disruptive to health. Ionizing radiation that results from x-rays, nuclear medicine, radiation therapy, and other sources can disrupt cellular activity and pose greater risks to health. The disposal and storage of radioactive waste from nuclear power plants pose potential public health problems.

POP QUIZ

LO 1 | Overpopulation: The Planet's Greatest Threat

1. The largest population that can be supported indefinitely given the resources available is the earth's
   a. maximum fertility rate.
   b. fertility capacity.
   c. maximum population growth.
   d. carrying capacity.

2. Human fertility rates fall when
   a. there is poverty and people can't afford to feed their families.
   b. governments subsidize families in the form of tax breaks.
   c. women have more education and power.
   d. environmental threats influence people to have fewer children.

LO 2 | Air Pollution

3. The air pollutant emitted primarily from motor vehicles is
   a. particulates.
   b. nitrogen dioxide.
   c. sulfur dioxide.
   d. carbon monoxide.

4. Which gas can become cancer causing when it seeps into a home?
   a. Radon
   b. Carbon monoxide
   c. Hydrogen sulfide
   d. Ozone

5. The barrier that protects us from the sun's harmful ultraviolet rays is
   a. photochemical smog.
   b. the ozone layer.
   c. gray air smog.
   d. the greenhouse effect.

LO 3 | Climate Change

6. When gases such as carbon dioxide and hydrocarbons form a layer in the atmosphere, trapping solar heat close to the surface to warm the planet, it is called
   a. photochemical smog.
   b. the ozone layer.
   c. gray air smog.
   d. the enhanced greenhouse effect.

LO 4 | Water Pollution and Shortages

7. Which of the following are major threats to our water supply?
   a. Agricultural use of herbicides and pesticides
   b. Contamination of groundwater and surface water from fracking
   c. Leaking home faucets, toilets, and lawn irrigation systems
   d. All of the above

LO 5 | Land Pollution

8. Buying products with little or no packaging is an example of reducing municipal solid waste by
   a. source reduction.
   b. recycling.
   c. cap and trade incentives.
   d. incineration.

LO 6 | Radiation

9. What is the recommended safe level of radiation exposure per year?
   a. 0.5 to 5 rads
   b. 6 to 100 rads
   c. 101 to 200 rads
   d. 201 to 350 rads

10. Which is a source of ionizing radiation?
   a. Diagnostic x-rays.
   b. TV
   c. Radio waves
   d. Microwaves

*Answers to the Pop Quiz can be found on page A-1. If you answered a question incorrectly, review the section identified by the Learning Outcome. For even more study tools, visit **Mastering Health**.*

THINK ABOUT IT!

LO 1 | Overpopulation: The Planet's Greatest Threat

1. How are the rapid increases in global population and consumption of resources related? Is population control the best solution? Why or why not?

LO 2 | Air Pollution

2. What are the primary sources of air pollution? What can be done to reduce air pollution?

LO 3 | Climate Change

3. What are the causes and consequences of global warming? What can individuals and communities do to reduce the threat of global warming?

LO 4 | Water Pollution and Shortages

4. What are point and nonpoint sources of water pollution? What can be done to reduce or prevent water pollution?

LO 5 | Land Pollution

5. How do you think communities and governments could encourage recycling efforts?

LO 6 | Radiation

6. What can you do to reduce your amount of radiation exposure? On the community level? On the national level?

ACCESS YOUR HEALTH ON THE INTERNET

Visit Mastering Health for links to the websites and RSS feeds.

The following websites explore further topics and issues related to environmental health.

Environmental Protection Agency (EPA). The EPA is the U.S. government agency responsible for overseeing environmental regulation and protection issues. **www.epa.gov**

National Center for Environmental Health (NCEH). This site provides information on a wide variety of environmental health issues, including a series of helpful fact sheets. **www.cdc.gov /nceh**

National Environmental Health Association (NEHA). This organization provides educational resources and opportunities for environmental health professionals. **www.neha.org**

APPENDIX A   POP QUIZ ANSWERS

Chapter 1
1. b; 2. b; 3. d; 4. b; 5. a; 6. c; 7. d; 8. a; 9. a; 10. a

Chapter 1a
1. b; 2. d; 3. c; 4. c

Chapter 2
1. b; 2. a; 3. b; 4. d; 5. c; 6. b; 7. b; 8. b; 9. b; 10. b

Chapter 2A
1. c; 2. b; 3. d

Chapter 3
1. c; 2. b; 3. c; 4. a; 5. d; 6. c; 7. d; 8. c; 9. b; 10. d

Chapter 4
1. a; 2. c; 3. a; 4. d; 5. d

Chapter 5
1. b; 2. a; 3. b; 4. d; 5. d; 6. c; 7. a; 8. b; 9. d; 10. c

Chapter 6
1. c; 2. d; 3. b; 4. c; 5. b; 6. a; 7. a; 8. d; 9. b; 10. d

Chapter 6a
1. c; 2. b; 3. d; 4. c

Chapter 7
1. c; 2. b; 3. d; 4. c; 5. a; 6. b; 7. d; 8. b; 9. a; 10. c; 11. a; 12. a

Chapter 8
1. b; 2. b; 3. c; 4. c; 5. d; 6. a; 7. a; 8. b; 9. d; 10. c

Chapter 9
1. c; 2. c; 3. b; 4. d; 5. b; 6. d; 7. c; 8. c; 9. b; 10. a

Chapter 10
1. a; 2. b; 3. b; 4. a; 5. c; 6. b; 7. b; 8. c; 9. b; 10. d

Chapter 11
1. b; 2. a; 3. c; 4. c; 5. b; 6. c; 7. b; 8. a; 9. d; 10. a

Chapter 11a
1. a; 2. b; 3. d

Chapter 12
1. d; 2. c; 3. c; 4. b; 5. b; 6. b; 7. a; 8. c; 9. b; 10. a

Chapter 13
1. d; 2. b; 3. b; 4. b; 5. c; 6. b; 7. b; 8. a; 9. c; 10. b

Chapter 13a
1. c; 2. d; 3. c

Chapter 14
1. c; 2. d; 3. a; 4. a; 5. c; 6. b; 7. d; 8. d; 9. a; 10. c

Chapter 14a
1. c; 2. c; 3. c; 4. a; 5. a

Chapter 15
1. c; 2. d; 3. a; 4. a; 5. d; 6. d; 7. b; 8. a; 9. c; 10. d

Chapter 15a
1. c; 2. c; 3. d; 4. a

Chapter 15b
1. b; 2. d; 3. c; 4. c; 5. b

Chapter 16
1. d; 2. c; 3. d; 4. a; 5. b; 6. d; 7. d; 8. a; 9. a; 10. a

REFERENCES

Chapter 1: Accessing Your Health

1. J. Xu et al., "Mortality in the United States, 2015," NCHS Data Brief, no. 267 (2016), Available at https://www.cdc.gov/nchs/products/databriefs/db267.htm.
2. Centers for Disease Control and Prevention, "Achievements in Public Health, 1900–1999: Control of Infectious Diseases," *Morbidity and Mortality Weekly Report* 48, no. 29 (1999): 621–29, www.cdc.gov/mmwr/preview/mmwrhtml/mm4829a1.htm.
3. R.A. Rudd, "Increases in Drug and Opioid-Involved Overdose Deaths—United States, 2010–2015," *Morbidity and Mortality Weekly Report* 65(2016):1445–1452, DOI: http://dx.doi.org/10.15585/mmwr.mm655051e1.
4. Organization for Economic Cooperation and Development, "Health at a Glance 2015," Accessed January 25, 2017, Available at: http://www.oecd.org/unitedstates/Health-at-a-Glance-2015-Key-Findings-UNITED-STATES.pdf.
5. U.S. Department of Health and Human Services (DHHS), "Health-Related Quality of Life & Well-Being," *Healthy People 2020* (Washington, DC: U.S. Government Printing Office), February 3, 2016, www.healthypeople.gov/2020/topics-objectives/topic/health-related-quality-of-life-well-being.
6. Centers for Disease Control and Prevention, "Adult Obesity Facts," September 1, 2016, http://www.cdc.gov/obesity/data/adult.html.
7. World Health Organization (WHO), "Constitution of the World Health Organization," *Chronicles of the World Health Organization* (Geneva: WHO, 1947), www.who.int/governance/eb/constitution/en/index.html.
8. R. Dubos, *So Human an Animal: How We Are Shaped by Surroundings and Events* (New York: Scribner, 1968), 15.
9. U.S. Department of Health and Human Services (DHHS), *Healthy People 2020*, 2016.
10. Ibid.
11. Centers for Disease Control and Prevention, "Chronic Disease Prevention and Health Promotion: Chronic Disease Overview," February 23, 2016, https://www.cdc.gov/chronicdisease/overview.
12. Ibid.
13. J.F. Sallis and Jordan A. Carlson, "Population Health: Behavioral and Social Science Insights Physical Activity: Numerous Benefits and Effective Interventions." Rockville, MD: Agency for Healthcare Research and Quality (2015), Available at http://www.ahrq.gov/professionals/education/curriculum-tools/population-health/sallis.html.
14. X. Wang et al., "Fruit and vegetable consumption and mortality from all causes, cardiovascular disease, and cancer: systematic review and dose-response meta-analysis of prospective cohort studies," *British Medical Journal* 349 (2014): g4490, doi:10.1136/bmj.g4490.
15. CDC, "Fact Sheets: Alcohol Use and Your Health," October 2016, https://www.cdc.gov/alcohol/fact-sheets/alcohol-use.htm.
16. CDC, "Smoking and Tobacco Use Fast Facts," December 2016, www.cdc.gov/tobacco/data_statistics/fact_sheets/fast_facts/index.htm#toll.
17. H. C. Gooding et al., "Optimal Lifestyle Components in Young Adulthood Are Associated with Maintaining the Ideal Cardiovascular Health Profile into Middle Age," *Journal of the American Heart Association* 4, no. 11 (2015): e002048.
18. President's Commission on Combatting Drug Addiction and the Opioid Crisis. "Preliminary Report." August 2017. https://www.whitehouse.gov/sites/whitehouse.gov/files/ondcp/commission-interim-report.pdf.
19. U.S. Department of Health and Human Services (DHHS), *Healthy People 2020*, 2016.
20. P. Pilkington, J. Powell, and A. Davis. "Evidence-Based Decision Making When Designing Environments for Physical Activity: The Role of Public Health," *Sports Medicine* (2016): 997–1002.
21. U.S. Department of Health and Human Services, "New Report Details Impact of the Affordable Care Act," December 13, 2016, https://www.hhs.gov/healthcare/facts-and-features/fact-sheets/new-report-details-impact-affordable-care-act.html#.
22. J. Kabat-Zinn, *Wherever You Go, There You Are: Mindfulness Meditation in Everyday Life* (New York: Hachette, 2014).
23. Rosenstock, "Historical Origins of the Health Belief Model," *Health Education Monographs* 2, no. 4 (1974): 328–35.
24. Bandura, "Human Agency in Social Cognitive Theory," *American Psychologist* 44, no. 9 (1989): 1175–84.
25. J.J. Annesi et al., "Effects of the Youth Fit 4 Life physical activity/nutrition protocol on body mass index, fitness and targeted social cognitive theory variables in 9- to 12-year-olds during afterschool care," *Journal of Paediatrics and Child Health* (2017), doi:10.1111/jpc.13447.
26. J. O. Prochaska and C. C. DiClemente, "Stages and Processes of Self-Change of Smoking: Toward an Integrative Model of Change," *Journal of Consulting and Clinical Psychology* 51 (1983): 390–95.
27. M. Jung, "Implications of Graphic Cigarette Warning Labels on Smoking Behavior: An International Perspective," *Journal of Cancer Prevention* 21, no. 1(2016): 21–25, doi:10.15430/JCP.2016.21.1.21.
28. Y. Kang et al., "Dispositional Mindfulness Predicts Adaptive Affective Responses to Health Messages and Increased Exercise Motivation," *Mindfulness* (2016): 1-11, doi:10.1007/s12671-016-0608-7.
29. G. Goldzweig et al., "Perceived Threat and Depression among Patients with Cancer: The Moderating Role of Health Locus of Control," *Psychology, Health, & Medicine* 21, no. 5 (2016): 601–607.
30. A. Ellis and M. Benard, *Clinical Application of Rational Emotive Therapy* (New York: Plenum, 1985).
31. National Institute on Drug Abuse, "Drugs, Brains, and Behavior: The Science of Addiction: Treatment and Recovery," July 2014, www.drugabuse.gov/publications/drugs-brains-behavior-science-addiction/treatment-recovery.
32. American Cancer Society, "Staying Tobacco-Free After You Quit Smoking," May 6, 2016, http://www.cancer.org/healthy/stay-away-from-tobacco/guide-quitting-smoking/staying-tobacco-free-after-you-quit-smoking.html.

Pulled Statistics:

page 03, J. Xu, S.L. Murphy, K.D. Kochanek, and E. Arias, "Mortality in the United States, 2015," *National Center for Health Statistics Data Brief*, no. 267, December, 2016. https://www.cdc.gov/nchs/products/databriefs/db267.htm.

page 08, Centers for Disease Control and Prevention, "Chronic Disease Prevention and Health Promotion: Chronic Disease Overview," February 23, 2016, https://www.cdc.gov/chronicdisease/overview/

Focus On: Difference, Disparity, and Health: Achieving Health Equity

1. K. Davis, K. Stremikis, D. Squires, and C. Schoen, "Mirror, Mirror on the Wall: How the Performance of the U.S. Health Care System Compares Internationally," 2014 Update, Commonwealth Fund, Available at www.commonwealthfund.org/publications/fund-reports/2014/jun/mirror-mirror.
2. U.S. Department of Health and Human Services, *Healthy People 2020*, "About Healthy People," 2017, Available at www.healthypeople.gov/2020/About-Healthy-People.
3. World Health Organization, "Health Systems: Equity," 2017, Available at www.who.int/healthsystems/topics/equity/en.
4. K. Chaturvedi and S.K. Chaturvedi, "Understanding Health Inequality," n.d., Available at www.pitt.edu/~super7/46011-47001/46661.ppt.
5. U.S. Department of Health and Human Services, *Healthy People 2020*, "Disparities," 2017, Available at www.healthypeople.gov/2020/about/foundation-health-measures/Disparities.
6. Ibid.
7. L. Farrer, C. Marinetti, Y. Cavaco, and C. Costongs, "Advocacy for Health Equity: A Synthesis Review." *Milbank Quarterly* 93, no. 2 (2015): 392–437, doi:10.1111/1468-0009.12112.
8. M.C. Arcaya, A.L. Arcaya, and S.V. Subramanian, "Inequalities in Health: Definitions, Concepts, and Theories." *Global Health Action* 8, no. 10 (2015), doi:10.3402/gha.v8.27106, Available at www.ncbi.nlm.nih.gov/pmc/articles/PMC4481045.
9. S.L. Colby and J.M. Ortman, "Projections of the Size and Composition of the U.S. Population: 2014–2060, U.S. Census Bureau, March 2015, Available at www.census.gov/content/dam/Census/library/publications/2015/demo/p25-1143.pdf.
10. J. Zong and J. Batalova, "Frequently Requested Statistics on Immigrants and Immigration in the United States," Migration Policy Institute, March 8, 2017, Available at http://www.migrationpolicy.org/article/frequently-requested-statistics-immigrants-and-immigration-united-states.
11. S.L. Colby and J.M. Ortman, "Projections of the Size and Composition of the U.S. Population: 2014-2060, U.S. Census Bureau, March, 2015, Available at www.census.gov/content/dam/Census/library/publications/2015/demo/p25-1143.pdf.
12. Harris Interactive, "The GLBT Market Research Leaders—Hands Down," 2013, Available at http://www.witeck.com/wp-content/uploads/2013/03/partnership-with-harris-interactive.pdf.
14. G.J. Gates, "In U.S., More Adults Identifying as LGBT," Gallup, January 11, 2017, Available at www.gallup.com/poll/201731/lgbt-identification-rises.aspx.
15. Pew Research Center, "America's Changing Religious Landscape," May 12, 2015, Available at http://www.pewforum.org/2015/05/12/americas-changing-religious-landscape.
16. Pew Research Center, "Nones on the Rise," October 9, 2012, Available at http://www.pewforum.org/2012/10/09/nones-on-the-rise.
17. Pew Research Center, "America's Changing Religious Landscape," May 12, 2015, Available at http://www.pewforum.org/2015/05/12/americas-changing-religious-landscape.
18. Ibid.
19. C.N. Adichie, *Americanah*, New York: Anchor Books, 2013.
20. Centers for Disease Control and Prevention, "CDC Health Disparities and Inequalities Report—United States, 2013," *Morbidity and Mortality Weekly Report* 62, Suppl. 3 (2013), Available at www.cdc.gov/minorityhealth/chdireport.html.
21. K.D. Kochanek, S.L. Murphy, J. Xu, and B. Tejada-Vera, "Deaths: Final Data for 2014," *National Vital Statistics Reports* 65, no. 4 (2016), Available at https://www.cdc.gov/nchs/data/nvsr/nvsr65/nvsr65_04.pdf.
22. A. Case and A. Deaton, "Rising Morbidity and Mortality in Midlife among White Non-Hispanic Americans in the 21st Century," *PNAS* 112 no. 49 (2015): 15078–83, Available at http://www.pnas.org/content/112/49/15078.

23. Centers for Disease Control and Prevention, "CDC Health Disparities and Inequalities Report—United States, 2013," *Morbidity and Mortality Weekly Report* 62, Suppl. 3 (2013), Available at www.cdc.gov/minorityhealth/chdireport.html.

24. Centers for Disease Control and Prevention, "Burden of Tobacco Use in the U.S.," April 11, 2017, Available at https://www.cdc.gov/tobacco/campaign/tips/resources/data/cigarette-smoking-in-united-states.html#lgbt.

25. S. Dejun et al., "Mental Health Disparities within the LGBT Population: A Comparison between Transgender and Nontransgender Individuals," *Transgender Health* 1, no. 1 (2016): 12–20, doi:10.1089/trgh.2015.0001.

26. T.R. Frieden, "Foreword: CDC Health Disparities and Inequalities Report—United States, 2013," *Morbidity and Mortality Weekly Report* 62, Suppl. 3 (2013), Available at www.cdc.gov/minorityhealth/chdireport.html.

27. J.Z. Ayanian, "The Costs of Racial Disparities in Health Care," *Harvard Business Review*, October 1, 2015, Available at https://hbr.org/2015/10/the-costs-of-racial-disparities-in-health-care.

28. U.S. Department of Health and Human Services), *Healthy People 2020*, "Disparities," 2017, Available at www.healthypeople.gov/2020/about/foundation-health-measures/Disparities.

29. K.L. Walters et al., "Health Equity: Eradicating Health Inequalities for Future Generations," American Academy of Social Work and Social Welfare, Working Paper No. 19, January 2016, Available at http://aaswsw.org/wp-content/uploads/2016/01/WP19-with-cover2.pdf.***

30. K. Chaturvedi and S.K. Chaturvedi, "Understanding Health Inequality," n.d. , Available at www.pitt.edu/~super7/46011-47001/46661.ppt.

31. C. Stone, D. Trisi, A. Sherman, and E. Horton, "A Guide to Statistics on Historical Trends in Income Inequality," Center on Budget and Policy Priorities, November 7, 2016, Available at http://www.cbpp.org/research/poverty-and-inequality/a-guide-to-statistics-on-historical-trends-in-income-inequality.

32. S. Artiga, "Disparities in Health and Health Care: Five Key Questions and Answers," Henry J. Kaiser Family Foundation, August 12, 2016, Available at http://kff.org/disparities-policy/issue-brief/disparities-in-health-and-health-care-five-key-questions-and-answers.

33. K.L. Walters et al., "Health Equity: Eradicating Health Inequalities for Future Generations," American Academy of Social Work and Social Welfare, Working Paper No. 19, January 2016, Available at http://aaswsw.org/wp-content/uploads/2016/01/WP19-with-cover2.pdf.

34. A. Coleman-Jensen, M. Rabbitt, C. Gregory, and A. Singh, "Household Food Security in the United States in 2015," Economic Research Report No. 215, September 2016, Available at https://www.ers.usda.gov/publications/pub-details/?pubid=79760.

35. Ibid.

36. P. Bravemen, S. Egerter, and D.R. Williams, "The Social Determinants of Health: Coming of Age," *Annual Review of Public Health*, 32 (2011): 381–98, doi:10.1146/annurev-publhealth-031210-101218.

37. Centers for Disease Control and Prevention, "CDC Health Disparities and Inequalities Report—United States, 2013," *Morbidity and Mortality Weekly Report* 62, Suppl. 3 (2013), Available at www.cdc.gov/minorityhealth/chdireport.html.

38. P.H. Wise, "Child Poverty and the Promise of Human Capacity: Childhood as a Foundation for Healthy Aging," *Academic Pediatrics* 3, Suppl. (2016): S37–S45, doi:10.1016/j.acap.2016.01.014.

39. B.P. Bosworth, G. Burtless, and K. Zhang, "What Growing Life Expectancy Gaps Mean for the Promise of Social Security," Brookings Institution, February 12, 2016, Available at https://www.brookings.edu/research/what-growing-life-expectancy-gaps-mean-for-the-promise-of-social-security/#recent.

40. M. Huynh, et al., "Spatial Social Polarization and Birth Outcomes: Preterm Birth and Infant Mortality, New York City, 2010–2014," *Scandinavian Journal of Public Health*, April 2017, doi:10.1177/1403494817701566.

41. N.L. Hair, J.L. Hanson, B.L. Wolfe, and S.D. Pollak, "Association of Child Poverty, Brain Development, and Academic Achievement," *JAMA Pediatrics* 169, no. 9 (2015): 822–29, Available at https://www.ncbi.nlm.nih.gov/pmc/articles/PMC4687959.

42. Centers for Disease Control and Prevention, "Table 3, Delay or Nonreceipt of Needed Medical Care, Nonreceipt of Prescription Drugs, or Nonreceipt of Needed Dental Care during the Past 12 Months Due to Cost, by Selected Characteristics: United States, Selected Years 1997–2014," April 27, 2016, Available at https://www.cdc.gov/nchs/hus/poverty.htm.

43. Centers for Disease Control and Prevention, "CDC Health Disparities and Inequalities Report—United States, 2013," *Morbidity and Mortality Weekly Report* 62, Suppl. 3 (2013), Available at www.cdc.gov/minorityhealth/chdireport.html.

44. Centers for Disease Control and Prevention, "Table 42, Disability Measures among Adults Aged 18 and Over, by Selected Characteristics: United States, Selected Years 1997–2014," April 27, 2016, Available at https://www.cdc.gov/nchs/data/hus/2015/042.pdf.

45. U.S. Department of Health and Human Services, *Healthy People 2020*, "Social Determinants of Health," April, 2017, Available at https://www.healthypeople.gov/2020/topics-objectives/topic/social-determinants-of-health.

46. American Psychological Association, "Stress in America: Impact of Discrimination," March 10, 2016, Available at www.stressinamerica.org.

47. Ibid.

48. Ibid.

49. National Library of Medicine, "Health Literacy: Definition," 2017, Available at https://nnlm.gov/professional-development/topics/health-literacy.

50. Ibid.

51. Ibid.

52. J.J. Wing, et al., "Change in Neighborhood Characteristics and Change in Coronary Artery Calcium," *Circulation* 134 (2016): 504–13, doi:10.1161/CIRCULATIONAHA.115.020534.

53. A.Y. Hansen, M.R. Umstattd Meyer, J.D. Lenardson, and D. Hartley, "Built .Environments and Active Living in Rural and Remote Areas: A Review of the Literature," *Current Obesity Reports* 4, no. 4 (2015): 484–93, doi:10.1007/s13679-015-0180-9.

54. A.J. Cohen et al., "Estimates and 25-Year Trends of the Global Burden of Disease Attributable to Ambient Air Pollution: An Analysis of Data from the Global Burden of Diseases Study 2015," *Lancet* April 10, 2017, pii: S0140-6736(17)30505-6, doi:10.1016/S0140-6736(17)30505-6.

55. Centers for Disease Control and Prevention, "Lead: Data, Statistics, and Surveillance," February 9, 2017, Available at www.cdc.gov/nceh/lead/default.htm.

56. Ibid.

57. K.P. Theall, E.A. Shirtcliff, A.R. Dismukes, M. Wallace, and S.S. Drury, "Association between Neighborhood Violence and Biological Stress in Children," *JAMA Pediatrics* 171, no. 1 (2017): 53–60, doi:10.1001/jamapediatrics.2016.2321.,

58. J. Nothling, S. Sulliman, L. Martin, C. Simmons, and S. Seedat, "Differences in Abuse, Neglect, and Exposure to Community Violence in Adolescents with and without PTSD and Depression," *Journal of Interpersonal Violence* October 24, 2016, pii: 0886260516674944.

59. S.A. Sumner, J.A. Mercy, L.L. Dahlberg, S.D. Hillis, J. Klevens, and D. Houry, "Violence in the United States: Status, Challenges, and Opportunities," *Journal of the American Medical Association* 31, no. 5 (2015): 478–88, doi:10.1001/jama.2015.8371.

60. K. Eldeirawi et al., "Association of Neighborhood Crime with Asthma and Asthma Morbidity among Mexican American Children in Chicago, Illinois," *Annals of Allergy and Asthma Immunology* 117, no. 5 (2016): 502–7, doi:10.1016/j.anal.2016.09.429.

61. S..A. Sumner, J.A. Mercy, L.L. Dahlberg, S.D. Hillis, J. Klevens, and D. Houry, "Violence in the United States: Status, Challenges, and Opportunities."

62. J. Pykett, R. Lilley, M. Whitehead, R. Howell, and R. Jones, "Mindfulness, Behaviour Change and Decision Making: An Experimental Trial," Economic and Social Research Council, January 2016, Available at http://www.sps.ed.ac.uk/staff/sociology/rachel_howell/Mindfulness_Behaviour_Change_and_Decision_Making_Final_Report.pdf.

63. A. Lueke and B. Gibson, "Mindfulness Meditation Reduces Implicit Age and Race Bias," *Social Psychology and Personality Science* 6, no. 3 (2015): 284–91, doi:10.1177/1948550614559651.

64. N. Torres, "Mindfulness Mitigates Biases You May Not Know You Have," *Harvard Business Review*, December 24, 2014, Available at https://hbr.org/2014/12/mindfulness-mitigates-biases-you-may-not-know-you-have.

65. A. Thompson and J.B. Cuseo, *Diversity and the College Experience: Research-Based Strategies for Appreciating Human Differences*, 2nd ed., Dubuque, Iowa: Kendall Hunt, 2014.

66. P. Gurin, B.A. Nagda, and X. Zuniga, *Dialogue across Difference: Practice, Theory, and Research on Intergroup Dialogue*, New York: Russell Sage Foundation, 2013.

67. U.S. Department of Health and Human Services, "National Prevention Strategy: Elimination of Health Disparities—A Report of the Surgeon General," May 2014, Available at https://www.surgeongeneral.gov/priorities/prevention/strategy/health-disparities.pdf.

68. A.S. Noonan, H.E. Velasco-Mondragon, and F.A. Wagner, "Improving the Health of African Americans in the USA: An Overdue Opportunity for Social Justice," *Public Health Reviews* 37, no. 12 (2016), doi:10.1186/s40985-016-0025-4.

69. U.S. Department of Health and Human Services, "National Prevention Strategy: Elimination of Health Disparities—A Report of the Surgeon General," May 2014, Available at https://www.surgeongeneral.gov/priorities/prevention/strategy/health-disparities.pdf.

70. Ibid.

71. S. Artiga, "Disparities in Health and Health Care: Five Key Questions and Answers," Henry J. Kaiser Family Foundation, August 12, 2016, Available at http://kff.org/disparities-policy/issue-brief/disparities-in-health-and-health-care-five-key-questions-and-answers.

72. Ibid.

73. U.S. Department of Health and Human Services, "National Prevention Strategy: Elimination of Health Disparities—A Report of the Surgeon General," May 2014, Available at https://www.surgeongeneral.gov/priorities/prevention/strategy/health-disparities.pdf.

74. U.S. Department of Health and Human Services, *Healthy People 2020*, "Healthy People: Section III: Historical Context for Developing Healthy People 2020," 2010, Available at http://www.healthypeople.gov/2010/hp2020/advisory/PhaseI/sec3.htm.

75. National Institutes of Health, "NIH Research Timelines: Health Disparities," March, 2013, Available at https://report.nih.gov/NIHfactsheets/ViewFactSheet.aspx?csid=124.

Pulled Statistics:

page 30, B.D. Proctor, J.L. Semega, and M.A. Kollar, "Income and Poverty in the United States: 2015," U.S. Census Bureau, Report Number P60-256, September 26, 2016, Available at https://www.census.gov/library/publications/2016/demo/p60-256.html.

Chapter 2: Promoting and Preserving Your Psychological Health

1. K. Neff, *Self Compassion: The Proven Power of Being Kind to Yourself* (New York: Harper-Collins, 2015).

2. H. Maslow, *Motivation and Personality*, 2nd ed. (New York: Harper and Row, 1970).

3. D. J. Anspaugh and G. Ezell, *Teaching Today's Health*, 10th ed. (Boston: Pearson, 2013).

4. Y. Yang et al., "Social Relationships and Physiological Determinants of Longevity across the Lifespan," *Proceedings of the National Academy of Sciences of the United States of America* 113, no. 3 (2016): 578–83; M. Ramsey and A. Gentzler, "An Upward Spiral: Bidirectional Associations between Positive Affect and Positive Aspects of Close Relationships across the Life Span," *Developmental Review* 36 (2015): 58–104.

5. D. Melkasha, *Friendship and Happiness across the Lifespan*, (New York: Springer, 2015).

6. S. Straussner and C. Fewel, "Children of Parents Who Abuse Alcohol and Drugs," in *Parental Psychiatric Disorder: Distressed Parents and Their Children*, 3rd ed., eds. A. Reupert, D. Mayberry, J. Nicholson, et al. (Cambridge, UK: Cambridge University Press, 2015), 138–53.

7. S. Levens et al., "The Role of Family Support and Perceived Stress Reactivity in Predicting Depression in College Freshman," *Journal of Social and Clinical Psychology* 35, no. 4 (2016): 342–55; D. Lamis et al., "Depressive Symptoms and Suicidal Ideation in College Students:

The Mediating and Moderating Roles of Hopelessness, Alcohol Problems, and Social Support," *Journal of Clinical Psychology* 72, no. 9 (2016): 919–32.

8. American College Health Association, *National College Health Assessment II: Reference Group Executive Summary, Fall, 2016*, (Baltimore: American College Health Association, 2017).

9. M. Weijs-Perree et al., "Factors Influencing Social Satisfaction and Loneliness: A Path Analysis," *Journal of Transport Geography* 45 (2015): 24–31.

10. J. Cacioppo et al., "Loneliness across Phylogeny and a Call for Comparative Studies and Animal Models," *Perspectives on Psychological Science* 10, no. 2 (2015): 202–12.

11. Ibid.

12. National Cancer Institute, "Spirituality in Cancer Care," May 18, 2015, www.cancer.gov/cancertopics/pdq/supportivecare/spirituality/patient.

13. T. Marshall, K. Lefringhausen, and N. Ferenczi, "The Big Five, Self-Esteem, Narcissism as Predictors of the Topics People Write about in Facebook Status Updates," *Personality and Individual Differences* 85 (2015): 35–40; A. Diddaway and E. Rafestesder, "Agenda for Conceptualizing and Researching Praise and Criticism," *Journal of Paediatrics and Child Health* 52, no.1 (2016): 99.

14. C. Dweck, "A for Effort," *Scientific American* 23 no. 5 (2015): 80, www.nature.com/scientificamerican/journal/v23/n5s/full/scientificamericangenius0115-80.html.

15. M. Seligman, *Helplessness: On Depression, Development, and Death* (New York: W. H. Freeman, 1975).

16. K. Huffman and C. A. Sanderson, *Real World Psychology* (Hoboken, NJ: Wiley, 2014).

17. P. Salovey and J. Mayer, "Emotional Intelligence," *Imagination, Cognition, and Personality* 9, no. 3 (1989): 185–211.

18. HBR 10 Must Reads, *On Emotional Intelligence* (Boston: Harvard Business Review Press, 2015).

19. D. Goleman et al., *Primal Leadership: Unleashing the Power of Emotional Intelligence* (Boston: Harvard Business Review Press, 2013); I. Tuhovasky, *Emotional Intelligence: A Practical Guide to Making Friends with Your Emotions and Raising Your EQ* (Ian Tuhovasky, 2015).

20. K. Huffman and C. A. Sanderson, *Real World Psychology* (Hoboken, NJ: Wiley, 2014).

21. Ibid.

22. M. Seligman et al., "White Paper: Positive Health and Heath Assets: Re-analysis of Longitudinal Datasets." *U Penn Positive Health* (2015), Available at https://ppc.sas.upenn.edu/sites/ppc.sas.upenn.edu/files/positivehealthassetspub.pdf.

23. Ibid.

24. M. Seligman, *Flourish: A Visionary New Understanding of Happiness and Well-Being* (New York: Free Press, 2011).

25. S. Donaldson et al., "Happiness, Excellence, and Optimal Human Functioning Revisited: Examining the Peer Reviewed Literature Linked to Positive Psychology," *Journal of Positive Psychology* 10, no. 3 (2015): 185–95.

26. M. Garaigordobil, "Predictor Variables of Happiness and Its Connection with Risk and Protective Factors for Health," *Frontiers in Psychology* 6 (2015): 1176.

27. Ibid.

28. P. de Souto Barreto and Y. Rolland, "Happiness and Unhappiness Have No Direct Effect on Mortality," *Lancet* 387, no. 10021 (2016): 822–23.

29. Mayo Clinic Staff, "Mental Illness: Causes," October 2015, www.mayoclinic.org/diseases-conditions/mental-illness/basics/causes/con-20033813.

30. Ibid.

31. Substance Abuse and Mental Health Services Administration, "Key Substance Use and Mental Health Indicators in the United States: Results from the 2015 National Survey on Drug Use and Health," September 2016, Available at https://www.samhsa.gov/data/sites/default/files/NSDUH-FFR1-2015/NSDUH-FFR1-2015/NSDUH-FFR1-2015.htm.

32. Ibid.

33. L. Szabo, "Cost of Not Caring: Nowhere to Go," *USA Today*, May 5, 2014, www.usatoday.com/story/news/nation/2014/05/12/mental-health-system-crisis/7746535; T. Insel, "Director's Blog: Mental Health Awareness Month: By the Numbers," *National Institute of Mental Health*, May 15, 2015, http://www.nimh.nih.gov/about/director/2015/mental-health-awareness-month-by-the-numbers.shtml.

34. R. P. Gallagher, "National Survey of College Counseling 2014," *International Association of Counseling Services, Inc. Monograph Series* 9V (2014), Available at http://0201.nccdn.net/1_2/000/000/088/0b2/NCCCS2014_v2.pdf.

35. American College Health Association, *American College Health Association–National College Health Assessment II (ACHA–NCHA II): Reference Group Data Report Fall, 2016* (Baltimore: American College Health Association, 2017), Available at http://www.acha-ncha.org/docs/NCHA-II_FALL_2016_REFERENCE_GROUP_DATA_REPORT.pdf.

36. Ibid.

37. Ibid.

38. U.S. National Library of Medicine, "Medline Plus: Mood Disorders," December 27, 2016, https://medlineplus.gov/mooddisorders.html.

39. National Institute of Mental Health, "Major Depression among Adults," Accessed April 2017, https://www.nimh.nih.gov/health/statistics/prevalence/major-depression-among-adults.shtml.

40. Ibid.

41. Ibid.

42. American College Health Association, *American College Health Association–National College Health Assessment II (ACHA–NCHA II): Reference Group Data Report Fall, 2016* (Baltimore: American College Health Association, 2017), Available at http://www.acha-ncha.org/docs/NCHA-II_FALL_2016_REFERENCE_GROUP_DATA_REPORT.pdf.

43. National Institute of Mental Health, "Dysthymic Disorder among Adults," Accessed April 2017, https://www.nimh.nih.gov/health/statistics/prevalence/dysthymic-disorder-among-adults.shtml.

44. Substance Abuse and Mental Health Services Administration, "Mental Disorders: Bipolar and Related Disorders," October 27, 2015, www.samhsa.gov/disorders/mental.

45. WebMD, "Seasonal Depression (Seasonal Affective Disorder)," Accessed February 23, 2015, www.webmd.com/depression/guide/seasonal-affective-disorder.

46. Cleveland Clinic, "Seasonal Depression," Accessed February 2016, https://my.clevelandclinic.org/services/neurological_institute/center-for-behavioral-health/-disease-conditions/hic-seasonal-depression.

47. Mayo Clinic Staff, MayoClinic.com, "Depression: Causes," 2015, www.mayoclinic.org/diseases-conditions/depression/basics/causes/con-20032977.

48. Substance Abuse and Mental Health Services Administration, "Mental Disorders: Anxiety Disorders," October 27, 2015, www.samhsa.gov/disorders/mental; R. Karg et al., "Past Year Mental Health Disorders among Adults in the U.S.," 2014, https://www.samhsa.gov/data/sites/default/files/NSDUH-DR-N2MentalDis-2014-1/Web/NSDUH-DR-N2MentalDis-2014.htm; K. R. Merikangas et al., "Lifetime Prevalence of Mental Disorders in U.S. Adolescents: Results from the National Comorbidity Survey Replication—Adolescent Supplement (NCS-A)," *Journal of the American Academy of Child and Adolescent Psychiatry* 49, no. 10 (2010): 980–89, doi:10.1016/j.jaac.2010.05.017.

49. American College Health Association, *American College Health Association–National College Health Assessment II (ACHA–NCHA II): Reference Group Data Report Fall, 2016* (Baltimore: American College Health Association, 2017), Available at http://www.acha-ncha.org/docs/NCHA-II_FALL_2016_REFERENCE_GROUP_DATA_REPORT.pdf.

50. National Institute of Mental Health, "Generalized Anxiety Disorder, GAD," Accessed April 2017, www.nimh.nih.gov/health/publications/anxiety-disorders/generalized-anxiety-disorder-gad.shtml.

51. American College Health Association, *American College Health Association–National College Health Assessment II (ACHA–NCHA II): Reference Group Data Report Fall, 2016* (Baltimore: American College Health Association, 2017., Available at http://www.acha-ncha.org/docs/NCHA-II_FALL_2016_REFERENCE_GROUP_DATA_REPORT.pdf.

52. Mayo Clinic Staff, "Panic Attacks and Panic Disorder: Symptoms," May 2015, www.mayoclinic.org/diseases-conditions/panic-attacks/basics/symptoms/con-20020825.

53. Web MD, "Anxiety and Panic Disorders Health Center: Specific Phobias," February 24, 2016, www.webmd.com/anxiety-panic/specific-phobias.

54. Ibid.

55. National Institute of Mental Health, "Anxiety Disorders," March 2016, https://www.nimh.nih.gov/health/topics/anxiety-disorders/index.shtml.

56. National Institute of Mental Health, "Obsessive Compulsive Disorder: Prevalence," Accessed February 23, 2015, www.nimh.nih.gov/health/statistics/prevalence/obsessive-compulsive-disorder-among-adults.shtml.

57. National Institute of Mental Health, "Obsessive Compulsive Disorder," January 2016, http://www.nimh.nih.gov/health/topics/obsessive-compulsive-disorder-ocd/index.shtml.

58. Anxiety and Depression Association of America, "Facts and Statistics," Accessed February 23, 2015, www.adaa.org/about-adaa/press-room/facts-statistics.

59. Ibid.; J. Gradus, "Epidemiology of PTSD," PTSD: National Center for PTSD," U.S. Department of Veterans Affairs, National Center for PTSD, February 23, 2016, http://www.ptsd.va.gov/professional/PTSD-overview/epidemiological-facts-ptsd.asp.

60. U.S. Department of Veterans Affairs, "PTSD: National Center for PTSD," October 3, 2016, www.ptsd.va.gov/public/PTSD-overview/basics/how-common-is-ptsd.asp.

61. National Institute of Mental Health, "Post-Traumatic Stress Disorder," February 2016, www.nimh.nih.gov/health/topics/post-traumatic-stress-disorder-ptsd/index.shtml#part4.

62. J. Gradus, "Epidemiology of PTSD," U.S. Department of Veterans Affairs, National Center for PTSD, February 23, 2016, www.ptsd.va.gov/professional/PTSD-overview/epidemiological-facts-ptsd.asp; S. Staggs, "Myths and Facts about PTSD," *PsychCentral*, February 2014, http://psychcentral.com/lib/myths-and-facts-about-ptsd.

63. American Psychiatric Association, *Diagnostic and Statistical Manual of Mental Disorders*, 5th ed. (Washington, DC: American Psychiatric Association, 2013).

64. National Institutes of Health, "Any Personality Disorder," National Institute of Mental Health, Accessed February 2016, www.nimh.nih.gov/health/statistics/prevalence/any-personality-disorder.shtml; P. Tyrer, F. Reed, and M. Crawford, "Classification, Assessment Prevalence, and Effect of Personality Disorder," *Lancet* 385, no. 9969 (2015): 717–26.

65. A.D.A.M. Medical Encyclopedia, "Antisocial Personality Disorder," PubMed Health (Bethesda, MD: U.S. National Library of Medicine, 2016).

66. Mayo Clinic Staff, MayoClinic.com, "Borderline Personality Disorder," July 2015, http://www.mayoclinic.org/diseases-conditions/borderline-personality-disorder/basics/-symptoms/con-20023204.

67. Mayo Clinic, "Borderline Personality Disorder," July 2015, www.mayoclinic.org/diseases-conditions/borderline-personality-disorder/basics/definition/con-20023204.

68. National Institutes of Health, "Borderline Personality Disorder," National Institute of Mental Health, Accessed February 2016, http://www.nimh.nih.gov/health/topics/borderline-personality-disorder/index.shtml.

69. Ibid.

70. National Institute of Mental Health, "Schizophrenia," February 2016, www.nimh.nih.gov/health/topics/schizophrenia/index.shtml.

71. Ibid.

72. Ibid.

73. World Health Organization, "Preventing Suicide: A Global Imperative," 2014, Available at www.who.int/mental_health/suicide-prevention/world_report_2014/en.

74. World Health Organization, "Suicide: Fact Sheet," 2017, Available at http://www.who.int/mediacentre/factsheets/fs398/en.

75. World Health Organization, "Preventing Suicide: A Global Imperative," 2014, Available at www.who.int/mental_health/suicide-prevention/world_report_2014/en.

76. M. Heron, "Deaths: Leading Causes for 2014," *National Vital Statistics Reports* 65, no. 5 (2016), Available

at https://www.cdc.gov/nchs/data/nvsr/nvsr65/nvsr65_05.pdf.

77. American College Health Association, *American College Health Association–National College Health Assessment II (ACHA–NCHA II): Reference Group Data Report Fall, 2016* (Baltimore: American College Health Association, 2017/, Available at http://www.acha-ncha.org/docs/NCHA-II_FALL_2016_REFERENCE_GROUP_DATA_REPORT.pdf.

78. Ibid.; Centers for Disease Control and Prevention, "Suicide Facts at a Glance 2015," Accessed February 2016, http://www.cdc.gov/violenceprevention/pdf/suicide-datasheet-a.pdf.

79. A. Haas et al., "Suicide Attempts among Transgender and Gender Non-Conforming Adults: Findings of the National Transgender Discrimination Survey," American Foundation for Suicide Prevention, January 2014.

80. Ibid.; E. Mereish, C. O'Cleirigh, and J. Bradford, "Interrelationships between LGBT-Based Victimization, Suicide, and Substance Use Problems in a Diverse Sample of Sexual and Gender Minority Men and Women," *Psychology, Health & Medicine* 19, no. 1 (2014): 1–13; A. Flynn et al., "Victimization of Lesbian, Gay, and Bisexual People in Childhood: Associations with Attempted Suicide," *Suicide and Life-Threatening Behavior* 46, no. 4 (2016):457–70; T. Hottes, "Lifetime Prevalence of Suicide Attempts Among Sexual Minority Adults by Study Sampling Strategies: A Systematic Review and Meta-Analysis," *American Journal of Public Health* 106, no. 5 (2016): e1–e12.

81. Centers for Disease Control and Prevention, "Suicide Facts at a Glance 2015," Accessed February 2016, http://www.cdc.gov/violenceprevention/pdf/suicide-data-sheet-a.pdf.

82. Ibid.

83. American Foundation for Suicide Prevention, "Warning Signs of Suicide," Accessed February 2016, www.afsp.org/preventing-suicide/risk-factors-and-warning-signs.

84. Ibid.

85. Befrienders Worldwide, "Helping a Suicidal Friend or Relative," Accessed February 2016, http://www.befrienders.org/helping-a-friend; and Befrienders Worldwide, "Suicidal Feelings," Accessed February 2016, http://www.befrienders.org/suicidal-feelings.

86. National Institute of Mental Health, "Use of Mental Health Services and Treatment among Adults," Accessed April 2017, https://www.nimh.nih.gov/health/statistics/prevalence/use-of-mental-health-services-and-treatment-among-adults.shtml.

87. MentalHealth.gov, "Mental Health Myths and Facts," Accessed February 2016, www.mentalhealth.gov/basics/myths-facts/.

88. S. Clement et al., "What Is the Impact of Mental Health-Related Stigma on Help-Seeking? A Systematic Review of Quantitative and Qualitative Studies," *Psychological Medicine* 45, no. 1 (2015): 11–27.

89. K. Huffman and C. A. Sanderson, *Real World Psychology* (Hoboken, NJ: Wiley, 2014).

90. Ibid.

91. Mayo Clinic, "Cognitive Behavioral Therapy," February 2016, http://www.mayoclinic.org/tests-procedures/cognitive-behavioral--therapy/home/ovc-20186868.

92. Drug Watch, "FDA Warnings for Antidepressants," October 12, 2015, http://www.drugwatch.com/ssri/fda-warnings; R. Friedman, "Antidepressants' Black-Box Warning—10 Years Later," *New England Journal of Medicine* 371, no. 18 (2014): 1666–68" http://www.drugwatch.com/ssri/fda-warnings; R. Friedman, "Antidepressants' Black-Box Warning—10 Years Later," *New England Journal of Medicine* 371, no. 18 (2014): 1666–68.

Pulled Statistics:

page 52, Centers for Disease Control and Prevention, "Suicide: Facts at a Glance, 2015," Accessed February 2016, Available at www.cdc.gov/violenceprevention/pdf/suicide-datasheet-a.pdf.

page 55, D. Eisenberg et al., "Data from the Healthy Minds Network: The Economic Case for Student Mental Health Services," DepressionCenter.org, March 13, 2014, www.depressioncenter.org/docc/2014/pdf/eisenberg-lipson-economic-case-for-student-mental-health.pdf.

Focus On: Cultivating Your Spiritual Health

1. K. Eagan et al., *The American Freshman: National Norms Fall 2015* (Los Angeles: Higher Education Research Institute, UCLA, 2015), Available at https://www.heri.ucla.edu/monographs/TheAmericanFreshman2015-Expanded.pdf.

2. Ibid.

3. H.G. Koenig, "Religion, Spirituality and Health: A Review and Update," *Advances in Mind–Body Medicine* 29, no. 3 (2015): 19–26.

4. Pew Research Center, *The Global Religious Landscape* (Washington, DC: Pew Research Center's Forum on Religion and Public Life, 2012), Available at http://www.pewforum.org/2012/12/18/global-religious-landscape-exec.

5. Ibid; K. Eagan et al., *The American Freshman: National Norms Fall 2015* (Los Angeles: Higher Education Research Institute, UCLA, 2015), Available at https://www.heri.ucla.edu/monographs/TheAmericanFreshman2015-Expanded.pdf.

6. B.A. Alper, "Millennials Are Less Religious Than Older Americans, but Just as Spiritual," Pew Research Center, November 23, 2015, www.pewresearch.org/fact-tank/2015/11/23/millennials-are-less-religious-than-older-americans-but-just-as-spiritual.

7. B. Brown, *Rising Strong* (New York: Random House, 2017); B. Brown, *The Gifts of Imperfection: Let Go of Who You Think You're Supposed to Be and Embrace Who You Are* (Center City, MN: Hazelden, 2010).

8. B.L. Seaward, *Managing Stress: Principles and Strategies for Health and Well Being*, 8th ed. (Sudbury, MA: Jones and Bartlett, 2015).

9. DanahZohar.com, "Learn the Qs," Accessed January 2014, http://dzohar.com/?page_id=622.

10. C. Wigglesworth, "Spiritual Intelligence and Why It Matters," Deep Change, 2011, www.deepchange.com/SpiritualIntelligenceEmotionalIntelligence2011.pdf.

11. National Institutes of Health, National Center for Complementary and Integrative Health, "2016 Strategic Plan," Accessed March 2017, https://nccih.nih.gov/about/strategic-plans/2016.

12. D. Fishbein et al., "Behavioral and Psychophysiological Effects of a Yoga Intervention on High-Risk Adolescents: A Randomized Control Trial," *Journal of Child and Family Studies* 25, no. 2 (2016): 518–29; H. Lu et al., "The Brain Structure Correlates of Individual Differences in Trait Mindfulness: A Voxel-Based Morphometry Study," *Neuroscience/* 272 (2014): 21–8; H. Huang et al., "A Meta-Analysis of the Benefits of Mindfulness-Based Stress Reduction (MBSR) on Psychological Function among Breast Cancer (BC) Survivors," *Breast Cancer* 23. no. 4 (2016); 568–76, http://link.springer.com/article/10.1007/s12282-015-0604-0#page1; E. Hoge et al., "Effects of Mindfulness Meditation on Occupational Functioning and Health Care Utilization in Individuals with Anxiety," *Journal of Psychosomatic Research* 95 (2017): 7–11.

13. National Cancer Institute, "Spirituality in Cancer Care," July 17, 2015, www.cancer.gov/cancertopics/pdq/supportivecare/-spirituality/HealthProfessional/page1.

14. M. Mollica et al., "Spirituality Is Associated with Better Prostate Cancer Treatment Decision Making Experiences," *Journal of Behavioral Medicine* 39, no. 1 (2016): 161–69.

15. P. Rajguru et al., "Use of Mindfulness Meditation in the Management of Chronic Pain: A Systematic Review of Randomized Controlled Trials," *American Journal of Lifestyle Medicine* 9, no 3 (2015): 176–84.

16. E. Singer, R. McElroy, and P. Muennig, "Social Capital and the Paradox of Poor but Healthy Groups in the United States," *Journal of Immigrant and Minority Health* 19, no. 3 (2017): 716–22, doi:10.1007/s10903-016-0396-0.

17. C. Aldwin et al., "Differing Pathways between Religiousness, Spirituality, and Health: A Self-Regulation Perspective," *Psychology of Religion and Spirituality* 6, no. 1 (2014): 9–21.

18. H. Jim et al., "Religion, Spirituality, and Physical Health in Cancer Patients: A Meta-Analysis," *Cancer* 121, no. 21 (2015): 3760–68.

19. S. Hooker, K. Masters, and K. Carey, "Multidimensional Assessment of Religiousness/Spirituality and Health Behaviors in College Students," *International Journal for the Psychology of Religion* 24, no. 3 (2014): 228–40; V. Kress et al., "Spirituality/Religiosity, Life Satisfaction, and Life Meaning as Protective Factors for Nonsuicidal Self-Injury in College Students," *Journal of College Counseling* 18, no. 2 (2015): 160–74.

20. National Cancer Institute, "Spirituality in Cancer Care," July 17, 2015, www.cancer.gov/cancertopics/pdq/supportivecare/-spirituality/HealthProfessional/page1.

21. L. Waters, A. Barsky, A. Ridd, and K. Allen, "Contemplative Education: A Systematic, Evidence-Based Review of the Effect of Meditation Interventions in Schools," *Educational Psychology Review* 27, no. 1 (2015): 103–34, doi:10.1007/s10648-014-9258-2.

22. National Center for PTSD, "Spirituality and Trauma: Professionals Working Together," February 23, 2016, www.ptsd.va.gov/-professional/provider-type/community/fs-spirituality.asp.

23. Ibid.; NCCAM, "Prayer and Spirituality in Health: Ancient Practices, Modern Science," *CAM at the NIH: Focus on Complementary and Alternative Medicine* 12, no. 1 (2005), www.jpsych.com/pdfs/NCCAM%20-%20Prayer%20and%20Spirituality%20in%20Health.pdf; NCI, "Spirituality in Cancer Care," July 17, 2015, www.cancer.gov/cancertopics/pdq/supportivecare/-spirituality/HealthProfessional/page1.

24. D.R. Vago and D.A. Silbersweig, "Self-Awareness, Self-Regulation, and Self-Transcendence (S-ART): A Framework for Understanding the Neurobiological Mechanisms of Mindfulness," *Human Neuroscience* 6 (2012): 296, Available at www.ncbi.nlm.nih.gov/pmc/articles/PMC3480633.

25. G. Desbordes et al., "Effects of Mindful-Attention and Compassion Meditation Training on Amygdala Response to Emotional Stimuli in an Ordinary, Non-meditative State," *Frontiers in Human Neuroscience* 6, no. 292 (2012): 292, doi:10.3389/fnhum.2012.00292.

26. B. Brown, "How to Listen to Pain," *Greater Good: The Science of a Meaningful Life*, February 17, 2016, http://greatergood.berkeley.edu/article/item/how_to_listen_to_pain.

27. D. Desteno, "The Kindness Cure," *Atlantic*, July 21, 2015, https://www.theatlantic.com/health/archive/2015/07/mindfulness-meditation-empathy-compassion/398867.

28. F. Zeidan et al., "Neural Correlates of Mindfulness Meditation-Related Anxiety Relief," *Social Cognitive and Affective Neuroscience* 9, no. 6 (2014): 751–59, doi:10.1093/scan/nst041; G. Desbordes et al., "Effects of Mindful-Attention and Compassion Meditation Training on Amygdala Response to Emotional Stimuli in an Ordinary, Non-meditative State," *Frontiers in Human Neuroscience* 6, no. 292 (2012): 292, doi:10.3389/fnhum.2012.00292; J.C. Ong et al., "A Randomized Controlled Trial of Mindfulness Meditation for Chronic Insomnia," *Sleep* 37, no. 9 (2013): 1553–63; NCCIH, "Research Spotlight," 2014.

29. E. Hoge et al., "Randomized Controlled Trial of Mindfulness Meditation for Generalized Anxiety Disorder: Effects on Anxiety and Stress Reactivity," *Journal of Clinical Psychiatry* 74, no. 8 (2013): 786–92; S. Jedel et al., "A Randomized Controlled Trial of Mindfulness-Based Stress Reduction to Prevent Flare-Up in Patients with Inactive Ulcerative Colitis," *Digestion* 89, no. 2 (2014): 142–55.

30. W. Marchand, "Neural Mechanisms of Mindfulness and Meditation: Evidence From Neuroimging Studies," *World Journal of Radiology* 6, no. 7 (2014): 471–79, doi:10.4329/wjr.v6.i7.471.

31. S. Keng et al., "Effects of Mindfulness on Psychological Health," *Clinical Psychology Review* 31, no. 6 (2011); 1041–56; M. Spijkerman, W. Pots, and E. Bohlmeijer, "Effectiveness of Online Mindfulness-Based Interventions in Improving Mental Health: A Review and Meta-Analysis of Randomised Controlled Trials," *Clinical Psychology Review* 45 (2016): 102–14.

32. W. Marchand, "Neural Mechanisms of Mindfulness and Meditation: Evidence From Neuroimging Studies," *World Journal of Radiology* 6, no. 7 (2014): 471–79, doi:10.4329/wjr.v6.i7.471; B. Holzel et al., "Neural Mechanisms of Symptom Improvements in Generalized Anxiety Disorder Following Mindfulness Training," *Neuroimage: Clinical* 2 (2013): 448–58; A.

Taren et al., "Mindfulness Meditation Training Alters Stress-Related Amygdala Resting State Functional Connectivity: A Randomized Controlled Trial," *Social Cognitive and Affective Neuroscience* 10, no. 12 (2015): 1758–68.

33. A. Lucette et al., "Spirituality and Religiousness Are Associated with Fewer Depressive Symptoms in Individuals with Medical Conditions," *Psychosomatics* (2016), doi:10.1016/j.psym.2016.03.005; University of Minnesota Center for Spirituality and Healing, "What Is Prayer?," August 2013, www.takingcharge.csh.umn.edu/explore-healing-practices/prayer.

34. L. Larkey et al., "Randomized Controlled Trial of Qigong/Tai Chi Easy on Cancer-Related Fatigue in Breast Cancer Survivors," *Annals of Behavioral Medicine* 49, no. 2 (2015): 165–76; American Tai Chi Association, "Psychiatric Expert: Tai Chi and Qigong Can Improve Mood in Older Adults," September 6, 2013, www.americantaichi.net/TaiChiQigongForHealthArticle.asp?cID=2&sID=10&article=chi_201309_1&subject=Mental Health.

35. M. Rudd and J. Aakers, "How to Be Happy by Giving to Others," *Scientific American*, July 8, 2014, www.scientificamerican.com/article/how-to-be-happy-by-giving-to-others.

36. K. Azzarelli, "Rethinking Happiness: Using Your Power for Purpose," *Annals of the New York Academy of Sciences* 1384 (2016): 32–5, doi:10.1111/nyas.13149.

Pulled Statistics:

page 62, K. Eagan et al., *The American Freshman: National Norms Fall 2015* (Los Angeles: Higher Education Research Institute, UCLA, 2015), Available at https://www.heri.ucla.edu/monographs/TheAmericanFreshman2015-Expanded.pdf.

page 68, H. Cramer et al., "Prevalence, Patterns, and Predictors of Yoga Use: Results of a US Nationally Representative Survey," *American Journal of Preventive Medicine* 50, no. 2 (2016): 230–35.

Chapter 3: Managing Stress and Coping with Life's Challenges

1. American Psychological Association, "Stress in America," 2015; American Psychological Association, "Stress in America Annual Survey: Are Teens Adopting Adults' Stress Habits?" February 11, 2014, Available at www.apa.org/news/press/releases/stress/2013/stress-report.pdf; American Psychological Association, "Stress in America, The Impact of Discrimination," 2015, http://www.apa.org/news/press/releases/stress/2015/impact-of-discrimination.pdf.

2. American Psychological Association, "A Stress Snapshot: Women Continue to Face an Uphill Battle with Stress," Accessed January 30, 2015, http://apa.org/news/press/releases/stress/2013/snapshot.aspx.

3. American Psychological Association, "Stress in Americaa, The Impact of Discrimination," 2015, http://www.apa.org/news/press/releases/stress/2015/impact-of-discrimination.pdf.

4. American Psychological Association, "A Stress Snapshot: Women Continue to Face an Uphill Battle with Stress," Accessed January 30, 2015, http://apa.org/news/press/releases/stress/2013/snapshot.aspx.

5. American Psychological Association, "Stress: The Different Kinds of Stress," Accessed February 2014, www.apa.org.

6. B.L. Seaward, *Managing Stress: Principles and Strategies for Health and Well-Being*, 8th ed. (Sudbury, MA: Jones and Bartlett, 2013), 8; National Institute of Mental Health (NIMH), "Fact Sheet on Stress," Accessed January 2017, www.nimh.nih.gov/health/publications/stress/index.shtml/index.shtml.

7. H. Selye, *Stress without Distress* (New York: Lippincott Williams & Wilkins, 1974), 28–29.

8. W.B. Cannon, *The Wisdom of the Body* (New York: Norton, 1932).

9. C. Fagundes and B. Way, "Early-Life Stress and Adult Inflammation," *Current Directions in Psychological Science* 23, no. 4 (2014): 277–83; J. Morey et al., "Current Directions in Stress and Human Immune Function," *Current Opinion in Psychology* 5 (2015): 13–17; Mayo Clinic, "Chronic Stress Puts Your Health at Risk," April 21, 2016, http://www.mayoclinic.org/healthy-lifestyle/stress-management/in-depth/stress/art-20046037; A. Marsland et al., "The Effects of Acute Psychological Stress on Circulating and Stimulated Inflammatory Markers: A Systematic Review and Meta-analysis," *Brain, Behavior and Immunity* (2017).

10. American Psychological Association, "Stress in America: The Impact of Discrimination," March 2016, https://www.apa.org/news/press/releases/stress/2016/impact-of-discrimination.pdf; M. Dentato, "The Minority Stress Perspective," *American Psychological Association*, Accessed January 2017, www.apa.org/pi/aids/resources/exchange/2012/04/minority-stress.aspx.

11. R. Yerkes and J. Dodson, "The Relation of Strength of Stimulus to Rapidity of Habit-Formation," *Journal of Comparative Neurology and Psychology* 18, no. 5 (1908): 459–82.

12. C. Cardoso and M.A. Ellenbogen, "Tend-and-Befriend Is a Beacon for Change in Stress Research: A Reply to Tops," *Psychoneuroendocrinology* 45 (2014): 212–13; J. Berger et al., "Cortisol Modulates Men's Affiliative Responses to Acute Social Stress," *Psychoneuroendocrinology* 63 (2016): 1–9.

13. N.K. Dess, "Tend and Befriend: Women Tend to Nurture and Men to Withdraw When Life Gets Hard," June 9, 2016, *Psychology Today*, https://www.psychologytoday.com/articles/200009/tend-and-befriend.

14. N. Rohleder, "Chapter 9: Chronic Stress and Disease," in *Insights to Neuroimmune Biology*, 2nd ed., edited by I. Berci (Amsterdam: Elsevier Publishing, 2016); E. Dalton et al. Dalton, "Pathways Maintaining Physical Health Problems from Childhood to Young Adulthood: The Role of Stress and Mood." *Psychology & Health* 31, no. 11 (2016): 1255–71; P. Gianaros and T. Wager, "Brain-Body Pathways Linking Psychological Stress and Physical Health," *Current Directions in Psychological Science* 24, no. 4 (2015): 313–21; K.M. Scott et al., "Associations between Lifetime Traumatic Events and Subsequent Chronic Physical Conditions: A Cross-National, Cross-Sectional Study," *PLoS ONE* 8, no. 11 (2013), e80573.

15. K.M. Scott et al., "Associations between Lifetime Traumatic Events and Subsequent Chronic Physical Conditions: A Cross-National, Cross-Sectional Study," *PLoS One* 8, no. 11 (2013), doi:10.1371/journal.pone.0080573.

16. A. Lansing et al., "Assessing Stress Related Treatment Needs among Girls at Risk for Poor Functional Outcomes: The Impact of Cumulative Adversity, Criterion Traumas and Non-Criterion Events," *Journal of Anxiety Disorders* (2016); R. Scaer, *The Body Bears the Burden: Trauma, Dissociation, and Disease*, 3rd ed. (New York: Routledge Press, 2014).

17. J. Sumner et al. "Associations of Trauma Exposure and Posttraumatic Stress Symptoms with Venous Thromboembolism over 22 Years in Women," *Journal of the American Heart Association* 5, no. 5 (2016): e003197; H.M. Lagraauw et al., "Acute and Chronic Psychological Stress as Risk Factors for Cardiovascular Disease: Insights Gained from Epidemiological, Clinical, and Experimental Studies," *Brain, Behavior, and Immunity* 50 (2015): 18–30; A. Marsland et al., "The Effects of Acute Psychological Stress on Circulating and Stimulated Inflammatory Markers: A Systematic Review and Meta-analysis," *Brain, Behavior and Immunity* (2017); J. Holt-Lunstad and T. Smith, "Loneliness and Social Isolation as Risk Factors for CVD: Implications for Evidence-Based Patient Care and Scientific Inquiry," *Heart* 102, no. 13 (2016): 967–89.

18. M. Kivimäki and I. Kawachi, "Work Stress as a Risk Factor for Cardiovascular Disease," *Current Cardiology Reports* 17, no. 9 (2015): 1–9; M. Skogstad et al., "Systematic Review of the Cardiovascular Effects of Occupational Noise," *Occupational Medicine* 66, no. 1 (2016): 10–16.

19. S. Garbarino and N. Magnavita, "Work Stress and Metabolic Syndrome in Police Officers: A Prospective Study," *PLoS ONE* 10, no. 12 (2015): e0144318; F. Bartoli et al., "Posttraumatic Stress Disorder and Risk of Obesity: Systematic Review and Meta-analysis," *Journal of Clinical Psychiatry* 76, no. 10 (2015): e1253–61.

20. R. Lin, et al. "Systemic Causes of Hair Loss," *Annals of Medicine* 48, no. 6 (2016): 393–402; A. Skrok and L. Rudnicka, "Stress-Related Hair Disorders," in *Stress and Skin Disorders*, edited by K. França and M. Jafferany (Cham, Switzerland: Springer International Publishing, 2017). 155–64.

21. D. Young-Hyman et al., "Psychosocial Care for People with Diabetes: A Position Statement of the American Diabetes Association," *Diabetes Care* 39, no. 12 (2016): 2126–40, Available at http://care.diabetesjournals.org/content/39/12/2126; S.A. Brown et al., "Biobehavioral Determinants of Glycemic Control in Type 2 Diabetes: A Systematic Review and Meta-analysis," *Patient Education and Counseling* 99, no. 10 (2016): 1558–67; American Diabetes Association, "How Stress Affects Diabetes," June 7, 2013, www.diabetes.org/living-with-diabetes/complications/mental-health/stress.html.

22. S.H. Ley et al. "Contribution of the Nurses' Health Studies to Uncovering Risk Factors for Type 2 Diabetes: Diet, Lifestyle, Biomarkers, and Genetics," *American Journal of Public Health* 106, no. 9 (2016): 1624–30.

23. M. Virtanen et al., "Psychological Distress and Incidence of Type 2 Diabetes in High Risk and Low Risk Populations: The Whitehall II Cohort Study," *Diabetes Care* 37, no. 8 (2014): 2091–97; C. Crump et al. "Stress Resilience and Subsequent Risk of Type 2 Diabetes in 1.5 Million Young Men," *Diabetologia* 5/9, no. 4 (2016): 728–33.

24. National Digestive Diseases Information Clearinghouse (NDDIC), "Irritable Bowel Syndrome: How Does Stress Affect IBS?" Accessed January 2017, http://digestive.niddk.nih.gov/ddiseases/pubs/ibs/#stress.

25. B. Bartosz, et al. "Mechanisms by Which Stress Affects the Experimental and Clinical Inflammatory Bowel Disease (IBD): Role of Brain-Gut Axis," *Current Neuropharmacology* 14, no. 8 (2016): 892–900; H.F. Herlong, "Digestive Disorders White Paper: 2013," *Johns Hopkins Health Alerts*, 2013, www.johnshopkinshealthalerts.com.

26. E. Carlsson et al., "Psychological Stress in Children May Alter the Immune Response," *Journal of Immunology* 192, no. 5 (2014): 2071–81; J. Morey et al., "Current Directions in Stress and Human Immune Function," 2015.

27. F.S. Dhabhar, "Effects of Stress on Immune Function: The Good, the Bad, and the Beautiful," *Immunologic Research* 58, no. 2–3 (2014): 193–210; J. Morey et al., "Current Directions in Stress and Human Immune Function," 2015.

28. American College Health Association (ACHA), American College Health Association–National College Health Assessment II (ACHA-NCHA II): Reference Group Data Report Fall, 2016 (Hanover, MD: American College Health Association, 2017).

29. Ibid.

30. O.T. Wolf et al., "Stress and Memory: A Selective Review on Recent Developments in the Understanding of Stress Hormone Effects on Memory and Their Clinical Relevance," *Journal of Neuroendocrinology* 28, no. 8 (2016); G. Shields et al., "The Effects of Acute Stress on Core Executive Functions: A Meta-analysis and Comparison with Cortisol," *Neuroscience & Biobehavioral Reviews* 68 (2016): 651–68.

31. J. Oliver et al., "Impairments of the Spatial Working Memory and Attention Following Acute Psychosocial Stress," *Stress and Health* 31, no. 2 (2015): 115–23; G. Shields et al., "The Effects of Acute Stress on Core Executive Functions: A Meta-analysis and Comparison with Cortisol," *Neuroscience & Biobehavioral Reviews* 68 (2016): 651–68.

32. D. Baglietto-Vargas et al., "Short-Term Modern Life-like Stress Exacerbates Ab-Pathology and Synapse Loss in 3xTg-AD Mice," *Journal of Neurochemistry* 134, no. 5 (2015): 915–26; E. Marcello, "Alzheimer's Disease and Modern Lifestyle: What Is the Role of Stress?," *Journal of Neurochemistry* 134, no. 5 (2015): 795–98.

33. L. Mah, C. Szabuniewicz, and A.J. Fiocco, "Can Anxiety Damage the Brain?" *Current Opinion in Psychiatry* 29, no. 1 (2016): 56–62; D. Toral-Rios, "Oxidative Stress, Metabolic Syndrome and Alzheimer's Disease," *Biochemistry of Oxidative Stress* 16 (2016): 361–74; A. Pole et al., "Oxidative Stress, Cellular Senescence and Ageing," *AIMS Molecular Science* 3, no. 3(2016).

34. American Psychological Association, "Stress in America: The Impact of Discrimination," March 2016, http://www.apa.org/news/press/releases/stress/2015/impact-of-discrimination.pdf; American Psychological Association, "Stress in America: Paying with Our Health," 2015, Accessed April 2015, http://www.apa.org/news/press/releases/stress/2014/stress-report.pdf.

35. American Psychological Association, "Stress in America: The Impact of Discrimination," March 2016, http://www.apa.org/news/press/releases/stress/2015/impact-of-discrimination.pdf.

36. Ibid.

37. K. Donahue, "Daily Hassles, Mental Health Outcome and Dispositional Mindfulness in Student Registered Nurse Anesthetists," Doctoral dissertation, Oregon Health and Science University OHSU Digital Commons, 2016; Y. Jeong et al., "Do Hassles and Uplifts Trajectories Predict Mortality? Longitudinal Findings from the VA Normative Aging Study," *Journal of Behavioral Medicine* 39, no. 3 (2016): 408–19; C. Aldwin et al., "Do Hassles Mediate between Life Events and Mortality in Older Men? Longitudinal Findings from the VA Normative Aging Study," *Experimental Gerontology* 59 (2014): 74–80.

38. Y. Jeong et al., "Do Hassles and Uplifts Trajectories Predict Mortality? Longitudinal Findings from the VA Normative Aging Study," *Journal of Behavioral Medicine* 39, no. 3 (2016): 408–19; C. Aldwin et al., "Do Hassles Mediate between Life Events and Mortality?," 2014.

39. J. Siegris and J. Li, "Associations of Extrinsic and Intrinsic Components of Work Stress with Health: A Systematic Review of Evidence on the Effort-Reward Imbalance Model," *International Journal of Environmental Research and Public Health* 13, no. 4 (2016): 432; K. Toren et al., "A Longitudinal General Population-Based Study of Job Strain and Risk for Coronary Heart Disease and Stroke in Swedish Men," *BMJ Open* 4, no. 3 (2014): e004355, doi:10.1136/bmjopen-2013-004355.

40. F. Powell, "10 Student Loan Facts College Grads Need to Know," *U.S. News and World Report*, May 9, 2016, http://www.usnews.com/education/best-colleges/paying-for-college/slideshows/10-student-loan-facts-college-grads-need-to-know.

41. American College Health Association, National College Health Assessment II: Reference Group Data Report Fall, 2016, 2017.

42. .American Psychological Association, "Stress in America: Paying with Our Health," 2015.

43. A. Gold, "Why Self Esteem Is Important for Mental Health," NAMI, July 12, 2016, http://www.nami.org/Blogs/NAMI-Blog/July-2016/Why-Self-Esteem-Is-Important-for-Mental-Health; K.N. Mossakowski, "Disadvantaged Family Background and Depression among Young Adults in the United States: The Roles of Chronic Stress and Self-esteem," *Stress and Health* 31, no. 1 (2015): 52–62; K.R. Conner et al., "Posttraumatic Stress Disorder and Suicide in 5.9 Million Individuals Receiving Care in the Veterans Health Administration Health System," *Journal of Affective Disorders* 166 (2014): 1–5.

44. J. Twenge, *Generation Me—Revised and Updated: Why Today's Young Americans Are More Confident, Assertive, Entitled and More Miserable Than Ever* (New York: Simon and Schuster, 2014).

45. E. Anderson, "Giving Negative Feedback to Millennials: How Can Managers Criticize the 'Most Praised' Generation," *Management Research Review* 39, no. 6 (2016): 692–705.

46. A. Peng, J. Schaubroeck, and J. Xie, "When Confidence Comes and Goes: How Variation in Self-Efficacy Moderates Stressor-Strain Relationships," *Journal of Occupational Health Psychology*, Jan. 19, 2015, http://dx.doi.org/10.1037/a0038588; R. Fida et al. "'Yes I Can'": The Protective Role of Personal Self Efficacy in Hindering Counterproductive Work Activity under Stressful Conditions," *Anxiety, Stress and Coping* 2014: 1–21, doi:10.1080/10615806.2014.969718.

47. P. Schonfeld et al., "The Effects of Daily Stress on Positive and Negative Mental Health: Mediation through Self-efficacy," *International Journal of Clinical and Health Psychology* 6, no. 1 (2016): 692–705.

48. A. Peng and J. Schaubroeck, "When Confidence Comes and Goes: How Variation in Self-efficacy Moderates Stressor-Strain Relationships," *Journal of Occupational Health Psychology* 20, no. 3 (2015): 359–76; M. Komarraju and D. Nadler, "Self Efficacy and Academic Achievement: Who Do Implicit Beliefs, Goals and Effort Regulation Matter?," *Learning and Individual Differences* 25 (2013): 67–72.

49. T. Honicke and J. Broadbent, "The Influence of Academic Self-efficacy on Academic Performance: A Systematic Review," *Educational Research Review* 17 (2016): 63–84; P.N. von der Embse and S. Witmer, "High-Stakes Accountability: Student Anxiety and Large-Scale Testing," *Journal of Applied School Psychology* 30, no. 2 (2014): 132–56, doi:10.1080/15377903.2014.888529.

50. .T. Honicke and J. Broadbent, "The Influence of Academic Self-efficacy on Academic Performance: A Systematic Review," *Educational Research Review* 17 (2016): 63–84.

51. M. Friedman and R.H. Rosenman, *Type A Behavior and Your Heart* (New York: Knopf, 1974).

52. S.C. Kobasa, "Stressful Life Events, Personality, and Health: An Inquiry into Hardiness," *Journal of Personality and Social Psychology* 37, no. 1 (1979): 1–11.

53. R. Graber, F. Pichon, and E. Carubine, "Psychological Resilience: State of Knowledge and Future Research Agendas: Working Paper 425," October 2015, Available at http://www.odi.org/sites/odi.org.uk/files/odi-assets/publications-opinion-files/9872.pdf.

54. M. Sarkar and D. Fletcher, "Ordinary Magic, Extraordinary Performance: Psychological Resilience and Thriving in High Achievers," *Sport, Exercise, and Performance Psychology* 3, no. 1 (2014): 46.

55. A. Duckworth and J.J. Gross, "Self-Control and Grit Related but Separable Determinants of Success," *Current Directions in Psychological Science* 23, no. 5 (2014): 319–25.

56. J. Gu et al., "How Do Mindfulness-Based Cognitive Therapy and Mindfulness-Based Stress Reduction Improve Mental Health and Well Being? A Systematic Review and Meta-analysis of Mediation Studies," *Clinical Psychology Review* 37 (2015): 1–12; A. Rosenberg et al., "Promoting Resilience in Stress Management: A Pilot Study of a Novel Resilience-Promoting Intervention for Adolescents and Young Adults with Serious Illness," *Journal of Pediatric Psychology* 40, no. 9 (2015): 992–99; J. Donald et al., "Daily Stress and the Benefits of Mindfulness: Examining the Daily and Longitudinal Relations between Present Moment Awareness and Stress Responses," *Journal of Research in Personality* 65 (2016): 30–47.

57. P. Pimple et al., "Association between Anger and Mental Stress–Induced Myocardial Ischemia," *American Heart Journal* 169, no. 1 (2015): 115–21.

58. American Heart Association. "Is Broken Heart Syndrome Real?," April 18, 2016, www.heart.org.

59. G. Mate, *When the Body Says No: Understanding the Stress-Disease Connection* (Hoboken, NJ: John Wiley and Sons, 2011).

60. J. Thayer et al., "Potential Biological Pathways Linking Type-D Personality and Poor Health: A Cross-Sectional Investigation," *Psychotherapy and Psychosomatics* 84 (2015); R. Garcia-Retamero et al., "On the Relationship between Type-D Personality and Cardiovascular Health," *European Health Psychologist* 17, Supplement (2015): 707.

61. E. Chen, K. C. McLean, and G.E. Miller, "Shift-and-Persist Strategies: Associations with Socioeconomic Status and the Regulation of Inflammation among Adolescents and Their Parents," *Psychosomatic Medicine* 77, no. 4 (2015): 371–82.

62. K. Eagan et al., "The American Freshman: Fifty-Year Trends, 1966–2015," Los Angeles Higher Education Research Institute, UCLA (2016), Available at https://www.heri.ucla.edu/monographs/50YearTrendsMonograph2016.pdf.

63. Higher Education Research Institute, "A Year of Change: First Year," Accessed January 31, 2015, www.heri.ucla.edu/infographics/YFCY-2014-Infographic.pdf; K. Eagen et al., *The American Freshman: National Norms Fall 2014—Expanded Edition* (Los Angeles: Higher Education Research Institute, 2015),www.heri.ucla.edu/monographs/TheAmericanFreshman2014-Expanded.pdf.

64. Higher Education Research Institute, "A Year of Change: First Year," Accessed January 31, 2015, www.heri.ucla.edu/infographics/YFCY-2014-Infographic.pdf; K. Eagen et al., *The American Freshman: National Norms Fall 2014—Expanded Edition* (Los Angeles: Higher Education Research Institute, 2015),www.heri.ucla.edu/monographs/TheAmericanFreshman2014-Expanded.pdf.

65. B.L. Seaward, *Managing Stress: Principles and Strategies for Health and Well-Being*, 8th ed. (Sudbury, MA: Jones and Bartlett, 2013), 8.

66. K. Donahue, "Daily Hassles, Mental Health Outcomes, and Dispositional Mindfulness in Student Registered Nurse Anesthetists," Doctoral dissertation. Oregon Health and Science University. OSU Digital Commons. Available at http://digitalcommons.ohsu.edu/cgi/viewcontent.cgi?article=16915&context=etd.

67. C.Y. Lee & S.E. Goldstein, "Loneliness, Stress, and Social Support in Young Adulthood: Does the Source of Support Matter?" *Journal of Youth and Adolescence* 45, no. 3 (2016): 568–80; C. Karatekin and R Ahluwalia, "Effects of Adverse Childhood Experiences, Stress and Social Support on the Health of College Students," *Journal of Interpersonal Violence* (2016): 0886260516681880.

68. B.L. Seaward, *Managing Stress: Principles and Strategies for Health and Well-Being*, 8th ed. (Sudbury, MA: Jones and Bartlett, 2013), 8.

69. W. Lovallo, *Stress and Health: Biological and Psychological Interactions*, 3rd ed. (Thousand Oaks, CA: Sage, 2016); A. Lurie and K. Monahan, "Humor, Aging, and Life Review: Survival through the Use of Humor," *Social Work in Mental Health* 13, no. 1 (2015): 82–91; C. Dormann, "Laughter as the Best Medicine: Exploring Humour-Mediated Health Applications," in *Distributed, Ambient, and Pervasive Interactions*, edited by N. Streitz (New York: Springer, 2015), 639–50.

70. W. Lovallo, *Stress and Health: Biological and Psychological Interactions*, 3rd ed. (Thousand Oaks, CA: Sage, 2016); D.A. Girdano, D.E. Dusek, and G.S. Everly, *Controlling Stress and Tension*, 9th ed. (San Francisco: Benjamin Cummings, 2013), 375.

71. W. Lovallo, *Stress and Health: Biological and Psychological Interactions*, 3rd ed. (Thousand Oaks, CA: Sage, 2016); R. Gotink, et al., "8-Week Mindfulness Based Stress Reduction Induces Brain Changes Similar to Traditional Long-Term Meditation Practice: A Systematic Review," *Brain and Cognition* 108 (2016): 32–41; M. A. Stults-Kolehmainen and R. Sinha, "The Effect of Stress on Physical Activity and Exercise," *Sports Medicine* 44, no. 1 (2014): 81–121.

72. P. Norman and A. Wrona-Clarke, "Combining Self-affirmation and Implementation Intentions to Reduce Heavy Episodic Drinking in University Students," *Psychology of Addictive Behaviors* 30, no. 4 (2016): 434–41; A. Toli, T. Webb, and G.E. Hardy, "Does Forming Implementation Intentions Help People with Mental Health Problems to Achieve Goals? A Meta-analysis of Experimental Studies with Clinical and Analogue Samples," *British Journal of Clinical Psychology* 55, no. 1 (2016): 69–90.

73. Yoga Journal and Yoga Alliance, "Yoga in America Study," January 2016, Available at https://www.yogaalliance.org/Home/Media_Inquiries/2016_Yoga_in_America_Study_Conducted_by_Yoga_Journal_and_Yoga_Alliance_Reveals_Growth_and_Benefits_of_the_Practice.

74. C. Lau, R. Yu, and J.Woo, "Effects of a 12-Week Hatha Yoga Intervention on Cardiorespiratory Endurance, Muscular Strength and Endurance, and Flexibility in Hong Kong Chinese Adults: A Controlled Clinical Trial," *Evidence-Based Complementary and Alternative Medicine* 2015 (2015); M.E. Papp et al., "Effects of High-Intensity Hatha Yoga on Cardiovascular Fitness, Adipocytokines, and Apolipoproteins in Healthy Students: A Randomized Controlled Study," *Journal of Alternative and Complementary Medicine* 22, no. 1 (2016): 81–87

75. H. Cramer et al., "Prevalence, Patterns and Predictors of Meditation Use among U.S. Adults: A Nationally Representative Survey," *Scientific Reports* 6 (2016).

76. S. Lu et al., "Meditation and Blood Pressure: A Meta-analysis of Randomized Clinical Trials," *Journal of Hypertension* (2016); S.R. Steinhubl et al., "Cardiovascular and Nervous System Changes during Meditation," *Frontiers in Human Neuroscience* 9 (2015): 145; R.D. Brook et al., "Beyond Medications and Diet: Alternative Approaches to Lowering Blood Pressure," Hypertension 61, no. 6 (2013): 1360–83.

77. National Center for Complementary and Integrative Health, "Massage Therapy for Health Purposes: What You Need to Know," Accessed February, 2017. http://nccam.nih.gov/health/massage/massageintroduction.htm.

Pulled Statistics:
page 82, American Psychological Association, "Stress in America," 2015.

page 87, American Psychological Association, "Stress in America," 2015.

Chapter 4: Improving Your Sleep

1. Centers for Disease Control and Prevention, "Insufficient Sleep Is a Public Health Problem," September 3, 2015, www.cdc.gov/features/dssleep; Y. Liu et al., "Prevalence of Healthy Sleep Duration among Adults—United States, 2014," *MMWR: Morbidity and Mortality Weekly Report* 65 (2016).

2. National Sleep Foundation, "2013 International Bedroom Poll: Summary of Findings," Accessed February 2016, Available at https://sleepfoundation.org/sites/default/files/RPT495a.pdf.

3. M. Hafner et al., *Why Sleep Matters—The Economic Costs of Insufficient Sleep: A Cross-Country Comparative Analysis* (Santa Monica, CA: RAND Corporation, 2016).

4. Centers for Disease Control and Prevention, "Insufficient Sleep Is a Public Health Problem," 2015.

5. Centers for Disease Control and Prevention, "Insufficient Sleep Is a Public Health Problem," September 3, 2015, www.cdc.gov/features/dssleep; Y. Liu et al., "Prevalence of Healthy Sleep Duration among Adults—United States, 2014," *MMWR: Morbidity and Mortality Weekly Report* 65 (2016).

6. National Highway Traffic Safety Administration, "Research on Drowsy Driving," Accessed February 2017, www.nhtsa.gov/Driving+Safety/Drowsy+Driving.

7. U.S. Department of Transportation, "NHTSA Drowsy Driving Research and Program Plan," March 2016, Available at https://www.nhtsa.gov/sites/nhtsa.dot.gov/files/drowsydriving_strategicplan_030316.pdf; National Sleep Foundation, "Drowsy Driving Facts and Stats," Accessed March 2017. Centers for Disease Control and Prevention, "Insufficient Sleep Is a Public Health Problem," 2015.

8. *American College Health Association, American College Health Association–National College Health Assessment II (ACHA–NCHA II): Reference Group Data Report Fall 2016* (Hanover, MD: American College Health Association, 2017), Available at www.achancha.org/reports_ACHA-NCHAII.html.

9. Ibid.

10. S. Hershner and R. Chevin, "Causes and Consequences of Sleepiness among College Students," *Nature and Science of Sleep* 6 (2014): 73–84; A. Wald et al., "Associations between Healthy Lifestyle Behaviors and Academic Performance in U.S. Undergraduates: A Secondary Analysis of the American College Health Association's National College Health Assessment II," *American Journal of Health Promotion* 28, no. 5 (2014): 298–305.

11. *American College Health Association, American College Health Association–National College Health Assessment II (ACHA–NCHA II): Reference Group Data Report Fall 2016* (Hanover, MD: American College Health Association, 2017, Available at www.achancha.org/reports_ACHA-NCHAII.html.

12. S. Hershner and R. Chevin, "Causes and Consequences of Sleepiness among College Students," 2014; A. Wald et al., "Associations between Healthy Lifestyle Behaviors," 2014.

13. *American College Health Association, American College Health Association–National College Health Assessment II (ACHA–NCHA II): Reference Group Data Report Fall 2016* (Hanover, MD: American College Health Association, 2017 Available at www.achancha.org/reports_ACHA-NCHAII.html.

14. National Sleep Foundation, "Excessive Sleepiness," Accessed February 2016, http://sleepfoundation.org/sleep-disorders-problems/excessive-sleepiness.

15. U.S. Department of Transportation, "NHTSA Drowsy Driving Research and Program Plan," March 2016, Available at https://www.nhtsa.gov/sites/nhtsa.dot.gov/files/drowsydriving_strategicplan_030316.pdf.

16. American Academy of Sleep Medicine, *The International Classification of Sleep Disorders: Diagnostic—Coding Manual*, 3rd ed. (Westchester, IL: American Academy of Sleep Medicine, 2015).

17. National Sleep Foundation, "Who's at Risk?," Accessed February 10, 2017, http://drowsydriving.org/about/whos-at-risk/; Harvard University, Radcliff Institute for Advanced Study, "Drowsy Driving," Accessed February 10, 2017, www.radcliffe.harvard.edu/news/radcliffe-magazine/drowsy-driving.

18. National Sleep Foundation, "Excessive Sleepiness and Industrial Accidents," Accessed March 2016, https://sleepfoundation.org/excessivesleepiness/content/the-relationship-between-sleep-and-industrial-accidents.

19. M. Lee et al., "High Risk of Near Crash Events Following Night Shift Work," *Proceedings of the National Academy of Sciences* 113, no. 1 (2016): 176–81.

20. Ibid.; Morris, Downing & Sherred, LLP, "Shift Work and the Effect on Worker Health," February 2, 2017, http://www.morrisdowningsherred.com/blog/2017/02/shift-work-and-the-effect-on-worker-health.shtml.

21. C. Sieber, "Long Haul Truck Driver Survey Results," Centers for Disease Control and Prevention, March 3, 2015, https://blogs.cdc.gov/niosh-science-blog/2015/03/03/truck-driver-health; National Sleep Foundation, "Who's at Risk?," Accessed February 2017, http://drowsydriving.org/about/whos-at-risk.

22. National Sleep Foundation, "Sleep and Pain: 2015 Sleep in America Poll," Accessed February 2017, https://sleepfoundation.org/sleep-polls-data/sleep-in-america-poll/2015-sleep-and-pain.

23. G. Hertz et al., "Sleep Dysfunction in Women," *Medscape*, 2014, http://emedicine.medscape.com/article/1189087-overview; National Sleep Foundation, "Why Are Women Sleepier Than Men? What's Up with Sleepiness in Women?," Accessed February 2016, https://sleepfoundation.org/sleep-news/why-are-women-sleepier-men-whats-sleepiness-women; ResMed, "Gender Differences in Sleep," July 25, 2016, http://splus.resmed.com/gender-differences-sleep.

24. C. Nugent and L. Black, "Sleep Duration, Quality of Sleep, and Use of Sleep Medication, by Sex and Family Type, 2013–2014," *NCHS Data Brief* 230 (2016), Available at www.cdc.gov/nchs/data/databriefs/db230.pdf.

25. S. Garbarino et al., "Co-Morbidity, Mortality, Quality of Life and Healthcare/Welfare/Social Costs of Disordered Sleep: A Rapid Review," *International Journal of Environmental Research and Public Health* 13, no. 8 (2016).

26. A. Ong et al., "Positive Affect and Sleep: A Systematic Review," *Sleep Medicine Reviews* (2016); L. Beattie et al., "Social Interactions, Emotion, and Sleep: A Systematic Review and Research Agenda," *Sleep Medicine Reviews* 24 (2015): 83–100.

27. N.F. Watson et al. "Transcriptional Signatures of Sleep Duration Discordance in Monozygotic Twins," *Sleep* 40, no. 1 (2017); N. Rod et al., "The Joint Effect of Sleep Duration and Disturbed Sleep on Cause-Specific Mortality: Results from the Whitehall II Cohort Study," *PLoS ONE* 9, no. 4 (2014): e91965, doi:10.1371/journal.pone.0091965.

28. K.M. Orzech et al., "Sleep Patterns Are Associated with Common Illness in Adolescents," *Journal of Sleep Research* 23, no. 2 (2013): 133–42; A. Prather et al., "Behaviorally Assessed Sleep and Susceptibility to the Common Cold," *Sleep* 38, no. 9 (2015): 1353–59.

29. R. Dumbell et al., "Circadian Clocks, Stress, and Immunity," *Frontiers in Endocrinology* 7 (2016); N. Labrecque and N. Cermakian, "Circadian Clocks in the Immune System," *Journal of Biological Rhythms* 30, no. 4 (2015): 277–90.

30. F. Heredia et al., "Self-Reported Sleep Duration, White Blood Cell Counts and Cytokine Profiles in European Adolescents: The Helena Study," *Sleep Medicine* 15, no. 10 (2014): 1251–58.

31. V. Aho et al., "Prolonged Sleep Restriction Induces Changes in Pathways Involved in Cholesterol Metabolism and Inflammatory Responses," *Scientific Reports* 6 (2016); M. Irwin et al., "Sleep Disturbance, Sleep Duration, and Inflammation: A Systematic Review and Meta-Analysis of Cohort Studies and Experimental Sleep Deprivation," *Biological Psychiatry* 80, no. 1 (2016): 40–52.

32. M. Irwin et al., "Sleep Disturbance, Sleep Duration, and Inflammation: A Systematic Review and Meta-Analysis of Cohort Studies and Experimental Sleep Deprivation," *Biological Psychiatry* 80, no. 1 (2016): 40–52; R. Yuan et al., "The Effect of Sleep Deprivation on Coronary Heart Disease," *Chinese Medical Sciences Journal* 31, no. 4 (2016): 247–53; R. Fukuoka et al., "Nocturnal Intermittent Hypoxia and Short Sleep Duration Were Independently Associated with Elevated C-reactive Protein Level in Patients with Coronary Artery Disease," *Circulation* 132, Suppl. 3 (2015): A17077; S. Nakamura et al., "Impact of Sleep-Disordered Breathing and Efficacy of Positive Airway Pressure on Mortality in Patients with Chronic Heart Failure and Sleep-Disordered Breathing: A Meta-Analysis," *Clinical Research in Cardiology* 104, no. 3 (2015): 208–16.

33. M. Irwin et al., "Sleep Disturbance, Sleep Duration, and Inflammation: A Systematic Review and Meta-Analysis of Cohort Studies and Experimental Sleep Deprivation," *Biological Psychiatry* 80, no. 1 (2016): 40–52; R. Yuan et al., "The Effect of Sleep Deprivation on Coronary Heart Disease," *Chinese Medical Sciences Journal* 31, no. 4 (2016): 247–53.

34. A. Cooper et al., "Sleep Duration and Cardio-metabolic Risk Factors among Individuals with Type 2 Diabetes," 2015; M.A. Miller et al., "Sustained Short Sleep and Risk of Obesity: Evidence in Children and Adults," in *Handbook of Obesity*, vol. 1, 3rd ed., edited by G. A. Bray and C. Bouchard (Boca Raton, FL: CRC Press, Taylor & Francis Group, 2014), 397–41; Q. Xiao et al., "A Large Prospective Investigation of Sleep Duration, Weight Change and Obesity in the NIH-AARP Diet and Health Study," *American Journal of Epidemiology* 178, no. 11 (2013): 1600–10.

35. M.A. Miller et al., "Sustained Short Sleep and Risk of Obesity," 2014; Q. Xiao et al., "A Large Prospective Investigation of Sleep Duration," 2013; National Sleep Foundation, "Obesity and Sleep," Accessed January 2016, www.sleepfoundation.org/article/sleep-topics/obesity-and-sleep.

36. M. Nagayoshi, et al. "Obstructive Sleep Apnea and Incident Type 2 Diabetes," *Sleep Medicine* 25 (2016): 156–61; A. Cooper et al., "Sleep Duration and Cardio-metabolic Risk Factors among Individuals with Type 2 Diabetes," *Sleep Medicine* 16, no. 1 (2015): 119–25; M. Kohasieh and A. Makaryrus, "Sleep Deficiency and Deprivation Leading to Cardiovascular Disease," *International Journal of Hypertension* 2015 (2015); Z. Shan et al., "Sleep Duration and Risk of Type 2 Diabetes: A Meta-analysis of Prospective Studies," *Diabetes Care* 38, no. 3 (2015): 529–37; J. Ferrie et al., "Change in Sleep Duration and Type 2 Diabetes: The Whitehall II Study," *Diabetes Care* 38, no. 8 (2015): 1467–72; A. Cooper et al., "Sleep Duration and Cardiometabolic Risk Factors among Individuals with Type 2 Diabetes," 2015.

37. L. Wise et al., "Sleep and Male Fecundity in a North American Preconception Cohort Study," *Fertility and Sterility* 106, no. 3 (2016): e79; N. White, "Influence of Sleep on Fertility in Women," *American Journal of Lifestyle Medicine* 10, no. 4 (2016): 239–41.

38. National Institutes of Health, "Information about Sleep," Accessed February 2016, http://science.education.nih.gov/supplements/nih3/sleep/guide/info-sleep.html; C. Peri, "What Lack of Sleep Does to Your Mind," *WebMD*, Accessed February 2017. www.webmd.com/sleep-disorders/excessive-sleepiness-10/emotions-cognitive.

39. A. Chatburn et al., "Complex Associative Memory Processing and Sleep: A Systematic Review and Meta-analysis of Behavioural Evidence and Underlying EEG Mechanisms." *Neuroscience and Biobehavioral Reviews* 47 (2014): 645–55; S. Hershner and R. Chervin, "Causes and Consequences of Sleepiness among College Students," 2014.

40. J. Hamilton, "Lack of Deep Sleep May Set the Stage for Alzheimer's," *NPR Morning Edition*, January 4, 2016, http://www.npr.org/sections/health-shots/2016/01/04/460620606/lack-of-deep-sleep-may-set-the-stage-for-alzheimers.

41. M. Boehm et al., "Depression, Anxiety, and Tobacco Use: Overlapping Impediments to Sleep in a National Sample of College Students," *Journal of American College Health* 64, no. 7 (2016): 565–74.

42. H. Fullagar et al., "Sleep and Athletic Performance: The Effects of Sleep Loss on Exercise Performance, and Physiological and Cognitive Responses to Exercise," *Sports Medicine* 45, no. 2 (2015): 161–86.

43. AAA Foundation for Traffic Safety, "Acute Sleep Deprivation and Crash Risk," Accessed February 2017, https://www.aaafoundation.org/acute-sleep-deprivation-and-crash-risk; National Highway Traffic Safety Administration, "Research on Drowsy Driving," Accessed February 2016, www.nhtsa.gov/Driving+Safety/Drowsy+Driving; National Sleep Foundation, "Healthy Sleep Project Urges Parents to Teach Teens to Avoid Drowsy Driving," April 7, 2015, Available at www.sleepeducation.org/docs/default--document-library/healthy-sleep-teen-drowsy-driving.pdf.

44. AAA Foundation for Traffic Safety, "Acute Sleep Deprivation and Crash Risk," Accessed February 2017, https://www.aaafoundation.org/acute-sleep-deprivation-and-crash-risk.

45. AAA Foundation for Traffic Safety, "Acute Sleep Deprivation and Crash Risk," Accessed February 2017, https://www.aaafoundation.org/acute-sleep-deprivation-and-crash-risk; National Highway Traffic Safety Administration, "Research on Drowsy Driving," Accessed February 2016, www.nhtsa.gov/Driving+Safety/Drowsy+Driving.

46. Centers for Disease Control and Prevention, "Insufficient Sleep is a Public Health Epidemic," January 13, 2014, www.cdc.gov/features/dssleep; National Highway Traffic Safety Administration, "Drowsy Driving and Automobile Crashes," February 2014, www.nhtsa.gov/people/injury/drowsy_driving1/Drowsy.html#NCSDR/NHTSA.

47. National Sleep Foundation, "Depression and Sleep," Accessed February 2016, https://sleepfoundation.org/sleep-disorders-problems/depression-and-sleep.

48. National Institute of General Medical Sciences, "Circadian Rhythms Fact Sheet," Accessed February 23, 2017, www.nigms.nih.gov/Education/Pages/Factsheet_CircadianRhythms.aspx.

49. A. Ramkisoengsing and J. Meijer, "Synchronization of Biological Clock Neurons by Light and Peripheral Feedback Systems Promotes Circadian Rhythms and Health," *Frontiers in Neurology* 6, no. 128 (2015): 128; M. Vitaterna, J. Takahashi, and F. Turek, "Overview of Circadian Rhythms," National Institute on Alcohol Abuse and Alcoholism, 2014, http://pubs.niaaa.nih.gov/publications/arh25-2/85-93.htm.

50. NIH, "Teacher's Guide—Information about Sleep," Accessed February 2017, http://science.education.nih.gov/supplements/nih3/sleep/guide/info-sleep.htm.

51. B. Rasch and J. Born, "About Sleep's Role in Memory," *Physiological Reviews* 93, no. 2 (2013): 681–766; R. Boyce and A. Adamantidis, "REM: Sleep on It!" *Neuropsychopharmacology* 42, no. 1 (2017): 375.

52. N. Watson et al., "Joint Consensus Statement of the American Academy of Sleep Medicine and Sleep Research Society on the Recommended Amount of Sleep for a Healthy Adult: Methodology and Discussion," *Journal of Clinical Sleep Medicine* 11, no. 8 (2015): 931–52; N.F. Watson et al., "Recommended Amount of Sleep for a Healthy Adult: A Joint Consensus Statement of the American Academy of Sleep Medicine and Sleep Research Society," *Sleep* 38, no. 6 (2015): 843–44.

53. Centers for Disease Control and Prevention, "Insufficient Sleep Is a Public Health Epidemic," 2014; C. Nugent and L. Black, "Sleep Duration, Quality of Sleep, and Use of Sleep Medication, by Sex and Family Type, 2013–2014," *NCHS Data Brief* 230 (2016); "Why Americans Can't Sleep," *Consumer Reports*, January 14, 2016, Available at www.consumerreports.org/sleep/why-americans-cant-sleep.

54. NIH, "Teacher's Guide—Information about Sleep," 2017.

55. E. Mezick et al., "Sleep Duration and Cardiovascular Responses to Stress in Undergraduate Men," *Psychophysiology* 51, no. 1 (2014): 88–96.

56. A. Ramkisoengsing and J. Meijer, "Synchronization of Biological Clock Neurons by Light and Peripheral Feedback Systems Promotes Circadian Rhythms and Health," 2015.

57. N. Rod et al., "The Joint Effect of Sleep Duration and Disturbed Sleep on Cause-Specific Mortality: Results from the Whitehall II Cohort Study," *PLoS ONE* 9, no. 4 (2014): e91965.

58. A. Prather et al., "Behaviorally Assessed Sleep and Susceptibility to the Common Cold," *Sleep* 38, no. 9 (2015): 1353–59.

59. P. Slobodanka et al., "Effects of Recovery Sleep after One Work Week of Mild Sleep Restriction on Interleukin-6 and Cortisol Secretion and Daytime Sleepiness and Performance," *American Journal of Physiology: Endocrinology and Metabolism* 305, no. 7 (2013): E890–96.

60. National Sleep Foundation, "Napping," Accessed February 5, 2015, http://sleepfoundation.org/sleep-topics/napping; National Sleep Foundation, "Drowsy Driving—Is There a Perfect Time to Take a Nap?," Accessed January 15, 2015.

61. Y.-H. Fu, "What Genes Tell Us about Sleep," TEDX Thatcher School Video Lecture Series, November 23, 2015.

62. Centers for Disease Control and Prevention, "Insufficient Sleep Is a Public Health Problem," 2015; A.

63. Ramkisoengsing and J. Meijer, "Synchronization of Biological Clock Neurons by Light and Peripheral Feedback Systems Promotes Circadian Rhythms and Health," 2015.

63. Centers for Disease Control and Prevention, "Insufficient Sleep Is a Public Health Problem," 2015; A. Ramkisoengsing and J. Meijer, "Synchronization of Biological Clock Neurons by Light and Peripheral Feedback Systems Promotes Circadian Rhythms and Health," 2015.

64. Centers for Disease Control and Prevention, "Insufficient Sleep Is a Public Health Problem," 2015; A. Ramkisoengsing and J. Meijer, "Synchronization of Biological Clock Neurons by Light and Peripheral Feedback Systems Promotes Circadian Rhythms and Health," 2015.

65. Centers for Disease Control and Prevention, "Insufficient Sleep Is a Public Health Problem," 2015; A. Ramkisoengsing and J. Meijer, "Synchronization of Biological Clock Neurons by Light and Peripheral Feedback Systems Promotes Circadian Rhythms and Health," 2015.

66. National Sleep Foundation, "Caffeine and Sleep," Accessed February 2016, https://sleepfoundation.org/sleep-topics/caffeine-and-sleep; *American College Health Association–National College Health Assessment II (ACHA–NCHA II): Reference Group Data Report Spring 2016* (Hanover, MD: American College Health Association, 2017, Available at www.achancha.org/reports_ACHA-NCHAII.html.

67. National Sleep Foundation, "Insomnia," Accessed February 5, 2017, http://sleepfoundation.org/sleep-disorders-problems/insomnia.

68. Ibid.

69. Ibid.

70. Ibid.

71. American College Health Association, *National College Health Assessment II (ACHA–NCHA II): Reference Group Data Report Fall 2017* (Hanover, MD: American College Health Association, 2017, Available at www.achancha.org/reports_ACHA-NCHAII.html.

72. Society of Behavioral Medicine, "Adult Insomnia," Accessed February 2016, www.behavioralsleep.org/index.php/sbsm/about-adult-sleep-disorders/adult-insomnia.

73. J.M. Trauer et al., "Cognitive Behavioral Therapy for Chronic Insomnia: A Systematic Review and Meta-analysis," *Annals of Internal Medicine* 163, no. 3 (2015): 191–204.

74. National Sleep Foundation, "Sleep Apnea and Sleep," Accessed February 2017, https://sleepfoundation.org/sleep-disorders-problems/sleep-related-breathing-disorders/obstructive-sleep-apnea.

75. Sleep Disorders Guide, "Sleep Apnea Statistics," Accessed January 2017, www.sleepdisordersguide.com/sleepapnea/sleep-apnea-statistics.html.

76. National Sleep Foundation, "Sleep Apnea and Sleep," 2017.

77. Ibid.

78. Ibid.

79. U.S. Food and Drug Administration, "Inspire Upper Airway Stimulation - P130008," January 11, 2016, www.fda.gov/Medical-Devices/ProductsandMedicalProcedures/DeviceApprovalsandClearances/Recently-ApprovedDevices/ucm398321.htm.

80. National Institute of Neurological Disorders and Stroke, "Restless Legs Syndrome Fact Sheet," July 27, 2015, www.ninds.nih.gov/disorders/restless_legs/detail_restless_legs.htm; How Sleep Works, "Sleep Disorders," Accessed March 2016, http://howsleepworks.com/disorders.html.

81. Ibid.

82. National Institute of Neurological Disorders and Stroke, "Narcolepsy Fact Sheet," updated January 5, 2015, www.ninds.nih.gov/disorders/narcolepsy/detail_narcolepsy.htm.

83. National Sleep Foundation, "Narcolepsy and Sleep," Accessed February 2017, https://sleepfoundation.org/sleep-disorders—problems/narcolepsy-and-sleep.

84. National Sleep Foundation, "Sleep Hygiene," Accessed February 2017, https://sleepfoundation.org/ask-the-expert/sleep-hygiene.

85. NIH, "Brain Basics: Understanding Sleep," April 17, 2015, www.ninds.nih.gov/disorders/brain_basics?understand_sleep.htm; J. Levenson et al., "The Pathophysiology of Insomnia," *CHEST Journal* 147, no. 4 (2015): 1179–92.

86. National Sleep Foundation, "What You Breathe While You Sleep Can Affect How You Feel the Next Day," Accessed February 5, 2015, http://sleepfoundation.org/bedroom/smell.php.

86. National Sleep Foundation, "What You Breathe While You Sleep Can Affect How You Feel the Next Day," Accessed February 5, 2015, http://sleepfoundation.org/bedroom/smell.php.

87. Vanderbilt University Medical Center Reporter, "Take a Walk in the Sun to Ease Time Change Woes, Sleep Expert Says," October 30, 2014, http://news.vanderbilt.edu/2014/10/take-a-walk-in-the-sun-to-ease-time-change-woes-says-vanderbilt-sleep-expert.

88. National Sleep Foundation, "Exercise and Sleep," Accessed February 2017, https://sleepfoundation.org/sleep-polls-data/sleep-in-america-poll/2013-exercise-and-sleep.

89. National Sleep Foundation, "Sleep Hygiene," 2017.

90. National Sleep Foundation, "Sleep Hygiene," 2017.

91. M. Thakkar et al., "Alcohol Disrupts Sleep Homeostasis," *Alcohol* 49, no. 4 (2015): 299–310.

Pulled Statistics:

page 101, AAA Foundation for Traffic Safety. "Acute Sleep Deprivation and crash risks". Accessed February 2017, https://www.aaafoundation.org/acute-sleep-deprivation-and-crash-risk.

page 102, "The Science of Sleep: Lack of Sleep Could Cost Americans $411 Billion a Year." *Popular Science Special Edition*, February 2017, Page 60–62.

Chapter 5: Preventing Violence and Injury

1. Voltaire, "Semiramis," V.1, translated by J.K. Hoyt, in *The Cyclopaedia of Practical Quotations* (New York: Funk & Wagnalls Company, 1896).

2. D. Prothrow-Stith, *Deadly Consequences* (New York: Harper Collins, 1992).

3. World Health Organization, *Global Status Report on Violence Prevention* (Geneva: World Health Organization, 2014), Available at www.undp.org/content/dam/undp/library/corporate/Reports/UNDP-GVA-violence-2014.pdf.

4. Centers for Disease Control and Prevention, "Ten Leading Causes of Death by Age Group, United States, 2014," Accessed March 2017, Available at https://www.cdc.gov/injury/wisqars/pdf/leading_causes_of_death_by_age_group_2014-a.pdf.

5. Federal Bureau of Investigation, *Crime in the United States, Preliminary Semiannual Uniform Crime Report for January–June 2016*, 2016, https://www.fbi.gov/about-us/cjis/ucr/crime-in-the-u.s/2016/preliminary-semiannual-uniform-crime-report-januaryjune-2016/tables/table-3.

6. L. Langton and J. Truman, "Criminal Victimization-2015," Bureau of Justice Statistics, October 20, 2016., https://www.bjs.gov/index.cfm?ty=pbdetail&iid=5804.

7. C. Barnett-Ryan, L. Langton, and M. Planty, "The Nation's Two Crime Measures," September 18, 2014, Bureau of Justice Statistics, www.bjs.gov/index.cfm?ty=pbdetail&iid=5112; Bureau of Justice Statistics, "Reporting Crimes to Police," February 11, 2015, www.bjs.gov/index.cfm?ty=tp&tid=96.

8. L. Langton and J. Truman, "Criminal Victimization, 2014," Bureau of Justice Statistics, August 27, 2015, http://www.bjs.gov/index.cfm?ty=pbdetail&iid=5366.

9. Ibid.

10. American College Health Association, *American College Health Association—National College Health Assessment II: Reference Group Data Report, Fall 2016* (Baltimore, MD: American College Health Association, 2017).

11. Ibid.

12. Ibid.

13. C. Krebs et al., "Campus Climate Survey Validation Study Final Technical Report," *Bureau of Justice Statistics Research and Development Series* (2016): 1–193, Available at http://www.bjs.gov/content/pnd.pdf/ccsvsftr.pdf.

14. National Center for Victims of Crime, "School and Campus Crime Fact Sheet," Accessed March 2017, https://ovc.ncjrs.gov/ncvrw2016/content/section-6/PDF/2016NCVRW_6_SchoolCrime-508.pdf.

15. World Health Organization Violence Prevention Alliance, "The Ecological Framework," Accessed June

2016, www.who.int/violenceprevention/approach/ecology/en/index.html; Centers for Disease Control and Prevention, National Center for Injury Prevention and Control, "Understanding School Violence: Fact Sheet—2015," Accessed June 2016, http://www.cdc.gov/violenceprevention/pdf/School_Violence_Fact_Sheet-a.pdf.

16. A. Martin et al., "Formal Controls, Neighborhood Disadvantage and Violent Crime in U.S. Cities: Examining (Un)intended Consequences," *Journal of Criminal Justice* 44 (2016): 58–65; Springer; American Psychological Association, "Violence and Socioeconomic Status," Accessed June 2014, www.apa.org/pi/ses/resources/publications/factsheet-violence.aspx.
17. C. Spencer et al., "Gender Differences in Risk Markers for Perpetration of Physical Partner Violence: Results from a Meta-analytic Review," *Journal of Family Violence* 31, no. 8 (2016): 981–84; E. Wright, "Less Social Support for Women in Disadvantaged Neighborhoods Means That They Are More Likely to Be the Victims of Intimate Partner Violence" *USApp—American Politics and Policy Blog*, May 12, 2016; World Health Organization Violence Prevention Alliance, "The Ecological Framework," Accessed June 2014, www.who.int/violenceprevention/approach/ecology/en/index.html.
18. M.L. Hunt, A.W. Hughey, and M.G. Burke, "Stress and Violence in the Workplace and on Campus: A Growing Problem for Business, Industry and Academia," *Industry and Higher Education* 26, no. 1 (2012): 43–51.
19. T. Dishion, "A Developmental Model of Aggression and Violence: Microsocial and Macrosocial Dynamic within an Ecological Framework," *Handbook of Developmental Psychology* (New York: Springer, 2014), 449–65.
20. K. Makin-Byrd and K.L. Bierman, "Individual and Family Predictors of the Perpetration of Dating Violence and Victimization in Late Adolescence," *Journal of Youth Adolescence* 42, no. 4 (2013): 536–50, doi:10.1007/s10964-012-9810-7; A. Ruddle, et al. "Aggression and Violent Behavior Domestic violence offending behaviors: A review of the literature examining childhood exposure, implicit theories, trait aggression and anger rumination as predictive factors." Aggression and Violent Behavior. Volume 34, May 2017, Pages 154-165. https://doi.org/10.1016/j.avb.2017.01.016; C. Cook et al., "Predictors of Bullying and Victimization in Childhood and Adolescence: A Meta-Analytic Investigation," *School Psychology Quarterly* 25, no. 2 (2010): 65–83.
21. R. Puff and J. Segher, *The Everything Guide to Anger Management: Proven Techniques to Understand and Control Anger* (Avon, MA: Adams Media,, 2014).
22. N. Fernandez-Castillo and B. Cormand, "Aggressive Behavior in Humans: Genes and Pathways Identified through Association Studies," *American Journal of Medical Genetics Part B: Neuropsychiatric Genetics* 171 (2016): 676–96; P. Asherson and B. Cormand, "The Genetics of Aggression: Where Are We Now?" *American Journal of Medical Genetics Part B: Neuropsychiatric Genetics* 171, no. 5 (2016): 559–61; D. Boisvert and J. Vaske, "Genetic Theories of Criminal Behavior," *The Encyclopedia of Criminology and Criminal Justice* (Boston, MA: Wiley-Blackwell, 2014), 1–6.
23. S. Swearer and S. Hymel, "Understanding the Psychology of Bullying: Moving toward a Social-ecological Diathesis-Stress Model," *American Psychologist* 70, no. 4 (2015): 344–53; M. Nielsen et al., "Post-traumatic Stress Disorder as a Consequence of Bullying at Work and at School: A Literature Review and Meta-analysis," *Aggression and Violent Behavior* 21 (2015): 17–24. doi:10.1016/j.avb.2015.01.001.
24. S. Swearer and S. Hymel, "Understanding the Psychology of Bullying: Moving Toward a Social-Ecological Diatheses-Stress Model," *American Psychologist* 70, no. 4 (2015): 344; W. Gunter and B. Newby, "From Bullied to Deviant: The Victim-Offender Overlap among Bullying Victims," *Youth Violence and Juvenile Justice* 13, no. 1(2015): 3–17.
25. K. Leonard and B.M. Quigley, "Thirty Years of Research Show Alcohol to Be a Cause of Intimate Partner Violence: Future Research Needs to Identify Who to Treat and How to Treat Them," *Drug and Alcohol Review* 36, no. 1 (2017): 7–9; K.M. Devries et al., "Intimate Partner Violence Victimization and Alcohol Consumption in Women: A Systematic Review and Meta-analysis," *Addiction* 109 (2014): 379–91, doi:10.1111/add.12393; A. Abbey, "Alcohol's Role in Sexual Violence Perpetration: Theoretical Explanations, Existing Evidence and Future Directions," *Drugs and Alcohol Review* 30, no. 5 (2012): 481–85; J.M. Boden, D.M. Fergusen, and L.J. Horwood, "Alcohol Misuse and Violent Behavior: Findings from a 30-Year Longitudinal Study," *Drugs and Alcohol Dependence* 122 (2012): 135–41; United Nations Office on Drugs and Crime, "World Drug Report," 2013, www.unodc.org/unodc/secured/wdr/wdr2013/World_Drug_Report_2013.pdf; A. Sanderlund et al., "The Association between Sports Participation, Alcohol Use and Aggression and Violence: A Systematic Review," *Journal of Science and Medicine in Sport* 17, no. 1 (2014): 2–7.
26. C. Cunradi, "Discrepant Patterns of Heavy Drinking, Marijuana Use, and Smoking and Intimate Partner Violence: Results from the California Community Health Study of Couples," *Journal of Drug Education* 45, no. 2 (2015): 73–95; K. Leonard and B.M. Quigley, "Thirty Years of Research Show Alcohol to be a Cause of Intimate Partner Violence: Future Research Needs to Identify Who to Treat and How to Treat Them," *Drug and Alcohol Review* 36, no. 1 (2017): 7–9
27. C. Cunradi, "Discrepant Patterns of Heavy Drinking, Marijuana Use, and Smoking and Intimate Partner Violence: Results from the California Community Health Study of Couples," *Journal of Drug Education* 45, no. 2 (2015): 73–95; K. Leonard and B.M. Quigley, "Thirty Years of Research Show Alcohol to be a Cause of Intimate Partner Violence: Future Research Needs to Identify Who to Treat and How to Treat Them," *Drug and Alcohol Review* 36, no. 1 (2017): 7–9
28. R. Stansfield, "Teen Involvement in Sports and Risky Behavior: A Cross-National and Gendered Analysis," *British Journal of Criminology* 57, no. 1 (2017): 172–93; A. Sanderlund et al., "The Association between Sports Participation, Alcohol Use and Aggression and Violence: A Systematic Review," *Journal of Science and Medicine in Sport* 17, no. 1 (2014): 2–7.
29. C. Love et al., "Understanding the Connection between Suicide and Substance Abuse: What the Research Tells Us," SAMHSA Webinar Series, September 11, 2014, http://captus.samhsa.gov/sites/default/files/capt_resource/webcast_suicide_and_substance_abuse_part_1_sept_11_2014_final.pdf; A. Agrawal et al., "Reciprocal Relationship between Substance Abuse and Disorders and Suicide Ideation and Suicide Attempts in the Collaborative Study of Genetics of Alcoholism," *Journal of Affective Disorders* 213 (2017): 96–104.
30. C. Ferguson, "Does Media Violence Predict Societal Violence? It Depends on What You Look at and When?" *Journal of Communication* 65, no. 1(2015): E1–E22; W. Gunter and K. Daley, "Causal or Spurious? Using Propensity Score Matching to Detangle the Relationship between Violent Video Games and Violent Behavior," *Computers in Human Behavior* 4, no. 28 (2012): 1348–55.
31. S. Calvert et al., "The American Psychological Association Task Force Assessment of Violent Video Games: Science in the Service of Public Interest," *American Psychologist* 72, no. 2(2017): 126.
32. ChildStats.Gov, "America's Children in Brief: Key National Indicators of Well-Being, 2012," Accessed June 2014, http://childstats.gov/pdf/ac2012/ac_12.pdf.
33. Centers for Disease Control and Prevention, "Youth Violence: Definitions," March 2016, www.cdc.gov/violenceprevention/youthviolence/definitions.html; L.L. Dahlberg and E.G. Krug, "Violence: A Global Public Health Problem," in *World Report on Violence and Health* (Geneva: World Health Organization, 2002), 1–21.
34. World Health Organization, "Definitions and Typology of Violence," 2015.
35. Centers for Disease Control and Prevention, "Health, United States, 2015," April 2016, http://www.cdc.gov/nchs/data/hus/hus15.pdf.
36. Federal Bureau of Investigation, "Crime in the United States, 2016 Preliminary Semi-annual Uniform Crime Report," June 2016, Available at https://ucr.fbi.gov/crime-in-the-u.s/2016/preliminary-semiannual-uniform-crime-report-januaryjune-2016/tables/table-3.
37. Ibid.
38. Centers for Disease Control and Prevention, "Health, United States, 2015," April 2016, http://www.cdc.gov/nchs/data/hus/hus15.pdf.
39. Bureau of Justice Statistics. "Hate Crime," February 11, 2016, http://www.bjs.gov/index.cfm?ty=tp&tid=37#summary.
40. Federal Bureau of Investigation, "Latest Hate Crime Statistics Available," November 16, 2015, https://www.fbi.gov/news/stories/2015/november/latest-hate-crime-statistics-available.
41. Bureau of Justice Statistics, "Hate Crime Victimization: 2004–2012 Statistical Tables," February 2014, www.bjs.gov/index.cfm?ty=pbdetail&iid=4883.
42. Ibid.
43. U.S. Department of Justice, "Juvenile Justice Fact Sheet—Highlights of the 2012 National Youth Gang Survey," December 2014, www .ojjdp.gov/pubs/248025.pdf; Federal Bureau of Investigation, "2013 National Gang Threat Assessment: Emerging Trends," February 2015, www.fbi.gov/stats-services/publications/national-gang-report-2013.
44. FBI, "National Gang Report, 2015," 2015, Available at https://www.fbi.gov/stats-services/publications/national-gang-report-2015.pdf; U.S. Department of Justice, "Juvenile Justice Fact Sheet—Highlights of the 2012 National Youth Gang Survey," December 2014, www.ojjdp.gov/pubs/248025.pdf; Federal Bureau of Investigation, "2013 National Gang Threat Assessment—Emerging Trends," February 2015, www.fbi.gov/stats-services/publications/national-gang-report-2013.
45. FBI, "2013 National Gang Threat Assessment: Emerging Trends," February 2015, www.fbi.gov/stats-services/publications/national-gang-report-2013.
46. Violence Prevention Institute, "Why People Join Gangs and What You Can Do," Accessed June 2016, http://www.violencepreventioninstitute.com/youngpeople.html.
47. FBI, "What We Investigate: Cyber Crime," Accessed March, 2017, https://www.fbi.gov/investigate/cyber.
48. Ibid.
49. U.S. Code of Federal Regulations, Title 28CFR0.85.
50. U.S. Department of Homeland Security, "The Internet as a Terrorist Tool for Recruitment and Radicalization of Youth—White Paper," April 24, 2009, Available at www.homelandsecurity.org/docs/reports/Internet_Radicalization.pdf.
51. Centers for Disease Control and Prevention-Injury Prevention and Control, "The National Intimate Partner and Sexual Violence Survey," May 2015, http://www.cdc.gov/violenceprevention/nisvs/index.html.
52. American Psychological Association, "Intimate Partner Violence—Facts and Resources," Accessed March 2017, http://www.apa.org/topics/violence/partner.aspx.
53. Ibid.
54. Centers for Disease Control and Prevention, "The National Intimate Partner and Sexual Violence Survey," May 2015, http://www.cdc.gov/violenceprevention/nisvs/index.html.
55. American Psychological Association, "Intimate Partner Violence—Facts and Resources," Accessed June 2016, http://www.apa.org/topics/violence/partner.aspx.
56. Ibid.
57. L. Walker, *The Battered Woman* (New York: Harper and Row, 1979).
58. L. Walker, *The Battered Woman Syndrome*, 3rd ed. (New York: Springer, 2009).
59. Child Welfare Information Gateway, *Definitions of Child Abuse and Neglect* (Washington, DC: U.S. Department of Health and Human Services, Children's Bureau, 2014), Available at www.childwelfare.gov/topics/systemwide/laws-policies/statutes/define; U.S. Department of Health and Human Services Administration for Children and Families, "Definitions of Child Abuse and Neglect," February 2011, www.childwelfare.gov/systemwide/laws_policies/statutes/define.cfm.
60. Childhelp, "Child Abuse Statistics and Facts," Accessed July 2016, www.childhelp.org/child-abuse-statistics.
61. U.S. Department of Health & Human Services, Administration for Children and Families, Administration on Children, Youth and Families, Children's Bureau. (2017). Child Maltreatment 2015. Available from http://www.acf.hhs.gov/programs/cb/research-data-technology/statistics-research/child-maltreatment.

62. T. Messman-Moore and P. Bhuptaini. "A Review of the Long-Term Impact of Child Maltreatment on Posttraumatic Stress Disorder and Its Comorbidities: An Emotion Dysregulation Perspective." Clinical Pscyhology Science and Practice. 2017. 24(2):154-179.

63. Ibid.

64. Centers for Disease Control and Prevention, "Understanding Elder Abuse, Fact Sheet 2016," Accessed March 2017. https://www.cdc.gov/violenceprevention/pdf/em-factsheet-a.pdf.

65. I. Quellet-Morin et al., "Intimate Partner Violence and New Onset Depression: A Longitudinal Study of Women's Childhood and Adult Histories of Abuse," Depression and Anxiety 32, no. 5 (2015): 316–24.

66. Federal Bureau of Investigation, "Preliminary Semiannual Uniform Crime Report: Data Declaration," 2015, https://www.fbi.gov/about-us/cjis/ucr/crime-in-the-u.s/2015/preliminary-semiannual-uniform-crime-report-januaryjune-2015/tables/table-3/table_3_january_to_june_2015_percent_change_for_consecutive_years.xls/@@template-layout-view?override-view=data-declaration.

67. Ibid.

68. Ibid.

69. White House Task Force to Protect Students from Sexual Assault, Not Alone: First Report of White House Task Force to Protect Students from Sexual Assault, April 2014, www.whitehouse.gov/sites/default/files/docs/report_0.pdf.

70. Jeanne Clery Act Information, "The Campus Sexual Violence Elimination Act," 2014, www.cleryact.info/campus-save-act.html.

71. White House Task Force to Protect Students from Sexual Assault, Not Alone: First Report of White House Task Force to Protect Students from Sexual Assault, April 2014, www.whitehouse.gov/sites/default/files/docs/report_0.pdf.

72. N. Anderson, "These Campuses Have the Most Reports of Rape," Washington Post, June 7, 2016, https://www.washingtonpost.com/news/grade-point/wp/2016/06/07/these-colleges-have-the-most-reports-of-rape.

73. SB-967, "Student Safety: Sexual Assault," 2013–2014, https://leginfo.legislature.ca.gov/faces/billNavClient.xhtml?bill_id=201320140SB967.

74. B. Chappell, "California Enacts 'Yes Means Yes' Law, Defining Sexual Consent," September 29, 2014, www.npr.org/blogs/thetwo-way/2014/09/29/352482932/california-enacts-yes-means-yes-law-defining-sexual-consent.

75. A. Jackson, "State Contexts and the Criminalization of Marital Rape across the United States," Social Science Research 51 (2015): 290–306.

76. Oregon State University, "Sexual Harassment and Sexual Violence," Accessed June 2016, http://eoa.oregonstate.edu/sexual-harassment-and-violence-policy.

77. P. Brady and L. Boufford, "Majoring in Stalking: Exploring Stalking Experiences between College Students and the General Public," Crime Victims Institute—Series on Stalking (2014), Available at http://dev.cjcenter.org/_files/cvi/Stalking%20Series3tInpdf.pdf.

78. D. Woodlock, "The Abuse of Technology in Domestic Violence and Stalking," Violence against Women 23, no. 5 (2017): 584–602.

79. P. Brady and L. Boufford, "Majoring in Stalking: Exploring Stalking Experiences between College Students and the General Public," Crime Victims Institute—Series on Stalking (2014), Available at http://dev.cjcenter.org/_files/cvi/Stalking%20Series3tInpdf.pdf.

80. Ibid.

81. M. Breiding et al., "Prevalence and Characteristics of Sexual Violence, Stalking, and Intimate Partner Violence Victimization," 2014.

82. Centers for Disease Control and Prevention, "Sexual Violence, Stalking, and Intimate Partner Violence Widespread in the US," 2011; Office of Justice Programs, "2014 NCVRW Resource Guide: Crime Victimization in the United States," Available at https://www.ncjrs.gov/ovc_archives/ncvrw/2014/pdf/StatisticalOverviews.pdf.

83. National Children's Alliance, "CAC Statistics," Accessed June 2016. http://www.nationalchildrensalliance.org/cac-statistics.

84. The Children's Assessment Center, "Child Sexual Abuse Facts," Accessed June 2016, http://cachouston.org/child-sexual-abuse-facts; RAIN, "Child Sexual Abuse," Accessed June 2016. https://www.rainn.org/articles/child-sexual-abuse; Childhelp, "Child Abuse in America—2014," Accessed June 2016; U.S. Department of Health and Human Services, Children's Bureau, "Child Maltreatment," 2013, www.acf.hhs.gov/sites/default/files/cb/cm2012.pdf.

85. Ibid.

86. M. Bouroughs et al., "Complexity of Childhood Sexual Abuse: Predictors of Current Post-Traumatic Stress Disorder, Mood Disorders, Substance Use, and Sexual Risk Behavior among Adult Men Who Have Sex with Men," Archives of Sexual Behavior 44, no. 7 (2015): 1891–1902; Childhelp, "Child Abuse in America—2014," Accessed June 2016; T. Hilberg, C. Hamilton-Giachrtsis, and L. Dixon, "Review of Meta-analyses on the Association between Child Sexual Abuse and Adult Mental Health Difficulties: A Systematic Approach," Trauma, Violence, & Abuse 12, no. 1 (2011): 38–49.

87. Childhelp, "Child Abuse in America—2014," Accessed June, 2016???.

88. National Safety Council, "What Are the Odds of Dying From . . . ," Accessed March 2017, http://www.nsc.org/learn/safety-knowledge/Pages/injury-facts-chart.aspx; Centers for Disease Control and Prevention, "10 Leading Causes of Death by Age Group, United States—2014," Accessed March 8, 2017, Available at http://www.cdc.gov/injury/wisqars/leadingcauses.html.

89. Ibid.

90. National Safety Council, "What Are the Odds of Dying From . . . ," Accessed March 2017, http://www.nsc.org/learn/safety-knowledge/Pages/injury-facts-chart.aspx.

91. Ibid.

92. National Highway Traffic Safety Administration, "Traffic Safety Facts, 2015 Data: Alcohol-Impaired Driving," December 2015, www.nrd.nhtsa.dot.gov/Pubs/812231.pdf.

93. Ibid.

94. Ibid.

95. Ibid.

96. National Institute on Drug Abuse, "Drug Facts: Drugged Driving," Revised June 2016, www.drugabuse.gov/publications/drugfacts/drugged-driving.

97. Ibid.

98. S. Salomonsen-Sautel et al., "Trends in Fatal Motor Vehicle Crashes before and after Marijuana Commercialized in Colorado," Drug and Alcohol Dependence 140 (2014): 137–44.

99. National Institute on Drug Abuse, "Drug Facts: Drugged Driving," Revised June 2016, www.drugabuse.gov/publications/drugfacts/drugged-driving.

100. Centers for Disease Control and Prevention, "Drowsy Driving: Asleep at the Wheel," November 5, 2015, www.cdc.gov/features/dsDrowsyDriving.

101. Centers for Disease Control and Prevention, "Distracted Driving," March 7, 2016, www.cdc.gov/motorvehiclesafety/-distracted_driving; National Safety Council, "Injury Facts," February 2017, http://www.nsc.org/learn/safety-knowledge/Pages/injury-facts.aspx.

102. National Highway Traffic Safety Administration. "Traffic Safety Facts: Crash Stats," March 2017; Distraction.gov, "Facts and Statistics," Accessed March 2017, https://www.distraction.gov/stats-research-laws/facts-and-statistics.html.

103. T. Johnson, "Distraction and Teen Crashes: Even Worse Than We Thought," AAA Newsroom, March 25, 2015, http://newsroom.aaa.com/2015/03/distraction-teen-crashes-even-worse-thought.

104. National Highway Traffic Safety Administration, "Injury Statistics," 2017.

105. National Highway Traffic Safety Administration, "Distracted Driving Research: Teens and Young Drivers," Accessed March 2017 , http://www.nsc.org/learn/NSC-Initiatives/Pages/distracted-driving-research-studies.aspx.

106. Centers for Disease Control and Prevention, "Distracted Driving," March 7, 2016, https://www.cdc.gov/motorvehiclesafety/distracted_driving.

107. Insurance Institute for Highway Safety-Highway Loss Data Institute, "Distracted Driving," April 2017, http://www.iihs.org/iihs/topics/laws/cellphonelaws/maptextingbans.

108. Centers for Disease Control and Prevention, "Policy Impact: Seat Belts," Updated January 2014, www.cdc.gov/Motorvehiclesafety/seatbeltbrief.

109. National Highway Traffic Safety Administration, "Traffic Safety Facts: 2014 Data," March 2016, www-nrd.nhtsa.dot.gov/Pubs/812246.pdf.

110. National Highway Traffic Safety Administration, "Quick Facts 2014," March 2016, Available at http://www-nrd.nhtsa.dot.gov/Pubs/812234.pdf.

111. National Highway Traffic Safety Administration, "Traffic Safety Facts 2014 Data," 2016.

112. National Highway Traffic Safety Administration, "Bicyclists and Other Cyclists," May 2015, www-nrd.nhtsa.dot.gov/Pubs/812151.pdf.

113. Insurance Institute for Highway Safety, "Pedestrians and Bicyclists," February 2016, http://www.iihs.org/iihs/topics/t/pedestrians-and-bicyclists/fatalityfacts/bicycles.

114. Centers for Disease Control and Prevention, "10 Leading Causes of Injury Deaths by Age Group Highlighting Unintentional Injury Deaths, United States, 2014," February 25, 2016, Available at www.cdc.gov/injury/wisqars/leadingcauses.html.

115. Ibid; Centers for Disease Control and Prevention, "Unintentional Drowning: Get the Facts," April 28, 2016, www.cdc.gov/HomeandRecreationalSafety/Water-Safety/waterinjuries-factsheet.html.

116. Ibid.

117. Ibid.

118. U.S. Coast Guard, "Coast Guard News: U.S. Coast Guard Releases 2015 Recreational Boating Statistics Report," May 17, 2015, http://www.uscgnews.com/go/doc/4007/2504554/US-Coast-Guard-releases-2015-Recreational-Boating-Statistics-Report.

119. Ibid.

120. Ibid.

121. U. S. Coast Guard, "Boating Safety Resource Center: BUI Initiatives," March, 2017, www.uscgboating.org/recreational-boaters/boating-under-the-influence.php

122. American Boating Association, "Boating Safety—It Could Mean Your Life," 2015, www.americanboating.org/safety.asp.

123. Centers for Disease Control and Prevention, "Opioid Overdose," March 16, 2016, www.cdc.gov/drugoverdose; American Society of Addiction Medicine, "Opioid Addiction 2016 Facts and Figures," Accessed March 2017, http://www.asam.org/docs/default-source/advocacy/opioid-addiction-disease-facts-figures.pdf; Centers for Disease Control and Prevention, "10 Leading Causes of Injury Deaths by Age Group Highlighting Unintentional Injury Deaths, United States, 2014," February 25, 2016, www.cdc.gov/injury/wisqars/leadingcauses.html.

124. Ibid.

125. Ibid.

126. J.B. Mowry et al., "2015 Annual Report of the American Association of Poison Control Centers' National Poison Data System (NPDS): 33nd Annual Report," Clinical Toxicology 54, no. 10 (2016): 924–1109, Available at https://aapcc.s3.amazonaws.com/pdfs/annual_reports/2015_AAPCC_NPDS_Annual_Report_33rd_PDF.pdf.

127. American Association of Poison Control Centers, "Prevention," February 2015, www.aapcc.org/prevention.

128. Centers for Disease Control and Prevention, "10 Leading Causes of Injury Deaths by Age Group Highlighting Unintentional Injury Deaths, United States, 2014," February 25, 2016, Available at www.cdc.gov/injury/wisqars/leadingcauses.html.

129. Centers for Disease Control and Prevention, "Important Facts about Falls," January 20, 2016, www.cdc.gov/homeandrecreationalsafety/falls/adultfalls.html.

130. U.S. Fire Administration, "U.S. Fire Deaths, Fire Death Rates, and Risks of Dying in a Fire," Accessed March 2017, www.usfa.fema.gov/data/statistics/fire_death_rates.html.

131. U.S. Fire Administration, "Campus Fire Fatalities in Residential Buildings (2000–2015)," November 2015, https://www.usfa.fema.gov/downloads/pdf/publications/campus_fire_fatalities_report.pdf.

132. Ibid.

133. Ibid.

Pulled Statistics:

page 122, National Safety Council. "Injury Facts," 2017. http://www.nsc.org/learn/safety-knowledge/Pages/injury-facts-chart.aspx

page 123, Childhelp, "Child Abuse Statistics and Facts," 2017, www.childhelp.org/child-abuse-statistics.

page 128, Page 120, White House Task Force to Protect Students from Sexual Assault, "Not Alone: First Report of White House Task Force to Protect Students from Sexual Assault, "April 2014, www.whitehouse.gov/sites/default/files/docs/report_0.

Chapter 6: Connecting and Communicating in the Modern World

1. J.T. Cacioppo, *Rewarding Social Connections Promote Successful Aging*, Annual Meeting of the American Association for the Advancement of Science, Chicago, Illinois, 2014.

2. J. Holt-Lunstad et al., "Loneliness and Social Isolation as Risk Factors for Mortality," *Perspectives on Psychological Science* 10, no. 2 (2015): 227–37.

3. J.T. Cacioppo and S. Cacioppo, "Social Relationships and Health: The Toxic Effects of Perceived Social Isolation," *Social and Personality Psychology Compass* 8, no. 2 (2014): 58–72.

4. J. Holt-Lunstad et al., "Loneliness and Social Isolation as Risk Factors for Mortality," *Perspectives on Psychological Science* 10, no. 2 (2015): 227–37; J.L. Kohn and S.L. Averett, "The Effect of Relationship Status on Health with Dynamic Health and Persistent Relationships," *Journal of Health Economics* 36 (2014): 69–83.

5. J. Holt-Lunstad et al., "Loneliness and Social Isolation as Risk Factors for Mortality," *Perspectives on Psychological Science* 10, no. 2 (2015): 227–37; L.C. Hawkley and J.P. Capitanio, "Perceived Social Isolation, Evolutionary Fitness and Health Outcomes: A Lifespan Approach," *Philosophical Transactions of the Royal Society B* 370, no. 1669 (2015): 20140114.

6. Y.C. Yang et al., "Social Relationships and Physiological Determinants of Longevity across the Human Life Span," *Proceedings of the National Academy of Sciences* 113, no. 3 (2016): 578–83.

7. S. Higgs and J. Thomas, "Social Influences on Eating," *Current Opinion in Behavioral Sciences* 9 (2016): 1–6.

8. J. Holt-Lunstad and B.N. Uchino, "Social Support and Health," in *Health Behavior and Health Education: Theory, Research, and Practice*, 5th ed., edited by K. Glanz, B.K. Rimer, and K. Viswanath (San Francisco, CA: Jossey-Bass, 2015), 183–204.

9. S. Schnall, K.D. Harber, J.K. Stefanucci, and D.R. Proffitt, "Social Support and the Perception of Geographical Slant," *Journal of Experimental Social Psychology*, 44, no. 5 (2008): 1246–55.

10. K. Hampton, L.S. Goulet, L. Rainie, and K. Purcell, "Social Networking Sites and Our Lives," *Pew Internet and American Life Project*, June 16, 2011, Available at www.pewinternet.org/files/old-media//Files/Reports/2011/PIP%20-%20Social%20networking%20sites%20and%20our%20lives.pdf.

11. L. Johnson, "What Is Social Capital?," in *Social Capital and Community Well-Being*, edited by A.G. Greenber, T.P. Gullotta, and M. Bloom (New York: Springer International, 2016), 53–66.

12. J.T. Cacioppo and B. Patrick, *Loneliness: Human Nature and the Need for Social Connection* (New York: W.W. Norton, 2008); O. Stavrova and M. Luhmann, "Social Connectedness as a Source and Consequence of Meaning in Life," *Journal of Positive Psychology* 11, no. 5 (2016): 470–79.

13. J.T. Cacioppo and B. Patrick, *Loneliness: Human Nature and the Need for Social Connection* (New York: W.W. Norton, 2008).

14. H.C. Espeleta et al., "The Impact of Child Abuse Severity on Adult Attachment Anxiety and Avoidance in College Women: The Role of Emotion Dysregulation," *Journal of Family Violence* (2016): 1–9.

15. R. Sternberg, "A Triangular Theory of Love," *Psychological Review* 93 (1986): 119–35.

16. R. Sternberg, *Cupid's Arrow: The Course of Love through Time* (Boston: Cambridge University Press, 1998).

17. H. Fisher, *Anatomy of Love: A Natural History of Mating, Marriage, and Why We Stray* (New York: W.W. Norton, 2016).

18. Ibid.

19. L. Festinger, S. Schachter, and K. Back, *Social Pressures in Informal Groups: A Study of Human Factors in Housing* (Stanford, CA: Stanford University Press, 1950); R.L. Crooks and K. Baur, *Our Sexuality*, 13th ed. (Boston: Cengage Learning, 2016).

20. R.L. Crooks and K. Baur, *Our Sexuality*, 13th ed. (Boston: Cengage Learning, 2016).

21. Ibid.

22. C. Finkenauer and A. Buyukcan-Tetik, "To Know You Is to Feel Intimate with You: Felt Knowledge Is Rooted in Disclosure, Solicitation, and Intimacy," *Family Science* 6, no. 1 (2015): 109–18; C.R. Rogers, "Interpersonal Relationship: The Core of Guidance," in *Person to Person: The Problem of Being Human*, edited by C.R. Rogers and B. Stevens (Lafayette, CA: Real People Press, 1967), 85–101.

23. D. Worthington and M. Fitch-Hauser, *Listening: Processes, Functions, and Competency* (London: Routledge, 2016).

24. Ibid.

25. Ibid.

26. J. Wood, *Interpersonal Communication: Everyday Encounters*, 8th ed. (Boston: Woodsworth Publishing, 2015).

27. Ibid.

28. M. Gendon et al., "Perceptions of Emotion from Facial Expressions Are Not Culturally Universal: Evidence from a Remote Culture," *Emotion* 14, no. 2 (2014): 251–62.

29. K. Hampton, L.S. Goulet, L. Rainie, and K. Purcell, "Social Networking Sites and Our Lives," *Pew Internet and American Life Project*, June 16, 2011, Available at www.pewinternet.org/files/old-media//Files/Reports/2011/PIP%20-%20Social%20networking%20sites%20and%20our%20lives.pdf.

30. Ibid.

31. Ibid.

32. Ibid.

33. E.C. Tandoc et al., "Facebook Use, Envy, and Depression among College Students: Is Facebooking Depressing?," *Computers in Human Behavior* 43 (2015): 139–46; H. Appel et al., "The Interplay between Facebook Use, Social Comparison, Envy, and Depression," *Current Opinion in Psychology* 9 (2016): 44–49.

34. Ibid.

35. K. Hampton et al., "Social Media and the Cost of Caring," Pew Research Center, January 15, 2015, http://www.pewinternet.org/2015/01/15/social-media-and-stress.

36. American Psychological Association, "Stress in America: Coping with Change," February 23, 2017, Available at http://www.apa.org/news/press/releases/stress/2017/technology-social-media.pdf.

37. K.M. Hertlein and K. Ancheta, "Advantages and Disadvantages of Technology in Relationships: Findings from an Open-Ended Survey," *The Qualitative Report* 19, no. 22 (2014): 1–11.

38. Y.T. Uhls et al., "Five Days at Outdoor Education Camp without Screens Improves Preteen Skills with Nonverbal Emotion Cues," *Computers in Human Behavior* 39 (2014): 387–92.

39. T. Worley, "Exploring the Association between Relational Uncertainty, Jealousy About Partner's Friendships, and Jealousy Expression in Dating Relationships," *Communication Studies* 65, no. 4 (2014): 370–88; B.D.L. Zandbergen and S.G. Brown, "Culture and Gender Differences in Romantic Jealousy," *Personality and Individual Differences* 72 (2015): 122–27.

40. U.S. Department of Labor, Bureau of Labor Statistics, "American Time Use Survey Summary–2015 Results," June 24, 2016, http://www.bls.gov/news.release/atus.pdf.

41. Gottman Institute, "Research FAQs," Accessed February 3, 2017, https://www.gottman.com/about/research/faq.

42. Ibid.

43. G.F. Kelly, *Sexuality Today*, 11th ed. (New York: McGraw-Hill, 2014).

44. F. Newport and J. Wilke, "Most in U.S. Want Marriage, but Its Importance Has Dropped," Gallup, August 2, 2013, www.gallup.com/poll/163802/marriage-importance-dropped.aspx.

45. G. Livingston and A. Caumont, "5 Facts on Love and Marriage in America," Pew Research Center, February 13, 2017, http://www.pewresearch.org/fact-tank/2017/02/13/5-facts-about-love-and-marriage.

46. Ibid.

47. U.S. Census Bureau, "Families and Living Arrangements: 2016, Table MS-2, Estimated Median Age at First Marriage, by Sex: 1890 to the Present," www.census.gov/hhes/families/data/marital.html.

48. S. Kennedy and S. Ruggles, "Breaking Up Is Hard to Count: The Rise of Divorce in the United States, 1980–2010," *Demography* 51, no. 2 (2014): 587–98.

49. K. Heller, "The Myth of the High Rate of Divorce," Psych Central, 2016, http://psychcentral.com/lib/the-myth-of-the-high-rate-of-divorce.

50. C.C. Miller, "The Divorce Surge Is Over, but the Myth Lives On," *New York Times*, December 2, 2014, www.nytimes.com/2014/12/02/upshot/the-divorce-surge-is-over-but-the-myth-lives-on.html.

51. Ibid.

52. P.N.E. Roberson, et al. "Do Differences Matter? A Typology of Emerging Adult Romantic Relationship," *Journal of Social and Personal Relationships* (2016): doi:0265407516661589.

53. R.G. Watt et al., "Social Relationships and Health Related Behaviors among Older US Adults," *BMC Public Health* 14, no. 1 (2014): 533; G.E. Miller and Y. Pylypchuk, "Marital Status, Spousal Characteristics, and the Use of Preventive Care," *Journal of Family and Economic Issues* 35, no. 3 (2014): 323–38.

54. C.C. Miller, "Study Finds More Reasons to Get and Stay Married," *New York Times*, January 8, 2015, www.nytimes.com/2015/01/08/upshot/study-finds-more-reasons-to-get-and-stay-married.html?rref=upshot&abt=0002&abg=0&_r=2.

55. R.G. Watt et al., "Social Relationships and Health Related Behaviors among Older US Adults," *BMC Public Health* 14, no. 1 (2014); G.E. Miller and Y. Pylypchuk, "Marital Status, Spousal Characteristics, and the Use of Preventive Care," *Journal of Family and Economic Issues* 35, no. 3 (2014): 323–38.

56. Ibid.

57. Ibid.

58. Ibid.

59. U.S. Census Bureau, "America's Families and Living Arrangements: 2016: Adults, Table AD-3," https://www.census.gov/hhes/families/data/adults.html.

60. U.S. Department of Health and Human Services, Division of Vital Statistics, "First Premarital Cohabitation in the United States: 2006–2010 National Survey of Family Growth," *National Health Statistics Report* 64 (2013), Available at www.cdc.gov/nchs/data/nhsr/nhsr064.pdf; U.S. Department of Health and Human Services, Center for Health Statistics, "Key Statistics from the National Survey of Family Growth," April 20, 2015, www.cdc.gov/nchs/nsfg/key_statistics/c.htm.

61. Ibid.

62. A. Kuperberg, "Age at Co-Residence, Premarital Cohabitation and Marriage Dissolution: 1985–2009," *Journal of Marriage and Family* 76 no. 2 (2014): 352–69.

63. J. Daugherty and C. Copen, "Trends in Attitudes about Marriage, Childbearing, and Sexual Behavior: United States, 2002, 2006–2010, and 2011–2013," *National Health Statistics Reports* 92 (2016): 1–10.

64. U.S. Department of Health and Human Services, Division of Vital Statistics, "First Premarital Cohabitation in the United States," 2013; U.S. Department of Health and Human Services, Center for Health Statistics, "Key Statistics from the National Survey of Family Growth," 2015.

65. U.S. Census Bureau, "Characteristics of Same-Sex Households: 2014," Accessed February 2017, www.census.gov/hhes/samesex/data/acs.html.

66. *Obergefell v. Hodges*, 576 U.S. (2015).

67. Ibid

68. Ibid.

69. U.S. Census Bureau, "Marital Status: 2007–2011 American Community Survey, 5-Year Estimates, Table S1201," http://factfinder2.census; U.S. Census Bureau, "Marital Status of the Population 15 Years Old and Over, by Sex, Race and Hispanic Origin: 1950 to Present, Table MS-1," Accessed February 2017, https://www.census.gov/hhes/families/data/marital.html.

70. U.S. Census Bureau, "Marital Status: 2007–2011 American Community Survey, 5-Year Estimates, Table S1201," http://factfinder2.census; U.S. Census Bureau, "Marital Status of the Population 15 Years Old and Over, by Sex, Race and Hispanic Origin: 1950 to Present, Table MS-1", Accessed February 2017, https://www.census.gov/hhes/families/data/marital.html.

71. N. Sarkisian and N. Gerstel, "Does Singlehood Isolate or Integrate? Examining the Link between Marital Status and Ties to Kin, Friends, and Neighbors," *Journal of Social and Personal Relationships* 33, no. 3 (2016): 361–84.

Pulled Statistics:
page 147, K. Parker, W. Wang, and M. Rohol, "Record Share of Americans Have Never Married," Pew Research, 2014, www.pewsocialtrends.org/files/2014/09/2014-09-24_never-Married-Americans.pdf.

page 152, A. Smith, "15% of American Adults Have Used Online Dating Sites or Mobile Dating Apps," Pew Research, 2016, www.pewinternet.org/2016/02/11/15-percent-of-american-adults-have-used-online-dating-sites-or-mobile-dating-apps/.

Focus On: Understanding Your Sexuality

1. Intersex Society of North America, "How Common Is Intersex?," Accessed March 2017, www.isna.org faq/frequency.

2. J.S. Greenberg, C.E. Bruess, and S.B. Oswalt, *Exploring the Dimensions of Human Sexuality*, 6th ed. (Burlington, MA: Jones and Bartlett, 2016).

3. W.J. Chambliss and D.S. Eglitis, *Discover Sociology*, 2nd ed. (Los Angeles: Sage Publications, 2015).

4. Ibid.

5. Human Rights Campaign, "Sexual Orientation and Gender Identity Definitions," Accessed March 2017, http://www.hrc.org/resources/sexual-orientation-and-gender-identity-terminology-and-definitions.

6. Ibid.

7. GLAAD, "GLAAD Media Reference Guide—Terms to Avoid," Accessed March 2017, http://www.glaad.org/reference/offensive.

8. M. Rosario and E. Schrimshaw, "Theories and Etiologies of Sexual Orientation," *APA Handbook of Sexuality and Psychology* 1 (2014): 555–96.

9. J. McCarthy, "Satisfaction with Acceptance of Gay in U.S. at New High," Gallup, January 18, 2016, http://www.gallup.com/poll/188657/satisfaction-acceptance-gays-new-high.aspx.

10. G.M. Herek, "Beyond 'Homophobia': Thinking More Clearly about Stigma, Prejudice, and Sexual Orientation," *American Journal of Orthopsychiatry* 85, no. 5S (2015): S29–S37.

11. Federal Bureau of Investigation, "Bias Breakdown," November 16, 2015, https://www.fbi.gov/news/stories/2015/november/latest-hate-crime-statistics-available.

12. S.M. Cabrera et al., "Age of Thelarche and Menarche in Contemporary U.S. Females: A Cross-Sectional Analysis," *Journal of Pediatric Endocrinology and Metabolism* 27, 1–2 (2014): 47–51.

13. J.S. Greenberg, C.E. Bruess, and S.B. Oswalt, *Exploring the Dimensions of Human Sexuality*, 6th ed. (Burlington, MA: Jones and Bartlett, 2016).

14. Womenshealth.gov, "Premenstrual Symptoms Fact Sheet," January 4, 2017, https://www.womenshealth.gov/a-z-topics/premenstrual-syndrome#e.

15. E.W. Freeman, "Epidemiology and Etiology of Premenstrual Syndromes," March 3, 2017, http://www.medscape.org/viewarticle/553603.

16. Womenshealth.gov, "Premenstrual Symptoms Fact Sheet," January 4, 2017, https://www.womenshealth.gov/a-z-topics/premenstrual-syndrome#e.

17. Ibid.

18. Womenshealth.gov, "Menstruation and the Menstrual Cycle," January 4, 2017, https://www.womenshealth.gov/a-z-topics/menstruation-and-menstrual-cycle.

19. Ibid.

20. MedlinePlus, "Menopause," February 17, 2017, https://www.nlm.nih.gov/medlineplus/menopause.html.

21. Ibid.

22. Ibid.

23. Ibid.

24. MedlinePlus, "Menopause," February 17, 2017, https://www.nlm.nih.gov/medlineplus/menopause.html; H. Levine, "Is Hormone Replacement Therapy Making a Comeback?," *Consumer Reports*, May 15, 2016, http://www.consumerreports.org/women-s-health/is-hormone-replacement-therapy-making-a-comeback.

25. Centers for Disease Control and Prevention, Division of STD Prevention, "2015 Sexually Transmitted Diseases Treatment Guidelines," June 4, 2015, https://www.cdc.gov/std/tg2015/clinical.htm; M. Owings, S. Uddin, and S. Williams, "Trends in Circumcision for Male Newborns in U.S. Hospitals: 1979–2010," August 2013, www.cdc.gov/nchs/data/hestat/circumcision_2013/circumcision_2013.pdf.

26. American Academy of Pediatrics, "2012 Technical Report, Male Circumcision," *Pediatrics* 130, no. 3 (2012): e756–e785, doi:10.1542/peds.2012-1990.

27. Ibid.

28. J.S. Greenberg et al., *Exploring the Dimensions of Human Sexuality*, 6th ed. (Burlington, MA: Jones and Bartlett, 2016).

29. G.F. Kelly, *Sexuality Today*, 11th ed. (New York: McGraw-Hill, 2014).

30. W. Maltz, "The CERTS Model for Health Sex," Healthysex.com, Accessed May 2016, http://healthysex.com/healthy-sexuality/part-one-understanding/the-certs-model-for-healthy-sex.

31. R.L. Crooks and K. Baur, *Our Sexuality*, 13th ed. (Wadsworth Publishing: Belmont, CA, 2016).

32. American College Health Association, *American College Health Association–National College Health Assessment II (ACHA-NCHA II) Reference Group Data Report, Fall, 2016* (Hanover, MD: American College Health Association, 2017), Available at http://www.acha-ncha.org/docs/NCHA-II%20SPRING%202016%20UNDERGRADUATE%20REFERENCE%20GROUP%20DATA%20REPORT.pdf.

33. Ibid.

34. Ibid.

35. Ibid.

36. D.G. Duryea, N.G. Calleja, and D.A. MacDonald, "Nonmedical Use of Prescription Drugs by College Students with Minority Sexual Orientations," *Journal of College Student Psychotherapy* 29, no. 2 (2015): 147–59.

37. T.M. Hall, S. Shoptaw, and C.J. Reback, "Sometimes Poppers Are Not Poppers: Huffing as an Emergent Health Concern among MSM Substance Users," *Journal of Gay and Lesbian Mental Health* 19, no. 1 (2015): 118–21; T. Kofler, et al. "Use of Poppers (Amyl Nitrite): Unpleasant Side Effects in a Brothel," *European Journal of Case Reports in Internal Medicine* 1, no. 1 (2014): doi:10.12890/2014_000139.

38. Rape, Abuse, and Incest National Network, "Drug-Facilitated Sexual Assault," Accessed February 2017, https://rainn.org/get-information/types-of-sexual-assault/drug-facilitated-assault.

39. SIECUS, "Life Behaviors of a Sexually Healthy Adult," Accessed May 2016, www.siecus.org.

Pulled Statistics:
page 172, Data from American College *Health Association, American College Health Association—National College Health Assessment II (ACHA-NCHA II) Reference Group Data Report Spring 2016* (Baltimore: American College Health Association, 2016).

Chapter 7: Considering Your Reproductive Choices

1. American College Health Association, *American College Health Association—National College Health Assessment III (ACHA-NCHA III): Reference Group Data Report, Spring 2016*

2. L.B. Finer and M.R. Zolna, "Declines in Unintended Pregnancy in the United States, 2008–2011," *New England Journal of Medicine* 374, no. 9 (2016): 843–52.

3. J. Trussell, "Contraceptive Efficacy," in *Contraceptive Technology*, 20th rev. ed., eds. R.A. Hatcher et al. (New York: Ardent Media, 2011).

4. World Health Organization, "Nonoxynol-9 Ineffective in Preventing HIV Infection," Accessed March 2017, www.who.int/mediacentre/news/notes/release55/en.

5. J. Trussell, "Contraceptive Efficacy," in *Contraceptive Technology*, 20th rev. ed., eds. R.A. Hatcher et al. (New York: Ardent Media, 2011).

6. Ibid.

7. Ibid.

8. Mayo Clinic Staff, "Spermicide," January 2016, http://www.mayoclinic.org/tests-procedures/spermicide/home/ovc-20168558; World Health Organization, "Nonoxynol-9 Ineffective in Preventing HIV Infection," Accessed March 2017, www.who.int/mediacentre/news/notes/release55/en.

9. Ibid.

10. J. Trussell, "Contraceptive Efficacy," in *Contraceptive Technology*, 20th rev. ed., eds. R.A. Hatcher et al. (New York: Ardent Media, 2011).

11. HPSRx Enterprises, "Caya: For Patients," Accessed March 2017, http://caya.us.com/services/for-patients.

12. Ibid.

13. Ibid.

14. Ibid.

15. American College Health Association, *National College Health Assessment III (ACHA-NCHA III): Reference Group Data Report, Spring 2016* (Hanover, MD: American College Health Association, 2016), Available at http://www.acha-ncha.org/reports_ACHA-NCHAIIc.html.

16. J. Trussell, "Contraceptive Efficacy," in *Contraceptive Technology*, 20th rev. ed., eds. R.A. Hatcher et al. (New York: Ardent Media, 2011).

17. Ibid.

18. O. Lidegaard, "The Risk of Arterial Thrombosis Increases with the Use of Combined Oral Contraceptives," *Evidence Based Medicine* 21, no. 1 (2016): 38; A. Weill et al, "Low Dose Oestrogen Combined Oral Contraception and Risk of Pulmonary Embolism, Stroke, and Myocardial Infarction in Five Million French Women: Cohort Study," *British Medical Journal* 353 (2016): i2002.

19. J. Trussell, "Contraceptive Efficacy," in *Contraceptive Technology*, 20th rev. ed., eds. R.A. Hatcher et al. (New York: Ardent Media, 2011).

20. E.G. Raymond, "Progestin-Only Pills," in *Contraceptive Technology*, 20th rev. ed., eds. R.A. Hatcher et al. (New York: Ardent Media, 2011).

21. Mylan Pharmaceuticals, "Xulane," Accessed March 2017, www.xulane.com; Drugs.com, "Xulane," March 2017, www.drugs.com/mtm/xulane_transdermal.html.

22. J. Trussell, "Contraceptive Efficacy," in *Contraceptive Technology*, 20th rev. ed., eds. R. A. Hatcher et al. (New York: Ardent Media, 2011).

23. Drugs.com, "Xulane," March 2017, http://www.drugs.com/pro/xulane.html.

24. Ibid.

25. J. Trussell, "Contraceptive Efficacy," in *Contraceptive Technology*, 20th rev. ed., eds. R.A. Hatcher et al. (New York: Ardent Media, 2011).

26. Ibid.

27. Pfizer, "Depo-subQ Provera U.S. Patient Product Information," Accessed March 2017, http://www.pfizer.com/products/product-detail/depo_subq_provera_104.

28. J. Trussell, "Contraceptive Efficacy," in *Contraceptive Technology*, 20th rev. ed., eds. R.A. Hatcher et al. (New York: Ardent Media, 2011).

29. Merck & Co., Inc., "Nexplanon," Accessed March 2017, www.nexplanon.com/en/-consumer.

30. K. Daniels et al., "Current Contraceptive Use and Variation by Selected Characteristics Among Women Aged 15–44: United States, 2011–2013," *National Health Statistics Reports* 86 (2015): 1–15.

31. American Congress of Obstetricians and Gynecologists, "ACOG Committee Opinion-Adolescents and Long-Acting Reversible Contraception: Implants and Intrauterine Devices," Number 539, October 2012, www.acog.org/Resources_And_Publications/Committee_Opinions/Committee_on_Adolescent_Health_Care/Adolescents_and_Long-Acting_Reversible_Contraception.

32. J. Trussell, "Contraceptive Efficacy," in *Contraceptive Technology*, 20th rev. ed., eds. R.A. Hatcher et al. (New York: Ardent Media, 2011).

33. American College Health Association, *National College Health Assessment III (ACHA-NCHA III): Reference Group Data Report Spring 2016* (Hanover, MD: American College Health Association, 2016).

34. J. Trussell, "Contraceptive Efficacy," in *Contraceptive Technology*, 20th rev. ed., eds. R.A. Hatcher et al. (New York: Ardent Media, 2011).

35. American College Health Association, *National College Health Assessment III (ACHA-NCHA III): Reference Group Data Report Spring 2015* (Hanover, MD: American College Health Association, 2015).

36. J. Trussell, "Contraceptive Efficacy," in *Contraceptive Technology*, 20th rev. ed., eds. R.A. Hatcher et al. (New York: Ardent Media, 2011).

37. Office of Population Research and Association of Reproductive Health Professionals, The Emergency Contraception Website, "Answers to Frequently Asked Questions about Effectiveness," Updated January 2017, http://ec.princeton.edu/questions/eceffect.html.

38. American College Health Association, *National College Health Assessment II: Undergraduate Students Reference Group Data Spring 2017* (Hanover, MD: American College Health Association, 2017).

39. A.R.A. Aiken et al., "Similarities and Differences in Contraceptive Use Reported by Women and Men in the National Survey of Family Growth," *Contraception*, 2016, http://dx.doi.org/10.1016/j.contraception.2016.10.008.

40. U.S. Food and Drug Administration, "Medical Devices, FDA Activities," November 16, 2016, https://www.fda.gov/MedicalDevices/ProductsandMedicalProcedures/ImplantsandProsthetics/EssurePermanentBirthControl/ucm452254.htm.

41. J. Trussell, "Contraceptive Efficacy," in *Contraceptive Technology*, 20th rev. ed., eds. R.A. Hatcher et al. (New York: Ardent Media, 2011).

42. Ibid.

43. Guttmacher Institute, "Fact Sheet: Induced Abortion in the United States," January 2017, www.guttmacher.org/fact-sheet/induced-abortion-united-states.

44. Ibid.

45. *Roe v. Wade*, 410 U.S. 113 (1973).

46. L. Saad, "Americans' Attitudes toward Abortion Unchanged," *Gallup Social Issues*, Blog, May 25, 2016, http://www.gallup.com/poll/191834/americans-attitudes-toward-abortion-unchanged.aspx.

47. Center for Reproductive Rights, "Standing Up for Our Reproductive Rights: A Look Back at the 114th Congress," Report, 2017, Available at https://www.reproductiverights.org/sites/crr.civicactions.net/files/documents/Standing-Up-for-Reproductive-Rights-A%20-Look-Back-at-the-114th-Congress.pdf.

48. M.A. Biggs et al., "Mental Health Diagnoses 3 Years after Receiving or Being Denied an Abortion in the United States," *American Journal of Public Health* 105, no. 12 (2015): 2557–63; J.R. Steinberg, C.E. McCulloch, and N.E. Adler, "Abortion and Mental Health: Findings from the National Comorbidity Survey-Replication," *Obstetrics & Gynecology* 123, no. 2 (2014): 263–70.

49. Ibid.

50. Ibid.

51. Guttmacher Institute, "Fact Sheet: Induced Abortion in the United States," 2017, https://www.guttmacher.org/fact-sheet/induced-abortion-united-states?gclid=CNKFrYXc79ICFc-6wAodb1wKcQ.

52. Ibid.

53. Guttmacher Institute, "Bans on Specific Abortion Methods Used after the First Trimester," March 2017, https://www.guttmacher.org/state-policy/explore/bans-specific-abortion-methods-used-after-first-trimester.

54. Ibid.

55. Ibid.

56. M.F. MacDorman et al., "Recent Increases in the U.S Maternal Mortality Rate: Disentangling Trends from Measurement Issues," *Obstetrics and Gynecology* 128, no. 3 (2016): 447–55.

57. Planned Parenthood, "The Abortion Pill," Accessed March 2017, https://www.plannedparenthood.org/learn/abortion/the-abortion-pill.

58. M.J. Chen and M.D. Creinin, "Mifepristone with Buccal Misoprostol for Medical Abortion: A Systematic Review," *Obstetrics & Gynecology* 126, no. 1 (2015): 12–21.

59. Ibid.

60. M. Lino et al., "Expenditures on Children by Families, 2015," Miscellaneous Publication No. 1528-2015 (Washington, DC: U.S. Department of Agriculture, Center for Nutrition Policy and Promotion, 2017), Available at https://www.cnpp.usda.gov/sites/default/files/crc2015_March2017_0.pdf.

61. Castlight Health, "New Study Shows Huge Cost Differences for Having a Baby, Often in Same City," June 2016, http://www.castlighthealth.com/press-releases/new-study-shows-huge-cost-differences-for-having-a-baby-often-in-the-same-city.

62. T.J. Mathews and B.E. Hamilton, "Mean Age of Mothers in on the Rise," *NCHS Data Brief* 232 (2016): 1–7, https://www.cdc.gov/nchs/data/databriefs/db232.pdf.

63. B.E. Hamilton et al., "Births: Preliminary Data for 2015," *National Vital Statistics Report* 65, no. 13 (2016), Available at https://www.cdc.gov/nchs/data/nvsr/nvsr65/nvsr65_03.pdf.

64. American Pregnancy Association, "Miscarriage," Updated August 2016, http://american pregnancy.org/pregnancy complications/miscarriage.html.

65. Committee on Gynecologic Practice of American College of Obstetricians and Gynecologists, "Female Age-Related Fertility Decline," *Committee Opinion* 589 (2014), Available at http://www.acog.org/Resources-And-Publications/Committee-Opinions/Committee-on-Gynecologic-Practice/Female-Age-Related-Fertility-Decline.

66. Centers for Disease Control and Prevention, "Preconception Health and Health Care: Women," September 2016, www.cdc.gov/preconception/women.html.

67. Ibid.

68. J.P. Bonde et al., "The Epidemiologic Evidence Linking Prenatal and Postnatal Exposure to Endocrine Disrupting Chemicals with Male Reproductive Disorders: A Systematic Review and Meta-analysis," *Human Reproduction Update* 23, no. 1 (2016): 104–25; G.C. Di Renzo et al., "International Federation of Gynecology and Obstetrics Opinion on Reproductive Health Impacts of Exposure to Toxic Environmental Chemicals," *International Journal of Gynecology & Obstetrics* 131, no. 3 (2015): 219–25; Centers for Disease Control and Prevention, "Preconception Health and Healthcare," September 2016, www.cdc.gov/preconception/careformen/exposures.html.

69. D. Malaspina et al., "Paternal Age and Mental Health of Offspring," *Fertility and Sterility* 103, no. 6 (2015): 1392–96.

70. Planned Parenthood, "Pregnancy Tests," Accessed March 2017, https://www.planned parenthood.org/learn/pregnancy/pregnancy-test.

71. American Congress of Obstetricians and Gynecologists, "ACOG Committee Opinion no. 548: Weight Gain during Pregnancy," *Obstetrics and Gynecology* 121, no. 1 (2013): 210–12, doi:10.1097/01.AOG.0000425668.87506.4c.

72. Ibid.

73. Ibid.

74. American Congress of Obstetricians and Gynecologists, "Tobacco, Alcohol, Drugs, and Pregnancy," December 2013, www.acog.org/~/media/For%20Patients/faq170.pdf?dmc=1&ts=20140516T2242271513.

75. National Center for Chronic Disease Prevention and Health Promotion, "Tobacco Use and Pregnancy," *Reproductive Health*, Updated July 2016, https://www.cdc.gov/reproductivehealth/maternalinfanthealth/tobaccousepregnancy/index.htm; American Congress of Obstetricians and Gynecologists, "Tobacco, Alcohol, Drugs, and Pregnancy," 2013, December 2013, www.acog.org/~/media/For%20Patients/faq170.pdf?dmc=1&ts=20140516T2242271513.

76. CDC, "Facts about Cleft Lip and Cleft Palate," 2015, www.cdc.gov/ncbddd/birthdefects/cleftlip.html.

77. B.E. Hamilton et al., "Births: Preliminary Data for 2015," *National Vital Statistics Report* 65, no. 13 (2016), Available at https://www.cdc.gov/nchs/data/nvsr/nvsr65/nvsr65_03.pdf.

78. M. Thielking, *Stat News*, "Sky-High C-section Rates in the US Don't Translate into Better Birth Outcomes," December 1, 2015, https://www.statnews.com/2015/12/01/cesarean-section-childbirth.

79. American Pregnancy Association, "Preeclampsia," Updated August 2015, http://americanpregnancy.org/pregnancy-complications/preeclampsia.

80. American Pregnancy Association, "Miscarriage," Updated August 2016, http://americanpregnancy.org/pregnancy-complications/miscarriage.

81. V.P. Sepilian et al., "Ectopic Pregnancy," *Medscape Reference*, Updated November 2015, http://emedicine.medscape.com/article/2041923-overview.

82. What to Expect, "Stillbirth," Accessed March 2017, www.whattoexpect.com/pregnancy/pregnancy-health/complications/stillbirth.aspx.

83. American Psychological Association, "What Is Postpartum Depression and Anxiety?," Accessed March 2017, http://www.apa.org/pi/women/resources/reports/postpartum-depression.aspx.

84. Ibid.

85. American Academy of Pediatrics, "Policy Statement: Breastfeeding and the Use of Human Milk," *Pediatrics* 129, no. 3 (2012): 496.

86. National Institute of Child Health and Human Development, "What Are the Benefits of Breastfeeding?," Accessed March 2017, https://www.nichd.nih.gov/health/topics/breastfeeding/conditioninfo/Pages/benefits.aspx.

87. Centers for Disease Control and Prevention, "Sudden Unexpected Infant Death and Sudden Infant Death Syndrome," February 2017, www.cdc.gov/sids/aboutsuidandsids.htm.

88. Ibid.

89. Ibid.

90. Centers for Disease Control and Prevention, "Infertility FAQs," Reproductive Health, February 2017, www.cdc.gov/reproductivehealth/Infertility.

91. MayoClinic.com, "Infertility: Causes," July 2014, www.mayoclinic.com/health/infertility/DS00310/DSECTION=causes.

92. U.S. Department of Health and Human Services, "Polycystic Ovary Syndrome (PCOS) Fact Sheet," June 2016, www.womenshealth.gov/publications/our-publications/fact-sheet/polycystic-ovary-syndrome.html.

93. A. Talmor and B. Dunphy, "Female Obesity and Infertility," *Best Practice & Research Clinical Obstetrics & Gynaecology* 29, no. 4 (2015): 498–506.

94. Centers for Disease Control and Prevention, "Pelvic Inflammatory Disease CDC Fact Sheet," Sexually Transmitted Diseases, May 2016, www.cdc.gov/std/PID/STDFact-PID.htm.

95. Centers for Disease Control and Prevention, "Infertility: FAQs," February 2017, www.cdc.gov/reproductivehealth/Infertility/index.htm#4.

96. National Infertility Association, "The Semen Analysis," Accessed March 2017, http://www.resolve.org/about-infertility/male-workup/the-semen-analysis.html.

97. Ibid.; Mayo Clinic Staff, "Low Sperm Count," July 2015, www.mayoclinic.org/diseases-conditions/low-sperm-count/basics/causes/con-20033441.

98. Centers for Disease Control and Prevention, "Infertility: FAQs," February 2017, www.cdc.gov/reproductivehealth/Infertility/index.htm#4.

99. Ibid.

100. WebMD Medical Reference, "Fertility Drugs," June 2015, www.webmd.com/infertility-and-reproduction/guide/fertility-drugs.

101. American Society for Reproductive Medicine, "Fertility Drugs and the Risk for Multiple Births," Accessed March 2017, www.asrm.org/uploadedFiles/ASRM_Content/Resources/Patient_Resources/Fact_Sheets_and_Info_Booklets/fertilitydrugs_multiple births.pdf.

102. WebMD, "Using a Surrogate Mother: What You Need to Know," September 2015, www.webmd.com/infertility-and-reproduction/guide/using-surrogate-mother.

103. R.M. Kreider and D.A. Loftquist, *Adopted Children and Stepchildren: 2010*, U.S. Census Bureau, April 2014, www.census.gov/content/dam/Census/library/publications/2014/demo/p20-572.pdf.

104. Intercountry Adoption, U.S. Department of State, "FY 2015 Annual Report on Intercountry Adoption," Accessed March 2017, https://travel.state.gov/content/adoptionsabroad/en/about-us/statistics.html.

105. Adoption.com, "Adoption Costs," Accessed March 2017, http://adoption.com_internaitonal_adoption_costs.

Pulled Statistics:

page 180, American College Health Association, *American College Health Association—National College Health Assessment III (ACHA-NCHA III): Reference Group Data Report, Spring 2016* (Hanover, MD: American College Health Association, 2016), Available at www.achancha.org/reports_ACHA_NCHAII.htm.

page 194, Gallup, "Abortion Edges Up as Important Voting Issue for Americans," 2015, http://www.gallup.com/poll/183449/abortion-edges-important-voting-issue-americans.

Chapter 8: Recognizing and Avoiding Addiction and Drug Abuse

1. Office of the Surgeon General, *Facing Addiction in America: The Surgeon General's Report on Alcohol, Drugs, and Health*, November, 2016, Washington, DC: U.S. Department of Health and Human Services.

2. M. Potenza, "Perspective: Behavioral Addictions Matter," *Nature* 522, Suppl. 62 (2015): doi:10.1038/522S62a; S. S. Alavi et al., "Behavioral Addiction versus Substance Addiction: Correspondence of Psychiatric and Psychological Views," *International Journal of Preventive Medicine* 3, no. 4 (2012): 290–94.

3. N. Volkow et al., "Neurobiologic Advances from the Brain Disease Model of Addiction," *New England Journal of Medicine* 374, no. 4 (2016): 363–71.

4. American Society of Addiction Medicine, "Definition of Addiction," April 2011, www.asam.org/for-the-public/definition-of-addiction

5. National Institute on Drug Abuse, *Drugs, Brains, and Behavior: The Science of Addiction*, NIH Publication No. 07-5605, Available at www.nida.nih.gov/-scienceofaddiction.

6. National Council on Problem Gambling, "March Madness and Gambling: Have the Conversation," March 9, 2016, Available at https://images.production.membersuite.com/7339289f-0004-c76f-a8b9-0b3842784d72/20987/7339289f-001c-c537-bd2e-0b3b1fb1a928; American Psychiatric Association, *Diagnostic and Statistical Manual of Mental Disorders*, 5th ed. (Arlington, VA: American Psychiatric Publishing, 2013), 585.

7. American Psychiatric Association, *Diagnostic and Statistical Manual of Mental Disorders*, 5th ed. (Arlington, VA: American Psychiatric Publishing, 2013), 585.

8. J. Grohol, "Four Phases and Steps of Gambling Addiction," *Psych Central*, July 17, 2016, https://psychcentral.com/lib/four-phases-and-steps-of-gambling-addiction.

9. D. Nutt et al., "The Dopamine Theory of Addiction: 40 Years of Highs and Lows," *Nature Reviews Neuroscience* 16, no. 5 (2015): 305–12.

10. Elements Behavioral Health, "Internet, Gambling Addicts Also Suffer from Withdrawal," Accessed March 2016, https://www.elementsbehavioralhealth.com/behavioral-process-addictions/internet-gambling-addicts-also-suffer-from-withdrawal.

11. D. V. Rinker et al., "Racial and Ethnic Differences in Problem Gambling among College Students," *Journal of Gambling Studies* 32, no. 2 (2015): 581–90; National Center for Responsible Gambling, "Fact Sheet: Gambling on College Campuses," Accessed February 2016, http://www.collegegambling.org/just-facts/gambling-college-campuses.

12. Ibid.

13. Ibid.

14. A. Muller et al., "Compulsive Buying," *American Journal on Addictions* 24, no. 2 (2015): 132–37.

15. A. Muller et al., "Compulsive Buying," *American Journal on Addictions* 24, no. 2 (2015): 132–37; A. Weinstein et al., "Compulsive Buying-Features and Characteristics of Addiction," *Neuropathology of Drug Addictions and Substance Misuse* 3 (2016), http://dx.doi.org/10.1016/B978-0-12-800634-4.00098-6.

16. A. Weinstein et al., "Compulsive Buying-Features and Characteristics of Addiction," *Neuropathology of Drug Addictions and Substance Misuse* 3 (2016), http://dx.doi.org/10.1016/B978-0-12-800634-4.00098-6; A. Muller et al., "Compulsive Buying," *American Journal on Addictions* 24, no. 2 (2015): 132–37.

17. A. Weinsten et al., "A Study Investigating the Association between Compulsive Buying with Measure of Anxiety and Obsessive-Compulsive Behavior among Internet Shoppers," *Comprehensive Psychiatry* 57 (2015): 46–50; P. Trotzke et al., "Pathological Buying Online as a Specific Form of Internet Addiction: A Model-Based Experimental Investigation," *PLoS ONE* 10, no. 10 (2015): e0140296; K. Deryshire et al., "Problematic Internet Use and Associated Risks in a College Sample," *Comprehensive Psychiatry* 54, no. 5 (2013): 415–22.

18. A. Weinstein et al., "Compulsive Buying-Features and Characteristics of Addiction," *Neuropathology of Drug Addictions and Substance Misuse* 3 (2016), http://dx.doi.org/10.1016/B978-0-12-800634-4.00098-6.

19. A. Szabo et al., "Methodological and Conceptual Limitations in Exercise Addiction Research," *Yale Journal of Biology and Medicine* 88, no. 3 (2015): 303–08; A. Weinstein and Y. Weinstein, "Exercise Addiction: Diagnosis, Bio-psychological Mechanisms, and Treatment Issues," *Current Pharmaceutical Design* 20, no. 25 (2014): 4062–69.

20. Net Addiction, "FAQs," Accessed March 2016, http://netaddiction.com/faqs/; H. Pontes, D. Kuss, and M. Griffiths, "Clinical Psychology of Internet Addiction: A Review of Its Conceptualization, Prevalence, Neuronal Processes, and Implications for Treatment," *Neuroscience and Neuroeconomics* 4 (2015): 11–23.

21. W. Li et al., "Characteristics of Internet Addiction: Pathological Internet Use in U.S. University Students: A Qualitative-Method Investigation," *PLoS ONE* 10, no. 2 (2015): e0117372.

22. American College Health Association, *American College Health Association—National College Health Assessment II: Reference Group Data Report Fall 2016* (Baltimore. MD: American College Health Association, 2017).

23. Signs and Symptoms of Work Addiction. Addiction Help Center. 2016. http://www.addictionhelpcenter.com/signs-and-symptoms-of-work-addiction/.

24. Ibid.

25. M. Clark, et al., "All Work and No Play?: A Meta-analytic Examination of the Correlates and Outcomes of Workaholism," *Journal of Management* 42, no. 7(2016): 1836–73.

26. L. Kravina et al., "Work Alcoholism and Work Engagement in the Family: The Relationship between Parents and Children as a Risk Factor," *European Journal of Work and Organizational Psychology* 23, no. 6 (2014): 875–83.

27. M. Clark et al., "All Work and No Play? A Meta-analytic Examination of the Correlates and Outcomes of Workaholism," *Journal of Management* 42, no. 7 (2016): 1836–73.

28. R. Weiss, "Hypersexuality: Symptoms of Sexual Addiction," *Psych Central*, March 2016, http://psychcentral.com/lib/hypersexuality-symptoms-of-sexual-addiction.

29. Ibid.

30. Centers for Disease Control and Prevention, "Therapeutic Drug Use," January 19, 2017, https://www.cdc.gov/nchs/fastats/drug-use-therapeutic.htm.

31. Ibid.

32. Ibid.

33. Consumer Health Care Products Association, "Statistics on OTC Use," Accessed May 2016, http://www.chpa.org/MarketStats.aspx.

34. U.S. National Library of Medicine, "Over-the-Counter Medicines," February 8, 2017, https://www.nlm.nih.gov/medlineplus/overthe counter medicines.html.

35. L. D. Johnston et al., *Monitoring the Future National Results on Drug Use* (Ann Arbor, MI: Institute for Social Research, University of Michigan, 2016).

36. Erowid, "The DXM Vault," Accessed June 2016, www.erowid.org.

37. Center for Behavioral Health Statistics and Quality, "Behavioral Health Trends in the United States: Results from the 2015 National Survey on Drug Use and Health," 2016, Available at https://www.samhsa.gov/data/sites/default/files/NSDUH-FFR1-2015/NSDUH-FFR1-2015/NSDUH-FFR1-2015.htm.

38. Ibid.

39. Ibid.

40. L. D. Johnston et al., *Monitoring the Future National Results on Drug Use* (Ann Arbor, MI: Institute for Social Research, University of Michigan, 2016).

41. American College Health Association, *American College Health Association–National College Health Assessment Fall 2016 Reference Group Executive Summary*, 2017, Available at http://www.acha-ncha.org/docs/NCHA-II_WEB_Fall_2016_REFERENCE_GROUP_EXECUTIVE_SUMMARY.pdf.

42. American College Health Association, *American College Health Association—National College Health Assessment Fall 2016 Reference Group Data Report*, 2017. Available at http://www.acha-ncha.org/docs/NCHA-II%20Fall%202016%20REFERENCE%20GROUP%20DATA%20REPORT.pdf.

43. Ibid.

44. Higher Education Center for Alcohol and Drug Misuse Prevention and Recovery, "College Prescription Drug Study," Accessed June 2016, Available at http://hecaod.osu.edu/wp-content/uploads/2015/10/CPDS-Key-Findings-Report-1.pdf.

45. Ibid.

46. Center for Behavioral Health Statistics and Quality, "Behavioral Health Trends in the United States: Results from the 2015 National Survey on Drug Use and Health," 2016, Available at https://www.samhsa.gov/data/sites/default/files/NSDUH-FFR1-2015/NSDUH-FFR1-2015/NSDUH-FFR1-2015.htm.

47. Ibid.

48. Ibid.

49. Ibid.

50. A. Arria, et al., "Drug Use Patterns and Continuous Enrollment in College: Results from a Longitudinal Study," *Journal of Studies on Alcohol and Drugs* 74 (2013): 71–83.

51. A. Arria et al., "Drug Use Patterns in Young Adulthood and Post-College Employment," *Drug and Alcohol Dependence* 127, no. 1–3 (2013): 23–30.

52. Higher Education Center for Alcohol and Drug Misuse Prevention and Recovery, "College Prescription Drug Study," Accessed June 2016, Available at http://hecaod.osu.edu/wp-content/uploads/2015/10/CPDS-Key-Findings-Report-1.pdf.

53. Center for Behavioral Health Statistics and Quality, "Behavioral Health Trends in the United States: Results from the 2015 National Survey on Drug Use and Health," 2016, Available at https://www.samhsa.gov/data/sites/default/files/NSDUH-FFR1-2015/NSDUH-FFR1-2015/NSDUH-FFR1-2015.htm.

54. American College Health Association, *American College Health Association–National College Health Assessment Fall 2016 Reference Group Executive Summary*, 2017, Available at http://www.acha-ncha.org/docs/NCHA-II_WEB_Fall_2016_REFERENCE_GROUP_EXECUTIVE_SUMMARY.pdf.

55. Addiction Center, "Drinking and Drug Abuse Is Higher among Greeks," February 15, 2015, www .addictioncenter.com/college/drinking-drug-abuse-greek-life.

56. Ibid.

57. Center for Behavioral Health Statistics and Quality, "Behavioral Health Trends in the United States: Results from the 2015 National Survey on Drug Use and Health," 2016, , Available at https://www.samhsa.gov/data/sites/default/files/NSDUH-FFR1-2015/NSDUH-FFR1-2015/NSDUH-FFR1-2015.htm.

58. L. D. Johnston et al., *Monitoring the Future National Results on Drug Use* (Ann Arbor, MI: Institute for Social Research, University of Michigan, 2016).

59. National Institute on Drug Abuse, "What Is Methamphetamine?" DrugFacts, February 2017, https://www.drugabuse.gov/publications/drugfacts/methamphetamine; Medscape, "Methamphetamine Use Triples Parkinson's Risk," *Multispecialty*, 2014, http://www.medscape.com/viewarticle/837025.

60. National Institute on Drug Abuse, "What Is Methamphetamine?" DrugFacts, February 2017, https://www.drugabuse.gov/publications/drugfacts/methamphetamine.

61. National Institute on Drug Abuse, "What Are Synthetic Cathinones?," DrugFacts, January 2016, https://www.drugabuse.gov/publications/drugfacts/synthetic-cathinones-bath-salts.

62. Ibid.

63. Ibid.

64. Ibid.

65. Ibid.

66. D. C. Mitchell et al., "Beverage Caffeine Intakes in the U.S.," *Food and Chemical Toxicology* 63 (2014): 136–42.

67. Ibid.

68. Ibid.

69. Caffeineinformer, "20 Harmful Effects of Caffeine," February 1, 2017, http://www.caffeineinformer.com/harmful-effects-of-caffeine.

70. Caffeineinformer, "Top 24 Caffeine Health Benefits" January 19, 2017, https://www.caffeineinformer.com/top-10-caffeine-health-benefits.

71. National Institute on Drug Abuse, "Marijuana," DrugFacts, March 2016, https://www.drugabuse.gov/publications/drugfacts/marijuana.

72. Center for Behavioral Health Statistics and Quality, "Behavioral Health Trends in the United States: Results from the 2015 National Survey on Drug Use and

Health," 2016, Available at https://www.samhsa.gov/data/sites/default/files/NSDUH-FFR1-2015/NSDUH-FFR1-2015/NSDUH-FFR1-2015.htm.

73. L. D. Johnston et al., *Monitoring the Future National Results on Drug Use* (Ann Arbor, MI: Institute for Social Research, University of Michigan, 2016).

74. Leaf Science, "A Beginner's Guide to Marijuana Edibles," October 27, 2015, http://www.leafscience.com/2015/10/27/beginners-guide-marijuana-edibles.

75. Ibid.

76. National Institute on Drug Abuse, "Marijuana," Drug-Facts, March 2016, https://www.drugabuse.gov/publications/drugfacts/marijuana.

77. National Institutes of Health, "Marijuana," March 2016, https://www.drugabuse.gov/sites/default/files/marijuananadrugfacts_march_2016.pdf.

78. Ibid.

79. AAA Foundation, "Impaired Driving and Cannabis," May 2016, https://www.aaafoundation.org/impaired-driving-and-cannabis.

80. T. Johnson, "Fatal Road Crashes Involving Marijuana Double after State Legalizes Drugs," AAA, May 10, 2016, http://newsroom.aaa.com/2016/05/fatal-road-crashes-involving-marijuana-double-state-legalizes-drug.

81. American Lung Association, "Marijuana and Lung Health," March 23, 2015, http://www.lung.org/stop-smoking/smoking-facts/marijuana-and-lung-health.html.

82. National Institute on Drug Abuse, "Marijuana," Drug-Facts, March 2016, https://www.drugabuse.gov/publications/drugfacts/marijuana.

83. G. Schauer, "Toking, Vaping, and Eating for Health or Fun," *American Journal of Preventive Medicine* 50, no. 1 (2016): 108.

84. D. Tashkin, "How Beneficial Is Vaping Cannabis to Respiratory Health Compared to Smoking?" *Addiction* 110, no. 11 (2015): 1706–07.

85. National Institute on Drug Abuse, "Marijuana," Drug-Facts, 2016, https://www.drugabuse.gov/publications/drugfacts/marijuana.

86. C. Blanco et al., "Cannabis Use and Risk of Psychiatric Disorders," *JAMA Psychiatry* 73, no. 4 (2016): 388–95.

87. Ibid.

88. American Academy of Pediatrics, "Marijuana Legalization," March 2016, https://www.aap.org/en-us/advocacy-and-policy/state-advocacy/Documents/Marijuana%20Legalization.pdf.

89. Ibid.

90. Ibid.

91. National Institute on Drug Abuse, "Marijuana: Facts for Teens," May 2015, www.drugabuse.gov/publications/marijuana-facts-teens; Science Daily, "Marijuana Use Prior to Pregnancy Doubles Risk of Premature Birth," July 17, 2012, www.sciencedaily.com.

92. National Institute on Drug Abuse, "Synthetic Cannabinoids," DrugFacts, November 2015, https://www.drugabuse.gov/publications/drugfacts/synthetic-cannabinoids.

93. L. D. Johnston et al., *Monitoring the Future National Survey Results on Drug Use* (Ann Arbor, MI: Institute for Social Research, University of Michigan, 2016).

94. K. L. Egan, et al., "K2 and Spice Use among a Cohort of College Students in the Southeast Region of the USA," *American Journal of Drug and Alcohol Abuse* 41 no. 4 (2015): 317–22.

95. L. D. Johnston et al., *Monitoring the Future National Survey Results on Drug Use* (Ann Arbor, MI: Institute for Social Research, University of Michigan, 2016).

96. National Institute on Drug Abuse, "Synthetic Cannabinoids," DrugFacts, 2015, https://www.drugabuse.gov/publications/drugfacts/synthetic-cannabinoids.

97. Ibid.

98. Ibid.

99. Substance Abuse and Mental Health Services Administration, "Not for Human Consumption: Spice and Bath Salts," March 3, 2015, http://newsletter.samhsa.gov/2015/03/03/not-for-human-consumption-spice-and-bath-salts.

100. National Institute on Drug Abuse, "What Are CNS Depressants?" 2016, https://www.drugabuse.gov/publications/research-reports/prescription-drugs/cns-depressants/what-are-cns-depressants.

101. Ibid.

102. WebMD, "Barbiturate Abuse Overview," 2016, http://www.webmd.com/mental-health/addiction/barbiturate-abuse.

103. Partnership for Drug-Free Kids, "GHB," Accessed June 2016, www.drugfree.org/drug-guide/ghb.

104. National Institute on Drug Abuse, "What Is Heroin?" DrugFacts, January 2017, https://www.drugabuse.gov/publications/drugfacts/heroin.

105. Ibid.

106. Center for Behavioral Health Statistics and Quality, "Behavioral Health Trends in the United States: Results from the 2015 National Survey on Drug Use and Health," 2016, Available at https://www.samhsa.gov/data/sites/default/files/NSDUH-FFR1-2015/NSDUH-FFR1-2015/NSDUH-FFR1-2015.htm; Healthline, "Prescription Drugs are Leading to Heroin Addiction," February 2016. http://www.healthline.com/health-news/prescription-drugs-lead-to-addiction.

107. Centers for Disease Control and Prevention, "Increases in Drug and Opioid Overdose Deaths—United States, 2000–2014," *Morbidity and Mortality Weekly Report* 64, no. 50 (2016): 1378–82.

108. R.A. Rudd et al., Increases in Drug and Opioid-Involved Overdose Deaths —United States, 2010–2015. *Morbidity and Mortality Weekly Report* 65 (2016):1445–52.

109. Centers for Disease Control and Prevention, "Vital Signs: Demographic and Substance Use Trends Among Heroin Users—United States 2002–2013," *Morbidity and Mortality Weekly Report* 64, no. 26 (2015): 719–25; T. Cicero, "The Changing Face of Heroin Use in the United States: A Retrospective Analysis of the Past 50 Years," *Journal of the American Medical Association* 71, no. 7 (2014): 821–26.

110. National Institute on Drug Abuse, "What Is Heroin?," DrugFacts, January 2017, https://www.drugabuse.gov/publications/drugfacts/heroin.

111. Center for Behavioral Health Statistics and Quality, "Behavioral Health Trends in the United States: Results from the 2015 National Survey on Drug Use and Health," 2016, Available at https://www.samhsa.gov/data/sites/default/files/NSDUH-FFR1-2015/NSDUH-FFR1-2015/NSDUH-FFR1-2015.htm.

112. L. D. Johnston et al., *Monitoring the Future National Survey Results on Drug Use* (Ann Arbor, MI: Institute for Social Research, University of Michigan, 2016).

113. National Institute on Drug Abuse, "Common Hallucinogens and Dissociative Drugs," 2015, https://www.drugabuse.gov/publications/research-reports/hallucinogens-dissociative-drugs/what-are-dissociative-drugs.

114. National Institute on Drug Abuse, "Hallucinogens," DrugFacts, 2016, https://www.drugabuse.gov/publications/drugfacts/hallucinogens.

115. Ibid.

116. National Institute on Drug Abuse, "What Is MDMA?" DrugFacts, 2016, https://www.drugabuse.gov/publications/drugfacts/mdma-ecstasymolly.

117. Ibid.

118. Partnership at DrugFree.org, "Experts: People Who Think They Are Taking "Molly" Don't Know What They Are Getting," June 24, 2013, www.drugfree.org/join-together/drugs/experts-people-who-think-they-are-taking-molly-dont-know-what-theyre-getting.

119. Drugs.com, "PCP (Phencyclidine)," http://www.drugs.com/illicit/pcp.html.

120. Ibid.

121. Drugs.com, "Mescaline," 2016, http://www.drugs.com/illicit/mescaline.html.

122. National Institute on Drug Abuse, "Hallucinogens," DrugFacts, 2016, https://www.drugabuse.gov/publications/drugfacts/hallucinogens.

123. National Institute on Drug Abuse, "Commonly Used Club Drugs," 2016, https://www.drugabuse.gov/drugs-abuse/commonly-abused-drugs-charts#ketamine; Drugs.com, "Ketamine," 2016, http://www.drugs.com/cdi/ketamine.html.

124. National Institute on Drug Abuse, "Hallucinogens," DrugFacts, January 2016, www.drugabuse.gov/publications/drugfacts/hallucinogens.

125. Ibid.

126. Ibid.

127. Ibid.

128. Partnership for Drug-Free Kids, "Inhalants," 2016, http://www.drugfree.org/drug-guide/inhalants.

129. Ibid.

130. National Collegiate Athletic Association, "NCAA National Study of Substance Use Habits of College Student Athletes—Final Report 2014," August 2014, www.ncaa.org/sites/default/files/Substance%20Use%20Final%20Report_FINAL.pdf.

131. Ibid.

132. National Collegiate Athletic Association, "Substance Use: National Study of Substance Use Trends among NCAA College Student-Athletes," 2012, www.ncaapublications.com/productdownloads/SAHS09.pdf.

133. American College Health Association, *American College Health Association-National College Health Assessment-Reference Group, Spring 2016*, 2016, http://www.acha-ncha.org/docs/NCHA-II%20SPRING%202016%20REFERENCE%20GROUP%20DATA%20REPORT.pdf.

134. H. G. Pope et al., "The Lifetime Prevalence of Anabolic-Androgenic Steroid Use and Dependence in Americans: Current Best Estimates," *American Journal on Addictions* 23, no. 4 (2014): 371–77.

135. National Institute on Drug Abuse, "What Are Anabolic Steroids," DrugFacts, 2016, https://www.drugabuse.gov/publications/drugfacts/anabolic-steroids.

136. Ibid.

137. Association Against Steroid Use, "Legal Ramifications of Steroid Use," http://www.steroidabuse.com/legal-ramifications-of-steroid-abuse.html.

138. Substance Abuse and Mental Health Services Administration, "Results from the 2015 National Survey," 2016; Office of the Surgeon General, *Facing Addiction in America: The Surgeon General's Report on Alcohol, Drugs, and Health* (Washington, DC: U.S. Department of Health and Human Services, 2016).

139. Office of the Surgeon General, *Facing Addiction in America: The Surgeon General's Report on Alcohol, Drugs, and Health* (Washington, DC: U.S. Department of Health and Human Services, 2016).

140. Ibid.

141. Ibid.

142. Alcoholics Anonymous "Over 80 Years of Growth," 2016, http://www.aa.org/pages/en_US/aa-timeline/to/1; Rehabs.com, "AA Success Rates," 2016, http://luxury.rehabs.com/12-step-programs/aa-success-rates.

143. Office of the Surgeon General, *Facing Addiction in America: The Surgeon General's Report on Alcohol, Drugs, and Health* (Washington, DC: U.S. Department of Health and Human Services, 2016).

144. M.L. Dennis et al., "A Pilot Study to Examine the Feasibility and Potential Effectiveness of Using Smartphones to Provide Recovery Support for Adolescents," *Substance Abuse* 36, no. 4 (2015): 486–92.

145. S. Gaidos, "Vaccines Could Counter Addictive Opioids," *Science News,* June 28, 2016, https://www.sciencenews.org/article/vaccines-could-counter-addictive-opioids.

146. S. Gaidos, "Vaccines Could Counter Addictive Opioids," *Science News,* June 28, 2016, https://www.sciencenews.org/article/vaccines-could-counter-addictive-opioids; National Institute on Drug Abuse, "Dr. Thomas Kosten Q & A: Vaccines to Treat Addiction," 2015, https://www.drugabuse.gov/news-events/nida-notes/2015/06/dr-thomas-kosten-q-vaccines-to-treat-addiction.

147. Substance Abuse and Mental Health Services Administration, "Naltrexone," 2016, http://www.samhsa.gov/medication-assisted-treatment/treatment/naltrexone.

148. A.B. Laudet et al., "Characteristics of Students Participating in Collegiate Recovery Programs: A National Survey," *Journal of Substance Abuse Treatment* 51 (2015): 38–46.

149. Office of National Drug Control Policy, "How Illicit Drug Use Affects Business and the Economy," Executive Office of the President, Accessed June 2016, www.whitehouse.gov/ondcp/ondcp-fact-sheets/how-illicit-drug-use-affects-business-and-the-economy.

150. Ibid.

151. Pew Research Center, "America's New Drug Policy Landscape," April 2, 2014, http://www.people-press.org/2014/04/02/americas-new-drug-policy-landscape; Substance Abuse and Mental Health Services

Administration, "Prevention of Substance Abuse and Mental Illness," 2016, http://www.samhsa.gov/prevention.

Pulled Statistics:

page 218, American College Health Association. *American College Health Association—National College Health Assessment II: Reference Group Executive Summary, Spring 2016* (Hanover, MD: American College Health Association, 2016).

page 225, Substance Abuse and Mental Health Services Administration, "Driving Under the Influence of Alcohol and Illicit Drugs," Short Report (December, 2016), https://www.samhsa.gov/data/sites/default/files/report_2688/ShortReport-2688.html

Chapter 9: Drinking Alcohol Responsibly and Ending Tobacco Use

1. M. Stahre et al., "Contribution of Excessive Alcohol Consumption to Death and Years of Potential Life Lost in the United States," *Prevention of Chronic Disease* 11 (2014): 130293, www.cdc.gov/pcd/issues/2014/13_0293.htm.

2. U.S. Department of Health and Human Services, *The Health Consequences of Smoking—50 Years of Progress: A Report of the Surgeon General* (Atlanta, GA: U.S. Centers for Disease Control and Prevention, Office on Smoking and Health, 2014), Available at www.surgeongeneral.gov/library/reports/50-years-of-progress/exec-summary.pdf; Centers for Disease Control and Prevention, "Current Cigarette Smoking among Adults—United States 2005–2015," *Morbidity and Mortality Weekly* 65, no. 45 (2016): 1205–11.

3. A. Giacosa et al., "Mediterranean Way of Drinking and Longevity," *Critical Reviews in Food Science and Nutrition* 56 (2016): 635–40; R. M. Lamuela-Raventos et al., "Mechanism of the Protective Effects of Wine Intake on Cardiovascular Disease," *Wine Safety, Consumer Preference and Human Health* (New York: Springer International Publishing, 2016), 231–39; T. Stockwell et al., "Do 'Moderate' Drinkers Have Reduced Mortality Risk," *Journal of Studies on Alcohol and Drugs* 77, no. 2 (2016): 185–98.

4. Center for Behavioral Health Statistics and Quality, "Key Substance Use and Mental Health Indicators in the United States: Results from the 2015 National Survey on Drug Use and Health, 2016, (HHS Publication No. SMA 16-4984, NASUH Series H-51), http://www.samhsa.gov/data.

5. Ibid.

6. National Institute on Alcohol Abuse and Alcoholism, "Beyond Hangovers: Understanding Alcohol's Impact on Your Health," October 2015, https://pubs.niaaa.nih.gov/publications/Hangovers/beyondHangovers.pdf.

7. National Institute on Alcohol Abuse and Alcoholism, "Alcohol's Effects on the Body," Accessed May 4, 2016, http://niaaa.nih.gov/alcohol-health/alcohols-effects-body.

8. Blowfish for Hangovers, "How It Works," Accessed May 2016, http://forhangovers.com/pages/about.

9. Centers for Disease Control and Prevention, "Unintentional Drowning: Get the Facts," April 28, 2016, http://www.cdc.gov/HomeandRecreationalSafety/Water-Safety/waterinjuries-factsheet.html.

10. Ibid.

11. Mental Health America, "Suicide," June 18, 2016, http://www.mentalhealthamerica.net/suicide.

12. K. Conner et al., "Alcohol and Suicidal Behavior: What Is Known and What Can Be Done," *American Journal of Preventive Medicine* 47, no. 3 (2014): S204–08.

13. N. Barnett et al., "Description and Predictors of Positive and Negative Alcohol-Related Consequences in the First Year of College," *Journal of Studies on Alcohol and Drugs* 75, no. 1 (2014): 103–14.

14. American College Health Association, *American College Health Association—National College Health Assessment II: Reference Group Executive Summary Spring 2016* (Hanover, MD: American College Health Association, 2016), http://www.acha-ncha.org/docs/NCHA-II%20FALL%202016%20REFERENCE%20GROUP%20EXECUTIVE%20SUMMARY.pdf.

15. N. Barnett et al., "Description and Predictors of Positive and Negative Alcohol-Related Consequences in the First Year of College," *Journal of Studies on Alcohol and Drugs* 75, no. 1 (2014): 103–14.

16. "Poll: One in Five Women Say They Have Been Sexually Assaulted in College," *Washington Post*, June 12, 2015, https://www.washingtonpost.com/graphics/local/sexual-assault-poll.

17. Ibid.

18. Ibid.

19. Ibid.

20. Centers for Disease Control and Prevention, "Ten Leading Causes of Death by Age Group," February 2016, www.cdc.gov/injury/wisqars/leadingcauses.html.

21. Centers for Disease Control and Prevention, "Impaired Driving: Get the Facts," January 26, 2017, http://www.cdc.gov/motorvehicle safety/impaired_driving/impaired-drv_factsheet.html.

22. Ibid.

23. American College Health Association, *National College Health Assessment II: Reference Group Data Report, Spring 2016*, 2016.

24. Insurance Institute for Highway Safety, "Alcohol-Impaired Driving 2015," November 2016, http://www.iihs.org/iihs/topics/t/alcohol-impaired-driving/fatalityfacts/alcohol-impaired-driving/2015.

25. Ibid.

26. Ibid.

27. Ibid.

28. L. Squeglia et al., "Brain Development in Heavy Drinking Adolescents," *American Journal of Psychiatry* 172, no. 6 (2015): 531–42.

29. Ibid.

30. R. Rettner, "Cheers?: Counting the Calories in Alcoholic Drinks," *Livescience*, December 7, 2015, http://www.livescience.com/52990-alcohol-calories-weight-loss-be-healthy.html.

31. J. H. O'Keefe et al., "Alcohol and Cardiovascular Health: The Dose Makes the Poison . . . or the Remedy," *Mayo Clinic Proceedings* 89, no. 3 (2014): 382–93; A. Artero et al., "The Impact of Moderate Wine Consumption on Health," *Maturitas* 80, no. 1 (2015): 3–13.

32. The American Heart Association, "Alcohol and Heart Health," 2015, www.heart.org.

33. Ibid.

34. Ibid.

35. Ibid.

36. National Toxicology Program, *Report on Carcinogens*, 13th ed. (Research Triangle Park, NC: U.S. Department of Health and Human Services, Public Health Service, 2014), http://ntp.niehs.nih.gov/pubhealth/roc/roc13.

37. Y. Cao et al., "Light to Moderate Intake of Alcohol, Drinking Patterns, and Risk of Cancer: Results from Two Prospective US Cohort Studies," *British Medical Journal* 351 (2015): h4238.

38. Ibid.

39. Ibid.

40. I. Romieu et al., "Alcohol Intake and Breast Cancer in the European Prospective Investigation into Cancer and Nutrition," *International Journal of Cancer* 137, no. 8 (2015): 1921–30.

41. Ibid.

42. Substance Abuse and Mental Health Services Administration, "Protect Your Unborn Baby," Accessed January 2016, http://www.samhsa.gov/sites/default/files/programs_campaigns/fasd/fasd-infographic.pdf.

43. Centers for Disease Control and Prevention, "FASDs: Alcohol and Pregnancy," July 21, 2016, https://www.cdc.gov/ncbddd/fasd/alcohol-use.html.

44. Ibid.

45. Centers for Disease Control and Prevention, "Fetal Alcohol Spectrum Disorders (FASDs): Data and Statistics," March 13, 2017, www.cdc.gov/ncbddd/fasd/data.html.

46. Ibid.

47. Centers for Disease Control and Prevention, "Alcohol and Pregnancy: Why Take the Risk?" *Vital Signs*, February 2, 2016, https://www.cdc.gov/vitalsigns/fasd.

48. Centers for Disease Control and Prevention, "FASDs: Alcohol and Pregnancy," July 21, 2016, https://www.cdc.gov/ncbddd/fasd/alcohol-use.html.

49. Ibid.

50. American College Health Association, *National College Health Assessment II: Reference Group Executive Summary Spring 2016*, 2016.

51. Ibid.

52. U.S. Department of Health and Human Services, National Institute on Alcohol Abuse and Alcoholism, "Moderate and Binge Drinking," Accessed May 2016, http://www.niaaa.nih.gov/alcohol-health/overview-alcohol-consumption/moderate-binge-drinking.

53. Ibid.

54. C. Foster et al., "National College Health Assessment Measuring Negative Alcohol-Related Consequences among College Students," *American Journal of Public Health Research* 2, no. 1 (2014): 1–5.

55. American College Health Association, *National College Health Assessment II: Reference Group Executive Summary Spring 2016*, 2016.

56. L. Fucito, et al., "Perceptions of Heavy Drinking College Students about a Sleep and Alcohol Health Intervention," *Behavioral Sleep Medicine* 13, no. 5 (2016): 395–411. doi:10.1080/15402002.2014.919919.

57. Ibid.

58. A. White and R. Hingson, "The Burden of Alcohol Use: Excessive Alcohol Consumption and Related Consequences among College Students," *Alcohol Research: Current Reviews* 35, no. 2 (2014): 201.

59. Ibid.

60. J. Merrill et al., "The Effect of Descriptive Norms on Pregaming Frequency: Tests of Five Moderators," *Substance Use & Misuse* 51, no. 8 (2016): 1002–12.

61. A. Fairlie et al., "Prepartying, Drinking Games, and Extreme Drinking among College Students: A Daily Level Investigation," *Addictive Behaviors* 42 (2015): 91–5. doi:10.1016/j.addbeh.2014.11.001.

62. J. Merrill and K. Carey, "Drinking over the Lifespan: A Focus on College Ages," *Alcohol Research* 38, no. 1 (2016): 103–14.

63. B. Zamboanga and P. Peake, "Moving House Parties to the Lab: A Call for Experimental Studies on Drinking Games" *Addictive Behaviors* 67 (2017): 18–19.

64. J. Merrill and K. Carey, "Drinking over the Lifespan: A Focus on College Ages," *Alcohol Research* 38, no. 1 (2016): 103–114.

65. Ibid.

66. B. Zamboanga et al., "Drinking Game Participation among High School and Incoming Students: A Narrative Review," *Journal of Addictions Nursing* 24, no. 1 (2016): 24–31.

67. R. Martin et al., "Hazardous Drinking and Weight-Conscious Drinking Behaviors in a Sample of College Students and College Student Athletes," *Substance Abuse* (2016). doi:10.1080/08897077.2016.1142922.

68. M. Eisenberg and C. Fitz, "'Drunkorexia': Exploring the Who and Why of a Disturbing Trend in College Students' Eating and Drinking Behaviors," *American Journal of College Health* 62, no. 8 (2014): 570–77.

69. Ibid.

70. Ibid.

71. J. Stogner et al., "Innovative Alcohol Use: Assessing the Prevalence of Alcohol without Liquid and Other Non-Oral Routes of Alcohol Administration," *Drug and Alcohol Dependence* 142, no. 1 (2014): 74–8.

72. M. Miguez, "The Need of Widening the Lens of Alcohol Research, but Sharpening the Focus on Type of Alcohol Beverage," *Journal of Alcoholism and Drug Dependence* (2014). doi:10.4172/2329-6488.1000e112.

73. National Institute on Alcohol Abuse and Alcoholism, "Planning Alcohol Interventions Using NIAAA's College AIM: Alcohol Intervention Matrix," September 2015, NIH Publication No. 15-AA-8017.

74. Ibid.

75. Medline Plus, "Alcoholism and Alcohol Abuse," March 2015, www.nlm.nih.gov/medlineplus/ency/article/000944.htm.

76. National Institute on Alcohol Abuse and Alcoholism, "College Drinking," December 2015, http://pubs.niaaa.nih.gov/publications/CollegeFactSheet/CollegeFactSheet.pdf.

77. A. Arria, "College Student Success: The Impact of Health Concerns and Substance Abuse," Lecture presented at NASPA Alcohol and Mental Health Conference, Fort Worth, TX, January 19, 2013.

78. S. Gupta, "Are You a Functioning Alcoholic?" *Everyday Health*, April 25, 2016, http://www.everydayhealth.com/news/are-you-someone-you-know-functional-alcoholic.

79. M. Waldron et al., "Parental Separation and Early Substance Involvement: Results from Children of Alcoholic and Cannabis Twins," *Drug and Alcohol Dependence* 134 (2014): 78–84.

80. M. Schuckit, "A Brief History of Research on the Genetics of Alcohol and Other Drug Use Disorders," *Journal of Studies on Alcohol and Drugs* 75, Suppl. 17 (2014): 59–67.

81. Ibid.

82. B. Taub, "Here's What Happens to Alcoholics' Brains When They Quit Drinking," *IFLScience*, March 3, 2016, http://www.iflscience.com/brain/what-happens-alcoholics-brains-when-they-quit-drinking.

83. NEW Centers for Disease Control and Prevention, Fact Sheet, "Excessive Alcohol Use and Risks to Women's Health," March 7, 2016, www.cdc.gov/alcohol/fact-sheets/womens-health.htm.

84. National Institute on Alcohol Abuse and Alcoholism, "Alcohol: A Women's Health Issue," 2015, NIH Publication No. 15-4956.

85. Centers for Disease Control and Prevention, "Excessive Drinking Is Draining the U.S. Economy," January 12, 2016, www.cdc.gov/features/CostsOfDrinking.

86. Ibid.

87. Ibid.

88. Ibid.

89. S. Finn, "Alcohol Consumption, Dependence, and Treatment Barriers: Perceptions among Nontreatment Seekers with Alcohol Dependence," *Substance Use and Misuse* 49, no. 6 (2014): 762–69.

90. A. Laudet et al., "Collegiate Recovery Community Programs: What Do We Know and What Do We Need to Know?," *Journal of Social Work Practice in the Addictions* 14 (2014): 84–100; A. Laudet et al., "Characteristics of Students Participating in Collegiate Recovery Programs: A National Survey," *Journal of Substance Abuse Treatment* 51 (2014): 38–46.

91. O. Manejwala, "How Often Do Long-Term Sober Alcoholics and Addicts Relapse?" *Psychology Today*, February 13, 2014, https://www.psychologytoday.com/blog/craving/201402/how-often-do-long-term-sober-alcoholics-and-addicts-relapse.

92. U.S. Department of Health and Human Services, *The Health Consequences of Smoking—50 Years of Progress*, 2014, https://www.surgeongeneral.gov/library/reports/50-years-of-progress.

93. Centers for Disease Control and Prevention, "Fast Facts and Fact Sheets: Smoking and Tobacco Use," December 2016, www.cdc.gov/tobacco/data_statistics/fact_sheets/fast_facts/index.htm.

94. Centers for Disease Control and Prevention, "Current Cigarette Smoking Among Adults—United States, 2005–2015," *Morbidity and Mortality Weekly Report* 64, no. 44 (2016): 1205–1211.

95. Ibid.

96. Campaign for Tobacco-Free Kids, "Toll of Tobacco in the United States of America," 2017, www.tobaccofreekids.org/research/factsheets/pdf/0072.pdf?utm_source=factsheets_finder&utm_medium=link&utm_campaign=analytics.

97. Ibid.

98. Ibid.

99. American Cancer Society, "Cancer Facts & Figures 2017," Accessed March 2017, www.cancer.org/research/cancerfactsstatistics/cancerfactsfigures2017.

100. Campaign for Tobacco-Free Kids, "Toll of Tobacco in the United States of America," 2017, www.tobaccofreekids.org/research/factsheets/pdf/0072.pdf?utm_source=factsheets_finder&utm_medium=link&utm_campaign=analytic.

101. U.S. Department of Health and Human Services, *The Health Consequences of Smoking—50 Years of Progress*, 2014, https://www.surgeongeneral.gov/library/reports/50-years-of-progress.

102. Campaign for Tobacco-Free Kids, "Toll of Tobacco in the United States of America," 2017, www.tobaccofreekids.org/research/factsheets/pdf/0072.pdf?utm_source=factsheets_finder&utm_medium=link&utm_campaign=analytic.

103. American College Health Association, *American College Health Association–National College Health Assessment II: Reference Group Data Report, Spring 2016* (Baltimore: American College Health Association, 2016), Available from www.achancha.org/reports_ACHA-NCHAII.html.

104. Ibid.

105. Ibid.

106. J. Rosa and P. Aloise-Young, "A Qualitative Study of Smoker Identity among College Student Smokers," *Substance Use and Misuse* 50, no. 12 (2015): 1510–17.

107. American Cancer Society, "Light Smoking as Risky as a Pack a Day?," January 2013, http://blogs.cancer.org/expertvoices/2013/01/02/light-smoking-as-risky-as-a-pack-a-day.

108. Mayo Clinic, "Estrogen and Progestin Oral Contraceptives (Oral Route)," 2015, http://www.mayoclinic.org/drugs-supplements/estrogen-and-progestin-oral-contraceptives-oral-route/side-effects/drg-20069422.

109. U.S. Department of Health and Human Services, *The Health Consequences of Smoking—50 Years of Progress*, 2014, https://www.surgeongeneral.gov/library/reports/50-years-of-progress.

110. Tobacco-Free Kids, "1998 State Tobacco Settlement 17 Years Later," December 2015, http://www.tobaccofreekids.org/microsites/statereport2016.

111. 111th Congress of the United States of America, *Family Smoking Prevention and Tobacco Control Act of 2009*, HR 1256, www.govtrack.us.

112. U.S. Department of Health and Human Services, *The Health Consequences of Smoking—50 Years of Progress*, 2014, https://www.surgeongeneral.gov/library/reports/50-years-of-progress; U.S. Department of Health and Human Services, "How Tobacco Smoke Causes Disease: The Biology and Behavioral Basis for Smoking Attributable Disease: A Report of the Surgeon General," 2010, Available at www.ncbi.nlm.nih.gov.

113. *Diagnostic and Statistical Manual of Mental Disorders*, Fifth Edition (Washington, DC: American Psychiatric Association, 2013).

114. Ibid.

115. U.S. Department of Health and Human Services, *E-Cigarette Use among Youth and Young Adults: A Report of the Surgeon General—Executive Summary* (Atlanta, GA: U.S. Department of Health and Human Services, Centers for Disease Control and Prevention, National Center for Chronic Disease Prevention and Health Promotion, Office on Smoking and Health, 2016).

116. American College Health Association, *American College Health Association—National College Health Assessment II: Reference Group Data Report, Spring 2016*, 2016.

117. A. Littlefield et al., "Electronic Cigarette Use among College Students: Links to Gender, Race/Ethnicity, Smoking and Heavy Drinking," *Journal of American College Health* 63, no. 8 (2015): 523–29.

118. American Cancer Society, "Cancer Facts & Figures 2016," 2016.

119. National Cancer Institute, "Cigar Smoking and Cancer," Accessed March 13, 2016, http://www.cancer.gov/about-cancer/causes-prevention/risk/tobacco/cigars-fact-sheet.

120. American Cancer Society, "Cancer Facts & Figures 2016," 2016, https://www.cancer.org/research/cancer-facts-statistics/all-cancer-facts-figures/cancer-facts-figures-2016.html.

121. National Cancer Institute, "Cigar Smoking and Cancer," Accessed March 13, 2016, http://www.cancer.gov/about-cancer/causes-prevention/risk/tobacco/cigars-fact-sheet.

122. Centers for Disease Control and Prevention, "Smoking and Tobacco Use: Bidis and Kreteks," December 1, 2016, www.cdc.gov/tobacco/data_statistics/fact_sheets/tobacco_industry/bidis_kreteks.

123. Centers for Disease Control and Prevention, "Smoking & Tobacco Use: Hookahs," December 1, 2016, https://www.cdc.gov/tobacco/data_statistics/fact_sheets/tobacco_industry/hookahs; Centers for Disease Control and Prevention, "CDC Features: Dangers of Hookah," November 9, 2015, https://www.cdc.gov/features/hookahsmoking.

124. Campaign for Tobacco-Free Kids, "Smokeless Tobacco in the United States," 2016, https://www.tobaccofreekids.org/research/factsheets/pdf/0231.pdf.

125. Campaign for Tobacco-Free Kids, "Toll of Tobacco in the United States of America," 2017, www.tobaccofreekids.org/research/factsheets/pdf/0072.pdf?utm_source=factsheets_finder&utm_medium=link&utm_campaign=analytics.

126. National Cancer Institute, "Lung Cancer Prevention," February 2016, www.cancer.gov/cancertopics/pdq/prevention/lung/HealthProfessional/page2.

127. American Cancer Society, "Cancer Facts & Figures 2017," 2017, Accessed March 2017, www.cancer.org/research/cancerfactsstatistics/cancerfactsfigures2017.

128. American Cancer Society, "What Are Oral Cavity and Oropharyngeal Cancers?," January 2016, www.cancer.org/cancer/oralcavityandoropharyngealcancer/detailedguide/oral-cavity-and-oropharyngeal-cancer-what-is-oral-cavity-cancer.

129. American Cancer Society, "Cancer Facts & Figures 2017," 2017, Accessed March 2017, www.cancer.org/research/cancerfactsstatistics/cancerfactsfigures2017.

130. Ibid.

131. American Heart Association, *Heart Disease and Stroke Statistics—2017 Update: A Report from the American Heart Association* (Dallas, TX: American Heart Association, 2016), Available at http://circ.ahajournals.org/content/early/2017/01/25/CIR.0000000000000485.

132. Ibid.

133. Ibid.

134. Ibid

135. U.S. Department of Health and Human Services, *The Health Consequences of Smoking—50 Years of Progress: A Report of the Surgeon General*, 2014, https://www.surgeongeneral.gov/library/reports/50-years-of-progress.

136. American Lung Association, "Lung Health Diseases: What Causes COPD," November 1, 2016, http://www.lung.org/lung-health-and-diseases/lung-disease-lookup/copd/symptoms-causes-risk-factors/what-causes-copd.html.

137. C. B. Harte et al., "Association between Cigarette Smoking and Erectile Tumescence: The Mediating Role of Heart Rate Variability," *International Journal of Impotence Research* 25, no. 4 (2013): 155–59. doi:10.1038/ijir.2012.43.

138. Centers for Disease Control and Prevention, "Tobacco Use and Pregnancy," September 2016, www.cdc.gov/reproductivehealth/TobaccoUsePregnancy.

139. Ibid.

140. American Academy of Periodontology, "Gum Disease Risk Factors," Accessed March 2017, www.perio.org/consumer/risk-factors; Centers for Disease Control and Prevention, "Smoking, Gum Disease, and Tooth Loss," September 2015, http://www.cdc.gov/tobacco/campaign/tips/diseases/periodontal-gum-disease.html.

141. S. Karama et al., "Cigarette Smoking and Thinning of the Brain's Cortex," *Molecular Psychiatry* 20 (2015): 778–85; I. Moreno-Gonzalez, et al., "Smoking Exacerbates Amyloid Pathology in a Mouse Model of Alzheimer's Disease," *Nature Communications* 4 (2013), www.nature.com/ncomms/journal/v4/n2/abs/ncomms2494.html.

142. Centers for Disease Control and Prevention, "Secondhand Smoke (SHS) Facts," February 21, 2017, https://www.cdc.gov/tobacco/data_statistics/fact_sheets/secondhand_smoke/general_facts/index.htm.

143. American Nonsmokers' Rights Foundation, "Overview List—How Many Smoke-Free Laws," April 4, 2016, www.no-smoke.org/pdf/mediaordlist.pdf.

144. Ibid.

145. Ibid.

146. American Lung Association, "Health Effects of Secondhand Smoke," Accessed April 2016, http://www.lung.org/stop-smoking/smoking-facts/health-effects-of-secondhand-smoke.html.

147. American Nonsmokers' Rights Foundation, "Overview List–How Many Smoke-Free Laws," April 4, 2016, www.no-smoke.org/pdf/mediaordlist.pdf.

148. Centers for Disease Control and Prevention, "Secondhand Smoke (SHS) Facts," February 21, 2017, https://www.cdc.gov/tobacco/data_statistics/fact_sheets/secondhand_smoke/general_facts/index.htm.

149. Centers for Disease Control and Prevention, "Health Effects of Secondhand Smoke Fact Sheet," February 2016, http://www.cdc.gov/tobacco/data_statistics/fact_sheets/second_hand_smoke/health_effects/index.htm.

150. Centers for Disease Control and Prevention, "Quitting Smoking among Adults–United States 2000-2015," *Morbidity and Mortality Weekly* 65 no. 52 (2017): 1457–64; Centers for Disease Control and Prevention,

"Tobacco Use: Smoking Cessation," February 2016, www.cdc.gov/tobacco/data_statistics/fact_sheets/cessation/quitting/index.htm#quitting.

151. American Lung Association, "Benefits of Quitting," Accessed March 2017, www.lung.org/stop-smoking/i-want-to-quit/benefits-of-quitting.html; Centers for Disease Control and Prevention, "Quitting Smoking," February 2017, www.cdc.gov/tobacco/data_statistics/fact_sheets/cessation/quitting/index.htm?utm_source=feedburner&utm_medium=feed&utm_campaign=Feed%3A+CdcSmoking AndTobaccoUse FactSheets+%28CDC+-+Smoking+and+Tobacco+Use+-+Fact+Sheets%29.

152. Ibid.

153. Ibid.

154. Ibid.

155. H. Holmes, "What a Pack of Cigarettes Costs Now, State by State," *The Awl*, July 6, 2016, https://theawl.com/what-a-pack-of-cigarettes-costs-in-every-state-266d285b8a68#.xhj2e7evz.

156. American Cancer Society, "How to Quit Smoking," November 16, 2016, https://www.cancer.org/latest-news/how-to-quit-smoking.html Drugs.com, "Nicotine Patch," Accessed March 2016, http://www.drugs.com/price-guide/nicotine.

157. Drugs.com, "Nicotine Patch," Accessed March 2016, http://www.drugs.com/price-guide/nicotine.

158. Ibid.

159. U.S. Food and Drug Administration, "FDA 101: Smoking Cessation Products," February 2016, http://www.fda.gov/ForConsumers/ConsumerUpdates/ucm198176.htm.

Pulled Statistics:

page 239, National Institute on Alcohol Abuse and Alcoholism, "Alcohol Facts and Statistics," 2017, www.niaaa.nih.gov/alcohol-health/overview-alcohol-consumption/alcohol-facts-and-statistics.

page 245, National Institute on Alcohol Abuse and Alcoholism, "Alcohol Facts and Statistics," 2017, www.niaaa.nih.gov/alcohol-health/overview-alcohol-consumption/alcohol-facts-and-statistics.

Chapter 10: Nutrition: Eating for a Healthier You

1. Institute of Medicine, *Dietary Reference Intakes: Applications in Dietary Planning* (Washington, DC: National Academies Press: 2003), Updated 2013, Available at http://fnic.nal.usda.gov.

2. U.S. Department of Agriculture, "Part D: Section 6: Sodium, Potassium, and Water," *Report of the Dietary Guidelines Advisory Committee on the Dietary Guidelines for Americans, 2010* (Washington, DC.: U.S. Department of Agriculture, Agricultural Research Service, 2010).

3. A.E. Carroll, "No, You Do Not Have to Drink 8 Glasses of Water a Day," *New York Times*, August 24, 2015, www.nytimes.com/2015/08/25/upshot/no-you-do-not-have-to-drink-8-glasses-of-water-a-day.html?_r=0.

4. S.C. Killer, A.K. Blannin, and A.E. Jeukendrup, "No Evidence of Dehydration with Moderate Daily Coffee Intake: A Counterbalanced Cross-Over Study in a Free-Living Population," *PLoS ONE* 9, no. 1 (2014): e84154, doi:10.1371/journal.pone.0084154.

5. American College of Sports Medicine (ACSM), "Selecting and Effectively Using Hydration for Fitness," 2011, www.acsm.org/docs/brochures/selecting-and-effectively-using-hydration-for-fitness.pdf.

6. U.S. Department of Agriculture, "What We Eat in America," NHANES 2011–2012, February 11, 2015, www.ars.usda.gov/SP2UserFiles/Place/80400530/pdf/1112/Table_1_NIN_GEN_11.pdf.

7. Food and Nutrition Board, Institute of Medicine, *Dietary Reference Intakes for Energy, Carbohydrate, Fiber, Fat, Fatty Acids, Cholesterol, Protein, and Amino Acids (Macronutrients)* (Washington, DC: National Academies Press, 2005), Available at www.nap.edu/openbook.php?isbn=0309085373.

8. Dietitians of Canada, the Academy of Nutrition and Dietetics, and the American College of Sports Medicine, "Nutrition and Athletic Performance: Position of Dietitians of Canada, the Academy of Nutrition and Dietetics, and the American College of Sports Medicine," February 2016, Available at https://www.dietitians.ca/Downloads/Public/noap-position-paper.aspx.

9. Institute of Medicine of the National Academies, "Dietary, Functional, and Total Fiber," *Dietary Reference Intakes for Energy, Carbohydrate, Fiber, Fat, Fatty Acids, Cholesterol, Protein, and Amino Acids* (Washington, DC: National Academies Press, 2005), 339–421, Available at www.nap.edu/openbook.php?isbn=0309085373.

10. Ibid.

11. C.E. Ramsden et al., "Use of Dietary Linoleic Acid for Secondary Prevention of Coronary Heart Disease and Death: Evaluation of Recovered Data from the Sydney Diet Heart Study and Updated Meta-Analysis," *British Medical Journal* 346 (2013): e8707; M.A. Leslie et al., "A Review of the Effect of Omega-3 Polyunsaturated Fatty Acids on Blood Triacylglycerol Levels in Normolipidemic and Borderline Hyperlipidemic Individuals," *Lipids in Health and Disease* 14, no. 1 (2015): 1.

12. W. Willet, "Dietary Fats and Coronary Heart Disease," *Journal of Internal Medicine* 272, no. 1 (2012): 13–24.

13. U.S. Food and Drug Administration, "FDA Targets Trans Fats in Processed Foods," FDA Consumer Updates, March 17, 2017, www.fda.gov/ForConsumers/ConsumerUpdates/ucm372915.htm.

14. Ibid.

15. Ibid.

16. H.J. Silver et al., "Consuming a Balanced High Fat Diet for 16 Weeks Improves Body Composition, Inflammation and Vascular Function Parameters in Obese Premenopausal Women," *Metabolism* 63, no. 4 (2014): 562–73; A. Trichopoulou et al., "Definitions and Potential Health Benefits of the Mediterranean Diet: Views from Experts around the World," *BMC Medicine* 12, no. 1 (2014): 112.

17. National Institutes of Health Office of Dietary Supplements, "Dietary Supplement Fact Sheet: Vitamin D," February 11, 2016, http://ods.od.nih.gov/factsheets/VitaminD-HealthProfessional.

18. Ibid.

19. Ibid.

20. U.S. Department of Agriculture, *What We Eat in America*, 2010.

21. U.S. Department of Health and Human Services and U.S. Department of Agriculture, *2015–2020 Dietary Guidelines for Americans*, 2015.

22. Ibid.

23. S.A. McNaughton et al., "An Energy-Dense, Nutrient-Poor Dietary Pattern Is Inversely Associated with Bone Health in Women," *Journal of Nutrition* 141, no. 8 (2011): 1516–23, doi:10.3945/jn.111.138271.

24. World Health Organization, "Micronutrient Deficiencies: Iron Deficiency Anemia," Accessed March 2017, http://www.who.int/nutrition/topics/ida/en.

25. Food and Nutrition Board, Institute of Medicine, *Dietary Reference Intakes for Vitamin A, Vitamin K, Arsenic, Boron, Chromium, Copper, Iodine, Iron, Manganese, Molybdenum, Nickel, Silicon, Vanadium, and Zinc* (Washington, DC: National Academies Press, 2001).

26. R. Gozzelino and P. Arosio, "Iron Homeostasis in Health and Disease," *International Journal of Molecular Sciences* 17, no. 1 (2016): 130.

27. Academy of Nutrition and Dietetics, "Position of the Academy of Nutrition and Dietetics: Functional Foods," *Journal of the Academy of Nutrition and Dietetics* 113 no. 8(2013): 1096–103.

28. Ibid.

29. J. Fiedor and K. Burda, "Potential Role of Carotenoids as Antioxidants in Human Health and Disease," *Nutrients* 6, no. 2 (2014): 466–88.

30. J. Harasym and R. Oledzki, "Effect of Fruit and Vegetable Antioxidants on Total Antioxidant Capacity of Blood Plasma," *Nutrition* 30, no. 5 (2014): 511–17.

31. M.E. Obrenovich et al., "Antioxidants in Health, Disease, and Aging," *CNS & Neurological Disorders Drug Targets* 10, no. 2 (2011): 192–207; V. Ergin et al., "Carbonyl Stress in Aging Process: Role of Vitamins and Phytochemicals as Redox Regulators," *Aging and Disease* 4, no. 5 (2013): 276–94.

32. H. Stutz et al., "Analytical Tools for the Analysis of Beta-Carotene And Its Degradation Products," *Free Radical Research* 49, no. 4 (2015): 650–80; M.J. Gostner et al., "The Good and Bad of Antioxidant Foods: An Immunological Perspective," *Food and Chemical Toxicology* 80 (2015): 72–79.

33. U.S. Department of Agriculture, "Food Availability (Per Capita) Data System," Accessed March 2017, https://www.ers.usda.gov/data-products/food-availability-per-capita-data-system.

34. U.S. Department of Health and Human Services and U.S. Department of Agriculture, *2015–2020 Dietary Guidelines for Americans*, 2015.

35. U.S. Department of Agriculture, "Empty Calories: How Do I Count the Empty Calories I Eat?" September 30, 2015, http://archive.rhizome.org/artbase/53981/www.choosemyplate.gov/food-groups/emptycalories_count_table.html. Accessed April 2017.

36. U.S. Food and Drug Administration, "Label Claims for Conventional Foods and Dietary Supplements," April 11, 2016, www.fda.gov/Food/IngredientsPackagingLabeling/LabelingNutrition/ucm111447.htm.

37. The Vegetarian Resource Group, "How Often Do Americans Eat Vegetarian Meals? And How Many Adults in the U.S. Are Vegan?" May 29, 2015, www.vrg.org/blog/2015/05/29/how-often-do-americans-eat-vegetarian-meals-and-how-many-adults-in-the-u-s-are-vegetarian-2.

38. Ibid.

39. Y. Yokoyama et al., "Vegetarian Diets and Blood Pressure: A Meta-Analysis," *Journal of the American Medical Association Internal Medicine* 174, no. 4 (2014): 577–87.

40. C.G. Lee et al., "Vegetarianism as a Protective Factor for Colorectal Adenoma and Advanced Adenoma in Asians," *Digestive Diseases and Science* 59, no. 5 (2014): 1025–35.

41. Council for Responsible Nutrition, "2015 CRN Consumer Survey on Dietary Supplements," October 23, 2015, www.crnusa.org/CRNPR15-CCSurvey102315.html.

42. Ibid.

43. Office of Dietary Supplements, "Frequently Asked Questions," July 2013, http://ods.od.nih.gov/Health_Information/ODS_-Frequently_Asked_Questions.aspx#; V.A. Moyer, "Vitamin, Mineral, and Multi-vitamin Supplements for the Primary Prevention of Cardiovascular Disease and Cancer: U.S. Preventive Services Task Force Recommendation Statement," *Annals of Internal Medicine* 160, no. 8 (2014): 558–64.

44. M.J. Krantz et al., "Effects of Omega-3 Fatty Acids on Arterial Stiffness in Patients with Hypertension: A Randomized Pilot Study," *Journal of Negative Results in Biomedicine* 14, no. 1 (2015): 21.

45. New York State Office of the Attorney General, "Attorney General Schneiderman Asks Major Retailers to Halt Sales of Certain Herbal Supplements as DNA Tests Fail to Detect Plant Materials Listed on Majority of Products Tested," February 3, 2015, www.ag.ny.gov/press-release/ag-schneiderman-asks-major-retailers-halt-sales-certain-herbal-supplements-dna-tests. Accessed March 2017.

46. U.S. Department of Health and Human Services, "Food Safety Modernization Act (FSMA)," November 2013, www.fda.gov/Food/GuidanceRegulation/FSMA/ucm304045.htm. Accessed March 2017.

47. U.S. Food and Drug Administration, "'Natural' on Food Labeling," December 24, 2015, www.fda.gov/Food/Guidance-Regulation/GuidanceDocumentsRegulatoryInformation/LabelingNutrition/ucm456090.htm. Accessed March 2017.

48. Organic Trade Association, "Market Analysis: U.S. Organic Industry Survey, 2015," https://www.ota.com/resources/market-analysis. Accessed March 2017.

49. Ibid.

50. K. Brandt et al., "Agroecosystem Management and Nutritional Quality of Plant Foods: The Case of Organic Fruits and Vegetables,"*Critical Reviews in Plant Sciences* 30, no. 1–2 (2011): 177–97; C. Smith-Spangler et al., "Are Organic Foods Safer or Healthier Than Conventional Alternatives? A Systematic Review," *Annals of Internal Medicine* 157, no. 5 (2012): 348–66, doi:10.7326/0003-4819-157-5-201209040-00009.

51. International Agency for Research on Cancer, "IARC Monographs Volume 112: Evaluation of Five Organophosphate Insecticides and Herbicides," March 20, 2015, Available at www.iarc.fr/en/media-centre/iarc-news/pdf/MonographVolume112.pdf. Accessed March 2017.

52. F. Galgano et al. "Conventional and Organic Foods: A Comparison Focused on Animal Products," *Cogent Food & Agriculture* 2, no. 1(2016): 1142818, http://www.tandfonline.com/doi/full/10.1080/23311932.2016.1142818?scroll=top&needAccess=tru.

53. J. Miquel, "Organic versus Conventional Food: A Comparison Regarding Food Safety," *Food Reviews International* 33, no. 4 (2017): 424–446, http://dx.doi.org/10.1080/87559129.2016.1196490.

54. U.S. Environmental Protection Agency, "Food and Pesticides," December 2015, www.epa.gov/safepestcontrol/food-and-pesticides.

55. J.L. Wood et al., "Microbiological Survey of Locally Grown Lettuce Sold at Farmers' Markets in Vancouver, British Columbia," *Journal of Food Protection* 78, no. 1 (2015): 203–08.

56. Centers for Disease C, "Burden of Food-Borne Illness: Findings," January 2016, www.cdc.gov/foodborneburden/index.html.

57. Centers for Disease Control and Prevention, *Foodborne Diseases Active Surveillance Network (FoodNet): FoodNet 2015 Surveillance Report (Final Data)* (Atlanta, GA: U.S. Department of Health and Human Services, Centers for Disease Control and Prevention, 2017).

58. Centers for Disease Control and Prevention, "Botulism," May 3, 2016, Available at https://www.cdc.gov/botulism.

59. U.S. Government Accountability Office, "Progress on Many High-Risk Areas, While Substantial Efforts Needed on Others," February 15, 2017, Available at www.gao.gov/products/GAO-17-317.

60. M. Jay-Russell et al., "Exploration of the Impact of Application Intervals for the Use of Raw Animal Manure as a Soil Amendment, on Tomato Contamination," Accessed March 2017, Available at www.wifss.ucdavis.edu/wp-content/uploads/2015/pdfs/OryangJayRussellPosterOFVMScienceaResearchConference_08_14.pdf.

61. Centers for Disease Control and Prevention, "Surveillance for Foodborne Disease Outbreaks—United States, 1998–2008," *Morbidity and Mortality Weekly Report* 62, no. SS2 (2013), www.cdc.gov/foodsafety/fdoss/data/annual-summaries/mmwr-questions-and-answers-1998-2008.html.

62. National Institute of Allergy and Infectious Diseases, "Food Allergy," January 2016, www.niaid.nih.gov/topics/foodallergy/Pages/default.aspx.

63. National Institute of Allergy and Infectious Diseases, "Guidelines for the Diagnosis and Management of Food Allergy: What's in It for Patients?" October 2016. https://www.niaid.nih.gov/diseases-conditions/food-allergy-guidelines-patients. Accessed April 2017.

64. U.S. Food and Drug Administration, "Food Allergies: What You Need to Know," April 5, 2017, www.fda.gov/food/resourcesforyou/consumers/ucm079311.htm.

65. National Institute of Diabetes and Digestive and Kidney Diseases, "Celiac Disease," Accessed March 2017, www.niddk.nih.gov/health-information/health-topics/digestive-diseases/celiac-disease/Pages/facts.aspx.

66. National Institute of Child Health and Human Development, "Lactose Intolerance," Accessed March 2017, https://www.nichd.nih.gov/health/topics/lactose/Pages/default.aspx.

67. W. Klumper and M Qaim, "A Meta-Analysis of the Impacts of Genetically Modified Crops," *PLoS ONE* 9, no. 11 (2014): e111629.

68. American Association for the Advancement of Science, "Statement by the AAAS Board of Directors on Labeling of Genetically Modified Foods," March 31, 2014, www.aaas.org/news/statement-aaas-board-directors-labeling-genetically-modified-foods.World Health Organization, "Frequently Asked Questions on Genetically Modified Foods," May 2014, http://www.who.int/foodsafety/areas_work/food-technology/faq-genetically-modified-food/en.

Pulled Statistics:

page 284, M. W. Eich, "Healthiest Yogurts: How Much Sugar is in Your Favorite Yogurt?—Updated March 2016," *Margaret Wertheim, MS, RDN, Nutrition for Fertility,* Pregnancy, and Beyond, April 27, 2015, http://margaretwertheimrd.com/healthiest-yogurts-how-much-added-sugar-is-in-your-favorite-yogurt/.

page 288, *American College Health Association–National College Health Assessment II: Reference Group Executive Summary Spring 2015* (Hanover, MD: American College Health Association, 2015).

Chapter 11: Reaching and Maintaining a Healthy Weight

1. M. Ng et al., "Global, Regional, and National Prevalence of Overweight and Obesity in Children and Adults during 1980–2013: A Systematic Analysis for the Global Burden of Disease Study 2013," *Lancet* 384, no. 9945 (2014): 766–81.

2. Ibid.

3. Ibid., C. L. Ogden et al., "Trends in Obesity Prevalence among Children and Adolescents in the United States, 1988 through 2013–2014," *Journal of the American Medical Association* 315, no. 21 (2016): 2292–99, doi:10.1001/jama.2016.636; K. Flegal et al., "Trends in Obesity among Adults in the United States, 2005–2014. *Journal of the American Medical Association* 315, no. 21 (2016): 2284–91.

4. Centers for Disease Control, National Center for Health Statistics, "Health, United States, 2014; Table 64, Healthy Weight, Overweight, and Obesity among Adults Aged 20 and Over, by Selected Characteristics: United States, Selected Years 1988–1994 through 2009–2012," May 2015, Available at www.cdc.gov/nchs/hus/contents2014.htm#064; K. Flegal et al., "Trends in Obesity among Adults in the United States, 2005–2014. *Journal of the American Medical Association* 315, no. 21 (2016): 2284–91.

5. K. Flegal et al. "Trends in Obesity among Adults in the United States, 2005–2014. *Journal of the American Medical Association* 315, no. 21 (2016): 2284–91.

6. C. L. Ogden et al., "Trends in Obesity Prevalence among Children and Adolescents in the United States.,1988 through 2013–2014," *Journal of the American Medical Association* 315, no. 21 (2016): 2292–99, doi:10.1001/jama.2016.636; E. J. Benjamin et al., "Heart Disease and Stroke Statistics—2017 Update: A Report from the American Heart Association," *Circulation* 135, no. 10 (2017): e146–e603.

7. E. J. Benjamin et al., "Heart Disease and Stroke Statistics—2017 Update: A Report from the American Heart Association," *Circulation* 135, no. 10 (2017): e146–e603.

8. Ibid.

9. Ibid.

10. Ibid.

11. World Health Organization, "Obesity and Overweight Fact Sheet," January 2015, www.who.int/mediacentre/factsheets/fs311/en.

12. Ibid.; International Obesity Taskforce, "Obesity: The Global Epidemic," 2014, www.iaso.org/iotf/obesity/obesitytheglobalepidemic; M. Ng et al., "Global, Regional, and National Prevalence of Overweight and Obesity in Children and Adults during 1980–2013: A Systematic Analysis for the Global Burden of Disease Study 2013," *Lancet* 384, no. 9945 (2014): 766–81.

13. S. Vandevijvere et al., "Increased Food Energy Supply as a Major Driver of the Obesity Epidemic: A Global Analysis," *Bulletin of the World Health Organization* 93, no. 7 (2015):446–56.

14. L. Ferrucci et al., "Age-Related Change in Mobility: Perspectives from Life Course Epidemiology and Geroscience," *Journals of Gerontology Series A: Biological Sciences and Medical Sciences* 71, no. 9 (2016): 1184–94.

15. K. M. Flegal et al., "Association of All-Cause Mortality with Overweight and Obesity Using Standard Body Mass Index Categories: A Systematic Review and Meta-Analysis," *Journal of the American Medical Association* 309, no. 1 (2013): 71–82: Centers for Disease Control and Prevention, "Adult Obesity Causes and Consequences," August 15, 2016, https://www.cdc.gov/obesity/adult/causes.html.

16. M. Simmonds et al., "Predicting Adult Obesity from Childhood Obesity: A Systematic Review and Meta-analysis," *Obesity Reviews* 17, no. 2 (2016): 95–107; A. Llewellyn et al., "Childhood Obesity as a Predictor of Morbidity in Adulthood: A Systematic Review and Meta-analysis," *Obesity Reviews* 17, no. 1 (2016): 56–7.

17. CDC, "At a Glance 2016, Diabetes: Working to Reverse the US Epidemic," Accessed March 2017, https://www.cdc.gov/chronicdisease/resources/publications/aag/pdf/2016/diabetes-aag.pdf; CDC, "Early Release of Selected Estimates Based on Data from the National Health Interview Survey," January–September 2016, Available at https://www.cdc.gov/nchs/data/nhis/earlyrelease/earlyrelease201702_06.pdf.

18. S. Uzogara, "Obesity Epidemic, Medical and Quality of Life Consequences: A Review," *International Journal of Public Health Research* 5, no. 1 (2017): 1–12.

19. S. Higgs and J. Thomas, "Social Influences on Eating," *Current Opinion in Behavioral Sciences* 9 (2016): 1–6; M. Gurnani, C. Birken, and J. Hamilton, "Childhood Obesity: Causes, Consequences, and Management," *Pediatric Clinics of North America* 62, no. 4 (2015): 821–40; J. A. Woo Baidal et al., "Risk Factors for Childhood Obesity in the First 1,000 Days: A Systematic Review," *American Journal of Preventive Medicine* 50, no. 6 (2016): 761–79, doi:10.1016/j.amepre.2016.11.012.

20. J. Buss et al., "Associations of Ghrelin with Eating Behaviors, Stress, Metabolic Factors, and Telomere Length among Overweight and Obese Women: Preliminary Evidence of Attenuated Ghrelin Effects in Obesity," *Appetite* 76, no. 1 (2014): 84–94; R. Boswell and H. Kober, "Food Cue Reactivity and Craving Predict Eating and Weight Gain: A Meta-analytic Review," *Obesity Reviews* 17, no. 2 (2015): 159–77.

21. Ibid.

22. Ibid.; L. Quan et al., "Association of Fat-Mass and Obesity-Associated Genet FTO rs9939609 Polymorphism with the Risk of Obesity among Children and Adolescents: A Meta-analysis," *European Review for Medical and Pharmacological Sciences* 19, no. 4 (2015): 614–23.

23. O. Al Massadi et al., "Current Understanding of the Hypothalamic Ghrelin Pathways Inducing Appetite and Adiposity," *Trends in Neurosciences* 40, no. 3 (2017): 167–80; HealthyChildren.org, "Organic Causes of Weight Gain and Obesity," November 21, 2015, https://www.healthychildren.org/English/health-issues/conditions/obesity/Pages/Organic-Causes-of-Weight-Gain-and-Obesity.aspx.

24. H. Feng et al., "Review: The Role of Leptin in Obesity and the Potential for Leptin Replacement Therapy," *Endocrine* 44, no. 1 (2013): 33–9; C. Llewelyn and J. Wardle, "Behavioral Susceptibility to Obesity: Gene-Environment Interplay in the Development of Weight," *Physiology & Behavior* 152, part B (2015): 494–501.

25. C. Llewelyn and J. Wardle, "Behavioral Susceptibility to Obesity: Gene-Environment Interplay in the Development of Weight," *Physiology & Behavior* 152, part B (2015): 494–501.

26. E. Horn et al., "Behavioral and Environmental Modification of the Genetic Influence on BMI: A Twin Study," *Behavior Genetics* 45, no. 4 (2015): 409–26.

27. M. Reinhart et al., "A Human Thrifty Phenotype Associated with Less Weight Loss during Caloric Restriction," *Diabetes* 64, no. 8 (2015): 2859–67.

28. R. L. Minster et al., "A Thrifty Variant in CREBRF Strongly Influences Body Mass Index in Samoans," *Nature Genetics* 48, no. 9 (2016): 1049–54.

29. H. Pontzer et al., "Constrained Total Energy Expenditure and Adaptation to Physical Activity in Adult Humans," *Current Biology* 26, no. 3 (2016): 410–17; E. Fothergill, "Persistent Metabolic Adaptation 6 Years after 'The Biggest Loser' Competition." *Obesity*, 2016. 24, no. 8 (2016): 1612–19.

30. E. Fothergill, "Persistent Metabolic Adaptation 6 Years after 'The Biggest Loser' Competition." *Obesity* 24, no. 8 (2016): 1612–19.

31. L. K. Mahan and J. Raymond, *Krause's Food and Nutrition Care Processes,* Fourteenth Edition. (St. Louis, MO: Elsevier, 2017).

32. USDA Economic Research Service, "Food Availability (per Capita) Data System," November 2016, https://www.ers.usda.gov/data-products/food-availability-per-capita-data-system.

33. CDC, "Early Release of Selected Estimates Based on Data from the National Health Interview Survey," January–September 2016, Available at https://www.cdc.gov/nchs/data/nhis/earlyrelease/earlyrelease201702_06.pdf.

34. Ibid.

35. S. Higgs and J. Thomas, "Social Influences on Eating," *Current Opinion in Behavioral Sciences* 9 (2016):1–6; W. Willett et al., *Thinfluence: The Powerful and Surprising Effect Friends, Family, Work and Environment Have on Weight* (Emmaus, PA: Rodale Press: 2014).

36. W. Willett et al., *Thinfluence: The Powerful and Surprising Effect Friends, Family, Work and Environment Have on Weight* (Emmaus, PA: Rodale Press: 2014).

37. Ibid.

38. J. Kolodziejczyk et al., "Influence of Specific Individual and Environmental Variables on the Relationship between Body Mass Index and Health-Related Quality of Life in Overweight and Obese Adolescents," *Quality of Life Research* 24, no. 1 (2015): 251–61.

39. A. Tambo et al., "The Microbial Hypothesis: Contributions of Adenovirus Infection and Metabolic Endotoxaemia to the Pathogenesis of Obesity," *International Journal of Chronic Diseases* 2016 (2016): 7030795, doi:10.1155/2016/7030795.

40. Y.-M. Lee et al., "Persistent Organic Pollutants in Adipose Tissue Should Be Considered in Obesity Research," *Obesity Reviews* 18, no. 2 (2017): 129–39.

41. H. Lawman et al., "The Role of Prescription Medications in the Association of Self-reported Sleep Duration and Obesity in U.S. Adults 2007–2012," *Obesity* 24, no. 10 (2016): 2210–16; V. Medici et al., "Common Medications Which Lead to Unintended Alterations in Weight Gain or Organ Lipotoxicity," *Current Gastroenterology Reports* 18, no. 1 (2016): 1.

42. A. W. McHill and K. P. Wright, "Role of Sleep and Circadian Disruption on Energy Expenditure and in Metabolic Predisposition to Human Obesity and Metabolic Disease," *Obesity Reviews* 18, Suppl. 1 (2017): 15–24.

43. CDC, "Defining Overweight and Obesity," June 16, 2016, https://www.cdc.gov/obesity/adult/defining.html.

44. Ibid.

44. Ibid.

46. Ibid.

47. K. M. Flegal. "Trends in Obesity among Adults in the United States, 2005–2016," *Journal of the American Medical Association* 315, no. 21 (2016): 2284–91; CDC, "Obesity Prevalence Maps," September 11, 2015, www.cdc.gov/obesity/data/prevalence-maps.html.

48. American Heart Association, "Body Composition Tests," August 19, 2016, www.heart.org/HEARTORG/GettingHealthy/NutritionCenter/Body-Composition-Tests_UCM_305883_Article.jsp; S. J. Mooney, A. Baecker, and A. G. Rundel, "Comparison of Anthropometric and Body Composition Measures as Predictors of Components of the Metabolic Syndrome in the Clinical Setting," *Obesity Research and Clinical Practice* 7, no. 1 (2013): e55–e66.

49. C. L. Ogden et al., "Trends in Obesity Prevalence among Children and Adolescents in the United States, 1988 through 2013–2014," *Journal of the American Medical Association* 315, no. 21 (2016): 2292–99, doi:10.1001/jama.2016.636.

50. B. Major et al., "The Ironic Effects of Weight Stigma," *Journal of Experimental Social Psychology* 51 (2014): 74–80; S. A. Mustillo, K. Budd, and K. Hendrix, "Obesity, Labeling, and Psychological Distress in Late-Childhood and Adolescent Black and White Girls: The Distal Effects of Stigma," *Social Psychology Quarterly* 76, no. 3 (2013): 268–89.

51. F. Ortega et al., "Obesity and Cardiovascular Disease," *Circulation* 118 (2016): 1752–70.

52. National Heart, Lung, and Blood Institute, "Classification of Overweight and Obesity by BMI, Waist Circumference and Associated Disease Risks," Accessed March 2017, www.nhlbi.nih.gov/health/public/heart/obesity/lose_wt/bmi_dis.htm.

53. University of Maryland Medical Center, Rush University, "Waist to Hip Ratio," February 7, 2016, http://umm.edu/health/medical/reports/images/waisttohip-ratio.

54. P. Brambilla et al., "Waist Circumference-to-Height Ratio Predicts Adiposity Better Than Body Mass Index in Children and Adolescents," *International Journal of Obesity* 37, no. 7 (2013): 943–46.

55. S. Vangsness, "Mastering the Mindful Meal," Brigham Health Nutrition and Wellness Hub, April 13, 2016, http://www.brighamandwomens.org/Patients_Visitors/pcs/nutrition/services/healtheweightforwomen/special_topics/intelihealth0405.aspx.

56. N. Alajmi et al., "Appetite and Energy Intake Response to Acute Energy Deficits in Females vs. Males," *Medicine and Science in Sports and Exercise* 48, no. 3 (2016): 412–20.

57. A. Saltiel, "New Therapeutic Approaches for the Treatment of Obesity," *Science Translational Medicine* 8, no. 323 (2016): 323rv2; J. Domecq et al., "Drugs Commonly Associated with Weight Change: A Systematic Review and Meta-analysis," *Journal of Clinical Endocrinology and Metabolism* 100, no. 2 (2015): 363–70.

58. Drugs.com "Medications for Obesity," Accessed March 2017, https://www.drugs.com/condition/obesity.html.

59. Mayo Clinic, "Gastric Bypass Surgery: Risks," Accessed March, 2017, www.mayoclinic.org/tests-procedures/bariatric-surgery/basics/risks/prc-20019138.

60. John's Hopkins Health Library, "BPD/DS Weight-Loss Surgery," Accessed March 2017, http://www.hopkinsmedicine.org/healthlibrary/test_procedures/gastroenterology/bpdds_weight-loss_surgery_135,64.

61. I. Lanza, "Enhancing the Metabolic Benefits of Bariatric Surgery: Tipping the Scales with Exercise," *Diabetes* 64, no. 11 (2015): 3656–58. J. Yu et al., "The Long Term Effects of Bariatric Surgery for Type 2 Diabetes: Systematic Review and Meta-Analysis of Randomized and Non-randomized Evidence," *Obesity Surgery* 25, no. 1 (2015): 143–58.

Pulled Statistics:

page 306, S. Vikraman et al., "Caloric Intake from Fast Food among Children and Adolescents in the U.S. 2011–2012," NCHS Data Brief No. 213 (2015), www.cdc.gov.

page 308, Centers for Disease Control and Prevention, National Health Statistics, "Obesity and Overweight," February 25, 2016, www.cdc.gov/nchs/Fastats/obesity-overweight.htm; CDC, "Health, United States, 2014," Accessed April 2016, Available at http://www.cdc.gov/nchs/data/hus/hus14.pdf#059.

Focus On: Enhancing Your Body Image

1. M. Dahl, "Stop Obsessing: Women Spend 2 Weeks a Year on Their Appearance, TODAY Survey Shows" *Today*, February 24, 2014, http://www.today.com/health/stop-obsessing-women-spend-2-weeks-year-their-appearance-today-2D12104866.

2. Ibid.

3. M. Bucchianeri et al., "Body Dissatisfaction from Adolescence to Young Adulthood: Findings from a 10-Year Longitudinal Study," *Body Image* 10, no. 1 (2013): 1–7.

4. M.M. Gillen, "Associations between Positive Body Image and Indicators of Men's and Women's Mental and Physical Health," *Body Image* 13 (2015): 67–74.

5. A. Conason, "Is Facebook Making Us Hate Our Bodies?," *Psychology Today*, June 9, 2015, https://www.psychologytoday.com/blog/eating-mindfully/201506/is-facebook--making-us-hate-our-bodies.

6. K. Schreiber, "Promoting a Thin and Ultra-Athletic Physique Has Unforeseen Consequences," *Psychology Today*, September 1, 2015, https://www.psychologytoday.com/articles/201509/mind-your-body-body-conscious.

7. Centers for Disease Control and Prevention, "FASTSTATS: Obesity and Overweight," February 25, 2016, www.cdc.gov/nchs/fastats/obesity-overweight.htm.

8. L. Choate, "Dads: What's Your Impact on Your Daughter's Body Image?," *Psychology Today*, July 3, 2015, https://www.psychologytoday.com/blog/girls-women-and-wellness/201507/dads-whats-your-impact-your-daughters-body-image.

9. L. Choate, "Moms: What Will Your Body Image Legacy Be?," *Psychology Today*, June 29, 2015, https://www.psychologytoday.com/blog/girls-women-and-wellness/201506/moms-what-will-your-body-image-legacy-be?collection=1076687.

10. R. Puhl et al., "Cross-National Perspectives about Weight-Based Bullying in Youth: Nature, Extent and Remedies," *Pediatric Obesity* (2015), doi:10.1111/ijpo.12051.

11. L. Rakhkovskaya et al., "Sociocultural and Identity Predictors of Body Dissatisfaction in Ethnically Diverse College Women," *Body Image* 16 (2016): 32–40.

12. Mayo Clinic, "Body Dysmorphic Disorder," May 2013, http://www.mayoclinic.org/diseases-conditions/body-dysmorphic-disorder/basics/causes/con-20029953.

13. S. Rossell et al., "Can Understanding the Neurobiology of Body Dysmorphic Disorder (BDD) Inform Treatment?," *Australasian Psychiatry* 23, no. 4 (2015), doi:10.1177/1039856215591327.

14. K. Phillips et al., "A Preliminary Candidate Gene Study in Body Dysmorphic Disorder," *Journal of Obsessive-Compulsive Related Disorders* 6 (2015): 72–6.

15. Ibid.

16. Body Image Health, "The Model for Healthy Body Image and Weight," Accessed February 2016, http://bodyimagehealth.org/model-for-healthy-body-image.

17. I. Ahmed et al., "Body Dysmorphic Disorder," *Medscape Reference*, August 2014, http://emedicine.medscape.com/article/291182-overview.

18. Mayo Clinic Staff, "Body Dysmorphic Disorder," 2013; KidsHealth, "Body Dysmorphic Disorder," February 2016, http://kidshealth.org/parent/emotions/feelings/bdd.html.

19. Ibid.

20. I. Ahmed et al., "Body Dysmorphic Disorder," *Medscape Reference*, August 2014, http://emedicine.medscape.com/article/291182-overview.

21. American Psychiatric Association, *Diagnostic and Statistical Manual of Mental Disorders*, 5th ed. (Washington, DC: American Psychiatric Association, 2013).

22. National Eating Disorders Association, "Get the Facts on Eating Disorders," Accessed February 2016, www.nationaleatingdisorders.org/get-facts-eating-disorders.

23. D.A. Gagne et al., "Eating Disorder Symptoms and Weight and Shape Concerns in a Large Web-Based Convenience Sample of Women Ages 50 and Above: Results of the Gender and Body Image (GABI) Study," *International Journal of Eating Disorders* 45, no. 7 (2012): 832–44.

24. American College Health Association, *National College Health Assessment II: Undergraduates Reference Group Executive Summary Spring 2015* (Hanover, MD: American College Health Association, 2015), Available at www.acha-ncha.org/reports_ACHA-NCHAII.html.

25. National Collegiate Athletic Association, "Disordered Eating in Student-Athletes: Understanding the Basics and What We Can Do about It," Accessed February 2016, http://www.ncaa.org/health-and-safety/nutrition-and-performance/disordered-eating-student-athletes-understanding-basics.

26. Alliance for Eating Disorder Awareness, "What Are Eating Disorders?," Accessed February 2016, http://www.allianceforeatingdisorders.com/portal/what-are-eating-disorders#.VrKmr5MrKRt.

27. Ibid.

28. National Eating Disorders Association, "Anorexia Nervosa," Accessed February 2016, www.nationaleatingdisorders.org/anorexia-nervosa.

29. Ibid.

30. B. Carrot et al. "Are Lifetime Affective Disorders Predictive of Long-Term Outcome in Severe Adolescent Anorexia Nervosa?," *European Child and Adolescent Psychiatry* (2017): doi:10.1007/s00787-017-0963-5.

31. C.M. Pearson et al. "Stability and Change in Patterns of Eating Disorder Symptoms from Adolescence to Young Adulthood." *International Journal of Eating Disorders* (2017): doi:10.1002/eat.22692.

32. U.S. National Library of Medicine, "Anorexia Nervosa," A.D.A.M. Medical Encyclopedia, March 10, 2014, https://www.nlm.nih.gov/medlineplus/ency/article/000362.htm; B. Suchan et al., "Reduced

Connectivity between the Left Fusiform Body Area and the Extrastriate Body Area in Anorexia Nervosa Is Associated with Body Image Distortion," *Behavioural Brain Research* 241 (2013): 80–5.

33. R. Kessler et al., "The Prevalence and Correlates of Binge Eating Disorder in the World Health Organization World Mental Health Surveys," *Biological Psychiatry* 73, no. 9 (2013): 904–14, doi:10.1016/j.biopsych.2012.11.020.

34. National Institute of Mental Health, "Eating Disorders," February 2016, www.nimh.nih.gov/health/topics/eating-disorders/index.shtml.

35. M. Skunde et al., "Neural Signature of Behavioural Inhibition in Women with Bulimia Nervosa," *Journal of Psychiatry & Neuroscience* 41, no. 5 (2016): E69.

36. Mayo Clinic, "Binge-Eating Disorder," February 9, 2016, http://www.mayoclinic.org/diseases-conditions/binge-eating-disorder/basics/definition/con-20033155.

37. R. Kessler et al., "The Prevalence and Correlates of Binge Eating Disorder in the World Health Organization World Mental Health Surveys," *Biological Psychiatry* 73, no. 9 (2013): 904–14.

38. National Eating Disorder Association, "Other Specified Feeding or Eating Disorder," March 2014, www.nationaleatingdisorders.org/other-specified-feeding-or-eating-disorder.

39. T. Insel, "Director's Blog: Spotlight on Eating Disorders," National Institute of Mental Health, February 24, 2012, http://www.nimh.nih.gov/about/director/2012/spotlight-on-eating-disorders.shtml#i; Mirasol Eating Disorder Recovery Centers, "Eating Disorder Statistics," Accessed March 2016, http://www.mirasol.net/learning-center/eating-disorder-statistics.php.

40. M. Smith, L. Robinson, and J. Segal, "Helping Someone with an Eating Disorder," Helpguide.org, February 2016, http://www.helpguide.org/articles/eating-disorders/helping-someone-with-an-eating-disorder.htm.

41. National Eating Disorder Association, "Find Help and Support," Accessed February 2016, www.nationaleating-disorders.org/find-help-support.

42. B. Cook, "Exercise Addiction and Compulsive Exercising: Relationship to Eating Disorders, Substance Use Disorders, and Addictive Disorders," in *Eating Disorders, Addictions and Substance Use Disorders*, edited by T.D. Brewerton and A.B. Dennis (New York: Springer, 2014), 127–44.

43. J.J. Waldron, "When Building Muscle Turns into Muscle Dysmorphia," Association for Sport Applied Psychology, Accessed February 2016, www.appliedsportpsych.org/resource-center/health-fitness-resources/when-building-muscle-turns-into-muscle-dysmorphia.

44. M. Silverman, "What Is Muscle Dysmorphia?" Massachusetts General Hospital, February 18, 2011, https://mghocd.org/what-is-muscle-dysmorphia/; J.J. Waldron, "When Building Muscle Turns into Muscle Dysmorphia," Association for Sport Applied Psychology, Accessed February 2016, www.appliedsportpsych.org/resource-center/health-fitness-resources/when-building-muscle-turns-into-muscle-dysmorphia.

45. L.M. Gottschlich et al., "Female Athlete Triad," *Medscape*, 2017, http://emedicine.medscape.com/article/89260-overview.

46. L. Bacon, *Health at Every Size: The Surprising Truth about Your Weight* (Dallas, TX: BenBella Books, 2010).

Pulled Statistics:

page 326, American College Health Association, National College Health Assessment II: Undergraduates Reference Group Executive Summary Spring 2015 (Hanover, MD: American College Health Association, 2015), Available at www.acha-ncha.org/reports_ACHA-NCHAII.html.

Chapter 12: Improving Your Personal Fitness

1. Centers for Disease Control and Prevention, "Data, Trend and Maps," Accessed May 08, 2017, https://www.cdc.gov/nccdphp/dnpao/data-trends-maps/index.html.

2. Ibid.

3. Ibid.

4. C. Bouchard, S.N. Blair, and P. Katzmarzyk, "Less Sitting, More Physical Activity, or Higher Fitness?," *Mayo Clinic Proceedings* 90, no. 11 (2015): 1–8; A. Biswas et al., "Sedentary Time and Its Association with Risk for Disease Incidence, Mortality, and Hospitalization in Adults," *Annals of Internal Medicine* 162, no. 2 (2015): 123–32.

5. American College Health Association, *National College Health Assessment II (ACHA-NCHA II): Reference Group Executive Summary, Fall 2016* (Hanover, MD: American College Health Association, 2017), Available at http://www.acha-ncha.org/docs/NCHA-II%20SPRING%202016%20US%20REFERENCE%20GROUP%20EXECUTIVE%20SUMMARY.pdf.

6. C. Bouchard, S.N. Blair, and P. T. Katzmarzyk, "Less Sitting, More Physical Activity, or Higher Fitness?," *Mayo Clinic Proceedings* 90, no. 11 (2015): 1–8.

7. L.R.S.M. Cart, "Letter to the Editor: Standardized Use of the Terms 'Sedentary' and 'Sedentary Behaviours,'" *Applied Physiology, Nutrition and Metabolism* 37 (2012): 540–42.

8. Ibid.

9. L.R.S.M. Cart, "Letter to the Editor: Standardized Use of the Terms 'Sedentary' and 'Sedentary Behaviours,'" *Applied Physiology, Nutrition and Metabolism* 37 (2012): 540–42.

10. N. Owen et al., "Too Much Sitting: The Population-Health Science of Sedentary Behavior," *Exercise and Sport Science Reviews* 38, no. 3 (2010): 105–13.

11. C. Bouchard, S.N. Blair, and P. Katzmarzyk, "Less Sitting, More Physical Activity, or Higher Fitness?," *Mayo Clinic Proceedings* 90, no. 11 (2015): 1–8; A. Biswas et al., "Sedentary Time and Its Association with Risk for Disease Incidence, Mortality, and Hospitalization in Adults," *Annals of Internal Medicine* 162, no. 2 (2015): 123–32.

12. A. Biswas et al., "Sedentary Time and Its Association with Risk for Disease Incidence, Mortality, and Hospitalization in Adults," *Annals of Internal Medicine* 162, no. 2 (2015): 123–32.

13. M. Böejesson, A. Onerup, S. Lundqvist, and B. Dahlöf, "Physical Activity and Exercise Lower Blood Pressure in Individuals with Hypertension: Narrative Review of 27 RTCs," *British Journal of Sports Medicine* 50, no. 6 (2016): 356–61.

14. M.L. Zwald et al., "Prevalence of Low High-Density Lipoprotein Cholesterol among Adults, by Physical Activity: United States, 2011–2014," *NCHS Data Brief* 276 (2017): 1; D.J. Elmer et al., "Inflammatory, Lipid and Body Composition Response to Interval Training or Moderate Aerobic Training," *European Journal of Applied Physiology* 116 (2016): 601–9; B.B. Gibbs et al., "Six-Month Changes in Ideal Cardiovascular Health vs. Framingham 10-Year Coronary Heart Disease Risk among Adults Enrolled in a Weight Loss Intervention," *Preventive Medicine* 86 (2016): 123–29.

15. D.J. Elmer et al., "Inflammatory, Lipid and Body Composition Response to Interval Training or Moderate Aerobic Training," *European Journal of Applied Physiology* 116 (2016): 601–9; B.B. Gibbs et al., "Six-Month Changes in Ideal Cardiovascular Health vs. Framingham 10-Year Coronary Heart Disease Risk among Adults Enrolled in a Weight Loss Intervention," *Preventive Medicine* 86 (2016): 123–29.

16. P. Perez-Martinez et al., "Lifestyle Recommendations for the Prevention and Management of Metabolic Syndrome: An International Panel Recommendation," *Nutrition Reviews* 75, no. 5 (2017): 307–26; S.I. Kseneva et al., "Effectiveness of Lifestyle Modification in Corrections of States Associated with Metabolic Syndrome," *Bulletin of Experimental Biology and Medicine* 162, no. 1 (2016): 38–41.

17. Ibid.

18. Ibid.

19. J. Henson et al., "Sedentary Behavior as a New Behavioural Target in the Prevention and Treatment of Type 2 Diabetes," *Diabetes Metabolism Research and Reviews* 32, Suppl. 1 (2016): 213–20; L. Pai et al., "The Effectiveness of Regular Leisure-Time Physical Activities on Long-Term Glycemic Control in People with Type 2 Diabetes: A Systemic Review and Meta-Analysis," *Diabetes Research and Clinical Practice* 113 (2016): 77–85.

20. E.M. Balk et al., "Combined Diet and Physical Activity Promotion Programs to Prevent Type 2 Diabetes among Persons at Increased Risk: A Systematic Review for the Community Preventive Task Force," *Annals of Internal Medicine* 163, no. 6 (2015): 437–51; M.J. Armstrong and R.J. Sigal, "Exercise Is Medicine: Key Concepts in Discussing Physical Activity with Patients Who Have Type 2 Diabetes," *Canadian Journal of Diabetes* 39 (2015): s129–s133.

21. J. Erdrich et al., "Proportion of Colon Cancer Attributable to Lifestyle in a Cohort of US Women," *Cancer, Causes and Control* (2015), doi:10.1007/s10552-015-0619-z; M. Harvie, A. Howell, and D. Evans, "Can Diet and Lifestyle Prevent Breast Cancer: What Is the Evidence?" *ASCO Educational Book* 35 (2015): e66–73, doi:10.14694/EdBook_AM.2015.35.e66.

22. L.F.M. Rezende et al., "All-Cause Mortality Attributable Risk to Sitting Time: Analysis of 54 Countries Worldwide," *American Journal of Preventive Medicine* 51, no. 2 (2016): 253–63; A. Biswas et al., "Sedentary Time and Its Association with Risk for Disease Incidence, Mortality, and Hospitalization in Adults," *Annals of Internal Medicine* 162, no. 2 (2015): 123–32.

23. American Cancer Society, "Diet and Physical Activity: What's the Cancer Connection?," April 2017, www.cancer.org/cancer/cancercauses/dietandphysicalactivity/diet-and-physical-activity; D.C. Whiteman and I.F. Wilson, "The Fractions of Cancer Attributable to Modifiable Risk Factors: A Global Review," *Cancer Epidemiology* 44 (2016): 203–21.

24. B.R. Beck et al., "Exercise and Sports Science Australia (ESSA) Position Statement on Exercise Prescription for the Prevention and Management of Osteoporosis," *Journal of Science and Medicine in Sport* 20 (2016): 438–45.

25. B.K. Greer et al., "EPOC Comparison between Isocaloric Bouts of Steady-State Aerobic, Intermittent Aerobic, and Resistance Training," *Research Quarterly for Exercise and Sport* 86, no. 2 (2015): 190–95.

26. J.E. Turner, "Is Immunosenescence Influenced by Our Lifetime 'Dose' of Exercise?," *Biogerontology* 17, no. 3 (2016): 581–602.

27. G.J. Koelwyn et al., "Exercise in Regulation of Inflammation-Immune Axis Function in Cancer Initiation and Progression," *Oncology*, December 15, 2015, www.cancernetwork.com/oncology-journal/exercise-regulation-inflammation-immune-axis-function-cancer-initiation-and-progression; N. Sallam and I. Laher, "Exercise Modulates Oxidative Stress and Inflammation in Aging and Cardiovascular Disease," *Oxidative Medicine and Cellular Longevity* (2016), doi:10.1155/2016/7239639.

28. K. Kruger et al., "The Immunomodulatory Effects of Physical Activity," *Current Pharmaceutical Design* 22, no. 24 (2016): 3730–48.

29. C. Jin et al., "Exhaustive Submaximal Endurance and Resistance Exercises Induce Temporary Immunosuppression via Physical and Oxidative Stress," *Journal of Exercise Rehabilitation* 11, no. 4 (2015): 198–203.

30. J. Richards et al., "Don't Worry, Be Happy: Cross-Sectional Associations between Physical Activity and Happiness in 15 European Countries," *BMC Public Health* 15, no. 1 (2015): 1.

31. H. Hausenblas and R. E. Rhodes, *Exercise Psychology, Physical Activity and Sedentary Behavior*, 2017.

32. Ibid.

33. E.A. Haapala, "Physical Activity and Sedentary Time in Relation to Academic Achievement in Children," *Journal of Science and Medicine in Sport* 20, no. 6 (2017): 583–89; S. Kao et al., "Muscular and Aerobic Fitness, Working Memory, and Academic Achievement in Children," *Medicine and Science in Sports and Exercise* 49, no. 3 (2017): 500–8.

34. J.D. de Vries et al., "Exercise as an Intervention to Reduce Study-Related Fatigue among University Students," 2016.

35. 67. A.N. Slade and S.M. Kies, "The Relationship between Academic Performance and Recreation Use Among First-Year Medical Students," *Medical Education Online* 20 (2015), doi:10.3404/meo.v20.25105.

36. Ibid.

37. M. Beckett et al., "A Meta-Analysis of Prospective Studies in the Role of Physical Activity and the Prevention of Alzheimer's Disease in Older Adults," *BMC Geriatrics* 15, no. 9 (2015), doi:10.10.1186/s12877-015-0007-2.

38. C. Bouchard, S.N. Blair, and P. Katzmarzyk, "Less Sitting, More Physical Activity, or Higher Fitness?," *Mayo Clinic Proceedings* 90, no. 11 (2015): 1–8.

39. C. Bouchard, S.N. Blair, and P. Katzmarzyk, "Less Sitting, More Physical Activity, or Higher Fitness?," *Mayo Clinic Proceedings* 90, no. 11 (2015): 1–8; L.F.M. Rezende et al., "All-Cause Mortality Attributable Risk to Sitting Time Analysis of 54 Countries Worldwide," *American Journal of Preventive Medicine* 51, no. 2 (2016): 253–63.

40. D. Dunlop et al., "Sedentary Time in US Older Adults Associated with Disability in Activities of Daily Living Independent of Physical Activity," *Journal of Physical Activity and Health* 12, no. 1 (2015): 93–101.

41. K. Brown and D. Stanforth, "Go Green with Outdoor Activity," *ACSM's Health & Fitness Journal* 21, no. 1 (2017), 10–15.

42. American College of Sports Medicine, *ACSM's Guidelines for Exercise Testing and Prescription*, 10th ed. (Baltimore, MD: Lippincott Williams & Wilkins, 2018).

43. Ibid.

44. Ibid.

45. Ibid.

46. Ibid.

47. V.H. Heyward, *Advanced Assessment and Exercise Prescription* (Champaign, IL: Human Kinetics, 2014).

48. D.G. Behm et al., "Acute Effects of Muscle Stretching on Physical Performance, Range of Motion, and Injury Incidence in Healthy Active Individuals: A Systematic Review," *Applied Physiology, Nutrition, and Metabolism* 41, no. 1 (2016): 1–11; S. Sadler et al., "Restriction in Lateral Bending Range of Motion, Lumbar Lordosis, and Hamstring Flexibility Predicts the Development of Low Back Pain: A Systematic Review of Prospective Cohort Studies," *BMC Musculoskeletal Disorders* 18, no. 1 (2017): 179

49. D.G. Behm et al., "Acute Effects of Muscle Stretching on Physical Performance, Range of Motion, and Injury Incidence in Healthy Active Individuals: A Systematic Review," *Applied Physiology, Nutrition, and Metabolism* 41, no. 1 (2016): 1–11; S. Sadler et al., "Restriction in Lateral Bending Range of Motion, Lumbar Lordosis, and Hamstring Flexibility Predicts the Development of Low Back Pain: A Systematic Review of Prospective Cohort Studies," *BMC Musculoskeletal Disorders* 18, no. 1 (2017): 179.

50. T.M. Manini et al., "Effect of Physical Activity on Self-reported Disability in Older Adults: Results from the LIFE Study," *Journal of the American Geriatrics Society* 65, no. 5 (2017): 980–88.

51. American College of Sports Medicine, *ACSM's Guidelines for Exercise Testing and Prescription*, 10th ed. (Baltimore, MD: Lippincott Williams& Wilkins, 2018).

52. Ibid.

53. D.G. Behm et al., "Acute Effects of Muscle Stretching on Physical Performance, Range of Motion, and Injury Incidence in Healthy Active Individuals: A Systematic Review," *Applied Physiology, Nutrition, and Metabolism* 41, no. 1 (2016): 1–11.

54. Ibid.

55. J. Calstayud et al., "Core muscle activity in a series of balance exercises with different stability conditions," *Gait & Posture* 42, no. 2 (2015): 186–92.

56. D.G. Behm et al., "Acute Effects of Muscle Stretching on Physical Performance, Range of Motion, and Injury Incidence in Healthy Active Individuals: A Systematic Review ," *Applied Physiology, Nutrition, and Metabolism* 41, no. 1 (2016): 1–11.

57. D. McCartney, "The Effect of Fluid Intake Following Dehydration on Subsequent Athletic and Cognitive Performance: a Systematic Review and Meta-analysis," *Sports Medicine-Open* 3, no. 1 (2017): 13.

58. Ibid.

59. J. Potter and B. Fuller, "The Effectiveness of Chocolate Milk as a Post-Climbing Recovery Aid," *Journal of Sports Medicine and Physical Fitness* 55, no. 12 (2015): 1438–44.

60. American Academy of Ophthalmology, "Eye Health in Sports and Recreation," March 2016, www.aao.org/eye-health/tips-prevention/injuries-sports.

61. Ibid.

62. Bicycle Helmet Safety Institute, "Helmet-Related Statistics from Many Sources," January 2016, www.helmets.org/stats.htm.

63. American College Health Association, *National College Health Assessment II (ACHA-NCHA II): Reference Group Data Report, Fall 2016* (Hanover, MD: American College Health Association, 2017).

64. Bicycle Helmet Safety Institute, "Helmet-Related Statistics from Many Sources," January 2016, www.helmets.org/stats.htm.

65. American College of Sports Medicine, *ACSM's Guidelines for Exercise Testing and Prescription*, 9th ed. (Baltimore, MD: Lippincott Williams & Wilkins, 2014).

66. Mayo Clinic, "Hypothermia: Definition," May 11, 2017, www.mayoclinic.org/diseases-conditions/hypothermia/basics/definition/con-20020453.

67. American College of Sports Medicine, *ACSM's Guidelines for Exercise Testing and Prescription*, 9th ed. (Baltimore, MD: Lippincott Williams & Wilkins, 2014).

68. Mayo Clinic, "Winter Fitness: Safety Tips for Exercising Outdoors," September 9, 2016, http://www.mayoclinic.org/healthy-lifestyle/fitness/in-depth/fitness/art-20045626.

Pulled Statistics:

page 339, Centers for Disease Control and Prevention, "Data, Trend and Maps," accessed May 08, 2017, https://www.cdc.gov/nccdphp/dnpao/data-trends-maps/index.html

page 347, Centers for Disease Control and Prevention–Division of Nutrition, Physical Activity and Obesity, "How Much Physical Activity Do Adults Need?" *Physical Activity for Everyone*, June 2015, www.cdc.gov/physicalactivity/basics/adults/index.htm.

Chapter 13: Reducing Your Risk of Cardiovascular Disease and Cancer

1. M. Naghavi et al., "Global, Regional, and National Age–Sex Specific All-Cause and Cause-Specific Mortality for 240 Causes of Death, 1990–2013: A Systematic Analysis for the Global Burden of Disease Study 2013," *Lancet* 117, no. 171 (2015): 385.

2. Ibid.

3. E. Benjamin et al., "Heart Disease and Stroke Statistics—2017 Update: A Report from the American Heart Association," *Circulation* 135, no. 10 (2017): e146–e603.

4. Ibid.

5. Ibid.

6. Ibid.

7. World Health Organization, "Cardiovascular Diseases (CVDs): Fact Sheet," September 2016, http://www.who.int/mediacentre/factsheets/fs317/en; E. Benjamin et al., "Heart Disease and Stroke Statistics—2017 Update: A Report from the American Heart Association," *Circulation* 135, no. 10 (2017): e146–e603.

8. Ibid.

9. American Heart Association, "2020 Cardiovascular Health Impact Goals," 2013, https://www.heart.org/idc/groups/heart-public/@wcm/@sop/@smd/documents/downloadable/ucm_319831.pdf; D. M. Lloyd-Jones et al., "Defining and Setting National Goals for Cardiovascular Health Promotion and Disease Reduction: The AHA's Strategic Impact Goal through 2020 and Beyond," *Circulation* 121 (2010): e14–e31.

10. E. Benjamin et al., "Heart Disease and Stroke Statistics—2017 Update: A Report from the American Heart Association," *Circulation* 135, no. 10 (2017): e146–e603; D.M. Lloyd-Jones et al., "Defining and Setting National Goals for Cardiovascular Health Promotion and Disease Reduction: The AHA's Strategic Impact Goal through 2020 and Beyond," *Circulation* 121 (2010): e14–e31.

11. E. Benjamin et al., "Heart Disease and Stroke Statistics—2017 Update: A Report from the American Heart Association," *Circulation* 135, no. 10 (2017): e146–e603.

12. American Heart Association, "Why Blood Pressure Matters," August 2014, www.heart.org/HEARTORG/Conditions/HighBloodPressure/WhyBloodPressureMatters/Why-Blood-Pressure-Matters_UCM_002051_Article.jsp.

13. P. Welton et al. 2017 ACC/AHA/AAPA/ABC/ACPM/AGS/APhA/ASH/NMA/PCNA Guidelines for the Prevention, Detection, Evaluation and Management of High Blood Pressure in Adults. Journal of the American College of Cardiology. 2017. doi:10.1016/j.jacc.2017.11.006.

14. Ibid.

15. Ibid.

16. Ibid.

17. L. Rutten-Jacobs et al., "Cardiovascular Disease Is the Main Cause of Long-Term Excess Mortality after Ischemic Stroke in Young Adults," *Hypertension* 65, no. 3 (2015): 670–75.

18. E. Benjamin et al., "Heart Disease and Stroke Statistics—2017 Update: A Report from the American Heart Association," *Circulation* 135, no. 10 (2017): e146–e603.

19. Ibid.

20. Centers for Disease Control and Prevention, "High Blood Pressure Facts," February 19, 2015, www.cdc.gov/bloodpressure/facts.htm.

21. E. Benjamin et al., "Heart Disease and Stroke Statistics—2017 Update: A Report from the American Heart Association," *Circulation* 135, no. 10 (2017): e146–e603.

22. Ibid.

23. H. Johnson et al., "They're Younger$ . . . $It's Harder: Primary Providers' Perspectives on Hypertension Management in Young Adults: A Multicenter Qualitative Study," *BMC Research Notes* 10, no. 9 (2017): 9.

24. American Heart Association, "Understand your Risk for PAD," February 17, 2017, https://www.heart.org/HEARTORG/Conditions/VascularHealth/PeripheralArteryDisease/Understand-Your-Risk-for-PAD_UCM_301304_Article.jsp.

25. American Heart Association, "About Peripheral Artery Disease," November 16, 2016. www.heart.org/HEARTORG/Conditions/More/PeripheralArteryDisease/About-Peripheral-Artery-Disease-PAD_UCM_301301_Article.jsp.

26. E. Benjamin et al., "Heart Disease and Stroke Statistics—2017 Update: A Report from the American Heart Association," *Circulation* 135, no. 10 (2017): e146–e603.

27. Ibid.

28. Ibid.

29. WebMD, " Pre-Ventricular Contractions," Accessed April 2017, http://www.webmd.com/heart-disease/tc/premature-ventricular-contractions-pvcs-topic-overview.

30. Ibid.; American Heart Association, "Angina (Chest Pain)," April 14, 2017, www.heart.org/HEARTORG/Conditions/HeartAttack/SymptomsDiagnosisofHeartAttack/Angina-Chest-Pain_UCM_450308_Article.jsp; American Heart Association, "Angina in Women Can Be Different Than Men," April 18, 2016, http://www.heart.org/HEARTORG/Conditions/HeartAttack/WarningSignsofaHeartAttack/Angina-in-Women-Can-Be-Different-Than-Men_UCM_448902_Article.jsp#.VzJHJmQrIfE.

31. E. Benjamin et al., "Heart Disease and Stroke Statistics—2017 Update: A Report from the American Heart Association," *Circulation* 135, no. 10 (2017): e146–e603.

32. Ibid.

33. U.K. Patel et al. "Trends in Acute Ischemic Stroke Hospitalizations and Risk Factors among Young Adults: 12 Years of Nationally Representative Data," *Stroke* 48, Suppl. 1 (2017): AWP182 D. Ingram and J. Montresor-Lopez, "Differences in Stroke Mortality, Adults Aged 45 and Over: United States 2010–2013," NCHS Data Brief No. 207, July 2015, Available at http://www.cdc.gov/nchs/data/databriefs/db207.pdf; E. Benjamin et al., "Heart Disease and Stroke Statistics—2017 Update: A Report from the American Heart Association," *Circulation* 135, no. 10 (2017): e146–e603.

34. M. Goyal et al., "Recent Endovascular Trials: Implications for Radiology Departments, Radiology Residency, and Neuro-radiology Fellowship Training at Comprehensive Stroke Centers," *Radiology* 278, no. 3 (2016): 642–45.

35. C.J.L. Murray et al., "The State of US Health, 1990–2010 Burden of Diseases, Injuries, and Risk Factors," *Journal of the American Medical Association* 310, no. 6 (2013): 591–608.

36. E. Benjamin et al., "Heart Disease and Stroke Statistics—2017 Update: A Report from the American

Heart Association," *Circulation* 135, no. 10 (2017): e146–e603; A. Noortie, "Ischaemic Stroke in Young Adults: Risk Factors and Long-Term Consequences," *Nature Reviews Neurology* 10, no. 6 (2014): 315–25; Y. Yano et al., "Isolated Systolic Hypertension in Young and Middle-Aged Adults and 31-Year Risk for Cardiovascular Mortality," *Journal of the American College of Cardiology* 65, no. 4 (2015): 327–33.

37. Ibid.

38. Ibid.

39. M. Aguilar et al., "Prevalence of the Metabolic Syndrome in the United States, 2003–2012," *Journal of the American Medical Association* 313, no. 19 (2015): 1973–74.

40. Ibid.

41. E. Benjamin et al., "Heart Disease and Stroke Statistics—2017 Update: A Report from the American Heart Association," *Circulation* 135, no. 10 (2017): e146–3603; S. Grundy et al., "Definition of Metabolic Syndrome. Report of the National Heart, Lung, and Blood Institute/American Heart Association Conference on Scientific Issues Related to Definition," *Circulation* 109, no. 2 (2011): 433–38.

42. N. Allen et al., "Blood Pressure Trajectories in Early Adulthood and Subclinical Atherosclerosis in Middle Age," *JAMA* 311, no. 5 (2014): 490–97; Y. Yano et al., "Isolated Systolic Hypertension in Young and Middle-Aged Adults and 31-Year Risk for Cardiovascular Mortality," *Journal of the American College of Cardiology* 65, no. 4 (2015): 327–33; P. Chu et al., "Comparative Effectiveness of Personalized Lifestyle Management Strategies for Cardiovascular Disease Risk Reduction," *Journal of the American Heart Association* 5, no. 3 (2016): e201937.

43. Centers for Disease Control and Prevention. "Current Cigarette Smoking Among Adults in the United States." Dec. 1, 2016. https://www.cdc.gov/tobacco/data_statistics/fact_sheets/adult_data/cig_smoking/index.htm

44. American College Health Association, *American College Health Association—National College Health Assessment II: Reference Group Executive Summary Fall 2016* (Hanover, MD: American College Health Association, 2017).

45. E. Benjamin et al., "Heart Disease and Stroke Statistics—2017 Update: A Report from the American Heart Association," *Circulation* 135, no. 10 (2017): e146–e603.

46. Ibid.

47. U.S. Department of Health and Human Services and U.S. Department of Agriculture, *2015–2020 Dietary Guidelines for Americans*, 8th ed., December 2015, Available at http://health.gov/dietaryguidelines/2015/guidelines.

48. Ibid.; K. Solid, "New Dietary Guidelines: What Changed and What Stayed the Same," International Food Information Council Foundation, August 24, 2016, http://www.foodinsight.org/new-dietary-guidelines-americans-2015-changes.

49. U.S. Department of Health and Human Services and U.S. Department of Agriculture, *2015–2020 Dietary Guidelines for Americans*, 8th ed., December 2015, Available at http://health.gov/dietaryguidelines/2015/guidelines.

50. Ibid.

51. G. Qiuping et al., "Prescription Cholesterol-Lowering Medication Use in Adults Aged 40 and Over: United States 2003–2012," NCHS Data Brief No. 177 (Hyattsville, MD: National Center for Health Statistics USDHHS, 2015); E. Benjamin et al., "Heart Disease and Stroke Statistics—2017 Update: A Report from the American Heart Association," *Circulation* 135, no. 10 (2017): e146–e603.

52. Ibid.

53. American Heart Association, "American Heart Association Survey Finds Patients Uncertain about How to Best Manage Their Cholesterol," April 10, 2017, http://newsroom.heart.org/news/american-heart-association-survey-finds-patients-uncertain-about-how-to-best-manage-their-cholesterol.

54. V. Papademetriou et al., "Effects of High Density Lipoprotein Raising Therapies on Cardiovascular Outcomes in Patients with Type 2 Diabetes Mellitus, with or without Renal Impairment: The Action to Control Cardiovascular Risk in Diabetes Study," *American Journal of Nephrology* 45, no. 2 (2017): 136–45; D. Keene et al., "Effect on Cardiovascular Risk of High Density Lipoprotein Targeted Drug Treatments Niacin, Fibrates, and CETP Inhibitors: Meta-analysis of Randomised Controlled Trials Including 117,411 Patients," *British Medical Journal* 349 (2014): g4379; T. Wood et al., "The Cardiovascular Risk Reduction Benefits of a Low-Carbohydrate Diet Outweigh the Potential Increase in LDL-Cholesterol," *British Journal of Nutrition* 115, no. 6 (2016): 1126–128.

55. N.J. Stone et al., "2013 ACC/AHA Guidelines on the Treatment of Blood Cholesterol to Reduce Atherosclerotic Cardiovascular Risk in Adults," *Circulation* 63, no. 25, pt. B (2014): 2889–934.

56. E. Benjamin et al., "Heart Disease and Stroke Statistics—2017 Update: A Report from the American Heart Association," *Circulation* 135, no. 10 (2017): e146–e603.

57. Ibid.

58. S. Wood and R. Valentino, "The Brain Norepinephrine System, Stress and Cardiovascular Vulnerability," *Neuroscience and Biobehavioral Reviews* (2016), doi:10.1016/j.neurbiorev.2016.04.018; N. Batelaan et al., "Anxiety and New Onset of Cardiovascular Disease: Critical Review and Meta-analysis," *British Journal of Psychiatry* 208, no. 3 (2016): 223–31.

59. Ibid.

60. E. Benjamin et al., "Heart Disease and Stroke Statistics—2017 Update: A Report from the American Heart Association," *Circulation* 135, no. 10 (2017): e146–e603.

61. Ibid.; T Huang and F. Hu, "Gene-Environmental Interactions and Obesity: Recent Developments and Future Directions," *BMC Medical Genomics* 8, Suppl. 1 (2015): S2.

62. E. Benjamin et al., "Heart Disease and Stroke Statistics—2017 Update: A Report from the American Heart Association," *Circulation* 135, no. 10 (2017): e146–e603.

63. Ibid.

64. P. Ridker, "A Test in Context: High Sensitivity C-Reactive Protein," *Journal of the American College of Cardiology* 67, no. 6 (2016): 712–23; M. Jimenez et al., "Association between High Sensitivity C-Reactive Protein and Total Stroke by Hypertensive Stroke among Men," *Journal of the American Heart Association* 4, no. 9 (2015): e002013.

65. "The PLAC Test: Predicting Heart Attack Risk in People with No Symptoms." *Scientific American—Health After 50* 27, no. 2 (2015): 1–2.

66. G. Ren et al., "Effect of Flaxseed Intervention on Inflammatory Marker C-Reactive Protein: A Systematic Review and Meta-analysis of Randomized Controlled Trials," *Nutrients* 8, no. 3(2016): 136; G. Colussi et al., "Impact of Omega-3 Polyunsaturated Fatty Acids on Vascular Function and Blood Pressure: Relevance for Cardiovascular Outcomes," *Nutrition, Metabolism, and Cardiovascular Diseases* 27, no. 3: 191–200.

67. D. Siscovick et al., "Omega-3 Polyunsaturated Fatty Acid (Fish Oil) Supplementation and the Prevention of Clinical Cardiovascular Disease: A Science Advisory from the American Heart Association," *Circulation* (2017): CIR-0000000000000482.

68. Ibid.

69. J. Lupton et al., "Serum Homocysteine Is Not Independently Associated with an Atherogenic Lipid Profile: The Very Large Database of Lipids (VLDL-21) Study," *Atherosclerosis* 249 (2016): 59–64.

70. Y. Li et al., "Folic Acid Supplementation and the Risk of Cardiovascular Diseases: A Meta-analysis of Randomized Controlled Trials," *Journal of the American Heart Association* 5, no. 8 (2016): e003768.

71. U.S. Preventive Services Task Force, "Understanding Task Force Recommendations: Aspirin Use for the Primary Prevention of Cardiovascular Disease and Colorectal Cancer," April 2016, http://www.uspreventiveservicestaskforce.org/Home/GetFile/11/218/aspr-cvccrc-finalrsfact/pdf; FDA, "Can an Aspirin a Day Help Prevent a Heart Attack?," February 22, 2016, www.fda.gov/For-Consumers/ConsumerUpdates/ucm390539.htm.

72. American Heart Association, "Prevention and Treatment of Heart Attack," February 10, 2016, http://www.heart.org/HEARTORG/Conditions/HeartAttack/PreventionTreatmentofHeartAttack/Prevention-and-Treatment-of-Heart-Attack_UCM_002042_Article.jsp#.VzJaa2QrIfE.

73. E. Benjamin et al., "Heart Disease and Stroke Statistics—2017 Update: A Report from the American Heart Association," *Circulation* 135, no. 10 (2017): e146–e603.

74. Ibid.

75. American Cancer Society, *Cancer Facts & Figures 2017* (Atlanta, GA: American Cancer Society, 2017), Available at https://www.cancer.org/content/dam/cancer-org/research/cancer-facts-and-statistics/annual-cancer-facts-and-figures/2017/cancer-facts-and-figures-2017.pdf.

76. American Cancer Society, "Cancer Statistics Center," Accessed April 2017, https://cancerstatisticscenter.cancer.org/#.

77. Ibid.

78. Ibid.

79. Ibid.

80. Ibid.

81. Ibid.

82. American Cancer Society, *Cancer Facts & Figures 2017* (Atlanta, GA: American Cancer Society, 2017), Available at https://www.cancer.org/content/dam/cancer-org/research/cancer-facts-and-statistics/annual-cancer-facts-and-figures/2017/cancer-facts-and-figures-2017.pdf.

83. Ibid.

84. U.S. Department of Health and Human Services, *The Health Consequences of Smoking: 50 Years of Progress: A Report of the Surgeon General* (Atlanta, GA: U.S. Department of Health and Human Services, Centers for Disease Control and Prevention, National Center for Chronic Disease Prevention and Health Promotion, Office on Smoking and Health, 2014).

85. World Health Organization, "Report on the Global Tobacco Epidemic, 2015," July 7, 2015, Available at www.who.int/tobacco/global_report/2015/en.

86. Cancer Research UK, "Worldwide Cancer," May 2015, http://publications.cancerresearchuk.org/downloads/Product/CS_KF_WORLDWIDE.pdf.

87. V. Bagnardi et al., "Alcohol Consumption and Site-Specific Cancer Risk: A Comprehensive Dose-Response Meta-analysis," *British Journal of Cancer* 112, no. 3 (2015): 580–93.

88. Centers for Disease Control and Prevention, "Fact Sheet—Alcohol Use and Your Health," February 29, 2016, http://www.cdc.gov/alcohol/fact-sheets/alcohol-use.htm; Centers for Disease Control and Prevention, "Fact Sheets—Excessive Alcohol Use and Risks to Men's Health," March 7, 2016, http://www.cdc.gov/alcohol/fact-sheets/mens-health.htm; National Cancer Institute, "Alcohol and Cancer Risk Sheet," June 24, 2013, www.cancer.gov/cancertopics/factsheet/Risk/alcohol.

89. American Cancer Society, *Cancer Facts and Figures 2017* (Atlanta, GA: American Cancer Society, 2017), Available at https://www.cancer.org/content/dam/cancer-org/research/cancer-facts-and-statistics/annual-cancer-facts-and-figures/2017/cancer-facts-and-figures-2017.pdf.

90. American Cancer Society, *Cancer Facts and Figures 2017* (Atlanta, GA: American Cancer Society, 2017), Available at https://www.cancer.org/content/dam/cancer-org/research/cancer-facts-and-statistics/annual-cancer-facts-and-figures/2017/cancer-facts-and-figures-2017.pdf; D. Aune et al., "Anthropometric Factors and Endometrial Cancer Risk: A Systematic Review and Dose–Response Meta-analysis of Prospective Studies," *Annals of Oncology* 26, no. 8 (2015): 1635–48.

91. Ibid.

92. Ibid.

93. A. Blanc-Lapierre, "Lifetime Report of Perceived Stress at Work and Cancer among Men: A Case Control Study in Montreal, Canada," *Preventive Medicine* 96 (2017): 28–35; K. Heikkila et al., "Work Stress and Risk of Cancer: Meta-analysis of 5700 Incident Cancer Events in 116,000 European Men and Women," *British Medical Journal* 346 (2013): 1165.

94. Cancer.net, "Hereditary Cancer-Related Syndromes," Accessed April 2017, http://www.cancer.net/navigating-cancer-care/cancer-basics/genetics/hereditary-cancer-related-syndromes; American Cancer Society, "Family Cancer Syndromes," April 19, 2017, www.cancer.org/cancer/cancercauses/geneticsandcancer/heredity-and-cancer.

95. American Cancer Society, "Family Cancer Syndromes," April 19, 2017, www.cancer.org/cancer/cancercauses/geneticsandcancer/heredity-and-cancer.

96. American Cancer Society, "Breast Cancer Overview: Do We Know What Causes Breast Cancer?," May 4, 2016, www.cancer.org/Cancer/BreastCancer/DetailedGuide/breast-cancer-what-causes; American Cancer Society, Cancer Facts and Figures 2016 (Atlanta, GA: American Cancer Society, 2016), Available at https://www.cancer.org/research/cancer-facts-statistics/all-cancer-facts-figures/cancer-facts-figures-2016.html.

97. American Cancer Society, "Cancer Facts and Figures for Hispanic/Latinos, 2012–2014," Accessed May 2014, www.cancer.org/acs/groups/content/@epidemiologysurveilance/documents/document/acspc-034778.pdf; M. Banegas et al., "The Risk of Developing Invasive Breast Cancer in Hispanic Women," Cancer 119, no. 7 (2013): 1373–80.

98. J. Godos, "Markers of Systemic Inflammation and Colorectal Adenoma Risk: Meta-analysis of Observational Studies," World Journal of Gastroenterology 23, no. 10 (2017): 1909; R. Francescone, V. Hou, and S. Grivennikov, "Microbiome, Inflammation, and Cancer," Cancer Journal 20, no. 3 (2014): 181–89.

99. R. Francescone, V. Hou, and S. Grivennikov, "Microbiome, Inflammation, and Cancer," Cancer Journal 20, no. 3 (2014): 181–89; T. Deng, "Obesity, Inflammation and Cancer," Annual Review of Pathology: Mechanisms of Disease 11 (2016): 421–49.

100. Crohn's and Colitis Foundation of America, "Bringing to Light the Risk of Colorectal Cancer among Crohn's & Ulcerative Colitis Patients," Accessed June 2016, http://www.ccfa.org/resources/risk-of-colorectal-cancer.html; S. Sebastian et al., "Colorectal Cancer in Inflammatory Bowel Disease: Results of the 3rd ECCO Pathogenesis Scientific Workshop (I)," Journal of Crohn's and Colitis 8, no. 1 (2014): 5–18.

101. J. Lin, "The NTP Cell Phone RF Radiation Health Effects Project," Health Matters, 2017, Available at http://ieeexplore.ieee.org/stamp/stamp.jsp?arnumber=7779288.

102. National Cancer Institute, "Cell Phones and Cancer Risk," March 2013, www.cancer.gov; S. Joachim et al., "Cellular Telephone Use and Cancer Risk: Update of a Nationwide Danish Cohort," Journal of the National Cancer Institute 98, no. 23 (2006): 1707–13.

103. American Cancer Society, "Can Infections Cause Cancer?," July 11, 2016. https://www.cancer.org/cancer/cancer-causes/infectious-agents/infections-that-can-lead-to-cancer/intro.html.

104. Ibid.

105. D. Saslow et al., "Human Papillomavirus Vaccination Guideline Update: American Cancer Society Guideline Endorsement," CA: A Cancer Journal for Clinicians 66, no. 5 (2016): 375–85; Centers for Disease Control and Prevention, "Put Vaccination on Your Back to School List," August 5, 2015, https://www.cdc.gov/features/hpvvaccine.

106. D. Saslow et al., "Human Papillomavirus Vaccination Guideline Update: American Cancer Society Guideline Endorsement," CA: A Cancer Journal for Clinicians 66, no. 5 (2016): 375–85; Centers for Disease Control and Prevention, "Put Vaccination on Your Back to School List," August 5, 2015, https://www.cdc.gov/features/hpvvaccine; American Cancer Society, Cancer Facts and Figures 2017 (Atlanta, GA: American Cancer Society, 2017), Available at https://www.cancer.org/content/dam/cancer-org/research/cancer-facts-and-statistics/annual-cancer-facts-and-figures/2017/cancer-facts-and-figures-2017.pdf; National Cancer Institute, "Fact Sheet–HPV and Cancer," February 19, 2015, https://www.cancer.gov/about-cancer/causes-prevention/risk/infectious-agents/hpv-fact-sheet.

107. American Cancer Society, Cancer Facts and Figures 2017 (Atlanta, GA: American Cancer Society, 2017), Available at https://www.cancer.org/content/dam/cancer-org/research/cancer-facts-and-statistics/annual-cancer-facts-and-figures/2017/cancer-facts-and-figures-2017.pdf.

108. Ibid.

109. American Cancer Society, "Infections That Can Lead to Cancer," Accessed April, 2017, www.cancer.org/cancer/cancercauses/othercarcinogens/infectiousagents/infectiousagentsandcancer/infectious-agents-and-cancer-toc.

110. American Cancer Society, Cancer Facts and Figures 2017 (Atlanta, GA: American Cancer Society, 2017), Available at https://www.cancer.org/content/dam/cancer-org/research/cancer-facts-and-statistics/annual-cancer-facts-and-figures/2017/cancer-facts-and-figures-2017.pdf.

111. American Lung Association, "Lung Cancer Fact Sheet," November 3, 2016, http://www.lung.org/lung-health-and-diseases/lung-disease-lookup/lung-cancer/learn-about-lung-cancer/lung-cancer-fact-sheet.html.

112. E. Benjamin et al., "Heart Disease and Stroke Statistics—2017 Update: A Report from the American Heart Association," Circulation 135, no. 10 (2017): e146–e603.

113. American Cancer Society, Cancer Facts and Figures, 2017 (Atlanta, GA: American Cancer Society, 2017), Available at https://www.cancer.org/content/dam/cancer-org/research/cancer-facts-and-statistics/annual-cancer-facts-and-figures/2017/cancer-facts-and-figures-2017.pdf.

114. Ibid.

115. Ibid.

116. American Cancer Society, "Benefits of Quitting over Time," November 13, 2105, http://www.cancer.org/healthy/stayawayfromtobacco/benefits-of-quitting-smoking-over-time.

117. Ibid.

118. Ibid.

119. American Cancer Society, Cancer Facts and Figures 2017 (Atlanta, GA: American Cancer Society, 2017), Available at https://www.cancer.org/content/dam/cancer-org/research/cancer-facts-and-statistics/annual-cancer-facts-and-figures/2017/cancer-facts-and-figures-2017.pdf.

120. Ibid.

121. Ibid.

122. American Cancer Society, "Breast MRI (Magnetic Resonance Imaging)," August 18, 2016, http://www.cancer.org/treatment/understandingyourdiagnosis/examsandtestdescriptions/mammogramsandotherbreastimagingprocedures/mammograms-and-other-breast-imaging-procedures-breast-m-r-i.

123. USPSTF, "Breast Cancer: Screening," January 2016, https://www.uspreventiveservicestaskforce.org/Page/Document/UpdateSummaryFinal/breast-cancer-screening1?ds=1&s=breast%20cancer%20screening.

124. American Cancer Society, Cancer Facts and Figures 2017 (Atlanta, GA: American Cancer Society, 2017), Available at https://www.cancer.org/content/dam/cancer-org/research/cancer-facts-and-statistics/annual-cancer-facts-and-figures/2017/cancer-facts-and-figures-2017.pdf.

125. Ibid.; M. Farvid, "Fruit and Vegetable Consumption in Adolescences and Early Adulthood and Risk of Breast Cancer: Population Based Cohort Study," BMJ 353 (2016): i2343.

126. Ibid.

127. H. Kyu et al., "Physical Activity and Risk of Breast Cancer, Colon Cancer, Diabetes, Ischemic Heart Disease, and Ischemic Stroke Events: Systematic Review and Dose-Response Meta-analysis for the Global Burden of Disease Study 2013," BMJ 354 (2016): i3857; I. Lahart et al., "Physical Activity, Risk of Death and Recurrence in Breast Cancer Survivors: A Systematic Review and Meta-analysis of Epidemiological Studies," Acta Oncologica 54, no. 5 (2015): 635–54, doi:10.3109/0284186X.2014.998275.

128. L.K. Juvet, "The Effect of Exercise on Fatigue and Physical Functioning in Breast Cancer Patients and after Treatment and at 6 Months Follow-up: a Meta-analysis," The Breast 33 (2017): 166–77; Y. Wu et al., "Meta-analysis of Studies on Breast Cancer Risk and Diet in Chinese Women," International Journal of Clinical and Experimental Medicine 8, no. 11 (2015): 73–85.

129. American Cancer Society, "Colorectal Cancer Facts and Figures, 2014–2016," Accessed June 2016, www.cancer.org/acs/groups/content/documents/document/acspc-042280.pdf; American Cancer Society, Cancer Facts and Figures 2017 (Atlanta, GA: American Cancer Society, 2017), Available at https://www.cancer.org/content/dam/cancer-org/research/cancer-facts-and-statistics/annual-cancer-facts-and-figures/2017/cancer-facts-and-figures-2017.pdf.

130. Ibid.

131. American Cancer Society, Cancer Facts and Figures 2017 (Atlanta, GA: American Cancer Society, 2017), Available at https://www.cancer.org/content/dam/cancer-org/research/cancer-facts-and-statistics/annual-cancer-facts-and-figures/2017/cancer-facts-and-figures-2017.pdf.

132. Ibid.

133. American Cancer Society, "Can Colorectal Cancer Be Prevented?" March 1, 2017, https://www.cancer.org/cancer/colon-rectal-cancer/causes-risks-prevention/prevention.html.

134. American Cancer Society, Cancer Facts and Figures 2017 (Atlanta, GA: American Cancer Society, 2017), Available at https://www.cancer.org/content/dam/cancer-org/research/cancer-facts-and-statistics/annual-cancer-facts-and-figures/2017/cancer-facts-and-figures-2017.pdf.

135. Ibid.

136. Skin Cancer Foundation, "Skin Cancer Facts," June 8, 2016, www.skincancer.org/skin-cancer-information/skin-cancer-facts.

137. UCSF School of Medicine, "Melanoma," May 4, 2007, http://www.dermatology.ucsf.edu/skincancer/general/types/melanoma.aspx.

138. American Cancer Society, Cancer Facts and Figures 2017 (Atlanta, GA: American Cancer Society, 2017), Available at https://www.cancer.org/content/dam/cancer-org/research/cancer-facts-and-statistics/annual-cancer-facts-and-figures/2017/cancer-facts-and-figures-2017.pdf.

139. Ibid.

140. Ibid.

141. Ibid.

142. Ibid.

143. Ibid.

144. Ibid.

145. K. Zu et al.. "Dietary Lycopene, Angiogenesis, and Prostate Cancer: A Prospective Study in the Prostate-Specific Antigen Era," Journal of the National Cancer Institute 106, no. 2 (2014): 1093–97.

146. Ibid.

147. Ibid.

148. Ibid.

149. Ibid.

150. Ibid.

151. National Cancer Institute, "Uterine Cancer," Accessed June 2016, www.cancer.gov/cancertopics/types/endometrial.

152. National Institutes of Health, National Cancer Institute, "SEER Stat Fact Sheets: Testis Cancer," February 2016, http://seer.cancer.gov/statfacts/html/testis.html.

153. Ibid.

154. American Cancer Society, "Testicular Cancer," February 12, 2016, www.cancer.org/cancer/testicularcancer/detailedguide/-testicular-cancer-risk-factors; American Cancer Society, "What Are the Key Statistics about Testicular Cancer?" February 12, 2016, http://www.cancer.org/cancer/testicularcancer/detailedguide/testicular-cancer-key-statistics.

155. Ibid.

156. American Cancer Society, Cancer Facts and Figures 2017 (Atlanta, GA: American Cancer Society, 2017), Available at https://www.cancer.org/content/dam/cancer-org/research/cancer-facts-and-statistics/annual-cancer-facts-and-figures/2017/cancer-facts-and-figures-2017.pdf.

Pulled Statistics:

page 364, D. Thompson, "Cost of Heart Disease in U.S. to Surpass $1 Trillion by 2035, Report Says ," HealthDay News, February 14, 2017, http://www.upi.com/Health_News/2017/02/14/Cost-of-heart-disease-in-US-to-surpass-1-trillion-by-2035-report-says/5891487126035.

page 369, E. Benjamin et al., "Heart Disease and Stroke Statistics—2017 Update: A Report from the American Heart Association," Circulation 135, no. 10 (2017): e146–e603.

Focus On: Minimizing Your Risk for Diabetes

1. Centers for Disease Control and Prevention, "Long Term Trends in Diabetes in the United States," April 2016, https://www.cdc.gov/diabetes/statistics/slides/long_term_trends.pdf.

2. Centers for Disease Control and Prevention, "At a Glance 2016 Diabetes," Accessed June 2017, www.cdc.gov/chronicdisease/resources/publications/aag/pdf/2016/diabetes-aag.pdf; American Diabetes Association, "Fast Facts," December 2015, http://professional.diabetes.org/sites/professional.diabetes.org/files/media/fast_facts_12-2015a.pdf.

3. Centers for Disease Control and Prevention, "National Diabetes Statistics Report, 2014," May 2015, https://www.cdc.gov/diabetes/data/statistics/2014statisticsreport.html; Centers for Disease Control and Prevention, "At a Glance 2016 Diabetes," Accessed June 2017, www.cdc.gov/chronicdisease/resources/publications/aag/pdf/2016/diabetes-aag.pdf.

4. Centers for Disease Control and Prevention. "Diabetes Surveillance Data," April 2016, https://www.cdc.gov/diabetes/data/statistics/faqs.html.

5. C. Bommer et al., "The Global Economic Burden of Diabetes in Adults Aged 20–79 Years: A Cost of Illness Study," Lancet Diabetes & Endocrinology 5, no. 6 (2017): 423–30; NCD Risk Factor Collaboration, "Worldwide Trends in Diabetes since 1980: A Pooled Analysis of 751 Population-based Studies with 4.4 Million Participants," Lancet 387, no. 10027 (2016): 1513–30.

6. T. Dall et al., "The Economic Burden of Elevated Blood Glucose Levels in 2012: Diagnosed and Undiagnosed Diabetes, Gestational Diabetes Mellitus, and Prediabetes," Diabetes Care 37, no. 12 (2014): 3172–79.

7. American Diabetes Association, "Type 1 Diabetes," Accessed May 2017, www.diabetes.org/diabetes-basics/type-1.

8. American Diabetes Association, "Genetics of Diabetes," Accessed May 2017, http://www.diabetes.org/diabetes-basics/genetics-of-diabetes.html?loc=db-slabnav.

9. Ibid.

10. Centers for Disease Control and Prevention, "National Diabetes Statistics Report, 2014," May 2015, https://www.cdc.gov/diabetes/data/statistics/2014statisticsreport.html; V. Lyssenko and M. Laakso, "Genetic Screening for the Risk of Type 2 Diabetes," Diabetes Care 36, Suppl. 2 (2013): S120–26.

11. American Diabetes Association, "Statistics about Diabetes," Accessed May 8, 2017, http://www.diabetes.org/diabetes-basics/statistics.

12. Centers for Disease Control and Prevention, "National Diabetes Statistics Report, 2014," May 2015, https://www.cdc.gov/diabetes/data/statistics/2014statisticsreport.html.

13. E. Mayor-Davis et al. "Increasing Trends of Type 1 and Type 2 Diabetes among Youth, 2002–2012," New England Journal of Medicine 376 (2017): 1419–29.

14. **A. Abbasi et al., "Body Mass Index and Incident Type 1 and Type 2 Diabetes in Children and Young Adults: A Retrospective Cohort Study," Journal of the Endocrine Society 1, no. 5 (2017): 524–37.**

15. E. Mayor-Davis et al. "Increasing Trends of Type 1 and Type 2 Diabetes among Youth, 2002–2012." New England Journal of Medicine 376 (2017): 1419–29.

16. American Diabetes Association, "Genetics of Diabetes," Accessed May 2017, http://www.diabetes.org/diabetes-basics/genetics-of-diabetes.html?loc=db-slabnav.

17. WHO, "Global Report on Diabetes," April 2016, http://apps.who.int/iris/bitstream/10665/204871/1/9789241565257_eng.pdf?ua=1.

18. F. He et al., "Abdominal Obesity and Metabolic Syndrome Burden in Adolescents—Penn State Children Cohort Study," Journal of Clinical Densitometry 18, no. 1 (2015): 30–6; T. Huang et al., "Genetic Predisposition to Central Obesity and Risk of Type 2 Diabetes," 2015.

19. Ibid.; S. Millar et al., "General and Central Obesity Measurement Associations with Markers of Chronic Low-Grade Inflammation and Type 2 Diabetes," Journal of Epidemiology and Community Health 69, Supplement 1(2015): A54–55.

20. P.L. Capers et al., "A Systematic Review and Meta-analysis of Randomized Controlled Trials of the Impact of Sleep Duration on Adiposity and Components of Energy Balance," Obesity Reviews 16, no. 9 (2015): 771–82; L. Bromley et al., "Sleep Restriction Decreases the Physical Activity of Adults at Risk for Type 2 Diabetes," Sleep 35, no. 7 (2012): 977–84.

21. Z. Shan et al., "Sleep Duration and Risk of Type 2 Diabetes: A Meta-analysis of Prospective Studies," Diabetes Care 38, no. 3 (2015): 529–37; H. C. Hung et al., "The Association between Self-Reported Sleep Quality and Metabolic Syndrome," PLoS ONE 8, no. 1 (2013): e54304, doi:10.1371/journal.pone.0054304.

22. T. Anothaisintawee et al., "Sleep Disturbances Compared to Traditional Risk Factors for Diabetes Development: Systematic Review and Meta-analysis," Sleep Medicine Reviews 30, (2016): 11–24; S. Kelly and M. Ismail, "Stress and Type 2 Diabetes: A Review of How Stress Contributes to the Development of Type 2 Diabetes," Annual Review of Public Health 36 (2015): 441–62.

23. T. Anothaisintawee et al., "Sleep Disturbances Compared to Traditional Risk Factors for Diabetes Development: Systematic Review and Meta-analysis," Sleep Medicine Reviews 30, (2016): 11–24; S. Kelly and M. Ismail, "Stress and Type 2 Diabetes: A Review of How Stress Contributes to the Development of Type 2 Diabetes," Annual Review of Public Health 36 (2015): 441–62.

24. L. Mongiello et al, "Many College Students Underestimate Diabetes Risk," Journal of Allied Health 45, no. 2 (2016): 81–6; N. Yahia et al., "Assessment of College Students' Awareness and Knowledge about Conditions Relevant to Metabolic Syndrome," Diabetology and Metabolic Syndrome 6, no. 1 (2014): 111; A. Lima et al., "Risk Factors for Type 2 Diabetes Mellitus in College Students: Association with Sociodemographic Variables," Revista Latino-Americana de Enfermagem 22, no. 3 (2014): 484–90.

25. M. Aguilar et al., "Prevalence of the Metabolic Syndrome in the United States, 2003–2012," Journal of the American Medical Association 313, no. 19 (2015): 1973–74.

26. Ibid.

27. Ibid.

28. Centers for Disease Control and Prevention, "What Is Prediabetes and Are You at Risk?," February 19, 2016, https://www.cdc.gov/diabetes/ndep/people-risk-diabetes/prediabetes.html; American Diabetes Association, "Diagnosing Diabetes and Learning about Prediabetes," November 21, 2016, www.diabetes.org/diabetes-basics/diagnosis; American Diabetes Association, "Diabetes Pro-Toolkit #3: All about Prediabetes," Accessed May 2017, Available at http://professional2.diabetes.org/content/PML/All_About_Prediabetes_24dee6ff-cbf0-4a55-80b7-9d5d29de0bd7/All_About_Prediabetes.pdf.

29. Centers for Disease Control and Prevention, "At a Glance 2016 Diabetes," Accessed June 2017, www.cdc.gov/chronicdisease/resources/publications/aag/pdf/2016/diabetes-aag.pdf; Centers for Disease Control and Prevention, "The Surprising Truth about Prediabetes," January 25, 2017, https://www.cdc.gov/features/diabetesprevention.

30. Z. Zou et al., "Influence of Primary Intervention of Exercise on Obese Type 2 Diabetes Mellitus: A Meta-analysis Review," Primary Care Diabetes 10, no. 3 (2016): 186–201.

31. American Diabetes Association, "What Is Gestational Diabetes?," November 21, 2016, www.diabetes.org/diabetes-basics/gestational/what-is-gestational-diabetes.html.

32. Ibid.; E. Noctor and F. Dunne, "Type 2 Diabetes after Gestational Diabetes: The Influence of Changing Diagnostic Criteria," World Journal of Diabetes 6, no. 2 (2015): 234–44.

33. National Healthy Mothers, Healthy Babies Coalition, "The Lasting Impact of Gestational Diabetes on Mother and Children," May 2015, www.hmhb.org/virtual-library/interviews-with-experts/gestational-diabetes; French National Research Agency, "The Impact of Gestational Diabetes Mellitus (GDM) on the Epigenetics of Mother and Newborn Infant and Long-Term Risk of Type 2 Diabetes," 2016, Available at http://www.agence-nationale-recherche.fr/?Project=ANR-16-CE17-0017.

34. P. Damm et al., "Gestational Diabetes Mellitus and Long-term Consequences for Mother and Offspring: A View from Denmark," Diabetologia 59, no. 7 (2016): 1396–99; Mayo Clinic, "Gestational Diabetes: Symptoms and Causes," April 28, 2017, http://www.mayoclinic.org/diseases-conditions/gestational-diabetes/symptoms-causes/dxc-20317176.

35. Centers for Disease Control and Prevention, "National Diabetes Statistics Report, 2014," May 2015, https://www.cdc.gov/diabetes/data/statistics/2014statisticsreport.html; American Diabetes Association, "Complications," May 2017, http://www.diabetes.org/living-with-diabetes/complications.

36. National Kidney Foundation, "Fast Facts," May 2016, www.kidney.org/news/newsroom/factsheets/FastFacts.cfm; U.S. Renal Disease Data System, "Annual Data Report, 2015," Available at https://www.usrds.org/adr.aspx.

37. Centers for Disease Control and Prevention, "National Diabetes Statistics Report, 2014," May 2015, https://www.cdc.gov/diabetes/data/statistics/2014statisticsreport.html.

38. Ibid.

39. Prevent Blindness America, "Diabetic Retinopathy Prevalence by Age," Accessed May 2017, www.visionproblemsus.org/diabetic-retinopathy/diabetic-retinopathy-by-age.html.

40. American Diabetes Association, "Diabetes and Oral Health Problems," Accessed May 2017, www.diabetes.org/living-with-diabetes/treatment-and-care/oral-health-and-hygiene/diabetes-and-oral-health.html; P. Eke et al., "Risk Indicators for Periodontitis in US Adults: NHANES 2009-2012," Journal of Periodontology 87, No. 10(2016): 1174–85.

41. Ibid.

42. American Diabetes Association, "Complications," May 2017, http://www.diabetes.org/living-with-diabetes/complications.

43. American Diabetes Association, "Standards of Medical Care in Diabetes—2016: Summary of Revisions," Diabetes Care 39, Suppl. 1 (2016): S4–S5.

44. Ibid.

45. Diabetes Prevention Program Research Group, "Reduction in the Incidence of Type 2 Diabetes with Lifestyle Intervention or Metformin," New England Journal of Medicine 345 (2002): 393–403.

46. Linus Pauling Institute, "Glycemic Index and Glycemic Load," Accessed May 2017, http://lpi.oregonstate.edu/infocenter/foods/grains/gigl.html.

47. American Diabetes Association, "Diabetes Superfoods," Accessed May 2017, http://www.diabetes.org/food-and-fitness/food/what-can-i-eat/making-healthy-food-choices/diabetes-superfoods.html.

48. Ibid.; A. Chanson-Rolle et al., "Systematic Review and Meta-analysis of Human Studies to Support a Quantitative Recommendation for Whole Grain Intake in Relation to Type 2 Diabetes," PLoS ONE 10, no. 6 (2015): e0131377.

49. S. Bhupathiraju et al., "Glycemic Index, Glycemic Load and Risk of Type 2 Diabetes: Results from 3 Large US Cohorts and an Updated Meta-Analysis," Circulation 129, Suppl. 1 (2014): AP 140 American Diabetes Association, "Diabetes Superfoods," Accessed May 2017, http://www.diabetes.org/food-and-fitness/food/what-can-i-eat/making-healthy-food-choices/diabetes-superfoods.html.

50. A. Wallin et al., "Fish Consumption and Frying of Fish in Relation to Type 2 Diabetes Incidence: A Prospective Cohort Study of Swedish Men," European Journal of Nutrition (2015): 1–10; Y. Kim et al., "Fish Consumption, Long-Chain Omega-3 Polyunsaturated Fatty Acid Intake and Risk of Metabolic Syndrome: A Meta-analysis," Nutrients 7, no. 4 (2015): 2085–2100.

51. A. Wallin et al., "Fish Consumption and Frying of Fish in Relation to Type 2 Diabetes Incidence: A Prospective Cohort Study of Swedish Men," European Journal of Nutrition (2015): 1–10; C. Jeppesen et al., "Omega-3 and Omega-6 Fatty Acids and Type 2 Diabetes," Current Diabetes Reports 13, no. 2 (2013): 279–88.

52. W. Cefalu et al., "Standards of Medical Care in Diabetes—2017," Diabetes Care 40, Suppl. 1 (2017), Available at http://care.diabetesjournals.org/content/diacare/suppl/2016/12/15/40.Supplement_1.DC1/DC_40_S1_final.pdf.

53. O. Farr and C. Mantzorous, "Treatment Options to Prevent Diabetes in Subjects with Prediabetes: Efficacy, Cost Effectiveness, and Future Outlook," Metabolism 70 (2017); A. Anabtawj and J. Miles, "Metformin: Nonglycemic Effects and Potential Novel Indications," Endocrine Practice 22,

no. 8 (2016): 999-1007; U. Hostalek et al., *"Therapeutic Use of Metformin in Prediabetes and Diabetes Prevention,"* Drugs 75, no. 10 (2015): 1071–94.

54. F. Rubino et al. "Metabolic Surgery in the Treatment Algorithm for Type 2 Diabetes: A Joint Statement by International Diabetes Organizations," *Surgery of Obesity and Related Diseases* 12, no. 6 (2016): 1144–62; D.E. Cummings et al., "Gastric Bypass Surgery vs Intensive Lifestyle and Medical Intervention for Type 2 Diabetes: The CROSSROADS Randomised Controlled Trial," *Diabetologia* 59, no. 5(2016): 945–53; J. Yu et al., "The Long Term Effects of Bariatric Surgery for Type 2 Diabetes: Systematic Review and Meta-analysis of Randomized and Non Randomized Evidence," *Obesity Surgery* 25, no. 1 (2015): 143–55.

55. Ibid.

56. M. Jenson et al., "2013 AHA/ACC/TOS Guideline for the Management of Overweight and Obesity in Adults: A Report of the American College of Cardiology/American Heart Association Task Force on Practice Guidelines and the Obesity Society," *Circulation* 25, Suppl. 2 (2014): S139–40.

57. **Medtronic, "Medtronic Gains Approval of First Artificial Pancreas Device System with Threshold Suspend Automation," September 2013,** http:// newsroom.medtronic.com/phoenix .zhtml?c=251324&p=irol-newsArticle&id=1859361; **S. Mukherjee, "An Artificial Pancreas for Diabetics Could Hit the Market Next Year,"** *Fortune* **, June 28, 2016,** http://fortune.com/2016/06/28/ medtronic-artificial-pancreas-diabetes.

Pulled Statistics:
page 401, National Kidney Foundation, "Diabetes and Kidney Disease," Accessed May 2017, www.kidney.org/ news/newsroom/factsheets/Diabetes-And-CKD.

Chapter 14: Protecting Against Infectious Diseases and Sexually Transmitted Infections

1. P. Damborg et al., "Bacterial Zoonoses Transmitted by Household Pets: State-of -the-Art and Future Perspectives for Targeted Research and Policy Actions," *Journal of Comparative Pathology* 155, no. 1 (2016): S27–S40; Go Pets America, "Diseases Transmissible between Dogs and People," Accessed May 2017, http://www.gopet-samerica.com/dog-health/zoonoses_dogs.aspx.

2. X. Wu et al., "Impact of Climate Change on Human Infectious Diseases: Empirical Evidence and Human Adaptation," *Environment International* 86 (2016): 14–23; L. Liang and P. Gong, "Climate Change and Human Infectious Diseases: A Synthesis of Research Findings from Global and Spatio-temporal Perspectives," *Environment International* 103 (2017): 99–108; World Health Organization, "Climate Change and Infectious Disease," May 2015, www.who.int/globalchange/publications/climatechangechap6.pdf; C. Heffernan, "Climate Change and Infectious Disease: Time for a New Normal?" *Lancet Infectious Diseases* 15, no. 2 (2015): 143–44

3. National Institute of Allergy and Infectious Diseases, "Autoimmune Diseases," January 5, 2016, http://www .niaid.nih.gov/topics/autoimmune/Pages/default.aspx.

4. Centers for Disease Control and Prevention, "Birth–18 years and 'Catch-Up' Immunization Schedules," March 29, 2016, www.cdc.gov/vaccines/schedules/hcp/child-adolescent.html.

5. Centers for Disease Control and Prevention, "Antibiotic/Antimicrobial Resistance," April 27, 2017. http:// www.cdc.gov/drugresistance.

6. Centers for Disease Control and Prevention, "Preventing Healthcare Associated Infections," Accessed May 2017, https://www.cdc.gov/washington/~cdcatWork/ pdf/infections.pdf; Centers for Disease Control and Prevention, "HAI Data and Statistics," October 25, 2016, www.cdc.gov/HAI/surveillance; S. Magill et al., "Multistate Point-Prevalence Survey of Health Care—Associated Infections," *New England Journal of Medicine* 370, no. 13 (2014): 1198–208.

7. Centers for Disease Control and Prevention, "General Information about MRSA in the Community," March 25, 2016, www.cdc.gov/mrsa/community/index.html.

8. Ibid.

9. Ibid.

10. P. Span, "Doctors See Gains against 'an Urgent threat,' C. Diff," *New York Times*, February 10, 2017, https:// www.nytimes.com/2017/02/10/health/clostridium-difficile-c-diff.html.

11. Centers for Disease Control and Prevention, "Clostridium Difficile Infection," March 2016, https://www .cdc.gov/HAI/organisms/cdiff/Cdiff_infect.html.

12. Centers for Disease Control and Prevention, "Group B Strep (GBS)," May 23, 2016, https://www.cdc.gov/ groupbstrep.

13. World Health Organization, "Global Health Observatory (GHO) Data: Meningococcal Meningitis," Accessed March 28, 2016, http://www.who.int/gho/epidemic_ diseases/meningitis/en; Centers for Disease Control and Prevention, "Meningococcal Disease: Surveillance," June 9, 2017, https://www.cdc.gov/meningococcal/ surveillance.

14. World Health Organization, "Global Health Observatory (GHO) Data: Meningococcal Meningitis," Accessed March 28, 2016, http://www.who.int/gho/epidemic_ diseases/meningitis/en; Centers for Disease Control and Prevention, "Meningococcal Disease: Surveillance," June 9, 2017, https://www.cdc.gov/meningococcal/ surveillance.

15. Ibid.

16. World Health Organization, "Media Centre: Tuberculosis Fact Sheet," March 2017, www.who.int/mediacentre/ factsheets/fs104/en.

17. K. Schmit et al., "Tuberculosis—United States, 2016," *MMWR Morbidity and Mortality Weekly Report* 66, no. 11 (2017): 289–94.

18. Ibid.

19. World Health Organization, "Tuberculosis and Women," 2015, http://www.who.int/tb/publications/ tb_women_factsheet_251013.pdf.

20. World Health Organization, "Tuberculosis and Women," 2015, http://www.who.int/tb/publications/ tb_women_factsheet_251013.pdf; Centers for Disease Control and Prevention, "New Treatment Regimen for Latent Tuberculosis Infection," March 25, 2016, http:// www.cdc.gov/tb/topic/treatment/12dose_video.htm; ScienceDaily, "Curcumin May Help Overcome Drug-Resistant Tuberculosis," March 25, 2016, www.science-daily.com/releases/2016/03/160325093704.htm.

21. Centers for Disease Control and Prevention, "TB Fact Sheet: BCG Vaccine," September 12, 2016, https://www .cdc.gov/tb/publications/factsheets/prevention/bcg .htm.

22. Centers for Disease Control and Prevention, "TB-MultiDrug Resistant," May 11, 2016, https://www. cdc.gov/tb/publications/factsheets/drtb/mdrtb.htm.

23. Centers for Disease Control and Prevention, "Common Colds: Protect Yourself and Others," February 6, 2017, www.cdc.gov/features/rhinoviruses.

24. Ibid.

25. C. DerSarkissian, "What's Causing My Cold?," January 23, 2017, http://www.webmd.com/cold-and-flu/ cold-guide/common_cold_causes.

26. Centers for Disease Control and Prevention, "Frequently Asked Flu Questions 2016–2017 Influenza Season," March 2017, https://www .cdc.gov/flu/about/season/flu-season-2016-2017.htm; Centers for Disease Control and Prevention, "FastStats: Leading Causes of Death, 2015," March 2017, https://www.cdc.gov/nchs/fastats/deaths.htm.

27. Centers for Disease Control and Prevention, "Frequently Asked Flu Questions 2016–2017 Influenza Season," March 2017, https://www.cdc.gov/flu/about/ season/flu-season-2016-2017.htm.

28. Centers for Disease Control and Prevention, "Selecting the Viruses in the Seasonal Influenza (Flu) Vaccine," October 20, 2015, www.cdc.gov/flu/about/season/ vaccine-selection.htm.

29. Centers for Disease Control and Prevention, "Seasonal Influenza Vaccine & Total Doses Distributed," March 15, 20176, http://www.cdc.gov/flu/professionals/ vaccination/vaccinesupply.htm.

30. Centers for Disease Control and Prevention, "ACIP Votes Down Use of LAIV for 2016–2017 Flu Season," June 2016, http://www.cdc.gov/media/releases/2016/ s0622-laiv-flu.html.

31. Centers for Disease Control and Prevention, "Hepatitis A Questions and Answers for Public," October 2016, https://www.cdc.gov/hepatitis/hav/afaq .htm#statistics; T.V. Murphy, "Progress toward Eliminating Hepatitis A Disease in the United States," *Morbidity and Mortality Weekly Report Supplements* 65, no. 1 (2016): 29–41.

32. D. Lavanchy and M. Kane, "Global Epidemiology of Hepatitis B Virus Infection," in *Hepatitis B Virus in Human Disease*, edited by Y.-F. Liaw and F. Zoulim (New York: Humana Press, 2016), 187–203; World Health Organization, "Hepatitis B," October 2016, http://www .who.int/immunization/monitoring_surveillance/ burden/vpd/surveillance_type/passive/hepatitis/en.

33. D. Lavanchy and M. Kane, "Global Epidemiology of Hepatitis B Virus Infection," in *Hepatitis B Virus in Human Disease*, edited by Y.-F. Liaw and F. Zoulim (New York: Humana Press, 2016), 187–203; World Health Organization, "Hepatitis B," October 2016, http://www .who.int/immunization/monitoring_surveillance/bur-den/vpd/surveillance_type/passive/hepatitis/en; Centers for Disease Control and Prevention, "Viral Hepatitis Surveillance United States—2015, June 19, 2017, https:// www.cdc.gov/hepatitis/statistics/2015surveillance/ pdfs/2015HepSurveillanceRpt.pdf.

34. Ibid.

35. Ibid.

36. Ibid.

37. D. Lavanchy and M. Kane, "Global Epidemiology of Hepatitis B Virus Infection," in *Hepatitis B Virus in Human Disease*, edited by Y.-F. Liaw and F. Zoulim (New York: Humana Press, 2016), 187–203; World Health Organization, "Hepatitis B," October 2016, http://www. who.int/immunization/monitoring_surveillance/bur-den/vpd/surveillance_type/passive/hepatitis/en; Centers for Disease Control and Prevention, "Viral Hepatitis Surveillance United States—2015, June 19, 2017, https:// www.cdc.gov/hepatitis/statistics/2015surveillance/ pdfs/2015HepSurveillanceRpt.pdf; Centers for Disease Control, "Hepatitis C FAQs for the Public," October 2016, https://www.cdc.gov/hepatitis/hcv/cfaq.htm.

38. Ibid.

39. Ibid.

40. Ibid.

41. World Health Organization, "Zika Virus and Complications," March 27, 2017, http://www.who.int/ emergencies/zika-virus/en; Centers for Disease Control and Prevention, "World Map of Areas with Risks of Zika," June 21, 2017, http://wwwnc.cdc .gov/travel/page/world-map-areas-with-zika.

42. R Seither et al., "Vaccination Coverage among Children in Kindergarten—United States, 2015–16 School Year," *Morbidity and Mortality Weekly*, https://www.cdc.gov/ nchs/nhis/releases/released201705; California Department of Public Health, "Vaccine Preventable Disease Surveillance in California: Annual Report—2015," 2016, www.cdph.ca.gov/programs/immunize/Documents/ VPD-Disease Summary2015.pdf.

43. Centers for Disease Control and Prevention, "West Nile Virus Disease Cases and Presumptive Viremic Blood Donors by State—United States, 2016," January 17, 2017, http://www.cdc.gov/westnile/statsmaps/ preliminarymapsdata/histatedate.html.

44. World Health Organization, "Cumulative Number of Confirmed Human Cases for Avian Influenza A(H5N1) Reported to WHO, 2003–2017," May 2017, who.int/ influenza/human_animal_interface/2017_05_16_ tableH5N1.pdf?ua=1ww.whd.

45. Ibid.

46. S. Shrestha et al., "Estimating the Burden of 2009 Pandemic Influenza A (H1N1) in the United States (April 2009–April 2010)," *Clinical Infectious Diseases* 52, Suppl. 1 (2011): S75–S82.

47. Centers for Disease Control and Prevention, "The 2009 H1N1 Pandemic," August 2010, www.cdc .gov/h1n1flu/cdcresponse.htm.

48. **D. Black and G. Slavich, "Mindfulness Meditation and the Immune System: A Systematic Review of Randomized Controlled Trials,"** *Annals of the New York Academy of Sciences* 1373 (2016): 13–24. doi:10.1111/nyas.1299.

49. M. Ewoenspoek, "The Effects of Early Life Adversity on the Immune System," *Psychoneuroendocrinology* 82 (2017): 140–54.

50. F. D'Acquisto, "Affective Immunology: Where Emotions and the Immune System Converge," *Dialogues in Clinical Neuroscience* 19, no. 1 (2017): 9–19.

51. Centers for Disease Control and Prevention, "Reported STDs at Unprecedented High in the U.S.," October 19, 2016, https://www.cdc.gov/nchhstp/newsroom/2016/std-surveillance-report-2015-press-release.html; U.S. Department of Health and Human Services, Office of Adolescent Health, "Sexually Transmitted Diseases," February 2016, http://www.hhs.gov/ash/oah/adolescent-health-topics/reproductive-health/stds.html.

52. Centers for Disease Control and Prevention, "Reported Cases of Sexually Transmitted Diseases on the Rise in United States," November 17, 2015, http://www.cdc.gov/nchhstp/newsroom/2015/std-surveillance-report-press-release.html.

53. Centers for Disease Control and Prevention, "Reported Cases of Sexually Transmitted Diseases on the Rise in United States," November 17, 2015, http://www.cdc.gov/nchhstp/newsroom/2015/std-surveillance-report-press-release.html; Centers for Disease Control and Prevention, "2015 Sexually Transmitted Disease Surveillance," October, 2016, Available at www.cdc.gov/std/stats15.

54. Centers for Disease Control and Prevention, "STDs: Adolescents and Young Adults," March, 2017, December 2014, www.cdc.gov/std/stats13/adol.htm.

55. U.S. Department of Health and Human Services. Office of Adolescent Health, "Sexually Transmitted Diseases, May 2016, http://www.hhs.gov/ash/oah/adolescent-health-topics/reproductive-health/stds.html.

56. Ibid.

57. Centers for Disease Control and Prevention, "10 Ways STDs Impact Women Differently from Men," Accessed June 2017, https://www.cdc.gov/std/health-disparities/stds-women.pdf.

58. U.S. Department of Health and Human Services. Office of Adolescent Health. "Sexually Transmitted Diseases, May 2016, http://www.hhs.gov/ash/oah/adolescent-health-topics/reproductive-health/stds.html.

59. Centers for Disease Control and Prevention, "2015 Sexually Transmitted Disease Surveillance," October 2016, Available at www.cdc.gov/std/stats15.

60. Centers for Disease Control and Prevention, "CDC Fact Sheet: Chlamydia (Detailed)," October 17, 2016, http://www.cdc.gov/std/chlamydia/stdfact-chlamydia-detailed.htm.

61. Centers for Disease Control and Prevention, "CDC Fact Sheet: Gonorrhea (Detailed)," May 19, 2016. http://www.cdc.gov/std/gonorrhea/stdfact-gonorrhea.htm.

62. Ibid.

63. Ibid.

64. Ibid.

65. Ibid.

66. Ibid.

67. Centers for Disease Control and Prevention, "CDC Fact Sheet: Genital Herpes (Detailed)," February 2017, https://www.cdc.gov/std/herpes/stdfact-herpes.htm.

68. Ibid.

69. American Sexual Health Association, "Herpes: Fast Facts," Accessed June 2017, www.ashasexualhealth.org/stdsstis/herpes/fast-facts-and-faqs; Centers for Disease Control and Prevention, "CDC Fact Sheet: Genital Herpes (Detailed)," February 2017, https://www.cdc.gov/std/herpes/stdfact-herpes.htm.

70. Ibid.

71. Ibid.

72. Ibid.

73. Centers for Disease Control and Prevention, "HPV Questions and Answers," November 2016, https://www.cdc.gov/hpv/parents/questions-answers.html.

74. Ibid.

75. Centers for Disease Control and Prevention, "Cervical Cancer," May 2017, http://www.cdc.gov/cancer/cervical/.

76. American Cancer Society, "Cancer Facts & Figures 2016" (Atlanta, GA: American Cancer Society, 2017), Available at http://www.cancer.org/acs/groups/content/@research/documents/document/acspc-047079.pdf.

77. Centers for Disease Control and Prevention, "Human Papillomavirus (HPV) and Oropharyngeal Cancer—Fact Sheet," January 2017, http://www.cdc.gov/std/hpv/stdfact-hpvandoropharyngealcancer.htm.

78. Centers for Disease Control and Prevention, "Trichomoniasis: CDC Fact Sheet," March 2017, www.cdc.gov/std/trichomonas/stdfact-trichomoniasis.htm.

79. Ibid.

80. UNAIDS "Fact Sheet," February, 2017, http://www.unaids.org/en/resources/fact-sheet; AMFAR, "Statistics World Wide," February 2017, http://www.amfar.org/About-HIV-and-AIDS/Facts-and-Stats/Statistics—Worldwide.

81. Ibid.

82. Ibid.

83. Ibid.

84. Ibid.

85. Centers for Disease Control and Prevention, "HIV in the United States: At a Glance" June 9, 2017, http://www.cdc.gov/hiv/statistics/overview/ataglance.html; Kaiser Family Foundation, "The HIV/AIDS Epidemic in the United States: The Basics," February 2, 2017, http://www.kff.org/hivaids/fact-sheet/the-hivaids-epidemic-in-the-united-states-the-basics.

86. Ibid.

87. AMFAR, "Basic Facts about HIV/AIDS," August 2016, http://www.amfar.org/About-HIV-and-AIDS/Basic-Facts-About-HIV; Centers for Disease Control and Prevention, "HIV in the United States—At a Glance," June 9, 2017, https://www.cdc.gov/hiv/statistics/overview/ataglance.html.

88. Centers for Disease Control and Prevention, "Today's HIV/AIDS Epidemic," August 2016, https://www.cdc.gov/nchhstp/newsroom/docs/factsheets/todaysepidemic-508.pdf; Centers for Disease Control and Prevention, "HIV in the United States—At a Glance," June 9, 2017, https://www.cdc.gov/hiv/statistics/overview/ataglance.html.

89. AVERT, "Women and Girls, HIV and AIDS," May 2017. https://www.avert.org/professionals/hiv-social-issues/key-affected-populations/women; Centers for Disease Control and Prevention, "HIV among Women," March 2016, www.cdc.gov/HIV/risk/gender/women/facts/index.html.

90. World Health Organization, "Mother to Child Transmission of HIV," July 2015, www.who.int/hiv/topics/mtct/en.

91. Ibid.

92. Centers for Disease Control and Prevention, "HIV/AIDS Testing," June 6, 2017, https://www.cdc.gov/hiv/basics/testing.html.

93. Pharmaceutical Research and Manufacturers of America, "Medicine in Development: 2014 Report," May 2015, www.phrma.org/sites/default/files/pdf/2014-meds-in-dev-hiv-aids.pdf.

94. U.S. Department of Health and Human Services, "Limitations to Treatment Safety and Efficacy: Cost Considerations and Antiretroviral Therapy," July 14, 2016, https://aidsinfo.nih.gov/guidelines/html/1/adult-and-adolescent-arv-guidelines/459/cost-considerations-and-antiretroviral-therapy.

95. Ibid.

96. U.S. Department of Health and Human Services, "HIV Prevention—Pre-Exposure Prophylaxis. (PrEP)," May, 2017, https://aidsinfo.nih.gov/understanding-hiv-aids/fact-sheets/20/85/pre-exposure-prophylaxis–prep; Centers for Disease Control and Prevention, "HIV-PrEP," May, 30, 2017, https://www.cdc.gov/hiv/basics/prep.html.

97. Ibid.

Pulled Statistics:
page 453, Centers for Disease Control and Prevention. Sexually Transmitted Disease Surveillance 2015. Atlanta: U.S. Department of Health and Human Services; 2016.

Focus On: Reducing Risks for Chronic Diseases and Conditions

1. American Lung Association, "Estimated Prevalence and Incidence of Lung Disease," May 2017, http://www.lung.org/our-initiatives/research/monitoring-trends-in-lung-disease/estimated-prevalence-and-incidence-of-lung-disease; Centers for Disease Control and Prevention, "Leading Causes of Death," March 17, 2017, https://www.cdc.gov/nchs/fastats/leading-causes-of-death.htm.

2. National Center for Health Statistics, "FastStats, Chronic Obstructive Pulmonary Disease (COPD) Includes: Chronic Bronchitis and Emphysema," March 31, 2017, https://www.cdc.gov/nchs/fastats/copd.htm.

3. Centers for Disease Control and Prevention, "Summary Health Statistics Tables for U.S. Adults: National Health Interview Survey, 2015: Table A-2," March 2017, Available at http://ftp.cdc.gov/pub/Health_Statistics/NCHS/NHIS/SHS/2014_SHS_Table_A-2.pdf.

4. Ibid.

5. Ibid.

6. National Center for Health Statistics, "FastStats: Asthma," March 31, 2017, https://www.cdc.gov/nchs/fastats/asthma.htm.

7. National Center for Health Statistics, "FastStats: Asthma," March 31, 2017, https://www.cdc.gov/nchs/fastats/asthma.htm; Centers for Disease Control and Prevention, "Data, Statistics and Surveillance: Asthma Surveillance Data," March 2017, https://www.cdc.gov/asthma/asthmadata.htm.

8. L.J. Akinbami and C.D. Fryar, "Asthma Prevalence by Weight Status among Adults: U.S 2001–2014," *NCHS Data Brief* 239 (2016): 1–8.

9. Centers for Disease Control and Prevention, "FastStats: Asthma," March 31, 2107, https://www.cdc.gov/nchs/fastats/asthma.htm.

10. Asthma and Allergy Foundation of America, "What Causes or Triggers Asthma?" September 2015, http://www.aafa.org/page/asthma-triggers-causes.aspx.

11. Ibid.

12. Asthma and Allergy Foundation of America, "What Causes or Triggers Asthma?" September 2015, http://www.aafa.org/page/asthma-triggers-causes.aspx; D. Morales et al., "NSAID-exacerbated Respiratory Disease: A Metaanalysis Evaluating Prevalence, Mean Provocative Dose of Aspirin and Increased Asthma Morbidity," *Allergy* 70, no. 7 (2015): 828–35; WebMD, "Aspirin and Other Drugs That Trigger Asthma," Accessed June 2017, http://www.webmd.com/asthma/guide/medications-trigger-asthma.

13. Centers for Disease Control and Prevention, "National Health Interview Survey (NHIS) Data, Table 4.1: Current Asthma Prevalence by Age and Race—United States, 2015," February 10, 2017, https://www.cdc.gov/asthma/nhis/2015/table4-1.htm.

14. National Institute of Allergy and Infectious Diseases, "Allergic Diseases," May 2016, https://www.niaid.nih.gov/topics/allergicdiseases/Pages/default.aspx; Asthma and Allergy Foundation of America, "Research—Allergy Facts and Figures," Accessed May 2017, http://www.aafa.org/page/allergy-facts.aspx.

15. W. Acker et al., "Prevalence of Food Allergies and Intolerance Documented in Electronic Health Records," *Journal of Allergy and Clinical Immunology*, epub ahead of print, May 2017, http://www.jacionline.org/article/S0091-6749%2817%2930672-3/pdf.

16. Ibid.

17. W. Acker et al., "Prevalence of Food Allergies and Intolerance Documented in Electronic Health Records," *Journal of Allergy and Clinical Immunology*, epub ahead of print, May 2017, http://www.jacionline.org/article/S0091-6749%2817%2930672-3/pdf; Centers for Disease Control and Prevention, "Allergies and Hay Fever," March 2017, https://www.cdc.gov/nchs/fastats/allergies.htm.

18. National Library of Medicine, "Neurological Diseases," *Medline Plus*, February 20117, https://www.nlm.nih.gov/medlineplus/neurologicdiseases.html.

19. R. Burch et al., "The Prevalence and Burden of Migraine and Severe Headache in the United States: Updated Statistics from Government Health Surveillance Studies," *Headache: The Journal of Head and Face Pain* 55, no. 1 (2015): 21–34, doi:10.1111/head.12482.

20. Ibid.

21. Ibid.

22. Ibid.

23. R. Burch et al., "The Prevalence and Burden of Migraine and Severe Headache in the United States: Updated Statistics from Government Health Surveillance Studies," *Headache: The Journal of Head and Face*

Pain 55, no. 1 (2015): 21–34, doi:10.1111/head.12482; American Migraine Foundation, "Types of Headache—Migraine," Accessed June 2017, https://americanmigrainefoundation.org/living-with-migraines/types-of-headachemigraine.

24. R. Burch et al., "The Prevalence and Burden of Migraine and Severe Headache in the United States," *Headache: The Journal of Head and Face Pain* 55, no. 1 (2015): 21–34; National Institute of Neurological Disorders and Stroke, "Migraine Information Page," Accessed June 2017, https://www.ninds.nih.gov/disorders/migraine/migraine.htm; American Migraine Foundation, "Types of Headache–Migraine," Accessed June 2017, https://americanmigrainefoundation.org/living-with-migraines/types-of-headachemigraine.

25. National Institute of Neurological Disorders and Stroke, "Migraine Information Page," Accessed June 2017, https://www.ninds.nih.gov/Disorders/All-Disorders/Migraine-Information-Page.

26. American Migraine Foundation, "Living with Migraines," Accessed June 2017, https://americanmigrainefoundation.org/living-with-migraines.

27. American Migraine Foundation, "Cluster Headaches," Accessed June 2017, https://americanmigrainefoundation.org/understanding-migraine/cluster-headache; American Migraine Foundation, "Types of Headache–Migraine," 2017.

28. American Migraine Foundation. "Cluster Headaches," Accessed June 2017, https://americanmigrainefoundation.org/living-with-migraines/types-of-headache-migraine/cluster-headaches; American Migraine Foundation, "Types of Headache-Migraine," Accessed June 2017, https://americanmigrainefoundation.org/living-with-migraines/types-of-headachemigraine.

29. Centers for Disease Control and Prevention, "Epilepsy Fast Facts," February 2016, https://www.cdc.gov/epilepsy/basics/fast_facts.htm.

30. National Institute of Diabetes and Digestive and Kidney Diseases, "Definition and Facts for Irritable Bowel Syndrome," Accessed June 2017, https://www.niddk.nih.gov/health-information/digestive-diseases/irritable-bowel-syndrome/definition-facts.

31. Ibid.

32. National Institute of Diabetes and Digestive and Kidney Diseases, "Definition and Facts for Irritable Bowel Syndrome," February 2015, https://www.niddk.nih.gov/health-information/digestive-diseases/irritable-bowel-syndrome/definition-facts; J. Cunha and B. Anand, "Irritable Bowel Syndrome (IBS)," Accessed June 2017, http://www.medicinenet.com/irritable_bowel_syndrome_ibs/article.htm#irritable_bowel_syndrome_ibs_definition_and_facts.

33. Crohn's and Colitis Foundation, "What Are Crohn's and Colitis?" Accessed June 2017, http://www.crohnscolitisfoundation.org/what-are-crohns-and-colitis.

34. Ibid.

35. Crohn's and Colitis Foundation, "What Is Ulcerative Colitis?" Accessed June 2017, http://www.crohnscolitisfoundation.org/what-are-crohns-and-colitis/what-is-ulcerative-colitis.

36. Ibid.

37. Ibid.

38. Crohn's and Colitis Foundation of American, "What Is Crohn's Disease?" Accessed June, 2017. http://www.ccfa.org/what-are-crohns-and-colitis/what-is-crohns-disease.

39. Ibid.

40. Ibid.

41. Centers for Disease Control and Prevention, "Arthritis, National Statistics," March 17, 2017 https://www.cdc.gov/arthritis/data_statistics/national-statistics.html.

42. Ibid.

43. Ibid.

44. Centers for Disease Control and Prevention, "Osteoarthritis Fact Sheet," February 2, 2017, https://www.cdc.gov/arthritis/basics/osteoarthritis.htm; Centers for Disease Control and Prevention, "National Arthritis Statistics: Future Arthritis Burden," March 6, 2017, https://www.cdc.gov/arthritis/data_statistics/national-statistics.html#FutureArthritisBurden; United States Bone and Joint Initiative, *The Burden of Musculoskeletal Diseases in the United States (BMUS)*, 3rd ed. 2015, Accessed June 2017, Available at http://www.boneandjointburden.org.

45. Centers for Disease Control and Prevention, "Arthritis, National Statistics" March 17, 2017, https://www.cdc.gov/arthritis/data_statistics/national-statistics.html; National Institute of Arthritis and Musculoskeletal and Skin Disease, "Handout on Health: Osteoarthritis," April 2015, http://www.niams.nih.gov/health_info/osteoarthritis.

46. Centers for Disease Control and Prevention, "Arthritis, National Statistics" March 17, 2017, https://www.cdc.gov/arthritis/data_statistics/national-statistics.html; Centers for Disease Control and Prevention, "National Arthritis Statistics: Future Arthritis Burden," March 6, 2017, https://www.cdc.gov/arthritis/data_statistics/national-statistics.html#FutureArthritisBurden; Arthritis Foundation, "What Is Rheumatoid Arthritis?" Accessed June 2017, http://www.arthritis.org/about-arthritis/types/rheumatoid-arthritis/what-is-rheumatoid-arthritis.php017.

47. Arthritis Foundation, "What Is Rheumatoid Arthritis?" Accessed June 2017, http://www.arthritis.org/about-arthritis/types/rheumatoid-arthritis/what-is-rheumatoid-arthritis.php.

48. National Institute of Neurological Disorders and Stroke, "Low Back Pain Fact Sheet," Accessed April 2017, https://www.ninds.nih.gov/Disorders/Patient-Caregiver-Education/Fact-Sheets/Low-Back-Pain-Fact-Sheet.

49. Ibid.

50. A. Searle et al., "Exercise Interventions for the Treatment of Chronic Low Back Pain: A Systematic Review and Meta-analysis of Randomized, Controlled Trials," *Clinical Rehabilitation* 29, no. 12 (2015): 1155–67.

51. A. Qaseem et al., "Noninvasive Treatments for Acute, Subacute, and Chronic Low Back Pain: A Clinical Practice Guideline From the American College of Physicians," *Annals of Internal Medicine* 166, no. 7 (2017): 514–30.

52. Ibid.

53. National Institute of Neurological Disorders, "Repetitive Motion Disorders Information Page," Accessed June, 2017, https://www.ninds.nih.gov/Disorders/All-Disorders/Repetitive-Motion-Disorders-Information-Page.

54. Centers for Disease Control and Prevention, "Chronic Disease Prevention and Health Promotion," May 24, 2016, https://www.cdc.gov/chronicdisease.

Pulled Statistics:
page 440, CDC, "Health United States. 2015," Accessed June 2017, Available at https://www.cdc.gov/nchs/data/hus/hus15.pdf#019.

Chapter 15: Making Smart Health Care Choices

1. National Center for Health Statistics, "Health Insurance Coverage: Estimates from the National Health Interview Survey, January–September 2016," February 2017, Available at https://www.cdc.gov/nchs/data/nhis/earlyrelease/insur201702.pdf.

2. M.A. Hillen et al., " How Can Communication by Oncologists Enhance Patients' Trust? An Experimental Study," *Annals of Oncology* 25, no. 4 (2014): 896–901.

3. Joint Commission, "About the Joint Commission," 2016, www.jointcommission.org.

4. M. Makary and M. Daniel, "Medical Error—The Third Leading Cause of Death in the US," *British Journal of Medicine* 353 (2016): i2139.

5. J. James, "New Evidence-Based Estimates of Patient Harms Associated with Hospital Care," *Journal of Patient Safety* 9, no. 3 (2013): 122–28.

6. Consumer Health, "Patient Rights: Informed Consent," September 2016, http://www.emedicinehealth.com/patient_rights/article_em.htm.

7. A. Lundh et al., "Industry Sponsorship and Research Outcome," *Cochrane Database System Review*, February 16, 2017, doi:10.1002/14651858.MR000033.pub, https://www.ncbi.nlm.nih.gov/pubmed/28207928.

8. Centers for Disease Control and Prevention, "Therapeutic Drug Use," January 19, 2017, www.cdc.gov/nchs/fastats/drug-use-therapeutic.htm.

9. Ibid.

10. U.S. Department of Health and Human Services, "Facts about Generic Drugs," June 28, 2016, https://www.fda.gov/Drugs/ResourcesForYou/Consumers/BuyingUsingMedicineSafely/UnderstandingGenericDrugs/ucm167991.htm.

11. MedlinePlus, "Managed Care," January 2016, https://www.nlm.nih.gov/medlineplus/managedcare.html.

12. U.S. Centers for Medicare and Medicaid -Services, "National Health Expenditure Projections 2014–2024," July 2015, www.cms.gov/Research-Statistics-Data-and-Systems/Statistics-Trends-and-Reports/NationalHealthExpendData/Downloads/Proj2014.pdf.

13. National Committee to Preserve Social Security and Medicare, "Fast Facts about Medicare," February 2017, www.ncpssm.org/Medicare.

14. Centers for Medicare and Medicaid Services, "NHE Fact Sheet," March 21, 2017, https://www.cms.gov/research-statistics-data-and-systems/statistics-trends-and-reports/nationalhealthexpenddata/nhe-fact-sheet.html.

15. Henry J. Kaiser Family Foundation, "Medicaid in the United States," January 2017, http://files.kff.org/attachment/fact-sheet-medicaid-state-US.

16. U.S. Department of Health & Human Services, "2016 Poverty Guidelines," January 2016, https://aspe.hhs.gov/poverty-guidelines.

17. U.S. Department of Health & Human Services, "The Affordable Care Act Is Working," June 2015, http://www.hhs.gov/healthcare/facts-and-features/fact-sheets/aca-is-working/index.html.

18. Centers for Medicare and Medicaid Services, "Children's Health Insurance Program," July 2015, www.medicaid.gov/chip/chip-program-information.html.

19. National Conference of State Legislators, "Health Insurance: Premiums and Increases," January 2017, www.ncsl.org/issues-research/health/health-insurance-premiums.aspx.

20. National Center for Health Statistics, "Health Insurance Coverage: Estimates from the National Health Interview Survey, January-September 2016," February 2017, Available at https://www.cdc.gov/nchs/data/nhis/earlyrelease/insur201702.pdf.

21. Ibid.

22. American College Health Association, *American College Health Association–National College Health Assessment II: Reference Group Executive Summary. Fall 2016* (Hanover, MD: American College Health Association, 2017).

23. Henry J. Kaiser Family Foundation, "State Health Facts: Totally Professionally Active Physicians," September 2016, http://kff.org/other/state-indicator/total-active-physicians/?currentTimeframe=0&sortModel=%7B%22colId%22:%22Location%22,%22sort%22:%22asc%22%7D.

24. American Hospital Association, "Fast Facts on U.S. Hospitals," January 2017, www.aha.org/research/rc/stat-studies/fast-facts.shtml.

25. Centers for Medicare and Medicaid Services, "National Health Expenditure—Fact Sheet" March 2017.

26. Ibid.

27. U.S. Centers for Medicare and Medicaid Services, "The 80/20 Rule: How Insurers Spend Your Health Insurance Premiums," February 2013, https://www.cms.gov/CCIIO/Resources/Files/Downloads/mlr-report-02-15-2013.pdf.

28. L. S. Dafny, "Evaluating the Impact of Health Insurance Industry Consolidation: Learning from Experience," Commonwealth Fund, November 20, 2015, http://www.commonwealthfund.org/publications/issue-briefs/2015/nov/evaluating-insurance-industry-consolidation.

29. Ibid.

30. Central Intelligence Agency, "Country Comparison: Life Expectancy at Birth, 2016 Estimates," *CIA World Factbook*, April 2017, https://www.cia.gov/library/publications/the-world-factbook/rankorder/2102rank.html.

31. Ibid.

32. Central Intelligence Agency, "Country Comparison: Infant Mortality Rate, 2016 Estimates," *CIA World Factbook*, April 2017, https://www.cia.gov/library/publications/the-world-factbook/rankorder/2091rank.html.

33. U.S. Department of Health and Human Services, "The National Quality Strategy: Fact Sheet," January 2017, https://www.ahrq.gov/workingforquality/about/nqs-fact-sheets/fact-sheet.html.

Pulled Statistics:
page 453, U. S. Centers for Disease Control and Prevention, "Hospital Utilization," March 2017, www.cdc.gov/nchs/fastats/hospital.htm.
page 454, M. Makary and M. Daniel, "Medical Error—The Third Leading Cause of Death in the US," *British Journal of Medicine* 353 (2016):i2139.

Focus On: Understanding Complementary and Integrative Health

1. National Center for Complementary and Integrative Health, "Complementary, Alternative, or Integrative Health: What's in a Name?," June 2016, https://nccih.nih.gov/health/integrative-health#types.
2. Ibid.
3. Ibid.
4. Ibid.
5. T.C. Clarke et al., "Trends in the Use of Complementary Health Approaches among Adults: United States, 2002–2012," *National Health Statistics Reports* 79 (Hyattsville, MD: National Center for Health Statistics), February 2015, Available at www.cdc.gov/nchs/data/nhsr/nhsr079.pdf.
6. Ibid.
7. J.E. Stahl et al., "Relaxation Response and Resiliency Training and Its Effect on Healthcare Resource Utilization," *PLOS ONE* 10, no. 10 (2015): e0140212; M.D. Klatt et al., "A Healthcare Utilization Cost Comparison between Employees Receiving a Worksite Mindfulness or a Diet/Exercise Lifestyle Intervention to Matched Controls 5 Years post Intervention," *Complementary Therapies in Medicine* 27 (2016): 139–44.
8. J.E. Stahl et al., "Relaxation Response and Resiliency Training and Its Effect on Healthcare Resource Utilization," *PLOS ONE* 10, no. 10 (2015): e0140212.
9. National Center for Complementary and Integrative Health, "Traditional Chinese Medicine: In Depth," March 2017, https://nccih.nih.gov/health/whatiscam/chinesemed.htm.
10. National Center for Complementary and Integrative Health, "Traditional Chinese Medicine: In Depth," March 2017, https://nccih.nih.gov/health/whatiscam/chinesemed.htm; U.S. Food and Drug Administration, "Information for Consumers on Using Dietary Supplements," July 2016, https://www.fda.gov/Food/DietarySupplements/UsingDietarySupplements/default.htm.
11. National Center for Complementary and Integrative Health, "Ayurvedic Medicine: In Depth," April 2016, http://nccih.nih.gov/health/ayurveda/introduction.htm.
12. Ibid.
13. Ibid.
14. National Center for Complementary and Integrative Health, "Homeopathy," April 2016, http://nccih.nih.gov/health/homeopathy.
15. Ibid.
16. National Center for Complementary and Integrative Health, "Naturopathy," February 2016, https://nccih.nih.gov/health/naturopathy.
17. Ibid.
18. National Center for Complementary and Integrative Health, "Complementary, Alternative, or Integrative Health: What's in a Name?," June 2016, www.nccih.nih.gov/health/integrative-health.
19. American Chiropractic Association, "Facts about Chiropractic," Accessed May 2017, http://www.acatoday.org/News-Publications/News/Facts-About-Chiropractic.
20. National Center for Complementary and Integrative Health, "Spinal Manipulation," April 2016, https://nccih.nih.gov/health/spinalmanipulation; N. Paige et al. "Association of Spinal Manipulative Therapy with Clinical Benefit and Harm for Acute Low Back Pain: Systematic Review and Meta-analysis." *JAMA* 2017;317(14):1451–60. doi:10.1001/jama.2017.308.
21. American Chiropractic Association, "Facts about Chiropractic," Accessed May 2017, http://www.acatoday.org/News-Publications/News/Facts-About-Chiropractic.
22. National Center for Complementary and Integrative Health, "Massage Therapy for Health Purposes," March 2017, https://nccih.nih.gov/health/massage/massageintroduction.htm.
23. Ibid.
24. Ibid.
25. Bureau of Labor Statistics, U.S. Department of Labor, "Massage Therapists," *Occupational Outlook Handbook, 2016–2017 Edition*, June 2017, http://www.bls.gov/ooh/healthcare/massage-therapists.htm.
26. National Center for Complementary and Integrative Health, "Acupuncture: In Depth," February 2017, https://nccih.nih.gov/health/acupuncture/introduction.
27. K. Linde et al., "Acupuncture for the Prevention of Tension-Type Headache," *Cochrane Database of Systematic Reviews* 48, Art No. CD007587 (2016).
28. C. Lowe et al., "Sham Acupuncture Is as Efficacious as True Acupuncture for the Treatment of IBS: A Randomized Placebo Controlled Trial," *Neurogastroenterology and Motility* (2017).
29. R.L. Nahin et al., "Evidence-Based Evaluation of Complementary Health Approaches for Pain Management in the United States," *Mayo Clinic Proceedings* 91, no. 9 (2016): 1292–1306.
30. National Center for Complementary and Integrative Health, "Acupuncture: In Depth," February 2017, https://nccih.nih.gov/health/acupuncture/introduction#hed2.
31. G.A. Kelley and K.S. Kelley, "Meditative Movement Therapies and Health-Related Quality-of-Life in Adults: A Systematic Review of Meta-Analyses," *PLOS ONE* 10, no. 6 (2015): e0129181, doi:10.1371/journal.pone.0129181.
32. S. Jain et al., "Clinical Studies of Biofield Therapies: Summary, Methodological Challenges, and Recommendations," *Global Advances in Health and Medicine* 4, Suppl (2015): 58–66; R. Hammerschlag et al., "Nontouch Biofield Therapy: A Systematic Review of Human Randomized Controlled Trials Reporting Use of Only Nonphysical Contact Treatment," *Journal of Alternative and Complementary Medicine* 20, no. 12 (2014): 881–92, doi:10.1089/acm.2014.0017.
33. U.S. Food and Drug Administration, "'Natural' on Food Labeling," September 2016, www.fda.gov/Food/GuidanceRegulation/GuidanceDocumentsRegulatoryInformation/LabelingNutrition/ucm456090.htm.
34. U.S. Pharmacopeial Convention, "USP-Verified Dietary Supplements," Accessed May 2017, http://www.usp.org/usp-verification-services/usp-verified-dietary-supplements.
35. National Center for Complementary and Integrative Health, "Alerts and Advisories, 2017," Accessed May 2017, https://nccih.nih.gov/news/alerts.
36. National Center for Complementary and Integrative Health, "Using Dietary Supplements Wisely," June 2016, https://nccih.nih.gov/health/supplements/wiseuse.htm.

Pulled Statistics:
page 470, T. C. Clarke et al., "Trends in the Use of Complementary Health Approaches among Adults: United States, 2002–2012," *National Health Statistics Reports* 79 (Hyattsville, MD: National Center for Health Statistics), February 2015. Available at www.cdc.gov/nchs/data/nhsr/nhsr079.pdf.

Focus On: Aging, Death, and Dying

1. Central Intelligence Agency, *World Factbook. Country Comparisons: Life Expectancy at Birth*, 2016, https://www.cia.gov/library/publications/the-world-factbook/rankorder/2102rank.html.
2. U.S. Department of Health and Human Services, "A Profile of Older Americans: 2016," March 2017, https://www.giaging.org/documents/A_Profile_of_Older_Americans_2016.pdf.
3. Ibid.
4. Administration on Aging, U.S. Department of Health and Human Services, "Projected Future Growth of the Older Population," 2014, http://www.aoa.acl.gov/Aging_Statistics/future_growth/future_growth.aspx.
5. U.S. Department of Health and Human Services, "Profile of Older Americans: 2016," March 2017, https://www.giaging.org/documents/A_Profile_of_Older_Americans_2016.pdf.
6. Ibid.
7. Ibid.
8. Ibid.
9. Genworth, "Compare Long-Term Care Costs across the United States," 2015, https://www.genworth.com/about-us/industry-expertise/cost-of-care.html.
10. Administration on Aging, "A Profile of Older Americans, 2016," March 2017, https://www.giaging.org/documents/A_Profile_of_Older_Americans_2016.pdf.
11. International Osteoporosis Foundation, "Epidemiology," Accessed April 2017, https://www.iofbonehealth.org/epidemiology.
12. Centers for Disease Control and Prevention, "Arthritis-Related Statistics," March 2017, www.cdc.gov/arthritis/data_statistics/arthritis_related_stats.htm.
13. N. Jaipaul, "Effects of Aging on Urinary Tract," *Merck Manual: Consumer Version*, 2017, http://www.merckmanuals.com/home/kidney-and-urinary-tract-disorders/biology-of-the-kidneys-and-urinary-tract/effects-of-aging-on-the-urinary-tract.
14. P. Roland et al., "Presbycusis," *Medscape*, November 24, 2015, http://reference.medscape.com/article/855989-overview#a6.
15. A. Goman et al., "Addressing Estimated Hearing Loss in Adults in 2060," *JAMA Otolaryngology—Head & Neck Surgery* 143, no. 7 (2017): 733–34. doi:10.1001/jamaoto.2016.4642.
16. Peak Fitness, "Tai Chi and Other Low-Impact Exercises May Be Ideal for Elderly People with Chronic Health Problems, October 2015, http://fitness.mercola.com/sites/fitness/archive/2015/10/09/tai-chi-benefits.aspx.
17. L. Stein, "Sex and Seniors: The 70-Year Itch," *HealthDay*, January 20, 2016, https://consumer.healthday.com/encyclopedia/aging-1/misc-aging-news-10/sex-and-seniors-the-70-year-itch-647575.html; M. N. Lochlainne et al., "Sexual Activity and Aging," *Journal of American Medical Directors Association* 14, no. 8 (2013): 565–72.
18. Alzheimer's Association, "Quick Facts: Prevalence," 2017, http://www.alz.org/facts/#prevalence.
19. Ibid.
20. L. McBee, " Be Here Now—And Age Mindfully," *Aging Today*, June 25, 2014, http://www.asaging.org/blog/be-here-now-and-age-mindfully.
21. Centers for Disease Control and Prevention, "Important Facts about Falls," January 2016, https://www.cdc.gov/homeandrecreationalsafety/falls/adultfalls.html.
22. I. Young Kim et al., "Quantity of Dietary Protein Intake, but Not Pattern of Intake, Affects Net Protein Balance Primarily Through Differences in Protein Synthesis in Older Adults," *American Journal of Physiology Endocrinology and Metabolism* 308, no. 1 (2015): E21–E28.
23. By permission. From *Merriam-Webster's Collegiate® Dictionary*, 11th Edition © 2016 by Merriam-Webster, Inc., Available at www.Merriam-Webster.com.
24. President's Commission on the Uniform Determination of Death, *Defining Death: Medical, Ethical and Legal Issues in the Determination of Death* (Washington, DC: U.S. Government Printing Office, 1981).
25. Ad Hoc Committee of the Harvard Medical School to Examine the Definition of Brain Death, "A Definition of Irreversible Coma," *Journal of the American Medical Association* 205 (1968): 377.
26. Elisabeth Kübler-Ross, *On Death and Dying* (New York: Scribner, 2014).
27. R. Perper, "Worden's Four Tasks of Grieving," *Therapy Changes*, May 26, 2015, http://therapychanges.com/blog/2015/05/review-wordens-four-tasks-of-grieving.
28. National Institute on Aging, "Health and Aging, Advance Care Planning," March 10, 2016, https://www.nia.nih.gov/health/publication/advance-care-planning.
29. Aging with Dignity, "Five Wishes," 2016, www.agingwithdignity.org.
30. National Hospice and Palliative Care Organization, "NHPCO Facts and Figures: Hospice Care in America, 2015 Edition," 2015, www.nhpco.org.
31. U.S. National Library of Medicine, "Organ Donation," February 6, 2017, https://www.nlm.nih.gov/medlineplus/organdonation.html.

Pulled Statistics:
page 479, Administration on Aging, U.S. Dept. of Health and Human Services, "A Profile of Older Americans: 2015," 2016 https://aoa.acl.gov/Aging_Statistics/Profile/2015/6.aspx.

Chapter 16: Managing Stress and Coping with Life's Challenges

1. World Wildlife Fund, "Living Planet Report," Accessed June 2017, http://wwf.panda.org/about_our_earth/all_publications/lpr_2016.
2. Ibid.

3. U.N. Department of Economic and Social Affairs, "World Population Projected to Reach 9.8 Billion in 2050, and 11.2 Billion in 2100," June 21, 2017, https://www.un.org/development/desa/en/news/population/world-population-prospects-2017.html; Worldwatch Institute, "As Global Population Surpasses 7 Billion, Two Clear Strategies for a Sustainable Future," July 20, 2017, http://www.worldwatch.org/global-population-surpasses-7-billion-two-clear-strategies-sustainable-future.

4. U.N. Department of Economic and Social Affairs, "World Population Projected to Reach 9.8 Billion in 2050, and 11.2 Billion in 2100," June 21, 2017, https://www.un.org/development/desa/en/news/population/world-population-prospects-2017.html.

5. U.N. Environmental Programme, "Rate of Environmental Damage Increasing across the Planet but There Is Still Time to Reverse Worst Impacts if Governments Act Now, UNEP Assessment Says," May 19, 2016, www.unep.org/newscentre/Default.aspx?DocumentID=27074&ArticleID=36180&l=en.

6. Central Intelligence Agency, The World Factbook: Country Comparison: Total Fertility Rate, Accessed June 2016, https://www.cia.gov/library/publications/the-world-factbook/rankorder/2127rank.html.

7. U.N. Department of Economic and Social Affairs, "World Population Projected to Reach 9.8 Billion in 2050, and 11.2 Billion in 2100," June 21, 2017, https://www.un.org/development/desa/en/news/population/world-population-prospects-2017.html.

8. Ibid.

9. U.S. Census Bureau, "U.S. and World Population Clock," June 28, 2017, http://www.census.gov/popclock.

10. World Wildlife Fund, "Living Planet Report," Accessed June 2017, http://wwf.panda.org/about_our_earth/all_publications/lpr_2016; Global Footprint Network, "Key Findings of the National Footprint Accounts, 2016 Edition," June 8, 2016, http://www.footprintnetwork.org/en/index.php/GFN/page/footprint_data_and_results.

11. World Wildlife Fund, "Living Planet Report," Accessed June 2017, http://wwf.panda.org/about_our_earth/all_publications/lpr_2016.

12. United Nations, "UNEP Annual Report 2016," Accessed June 2017, http://www.unep.org/annualreport/2016/index.php?page=0&lang=en.

13. G. Ceballos et al., "Accelerated Modern Human-induced Species Losses: Entering the Sixth Mass Extinction," Science Advances 1, no. 5 (2015): e1400253, doi:10.1126/sciadv.1400253.

14. IUCN Red List of Threatened Species, "IUCN Red List Status: Mammals," July 2017, www.iucnredlist.org/initiatives/mammals/analysis/red-list-status.

15. World Wildlife Fund, "Living Planet Report," Accessed June 2017, http://wwf.panda.org/about_our_earth/all_publications/lpr_2016.

16. IUCN Red List of Threatened Species, "IUCN Red List Status: Amphibians," 2004, http://www.iucnredlist.org/initiatives/amphibians.

17. United Nations, Global Environment Outlook, Accessed July 2016, http://www.unep.org/geo.

18. United Nations, "UNEP Frontiers: 2016 Report: Emerging Issues of Environmental Concern," Accessed July 2017, http://www.unep.org/frontiers/sites/unep.org.frontiers/files/documents/unep_frontiers_2016.pdf.

19. Ibid.

20. C. Golden et al., "Fall in Fish Catch Threatens Human Health," Nature 534, no. 7607 (2016): 317–20; V. Christenson et al., "A Century of Fish Biomass Decline in the Ocean," Marine Ecology Program Series 512 (2014): 155–66, doi:10.3354/meps10946.

21. World Wildlife Fund, "Living Planet Report," Accessed June 2017, http://wwf.panda.org/about_our_earth/all_publications/lpr_2016; U.S. Department of Agriculture, "Overview: Agricultural Water Use," April 18, 2017, https://www.ers.usda.gov/topics/farm-practices-management/irrigation-water-use.aspx.

22. World Wildlife Fund, "Living Planet Report," Accessed June 2017, http://wwf.panda.org/about_our_earth/all_publications/lpr_2016; U.S. Department of Agriculture,

"Overview: Agricultural Water Use," April 18, 2017, https://www.ers.usda.gov/topics/farm-practices-management/irrigation-water-use.aspx; U.S. Environmental Protection Agency, "Case Study Analysis of the Impacts of Water Acquisition for Hydraulic Fracturing on Local Water Availability," May 2015, Available at https://www.epa.gov/sites/production/files/2015-07/documents/hf_water_acquisition_report_final_6-3-15_508_km.pdf.

23. U.S. Energy Information Administration, "Independent Statistics and Analysis," July 2017, www.eia.gov.

24. J.P. Deaton, "Who Consumes the Most Fossil Fuels per Capita?" HowStuffWorks, auto.howstuffworks.com/fuel-efficiency/fuel-consumption/consumes-most-fossil-fuel.htm.

25. U.S. Environmental Protection Agency, "Air Enforcement," January 2017, https://www.epa.gov/enforcement/air-enforcement.

26. U.S. Environmental Protection Agency, "Overview of Greenhouse Gases: Carbon Dioxide Emissions," April 2017, https://www3.epa.gov/climatechange/ghgemissions/gases/co2.html.

27. Ibid.

28. American Lung Association, "State of the Air: 2017," Accessed July 2017, http://www.lung.org/assets/documents/healthy-air/state-of-the-air/state-of-the-air-2017.pdf.

29. Ibid.

30. U.S. Environmental Protection Agency, "Effects of Acid Rain," July 2017, https://www.epa.gov/acidrain/effects-acid-rain.

31. U.S. Environmental Protection Agency, "An Introduction to Indoor Air Quality," January 27, 2017, https://www.epa.gov/indoor-air-quality-iaq/introduction-indoor-air-quality.

32. Ibid.

33. Ibid.

34. U.S. Environmental Protection Agency, "Overview of Greenhouse Gases: Emissions and Trends: Carbon Dioxide," Accessed July 2017; National Aeronautics and Space Administration, "Ozone Hole Watch," July 2016, http://ozonewatch.gsfc.nasa.gov.

35. American Association for the Advancement of Science, "What We Know: The Reality, Risks, and Response to Climate Change," Accessed July 2017, Available at http://whatweknow.aaas.org/wp-content/uploads/2014/07/whatweknow_website.pdf; J. Cook et al., "Consensus on Consensus: A Synthesis of Consensus Estimates on Human-caused Global Warming," Environmental Research Letters 11, no. 4 (2016): 048002.

36. U.S. Global Research Program, "Understand Climate Change," Accessed July 2017, http://www.globalchange.gov/climate-change; American Association for the Advancement of Science, "What We Know: The Reality, Risks, and Response to Climate Change," Accessed July 2017, Available at http://whatweknow.aaas.org/wp-content/uploads/2014/07/whatweknow_website.pdf; J. Cook et al., "Consensus on Consensus: A Synthesis of Consensus Estimates on Human-caused Global Warming," Environmental Research Letters 11, no. 4 (2016): 048002.

37. A. Crimmins and the U.S. Global Change Research Group, "The Impacts of Climate Change on Human Health in the United States: A Scientific Assessment," June 2016, https://health2016.globalchange.gov/downloads; National Aeronautics and Space Administration, "Climate Change: How Do We Know?," Accessed July 2016, http://climate.nasa.gov/evidence; U.S. Global Change Research Program, "The Impacts of Climate Change on Human Health in the United States: A Scientific Assessment," April 2016, https://health2016.globalchange.gov.

38. Environmental Protection Agency, "Climate Change Facts: Answers to Common Questions," February 2016, https://www3.epa.gov/climatechange/basics/facts.html; National Academy of Sciences, "Attribution of Extreme Weather Events in the Context of Climate Change," 2016, https://nas-sites.org/americasclimatechoices/other-reports-on-climate-change/2016-2/attribution-of-extreme-weather-events-in-the-context-of-climate-change.

39. J. Olivier et al., "Trends in Global CO2 Emissions: 2016 Report," PBL Netherlands

Environmental Assessment Agency, 2016, http://www.pbl.nl/sites/default/files/cms/publicaties/pbl-2016-trends-in-global-co2-emissions-2016-report.

40. **National Aeronautics and Space Administration, "NASA, NOAA Data Show 2016 Warmest Year on Record Globally,"** January 18, 2017, https://www.nasa.gov/press-release/nasa-noaa-data-show-2016-warmest-year-on-record-globally; Environmental Protection Agency, "Climate Change Facts: Answers to Common Questions," 2016; J. Olivier et al., "Trends in Global CO2 Emissions: 2016 Report," PBL Netherlands Environmental Assessment Agency, 2016, http://www.pbl.nl/sites/default/files/cms/publicaties/pbl-2016-trends-in-global-co2-emissions-2016-report; National Aeronautics and Space Administration, "Global Climate Change: A Blanket around the Earth," Accessed July 2017, http://climate.nasa.gov/causes; NOAA, "Greenhouse Gases," Accessed July 2017, https://www.ncdc.noaa.gov/monitoring-references/faq/greenhouse-gases.php.

41. J. Cook et al., "Consensus on Consensus: A Synthesis of Consensus Estimates on Human-Caused Global Warming," Environmental Research Letters 11, no. 4 (2016): 048002; National Aeronautics and Space Administration, "Global Climate Change: A Blanket around the Earth," Accessed July 2017, http://climate.nasa.gov/causes.

42. J. Cook et al., "Consensus on Consensus: A Synthesis of Consensus Estimates on Human-Caused Global Warming," Environmental Research Letters 11, no. 4 (2016): 048002; National Aeronautics and Space Administration, "Global Climate Change: A Blanket around the Earth," Accessed July 2017, http://climate.nasa.gov/causes; J. Olivier et al., "Trends in Global CO2 Emissions: 2016 Report," PBL Netherlands Environmental Assessment Agency, 2016, http://www.pbl.nl/sites/default/files/cms/publicaties/pbl-2016-trends-in-global-co2-emissions-2016-report.

43. J. Cook et al., "Consensus on Consensus: A Synthesis of Consensus Estimates on Human-Caused Global Warming," Environmental Research Letters 11, no. 4 (2016): 048002; National Aeronautics and Space Administration, "Global Climate Change: A Blanket around the Earth," Accessed July 2017, http://climate.nasa.gov/causes; J. Olivier et al., "Trends in Global CO2 Emissions: 2016 Report," PBL Netherlands Environmental Assessment Agency, 2016, http://www.pbl.nl/sites/default/files/cms/publicaties/pbl-2016-trends-in-global-co2-emissions-2016-report; U.S. Environmental Protection Agency, " Inventory of U.S. Greenhouse Gas Emissions and Sinks: 1990-2015," 2017, https://www.epa.gov/sites/production/files/2017-02/documents/2017_complete_report.pdf.

44. J. Cook et al., "Consensus on Consensus: A Synthesis of Consensus Estimates on Human-Caused Global Warming," Environmental Research Letters 11, no. 4 (2016): 048002; National Aeronautics and Space Administration, "Global Climate Change: A Blanket around the Earth," Accessed July 2017, http://climate.nasa.gov/causes; J. Olivier et al., "Trends in Global CO2 Emissions: 2016 Report," PBL Netherlands Environmental Assessment Agency, 2016, http://www.pbl.nl/sites/default/files/cms/publicaties/pbl-2016-trends-in-global-co2-emissions-2016-report; U.S. Environmental Protection Agency, " Inventory of U.S. Greenhouse Gas Emissions and Sinks: 1990–2015," 2017, https://www.epa.gov/sites/production/files/2017-02/documents/2017_complete_report.pdf. Population increases and human destruction pose additional threats.

45. U.N. Sustainable Development Goals: 17 Goals to Transform Our World, Accessed June 2017, http://www.un.org/sustainabledevelopment.

46. D. Vine, Center for Climate and Energy Solutions, "Achieving the United States' Intended National Determined Contributions," April 2016, http://www.c2es.org/docUploads/achieving-us-indc.pdf.

47. Ibid.

48. Environmental Defense Fund, "Cap and Trade—How Cap and Trade Works, Accessed July 2017, www.edf.org/climate/how-cap-and-trade-works.

49. Ibid.

50. The Water Information Program, "Water Facts," Accessed July 2017, www.waterinfo.org/resources/water-facts.

51. Ibid.

52. Ibid.

53. Ibid.

54. Pacific Institute, "Water Use Trends in the United States," April 2015, http://pacinst .org/wp-content/uploads/sites/21/2015/04/Water-Use-Trends-Report.pdf.

55. Pacific Institute, "Water Use Trends in the United States," April 2015, http://pacinst.org/wp-content/ uploads/sites/21/2015/04/Water-Use-Trends-Report.pdf; U.S. Geological Survey, "Water Questions & Answers: How Much Water Does the Average Person Use at Home per Day?" May 2016, http://water.usgs .gov/edu/qa-home-percapita.html.

56. Pacific Institute, "Water Use Trends in the United States," April 2015, http://pacinst.org/wp-content/ uploads/sites/21/2015/04/Water-Use-Trends-Report .pdf.

57. Water Information Program, "Water Facts," June 2015, www.waterinfo.org/resources/water-facts.

58. Milken Institute Global Conference, "Solving the Global Water Challenge," May 3, 2016, http://www .milkeninstitute.org/events/conferences/global-conference/2016/panel-detail/6175; Water Information Program. "Water Facts," June 2015, www.waterinfo.org/ resources/water-facts.

59. M. Kostich et al., "Concentrations of Prioritized Pharmaceuticals in Effluents from 50 Large Wastewater Treatment Plants in the U.S. and Implications for Risk Estimation," *Environmental Pollution* 184 (2014): 354–59.

60. J. Donn et al., "Pharmaceuticals Found in Drinking Water, Affecting Wildlife and Maybe Humans," Associated Press, Accessed July 2016, http://hosted.ap.org/ specials/interactives/pharmawater_site/day1_01.html.

61. Environmental Protection Agency, "Advancing Sustainable Materials Management 2014—Fact Sheet: Assessing Trends in Material Generation, Recycling, Composting, Combustion with Energy Recovery and Landfilling in the United States," November 2016, https://www.epa. gov/sites/production/files/2016-11/documents/2014_ smmfactsheet_508.pdf.

62. Ibid.

63. Ibid.

64. Environmental Protection Agency, "Hazardous Waste," May 2016. www.epa.gov/osw/basic-hazard.htm; U.S. Environmental Protection Agency, "Household Hazardous Waste," April 2016, http://www.epa.gov/osw/ conserve/materials/hhw.htm.

65. Environmental Protection Agency, "Superfund: Superfund National Accomplishments Summary, Fiscal Year 2016," May 2017, https://www.epa.gov/superfund/ superfund-remedial-annual-accomplishments;

Environmental Protection Agency, "Superfund National Priorities List (NPL) Sites by State," July 2017, https://www.epa.gov/superfund/ superfund-national-priorities-list-npl.

66. U.S. Nuclear Regulatory Commission, "Radiation Basics," 2014, www.nrc.gov/about-nrc/radiation/ health-effects/radiation-basics.html.

67. Ibid.

68. International Atomic Energy Agency, "Climate Change and Nuclear Power 2016," September 2016, http://www-pub.iaea.org/MTCD/Publications/PDF/ CCANP16web-86692468.pdf.

69. Ibid.

70. World Nuclear Association, "Fukushima Accident," April 2017, http://www.world-nuclear.org/infor-mation-library/safety-and-security/safety-of-plants/ fukushima-accident.aspx.

Pulled Statistics:

page 493, Population Reference Bureau, "2016 World Population Data Sheet," 2016, http://www.prb.org/pdf13/2013-population-data-sheet_eng.pdf.

page 503, U.S. Environmental Protection Agency, "Advancing Sustainable Materials Management, 2014 Fact Sheet," November 2016, Available at https://www.epa.gov/sites/ production/files/2016-11/documents/2014_smmfact-sheet_508.pdf.

PHOTO CREDITS

INDEX